BRITISH NATIONAL FORMULARY

Number 35
(March 1998)

British Medical Association
and
Royal Pharmaceutical Society of Great Britain

Copies may be obtained through any bookseller or, in case of difficulty, direct from the publishers:

British Medical Association
Tavistock Square
London WC1H 9JP, England

The Pharmaceutical Press
PO Box 151
Wallingford
Oxon OX10 8QU, England
E-mail: rpsgb@cabi.org

ISBN: 0 85369 411 7. ISSN: 0260–535X

The text for this edition was generated from an in-house database (designed by Quartet Software Ltd). Printed and bound in Great Britain by William Clowes, Beccles, Suffolk.

Joint Formulary Committee
1997–98

Chairman
Charles F. George, BSc, MD, FRCP, FFPM

Deputy Chairman
Nicholas L. Wood, BPharm, FRPharmS

Committee Members

Alison Blenkinsopp, PhD,
BPharm, MRPharmS
Peter Clappison, MB, ChB
Joy B. Edelman, MB BS, FRCP
MRCS, D(Obst)RCOG
Ann Lewis, OBE, Hon DSc, LLB,
FRPharmS, MCPP, MHSM,
Barrister

Frank P. Marsh, MA, MB, BChir,
FRCP
Jane Richards, OBE, MB BS, MRCS,
LRCP, FRCGP,
D(Obst)RCOG, DCH
James Smith, BPharm, PhD,
MRPharmS, MCPP, MIInfSc
Patrick C. Waller, MD, FRCP (Ed),
FFPM, MPH

Joint Secretaries
José L. García de Ancos LMS, MSc(Econ)

Stella R. Lowry, MB, ChB, BSc (until August 1997)

James E. F. Reynolds, PhD, FRPharmS, MIInfSc

Executive Secretary
Susan M. Thomas, BSc(Econ), MA

BNF Editorial Staff

Executive Editor
Dinesh K. Mehta, BPharm, MSc, MRPharmS

Senior Assistant Editors
John Martin, BPharm, PhD, MRPharmS

Staff Editors
Ann M. Hargreaves, MRPharmS
Bryony Jordan, BSc, DipPharmPract, MRPharmS
Craig A. Patterson, BPharm, DipHospPharm, MRPharmS
Rachel S. M. Ryan, BPharm, MRPharmS
Sunayana A. Shah, BPharm, MRPharmS
Louise J. Whitley, BSc, MSc, MRPharmS

Editorial Assistant
Abimbola Sogbetun, BPharm, MSc
Louise M. E. Wykes, BSc

Contents

Arrangement of Information

Guidance on prescribing
This part includes information on prescription writing, controlled drugs and dependence, prescribing for children and the elderly, and prescribing in palliative care. Advice is given on the reporting of adverse reactions.

Emergency treatment of poisoning
The main intention of this chapter is to provide information on the management of acute poisoning when first seen in the home, although aspects of hospital-based treatment are mentioned.

Classified notes on drugs and preparations
The main text consists of classified notes on drugs and preparations. These notes are divided into 15 chapters, each of which is related to a particular system of the human body or to an aspect of medical care. Each chapter is then divided into sections which begin with appropriate *notes for prescribers*. These notes are intended to provide information to doctors, pharmacists, nurses, and other health professionals to facilitate the selection of suitable treatment. The notes are followed by details of relevant drugs and preparations.

DRUGS appear under pharmacopoeial or other non-proprietary titles. When there is an *appropriate current monograph* (Medicines Act 1968, Section 65) preference is given to a name at the head of that monograph; otherwise a British Approved Name (BAN), if available, is used. If the International Non-proprietary Name (INN) differs from the British Approved Name it follows the title in brackets.

PREPARATIONS usually follow immediately after the drug which is their main ingredient. They are printed in text-sized type but those considered by the Committee to be less suitable for prescribing are described in smaller type. Small type is also used for the entries describing foods for special diets, stoma and urinary appliances, and wound management products. Preparations are included under a non-proprietary title if:

    (a) they are marketed under such a title,
    (b) they are not otherwise prescribable under the NHS, or
    (c) they may be prepared extemporaneously.

    If proprietary preparations are of a distinctive colour this is stated, but flavour is not usually mentioned.
    In the case of compound preparations the indications, cautions, contra-indications, side-effects, and interactions of all constituents should be taken into account in prescribing.

PREPARATIONS NOT AVAILABLE FOR NHS PRESCRIPTION. The symbol NHS has been placed against those preparations included in the BNF that are not prescribable under the NHS. Those prescribable only for specific disorders have a foot-note specifying the condition(s) for which the preparation remains available. Prescribers are reminded that some preparations which are not *prescribable* by brand name under the NHS may nevertheless be *dispensed* using the brand name in question providing that the prescription has been written in the form of an appropriate non-proprietary name.

PRESCRIPTION-ONLY MEDICINES. The symbol PoM has been placed against those preparations that are available only on medical or dental prescription. For more detailed information see *Medicines, Ethics and Practice*, No. 19, London, Pharmaceutical Press, 1998 (and subsequent editions as available). The symbol CD indicates that the preparation is subject to the prescription requirements of the Misuse of Drugs Act. For regulations governing prescriptions for such preparations see pages 7–9.

PRICES have been calculated from the basic cost used in pricing NHS prescriptions dispensed in October 1997 or later, see p. 1 for further details.

Appendixes and indexes
The appendixes include information on interactions, liver disease, renal impairment, pregnancy, breast-feeding, intravenous additives, borderline substances, appliances, and cautionary and advisory labels for dispensed medicines. They are designed for use in association with the main body of the text.

    The Dental Practitioners' List and the Nurse Prescribers' List are also included in this section. The indexes consist of the Index of Manufacturers and the Main Index.

Preface

The BNF is a joint publication of the British Medical Association and the Royal Pharmaceutical Society of Great Britain. It is published under the authority of a Joint Formulary Committee which comprises representatives of the two professional bodies and of the Department of Health. It is available both as a pocket book version and as an identical electronic version.

The Joint Formulary Committee acknowledges the help of individuals and organisations that provided information or advised on specific matters. The principal contributors for this edition were J. M. Aitken, K. G. M. M. Alberti, S. P. Allison, D. G. Arkell, M. J. P. Arthur, L. Beeley, R. H. Behrens, R. J. Buckley, I. Burgess, A. J. Camm, C. M. Castleden, D. W. Chadwick, D. A. Chamberlain, M. C. Colquhoun, B. T. Colvin, W. J. Cunliffe, W. A. M. Cutting, S. Dewar, C. Diamond, R. Dinwiddie, A. J. Duxbury, G. H. Elder, T. W. Evans, R. O. Feneck, R. G. Finch, B. G. Gazzard, A. M. Geddes, A. H. Ghodse, P. W. Golightly, E. C. Gordon-Smith, M. W. Greaves, I. A. Greer, J. Guillebaud, C. H. Hawkes, D. F. Hawkins, C. J. Hinds, R. M. Jones, J. R. Kirwan, P. G. Kopelman, M. J. S. Langman, P. Lawler, T. H. Lee, P. N. Leigh, L. Luzzatto, G. M. Mead, D. E. Neal, J. M. Neuberger, A. J. Nunn, D. J. Oliver, L. P. Ormerod, M. R. Partridge, P. A. Poole-Wilson, L. E. Ramsay, F. Reynolds, A. Richens, P. A. Routledge, R. S. Sawers, P. Sleight, M. C. Sheppard, S. D. Shorvon, I. Stockley, A. Tattersfield, R. N. Thin, S. Thomas, G. R. Thompson, D. G. Waller, D. A. Warrell, P. J. Watkins, G. B. Wyatt. The Committee wishes to record its particular thanks to members of the British Association of Dermatologists Therapy Guidelines and Audit Working Party, C. E. M. Griffiths (Chairman), S. M. Burge, C. B. Bunker, N. H. Cox, C. A. Holden, M. R. Judge, H. C. Williams, M. Benham (Secretariat), for invaluable discussions and advice. The Committee also wishes to express its thanks to K. Parfitt and staff, for valuable access to the *Martindale* data bank and files, and to E. I. Connor for assistance with the development of the electronic BNF. A. B. Prasad has provided valuable advice and guidance in the preparation of this edition. The help of M. Davis and S. M. Townsend-Smith for checks on BNF data is also acknowledged; the Committee is also grateful to J. Goodway for administrative assistance. P. D. Johnson and B. Thomas of Quartet Software Ltd have continued to support production of the electronic BNF. The Committee also wishes to express its thanks to correspondents in the pharmaceutical industry who provided information and made numerous comments on points of detail and to colleagues who have advised members of the Committee and the editorial staff on specific matters. Finally, the Committee would like to thank those doctors, pharmacists, nurses, and others who sent comments and suggestions.

The BNF is intended for rapid reference and cannot always contain all the information necessary for prescribing and dispensing. It should be supplemented as necessary from specialised publications and by reference to the manufacturers' product literature. Within the space available the monographs in the BNF reflect the information in the manufacturers' data sheets or Summaries of Product Characteristics, which are prepared in accordance with statutory requirements; they are available for most proprietary medicines. Less detail is given in some areas such as those dealing with obstetrics, malignant disease, and anaesthesia, since it is expected that those undertaking treatment will have specialised knowledge and will consult specialist literature. Supplementary information may be available from local drug information services.

Comments and constructive criticism will be welcome, and should be sent to:
Executive Editor, British National Formulary,
c/o Royal Pharmaceutical Society of Great Britain,
1 Lambeth High Street, London SE1 7JN.
Email: editor@bnf.rpsgb.org.uk

Changes

The BNF is revised twice yearly and numerous changes are made between issues. All copies of BNF No. 34 (September 1997) should therefore be withdrawn and replaced by BNF No. 35 (March 1998).

Significant changes have been made in the following sections for BNF No. 35:

Atrial fibrillation, section 2.3.1

ACE Inhibitors [reorganisation], section 2.5.5.1

Stable angina [new text], section 2.6

Antihistamines [reorganisation and revision of text], section 3.4.1

Antipsychotics [reorganisation], section 4.2.1

Notifiable diseases [new text], Chapter 5

Treatment of tuberculosis, section 5.1.9

Malaria prophylaxis [advice amended to reflect new guidelines], section 5.4.1

Glucose tolerance test [revised recommendations], section 6.1.6

Hormone replacement therapy [new text on risk of breast cancer], section 6.4.1.1

Combined oral contraceptives [clarification of risk factors for arterial disease and migraine], section 7.3.1

Head lice and scabies [revised text], section 13.10.4

Prophylaxis of acid aspiration [new text], section 15.1

Muscle relaxants [reorganisation and revision of text], section 15.1.5

Dose Changes

Preparations affected by changes in dose statements introduced into BNF No. 35:

Allopurinol, p. 442

Colchicine [familial Mediterranean fever], p. 441

Dermestril, p. 321

Diazepam rectal solution, pp. 160, 218

Filgrastim [no longer licensed in advanced HIV infection], p. 399

Fusafungine, p. 471

Hydorxocobalamin, p. 395

Ipratropium nasal spray, p. 470

Mifepristone, p. 345

Niferex preparations, p. 392–3

Suxamethonium, p. 548

Classification Changes

2.12   Lipid-regulating drugs [title change]

11.8.1   Tear deficiency, ocular lubricants and astringents [title change]

11.8.2   Ocular diagnostic and peri-operative preparations [title change]

12.2.3   Nasal preparations for infection and epistaxis [title change]

Electronic BNF

An electronic BNF Browser is also available in parallel with the paper BNF; information is presented in the familiar layout of the paper BNF. The eBNF allows rapid access to the data and contains hot links to facilitate navigation. It also includes a facility for adding user-defined annotations and bookmarks. Further features have been added to eBNF 35 to enhance access, navigation and printing.

An annual subscription to the eBNF Browser (two editions of the BNF) costs £60 for a single user; network versions are also available.

Hardware requirements:

Microsoft Windows 3.1 or higher and at least a 486 processor with 8 megabytes of RAM (16 megabytes recommended) and takes up 25 megabytes of hard disk space (extra space may be needed during installation). It can be networked and will operate on any Windows supported network.

Name Changes

Directive 92/27/EEC requires use of the Recommended International Non-proprietary Name (rINN) for medicinal substances. In the majority of cases the British Approved Name (BAN) and rINN are identical; where the names differ, the procedure for transition to rINNs is to be announced by the MCA. Those substances that appear in the BNF and are affected by the transition are listed below.

List 1[1] includes those substances where a change of name is considered to pose the highest potential risk to public health—both names will be required to appear on manufacturers'

labels and leaflets (giving precedence to the rINN) for a period of at least 5 years.

List 2[1] includes those substances where the rINN will be required to appear exclusively on manufacturers' labels and leaflets.

1. These lists are subject to change following completion of a consultation process.

List 1—Both names to appear

UK name	rINN
adrenaline	epinephrine
amethocaine	tetracaine
bendrofluazide	bendroflumethiazide
benzhexol	trihexyphenidyl
chlorpheniramine	chlorphenamine
dicyclomine	dicycloverine
dothiepin	dosulepin
flurandrenolone	fludroxycortide
frusemide	furosemide

UK name	rINN
mitozantrone	mitoxantrone
mustine	chlormethine
noradrenaline	norepinephrine
oxpentifylline	pentoxifylline
procaine penicillin	procaine benzylpenicillin
salcatonin	calcitonin (salmon)
thymoxamine	moxisylyte
trimeprazine	alimemazine

List 2—rINN to appear exclusively

UK name	rINN
amoxycillin	amoxicillin
amphetamine	amfetamine
amylobarbitone	amobarbital
amylobarbitone sodium	amobarbital sodium
beclomethasone	beclometasone
benorylate	benorilate
bethanidine	betanidine
busulphan	busulfan
butobarbitone	butobarbital
cephalexin	cefalexin
cephamandole nafate	cefamandole nafate
cephazolin	cefazolin
cephradine	cefradine
chloral betaine	cloral betaine
chlorbutol	chlorobutanol
chlormethiazole	clomethiazole
chlorthalidone	chlortalidone
cholecalciferol	colecalciferol
cholestyramine	colestyramine
clomiphene	clomifene
colistin sulphomethate sodium	colistimethate sodium
corticotrophin	corticotropin
danthron	dantron
desoxymethasone	desoximetasone
dexamphetamine	dexamfetamine
dienoestrol	dienestrol
dimethicone(s)	dimeticone
dimethyl sulphoxide	dimethyl sulfoxide
doxycycline hydrochloride (hemihydrate hemiethanolate)	doxycycline hyclate
ethacrynic acid	etacrynic acid
ethamsylate	etamsylate
ethinyloestradiol	ethinylestradiol
ethynodiol	etynodiol
flumethasone	flumetasone
flupenthixol	flupentixol
guaiphenesin	guaifenesin
hexamine hippurate	methenamine hippurate
hydroxyprogesterone hexanoate	hydroxyprogesterone caproate
hydroxyurea	hydroxycarbamide
indomethacin	indometacin
lignocaine	lidocaine

UK name	rINN
lysuride	lisuride
methohexitone	methohexital
methotrimeprazine	levomepromazine
methyl cysteine	mecysteine
methylene blue	methylthioninium chloride
methylphenobarbitone	methylphenobarbital
nicoumalone	acenocoumarol
oestradiol	estradiol
oestriol	estriol
oestrone	estrone
oxethazaine	oxetacaine
oxyphenisatin	oxyphenisatine
pentaerythritol tetranitrate	pentaerithrityl tetranitrate
phenobarbitone	phenobarbital
pipothiazine	pipotiazine
polyhexanide	polihexanide
potassium clorazepate	dipotassium clorazepate
pramoxine	pramocaine
prothionamide	protionamide
quinalbarbitone	secobarbital
riboflavine	riboflavin
sodium calciumedetate	sodium calcium edetate
sodium cromoglycate	sodium cromoglicate
sodium ironedetate	sodium feredetate
sodium picosulphate	sodium picosulfate
sorbitan monostearate	sorbitan stearate
stilboestrol	diethylstilbestrol
sulphacetamide	sulfacetamide
sulphadiazine	sulfadiazine
sulphadimidine	sulfadimidine
sulphaguanidine	sulfaguanidine
sulphamethoxazole	sulfamethoxazole
sulphasalazine	sulfasalazine
sulphathiazole	sulfathiazole
sulphinpyrazone	sulfinpyrazone
tetracosactrin	tetracosactide
thiabendazole	tiabendazole
thioguanine	tioguanine
thiopentone	thiopental
thyroxine sodium	levothyroxine sodium
urofollitrophin	urofollitropin
vitamin A	retinol

New Preparations

PoM **Asmasal Clickhaler®** (Evans)
Dry powder for inhalation, salbutamol (as sulphate) 95 micrograms/metered inhalation, net price 200-dose breath-actuated unit = £6.32. Counselling, dose (*see* p. 127). BNF section 3.1.1.1
For asthma and other conditions associated with reversible airways obstruction

PoM **Domperamol®** (Servier)
Tablets, f/c, paracetamol 500 mg, domperidone (as maleate) 10 mg, net price 16-tab pack = £7.00. Label: 17, 30. BNF section 4.7.4.1
For acute attacks of mild to moderate migraine

PoM **Elleste Solo® MX** (Searle)
Patches, self-adhesive, oestradiol, *MX 40 patch* (releasing approx. 40 micrograms/24 hours), net price 8-patch pack = £5.96; *MX 80 patch* (releasing approx. 80 micrograms/24 hours), 8-patch pack = £6.56. Counselling, administration. BNF section 6.4.1.1
For menopausal symptoms (and osteoporosis prophylaxis in case of *Elleste Solo MX 80®* **only**)

PoM **Epogam® 80** (Searle)
Capsules, gamolenic acid 80 mg in evening primrose oil, net price 120-cap pack = £24.41. BNF section 13.5.1
Additives: include vitamin E
For symptomatic relief of atopic eczema

▼ PoM **Raxar®** (A&H)
Tablets, grepafloxacin (as hydrochloride), 400 mg, net price 5-tab pack = £12.00, 10-tab pack = £24.00; 600 mg, 5-tab pack = £17.00, 10-tab pack = £34.00. Label: 6, 9, 11, counselling, driving. BNF section 5.1.12
For community-acquired pneumonia; acute exacerbation of chronic bronchitis; uncomplicated gonorrhoea; urethritis and cervicitis caused by *Chlamydia trachomatis*
DRIVING. May affect performance of skilled tasks e.g. driving

▼ PoM **Singulair®** (MSD)
Paediatric Chewable Tablets, pink, montelukast (as sodium) 5 mg, net price 28-tab pack = £25.69. Label: 24, counselling, see below
Additives: contains aspartame equivalent to phenylalanine 0.842 mg per tablet (section 9.4.1)
COUNSELLING. Tablet to be taken 1 hour before or 2 hours after food
Tablets, beige, f/c, montelukast (as sodium) 10 mg, net price 28-tab pack = £25.69.
BNF section 3.3
For prophylaxis of mild to moderate asthma (including exercise-induced bronchospasm) as add-on therapy in patients not controlled on inhaled corticosteroids and short-acting beta$_2$-stimulants

▼ PoM **Zanidip®** (Napp)
Tablets, yellow, f/c, lercanidipine hydrochloride 10 mg, net price 28-tab pack = £10.20. Label: 22. BNF section 2.6.2
For mild to moderate essential hypertension

Preparations included in relevant sections of BNF No. 35

Ambre Solaire®, p. 500
Amias®, p. 91
Aprovel®, p. 92
Bismuth Subnitrate and Iodoform Paste, p. 471
Colazide®, p. 44
Creon® 10 000, p. 57
Crinone®, p. 325
Dioralyte® Relief, p. 403
Elleste-Duet® Conti, p. 320
Erecnos®, p. 366
Evorel® Conti and Sequi, p. 320
E-Z Spacer®, p. 134
Isocard®, p. 95
Malarone®, p. 289
Menogon®, p. 330
Monosorb XL®, p. 96

NeoRecormon®, p. 397
Oxis®, p. 128
Posicor®, p. 99
Seroquel®, p. 172
Solian®, p. 170
Tarka®, p. 91
Tasmar®, p. 225
Urdox®, p. 57
Ursogal®, p. 57
Vaqta®, p. 523
Vistide®, p. 280
Zanaflex®, p. 446
Zidoval®, p. 350
Zorac®, p. 491

Discontinued Preparations

Preparations discontinued during the compilation of BNF No. 35

Adifax®
Adizem-XL Plus®
Alimix®
Bactrim®
Carbo-Cort®
Chloromycetin® injection
Choledyl®
Clinicide®
Daneral SA®
Diabinese®
Fefol Z®
Ferrocontin Continus®
Ferrocontin Folic Continus®
Glaucol®
Gonadotraphon LH®

Iduridin®
Imtack® Spray
Lasix + K®
Lithofalk®
Macrodex®
Medihaler-epi®
Monuril®
Ponderax®
Prestim Forte®
Rapitard MC®
Robaxisal Forte®
Semitard MC®
Tagamet Dual Action®
Tobralex®
Tolectin®

Drug Information Services

Information on any aspect of drug therapy can be obtained from Regional and District Drug Information Services. Details regarding the *local* services provided within your Region can be obtained by telephoning the following numbers.

England

Birmingham		0121-311 1974	Direct Line
	or	0121-378 2211	Extn 2296/2297
Bristol		(0117) 928 2867	Direct Line
Ipswich		(01473) 704430	Direct Line
	or	(01473) 704431	Direct Line
Leeds		(0113) 243 0715	Direct Line
Leicester		(0116) 255 5779	Direct Line
Liverpool		0151-794 8113/4/5/7	Direct Line
London			
Guy's Hospital		0171-955 5000	Extn 3594/5892
	or	0171-378 0023	Direct Line
Northwick Park Hospital		0181-869 3973	Direct Line
Manchester		0161-225 2063	Direct Line
	or	0161-276 6270	Direct Line
Newcastle		0191-232 1525	Direct Line
Southampton		(01703) 796908	Direct Line
	or	(01703) 796909	Direct Line

Wales

Cardiff	(01222) 742979	Direct Line

Scotland

Aberdeen	(01224) 681818	Extn 52316
Dundee	(01382) 60111	Extn 2351
Edinburgh	0131-536 2843	Direct Line
Glasgow	0141-552 4726	Direct Line

Northern Ireland

Belfast	(01232) 248095	Direct Line

Republic of Ireland

Dublin		Dublin 473 0589	Direct Line
	or	Dublin 453 7941	Extn 2348

National Teratology Information Services
0191-232 1525

Poisons Information Services

Belfast	(01232) 240503
Birmingham	0121-507 5588/9
Cardiff	(01222) 709901
Dublin	Dublin 837 9964 *or* Dublin 837 9966
Edinburgh	0131-536 2300
Leeds	(0113) 243 0715 *or* (0113) 292 3547
London	0171-635 9191 *or* 0171-955 5095
Newcastle	0191-232 5131

Note. Some of these centres also advise on laboratory analytical services which may be of help in the diagnosis and management of a small number of cases

Patient Packs

On January 1 1994, EC Directive 92/27/EEC came into force, outlining requirements for the labelling of medicines and for the format and content of user leaflets to be supplied with each medicine.

In the UK, packs which conform to the Directive are termed **patient packs**. They consist of a ready-to-dispense pack containing a patient information leaflet approved by the Medicines Control Agency (MCA).

All new medicines are required to comply with the Directive and when the licences of established medicines are renewed, they too will be required to comply with the Directive. It is anticipated that all medicines in the UK will comply by mid-1999.

The MCA has been approving patient packs according to a phased programme based on therapeutic categories.

Many medicines are already available in a manufacturer's original pack (often complete with a patient information leaflet). Amounts listed in the BNF correspond to these packs.

During the revision of each edition of the BNF careful note is taken of the information that appears on the patient information leaflets. Where it is considered appropriate to alert a prescriber to some specific limitation appearing on the patient information leaflet (for example, in relation to pregnancy) this advice now appears in the BNF.

The patient information leaflet also includes details of all inactive ingredients in the medicine. A list of common E numbers and the inactive ingredients to which they correspond is now therefore included in the BNF (see *inside back cover*).

Guidance on Prescribing

Prices in the BNF

Basic **net prices** are given in the BNF to provide an indication of relative cost. Where there is a choice of suitable preparations for a particular disease or condition the relative cost may be used in making a selection. Cost-effective prescribing must, however, take into account other factors (such as dose frequency and duration of treatment) that affect the total cost. The use of more expensive drugs is justified if it will result in better treatment of the patient or a reduction of the length of an illness or the time spent in hospital.

Prices have generally been calculated from the net cost used in pricing NHS prescriptions dispensed in October 1997, but where available later prices have been included; unless an original pack is available these prices are based on the largest pack size of the preparation in use in community pharmacies. The price for an extemporaneously prepared preparation has been omitted where the net cost of the ingredients used to make it would give a misleadingly low impression of the final price.

The unit of 20 is still sometimes used as a basis for comparison, but where suitable original packs or patient packs are available these are priced instead.

Gross prices vary as follows:

1. Costs to the NHS are greater than the net prices quoted and include professional fees and overhead allowances;

2. Private prescription charges are calculated on a separate basis;

3. Over-the-counter sales are at retail price, as opposed to basic net price, and include VAT.

BNF prices are NOT, therefore, suitable for quoting to patients seeking private prescriptions or contemplating over-the-counter purchases.

A fuller explanation of costs to the NHS may be obtained from the Drug Tariff.
It should be noted that separate Drug Tariffs are operative in England and Wales, Scotland, and Northern Ireland. Prices in the different tariffs may vary.

PACT and SPA

PACT (Prescribing Analyses and Cost) and SPA (Scottish Prescribing Analysis) automatically provide general practitioners with information about their prescribing. The information is sent on a quarterly basis direct from the Prescription Pricing Authority (and may be obtained for individual months on request). It is now available as a 'standard report' which replaces the previous *level 1* and *level 2 reports*. The previous *level 3 report* is replaced by a 'catalogue' which provides the data in a more helpful manner and is available on request for periods of one or more months.

General Guidance

Medicines should be prescribed only when they are necessary, and in all cases the benefit of administering the medicine should be considered in relation to the risk involved. This is particularly important during pregnancy where the risk to both mother and fetus must be considered (for further details see Prescribing in Pregnancy, Appendix 4).

ABBREVIATION OF TITLES. In general, titles of drugs and preparations should be written *in full*. Unofficial abbreviations should not be used as they may be misinterpreted; obsolete titles, such as Mist. Expect. should not be used.

NON-PROPRIETARY TITLES. Where non-proprietary ('generic') titles are given, they should be used in prescribing. This will enable any suitable product to be dispensed, thereby saving delay to the patient and sometimes expense to the health service. The only exception is where bioavailability problems are so important that the patient should always receive the same brand; in such cases, the brand name or the manufacturer should be stated. Non-proprietary titles should **not** be invented for the purposes of prescribing generically since this can lead to confusion, particularly in the case of compound and modified-release preparations.

Titles used as headings for monographs may be used freely in Great Britain and Northern Ireland but in other countries may be subject to restriction.

Many of the non-proprietary titles used in this book are titles of monographs in the European Pharmacopoeia, British Pharmacopoeia or British Pharmaceutical Codex 1973. In such cases the preparations must comply with the standard (if any) in the appropriate publication, as required by the Medicines Act (section 65).

PROPRIETARY TITLES. Names followed by the symbol ® are or have been used as proprietary names in the United Kingdom. These names may in general be applied only to products supplied by the owners of the trade marks.

DOSES. The doses stated in the BNF are intended for general guidance and represent, unless otherwise stated, the usual range of doses that are generally regarded as being suitable for adults. In general the *doses, indications, cautions, contra-indications and side-effects* in the BNF reflect those in the manufacturers' data sheets or Summaries of Product Characteristics (SPCs) which, in turn, reflect those in the corresponding Marketing Authorisations (formerly known as Product Licences). On the few occasions that an unlicensed drug is included in the BNF, this is now indicated in brackets after the entry. Where a use (or route) is recommended outside the licensed indication of an available product this too is indicated. It has been noted (*Drug and Therapeutics Bulletin*, 1992, *30*, 97–99) that prescribing of licensed medicines outside the recommendations of the Marketing Authorisation alters (and probably increases) the doctor's professional responsibility.

ORAL SYRINGES. An **oral syringe** is supplied when oral liquid medicines are prescribed in doses other than multiples of 5 mL. The oral syringe is marked in 0.5-mL divisions from 1 to 5 mL to measure doses of less than 5 mL. It is provided with an adaptor and an instruction leaflet. The *5-mL spoon* is used for doses of 5 mL (or multiples thereof).

STRENGTHS AND QUANTITIES. The strength or quantity to be contained in capsules, lozenges, tablets, etc. should be stated by the prescriber.

If a pharmacist receives an incomplete prescription for a systemically administered preparation other than a prescription for a controlled drug and considers it would not be appropriate for the patient to return to the doctor, the following procedures will apply:

(a) an attempt must always be made to contact the prescriber to ascertain the intention;

(b) if the attempt is successful the pharmacist must, where practicable, subsequently arrange for details of quantity, strength where applicable, and dosage to be inserted by the prescriber on the incomplete form;

(c) where, although the prescriber has been contacted, it has not proved possible to obtain the written intention regarding an incomplete prescription, the pharmacist may endorse the form 'p.c.' (prescriber contacted) and add details of the quantity and strength where applicable of the preparation supplied, and of the dose indicated. The endorsement should be initialled and dated by the pharmacist;

(d) where the prescriber cannot be contacted and the pharmacist has sufficient information to make a professional judgment the preparation may be dispensed. If the quantity is missing the pharmacist may supply sufficient to complete up to 5 days' treatment; except that where a combination pack (i.e. a proprietary pack containing more than one medicinal product) or oral contraceptive is prescribed by name only, the smallest pack shall be dispensed. In all cases the prescription must be endorsed 'p.n.c.' (prescriber not contacted) the quantity, the dose, and the strength (where applicable) of the preparation supplied must be indicated, and the endorsement must be initialled and dated;

(e) if the pharmacist has any doubt about exercising discretion, an incomplete prescription must be referred back to the prescriber.

ADDITIVES. Oral liquid preparations that do not contain *fructose, glucose* or *sucrose* are described as 'sugar-free' in the BNF. Preparations containing hydrogenated glucose syrup, mannitol, or sorbitol are also marked 'sugar-free' since there is evidence that they do not cause dental caries.

Where information on the presence of *aspartame, gluten, tartrazine, arachis (peanut) oil* or *sesame oil* is available, this is indicated in the BNF against the relevant preparation; the manufacturer should be contacted in the absence of information on additives in the BNF and in the product literature, if it is essential to check details.

Information is provided on *preservatives* in eye-drops and on *selected additives* in skin preparations (see section 13.1). Pressurised metered aerosols containing *chlorofluorocarbons* (CFCs) have also been identified throughout the BNF (see also section 3.1.1.1)

EXTEMPORANEOUS PREPARATION. The BP direction that a preparation must be *freshly prepared* indicates that it must be made not more than 24 hours before it is issued for use. The direction that a preparation should be *recently prepared* indicates that deterioration is likely if the preparation is stored for longer than about 4 weeks at 15° C to 25° C.

DRUGS AND DRIVING. Prescribers should advise patients if treatment is likely to affect their ability to drive motor vehicles. This applies particularly to drugs with sedative effects and patients should be warned that these effects are increased by alcohol. See also Appendix 10.

NOTICE CONCERNING PATENTS. In the BNF certain drugs have been included notwithstanding the existence of actual or potential patent rights. In so far as such substances are protected by Letters Patent, their inclusion in this Formulary neither conveys, nor implies, licence to manufacture.

HEALTH AND SAFETY. When handling chemical or biological materials particular attention should be given to the possibility of allergy, fire, explosion, radiation, or poisoning. Some substances, including corticosteroids, antibiotics, phenothiazines, and many cytotoxics, are irritant or very potent and should be handled with caution. Contact with the skin and inhalation of dust should be avoided.

SAFETY IN THE HOME. Patients must be warned to keep all medicines out of the reach of children. All solid dose and all oral and external liquid preparations must be dispensed in a reclosable *child-resistant container* unless:

(i) the medicine is in an original pack or patient pack such as to make this inadvisable;
(ii) the patient will have difficulty in opening a child-resistant container;
(iii) a specific request is made that the product shall not be dispensed in a child-resistant container;
(iv) no suitable child-resistant container exists for a particular liquid preparation.

All patients should be advised to dispose of *unwanted medicines* by returning them to a supplier for destruction.

NAME OF MEDICINE. The name of the medicine should appear on the label unless the prescriber indicates otherwise.

1. Subject to the conditions of paragraphs 4 and 6 below, the name of the prescribed medicine is stated on the label unless the prescriber deletes the letters 'NP' which appear on NHS prescription forms.

2. The strength is also stated on the label in the case of tablets, capsules, and similar preparations that are available in different strengths.

3. If it is the wish of the prescriber that a description such as 'The Sedative Tablets' should appear on the label, the prescriber should write the desired description on the prescription form.

4. The arrangement will extend to approved names, proprietary names or titles given in the BP, BPC, BNF, or DPF. The arrangement does not apply when a prescription is written so that several ingredients are given.

5. The name written on the label is that used by the prescriber on the prescription.

6. If more than one item is prescribed on one form and the prescriber does not delete the letters 'NP', each dispensed medicine is named on the label, subject to the conditions given above in paragraph 4. If the prescriber wants only selected items on such a prescription to be so labelled this should be indicated by deleting the letters 'NP' on the form and writing 'NP' alongside the medicines to be labelled.

7. When a prescription is written other than on an NHS prescription form the name of the prescribed preparation will be stated on the label of the dispensed medicine unless the prescriber indicates otherwise.

8. The Council of the Royal Pharmaceutical Society advises that the labels of dispensed medicines should indicate the total quantity of the product dispensed in the container to which the label refers. This requirement applies equally to solid, liquid, internal, and external preparations. If a product is dispensed in more than one container, the reference should be to the amount in each container.

Scope of the BNF

The BNF is intended for the guidance of medical practitioners, pharmacists, dentists, nurses, and others who have the necessary training and experience to interpret the information it provides. It is intended as a reference for the pocket, and should be supplemented by a study of more detailed publications when required.

Security and validity of prescriptions

The Councils of the British Medical Association and the Royal Pharmaceutical Society have issued a joint statement on the security and validity of prescriptions.
In particular, prescription forms should:
(i) not be left unattended at reception desks;
(ii) not be left in a car where they may be visible; and
(iii) when not in use, be kept in a locked drawer within the surgery and at home.
Where there is any doubt about the authenticity of a prescription, the pharmacist should contact the prescriber. If this is done by telephone, the number should be obtained from the directory rather than relying on the prescription form information, which may be false.

Prescription Writing

Shared care

In its guidelines on responsibility for prescribing between hospitals and general practitioners, the Department of Health has advised that legal responsibility for prescribing lies with the doctor who signs the prescription.

Prescriptions[1] should be written legibly in ink or otherwise so as to be indelible[2], should be dated, should state the full name and address of the patient, and should be signed in ink by the prescriber[3]. The age of the patient should preferably be stated, and is a legal requirement in the case of prescription-only medicines for children under 12 years of age.

The following should be noted:

(a) The unnecessary use of decimal points should be avoided, e.g. 3 mg, not 3.0 mg.

Quantities of 1 gram or more should be written as 1 g etc.

Quantities less than 1 gram should be written in milligrams, e.g. 500 mg, not 0.5 g.

Quantities less than 1 mg should be written in micrograms, e.g. 100 micrograms, not 0.1 mg.

When decimals are unavoidable a zero should be written in front of the decimal point where there is no other figure, e.g. 0.5 mL, not .5 mL.

Use of the decimal point is acceptable to express a range, e.g. 0.5 to 1 g.

(b) 'Micrograms' and 'nanograms' should **not** be abbreviated. Similarly 'units' should **not** be abbreviated.

(c) The term 'millilitre' (ml or mL)[4] is used in medicine and pharmacy, and cubic centimetre, c.c., or cm^3 should not be used.

(d) Dose and dose frequency should be stated; in the case of preparations to be taken 'as required' a **minimum dose interval** should be specified.

When doses other than multiples of 5 mL are prescribed for *oral liquid preparations* the dose-volume will be provided by means of an **oral syringe**, see p. 2 (except for preparations intended to be measured with a pipette).

Suitable quantities:

Elixirs, Linctuses, and Paediatric Mixtures (5-mL dose), 50, 100, or 150 mL

Adult Mixtures (10-mL dose), 200 or 300 mL

Ear Drops, Eye-drops, and Nasal Drops, 10 mL (or the manufacturer's pack)

Eye Lotions, Gargles, and Mouth-washes, 200 mL

(e) For suitable quantities of dermatological preparations, see section 13.1.

(f) The names of drugs and preparations should be written clearly and **not** abbreviated, using approved titles **only** (see also advice in box on p. 5 to **avoid** creating generic titles for modified-release preparations).

(g) The symbol 'NP' on NHS forms should be deleted if it is required that the name of the preparation should not appear on the label. For full details see p. 3.

(h) The quantity to be supplied may be stated by indicating the number of days of treatment required in the box provided on NHS forms. In most cases the exact amount will be supplied. This does not apply to items directed to be used as required—if the dose and frequency are not given the quantity to be supplied needs to be stated.

When several items are ordered on one form the box can be marked with the number of days of treatment providing the quantity is added for any item for which the amount cannot be calculated.

(i) Although directions should preferably be in **English without abbreviation**, it is recognised that some Latin abbreviations are used (for details see Inside Back Cover).

(j) A prescription for a preparation that has been withdrawn or needs to be specially imported for a named patient should be handwritten. The name of the preparation should be endorsed with the prescriber's signature and the letters 'WD' (withdrawn or specially-imported drug); there may be considerable delay in obtaining a withdrawn medicine.

---

1. The above recommendations are acceptable for **prescription-only medicines** (PoM). For items marked **CD** see also Controlled Drugs and Drug Dependence p. 7.

2. It is permissible to issue carbon copies of NHS prescriptions as long as they are signed in ink.

3. Computer-generated facsimile signatures do not meet the legal requirement.

4. The use of capital 'L' in mL is a printing convention throughout the BNF; both mL and ml are recognised abbreviations for SI units.

Computer-issued Prescriptions

For computer-issued prescriptions the following recommendations of the Joint Computing Group of the General Medical Services Committee and the Royal College of General Practitioners should also be noted:

1. The computer must print out the date[1], the patient's surname, one forename, other initials, and address, and may also print out the patient's title. The age of children under 12 years must be printed in the box available; a facility may exist to print out the age of older children and adults as well.

2. The doctor's name[2] must be printed at the bottom of the prescription form; this will be the name of the doctor responsible for the prescription (who will normally sign it). The doctor's surgery address, reference number, and Health Authority (HA)[3] are also necessary. In addition, the surgery telephone number should be printed.

3. When prescriptions are to be signed by trainees, assistants, locums, or deputising doctors, the name of the doctor printed at the bottom of the form must still be that of the responsible principal. To avoid difficulties for the pharmacist checking the prescription, the name of the signing doctor may be printed in the signature box, to be signed over on prescribing.

4. Names of medicines must come from a dictionary held in the computer memory, to provide a check on the spelling and ensure that the name is written in full. The computer can be programmed to recognise both the non-proprietary and the proprietary name of a particular drug and to print out the preferred choice, but must not print out both names. For medicines not in the dictionary, separate checking mechanisms are required—the user must be warned that no check was possible and the entire prescription must be entered in the lexicon.

5. The dictionary may contain information on the usual doses, formulations, and (where relevant) pack sizes to produce standard predetermined prescriptions for common preparations, and to provide a check on the validity of an individual prescription on entry.

6. The prescription must be printed in English without abbreviation; information may be entered or stored in abbreviated form. The dose must be in numbers, the frequency in words, and the quantity in numbers in brackets, thus: 40 mg four times daily (112). It must also be possible to prescribe by indicating the length of treatment required, see (h) above.

7. The BNF recommendations should be followed as in (a), (b), (c), (d), and (e) above.

8. Checks may be incorporated to ensure that all the information required for dispensing a particular drug has been filled in. Instructions such as 'as directed' should be avoided. For the instruction 'when required' the maximum daily dose should normally be specified.

9. Numbers and codes used in the system for organising and retrieving data must never appear on the form.

10. Supplementary warnings or advice should be written in full, should not interfere with the clarity of the prescription itself, and should be in line with any warnings or advice in the BNF; numerical codes should not be used.

11. A mechanism (such as printing a series of non-specific characters) may be incorporated to cancel out unused space, or wording such as 'no more items on this prescription' may be added after the last item. Otherwise the doctor should delete the space manually.

12. To avoid forgery the computer may print on the form the number of items to be dispensed (somewhere separate from the box for the pharmacist). The number of items per form need be limited only by the ability of the printer to produce clear and well-demarcated instructions with sufficient space for each item and a spacer line before each fresh item.

13. Handwritten alterations should only be made in exceptional circumstances—it is preferable to print out a new prescription. Any alterations that are made must be written in the doctor's own handwriting and countersigned.

14. Prescriptions for controlled drugs cannot be produced by a printer[4]. If there is a record of such a prescription in the computer, it must not be printed. Instead the computer may print out a blank form with the doctor's name[1] and other details printed at the bottom.

15. The strip of paper on the side of the FP10[5](Comp) may be used for various purposes but care should be taken to avoid including confidential information. It may be advisable for the patient's name to appear at the top, but this should be preceded by 'confidential'.

16. In rural dispensing practices prescription requests (or details of medicines dispensed) will normally be entered in one surgery. The prescriptions (or dispensed medicines) may then need to be delivered to another surgery or location; if possible the computer should hold up to 10 alternatives.

Generic names of **compound preparations** which appear in the BNF are those approved by the British Pharmacopoeia Commission; whenever possible they reflect the names of the active ingredients.

Prescribers should avoid creating their own compound names for the purposes of generic prescribing; such names do not have an approved definition and can be misinterpreted.

Special care should be taken to avoid errors when prescribing compound preparations; in particular the hyphen in the prefix 'co-' should be retained.

Special care should also be taken to avoid creating generic names for **modified-release** preparations where the use of these names could lead to confusion between formulations with different lengths of action.

---

1. The exemption for own handwriting regulations for phenobarbitone does not apply to the date; a computer-generated date need not be deleted but the date must also be added by the prescriber.
2. Except in Scotland where it does not appear.
3. Health Board in Scotland.
4. Except in the case of phenobarbitone (but see also footnote 1) or where the prescriber has been exempted from handwriting requirements, for details see Controlled Drugs and Drug Dependence p. 7.
5. GP10 in Scotland.

Emergency Supply of PoM at Patient's Request[1]

The Medicines (Products Other Than Veterinary Drugs) (Prescription Only) Order 1983, as amended, allows exemptions from the Prescription Only requirements for emergency supply to be made by a person lawfully conducting a retail pharmacy business provided:

(a) that the pharmacist has interviewed the person requesting the prescription-only medicine and is satisfied:
  (i) that there is immediate need for the prescription-only medicine and that it is impracticable in the circumstances to obtain a prescription without undue delay;
  (ii) that treatment with the prescription-only medicine has on a previous occasion been prescribed by a doctor[2] for the person requesting it;
  (iii) as to the dose which it would be appropriate for the person to take;
(b) that no greater quantity shall be supplied than will provide five days' treatment except when the prescription-only medicine is:
  (i) an ointment, cream, or preparation for the relief of asthma in an aerosol dispenser when the smallest pack can be supplied;
  (ii) an oral contraceptive when a full cycle may be supplied;
  (iii) an antibiotic in liquid form for oral administration when the smallest quantity that will provide a full course of treatment can be supplied;
(c) that an entry shall be made in the prescription book stating:
  (i) the date of supply;
  (ii) the name, quantity and, where appropriate, the pharmaceutical form and strength;
  (iii) the name and address of the patient;
  (iv) the nature of the emergency;
(d) that the container or package must be labelled to show:
  (i) the date of supply;
  (ii) the name, quantity and, where appropriate, the pharmaceutical form and strength;
  (iii) the name of the patient;
  (iv) the name and address of the pharmacy;
  (v) the words 'Emergency supply'.

(e) that the prescription-only medicine is not a substance specifically excluded from the emergency supply provision, and does not contain a Controlled Drug specified in schedules 1, 2, or 3 to the Misuse of Drugs Regulations 1985 except for phenobarbitone or phenobarbitone sodium for the treatment of epilepsy: for details see *Medicines, Ethics and Practice*, No. 19, London, Pharmaceutical Press, 1998 (and subsequent editions as available).

ROYAL PHARMACEUTICAL SOCIETY'S GUIDELINES

(1) The pharmacist should consider the medical consequences of *not* supplying.

(2) If the patient is not known to the pharmacist, the patient's identity should be established by way of appropriate documentation.

(3) It may occasionally be desirable to contact the prescriber, e.g. when the medicine requested has a potential for misuse or the prescriber is not known to the pharmacist.

(4) Care should be taken to ask whether the patient's doctor has stopped the treatment, or whether the patient is taking any other medication.

(5) Except for conditions which occur infrequently (e.g. hay fever, asthma attack or migraine), a supply should not be made if the item requested was last prescribed more than 6 months ago.

(6) Consideration should be given to supplying less than 5 days' quantity if this is justified.

(7) Where a prescription is to be provided later, a record of emergency supply as required by law must still be made. It is good practice to add to the record the date that the prescription is received on. Payment for the medicine supplied is not a legal requirement, but may help to minimise the abuse of the emergency supply exemption. If an NHS prescription is to be provided, a refundable charge may be made.

1. For emergency supply at the request of a doctor see *Medicines, Ethics and Practice*, No. 19, London, Pharmaceutical Press, 1998 (and subsequent editions as available).
2. The doctor must be a UK-registered doctor.

Plasma concentrations in the BNF are expressed in mass units per litre (e.g. mg/litre). The approximate equivalent in terms of amount of substance units (e.g. micromol/litre) is given in brackets.

Approximate Conversions and Units

lb	kg	stones	kg	ml	fl. oz
1	0.45	1	6.35	50	1.8
2	0.91	2	12.70	100	3.5
3	1.36	3	19.05	150	5.3
4	1.81	4	25.40	200	7.0
5	2.27	5	31.75	500	17.6
6	2.72	6	38.10	1000	35.2
7	3.18	7	44.45		
8	3.63	8	50.80		
9	4.08	9	57.15		
10	4.54	10	63.50		
11	4.99	11	69.85		
12	5.44	12	76.20		
13	5.90	13	82.55		
14	6.35	14	88.90		
		15	95.25		

Mass

1 kilogram (kg)	= 1000 grams (g)
1 gram (g)	= 1000 milligrams (mg)
1 milligram (mg)	= 1000 micrograms
1 microgram	= 1000 nanograms
1 nanogram	= 1000 picograms

Volume

1 litre	= 1000 millilitres (mL)
1 millilitre	= 1000 microlitres
1 pint	$\approx$ 568 mL

Other units

1 kilocalorie (kcal)	= 4186.8 joules (J)
1000 kilocalories (kcal)	= 4.1868 megajoules (MJ)
1 megajoule (MJ)	= 238.8 kilocalories (kcal)
1 millimetre of mercury (mmHg)	= 133.3 pascals (Pa)
1 kilopascal (kPa)	= 7.5 mmHg (pressure)

Controlled Drugs and Drug Dependence

PRESCRIPTIONS. Preparations which are subject to the prescription requirements of the Misuse of Drugs Regulations 1985, i.e. preparations specified in schedules 2 and 3, are distinguished throughout the BNF by the symbol **CD** (Controlled Drugs). The principal legal requirements relating to medical prescriptions are listed below.

Prescriptions ordering Controlled Drugs subject to prescription requirements must be *signed* and *dated*[1] by the prescriber and specify the prescriber's *address*. The prescription must always state *in the prescriber's own handwriting*[2] in ink or otherwise so as to be indelible:

1. The name and address of the patient;
2. In the case of a preparation, the form[3] and where appropriate the strength[4] of the preparation;
3. The total quantity of the preparation, or the number of dose units, *in both words and figures;*[5]
4. The dose.[6]

A prescription may order a Controlled Drug to be dispensed by instalments; the amount of the instalments and the intervals to be observed must be specified.[7] Prescriptions ordering 'repeats' on the same form are **not** permitted.

It is an offence for a doctor to issue an incomplete prescription and a pharmacist is **not** allowed to dispense a Controlled Drug unless all the information required by law is given on the prescription. Failure to comply with the regulations concerning the writing of prescriptions will result in inconvenience to patients and delay in supplying the necessary medicine.

DEPENDENCE AND MISUSE. The most serious drugs of addiction are **cocaine**, **diamorphine** (heroin), **morphine**, and the **synthetic opioids**. For arrangements for prescribing of diamorphine, dipipanone or cocaine for addicts, see p. 9.

Despite marked reduction in the prescribing of **amphetamines** there is concern that abuse of illicit amphetamine and related compounds is widespread.

Owing to problems of widespread abuse additional controlled drug requirements have been placed on **temazepam** (but it remains exempt from the additional prescribing requirements).

The principal **barbiturates** are now Controlled Drugs, but phenobarbitone and phenobarbitone sodium or a preparation containing either of these are exempt from the handwriting requirement but must fulfil all other controlled drug prescription requirements (**important**: the own handwriting exemption does **not** apply to the date; a computer-generated date need not be deleted but the date must also be added by the prescriber). Moreover, for the treatment of epilepsy phenobarbitone and phenobarbitone sodium are available under the emergency supply regulations (p. 6).

Cannabis (Indian hemp) has no approved medicinal use and cannot be prescribed by doctors. Its use is illegal but has become widespread. Cannabis is a mild hallucinogen seldom accompanied by a desire to increase the dose; withdrawal symptoms are unusual. **Lysergide** (lysergic acid diethylamide, LSD) is a much more potent hallucinogen; its use can lead to severe psychotic states in which life may be at risk.

1. A prescription is valid for 13 weeks from the date stated thereon.
2. Does not apply to prescriptions for temazepam. Otherwise applies unless the prescriber has been specifically exempted from this requirement or unless the prescription contains no controlled drug other than phenobarbitone or phenobarbitone sodium or a preparation containing either of these; the exemption does **not** apply to the date—a computer-generated date need not be deleted but the date must also be added by the prescriber.
3. The dosage form (e.g. tablets) must be included on a Controlled Drugs prescription irrespective of whether it is implicit in the proprietary name (e.g. *MST Continus*) or of whether only one form is available.
4. When more than one strength of a preparation exists the strength required must be specified.
5. Does not apply to prescriptions for temazepam.
6. The instruction 'one as directed' constitutes a dose but 'as directed' does not.
7. A special form, FP10(HP)(ad), in Scotland HBP(A), is available to doctors in NHS drug treatment centres for prescribing cocaine, dextromoramide, diamorphine, dipipanone, methadone, morphine, or pethidine by instalments for addicts (see also Terms of Service, paragraph 43). In Scotland general practitioners can prescribe by instalments on form GP10. In England and Wales forms FP10 and FP10(HP) are not suitable for this purpose but form FP10(MDA) is available. **Important**: in all cases a special licence is necessary to prescribe cocaine, diamorphine, or dipipanone for addicts except for treatment of organic disease or injury, for details see p. 9.

PRESCRIBING DRUGS LIKELY TO CAUSE DEPENDENCE OR MISUSE. The prescriber has three main responsibilities:

1. To avoid creating dependence by introducing drugs to patients without sufficient reason. In this context, the proper use of the morphine-like drugs is well understood. The dangers of other controlled drugs are less clear because recognition of dependence is not easy and its effects, and those of withdrawal, are less obvious. Perhaps the most notable result of uninhibited prescribing is that a very large number of patients in the country take tablets which do them neither much good nor much harm, but are committed to them indefinitely because they cannot readily be stopped.

2. To see that the patient does not gradually increase the dose of a drug, given for good medical reasons, to the point where dependence becomes more likely. This tendency is seen especially with hypnotics and anxiolytics (for CSM advice see section 4.1). The prescriber should keep a close eye on the amount prescribed to prevent patients from accumulating stocks that would enable them to arrange their own dosage or even that of their families and friends. A minimal amount should be prescribed in the first instance, or when seeing a new patient for the first time.

3. To avoid being used as an unwitting source of supply for addicts. Methods include visiting more than one doctor, fabricating stories, and forging prescriptions.

Patients under temporary care should be given only small supplies of drugs unless they present an unequivocal letter from their own doctors. Doctors should also remember that their own patients may be doing a collecting round with other doctors, especially in hospitals. It is sensible to decrease dosages steadily or to issue weekly or even daily prescriptions for small amounts if it is apparent that dependence is occurring.

The stealing and misuse of prescription forms could be minimised by the following precautions:

(a) do not leave unattended if called away from the consulting room or at reception desks; do not leave in a car where they may be visible; when not in use, keep in a locked drawer within the surgery and at home;

(b) draw a diagonal line across the blank part of the form under the prescription;

(c) write the quantity in words and figures when prescribing drugs prone to abuse; this is obligatory for controlled drugs (see Prescriptions, above);

(d) alterations are best avoided but if any are made they should be clear and unambiguous; add initials against altered items;

(e) if prescriptions are left for collection they should be left in a safe place in a sealed envelope.

TRAVELLING ABROAD. Prescribed drugs listed in schedules 4 and 5 to the Misuse of Drugs Regulations 1985 are not subject to import or export licensing but doctors are advised that patients intending to carry Schedule 2 and 3 drugs abroad may require an export licence. This is dependent upon the amount of drug to be exported and further details may be obtained from the Home Office by telephoning 0171-273 3806. Applications for licences should be sent to the Home Office, Drugs Branch, Queen Anne's Gate, London SW1H 9AT.

There is no standard application form but applications must be supported by a letter from a doctor giving details of:

the patient's name and current address;
the quantities of drugs to be carried;
the strength and form in which the drugs will be dispensed;
the dates of travel to and from the United Kingdom.

Ten days should be allowed for processing the application.

Individual doctors who wish to take Controlled Drugs abroad while accompanying patients, may similarly be issued with licences. Licences are not normally issued to doctors who wish to take Controlled Drugs abroad solely in case a family emergency should arise.

These import/export licences for named individuals do not have any legal status outside the UK and are only issued to comply with the Misuse of Drugs Act and facilitate passage through UK Customs control. For clearance in the country to be visited it would be necessary to approach that country's embassy or High Commission in the UK.

Misuse of Drugs Act

The Misuse of Drugs Act, 1971 prohibits certain activities in relation to 'Controlled Drugs', in particular their manufacture, supply, and possession. The penalties applicable to offences involving the different drugs are graded broadly according to the *harmfulness attributable to a drug when it is misused* and for this purpose the drugs are defined in the following three classes:

Class A includes: alfentanil, cocaine, dextromoramide, diamorphine (heroin), dipipanone, lysergide (LSD), methadone, morphine, opium, pethidine, phencyclidine, and class B substances when prepared for injection

Class B includes: oral amphetamines, barbiturates, cannabis, cannabis resin, codeine, ethylmorphine, glutethimide, pentazocine, phenmetrazine, and pholcodine

Class C includes: certain drugs related to the amphetamines such as benzphetamine and chlorphentermine, buprenorphine, diethylpropion, mazindol, meprobamate, pemoline, pipradrol, most benzodiazepines, androgenic and anabolic steroids, clenbuterol, chorionic gonadotrophin (HCG), non-human chorionic gonadotrophin, somatotropin, somatrem, and somatropin

The Misuse of Drugs Regulations 1985 define the classes of person who are authorised to supply and possess controlled drugs while acting in their professional capacities and lay down the conditions under which these activities may be carried out. In the regulations drugs are divided into five schedules each specifying the requirements governing such activities as import, export, production, supply, possession, prescribing, and record keeping which apply to them.

Schedule 1 includes drugs such as cannabis and lysergide which are not used medicinally. Possession and supply are prohibited except in accordance with Home Office authority.

Schedule 2 includes drugs such as diamorphine (heroin), morphine, pethidine, quinalbarbitone, glutethimide, amphetamine, and cocaine and are subject to the full controlled drug requirements relating to prescriptions, safe custody (except for quinalbarbitone), the need to keep registers, etc. (unless exempted in schedule 5).

Schedule 3 includes the barbiturates (except quinalbarbitone, now schedule 2), buprenorphine, diethylpropion, mazindol, meprobamate, pentazocine, phentermine, and temazepam. They are subject to the special prescription requirements (except for phenobarbitone and temazepam, see p. 7) but not to the safe custody requirements (except for buprenorphine, diethylpropion, and temazepam) nor to the need to keep registers (although there are requirements for the retention of invoices for 2 years).

Schedule 4 includes in Part II 33 benzodiazepines (temazepam is now in schedule 3) and pemoline which are subject to minimal control. Part I includes androgenic and anabolic steroids, clenbuterol, chorionic gonadotrophin (HCG), non-human chorionic gonadotrophin, somatotropin, somatrem, and somatropin. Controlled drug prescription requirements do not apply and Schedule 4 Controlled Drugs are not subject to safe custody requirements.

Schedule 5 includes those preparations which, because of their strength, are exempt from virtually all Controlled Drug requirements other than retention of invoices for two years.

Notification of Drug Misusers

In May 1997, the Misuse of Drugs (Supply to Addicts) Regulations 1997 revoked the requirement for doctors to send to the Home Office particulars of drug addicts.

The Addicts Index, which was held by the Home Office, has now been closed. However, doctors are expected to continue to report treatment demands of all drug misusers by returning the local drug misuse database reporting forms, which provide anonymised data, to the appropriate national or regional Drug Misuse Database (DMD). Information in the database is not limited, as was the Addicts Index, to opioid and cocaine misuse, but includes any misused drug that generates treatment demand.

Enquiries regarding regional and national DMDs can be made to database managers at the following contact telephone numbers.

ENGLAND

Anglia and Oxford
telephone 01865 226734; fax 01865 226652
North Thames
telephone 0181 846 6563; fax 0181 846 6555
North West
Merseyside and Cheshire: telephone 0151 794 5821; fax 0151 794 5488
North Western: telephone 0161 772 3782; fax 0161 772 3445
Northern and Yorkshire
Northern: telephone 0191 333 3245; fax 0191 333 3233
Yorkshire: telephone 0113 292 6960; fax 0113 292 6950
South and West
Wessex: telephone 01962 863511 ext 455; fax 01962 844759
South Western: telephone 0117 958 4384

South Thames
East: telephone 01273 323395; fax 01273 748178
West: telephone 0181 725 5352; fax 0181 725 2914
Trent
North: telephone 0114 279 5698; fax 0114 276 1401
South: telephone 0116 286 3267; fax 0116 275 2840
West Midlands
telephone 0121 627 2059; fax 0121 627 2051

SCOTLAND
telephone 0131 551 8715; fax 0131 551 1392

WALES
telephone 01222 667766; fax 01222 665940

In **Northern Ireland**, the Misuse of Drugs (Notification of and Supply to Addicts) (Northern Ireland) Regulations 1973 require doctors to send particulars of persons whom they consider to be addicted to certain controlled drugs to

Chief Medical Officer
Department of Health and Social Services
Block C.5.15
Castle Buildings
Belfast BT4 3PP
telephone 01232 520000 ext 20563

Enquiries should also be made to that department.

Prescribing of diamorphine (heroin), dipipanone, and cocaine for addicts

The Misuse of Drugs (Supply to Addicts) Regulations 1997 require that only medical practitioners who hold a special licence issued by the Home Secretary may prescribe, administer or supply diamorphine, dipipanone[1] (*Diconal®*) or cocaine in the treatment of drug addiction; other practitioners must refer any addict who requires these drugs to a treatment centre. Whenever possible the addict will be introduced by a member of staff from the treatment centre to a pharmacist whose agreement has been obtained and whose pharmacy is conveniently sited for the patient. Prescriptions for weekly supplies will be sent to the pharmacy by post and will be dispensed on a daily basis as indicated by the doctor. If any alterations of the arrangements are requested by the addict, the portion of the prescription affected must be represcribed and not merely altered. *General practitioners and other doctors may still prescribe diamorphine, dipipanone, and cocaine for patients (including addicts) for relief of pain due to organic disease or injury without a special licence.*

For prescription-writing guidelines, see p. 7.

---

1. Dipipanone in *Diconal®* tablets has been much misused by opioid addicts in recent years. Doctors and others should be suspicious of people who ask for the tablets, especially if temporary residents.

Adverse Reactions to Drugs

Any drug may produce unwanted or unexpected adverse reactions. Detection and recording of these is of vital importance. Doctors[1] and hospital pharmacists are urged to help by reporting adverse reactions to:

Medicines Control Agency
CSM Freepost
London SW8 5BR
(0800 731 6789)

Prepaid Yellow Cards for reporting are available from the above address; forms for doctors are bound in this book (inside back cover).

A 24-hour Freefone service is available to all parts of the UK for advice and information on suspected adverse drug reactions; contact the National Yellow Card Information Service at the MCA on 0800 731 6789. Outside office hours a telephone-answering machine will take messages.

The following regional centres also collect data:

CSM Mersey	CSM Wales
Freepost	Freepost
Liverpool L3 3AB	Cardiff CF4 1ZZ
(0151-794 8113)	(01222 744181
	Direct Line)
CSM Northern	CSM West Midlands
Freepost 1085	Freepost SW2991
Newcastle upon Tyne	Birmingham B18 7BR
NE1 1BR	[No telephone number]
(0191-232 1525 Direct Line)	

The CSM's Adverse Drug Reactions On-line Information Tracking (ADROIT) facilitates the monitoring of adverse drug reactions.

Suspected adverse reactions to *any* therapeutic agent should be reported, including drugs (*self-medication* as well as *prescribed* ones), blood products, vaccines, X-ray contrast media, dental or surgical materials, intra-uterine devices, herbal products, and contact lens fluids.

NEWER DRUGS. These are indicated by the symbol ▼. Doctors[1] and hospital pharmacists are asked to report *all* suspected reactions (i.e. any adverse or any unexpected event, however minor, which could conceivably be attributed to the drug). Reports should be made despite uncertainty about a causal relationship, irrespective of whether the reaction is well recognized, and even if other drugs have been given concurrently.

ESTABLISHED DRUGS AND VACCINES. Doctors[1] and hospital pharmacists are asked to report *all* serious suspected reactions, including those that are fatal, life-threatening, disabling, incapacitating, or which result in or prolong hospitalisation; they should be reported even if the effect is well recognised.

Examples include anaphylaxis, blood disorders, endocrine disturbances, effects on fertility, haemorrhage from any site, renal impairment, jaundice, ophthalmic disorders, severe CNS effects, severe skin reactions, reactions in pregnant women, and any drug interactions. Reports of serious adverse reactions are required to enable comparison with other drugs of a similar class. For established drugs doctors are asked not to report well-known, relatively minor side-effects, such as dry mouth with tricyclic antidepressants, constipation with opioids, or nausea with digoxin.

Special problems

Delayed drug effects. Some reactions (e.g. cancers, chloroquine retinopathy, and retroperitoneal fibrosis) may become manifest months or years after exposure. Any suspicion of such an association should be reported.

The elderly. Doctors are asked to be particularly alert to adverse reactions in the elderly.

Congenital abnormalities. When an infant is born with a congenital abnormality or there is a malformed aborted fetus doctors are asked to consider whether this might be an adverse reaction to a drug and to report all drugs (including self-medication) taken during pregnancy.

Prevention of adverse reactions

Adverse reactions may be prevented as follows:

1. Never use any drug unless there is a good indication. If the patient is pregnant do not use a drug unless the need for it is imperative.

2. Allergy and idiosyncrasy are important causes of adverse drug reactions. Ask if the patient had previous reactions.

3. Ask if the patient is already taking other drugs *including self-medication drugs*; interactions may occur.

4. Age and hepatic or renal disease may alter the metabolism or excretion of drugs, so that much smaller doses may be needed. Genetic factors may also be responsible for variations in metabolism, notably of isoniazid and the tricyclic antidepressants.

5. Prescribe as few drugs as possible and give very clear instructions to the elderly or any patient likely to misunderstand complicated instructions.

6. When possible use a familiar drug. With a new drug be particularly alert for adverse reactions or unexpected events.

7. If serious adverse reactions are liable to occur warn the patient.

Defective Medicines

During the manufacture or distribution of a medicine an error or accident may occur whereby the finished product does not conform to its specification. While such a defect may impair the therapeutic effect of the product and could adversely affect the health of a patient, it should **not** be confused with an Adverse Drug Reaction where the product conforms to its specification.

The Defective Medicines Report Centre assists with the investigation of problems arising from licensed medicinal products thought to be defective and co-ordinates any necessary protective action. Reports on suspect defective medicinal products should include the brand or the non-proprietary name, the name of the manufacturer or supplier, the strength and dosage form of the product, the product licence number, the batch number or numbers of the product, the nature of the defect, and an account of any action already taken in consequence. The Centre can be contacted at:

The Defective Medicines Report Centre
Medicines Control Agency
Room 1801, Market Towers
1 Nine Elms Lane
London SW8 5NQ
0171-273 0574 (weekdays 9.00 am–5.00 pm)
or 0171-210 3000 or 5371 (any other time)

---

1. A demonstration scheme also allows community pharmacists within the CSM's Monitoring Centres in Cardiff, Birmingham, Liverpool, and Newcastle to report suspected reactions. All pharmacists must discuss the particular case with the patient's doctor before sending a yellow card report. Whilst it is not recommended for a report to be made against the advice of the patient's doctor, the pharmacist may wish to exercise professional judgement in sending such a report.

Prescribing for Children

All children, and particularly neonates, differ from adults in their response to drugs. Special care is needed in the neonatal period (first 30 days of life) and doses should always be calculated according to weight. At this age, the risk of toxicity is increased by inefficient renal filtration, relative enzyme deficiencies, differing target organ sensitivity, and inadequate detoxifying systems causing delayed excretion. In childhood dosage should be adjusted for weight until 50 kg or puberty is reached.

Whenever possible painful intramuscular injections should be **avoided** in children.

PRESCRIPTION WRITING. Prescriptions should be written according to the guidelines in Prescription Writing (p. 4). Inclusion of age is a legal requirement in the case of prescription-only medicines for children under 12 years of age, but it is preferable to state the age for **all** prescriptions for children.

It is particularly important to state the strengths of capsules or tablets. Although liquid preparations are particularly suitable for children, many contain sucrose which encourages dental decay. When taken over a long period, sugar-free tablets and liquid medicines should be used when possible.

When a prescription for a liquid oral preparation is written and the dose ordered is smaller than 5 mL, the preparation will no longer be diluted. Instead an **oral syringe** will be supplied, for full details, see p. 2. Parents should be advised not to add any medicines to the contents of the infant's feeding bottle, since the drug may interact with the milk or other liquid in it; moreover the ingested dosage may be reduced, if the child does not drink all the contents.

Parents must be warned to keep **all** medicines out of the reach of children, see Safety in the Home, p. 3.

Rare paediatric conditions

Information on substances such as *biotin* and *sodium benzoate* used in rare metabolic conditions can be obtained from:

Drug Information Centre, Alder Hey Children's Hospital, Liverpool L12 2AP (Tel. 0151-252 5381);

Pharmacy, Hospital for Sick Children, Great Ormond St, London, WC1N 3JH (Tel. 0171-405 9200)

Dosage in Children

Children's doses in the BNF are stated in the individual drug entries as far as possible, except where paediatric use is not recommended or there are special hazards.

Doses are generally based on body-weight (in kilograms) or the following age ranges:

first month (neonate)
up to 1 year (infant)
1–5 years
6–12 years

DOSE CALCULATION. Children's doses may be calculated from adult doses by using age, body-weight, or body-surface area, or by a combination of these factors. The most reliable methods are those based on body-surface area.

Body-weight may be used to calculate doses expressed in mg/kg. Young children may require a higher dose per kilogram than adults because of their higher metabolic rates. Other problems need to be considered. For example, calculation by body-weight in the obese child would result in much higher doses being administered than necessary; in such cases, dose should be calculated from an ideal weight, related to height and age.

Body-surface area (BSA) estimates are more accurate for calculation of paediatric doses than body-weight since many physical phenomena are more closely related to body-surface area. The average body-surface area of a 70-kilogram human is about 1.8 m². Thus, to calculate the dose for a child the following formula may be used:

Approximate dose for patient =

$$\frac{\text{surface area of patient (m}^2) \times \text{adult dose}}{1.8}$$

The **percentage method** below may be used to calculate paediatric doses of commonly prescribed drugs that have a wide margin between the therapeutic and the toxic dose

Age	Ideal body-weight kg	lb	Height cm	in	Body-surface m²	Percentage of adult dose
Newborn*	3.4	7.5	50	20	0.23	12.5
1 month*	4.2	9	55	22	0.26	14.5
3 months*	5.6	12	59	23	0.32	18
6 months	7.7	17	67	26	0.40	22
1 year	10	22	76	30	0.47	25
3 years	14	31	94	37	0.62	33
5 years	18	40	108	42	0.73	40
7 years	23	51	120	47	0.88	50
12 years	37	81	148	58	1.25	75
Adult						
Male	68	150	173	68	1.80	100
Female	56	123	163	64	1.60	100

* The figures relate to full term and not preterm infants who may need reduced dosage according to their clinical condition.

More precise body-surface values may be calculated from height and weight by means of a nomogram (e.g. J. Insley, *A Paediatric Vade-Mecum*, 13th Edition, London, Arnold, 1996).

DOSE FREQUENCY. Doses for antibiotics are usually stated as every 6 hours. Some flexibility should be allowed in children to avoid waking them during the night. For example, the night-time dose may be given at the parent's bedtime.

Where new or potentially toxic drugs are used, the manufacturers' recommended doses should be carefully followed.

Prescribing in Palliative Care

Palliative care is the active total care of patients whose disease is not responsive to curative treatment. Control of pain, of other symptoms, and of psychological, social and spiritual problems, is paramount to provide the best quality of life for patients and their families. Careful assessment of symptoms and needs of the patient should be undertaken by a multidisciplinary team.

Specialist palliative care is available in most areas as day hospice care, home care teams (often known as Macmillan teams), in-patient hospice care, and hospital teams. Many acute hospitals and teaching centres now have consultative, hospital-based teams.

Hospice care of terminally ill patients has shown the importance of symptom control and psychosocial support of the patient and family. Families should be included in the care of the patient if they wish.

Many patients wish to remain at home with their families. Although some families may at first be afraid of caring for the patient at home, support can be provided by community nursing services, social services, voluntary agencies and hospices together with the general practitioner. The family may be reassured by the knowledge that the patient will be admitted to a hospital or hospice if the family cannot cope.

DRUG TREATMENT. The number of drugs should be as few as possible, for even the taking of medicine may be an effort. Oral medication is usually satisfactory unless there is severe nausea and vomiting, dysphagia, weakness, or coma, in which case parenteral medication may be necessary.

PAIN

Analgesics are always more effective in preventing the development of pain than in the relief of established pain.

The non-opioid analgesics **aspirin** or **paracetamol** given regularly will often make the use of opioids unnecessary. Aspirin (or other NSAIDs if preferred) may also control the pain of *bone secondaries*; naproxen, flurbiprofen, and indomethacin (section 10.1.1) are valuable and if necessary can be given rectally. Radiotherapy, radioactive isotopes of **strontium** (*Metastron*® available from Amersham) and bisphosphonates (section 6.6.2) may also be useful for pain due to bone metastases.

An opioid such as **codeine** or **dextropropoxyphene**, alone or in combination with a non-opioid analgesic at adequate dosage, may be helpful in the control of moderate pain if non-opioids alone are not sufficient. If these preparations are not controlling the pain, **morphine** is the most useful opioid analgesic.

ORAL ROUTE. Morphine is given *by mouth* as an oral solution regularly every 4 hours, the initial dose depending largely on the patient's previous treatment. A dose of 5–10 mg is enough to replace a weaker analgesic (such as paracetamol or co-proxamol), but 10–20 mg or more is required to replace a strong one (comparable to morphine itself). If the first dose of morphine is no more effective than the previous analgesic it should be increased by 50%, the aim being to choose the lowest dose which prevents pain. Although a dose of 5–20 mg is usually adequate there should be no hesitation in increasing it stepwise according to response to 100 mg or occasionally up to 500 mg or higher if necessary. If pain occurs between doses the next dose due is increased; in the interim an additional dose is given. The dose should be adjusted with careful assessment of the pain and the use of other drugs (such as NSAIDs) should also be considered.

Modified-release preparations of morphine are an alternative to the oral solution. Depending on the formulation of the modified-release preparation, the total daily morphine requirement may be given in two equal doses or as a single dose.

Preparations suitable for twice daily administration include *MST Continus*® tablets or suspension, *Oramorph*® SR tablets, and *Zomorph*® capsules. Preparations that allow administration of the total daily morphine requirement as a single dose include *MXL*® capsules. *Morcap SR*® capsules may be given either twice daily or as a single daily dose.

The starting dose of modified-release preparations designed for twice daily administration is usually 10–20 mg every 12 hours if no other analgesic (or only paracetamol) has been taken previously, but to replace a weaker opioid analgesic (such as co-proxamol) the starting dose is usually 20–30 mg every 12 hours. Increments should be made to the dose, not to the frequency of administration, which should remain at every 12 hours.

The effective dose of modified-release preparations can alternatively be determined by giving the oral solution of morphine every 4 hours in increasing doses until the pain has been controlled, and then transferring the patient to the same total 24-hour dose of morphine given as the modified-release preparation (divided into two portions for 12-hourly administration). The first dose of the modified-release preparation is given 4 hours after the last dose of the oral solution.[1]

Morphine, as oral solution or standard formulation tablets, should be prescribed for breakthrough pain.

PARENTERAL ROUTE. If the patient becomes unable to swallow, the equivalent intramuscular dose of morphine is half the oral solution dose; in the case of the modified-release tablets it is half the total 24-hour dose (which is then divided into 6 portions to be given every 4 hours). **Diamorphine** is preferred for injection because being more soluble it can be given in a smaller volume. The equivalent intramuscular (or subcutaneous) dose of diamorphine is only about a quarter to a third of the oral dose of morphine; *subcutaneous infusion via syringe driver* can be useful (for details, see p. 14).

---

1. Studies have indicated that administration of the last dose of the *oral solution* with the first dose of the *modified-release tablets* is not necessary.

RECTAL ROUTE. Morphine is also available for *rectal administration* as suppositories; alternatively **oxycodone** suppositories can be obtained on special order.

TRANSDERMAL ROUTE. Transdermal preparations of fentanyl are available (section 4.7.2). Careful conversion from oral morphine to transdermal fentanyl is necessary; a 25 micrograms/hr patch is equivalent to a total dose of morphine up to 135 mg/24 hours

GASTRO-INTESTINAL PAIN. The pain of *bowel colic* may be reduced by loperamide 2–4 mg 4 times daily. Hyoscine hydrobromide may also be helpful, given sublingually at a dose of 300 micrograms 3 times daily as *Kwells*® (Roche Consumer Health) tablets. For the dose by subcutaneous infusion using a syringe driver, see p. 14.

Gastric distension pain due to pressure on the stomach may be helped by a preparation incorporating an antacid with an antiflatulent (section 1.1.1) and by domperidone 10 mg 3 times daily before meals.

MUSCLE SPASM. The pain of muscle spasm can be helped by a muscle relaxant such as diazepam 5–10 mg daily or baclofen 5–10 mg 3 times daily.

NERVE PAIN. Pain due to nerve compression may be reduced by a corticosteroid such as dexamethasone 8 mg daily, which reduces oedema around the tumour, thus reducing compression.

Dysaesthetic or stabbing pain resulting from nerve irritation may be reduced by amitriptyline 25–75 mg at night, or by carbamazepine 200 mg 3 times daily.

Nerve blocks may be considered when pain is localised to a specific area. **Transcutaneous electrical nerve stimulation** (TENS) may also provide useful relief of pain.

MISCELLANEOUS CONDITIONS

Non-licensed indications or routes

Several recommendations in this section involve non-licensed indications or routes.

RAISED INTRACRANIAL PRESSURE. Headache due to raised intracranial pressure often responds to a high dose of a corticosteroid, such as dexamethasone 16 mg daily for 4 to 5 days, subsequently reduced to 4–6 mg daily if possible.

INTRACTABLE COUGH. Intractable cough may be relieved by moist inhalations or may require regular administration of an oral morphine hydrochloride (or sulphate) solution in an initial dose of 5 mg every 4 hours. Methadone linctus should be avoided as it has a long duration of action and tends to accumulate.

DYSPNOEA. Dyspnoea may be relieved by regular oral morphine hydrochloride (or sulphate) solution in carefully titrated doses, starting at 5 mg every 4 hours. Diazepam 5–10 mg daily may be helpful; a corticosteroid, such as dexamethasone 4–8 mg daily, may also be helpful if there is bronchospasm or partial obstruction.

EXCESSIVE RESPIRATORY SECRETION. Excessive respiratory secretion (death rattle) may be reduced by subcutaneous injection of hyoscine hydrobromide 400–600 micrograms every 4 to 8 hours; care must however be taken to avoid the discomfort of dry mouth. For the dose by subcutaneous infusion using a syringe driver, see next page.

RESTLESSNESS AND CONFUSION. Restlessness and confusion may require treatment with haloperidol 1–3 mg by mouth every 8 hours. Chlorpromazine 25–50 mg by mouth every 8 hours is an alternative, but causes more sedation. Methotrimeprazine is also used occasionally for restlessness. For the dose by subcutaneous infusion using a syringe driver, see next page

HICCUP. Hiccup due to gastric distension may be helped by a preparation incorporating an antacid with an antiflatulent (see section 1.1.1). If this fails, metoclopramide 10 mg every 6 to 8 hours by mouth or by intramuscular injection can be added; if this also fails, chlorpromazine 10–25 mg every 6 to 8 hours can be tried.

ANOREXIA. Anorexia may be helped by prednisolone 15–30 mg daily or dexamethasone 2–4 mg daily.

CONSTIPATION. Constipation is a very common cause of distress and is almost invariable after administration of an opioid. It should be prevented if possible by the regular administration of laxatives; a faecal softener with a peristaltic stimulant (e.g. co-danthramer), or lactulose solution with a senna preparation should be used (section 1.6.2 and section 1.6.3).

FUNGATING GROWTH. Fungating growth may be treated by cleansing with a mixture of 1 part of 4% povidone–iodine skin cleanser solution and 4 parts of liquid paraffin. Oral administration of metronidazole (section 5.1.11) may eradicate the anaerobic bacteria responsible for the odour of fungating tumours; topical application (section 13.10.1.2) is also used.

CAPILLARY BLEEDING. Capillary bleeding may be reduced by applying gauze soaked in adrenaline solution 1 mg/mL (1 in 1000).

DRY MOUTH. Dry mouth may be relieved by good mouth care and measures such as the sucking of ice or pineapple chunks or the use of artificial saliva (section 12.3.5); dry mouth associated with candidiasis can be treated by oral preparations of nystatin or miconazole (section 12.3.2); alternatively, fluconazole can be given by mouth (section 5.2). Dry mouth may be caused by certain medication including opioids, antimuscarinic drugs (e.g. hyoscine), antidepressants and some anti-emetics; if possible, an alternative preparation should be considered.

PRURITUS. Pruritus, even when associated with obstructive jaundice, often responds to simple measures such as emollients. In the case of obstructive jaundice, further measures include administration of cholestyramine or an anabolic steroid, such as stanozolol 5–10 mg daily; antihistamines can be helpful (section 3.4.1).

CONVULSIONS. Patients with cerebral tumours or uraemia may be susceptible to convulsions. Prophylactic treatment with phenytoin or carbamazepine (section 4.8.1) should be considered. When oral medication is no longer possible, diazepam as suppositories 10–20 mg every 4 to 8 hours, or phenobarbitone by injection 50–200 mg twice daily is continued as prophylaxis. For the use of midazolam by subcutaneous infusion using a syringe driver, see below.

DYSPHAGIA. A corticosteroid such as dexamethasone 8 mg daily may help, temporarily, if there is an obstruction due to tumour. See also under Dry Mouth.

NAUSEA AND VOMITING. Nausea and vomiting are very common in patients with advanced cancer. The cause should be diagnosed before treatment with anti-emetics (section 4.6) is started. Octreotide (section 8.3.4.3), which stimulates water and electrolyte absorption and inhibits water secretion in the small bowel, can be used by subcutaneous infusion, in a dose of 300–600 micrograms/24 hours to reduce intestinal secretions and vomiting.

Nausea and vomiting may also occur in the initial stages of morphine therapy but can be prevented by giving an anti-emetic such as haloperidol 1.5 mg daily (or twice daily if nausea continues) or prochlorperazine (section 4.6). An anti-emetic is usually only necessary for the first 4 or 5 days therefore fixed-combination opioid preparations containing an anti-emetic are not recommended since they lead to unnecessary anti-emetic therapy (often with undesirable drowsiness). For the administration of anti-emetics by subcutaneous infusion using a syringe driver, see below.

For the treatment of nausea and vomiting associated with cancer chemotherapy, see section 8.1.

INSOMNIA. Patients with advanced cancer may not sleep because of discomfort, cramps, night sweats, joint stiffness, or fear. There should be appropriate treatment of these problems before hypnotics are used. Benzodiazepines, such as temazepam, may be useful (section 4.1.1).

HYPERCALCAEMIA. See section 9.5.1.2.

SYRINGE DRIVERS

Although drugs can usually be administered by mouth to control the symptoms of advanced cancer, the parenteral route may sometimes be necessary. If the parenteral route is necessary, repeated administration of intramuscular injections can be difficult in a cachectic patient. This has led to the use of a portable syringe driver to give a continuous subcutaneous infusion, which can provide good control of symptoms with little discomfort or inconvenience to the patient.

Indications for the parenteral route are:

the patient is unable to take medicines by mouth owing to nausea and vomiting, dysphagia, severe weakness, or coma;

there is malignant bowel obstruction in patients for whom further surgery is inappropriate (avoiding the need for an intravenous infusion or for insertion of a nasogastric tube);

occasionally when the patient does not wish to take regular medication by mouth.

NAUSEA AND VOMITING. Haloperidol is given in a subcutaneous infusion dose of 2.5–10 mg/24 hours.

Methotrimeprazine causes sedation in about 50% of patients; it is given in a subcutaneous infusion dose of 25–200 mg/24 hours, although lower doses of 5–25 mg/24 hours may be effective with less sedation.

Cyclizine is particularly liable to precipitate if mixed with diamorphine or other drugs (see under Mixing and Compatibility, below); it is given in a subcutaneous infusion dose of 150 mg/24 hours.

Metoclopramide may cause skin reactions; it is given in a subcutaneous infusion dose of 30–60 mg/24 hours.

BOWEL COLIC AND EXCESSIVE RESPIRATORY SECRETIONS. Hyoscine hydrobromide effectively reduces respiratory secretions and is sedative (but occasionally causes paradoxical agitation); it is given in a subcutaneous infusion dose of 0.6–2.4 mg/24 hours.

Hyoscine butylbromide is effective in bowel colic, is less sedative than hyoscine hydrobromide, but is not always adequate for the control of respiratory secretions; it is given in a subcutaneous infusion dose of 20–60 mg/24 hours (important: this dose of hyoscine butylbromide must not be confused with the much lower dose of hyoscine hydrobromide, above).

RESTLESSNESS AND CONFUSION. Haloperidol has little sedative effect; it is given in a subcutaneous infusion dose of 5–30 mg/24 hours.

Methotrimeprazine has a sedative effect; it is given in a subcutaneous infusion dose of 50–200 mg/24 hours.

Midazolam is a sedative and an antiepileptic, and is therefore suitable for a very restless patient; it is given in a subcutaneous infusion dose of 20–100 mg/24 hours.

CONVULSIONS. If a patient has previously been receiving an antiepileptic or has a primary or secondary cerebral tumour or is at risk of convulsion (e.g. owing to uraemia) antiepileptic medication should not be stopped. Midazolam is the benzodiazepine antiepileptic of choice for continuous subcutaneous infusion, and is given in a dose of 20–40 mg/24 hours.

PAIN CONTROL. Diamorphine is the preferred opioid since its high solubility permits a large dose to be given in a small volume (see under Mixing and Compatibility, below). The table on the next page gives the approximate doses of morphine by mouth (as oral solution or standard tablets or as modified-release tablets) equivalent to diamorphine by injection (intramuscularly or by subcutaneous infusion).

MIXING AND COMPATIBILITY. The general principle that injections should be given into separate sites (and should not be mixed) does not apply to the use of syringe drivers in palliative care. Provided that there is evidence of compatibility, selected injections can be mixed in syringe drivers. Not all types of medication can be used in a subcutaneous infusion. In particular, chlorpromazine, prochlorperazine and diazepam are contra-indicated as they cause skin reactions at the injection site; to a lesser extent **cyclizine** and **methotrimeprazine** may also sometimes cause local irritation.

In theory injections dissolved in **water for injections** are more likely to be associated with pain (possibly owing to their hypotonicity). The use of **physiological saline** (sodium chloride 0.9%) however increases the likelihood of precipitation when more than one drug is used; moreover subcutaneous infusion rates are so slow (0.1–0.3 mL/hour) that pain is not usually a problem when water is used as a diluent.

Diamorphine can be given by subcutaneous infusion in a strength of up to 250 mg/mL; up to a strength of 40 mg/mL either *water for injections* or *physiological saline* (sodium chloride 0.9%) is a suitable diluent—above that strength only *water for injections* is used (to avoid precipitation).

The following can be mixed with *diamorphine:*
Cyclizine[1]
Dexamethasone[2]
Haloperidol[3]
Hyoscine butylbromide
Hyoscine hydrobromide
Methotrimeprazine
Metoclopramide[4]
Midazolam

Subcutaneous infusion solution should be monitored regularly both to check for precipitation (and discoloration) and to ensure that the infusion is running at the correct rate.

PROBLEMS ENCOUNTERED WITH SYRINGE DRIVERS. The following are problems that may be encountered with syringe drivers and the action that should be taken:

if the subcutaneous infusion runs *too quickly* check the rate setting and the calculation;

if the subcutaneous infusion runs *too slowly* check the start button, the battery, the syringe driver, the cannula, and make sure that the injection site is not inflamed;

if there is an *injection site reaction* make sure that the site does *not* need to be changed—firmness or swelling at the site of injection is not in itself an indication for change, but pain or obvious inflammation is.

Syringe driver rate settings. Staff using syringe drivers should be **adequately trained** and different rate settings should be **clearly identified** and **differentiated**; incorrect use of syringe drivers is a common cause of drug errors.

1. Cyclizine may precipitate at concentrations above 10 mg/mL *or* in the presence of physiological saline *or* as the concentration of diamorphine relative to cyclizine increases; mixtures of diamorphine and cyclizine are also liable to precipitate after 24 hours.
2. Special care is needed to avoid precipitation of dexamethasone when preparing.
3. Mixtures of haloperidol and diamorphine are liable to precipitate after 24 hours if haloperidol concentration is above 2 mg/mL.
4. Under some conditions metoclopramide may become discoloured; such solutions should be discarded.

Equivalent doses of morphine sulphate by mouth (as oral solution or standard tablets or as modified-release tablets) *or* of diamorphine hydrochloride by intramuscular injection *or by* subcutaneous infusion

These equivalences are approximate only and may need to be adjusted according to response

ORAL MORPHINE		PARENTERAL DIAMORPHINE	
Morphine sulphate oral solution or standard tablets	Morphine sulphate modified-release tablets	Diamorphine hydrochloride by intramuscular injection	Diamorphine hydrochloride by subcutaneous infusion
every 4 hours	**every 12 hours**	**every 4 hours**	**every 24 hours**
5 mg	20 mg	2.5 mg	15 mg
10 mg	30 mg	5 mg	20 mg
15 mg	50 mg	5 mg	30 mg
20 mg	60 mg	7.5 mg	45 mg
30 mg	90 mg	10 mg	60 mg
40 mg	120 mg	15 mg	90 mg
60 mg	180 mg	20 mg	120 mg
80 mg	240 mg	30 mg	180 mg
100 mg	300 mg	40 mg	240 mg
130 mg	400 mg	50 mg	300 mg
160 mg	500 mg	60 mg	360 mg
200 mg	600 mg	70 mg	400 mg

If breakthrough pain occurs give a subcutaneous (preferable) or intramuscular injection of diamorphine equivalent to one-sixth of the total 24-hour subcutaneous infusion dose. It is kinder to give an intermittent bolus injection *subcutaneously*—absorption is smoother so that the risk of adverse effects at peak absorption is avoided (an even better method is to use a subcutaneous butterfly needle).

To minimise the risk of infection no individual subcutaneous infusion solution should be used for longer than 24 hours.

Prescribing for the Elderly

Old people, especially the very old, require special care and consideration from prescribers.

POLYPHARMACY. Elderly patients are apt to receive multiple drugs for their multiple diseases. This greatly increases the risk of drug interactions as well as other adverse reactions. Moreover, symptoms such as headache, sleeplessness, and light-headedness which may be associated with social stress, as in widowhood, loneliness, and family dispersal can lead to further prescribing, especially of psychotropics. The use of drugs in such cases can at best be a poor substitute for effective social measures and at worst pose a serious threat from adverse reactions.

FORM OF MEDICINE. Elderly patients may have difficulty swallowing tablets; if left in the mouth, ulceration may develop. They should always be encouraged to take their tablets or capsules with enough fluid, and in some cases it may be advisable to prescribe liquid if available.

MANIFESTATIONS OF AGEING. In very old subjects, manifestations of normal ageing may be mistaken for disease and lead to inappropriate prescribing. For example, drugs such as prochlorperazine are commonly misprescribed for giddiness due to age-related loss of postural stability. Not only is such treatment ineffective but the patient may experience serious side-effects such as drug-induced parkinsonism, postural hypotension, and mental confusion.

SELF-MEDICATION. Self-medication with over-the-counter products or with drugs prescribed for a previous illness (or even for another person) may be an added complication. Discussion with relatives and a home visit may be needed to establish exactly what is being taken.

SUSCEPTIBILITY. The ageing nervous system shows increased *susceptibility* to many commonly used drugs, such as opioid analgesics, benzodiazepines, and antiparkinsonian drugs, all of which must be used with caution.

PHARMACOKINETICS

While drug distribution and metabolism may be significantly altered, the most important effect of age is reduction in renal clearance, frequently aggravated by the effects of prostatism, nephrosclerosis, or chronic urinary tract infection. Many aged patients thus possess only *limited reserves of renal function, excrete drugs slowly,* and are *highly susceptible to nephrotoxic drugs.* Acute illness may lead to rapid reduction in renal clearance, especially if accompanied by dehydration. Hence, a patient stabilised on a drug with a narrow margin between the therapeutic and the toxic dose (e.g. digoxin) may rapidly develop adverse effects in the aftermath of a myocardial infarction or a respiratory tract infection.

The net result of pharmacokinetic changes is that tissue concentrations are commonly increased by over 50%, and aged and debilitated patients may show even larger changes.

ADVERSE REACTIONS

Adverse reactions often present in the elderly in a vague and non-specific fashion. *Mental confusion* is often the presenting symptom (caused by almost any of the commonly used drugs). Other common manifestations are *constipation* (with antimuscarinics and many tranquillisers) and postural *hypotension* and *falls* (with diuretics and many psychotropics).

HYPNOTICS. Many hypnotics with long half-lives have serious hangover effects of drowsiness, unsteady gait, and even slurred speech and confusion. Those with short half-lives should be used but they too can present problems (section 4.1.1). Short courses of hypnotics are occasionally useful for helping a patient through an acute illness or some other crisis but every effort must be made to avoid dependence.

DIURETICS. Diuretics are overprescribed in old age and should **not** be used on a long-term basis to treat simple gravitational oedema which will usually respond to increased movement, raising the legs, and support stockings. A few days of diuretic treatment may speed the clearing of the oedema but it should rarely need continued drug therapy.

NSAIDs. Bleeding associated with *aspirin* and *other NSAIDs* is more common in the elderly who are more likely to have a fatal or serious outcome. NSAIDs are also a special hazard in patients with cardiac disease or renal impairment which may again place the elderly at particular risk.

Owing to the *increased susceptibilty of the elderly* to the *side-effects of NSAIDs* the following recommendations are made:

for *osteoarthritis, soft-tissue lesions and back pain* first try measures such as weight reduction, warmth, exercise and use of a walking stick;

for *osteoarthritis, soft tissue lesions, back pain and rheumatoid arthritis* avoid giving an NSAID unless *paracetamol* (alone or with a *low dose* of an opioid analgesic as in co-codamol 8/500 or co-dydramol 10/500) has failed to relieve the pain adequately;

where a paracetamol preparation has failed to relieve the pain adequately *add a very low dose of an NSAID* to the paracetamol preparation (starting with ibuprofen). For advice on prophylaxis of NSAID-induced peptic ulcers (where continued treatment with NSAIDs is necessary), see section 1.3.

if an NSAID is considered necessary monitor the patient for gastro-intestinal bleeding for 4 weeks (and for a similar time on switching to another NSAID). For the management of NSAID-associated peptic ulcers, see section 1.3.

do **not** give two NSAIDs at the same time.

OTHER DRUGS. Other drugs which commonly cause adverse reactions are *antiparkinsonian drugs, antihypertensives, psychotropics*, and *digoxin*; the usual maintenance dose of digoxin in very old patients is 125 micrograms daily (62.5 micrograms is often inadequate, and toxicity is common in those given 250 micrograms).

Drug-induced blood disorders are much more common in the elderly. Therefore drugs with a tendency to cause bone marrow depression (e.g. *co-trimoxazole, mianserin*) should be avoided unless there is no acceptable alternative.

The elderly generally require a lower maintenance dose of *warfarin* than younger adults; once again, the outcome of bleeding tends to be more serious.

GUIDELINES

First always question whether a drug is indicated at all.

LIMIT RANGE. It is a sensible policy to prescribe from a limited range of drugs and to be thoroughly familiar with their effects in the elderly.

REDUCE DOSE. Dosage should generally be substantially lower than for younger patients and it is common to start with about 50% of the adult dose. Some drugs (e.g. chlorpropamide) should be avoided altogether.

REVIEW REGULARLY. Review repeat prescriptions regularly. It may be possible to stop the drug (e.g. digoxin can often be withdrawn) or it may be necessary to reduce the dose to match diminishing renal function.

SIMPLIFY. Simplify regimens. Elderly patients cannot normally cope with more than three different drugs and, ideally, these should not be given more than twice daily. In particular, regimens which call for a confusing array of dosage intervals should be avoided.

EXPLAIN CLEARLY. Write full instructions on every prescription (*including* repeat prescriptions) so that containers can be properly labelled with full directions. Avoid imprecisions like 'as directed'. Child-resistant containers may be unsuitable.

REPEATS AND DISPOSAL. Instruct patients what to do when drugs run out, and also how to dispose of any that are no longer necessary. Try to prescribe matching quantities.

If these guidelines are followed most elderly people will cope adequately with their own medicines. If not then it is essential to enrol the help of a third party, usually a relative or a friend.

Emergency Treatment of Poisoning

TOXBASE is an on-line database which provides information about routine diagnosis, treatment and management of patients exposed to drugs, household products, and industrial and agricultural chemicals. It is available via a Viewdata system to authorised users including Accident and Emergency Departments (contact 0131-536 2303 for further information). **Important:** for more specialised information telephone the Poisons Information Centres.

TICTAC is a computer-aided tablet and capsule identification system. It is available to authorised users including Regional Drug Information Centres (see p. xiii) and Poisons Information Centres.

POISONS INFORMATION CENTRES (consult day and night)

Belfast	(01232) 240503
Birmingham	0121-507 5588
or	0121-507 5589
Cardiff	(01222) 709901
Dublin	Dublin 837 9964
or	Dublin 837 9966
Edinburgh	0131-536 2300
Leeds	(0113) 243 0715
or	(0113) 292 3547
London	0171-635 9191
or	0171-955 5095
Newcastle	0191-232 5131

Note. Some of these centres also advise on laboratory analytical services which may be of help in the diagnosis and management of a small number of cases

These notes are only guidelines and it is strongly recommended that **poisons information centres** (see above) be consulted in cases where there is doubt about the degree of risk or about appropriate management.

HOSPITAL ADMISSION. All patients who show features of poisoning should generally be admitted to hospital. Patients who have taken poisons with delayed actions should also be admitted, even if they appear well; delayed-action poisons include aspirin, iron, paracetamol, tricyclic antidepressants, co-phenotrope (diphenoxylate with atropine, *Lomotil*®), and paraquat; this also applies to modified-release preparations. A note should be sent of what is known and what treatment has been given.

It is often impossible to establish with certainty the identity of the poison and the size of the dose. Fortunately this is not usually important because only a few poisons (such as opioids, paracetamol, and iron) have specific antidotes and few patients require active removal of the poison. Most patients must be treated symptomatically. Nevertheless, knowledge of the type of poisoning does help in anticipating the course of events. Patients' reports may be of little help, as they may be confused or may only be able to say that they have taken an undefined amount, possibly of mixed drugs. Parents may think a child has taken something which could be poisonous and may exaggerate or underplay the risks out of anxiety or guilt. Sometimes symptoms are due to an illness such as appendicitis. Accidents can arise from a number of domestic and industrial products (the contents of which are not generally known).

General care

The **poisons information centres** (see above) will provide advice on all aspects of poisoning day and night

RESPIRATION

Respiration is often impaired in unconscious patients. An obstructed airway requires immediate attention. Pull the tongue forward, remove dentures and oral secretions, hold the jaw forward, insert an oropharyngeal airway if one is available, and turn the patient semiprone. The risk of inhaling vomit is minimised with the patient positioned semiprone and head down.

Most poisons that impair consciousness also depress respiration. Assisted ventilation by mouth-to-mouth or Ambu-bag inflation may be needed. Oxygen is not a substitute for adequate ventilation, though it should be given in the highest concentration possible in poisoning with carbon monoxide and irritant gases.

Respiratory stimulants do not help and are **potentially dangerous**.

BLOOD PRESSURE

Hypotension is common in severe poisoning with central nervous system depressants. A systolic blood pressure of less than 70 mmHg may lead to irreversible brain damage or renal tubular necrosis. The patient should be carried head downwards on a stretcher and nursed in this position in the ambulance. Oxygen should be given to correct hypoxia and an intravenous infusion should be set up if at all practicable. Vasopressor drugs should **not** be used.

Fluid depletion without hypotension is common after prolonged coma and after aspirin poisoning due to vomiting, sweating, and hyperpnoea.

Hypertension, often transient, is less frequent in poisoning; it may be associated with sympathomimetic drugs such as amphetamines, phencyclidine, and cocaine.

HEART

Cardiac conduction defects and arrhythmias may occur in acute poisoning, notably with tricyclic antidepressants. Arrhythmias often respond to correction of underlying hypoxia or acidosis. Ventricular arrhythmias that have been confirmed by emergency ECG and which are causing serious hypotension may require treatment with lignocaine (see p. 73). Supraventricular arrhythmias are seldom life-threatening and drug treatment is best withheld until the patient reaches hospital.

BODY TEMPERATURE

Hypothermia may develop in patients of any age who have been deeply unconscious for some hours particularly following overdose with barbiturates or phenothiazines. It may be missed unless temperature is measured rectally using a low-reading rectal thermometer. It is best treated by wrapping the patient (e.g. in a 'space blanket') to conserve body heat. A *mild* source of heat (such as water bottles heated to 42°C) may be used and care must be taken to avoid causing burns.

CONVULSIONS

Single short-lived convulsions do not require treatment. Diazepam, up to 10 mg by slow intravenous injection, preferably in emulsion form, should be given if convulsions are protracted or recur frequently; it should not be given intramuscularly.

Removal and elimination

REMOVAL FROM THE STOMACH

The dangers of attempting to empty the stomach have to be balanced against the toxicity of the ingested poison, as assessed by the quantity ingested, the inherent toxicity of the poison, and the time since ingestion. Gastric emptying is clearly unnecessary if the risk of toxicity is small or if the patient presents too late.

Emptying the stomach by **gastric lavage** is of doubtful value if attempted more than 1–2 hours after ingestion. However, a worthwhile recovery of salicylates may be achieved up to 4 hours after ingestion. The chief danger of gastric aspiration and lavage is inhalation of stomach contents, and it should **not** be attempted in drowsy or comatose patients unless there is a good enough cough reflex or the airway can be protected by a cuffed endotracheal tube. Stomach tubes should **not** be passed after corrosive poisoning.

Petroleum products are more dangerous in the lungs than in the stomach and therefore removal from the stomach is **not** advised because of the risk of inhalation.

On balance gastric lavage is seldom practicable or desirable before the patient reaches hospital.

Emesis induced by **ipecacuanha** (Paediatric Ipecacuanha Emetic Mixture BP) has been used in adults and children, but is of very limited value. There is no evidence that it prevents clinically significant absorption (even if used within 1–2 hours) and its adverse effects may often complicate diagnosis particularly in iron poisoning. It should only be considered if the patient is fully conscious, if the poison ingested is neither corrosive nor a petroleum distillate, if it is not adsorbed by activated charcoal, or if gastric lavage is inadvisable or refused (for advice call a poisons information centre).

Salt solutions, copper sulphate, apomorphine, and mustard are dangerous and should **not** be used.

IPECACUANHA

Indications: induction of emesis in selected patients, see notes above

Cautions: avoid in poisoning with corrosive or petroleum products owing to risk of aspiration (see notes above); also avoid if risk of aspiration, in shock, or if risk of convulsions; cardiovascular disease

Side-effects: excessive vomiting and mucosal damage; cardiac effects if absorbed

Dose: see under preparation below

Ipecacuanha Emetic Mixture, Paediatric (BP)
Paediatric Ipecacuanha Emetic

> *Note.* Paediatric Ipecacuanha Emetic Mixture is equivalent in strength to Ipecac Syrup USP
> *Mixture,* ipecacuanha liquid extract 0.7 mL, hydrochloric acid 0.025 mL, glycerol 1 mL, syrup to 10 mL
> *Dose:* ADULT 30 mL; CHILD 6–18 months 10 mL, older children 15 mL; the dose is followed by a tumblerful of water and repeated after 20 minutes if necessary

PREVENTION OF ABSORPTION

Given by mouth, **activated charcoal** can bind many poisons in the stomach, thereby *reducing their absorption*. The **sooner** it is given the **more effective** it is, but it may still be effective up to 2 hours after ingestion—longer in the case of modified-release preparations or of drugs with antimuscarinic (anticholinergic) properties. It is relatively safe and is particularly useful for the prevention of absorption of poisons which are toxic in small amounts, e.g. antidepressants.

For the use of charcoal in active elimination techniques, see below.

Carbomix® (Penn)

Powder, activated charcoal, net price 25-g pack = £8.50, 50-g pack = £11.90

Dose: reduction of absorption, 50 g; CHILD, 25 g (50 g in severe poisoning)

Active elimination, see below

Medicoal® (Concord)

Granules, effervescent, activated charcoal 5 g/ sachet. Contains Na+ 17.9 mmol/sachet. Net price 5-sachet pack = £6.52, 30-sachet pack = £30.16

Dose: reduction of absorption, initially 2 sachets repeated every 15–20 minutes until dose of charcoal given is 10 times that of poison ingested (if amount known) or until max. 10 sachets/24 hours have been given; each sachet suspended in approx. 100 mL water (may be administered in divided doses for children)

ACTIVE ELIMINATION TECHNIQUES

Repeated doses of **activated charcoal** by mouth *enhance the elimination* of some drugs after they have been absorbed; repeated doses are given after overdosage with:

Aspirin	Phenobarbitone
Carbamazepine	Quinine
Dapsone	Theophylline

The usual adult dose of activated charcoal is 50 g initially then 50 g every 4 hours. Vomiting should be treated (e.g. with an anti-emetic drug) since it may reduce the efficacy of charcoal treatment. In cases of intolerance, the dose may be reduced and the frequency increased (e.g. 25 g every 2 hours *or* 10 g every hour) but this may compromise efficacy.

Other techniques intended to enhance the elimination of poisons after absorption are only practicable in hospital and are only suitable for a small number of severely poisoned patients. Moreover, they only apply to a limited number of poisons. Examples include:

Haemodialysis for salicylates, phenobarbitone, methyl alcohol (methanol), ethylene glycol, and lithium

Haemoperfusion for medium- and short-acting barbiturates, chloral hydrate, meprobamate, and theophylline.

Forced alkaline diuresis is no longer recommended.

Specific drugs

ALCOHOL

Acute intoxication with alcohol (ethanol) is common in adults but also occurs in children. The features include ataxia, dysarthria, nystagmus, and drowsiness, which may progress to coma, with hypotension and acidosis. Aspiration of vomit is a special hazard and hypoglycaemia may occur in children and some adults. Patients are managed supportively with particular attention to maintaining a clear airway and measures to reduce the risk of aspiration of gastric contents. The blood glucose is measured and glucose given if indicated.

ANALGESICS (NON-OPIOID)

ASPIRIN. Absorption of aspirin and other salicylates may be delayed, especially if enteric-coated tablets have been taken; blood concentrations taken within the first 6 hours may therefore be misleadingly low.

The chief features of poisoning are hyperventilation, tinnitus, deafness, vasodilatation, and sweating. Coma is uncommon but indicates very severe poisoning. The associated acid-base disturbances are complex.

Gastric emptying can achieve a worthwhile recovery of salicylates up to 4 hours after ingestion.

Treatment must be in hospital where plasma salicylate, pH, and electrolytes can be measured. Fluid losses are replaced and sodium bicarbonate (1.26%) given to enhance urinary salicylate excretion when the plasma-salicylate concentration is greater than

500 mg/litre (3.6 mmol/litre) in adults *or*
350 mg/litre (2.5 mmol/litre) in children.

Haemodialysis is the treatment of choice for severe poisoning and should be seriously considered when the plasma salicylate concentration is greater than 700 mg/litre (5.1 mmol/litre).

NSAIDs. Mefenamic acid is an important member of this group encountered in overdosage. Convulsions are the most important feature of toxicity and are treated with diazepam.

Ibuprofen may cause nausea, vomiting, and tinnitus, but more serious toxicity is very uncommon. Gastric emptying is indicated if more than 100 mg/ kg has been ingested within the preceding 2 hours, followed by symptomatic measures.

PARACETAMOL. As little as 10–15 g (20–30 tablets) of paracetamol may cause severe hepatocellular necrosis and, less frequently, renal tubular necrosis. Nausea and vomiting, the only early features of poisoning, usually settle within 24 hours. Persistence beyond this time, often associated with the onset of right subcostal pain and tenderness, usually indicates development of hepatic necrosis. Liver damage is maximal 3–4 days after ingestion and may lead to encephalopathy, haemorrhage, hypoglycaemia, cerebral oedema, and death.

Therefore, despite a lack of significant early symptoms, patients who have taken an overdose of paracetamol should be transferred to hospital urgently.

Gastric emptying is carried out if the overdose was taken within 2 hours of admission.

Antidotes such as **acetylcysteine** and **methionine** protect the liver if given within 10–12 hours of ingestion; acetylcysteine is effective up to and possibly beyond 24 hours but expert advice is **essential**.

Patients at risk of liver damage and therefore requiring treatment can be identified from a single measurement of the plasma-paracetamol concentration, related to the time from ingestion, provided this time interval is not less than 4 hours; earlier samples may be misleading. The concentration is plotted on a paracetamol treatment graph of a reference line ('normal treatment line') joining plots of 200 mg/litre (1.32 mmol/litre) at 4 hours and 6.25 mg/litre (0.04 mmol/litre) at 24 hours (see below). Those whose plasma-paracetamol concentrations are above the *normal treatment line* are treated with acetylcysteine by intravenous infusion (or, provided the overdose has been taken **within 10–12 hours**, with methionine by mouth). Patients

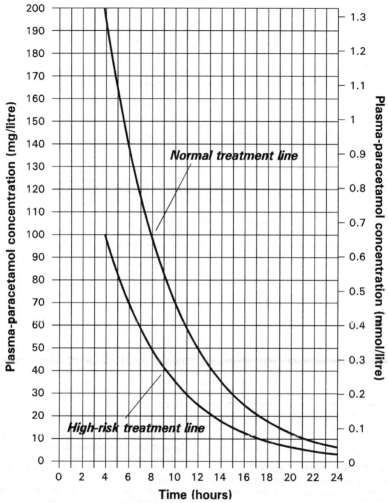

Time (hours)

Patients whose plasma-paracetamol concentrations are above the **normal treatment line** should be treated with acetylcysteine by intravenous infusion (or, provided the overdose has been taken **within 10–12 hours**, with methionine by mouth). Patients on enzyme-inducing drugs (e.g. carbamazepine, phenobarbitone, phenytoin, rifampicin, and alcohol) or who are malnourished (e.g. in anorexia, in alcoholism, or those who are HIV-positive) should be treated if their plasma-paracetamol concentrations are above the **high-risk treatment line**.

on enzyme-inducing drugs (e.g. carbamazepine, phenobarbitone, phenytoin, rifampicin, and alcohol) or who are malnourished (e.g. in anorexia, in alcoholism, or those who are HIV-positive) may develop toxicity at **lower** plasma-paracetamol concentrations and should be treated if concentrations are above the *high-risk treatment line* (which joins plots that are at 50% of the plasma-paracetamol concentrations of the normal treatment line).

In remote areas methionine (2.5 g) should be given by mouth since it is seldom practicable to give acetylcysteine outside hospital. Once the patient reaches hospital the need to continue treatment with the antidote will be assessed from the

plasma-paracetamol concentration (related to the time from ingestion).

See also Co-proxamol, under Analgesics (opioid).

ACETYLCYSTEINE

Indications: paracetamol overdosage (see notes above)

Cautions: asthma

Side-effects: rashes, anaphylaxis

Dose: by intravenous infusion, in glucose intravenous infusion 5%, initially 150 mg/kg in 200 mL over 15 minutes, followed by 50 mg/kg in 500 mL over 4 hours, then 100 mg/kg in 1000 mL over 16 hours

PoM **Parvolex®** (Evans)

Injection, acetylcysteine 200 mg/mL. Net price 10-mL amp = £2.65

METHIONINE

Indications: paracetamol overdosage, see notes above

Dose: by mouth, 2.5 g initially, followed by 3 further doses of 2.5 g every 4 hours

Methionine (Non-proprietary)

Tablets, DL-methionine 250 mg. Net price course of 40 tabs = £12.27
Available from Norton

ANALGESICS (OPIOID)

Opioids (narcotic analgesics) cause varying degrees of coma, respiratory depression, and pinpoint pupils. The specific antidote **naloxone** is indicated if there is coma or bradypnoea. Since naloxone has a shorter duration of action than many opioids, close monitoring and repeated injections are necessary according to the respiratory rate and depth of coma. Alternatively, it may be given by continuous intravenous infusion, the rate of administration being adjusted according to response.

CO-PROXAMOL. Combinations of dextropropoxyphene and paracetamol (co-proxamol) are frequently taken in overdosage. The initial features are those of acute opioid overdosage with coma, respiratory depression, and pinpoint pupils. Patients may die of acute cardiovascular collapse before reaching hospital (particularly if alcohol has also been consumed) unless adequately resuscitated or given **naloxone** as antidote to the dextropropoxyphene. Paracetamol hepatotoxicity may develop later and should be anticipated and treated as indicated above.

NALOXONE HYDROCHLORIDE

Indications: overdosage with opioids; for postoperative respiratory depression, see section 15.1.7

Cautions: physical dependence on opioids; cardiac irritability; naloxone is short-acting, see notes above

Dose: by intravenous injection, 0.8–2 mg repeated at intervals of 2–3 minutes to a max. of 10 mg if respiratory function does not improve (then question diagnosis); CHILD 10 micrograms/kg; subsequent dose of 100 micrograms/kg if no response

By subcutaneous or intramuscular injection, as intravenous injection but only if intravenous route not feasible (onset of action slower)

By continuous intravenous infusion, 2 mg diluted in 500 mL intravenous infusion solution at a rate adjusted according to the response

IMPORTANT. Doses used in acute opioid overdosage may not be appropriate for the management of opioid-induced respiratory depression and sedation in those receiving palliative care and in chronic opioid use, see also section 15.1.7 for management of postoperative respiratory depression

PoM **Naloxone** (Non-proprietary)

Injection, naloxone hydrochloride 400 micrograms/mL. Net price 1-mL amp = 74p
Available from Antigen, Faulding DBL

PoM **Min-I-Jet® Naloxone** (IMS)

Injection, naloxone hydrochloride 400 micrograms/mL. Net price 1-mL disposable syringe = £5.23; 2-mL disposable syringe = £9.74

PoM **Narcan®** (Du Pont)

Injection, naloxone hydrochloride 400 micrograms/mL, net price 1-mL amp = £4.79

Neonatal preparations —section 15.1.7

ANTIDEPRESSANTS

Tricyclic and related antidepressants cause dry mouth, coma of varying degree, hypotension, hypothermia, hyperreflexia, extensor plantar responses, convulsions, respiratory failure, cardiac conduction defects, and arrhythmias. Dilated pupils and urinary retention also occur. Metabolic acidosis may complicate severe poisoning; delirium with confusion, agitation, and visual and auditory hallucinations, is common during recovery.

Symptomatic treatment and activated charcoal by mouth may reasonably be given in the home before transfer but hospital admission is strongly advised, and supportive measures to ensure a patent airway and adequate ventilation during transfer are mandatory. Intravenous diazepam may be required for control of convulsions (preferably in emulsion form). Although arrhythmias are worrying, some will respond to correction of hypoxia and acidosis; the use of anti-arrhythmic drugs is best avoided. Diazepam given by mouth is usually adequate to sedate delirious patients but large doses may be required.

ANTIMALARIALS

Overdosage with chloroquine and hydroxychloroquine is extremely hazardous and difficult to treat. Urgent advice from a poisons information centre is essential. Life-threatening features include arrhythmias (which can have a very rapid onset) and convulsions (which can be intractable). Quinine overdosage is also a severe hazard and calls for urgent advice from a poisons information centre.

BETA-BLOCKERS

Therapeutic overdosages with beta-blockers may cause lightheadedness, dizziness, and possibly syncope due to impaired circulation secondary to bradycardia and hypotension; heart failure may be precipitated or exacerbated. These complications are most likely in patients with pre-existing conduction system disorders or impaired myocardial function. Bradycardia is the most common arrhythmia caused by beta-blockers, but sotalol occasionally induces ventricular tachyarrhythmias (sometimes of the torsades de pointes type). The effects of massive overdosage may vary from one beta-blocker to another; propranolol overdosage in particular may cause coma and convulsions.

Acute massive overdosage must be managed in hospital and expert advice should be obtained. Maintenance of a clear airway and adequate ventilation is mandatory. An intravenous injection of atropine is required to treat bradycardia and hypotension (3 mg for an adult, 40 micrograms/kg for a child). Cardiogenic shock unresponsive to atropine is probably best treated with an intravenous injection of glucagon 50–150 micrograms/kg [unlicensed indication and dose] in glucose 5% (with precautions to protect the airway in case of vomiting). A further dose of glucagon (or an intravenous infusion) may be required if the response is not maintained. If glucagon is not available, intravenous isoprenaline or intravenous prenalterol [not on UK market] are alternatives to glucagon.

HYPNOTICS AND ANXIOLYTICS

BARBITURATES. These cause drowsiness, coma, respiratory depression, hypotension, and hypothermia. The duration and depth of cerebral depression vary greatly with the drug, the dose, and the tolerance of the patient. The severity of poisoning is often greater with a large dose of barbiturate hypnotics than with the longer-acting phenobarbitone. The majority of patients survive with supportive measures alone. Charcoal haemoperfusion is the treatment of choice for the small minority of patients with very severe barbiturate poisoning who fail to improve, or who deteriorate despite good supportive care.

BENZODIAZEPINES. Benzodiazepines taken alone cause drowsiness, ataxia, dysarthria, and occasionally minor and short-lived depression of consciousness. They potentiate the effects of other central nervous system depressants taken concomitantly Flumazenil, a benzodiazepine antagonist, may be used in the *differential diagnosis* of unclear cases of multiple drug overdose but expert advice is **essential** since adverse effects may occur (e.g. convulsions in patients dependent on benzodiazepines).

IRON SALTS

Iron poisoning is commonest in childhood and is usually accidental. The symptoms are nausea, vomiting, abdominal pain, diarrhoea, haematemesis, and rectal bleeding. Hypotension, coma, and hepatocellular necrosis occur later. Mortality is reduced with intensive and specific therapy with **desferrioxamine**, which chelates iron. The stomach should be emptied at once by gastric lavage. The serum-iron concentration is measured as an emergency and intravenous desferrioxamine given to chelate absorbed iron in excess of the expected iron binding capacity. In **severe toxicity** intravenous desferrioxamine should be given *immediately* without waiting for the result of the serum-iron measurement (contact a poisons information centre for advice).

DESFERRIOXAMINE MESYLATE
(Deferoxamine Mesilate)

Indications: removal of iron from the body in poisoning; for use in chronic iron overload, see section 9.1.3

Cautions: avoid prochlorperazine

Side-effects: anaphylactic reactions, and hypotension when given too rapidly by intravenous injection

Dose: by continuous intravenous infusion, up to 15 mg/kg/hour; max. 80 mg/kg in 24 hours

PoM **Desferal®** (Novartis)
Injection, powder for reconstitution, desferrioxamine mesylate. Net price 500-mg vial = £3.70

LITHIUM

Most cases of lithium intoxication occur as a complication of long-term therapy and are caused by reduced excretion of the drug due to a variety of factors including dehydration, deterioration of renal function, infections, and co-administration of diuretics or NSAIDs (or other drugs that interact). Acute deliberate overdoses may also occur with delayed onset of symptoms (12 hours or more) due to slow entry of lithium into the tissues and continuing absorption from modified-release formulations.

The early clinical features are non-specific and may include apathy and restlessness which could be confused with mental changes due to the patient's depressive illness. Vomiting, diarrhoea, ataxia, weakness, dysarthria, muscle twitching, and tremor may follow. Severe poisoning is associated with convulsions, coma, renal failure, electrolyte imbalance, dehydration, and hypotension.

Therapeutic lithium concentrations are within the range of 0.4–1.0 mmol/litre; concentrations in excess of 2.0 mmol/litre are usually associated with serious toxicity and such cases may need treatment with haemodialysis (if there is renal failure). In acute overdosage much higher serum concentrations may be present without features of toxicity and measures to increase urine production are usually all that are necessary. Otherwise treatment is supportive with special regard to electrolyte balance, renal function, and control of convulsions.

PHENOTHIAZINES AND RELATED DRUGS

Phenothiazines cause less depression of consciousness and respiration than other sedatives. Hypotension, hypothermia, sinus tachycardia, and arrhythmias (particularly with thioridazine) may complicate poisoning. Dystonic reactions can occur with therapeutic doses, (particularly with prochlorperazine and trifluoperazine) and convulsions may occur in severe cases. Arrhythmias may respond to correction of hypoxia and acidosis but anti-arrhythmic drugs may also be needed. Dystonic reactions are rapidly abolished by injection of drugs such as benztropine or procyclidine (see section 4.9.2).

STIMULANTS

AMPHETAMINES. These cause wakefulness, excessive activity, paranoia, hallucinations, and hypertension followed by exhaustion, convulsions, hyperthermia, and coma. The early stages can be controlled by chlorpromazine and, if necessary, beta-blockers. Later, tepid sponging, anticonvulsants, and artificial respiration may be needed. Amphetamine excretion can be increased by forced acid diuresis but this is seldom necessary.

COCAINE. Cocaine can be smoked, sniffed, or injected. It stimulates the central nervous system causing agitation, dilated pupils, tachycardia, hypertension, hallucinations, hypertonia, and hyperreflexia. Convulsions, coma and metabolic acidosis may develop in the worst cases. Sedation, with intravenous diazepam, may be all that is necessary (and will also control convulsions); intravenous propranolol may be indicated for severe arrhythmias (labetalol may be preferred if there is associated hypertension).

ECSTASY. Ecstasy (methylenedioxymethamphetamine) may cause severe reactions, even at doses that were previously tolerated. The most serious effects are delirium, coma, convulsions, ventricular arrhythmias, hyperpyrexia, rhabdomyolysis, acute renal failure, acute hepatitis, disseminated intravascular coagulation, adult respiratory distress syndrome, hyperreflexia, hypotension and intracerebral haemorrhage; hyponatraemia has also been associated with ecstasy use.

Treatment is supportive, with diazepam to control severe agitation or persistent convulsions and close monitoring including ECG.

THEOPHYLLINE

Theophylline and related drugs are often prescribed as modified-release formulations and toxicity may therefore be delayed. They cause vomiting (which may be severe and intractable), agitation, restlessness, dilated pupils, and sinus tachycardia. More serious effects are haematemesis, convulsions, and supraventricular and ventricular arrhythmias. **Profound hypokalaemia** may develop rapidly.

The stomach should be emptied if the patient presents within 2 hours. Elimination of theophylline may be enhanced by repeated doses of activated charcoal by mouth (see also under Active Elimination Techniques). Hypokalaemia is corrected by intravenous infusion of potassium chloride and may be so severe as to require 60 mmol/hour (high doses under ECG monitoring). Convulsions should be controlled by intravenous administration of diazepam (emulsion preferred). Sedation with diazepam may be necessary in agitated patients.

Providing the patient is **not** an asthmatic, extreme tachycardia, hypokalaemia, and hyperglycaemia may be reversed by intravenous administration of propranolol (see section 2.4).

Other poisons

Consult poisons information services day and night—p. 18.

CYANIDES

Cyanide antidotes include dicobalt edetate, given alone, and sodium nitrite, followed by sodium thiosulphate. These antidotes are held for emergency use in hospitals as well as in centres where cyanide poisoning is a risk such as factories and laboratories.

DICOBALT EDETATE

Indications: acute poisoning with cyanides
Cautions: owing to toxicity to be used only when patient tending to lose, or has lost, consciousness; not to be used as a precautionary measure
Side-effects: hypotension, tachycardia, and vomiting
Dose: by intravenous injection, 300 mg (20 mL) over 1 minute (5 minutes if condition less serious) followed immediately by 50 mL of glucose intravenous infusion 50%; if response inadequate a second dose of both may be given; if no response after further 5 minutes a third dose of both may be given

PoM **Dicobalt Edetate** (Cambridge)
Injection, dicobalt edetate 15 mg/mL. Net price 20-mL (300-mg) amp = £6.88
Note. The brand name Kelocyanor® was formerly used for dicobalt edetate injection

SODIUM NITRITE

Indications: poisoning with cyanides (used in conjunction with sodium thiosulphate)
Side-effects: flushing and headache due to vasodilatation

PoM **Sodium Nitrite Injection**
Injection, sodium nitrite 3% (30 mg/mL) in water for injections
Dose: 10 mL by intravenous injection over 3 minutes, followed by 25 mL of sodium thiosulphate injection 50%, by intravenous injection over 10 minutes
'Special-order' [unlicensed] product: contact Martindale or regional hospital manufacturing unit

SODIUM THIOSULPHATE

Indications: poisoning with cyanides (used in conjunction with sodium nitrite)

PoM **Sodium Thiosulphate Injection**
Injection, sodium thiosulphate 50% (500 mg/mL) in water for injections
Dose: see above under Sodium Nitrite Injection
'Special-order' [unlicensed] product: contact Martindale or regional hospital manufacturing unit

---

HEAVY METALS

Heavy metal antidotes include dimercaprol, penicillamine, and sodium calciumedetate.

DIMERCAPROL
(BAL)
Indications: poisoning by antimony, arsenic, bismuth, gold, mercury, possibly thallium; adjunct (with sodium calciumedetate) in lead poisoning
Cautions: hypertension, renal impairment (discontinue or use with extreme caution if impairment develops during treatment), elderly, pregnancy and breast-feeding
Contra-indications: not indicated for iron, cadmium, or selenium poisoning; severe hepatic impairment (unless due to arsenic poisoning)
Side-effects: hypertension, tachycardia, malaise, nausea, vomiting, salivation, lachrymation, sweating, burning sensation (mouth, throat, and

eyes), feeling of constriction of throat and chest, headache, muscle spasm, abdominal pain, tingling of extremities; pyrexia in children; local pain and abscess at injection site

Dose: by intramuscular injection, 2.5–3 mg/kg every 4 hours for 2 days, 2–4 times on the third day, then 1–2 times daily for 10 days or until recovery

PoM **Dimercaprol** (Knoll)
Injection, dimercaprol 50 mg/mL. Net price 2-mL amp = £16.50
Note. Contains arachis (peanut) oil as solvent

PENICILLAMINE

Indications: poisoning by certain toxic metal ions, particularly by copper and lead
Cautions; Contra-indications; Side-effects: see section 10.1.3
Dose: 1–2 g daily in divided doses before food until urinary lead is stabilised at less than 500 micrograms/day; CHILD 20 mg/kg daily

Preparations
See section 10.1.3

SODIUM CALCIUMEDETATE
(Sodium Calcium Edetate)

Indications: poisoning by heavy metals, especially lead
Cautions: renal impairment
Side-effects: nausea, cramp; in overdosage renal damage
Dose: by intravenous infusion, adults and children up to 40 mg/kg twice daily in sodium chloride intravenous infusion 0.9% or glucose intravenous infusion 5% for up to 5 days, repeated if necessary after 48 hours

PoM **Ledclair®** (Sinclair)
Injection, sodium calciumedetate 200 mg/mL. Net price 5-mL amp = £4.38

NOXIOUS GASES

CARBON MONOXIDE. Carbon monoxide poisoning is now usually due to inhalation of smoke, car exhaust, or fumes caused by blocked flues or incomplete combustion of fuel gases in confined spaces. Its toxic effects are entirely due to hypoxia.

Immediate treatment is essential. The person should be removed into the fresh air, the airway cleared, and **oxygen** 100% administered as soon as available. Artificial respiration should be given as necessary and continued until adequate spontaneous breathing starts, or stopped only after persistent and efficient treatment of cardiac arrest has failed. Admission to hospital is desirable because complications may arise after a delay of hours or days. Cerebral oedema should be anticipated in severe poisoning and is treated with an intravenous infusion of mannitol (section 2.2.5). Referral for hyperbaric oxygen treatment should be discussed with the poisons information services if the victim is or has been unconscious, or has a blood carboxyhaemoglobin concentration of more than 20%, or is pregnant.

SULPHUR DIOXIDE, CHLORINE, PHOSGENE, AMMONIA. All of these gases can cause upper respiratory tract and conjunctival irritation to a greater or lesser degree. Pulmonary oedema, with severe breathlessness and cyanosis may develop suddenly up to 36 hours after exposure. Death may occur. Patients are kept under observation and those who develop pulmonary oedema are given corticosteroids and oxygen. Assisted ventilation may be necessary in the most serious cases.

PESTICIDES

PARAQUAT. Concentrated liquid paraquat preparations (e.g. *Gramoxone®*), available to farmers and horticulturists, contain 10–20% paraquat and are extremely toxic. Granular preparations, for garden use, contain only 2.5% paraquat and have caused few deaths.

Paraquat has local and systemic effects. Splashes in the eyes irritate and ulcerate the cornea and conjunctiva. Copious washing of the eye and instillation of antibacterial eye-drops, should aid healing but it may be a long process. Skin irritation, blistering, and ulceration can occur from prolonged contact both with the concentrated and dilute forms. Inhalation of spray, mist, or dust containing paraquat may cause nose bleeding and sore throat but not systemic toxicity.

Ingestion of concentrated paraquat solutions is followed by nausea, vomiting, and diarrhoea. Painful ulceration of the tongue, lips, and fauces may appear after 36 to 48 hours together with renal failure. Some days later there may be dyspnoea with pulmonary fibrosis due to proliferative alveolitis and bronchiolitis.

Treatment should be started immediately. The single most useful measure is oral administration of repeat-dose **activated charcoal**[1]; the first dose of 100 g is given with a laxative (e.g. magnesium sulphate), followed by activated charcoal 50 g every 4 hours (or more frequently if tolerated) until the charcoal is seen in the stool. Vomiting may preclude the use of activated charcoal and an anti-emetic may be required. Gastric lavage is of doubtful value. Intravenous fluids and analgesics are given as necessary. Oxygen therapy should be avoided in the early stages of management since this may exacerbate damage to the lungs, but oxygen may be required in the late stages to palliate symptoms. Measures to enhance elimination of absorbed paraquat are probably valueless but should be discussed with the poisons information services who will also give guidance on predicting the likely outcome from plasma concentrations. Paraquat absorption can be confirmed by a simple qualitative urine test.

ORGANOPHOSPHORUS INSECTICIDES. Organophosphorus insecticides are usually supplied as powders or dissolved in organic solvents. All are absorbed through the bronchi and intact skin as well as

---

1. **Fuller's earth** and **bentonite** given by mouth have also been used as adsorbents. A suspension of Fuller's earth 30% was used in three doses of 200–500 mL given at two-hour intervals; magnesium sulphate or mannitol were given with Fuller's earth to promote diarrhoea and empty the gut.

through the gut and inhibit cholinesterase activity thereby prolonging and intensifying the effects of acetylcholine. Toxicity between different compounds varies considerably, and onset may be delayed after skin exposure.

Anxiety, restlessness, dizziness, headache, miosis, nausea, hypersalivation, vomiting, abdominal colic, diarrhoea, bradycardia, and sweating are common. Muscle weakness and fasciculation may develop and progress to generalised flaccid paralysis including the ocular and respiratory muscles. Convulsions, coma, pulmonary oedema with copious bronchial secretions, hypoxia, and arrhythmias occur in severe cases. Hyperglycaemia and glycosuria without ketonuria may also be present.

Further absorption should be prevented by emptying the stomach, removing the patient to fresh air, or removing soiled clothing and washing contaminated skin. In severe poisoning it is vital to ensure a clear airway, frequent removal of bronchial secretions, and adequate ventilation and oxygenation. **Atropine** will reverse the muscarinic effects of acetylcholine and is given in a dose of 2 mg as atropine sulphate injection (intramuscularly or intravenously according to the severity of poisoning) every 20 to 30 minutes until the skin becomes flushed and dry, the pupils dilate, and tachycardia develops.

Pralidoxime mesylate (P2S), a cholinesterase reactivator, is indicated, as an adjunct to atropine, in moderate or severe poisoning but is only effective if given within 24 hours. It may be obtained from designated centres, the names of which are held by the poisons information centres (see p. 18). A dose of 30 mg/kg (diluted with 10–15 mL water for injections) by slow intravenous injection should produce improvement in muscle power within 30 minutes but repeated doses or, in severe cases, an intravenous infusion of up to 500 mg/hour may be required.

PRALIDOXIME MESYLATE
(P2S)

Indications: adjunct to atropine in the treatment of organophosphorus poisoning

Cautions: renal impairment, myasthenia gravis

Contra-indications: poisoning due to carbamates and to organophosphorus compounds without anticholinesterase activity

Side-effects: drowsiness, dizziness, disturbances of vision, nausea, tachycardia, headache, hyperventilation, and muscular weakness

Dose: by slow intravenous injection (diluted to 10–15 mL with water for injections and given over 5–10 minutes), 30 mg/kg initially followed by 1–2 further doses if necessary; usual max. 12 g in 24 hours

CHILD 20–60 mg/kg as required depending on severity of poisoning and response

Note. Pralidoxime mesylate doses in BNF may differ from those in product literature

PoM **Pralidoxime Mesylate**

Injection, pralidoxime mesylate 200 mg/mL

Available as 5-mL amps (from designated centres)

SNAKE BITES AND INSECT STINGS

SNAKE BITE. Acute envenoming from snake bite is rare in the UK and the only indigenous venomous snake is the adder (*Vipera berus*). The bite may cause local and systemic effects. Local effects include pain, swelling, bruising, and tender enlargement of regional lymph nodes. Systemic effects include early transient hypotension with syncope, angioedema, abdominal colic, diarrhoea, and vomiting, with later persistent or recurrent hypotension, ECG abnormalities, spontaneous systemic bleeding, coagulopathy, adult respiratory distress syndrome, and acute renal failure. There is a small risk of fatal envenoming especially in children and the elderly.

Indications for antivenom treatment include systemic envenoming, especially hypotension (see above), ECG abnormalities, vomiting, haemostatic abnormalities, polymorphonuclear leucocytosis, elevated serum creatine kinase and local envenoming if, after bites on the hand or foot, swelling extends beyond the wrist or ankle within 4 hours of the bite. For both **adults** and **children**, the contents of one vial (10 mL) of **European viper venom antiserum** (available from Farillon) is given *by intravenous injection* over 10–15 minutes or *by intravenous infusion* over 30 minutes after diluting in sodium chloride intravenous infusion 0.9% (use 5 mL diluent/kg body-weight). The **same dose** should be used for **adults** and **children**. The dose can be repeated in 1–2 hours if symptoms of **systemic envenoming** persist. Adrenaline injection must be immediately to hand for treatment of anaphylactic reactions to the antivenom (for full details see section 3.4.3).

Antivenom is available for certain foreign snakes, spiders and scorpions. For information on identification, management, and supply, telephone:

Oxford	(01865) 220968
or	(01865) 221332
or	(01865) 741166
Liverpool	0151-708 9393
Liverpool (Fazakerley Hospital Pharmacy)	
(supply only)	0151-525 5980
London	0171-635 9191

INSECT STINGS. Stings from ants, wasps, hornets, and bees cause local pain and swelling but seldom cause severe direct toxicity unless many stings are inflicted at the same time. If the sting is in the mouth or on the tongue marked swelling may cause respiratory distress. The stings from these insects are usually treated by cleaning the area, applying a cooling lotion (such as a calamine preparation), and giving an antihistamine by mouth. Bee stings should be removed by scraping them off with a finger nail or knife before cleaning the area. Anaphylactic reactions require treatment with intramuscular **adrenaline**; self-administered intramuscular adrenaline (e.g. *EpiPen*®) is the best first-aid treatment for patients with severe hypersensitivity. For full details of the management of anaphylaxis, see section 3.4.3.

Classified Notes on Drugs and Preparations

Doping Classes and Methods of the International Olympic Committee Medical Commission 1997

The following are examples of classes and methods prohibited in sport:

Classes	**Stimulants** eg. amphetamine, bromantan, caffeine (above 12mcg/mL), cocaine, ephedrine, certain ß2 agonists. **Narcotics** eg. diamorphine (heroin), morphine, methadone, pethidine. **Anabolic agents** eg. methandienone, nandrolone, stanozolol, testosterone, clenbuterol, DHEA. **Diuretics** eg. acetazolamide, frusemide, hydrochlorothiazide, triamterene. **Peptide & Glycoprotein Hormones & Analogues** eg. growth hormone, corticotrophin, chorionic gonadotrophin, erythropoietin.
Methods	**Blood Doping** **Pharmacological, Chemical & Physical Manipulation** eg. substances and methods that alter the integrity and validity of the urine; e.g. probenecid, catheterisation, urine substitutes.
Classes of drugs subject to certain restrictions	**Alcohol & Marijuana;** Restricted in certain sports. Refer to regulations of national or international federations. **Local Anaesthetics;** route of administration restricted to local or intra-articular injection. **Corticosteroids;** route of administration restricted to topical, inhalation*, local or intra-articular injection. **Beta-blockers;** restricted in certain sports. Refer to regulations of international sports federations.

*Written notification of administration should be given to relevant medical authority eg. governing body medical officer

Treatment Guidelines
Examples of permitted & prohibited substances

	ALLOWED	**BANNED**
ASTHMA	salbutamol*, terbutaline*, salmeterol*, beclomethasone*, fluticasone*, theophylline* (*by inhalation only) sodium cromoglycate.	products containing sympathomimetics eg. ephedrine, isoprenaline, fenoterol, rimiterol, orciprenaline.
COLD/ COUGH	all antibiotics, steam & menthol inhalations, permitted antihistamines, terfenadine, astemizole, pholcodine, guaiphenesin, dextromethorphan, paracetamol.	products containing sympathomimetics eg. ephedrine, pseudoephedrine, phenylpropanolamine.
DIARRHOEA	diphenoxylate, loperamide, products containing electrolytes (eg. Dioralyte, Rehidrat).	products containing opioids (eg. morphine).
HAY FEVER	antihistamines, nasal sprays containing a corticosteroid or xylometazoline, eye drops containing sodium cromoglycate.	products containing ephedrine, pseudoephedrine
PAIN	aspirin, codeine, dihydrocodeine, ibuprofen, paracetamol, all non-steroidal anti-inflammatories, dextropropoxyphene	products containing opioids, caffeine.
VOMITING	domperidone, metoclopramide.	

WARNING. Some vitamin, herbal and nutritional substances may contain prohibited substances, such as Guarana, Ma Huang, Chinese Ephedra.

The substances listed are only examples of substances permitted or prohibited by the IOC. Not all sports adopt the IOC Medical Code. If in doubt check with your governing body or with the UKSC Drug Information Line 0171-380 8030

Supplies of this card are available from: UK Sports Council, Ethics & Anti-Doping Directorate, Walkden House, 10 Melton Street, London NW1 2EB

Similar cards detailing classes of drugs and doping methods prohibited by the Football Association and the Lawn Tennis Association are also available

1: Drugs acting on the
GASTRO-INTESTINAL SYSTEM

The drugs and preparations in this chapter are described under the following sections:

1.1 Antacids and other drugs for dyspepsia

Antacids (usually containing aluminium or magnesium compounds) are useful for treating gastro-intestinal disease; they can often relieve symptoms in both ulcer and non-ulcer dyspepsia, and in gastro-oesophageal reflux disease (reflux oesophagitis). They are best given when symptoms occur or are expected, usually between meals and at bedtime, 4 or more times daily; additional doses may be required up to once an hour. Conventional doses e.g. 10 mL 3 or 4 times daily of liquid magnesium–aluminium antacids promote ulcer healing, but less well than antisecretory drugs (section 1.3); proof of a relationship between healing and neutralising capacity is lacking. Liquid preparations are more effective than solids.

Bismuth-containing antacids (unless chelates) are best avoided because absorbed bismuth can be neurotoxic, causing encephalopathy; they tend to be constipating. Calcium-containing antacids can induce rebound acid secretion: with modest doses the clinical significance is doubtful, but prolonged high doses also cause hypercalcaemia and alkalosis, and can precipitate the milk alkali syndrome. For **preparations** on sale to the public (not prescribable on the NHS), see p. 31

See also section 1.3 for drugs used in the treatment of peptic ulcer.

INTERACTIONS. Antacids should preferably not be taken at the same time as other drugs since they may impair absorption. Antacids may also damage enteric coatings designed to prevent dissolution in the stomach. See also **Appendix 1** (antacids and adsorbents).

1.1.1 Aluminium- and magnesium-containing antacids

Aluminium- and **magnesium-containing** antacids, such as magnesium carbonate, hydroxide and tri-silicate, and aluminium glycinate and hydroxide, being relatively insoluble in water, are long-acting if retained in the stomach. They are suitable for most antacid purposes. Magnesium-containing antacids tend to be laxative whereas aluminium-containing antacids may be constipating. Aluminium accumulation does not appear to be a risk if renal function is normal (see also Appendix 3).

Compound preparations have no clear advantages over simpler preparations: neutralising capacity may be the same.

Complexes such as **hydrotalcite** confer no special advantage.

Activated **dimethicone** (simethicone) is added to an antacid as an antifoaming agent to relieve flatulence. These preparations may be useful for the relief of hiccup in palliative care. **Alginates** added as protectants against gastro-oesophageal reflux disease (section 1.1.3) may be useful, but surface anaesthetics (e.g. oxethazaine) added to improve symptom relief are of doubtful efficacy. The amount of additional ingredient or antacid in individual preparations varies widely, as does their sodium content, so that preparations may not be freely interchangeable.

> **Low Na$^+$**
> The words low Na$^+$ added after some preparations indicate a sodium content of less than 1 mmol per tablet or 10-mL dose.

ALUMINIUM HYDROXIDE

Indications: dyspepsia; for use in hyperphosphataemia, see section 9.5.2.2

Cautions: see notes above; porphyria, see section 9.8.2; **interactions:** Appendix 1 (antacids and adsorbents)

Contra-indications: hypophosphataemia

Aluminium-only preparations
Aluminium Hydroxide (Non-proprietary)
Tablets, dried aluminium hydroxide 500 mg. Net price 20 = 15p
Dose: 1–2 tablets chewed 4 times daily and at bedtime or as required
Mixture (gel), about 4% w/w Al_2O_3 in water, with a peppermint flavour. Net price 200 mL = 41p
Dose: antacid, 5–10 mL 4 times daily between meals and at bedtime or as required; CHILD 6–12 years, up to 5 mL 3 times daily
Note. The brand name NHS Aludrox® (Pfizer Consumer) is used for aluminium hydroxide mixture; net price 200 mL = £1.18. NHS Aludrox® tablets also contain magnesium.

Alu-Cap® (3M)
Capsules, green/red, dried aluminium hydroxide 475 mg (low Na+). Net price 120-cap pack = £4.22
Dose: antacid, 1 capsule 4 times daily and at bedtime; CHILD not recommended for antacid therapy

Co-magaldrox
Co-magaldrox is a mixture of aluminium hydroxide and magnesium hydroxide; the proportions are expressed in the form *x/y* where *x* and *y* are the strengths in milligrams per unit dose of magnesium hydroxide and aluminium hydroxide respectively

Maalox® (Rhône-Poulenc Rorer)
Suspension, sugar-free, co-magaldrox 195/220 (magnesium hydroxide 195 mg, dried aluminium hydroxide 220 mg/5 mL (low Na+)). Net price 500 mL = £1.97
Dose: 10–20 mL 20 minutes–1 hour after meals and at bedtime or when required; CHILD under 14 years not recommended

Maalox TC® (Rhône-Poulenc Rorer)
Tablets, co-magaldrox 300/600 (magnesium hydroxide 300 mg, dried aluminium hydroxide 600 mg (low Na+)). Net price 100 = £3.86
Suspension, sugar-free, co-magaldrox 300/600 (magnesium hydroxide 300 mg, dried aluminium hydroxide 600 mg/5 mL (low Na+)). Net price 500 mL = £3.86
Dose: antacid, 1–2 tablets chewed or 5–10 mL suspension 4 times daily 20 minutes–1 hour after meals and at bedtime; duodenal ulcer, 3 tablets or 15 mL suspension 4 times daily (treatment) *or* twice daily (prevention of recurrence)

Mucogel® (Pharmax)
Suspension, sugar-free, co-magaldrox 195/220 (magnesium hydroxide 195 mg, dried aluminium hydroxide 220 mg/5 mL (low Na+)). Net price 500 mL = £1.91
Dose: 10–20 mL 3 times daily, 20 minutes–1 hour after meals, and at bedtime or when required; CHILD under 12 years not recommended

For **preparations** containing aluminium and magnesium on sale to the public and not prescribable on the NHS, see p. 31

MAGNESIUM CARBONATE
Indications: dyspepsia
Cautions: renal impairment; see also notes above; **interactions:** Appendix 1 (antacids and adsorbents)
Contra-indications: hypophosphataemia
Side-effects: diarrhoea; belching due to liberated carbon dioxide

Aromatic Magnesium Carbonate Mixture, BP
(Aromatic Magnesium Carbonate Oral Suspension)
Oral suspension, light magnesium carbonate 3%, sodium bicarbonate 5%, in a suitable vehicle containing aromatic cardamom tincture. Extemporaneous preparations should be recently prepared according to the following formula: light magnesium carbonate 300 mg, sodium bicarbonate 500 mg, aromatic cardamom tincture 0.3 mL, double-strength chloroform water 5 mL, water to 10 mL. Contains about 6 mmol Na+/10 mL. Net price 200 mL = 59p
Dose: 10 mL 3 times daily in water

For **preparations** also containing aluminium, see above and section 1.1.3.

MAGNESIUM TRISILICATE
Indications: dyspepsia
Cautions: see under Magnesium Carbonate
Contra-indications: see under Magnesium Carbonate
Side-effects: diarrhoea

Magnesium Trisilicate Tablets, Compound, BP
Tablets, magnesium trisilicate 250 mg, dried aluminium hydroxide 120 mg
Dose: 1–2 tablets chewed when required

Magnesium Trisilicate Mixture, BP
(Magnesium Trisilicate Oral Suspension)
Oral suspension, 5% each of magnesium trisilicate, light magnesium carbonate, and sodium bicarbonate in a suitable vehicle with a peppermint flavour. Extemporaneous preparations should be recently prepared according to the following formula: magnesium trisilicate 500 mg, light magnesium carbonate 500 mg, sodium bicarbonate 500 mg, concentrated peppermint emulsion 0.25 mL, double-strength chloroform water 5 mL, water to 10 mL. Contains about 6 mmol Na+/10 mL
Dose: 10 mL 3 times daily in water

Magnesium Trisilicate Oral Powder, Compound, BP
Oral powder, magnesium trisilicate 250 mg, chalk 250 mg, heavy magnesium carbonate 250 mg, sodium bicarbonate 250 mg/g. Contains about 3 mmol Na+/g. Label: 13
Dose: 1–5 g in liquid when required

For **preparations** also containing aluminium, see above and section 1.1.3.

ALUMINIUM-MAGNESIUM COMPLEXES

HYDROTALCITE
Aluminium magnesium carbonate hydroxide hydrate
Indications: dyspepsia
Cautions: see notes above; **interactions:** Appendix 1 (antacids and adsorbents)

Hydrotalcite (Hoechst Marion Roussel)
Tablets, hydrotalcite 500 mg (low Na+). Net price 56-tab pack = 81p
Dose: 2 tablets chewed between meals and at bedtime; CHILD under 6 years not recommended, 6–12 years 1 tablet
Suspension, hydrotalcite 500 mg/5 mL (low Na+). Net price 500-mL pack = £1.96
Dose: 10 mL between meals and at bedtime; CHILD under 6 years not recommended, 6–12 years 5 mL
Note. The brand name NHS Altacite® was formerly used for hydrotalcite suspension and tablets; for Altacite Plus® preparations, see below and p. 31

OTHER COMPOUND ANTACID PREPARATIONS

Altacite Plus® (Hoechst Marion Roussel)
Suspension, sugar-free, co-simalcite 125/500 (activated dimethicone 125 mg, hydrotalcite 500 mg)/5 mL (low Na+). Net price 500 mL = £1.85
Dose: 10 mL between meals and at bedtime when required; CHILD 8–12 years 5 mL
NHS *Tablets*, see p. 31

Asilone® (Seton)

Suspension, sugar-free, dried aluminium hydroxide 420 mg, activated dimethicone 135 mg, light magnesium oxide 70 mg/5 mL (low Na⁺). Net price 500 mL = £1.95

Dose: 5–10 mL after meals and at bedtime or when required up to 4 times daily; CHILD under 12 years not recommended

~~NHS~~ *Tablets*, see p. 31
~~NHS~~ *Liquid*, see p. 31

Diovol® (Pharmax)

Suspension, sugar-free, aluminium hydroxide 200 mg, activated dimethicone 25 mg, magnesium hydroxide 200 mg/5 mL (low Na⁺). Net price 300 mL = £1.13

Dose: 5–10 mL 3 times daily between meals and at bedtime or when required

Maalox Plus® (Rhône-Poulenc Rorer)

Suspension, sugar-free, dried aluminium hydroxide 220 mg, activated dimethicone 25 mg, magnesium hydroxide 195 mg/5 mL (low Na⁺). Net price 500 mL = £1.97

Dose: 5–10 mL 4 times daily (after meals and at bedtime or when required); CHILD under 5 years 5 mL 3 times daily, over 5 years appropriate proportion of adult dose

~~NHS~~ *Tablets*, see p. 31

PoM **Mucaine®** (Wyeth)

Suspension, sugar-free, aluminium hydroxide mixture 4.75 mL, magnesium hydroxide 100 mg, oxethazaine 10 mg/5 mL. Net price 200-mL pack = 76p

Dose: 5–10 mL (without fluid) 3–4 times daily (15 minutes before meals and at bedtime or when required); CHILD not recommended

> For **preparations** containing aluminium and magnesium on sale to the public and not prescribable on the NHS, see p. 31

1.1.2   Sodium bicarbonate

Sodium bicarbonate, being soluble in water, is rapid-acting, but absorbed bicarbonate can cause alkalosis in excessive doses. Like other carbonate-containing antacids it liberates carbon dioxide which causes belching. Sodium bicarbonate and antacid preparations with a high sodium content, such as magnesium trisilicate mixture, should be avoided in patients on salt-restricted diets (in heart failure and in hepatic and renal impairment).

SODIUM BICARBONATE

Indications: rapid relief of dyspepsia; urinary tract, section 7.4.3; acidosis, sections 9.2.1.3 and 9.2.2

Cautions: hepatic and renal impairment, cardiac disease, pregnancy; patients on sodium-restricted diet; elderly; avoid prolonged use; **interactions:** Appendix 1 (antacids and adsorbents)

Side-effects: belching, alkalosis on prolonged use

Dose: see under preparation, below

Sodium Bicarbonate Tablets, Compound, BP,

(Soda Mint Tablets), sodium bicarbonate 300 mg. Contains about 4 mmol Na⁺/tab

Dose: 2–6 tablets sucked when required

1.1.3   Other drugs for dyspepsia and gastro-oesophageal disease

Gastro-oesophageal reflux disease (reflux oesophagitis) results from reflux of gastric or duodenal contents into the oesophagus and causes symptoms, which include heartburn, acid regurgitation, and difficulty in swallowing (dysphagia); oesophageal inflammation, ulceration, and stricture formation may occur and there may be an association with asthma.

Initial management includes lifestyle changes (raising the head of the bed, weight reduction, avoidance of alcohol, cessation of smoking, and avoidance of aggravating foods such as fats) and treatment with **antacids** and **alginates**. Alginate-containing antacids form a 'raft' that floats on the surface of the stomach contents to reduce reflux and protect the oesophageal mucosa.

For those who do not respond to these measures, suppression of gastric acid secretion with a **histamine H₂-antagonist** (section 1.3.1) may relieve symptoms and reduce antacid consumption. Alternatively, a prokinetic agent such as **metoclopramide** (section 4.6) or **cisapride** (section 1.2) may improve gastro-oesophageal sphincter function and accelerate gastric emptying. The extent of oesophageal healing depends on the severity of the disease and duration of therapy. Endoscopically confirmed erosive, ulcerative, or stricturing disease responds best to treatment with a proton pump inhibitor (section 1.3.5) which usually needs to be maintained.

COMPOUND ALGINIC ACID PREPARATIONS

Algicon® (Rhône-Poulenc Rorer)

Tablets, aluminium hydroxide-magnesium carbonate co-gel 360 mg, magnesium alginate 500 mg, heavy magnesium carbonate 320 mg, potassium bicarbonate 100 mg, sucrose 1.5 g (low Na⁺). Net price 60-tab pack = £2.40

Caution: diabetes mellitus (high sugar content)

Dose: 1–2 tablets 4 times daily (chewed after meals and at bedtime); CHILD under 12 years not recommended

Suspension, yellow, aluminium hydroxide-magnesium carbonate co-gel 140 mg, magnesium alginate 250 mg, magnesium carbonate 175 mg, potassium bicarbonate 50 mg/5 mL (low Na⁺). Net price 500 mL (lemon and mint-flavoured) = £2.79

Dose: 10–20 mL 4 times daily (after meals and at bedtime); CHILD under 12 years not recommended

Gastrocote® (Seton)

Tablets, alginic acid 200 mg, dried aluminium hydroxide 80 mg, magnesium trisilicate 40 mg, sodium bicarbonate 70 mg. Contains about 1 mmol Na⁺/tablet. Net price 100-tab pack = £3.67

Dose: 1–2 tablets chewed 4 times daily (after meals and at bedtime); CHILD under 6 years not recommended

Caution: diabetes mellitus (high sugar content)

Liquid, sugar-free, peach-coloured, dried aluminium hydroxide 80 mg, magnesium trisilicate 40 mg, sodium alginate 220 mg, sodium bicarbonate 70 mg/5 mL. Contains 1.8 mmol Na⁺/5 mL. Net price 500 mL = £2.79

Dose: 5–15 mL 4 times daily (after meals and at bedtime)

Gaviscon® (R&C)

Tablets, sugar-free, alginic acid 500 mg, dried aluminium hydroxide 100 mg, magnesium trisilicate

25 mg, sodium bicarbonate 170 mg. Contains 2 mmol Na+/tablet. Net price 60-tab pack (peppermint or lemon flavour) = £2.25

Dose: 1–2 tablets chewed after meals and at bedtime, followed by water; CHILD 2–6 years 1 tablet (on doctor's advice only) and 6–12 years 1 tablet

Liquid, sugar-free, sodium alginate 250 mg, sodium bicarbonate 133.5 mg, calcium carbonate 80 mg/5 mL. Contains about 3 mmol Na+/5 mL. Net price 500 mL (aniseed- or peppermint-flavour) = £2.70

Dose: 10–20 mL after meals and at bedtime; CHILD 2–6 years (on doctor's advice only) and 6–12 years 5–10 mL

NHS *Gaviscon 250® and Gaviscon 500® Tablets,* see below

Gaviscon® Advance (R&C)

Suspension, sugar-free, sodium alginate 500 mg, potassium bicarbonate 100 mg/5 mL. Contains 2.3 mmol Na+, 1 mmol K+/5 mL. Net price 500 mL = £5.40

Dose: ADULT and CHILD over 12 years, 5–10 mL after meals and at bedtime

Infant Gaviscon® (R&C)

Oral powder, sugar-free, sodium alginate 225 mg, magnesium alginate 87.5 mg, dried aluminium hydroxide 112.5 mg with colloidal silica and mannitol/dose (half dual-sachet). Contains 0.92 mmol Na+/dose. Net price 15 dual-sachets (30 doses) = £2.46

Dose: INFANT under 4.5 kg 1 dose (half dual-sachet) mixed with feeds (or water in breast-fed infants) when required; over 4.5 kg 2 doses (1 dual-sachet); CHILD 2 doses (1 dual-sachet) in water after each meal

Note. Not to be used in premature infants, or where excessive water loss likely (e.g. fever, diarrhoea, vomiting, high room temperature), or if intestinal obstruction

IMPORTANT. Each half of the dual-sachet is identified as 'one dose'. To avoid errors prescribe as 'dual-sachet' with directions in terms of 'dose'

Topal® (Novex)

Tablets, alginic acid 200 mg, dried aluminium hydroxide 30 mg, light magnesium carbonate 40 mg with lactose 220 mg, sucrose 880 mg, sodium bicarbonate 40 mg (low Na+). Net price 42-tab pack = £1.67

Dose: 1–3 tablets chewed 4 times daily (after meals and at bedtime); CHILD half adult dose

Caution: diabetes mellitus (high sugar content)

ACTIVATED DIMETHICONE ALONE

Activated dimethicone (also known as simethicone) is an antifoaming agent.

Dentinox® (DDD)

Colic drops (= emulsion), activated dimethicone 21 mg/2.5-mL dose. Net price 100 mL = £1.30

Dose: gripes, colic or wind pains, INFANT 2.5 mL with or after each feed (max. 6 doses in 24 hours), may be added to bottle feed

Note. The brand name *Dentinox®* is also used for other preparations including teething gel

Infacol® (Pharmax)

Liquid, sugar-free, activated dimethicone 40 mg/mL (low Na+). Net price 50 mL = £1.76. Counselling, use of dropper

Dose: gripes, colic or wind pains, INFANT 0.5–1 mL before feeds

Indigestion **preparations** on sale to the public (not prescribable on the NHS) include:

Actal® (alexitol = aluminium), **Actonorm Gel®** (aluminium, magnesium, activated dimethicone, peppermint oil), **Actonorm Powder®** (see section 1.2), **Altacite®** (hydrotalcite = aluminium, magnesium), **Altacite Plus Tablets®** (co-simalcite = aluminium, magnesium, activated dimethicone; suspension is prescribable), **Aludrox Liquid®** (aluminium), **Aludrox Tablets®** (aluminium, magnesium), **Aluhyde®** (see section 1.2), **Andrews Antacid®** (calcium, magnesium), **APP®** (see section 1.2), **Asilone Antacid Liquid®** (aluminium, activated dimethicone, magnesium; suspension is prescribable), **Asilone Antacid Tablets®** (aluminium, activated dimethicone)

Barum Antacid® (calcium), **Bellocarb®** (see section 1.2), **Birley®** (aluminium, magnesium), **Bismag®** (magnesium, sodium bicarbonate), **Bisma-Rex®** (bismuth, calcium, magnesium, peppermint oil), **Bisodol Extra Tablets®** (calcium, magnesium, sodium bicarbonate, activated dimethicone), **Bisodol Heartburn Tablets®** (alginic acid, magaldrate, sodium bicarbonate), **Bisodol Powder®** (magnesium, sodium bicarbonate), **Bisodol Tablets®** and **Bisodol Extra Strong Mint Tablets®** (calcium, magnesium, sodium bicarbonate), **Boots Heartburn Relief®** (alginic acid, calcium, sodium bicarbonate), **Boots Indigestion Relief Tablets®** (aluminium, magnesium, activated dimethicone), **Boots Indigestion Tablets®** (calcium, magnesium, sodium bicarbonate), **Boots Infant S/F Gripe Mixture®** (sodium bicarbonate)

Carbellon® (magnesium, charcoal, peppermint oil)

De Witt's Antacid Powder® (calcium, magnesium, sodium bicarbonate, light kaolin, peppermint oil), **De Witt's Antacid Tablets®** (calcium, magnesium, peppermint oil), **Dijex®** (aluminium, magnesium), **Dynese®** (magaldrate = aluminium, magnesium)

Entrotabs® (aluminium, attapulgite, pectin)

Gaviscon 250® and **500® Tablets** (alginic acid, aluminium, magnesium, sodium bicarbonate; **Gaviscon® Tablets** are prescribable), **Gelusil®** (aluminium, magnesium)

Maalox Plus Tablets® (aluminium, magnesium, activated dimethicone; suspension is prescribable), **Maclean®** (aluminium, calcium, magnesium), **Magnatol®** (alexitol, magnesium, potassium bicarbonate, xanthan gum), **Milk of Magnesia Tablets®** (magnesium; liquid is prescribable), **Moorland®** (aluminium, bismuth, calcium, magnesium, light kaolin)

Nulacin® (calcium, magnesium, peppermint oil; *contains gluten*)

Opas® (calcium, magnesium, sodium bicarbonate)

Pepto-Bismol® (bismuth), **Premiums®** (aluminium, calcium, magnesium, peppermint oil)

Rap-eze® (calcium), **Remegel®** (calcium), **Rennie®** (calcium, magnesium), **Rennie Deflatine®** (calcium, magnesium, activated dimethicone), **Roter®** (bismuth, magnesium, sodium bicarbonate, frangula)

Setlers Antacid® (calcium), **Setlers Wind-eze®** (activated dimethicone), **Simeco®** (aluminium, magnesium, activated dimethicone), **Sovol®** (aluminium, magnesium, activated dimethicone)

Tums® (calcium)

Unigest® (aluminium, activated dimethicone)

Windcheaters® (activated dimethicone)

1.2   Antispasmodics and other drugs altering gut motility

The smooth muscle relaxant properties of antimuscarinic and other antispasmodic drugs may be useful as adjunctive treatment in *non-ulcer dyspepsia*, in the *irritable bowel syndrome*, and in *diverticular disease.* The gastric antisecretory effects of conventional antimuscarinic drugs are of little practical significance since dosage is limited by atropine-like side-effects. Moreover, they have been superseded by more powerful and specific antisecretory drugs, including the histamine H_2-receptor antagonists and the selective antimuscarinic pirenzepine.

The dopamine-receptor antagonists metoclopramide and domperidone, and the acetylcholine-release promoter cisapride all tend to stimulate transit in the gut.

ANTIMUSCARINICS

The antimuscarinics (less correctly termed 'anticholinergics') can be divided into atropine and its related alkaloids (including the belladonna alkaloids), and synthetic antimuscarinics. The synthetic antimuscarinics can, in turn, be divided into **tertiary amine** (dicyclomine hydrochloride) and **quaternary ammonium compounds** (propantheline bromide). Dicyclomine hydrochloride has a much less marked antimuscarinic action than atropine and may also have some direct action on smooth muscle.

Quaternary ammonium compounds are less lipid soluble than atropine and so may be less likely to cross the blood–brain barrier; they are also less well absorbed. Although central atropine-like side-effects, such as confusion, are thereby reduced, peripheral atropine-like side-effects remain common with dry mouth, difficult visual accommodation, hesitant micturition, and constipation at doses which act as gut neuromuscular relaxants or inhibitors of acid secretion. The elderly are particularly susceptible; glaucoma and urinary retention may occur.

Antimuscarinics tend to relax the oesophageal sphincter and should be avoided in patients with symptomatic reflux; all antispasmodics should be avoided in paralytic ileus. Despite these side-effects antimuscarinics are nevertheless useful in some *dyspeptics*, in the *irritable bowel syndrome*, and in *diverticular disease*. Nonselective antimuscarinics (e.g. belladonna alkaloids) are outmoded as ulcer treatments, any clinical virtues being outweighed by atropinic side-effects.

The quaternary ammonium compound, **hyoscine butylbromide** is advocated as a gastro-intestinal antispasmodic, but it is poorly absorbed; the injection is useful in endoscopy and radiology.

ATROPINE SULPHATE and BELLADONNA ALKALOIDS

Indications: see notes above; atropine sulphate, see also section 15.1.3

Cautions: elderly; urinary retention, prostatic enlargement, tachycardia, cardiac insufficiency, paralytic ileus, ulcerative colitis, and pyloric stenosis; may aggravate gastro-oesophageal reflux; pregnancy and breast-feeding; **interactions:** Appendix 1 (antimuscarinics)

Contra-indications: closed-angle glaucoma; see also notes above

Side-effects: dry mouth with difficulty in swallowing and thirst, dilatation of the pupils with loss of accommodation and sensitivity to light, increased intra-ocular pressure, flushing, dry skin, bradycardia followed by tachycardia, palpitations and arrhythmias, difficulty with micturition, and constipation; rarely fever, confusional states and rashes

PoM **Atropine** (Non-proprietary)
Tablets, atropine sulphate 600 micrograms. Net price 28-tab pack = £4.67
Available from CP
Dose: 0.6–1.2 mg at night

Indigestion **preparations** on sale to the public (not prescribable on the NHS) containing belladonna and related alkaloids include:

Actonorm Powder® (atropine, aluminium, calcium, magnesium, sodium bicarbonate, peppermint oil), **Aluhyde**® (belladonna, aluminium, magnesium), **APP**® (homatropine, aluminium, bismuth, calcium, magnesium)
Bellocarb® (belladonna, magnesium)
Enterosan® (belladonna, morphine, kaolin)
Opazimes® (belladonna, morphine, aluminium, kaolin)

DICYCLOMINE HYDROCHLORIDE
(Dicycloverine Hydrochloride)
Indications: adjunct in gastro-intestinal disorders characterised by smooth muscle spasm
Cautions: see under Atropine Sulphate
Contra-indications: see under Atropine Sulphate; infants under 6 months
Side-effects: see under Atropine Sulphate
Dose: 10–20 mg 3 times daily; CHILD 6–24 months 5–10 mg up to 3–4 times daily, 15 minutes before feeds, 2–12 years 10 mg 3 times daily

PoM ¹ **Merbentyl**® (Hoechst Marion Roussel)
Tablets, dicyclomine hydrochloride 10 mg. Net price 20 = £1.14
Syrup, dicyclomine hydrochloride 10 mg/5 mL. Net price 500 mL = £8.62
1. Dicyclomine hydrochloride can be sold to the public provided that the maximum single dose is 10 mg and the maximum daily dose is 60 mg
PoM **Merbentyl 20**® (Hoechst Marion Roussel)
Tablets, dicyclomine hydrochloride 20 mg. Net price 84-tab pack = £9.54

Compound preparations
Kolanticon® (Hoechst Marion Roussel)
Gel, sugar-free, dicyclomine hydrochloride 2.5 mg, dried aluminium hydroxide 200 mg, light magnesium oxide 100 mg, activated dimethicone (simethicone USP) 20 mg/5 mL. Net price 200 mL = £1.52; 500 mL = £1.85
Dose: 10–20 mL every 4 hours when required

HYOSCINE BUTYLBROMIDE
Indications: adjunct in gastro-intestinal disorders characterised by smooth muscle spasm (but see notes above); dysmenorrhoea (but see section 4.7.1)
Cautions: see under Atropine Sulphate and notes above
Contra-indications: see under Atropine Sulphate and notes above; avoid in porphyria (see section 9.8.2)
Side-effects: see under Atropine Sulphate and notes above
Dose: by mouth, 20 mg 4 times daily; CHILD 6–12 years, 10 mg 3 times daily
By intramuscular or intravenous injection (acute spasm), 20 mg, repeated after 30 minutes if necessary

---

PoM ¹ **Buscopan®** (Boehringer Ingelheim)

Tablets, coated, hyoscine butylbromide 10 mg. Net price 56-tab pack = £2.59 (not recommended, see notes above)

1. Can be sold to the public provided single dose does not exceed 20 mg, daily dose does not exceed 80 mg, and pack does not contain a total of more than 240 mg. Net price 20 × 10 mg-tab pack = £2.17

Injection, hyoscine butylbromide 20 mg/mL. Net price 1-mL amp = 20p

PROPANTHELINE BROMIDE

Indications: adjunct in gastro-intestinal disorders characterised by smooth muscle spasm; for use in urinary frequency, see section 7.4.2

Cautions; Contra-indications; Side-effects: see under Atropine Sulphate and notes above

Dose: 15 mg 3 times daily at least 1 hour before meals and 30 mg at night, max. 120 mg daily; CHILD not recommended

PoM **Pro-Banthine®** (Baker Norton)

Tablets, pink, s/c, propantheline bromide 15 mg. Net price 100-tab pack = £4.56. Label: 23

OTHER ANTISPASMODICS

Alverine, **mebeverine**, and **peppermint oil** are believed to be direct relaxants of intestinal smooth muscle and may relieve pain in the *irritable bowel syndrome* and *diverticular disease*. They have no serious adverse effects but, like all antispasmodics, should be avoided in paralytic ileus. Peppermint oil occasionally causes heartburn.

ALVERINE CITRATE

Indications: adjunct in gastro-intestinal disorders characterised by smooth muscle spasm; dysmenorrhoea

Contra-indications: intestinal obstruction, colonic atony, faecal impaction, combination with sterculia also contra-indicated if difficulty in swallowing; pregnancy and breast-feeding

Side-effects: nausea, headache, pruritus, rash and dizziness reported

Dose: see under preparations

Spasmonal® (Norgine)

Capsules, blue/grey, alverine citrate 60 mg. Net price 20 = £2.18

Dose: 1–2 capsules 1–3 times daily; CHILD not recommended

Note. A proprietary brand of alverine citrate 60 mg (Relaxyl®) is on sale to the public for irritable bowel syndrome

Compound preparations
Alvercol® (Norgine)

Granules, beige, coated, sterculia 62%, alverine citrate 0.5%. Net price 500 g = £12.19. Label: 25, 27, counselling, see below

Dose: irritable bowel syndrome, 1–2 heaped 5-mL spoonfuls swallowed without chewing with water once or twice daily after meals; CHILD 6–12 years, half adult dose

COUNSELLING. Preparations that swell in contact with liquid should always be carefully swallowed with water and should not be taken immediately before going to bed

MEBEVERINE HYDROCHLORIDE

Indications: adjunct in gastro-intestinal disorders characterised by smooth muscle spasm

Cautions: paralytic ileus; pregnancy and breast-feeding; avoid in porphyria (see section 9.8.2.)

PoM ¹ **Colofac®** (Solvay)

Tablets, s/c, mebeverine hydrochloride 135 mg. Net price 20 = £1.67

Dose: ADULT and CHILD over 10 years, 1 tablet 3 times daily preferably 20 minutes before meals

Note. Tablets containing mebeverine hydrochloride 135 mg also available from APS, Berk (Fomac®), Cox, Evans, Generics, Hillcross, Lagap, Norton

1. Mebeverine hydrochloride can be sold to the public provided that the max. single dose is 135 mg and the max. daily dose is 405 mg; proprietary brands on sale to the public include *Boots IBS Relief®*, *Colofac® IBS*, *Equilon®*

Liquid, yellow, sugar-free, mebeverine hydrochloride 50 mg (as embonate)/5 mL. Net price 300 mL = £3.50

Dose: ADULT and CHILD over 10 years, 15 mL 3 times daily preferably 20 minutes before meals

Compound preparations
PoM **Fybogel® Mebeverine** (R&C)

Granules, buff, effervescent, ispaghula husk 3.5 g, mebeverine hydrochloride 135 mg/sachet. Contains 7 mmol K⁺/sachet (caution in renal impairment). Net price 60 sachets = £15.00. Label: 13, 22, counselling, see below

Dose: irritable bowel syndrome, ADULT, 1 sachet in water morning and night 30 minutes before food; an additional sachet may also be taken before the midday meal if necessary; CHILD not recommended

COUNSELLING. Preparations that swell in contact with liquid should always be carefully swallowed with water and should not be taken immediately before going to bed

PEPPERMINT OIL

Indications: relief of abdominal colic and distension, particularly in irritable bowel syndrome

Cautions: rarely sensitivity to menthol

Side-effects: heartburn, rarely, allergic reactions (including rash, headache, bradycardia, muscle tremor, ataxia)

LOCAL IRRITATION. Capsules should not be broken or chewed because peppermint oil may irritate mouth or oesophagus

Colpermin® (Pharmacia & Upjohn)

Capsules, m/r, e/c, light blue/dark blue, blue band, peppermint oil 0.2 mL. Net price 100-cap pack = £10.96. Label: 5, 22, 25

Ingredients: include arachis (peanut) oil

Dose: 1–2 capsules, swallowed whole with water, 3 times daily 30–60 minutes before meals for up to 2–3 months if necessary; CHILD under 15 years not recommended

Mintec® (Monmouth)

Capsules, e/c, green/ivory, peppermint oil 0.2 mL.
Net price 100-cap pack = £12.80. Label: 5, 22, 25
Dose: 1–2 capsules swallowed whole with water, 3
times daily before meals for up to 2–3 months if necessary; CHILD not recommended

MOTILITY STIMULANTS

Metoclopramide and **domperidone** (section 4.6)
are dopamine antagonists which stimulate gastric
emptying and small intestinal transit, and enhance
the strength of oesophageal sphincter contraction.
Metoclopramide is used in some patients with *non-
ulcer dyspepsia*, to speed the transit of barium during intestinal follow-through examination, and as
accessory treatment for *oesophageal reflux*; domperidone is also used in *non-ulcer dyspepsia*. Metoclopramide and domperidone are useful in non-
specific and in cytotoxic-induced nausea and vomiting. Metoclopramide and occasionally domperidone may induce an acute dystonic reaction,
particularly in young women and children—for further details of this and other side-effects, see section
4.6.

Cisapride is a motility stimulant believed to promote release of acetylcholine in the gut wall; it does
not have dopamine-antagonist properties. It is of
use in treating *oesophageal reflux* and *gastric stasis*
and in the short-term management of *non-ulcer dyspepsia*. Concomitant administration with drugs
which inhibit the metabolism of cisapride can
increase plasma concentration of cisapride leading
to disturbances of cardiac rhythm (see under Cisapride below for recommendations).

CISAPRIDE

Indications: see under dose

Cautions: halve dose initially in hepatic and renal
impairment; elderly; cardiac disorders; **interactions:** Appendix 1 (cisapride); **important:** see
also Arrhythmias, below

ARRHYTHMIAS. Concomitant administration of cisapride
with drugs that inhibit its metabolism can raise plasma-
cisapride concentrations, which may result in QT prolongation and serious ventricular arrhythmias (including
torsades de pointes).
Recommendations are: *not to exceed* recommended dose
of cisapride, *to use with caution* in conditions leading to
QT prolongation such as uncorrected electrolyte disturbances (particularly hypokalaemia and hypomagnesaemia), *to use with caution* in congenital QT
prolongation, *to use with caution* in patients taking medication known to prolong QT interval; and *to avoid* concomitant administration of cisapride with oral or
parenteral formulations of clarithromycin, erythromycin, fluconazole, itraconazole, ketoconazole, or
miconazole.

Contra-indications: where gastro-intestinal stimulation dangerous; pregnancy and breast-feeding

Side-effects: abdominal cramps and diarrhoea,
occasional headaches and lightheadedness; convulsions, extrapyramidal effects and increased
urinary frequency; liver function abnormalities
(and possibly cholestasis) also reported; **important:** ventricular arrhythmias (including torsades

de pointes) have been reported, for recommendations see Arrhythmias above

Dose: ADULT and CHILD over 12 years

Symptoms and mucosal lesions associated with
gastro-oesophageal reflux, 10 mg 3–4 times daily
or 20 mg twice daily (12-week course recommended); maintenance treatment, 20 mg at bedtime *or* 10 mg twice daily (20 mg twice daily if
initial lesions were very severe) (halve 20-mg
dose and double frequency of administration if
severe abdominal cramps)

Symptoms of impaired gastric motility secondary
to disturbed and delayed gastric emptying associated with diabetes, systemic sclerosis and autonomic neuropathy, 10 mg 3–4 times daily initially
for 6 weeks (but longer treatment may be necessary)

Symptoms of dyspepsia (peptic ulcer or other
lesions excluded), 10 mg 3 times daily (usual
course 4 weeks)

COUNSELLING. Advise patient to take 15–30 minutes
before meals and at bedtime (for night symptoms)

PoM **Prepulsid®** (Janssen-Cilag)

Tablets, scored, cisapride (as monohydrate) 10 mg,
net price 120-tab pack = £37.60. Counselling,
administration, see above

Suspension, cisapride (as monohydrate) 5 mg/
5 mL. Net price 500 mL = £15.60. Counselling,
administration, see above

1.3   Ulcer-healing drugs

1.3.1	H₂-receptor antagonists
1.3.2	Selective antimuscarinics
1.3.3	Chelates and complexes
1.3.4	Prostaglandin analogues
1.3.5	Proton pump inhibitors
1.3.6	Other ulcer-healing drugs

Peptic ulceration commonly involves the stomach,
duodenum, and lower oesophagus; after gastric surgery it involves the gastro-enterostomy stoma.

Healing can be promoted by general measures,
stopping smoking and taking antacids and by
antisecretory drug treatment, but relapse is common
when treatment ceases. Nearly all duodenal ulcers
and most gastric ulcers not associated with NSAIDs
are caused by *Helicobacter pylori*. Long-term healing of duodenal and gastric ulcers can be achieved
by eradicating *H. pylori*; it is recommended that the
presence of *H. pylori* is confirmed before starting
eradication treatment.

The management of *H. pylori* infection and of
NSAID-associated ulcers is discussed below.

HELICOBACTER PYLORI INFECTION

Acid inhibition combined with antibiotic treatment
is highly effective in the eradication of *Helicobacter pylori*. Eradication commonly results in
long-term ulcer remission; *H. pylori* reinfection is
rare.

A proton pump inhibitor *and* clarithromycin (or another macrolide antibiotic) plus *either* amoxycillin *or* metronidazole given for one week produce *H. pylori* eradication in 90% of patients; treatment failure may reflect poor compliance, metronidazole resistance or, less commonly, clarithromycin resistance. Triple therapy and two-week regimens provide high eradication rates, but adverse effects are common and compliance is a problem.

Dual therapy regimens that include a proton pump inhibitor and a single antibiotic produce poor eradication rates and are not recommended.

Antibiotic-induced colitis is a possible (but uncommon) risk.

EXAMPLES OF HELICOBACTER PYLORI-ERADICATION REGIMENS

Triple therapy (one-week regimens)

Amoxycillin 500 mg 3 times daily
plus
Metronidazole 400 mg 3 times daily
plus
Omeprazole 20 mg twice daily *or* 40 mg once daily
for 7 days
Total net price = £17.18
  Note. Substitute clarithromycin 250 mg 3 times daily where metronidazole has been used before

Clarithromycin 250 mg twice daily
plus
Metronidazole 400 mg (*or* tinidazole 500 mg) twice daily
plus
Omeprazole 20 mg twice daily *or* 40 mg once daily
for 7 days
Total net price = £26.99 (metronidazole-containing regimen), £34.36 (tinidazole-containing regimen)

Amoxycillin 1 g twice daily
plus
Clarithromycin 500 mg twice daily
plus
[1] Omeprazole 20 mg twice daily *or* 40 mg once daily
for 7 days
Total net price = £39.03
1. Omeprazole 20 mg once daily has also been used as part of a 10-day regimen

Lansoprazole 30 mg twice daily
plus two of the following:
Amoxycillin 1 g twice daily
Clarithromycin 250 mg twice daily
Metronidazole 400 mg twice daily
for 7 days
Total net price = £27.56 (regimen containing amoxycillin and clarithromycin), £16.99 (regimen containing amoxycillin and metronidazole), £26.77 (regimen containing clarithromycin and metronidazole)
  Note. These regimens are also licensed for eradication of *H. pylori* associated with gastritis

Triple therapy (two-week regimens)

Tetracycline 500 mg 4 times daily
plus
Metronidazole 400 mg 3 times daily
plus
Tripotassium dicitratobismuthate 120 mg 4 times daily
for 14 days
Total net price = £18.52
  Note. May be poorly tolerated; amoxycillin 500 mg 4 times daily has been substituted for tetracycline

Amoxycillin 750 mg 3 times daily
plus
Metronidazole 500 mg 3 times daily
plus
Ranitidine 300 mg at night (or 150 mg twice daily)
for 14 days
Total net price = £24.47

Dual therapy (two-week regimens)
Note. Dual therapy regimens consisting of *either* clarithromycin and omeprazole *or* amoxycillin and omeprazole are licensed, but produce low rates of *H. pylori* eradication and are not recommended.

Ranitidine bismuth citrate 400 mg twice daily
plus either
Amoxycillin 500 mg 4 times daily
or
Clarithromycin 250 mg 4 times daily (*or* 500 mg 3 times daily)
for 14 days
Total net price = £28.93 (amoxycillin-containing regimen), £70.96–£93.47 (clarithromycin-containing regimens)
  Note. This regimen is also licensed for gastric ulcer disease; lower eradication rates than with triple therapy regimens

A total of 4–8 weeks of antisecretory treatment (with a H_2-receptor antagonist or omeprazole) may be considered for ulcer healing

NSAID-ASSOCIATED ULCERS

Gastro-intestinal bleeding and ulceration may occur with NSAID use (section 10.1.1).

Omeprazole or misoprostol may be used to prevent NSAID-associated peptic ulcers; colic and diarrhoea may limit the dose of misoprostol. H_2-receptor antagonists may be effective in preventing NSAID-associated duodenal ulcers.

In patients who need to continue NSAID treatment, NSAID-associated ulcers may be treated with H_2-receptor antagonists, proton pump inhibitors or misoprostol; omeprazole may produce more rapid healing since the rate of healing probably correlates with the intensity of acid suppression.

1.3.1 H₂-receptor antagonists

All H₂-receptor antagonists heal *gastric and duodenal ulcers* by reducing gastric acid output as a result of H₂-receptor blockade; like cimetidine and ranitidine, the newer ones (famotidine and nizatidine) can also be expected to relieve *peptic oesophagitis*. High doses of H₂-receptor antagonists have been used in the *Zollinger–Ellison syndrome*, but omeprazole may now be preferred.

Maintenance treatment with low doses reduces the rate of *ulcer relapse*, but does not modify the natural course of the disease when treatment has ceased and *H. pylori* eradication should be considered instead. Maintenance treatment is best suited to those with frequent severe recurrences and to the elderly who suffer ulcer complications.

Treatment of *undiagnosed dyspepsia* with H₂-receptor antagonists may be acceptable in younger patients but is undesirable in older people because the diagnosis of gastric cancer may be delayed.

Therapy can promote healing of *NSAID-associated ulcers* (section 1.3).

Treatment has not been shown to be beneficial in *haematemesis* and *melaena*, but prophylactic use reduces the frequency of bleeding from gastroduodenal erosions in *hepatic coma*, and possibly in other conditions requiring *intensive care*. Treatment also reduces the frequency of *acid aspiration* in obstetric patients at delivery (Mendelson's syndrome).

SIDE-EFFECTS. H₂-receptor antagonists are well tolerated and side-effects are uncommon with few significant differences between available drugs. Dizziness, somnolence or fatigue, and rash have occasionally been reported with all of them, and there are rare reports of headache, liver dysfunction, and blood disorders. Other rare reports include bradycardia or AV block, confusion, interstitial nephritis (cimetidine), and urticaria and angio-edema. Cimetidine is also associated with occasional gynaecomastia and rare reports of impotence and myalgia. Causal relationships of other reports, such as pancreatitis, are unclear.

INTERACTIONS. Cimetidine retards oxidative hepatic drug metabolism by binding to microsomal cytochrome P450. It should be avoided in patients stabilised on warfarin, phenytoin, and theophylline (or aminophylline), but other interactions (see **Appendix 1**) may be of less clinical relevance. Famotidine, nizatidine, and ranitidine do not share the drug metabolism inhibitory properties of cimetidine.

CIMETIDINE

Indications: benign gastric and duodenal ulceration, stomal ulcer, reflux oesophagitis, Zollinger-Ellison syndrome, other conditions where gastric acid reduction is beneficial (see notes above and section 1.9.4)

Cautions: see notes above; renal and hepatic impairment (reduce doses, see Appendixes 2 and 3); pregnancy and breast-feeding; preferably avoid intravenous injection (infusion is preferable) particularly in high dosage (may rarely cause arrhythmias) and in cardiovascular impairment; **interactions:** Appendix 1 (histamine H₂-antagonists) and notes above

Side-effects: altered bowel habit, dizziness, rash, tiredness; reversible confusional states, reversible liver damage, headache; rarely, blood disorders (including thrombocytopenia, agranulocytosis, and aplastic anaemia), muscle or joint pain, hypersensitivity, bradycardia and AV block; interstitial nephritis and acute pancreatitis reported; gynaecomastia is also an occasional problem with cimetidine (but usually only in high dosage), and reversible impotence has also been reported (see also notes above)

Dose: by mouth, 400 mg twice daily (with breakfast and at night) *or* 800 mg at night (benign gastric and duodenal ulceration) for at least 4 weeks (6 weeks in gastric ulceration, 8 weeks in ulcer associated with continued NSAID); when necessary the dose may be increased to 400 mg 4 times daily or rarely (e.g. as in stress ulceration) to a max. of 2.4 g daily in divided doses; INFANT under 1 year, 20 mg/kg daily in divided doses has been used; CHILD over 1 year, 25–30 mg/kg daily in divided doses

Maintenance, 400 mg at night *or* 400 mg morning and night

Reflux oesophagitis, 400 mg 4 times daily for 4–8 weeks

Zollinger–Ellison syndrome (but see notes above), 400 mg 4 times daily or occasionally more

Gastric acid reduction (prophylaxis of acid aspiration; do not use syrup), obstetrics 400 mg at start of labour, then up to 400 mg every 4 hours if required (max. of 2.4 g daily); surgical procedures 400 mg 90–120 minutes before induction of general anaesthesia

Short-bowel syndrome, 400 mg twice daily (with breakfast and at bedtime) adjusted according to response

To reduce degradation of pancreatic enzyme supplements, 0.8–1.6 g daily in 4 divided doses according to response 1–1½ hours before meals

By intramuscular injection, 200 mg every 4–6 hours; max. 2.4 g daily

By slow intravenous injection, 200 mg given over at least 2 minutes; may be repeated every 4–6 hours; if a larger dose is needed or there is cardiovascular impairment, the dose should be diluted and given over at least 10 minutes (infusion is preferable); max. 2.4 g daily

By intravenous infusion, 400 mg in 100 mL of sodium chloride 0.9% intravenous infusion infused over ½–1 hour (may be repeated every 4–6 hours) *or* by continuous infusion at an average rate of 50–100 mg/hour over 24 hours, max. 2.4 g daily; INFANT under 1 year, *by intramuscular injection or slow intravenous injection or infusion*, 20 mg/kg daily in divided doses has been used; CHILD over 1 year, 25–30 mg/kg daily in divided doses

---

PoM ¹ **Cimetidine** (Non-proprietary)

Tablets, cimetidine 200 mg, net price 120-tab pack = £10.27; 400 mg, 60-tab pack = £7.50; 800 mg, 30-tab pack = £7.81

Available from APS, Ashbourne (Peptimax®), Berk (Ultec®), BHR (Phimetin®), Bioglan, Cox, CP, Dexcel Pharma, Eastern (Zita®), Ethical Generics Ltd, Galen (Galenamet®), Lagap, Norton, Opus (Acitak®)

1. Cimetidine can be sold to the public for adults and children over 16 years (provided packs do not contain more than 2 weeks' supply) for the short-term symptomatic relief of heartburn, dyspepsia, and hyperacidity (max. single dose 200 mg, max. daily dose 800 mg), and for the prophylactic management of nocturnal heartburn (single night-time dose 100 mg); a proprietary brand (Tagamet 100® containing cimetidine 100 mg) is on sale to the public

PoM **Dyspamet®** (SK&F)

Chewtab® (chewable tablets), sugar-free, cimetidine 200 mg. Net price 120-tab pack – £18.40. Counselling, chew thoroughly

Note. Each chewable tablet contains aspartame 3 mg (see section 9.4.1)

Suspension, sugar-free, cimetidine 200 mg/5 mL. Contains sorbitol 2.79 g/5 mL. Net price 600 mL = £24.08

PoM **Tagamet®** (SK&F)

Tablets, all green, f/c, cimetidine 200 mg, net price 120-tab pack = £19.58; 400 mg, 60-tab pack = £22.62; 800 mg, 30-tab pack = £22.62

Effervescent tablets, sugar-free, cimetidine 400 mg. Contains 17.6 mmol Na⁺/tablet. Net price 60-tab pack = £20.56. Label: 13

Note. Each effervescent tablet contains aspartame 70 mg (see section 9.4.1)

Syrup, orange, cimetidine 200 mg/5 mL. Net price 600 mL = £28.49

Injection, cimetidine 100 mg/mL. Net price 2-mL amp = 36p

Cimetidine with alginate

PoM **Algitec®** (SK&F)

Chewtab® (chewable tablets), off-white, cimetidine 200 mg, alginic acid 500 mg. Contains 2.05 mmol Na⁺/tablet. Net price 120-tab pack = £22.50. Counselling, chew thoroughly

Note. Each chewable tablet contains aspartame 5 mg (see section 9.4.1)

Suspension, sugar-free, cimetidine 100 mg, sodium alginate 250 mg/5 mL. Contains 1.43 mmol Na⁺/5 mL. Net price 600 mL = £15.41

Dose: gastro-oesophageal reflux disease, 1 tablet chewed or 10 mL suspension 4 times daily (after meals and at bedtime), increased if necessary to 2 tablets or 20 mL suspension 4 times daily; to be taken for 4–8 weeks

FAMOTIDINE

Indications: see under Dose

Cautions: see under Cimetidine; does not inhibit hepatic microsomal drug metabolism

Side-effects: see under Cimetidine and notes above

Dose: benign gastric and duodenal ulceration, treatment, 40 mg at night for 4–8 weeks; maintenance (duodenal), 20 mg at night; CHILD not recommended

Reflux oesophagitis, 20–40 mg twice daily for 6–12 weeks; maintenance, 20 mg twice daily

Zollinger–Ellison syndrome (but see notes above), 20 mg every 6 hours (higher dose in those who have previously been receiving another H₂-antagonist); doses up to 800 mg daily in divided doses have been used

PoM ¹ **Pepcid®** (Morson)

Tablets, f/c, famotidine 20 mg (beige), net price 28-tab pack = £14.00; 40 mg (brown), 28-tab pack = £26.60

1. Famotidine can be sold to the public for adults and children over 16 years (provided packs do not contain more than 2 weeks' supply) for the short-term symptomatic relief of heartburn, dyspepsia, and hyperacidity (max. single dose 10 mg, max. daily dose 20 mg); proprietary brands (*Boots Excess Acid Control®*, *Pepcid® AC*, *Pepcid® AC Chewable* all containing famotidine 10 mg) are on sale to the public

NIZATIDINE

Indications: see under Dose

Cautions: see under Cimetidine; does not inhibit hepatic microsomal drug metabolism

Side-effects: see under Cimetidine and notes above; sweating also reported; rare reports of gynaecomastia

Dose: by mouth, benign gastric, duodenal or NSAID-associated ulceration, treatment, 300 mg in the evening *or* 150 mg twice daily for 4–8 weeks; maintenance, 150 mg at night; CHILD not recommended

Gastro-oesophageal reflux disease, 150–300 mg twice daily for up to 12 weeks

By intravenous infusion, for short-term use in peptic ulcer hospital inpatients as alternative to oral route, *by intermittent intravenous infusion* over 15 minutes, 100 mg 3 times daily, *or by continuous intravenous infusion*, 10 mg/hour; max. 480 mg daily; CHILD not recommended

PoM **Axid®** (Lilly)

Capsules, nizatidine 150 mg (pale yellow/dark yellow), net price 30-cap pack = £11.34; 300 mg (pale yellow/brown), 30-cap pack = £21.74

Note. Capsules containing nizatidine 150 mg and 300 mg also available from Ashbourne (Zinga®)

Injection, nizatidine 25 mg/mL. For dilution and use as an intravenous infusion. Net price 4-mL amp = £1.20

RANITIDINE

Indications: see under Dose, other conditions where reduction of gastric acidity is beneficial (see notes above and section 1.9.4)

Cautions: see under Cimetidine; does not significantly inhibit hepatic microsomal drug metabolism; avoid in porphyria (section 9.8.2)

Side-effects: see under Cimetidine and notes above; rare reports of breast swelling and tenderness in men; erythema multiforme reported

Dose: by mouth, 150 mg twice daily (morning and night) *or* 300 mg at night (benign gastric and duodenal ulceration) for 4 to 8 weeks, up to 6 weeks in chronic episodic dyspepsia, and up to 8 weeks in NSAID-associated ulceration; in duodenal ulcer 300 mg can be given twice daily for 4 weeks to achieve a higher healing rate; CHILD (peptic ulcer) 2–4 mg/kg twice daily, max. 300 mg daily Maintenance, 150 mg at night

Duodenal ulcer associated with *H. pylori*, see eradication regimens on p. 35; ranitidine treatment should be continued for a further 2 weeks

Prophylaxis of NSAID-induced duodenal ulcer, 150 mg twice daily

Reflux oesophagitis, 150 mg twice daily *or* 300 mg at night for up to 8 weeks, or if necessary 12 weeks (moderate to severe, 150 mg 4 times daily for up to 12 weeks); long-term treatment of healed oesophagitis, 150 mg twice daily

Zollinger–Ellison syndrome (but see notes above), 150 mg 3 times daily; doses up to 6 g daily in divided doses have been used

Gastric acid reduction (prophylaxis of acid aspiration) in obstetrics, *by mouth*, 150 mg at onset of labour, then every 6 hours; surgical procedures, *by intramuscular or slow intravenous injection*, 50 mg 45–60 minutes before induction of anaesthesia (intravenous injection diluted to 20 mL and given over at least 2 minutes), or *by mouth*, 150 mg 2 hours before induction of anaesthesia, and also, when possible on the preceding evening

By intramuscular injection, 50 mg every 6–8 hours

By slow intravenous injection, 50 mg diluted to 20 mL and given over at least 2 minutes; may be repeated every 6–8 hours

By intravenous infusion, 25 mg/hour for 2 hours; may be repeated every 6–8 hours

Prophylaxis of stress ulceration, initial slow intravenous injection of 50 mg (as above) then *continuous infusion*, 125–250 micrograms/kg per hour (may be followed by 150 mg twice daily *by mouth* when oral feeding commences)

PoM [1]**Ranitidine** (Non-proprietary)

Tablets, ranitidine (as hydrochloride) 150 mg, net price 60-tab pack = £26.89; 300 mg, 30-tab pack = £26.45

Available from Cox, CP, Ethical Generics Ltd, Galen, Generics, Genus, Hillcross, Norton, Ranbaxy

1. Ranitidine can be sold to the public for adults and children over 16 years (provided packs do not contain more than 2 weeks' supply) for the short-term symptomatic relief of heartburn, dyspepsia, and hyperacidity (max. single dose 75 mg, max. daily dose 300 mg); a proprietary brand (Zantac® 75 containing ranitidine (as hydrochloride) 75 mg) is on sale to the public

PoM **Zantac**® (GlaxoWellcome)

Tablets, f/c, ranitidine (as hydrochloride) 150 mg, net price 60-tab pack = £27.89; 300 mg, 30-tab pack = £27.43

Effervescent tablets, pale yellow, ranitidine (as hydrochloride) 150 mg (contains 14.3 mmol Na+/tablet), net price 60-tab pack = £27.88; 300 mg (contains 20.8 mmol Na+/tablet), 30-tab pack = £27.42. Label: 13

Note. The effervescent tablets contain aspartame (see section 9.4.1)

Syrup, sugar-free, ranitidine (as hydrochloride) 75 mg/5 mL. Net price 300 mL = £22.32

Injection, ranitidine 25 mg (as hydrochloride)/mL. Net price 2-mL amp = 64p

RANITIDINE BISMUTH CITRATE

(Ranitidine Bismutrex)

Indications: see under Dose

Cautions: see under Cimetidine; does not significantly inhibit hepatic microsomal drug metabolism; **interactions:** Appendix 1 (histamine H₂-antagonists)

Contra-indications: severe renal impairment; porphyria (section 9.8.2)

Side-effects: see under Ranitidine and notes above; rare reports of breast tenderness and swelling in men; see also under Tripotassium Dicitratobismuthate

Dose: 400 mg twice daily for 8 weeks in benign gastric ulceration or 4–8 weeks in duodenal ulceration; CHILD not recommended

Duodenal ulceration associated with *H. pylori*, see eradication regimens on p. 35; ranitidine bismuth citrate treatment should be continued for a further 2 weeks; long-term (maintenance) treatment not recommended (max. total of 16 weeks treatment in any 1 year); CHILD not recommended

COUNSELLING. May darken tongue and blacken faeces

▼ PoM **Pylorid**® (GlaxoWellcome)

Tablets, blue, f/c, ranitidine bismuth citrate 400 mg. Net price 28-tab pack = £26.00; 56-tab pack = £52.00. Counselling (discoloration tongue and faeces)

1.3.2   Selective antimuscarinics

Pirenzepine is a selective antimuscarinic drug which was used for the treatment of gastric and duodenal ulcers. It has now been discontinued.

1.3.3   Chelates and complexes

Tripotassium dicitratobismuthate is a bismuth chelate effective in healing gastric and duodenal ulcers, but not on its own in maintaining remission. It may be given in combination with two antibiotics (typically metronidazole and amoxycillin) to eradicate *Helicobacter pylori*, but other regimens are preferable (section 1.3).

The bismuth content is low but absorption has been reported; encephalopathy (described with older high-dose bismuth preparations) has not been reported. Tablets are as effective as the liquid and more palatable.

Ranitidine bismuth citrate (section 1.3.1) is used in the management of peptic ulcer, and in combination with an antibiotic for the eradication of *H. pylori* (section 1.3).

Sucralfate may act by protecting the mucosa from acid-pepsin attack in gastric and duodenal ulcers. It is a complex of aluminium hydroxide and sulphated sucrose but has minimal antacid properties.

TRIPOTASSIUM DICITRATOBISMUTHATE
(Bismuth Chelate)

Indications: benign gastric and duodenal ulceration; see also *Helicobacter pylori* eradication regimens on p. 35

Cautions: see notes above; **interactions:** Appendix 1 (tripotassium dicitratobismuthate)

Contra-indications: renal impairment, pregnancy

Side-effects: may darken tongue and blacken faeces; nausea and vomiting reported

De-Nol® (Yamanouchi)

Liquid, red, tripotassium dicitratobismuthate 120 mg/5 mL. Net price 560 mL = £20.51. Counselling, see below

Dose: 10 mL twice daily *or* 5 mL 4 times daily; taken for 28 days, followed by further 28 days if necessary; maintenance not indicated but course may be repeated after interval of 1 month; CHILD, not recommended

COUNSELLING. Each dose to be diluted with 15 mL of water; twice daily dosage to be taken 30 minutes before breakfast and main evening meal; four times daily dosage to be taken as follows: one dose 30 minutes before breakfast, midday meal and main evening meal, and one dose 2 hours after main evening meal; milk should not be drunk by itself during treatment but small quantities may be taken in tea or coffee or on cereal; antacids should not be taken half an hour before or after a dose; may darken tongue and blacken faeces

De-Noltab® (Yamanouchi)

Tablets, f/c, tripotassium dicitratobismuthate 120 mg. Net price 112-tab pack = £29.40. Counselling, see below

Dose: 2 tablets twice daily *or* 1 tablet 4 times daily; taken for 28 days followed by further 28 days if necessary; maintenance not indicated but course may be repeated after interval of 1 month; CHILD, not recommended

COUNSELLING. Each dose to be swallowed with half a tumblerful of water then as above under De-Nol®

SUCRALFATE

Indications: see under dose

Cautions: renal impairment (avoid if severe, see Appendix 3); pregnancy and breast-feeding; **interactions:** Appendix 1 (sucralfate)

Side-effects: constipation; diarrhoea, nausea, indigestion, gastric discomfort, dry mouth, rash, pruritus, back pain, dizziness, headache, vertigo and drowsiness

Dose: 2 g twice daily (on rising and at bedtime) *or* 1 g 4 times daily 1 hour before meals and at bedtime, taken for 4–6 weeks or in resistant cases 12 weeks; max. 8 g daily; CHILD not recommended

Prophylaxis of stress ulceration (suspension), 1 g 6 times daily (max. 8 g daily)

COUNSELLING. Tablets may be dispersed in 10–15 mL of water; antacids should not be taken half an hour before or after a dose

PoM **Antepsin®** (Wyeth)

Tablets, scored, sucralfate 1 g. Net price 112-tab pack = £9.80. Label: 5, counselling, see dose above

Suspension, sucralfate, 1 g/5 mL. Net price 560 mL = £9.80. Label: 5, counselling, antacids

1.3.4   Prostaglandin analogues

Misoprostol, a synthetic prostaglandin analogue has antisecretory and protective properties, promoting *gastric and duodenal ulcer* healing. It can prevent NSAID-associated ulcers, its use being most appropriate for the frail or very elderly from whom NSAIDs cannot be withdrawn.

MISOPROSTOL

Indications: see notes above and under Dose

Cautions: conditions where hypotension might precipitate severe complications (e.g. cerebrovascular disease, cardiovascular disease); **interactions:** Appendix 1 (misoprostol)

Contra-indications: pregnancy or planning pregnancy (increases uterine tone)—**important:** women of childbearing age, see also below, and breast-feeding

WOMEN OF CHILDBEARING AGE. Manufacturer advises that misoprostol should not be used in women of childbearing age unless the patient requires non-steroidal anti-inflammatory (NSAID) therapy and is at high risk of complications from NSAID-induced ulceration. In such patients it is advised that misoprostol should only be used if the patient takes *effective contraceptive measures* and has been advised of the *risks of taking misoprostol if pregnant*.

Side-effects: diarrhoea (may occasionally be severe and require withdrawal, reduced by giving single doses not exceeding 200 micrograms and by avoiding magnesium-containing antacids); also reported: abdominal pain, dyspepsia, flatulence, nausea and vomiting, abnormal vaginal bleeding (including intermenstrual bleeding, menorrhagia, and postmenopausal bleeding), rashes, dizziness

Dose: benign gastric and duodenal ulceration and NSAID-associated ulceration, 800 micrograms daily (in 2–4 divided doses) with breakfast (or main meals) and at bedtime; treatment should be continued for at least 4 weeks and may be continued for up to 8 weeks if required

Prophylaxis of NSAID-induced gastric and duodenal ulcer, 200 micrograms 2–4 times daily taken with the NSAID

CHILD not recommended

PoM **Cytotec**® (Searle)

Tablets, scored, misoprostol 200 micrograms, net price 60-tab pack = £11.14. Label: 21

With diclofenac or naproxen
See section 10.1.1

1.3.5   Proton pump inhibitors

The proton pump inhibitors **omeprazole**, **lansoprazole** and **pantoprazole** inhibit gastric acid by blocking the hydrogen-potassium adenosine triphosphatase enzyme system (the 'proton pump') of the gastric parietal cell. They are the treatment of choice for *stricturing and erosive oesophagitis*, lesser degrees usually responding to life-style change, H_2-receptor antagonists, antacids, or motility stimulants. Proton pump inhibitors are effective short-term treatments for *gastric and duodenal ulcer*; they are also used in combination with antibiotics for the eradication of *H. pylori* (see p. 35 for specific regimens); omeprazole is effective in the treatment of the *Zollinger-Ellison syndrome* (including cases resistant to other treatment).

CAUTIONS. Proton pump inhibitors should be used with caution in patients with liver disease (see Appendix 2), in pregnancy and breast-feeding; before treatment the presence of gastric malignancy should be excluded.

SIDE-EFFECTS. Side-effects of the proton pump inhibitors include headache, diarrhoea, rashes, pruritus, and dizziness.

Side-effects reported for omeprazole and lansoprazole include urticaria, nausea and vomiting, constipation, flatulence, abdominal pain, malaise, paraesthesia, muscle and joint pain, blurred vision, peripheral oedema, haematological changes (including eosinophilia, thrombocytopenia, leucopenia), liver enzyme changes and liver dysfunction also reported, depression and dry mouth.

OMEPRAZOLE

Indications: see under Dose
Cautions: see notes above; **interactions:** Appendix 1 (proton pump inhibitors)
Side-effects: see notes above; also reported, bullous eruption, erythema multiforme, angioedema, fever, bronchospasm, photosensitivity, interstitial nephritis, alopecia, somnolence, insomnia, increased sweating, gynaecomastia, rarely impotence, taste disturbance, stomatitis, gastro-intestinal candidiasis, encephalopathy in pre-existing severe liver disease; reversible mental confusion, agitation, and hallucinations in the severely ill
Dose: benign gastric and duodenal ulcers, 20 mg once daily for 4 weeks in duodenal ulceration or 8 weeks in gastric ulceration; in severe or recurrent cases increase to 40 mg daily; maintenance for recurrent duodenal ulcer, 20 mg once daily; prevention of relapse in duodenal ulcer, 10 mg daily increasing to 20 mg once daily if symptoms return

NSAID-associated peptic ulcer and gastroduodenal erosions, 20 mg once daily for 4 weeks, followed by a further 4 weeks if not fully healed; prophylaxis in patients with a history of NSAID-associated gastroduodenal lesions who require continued NSAID treatment, 20 mg once daily

Duodenal ulcer associated with *H. pylori*, see eradication regimens on p. 35 (amoxicillin with omeprazole regimen also licensed for benign gastric ulcer disease)

Zollinger-Ellison syndrome, initially 60 mg once daily; usual range 20–120 mg daily (above 80 mg in 2 divided doses)

Gastric acid reduction during general anaesthesia (prophylaxis of acid aspiration), 40 mg on the preceding evening then 40 mg 2–6 hours before surgery

Gastro-oesophageal reflux disease, 20 mg once daily for 4 weeks, followed by a further 4–8 weeks if not fully healed; 40 mg once daily has been given for 8 weeks in gastro-oesophageal reflux disease refractory to other treatment; may be continued at 20 mg once daily

Acid reflux disease (long-term management), 10 mg daily increasing to 20 mg once daily if symptoms return

Acid-related dyspepsia, 10–20 mg once daily for 2–4 weeks according to response

CHILD not recommended

COUNSELLING. Swallow whole or open capsule and mix contents with fruit juice or yoghurt

PoM **Losec**® (Astra)

Capsules, enclosing e/c granules, omeprazole 10 mg (pink), net price 28-cap pack = £19.95 (also 7-cap pack, hosp. only); 20 mg (pink/brown), 28-cap pack = £30.13 (also 7-cap pack, hosp. only); 40 mg (brown), 7-cap pack = £15.06. Counselling, administration

Note. Should be dispensed in original container (bottles contain a desiccant)

LANSOPRAZOLE

Indications: see under Dose
Cautions: see notes above; **interactions:** Appendix 1 (proton pump inhibitors)
Side-effects: see notes above; also reported, bruising, purpura and petechiae
Dose: benign gastric ulcer, 30 mg daily in the morning for 8 weeks
Duodenal ulcer, 30 mg daily in the morning for 4 weeks; maintenance 15 mg daily
Duodenal ulcer or gastritis associated with *H. pylori*, see eradication regimens on p. 35.
Gastro-oesophageal reflux disease, 30 mg daily in the morning for 4 weeks, followed by a further 4 weeks if not fully healed; maintenance 15–30 mg daily
Acid-related dyspepsia, 15–30 mg daily in the morning for 2–4 weeks
CHILD not recommended

PoM **Zoton**® (Lederle)
Capsules, enclosing e/c granules, lansoprazole
15 mg (yellow), net price 28-cap pack = £18.95,
56-cap pack = £37.90; 30 mg (lilac/purple), 14-
cap pack = £14.85, 28-cap pack = £29.69, 56-cap
pack = £59.38 (also 7-cap pack, hosp. only).
Label: 5, 23, 25

PANTOPRAZOLE
Indications: see under Dose
Cautions: see notes above
Side-effects: see notes above
Dose: benign gastric ulcer or gastro-oesophageal
reflux disease, 40 mg daily in the morning for 4
weeks, followed by further 4 weeks if not fully
healed
Duodenal ulcer, 40 mg daily in the morning for 2
weeks, followed by further 2 weeks if not fully
healed
In hepatic impairment, treatment given on alternate days

▼ PoM **Protium**® (Knoll)
Tablets, e/c, pantoprazole (as sodium sesquihy-
drate) 40 mg. Net price 28-tab pack = £29.76.
Label: 25

1.3.6 Other ulcer-healing drugs
Carbenoxolone is a synthetic derivative of glycyrrhizinic
acid (a constituent of liquorice).
The only oral preparation of carbenoxolone remaining
on the UK market is in the form of a combination with
antacids for *oesophageal ulceration and inflammation.*
Side-effects of carbenoxolone (commonly sodium and
water retention and occasionally hypokalaemia) may cause
or exacerbate hypertension, oedema, cardiac failure, and
muscle weakness. For these reasons other drugs are preferred; if used, regular monitoring of weight, blood pressure, and electrolytes is advisable during treatment.
Carbenoxolone may act by protecting the mucosal barrier
from acid–pepsin attack and increasing mucosal mucin
production.

CARBENOXOLONE SODIUM
Indications: benign gastric ulceration in young and middle-aged adults (see also under preparation)
Cautions: cardiac disease, hypertension, hepatic and
renal disease (see contra-indications); elderly (see under
preparation); not recommended in children. See also
notes above; **interactions:** Appendix 1 (carbenoxolone)
Contra-indications: hypokalaemia, cardiac failure and in
those receiving cardiac glycosides (unless electrolyte
levels monitored weekly and measures taken to avoid
hypokalaemia); hepatic and renal impairment (see
Appendixes 2 and 3); pregnancy
Side-effects: sodium and water retention (provoking
hypertension and cardiac failure), hypokalaemia (leading to impaired neuromuscular function and muscle
damage and to renal damage if prolonged)

Compound preparation
PoM **Pyrogastrone**® (Sanofi Winthrop)
Tablets, chewable, carbenoxolone sodium 20 mg, alginic
acid 600 mg, dried aluminium hydroxide 240 mg,
magnesium trisilicate 60 mg, sodium bicarbonate
210 mg (Na⁺ 3 mmol/tablet). Net price 100-tab pack =
£24.85. Label: 21, 24

Liquid, carbenoxolone sodium 10 mg, dried aluminium
hydroxide 150 mg (Na⁺ 0.85 mmol, K⁺ 1.5 mmol)/5 mL
when reconstituted with water. Net price 500 mL =
£12.39. Label: 21
Dose: for oesophageal inflammation and ulceration, 1
tablet, chewed, 3 times daily after meals, and 2 at night,
for 6–12 weeks or 10 mL liquid 3 times daily after meals
and 20 mL at night, for 6–12 weeks; not recommended
for children or for adults over 75 years

1.4 Antidiarrhoeal drugs
1.4.1   Adsorbents and bulk-forming drugs
1.4.2   Antimotility drugs

The **first line** of treatment in acute diarrhoea, as in
gastro-enteritis, is prevention or treatment of fluid
and electrolyte depletion. This is particularly
important in infants and in frail and elderly patients.
For details of **oral rehydration preparations**, see
section 9.2.1.2. Severe dehydration requires immediate admission to hospital and urgent replacement
of fluid and electrolytes.

Antispasmodics (section 1.2) are occasionally of
value in treating abdominal cramp associated with
diarrhoea but they should **not** be used for primary
treatment. Antispasmodics and antiemetics should
be **avoided** in young children with gastro-enteritis
since they are rarely effective and have troublesome
side-effects.

Antibacterial drugs are generally unnecessary in
simple gastro-enteritis, even when a bacterial cause
is suspected, because the complaint will usually
resolve quickly without such treatment, and infective diarrhoeas in the UK are often caused by viral
infections. Systemic bacterial infection does, however, need appropriate systemic treatment.
Erythromycin (see section 5.1.5) or **ciprofloxacin**
(see section 5.1.12) can be used for treating
Campylobacter enteritis. For drugs for shigellosis
and salmonellosis, see section 5.1, table 1. Ciprofloxacin is occasionally used for prophylaxis
against travellers' diarrhoea, but this is not recommended. Poorly absorbed drugs such as dihydros-
treptomycin, neomycin, and sulphaguanidine
should be **avoided** altogether in gastro-intestinal
infection. They prolong rather than shorten the time
taken to control diarrhoea by causing masked bacterial diarrhoea, carrier states, or antibiotic-associated colitis (pseudomembranous colitis). Clioquinol
should also be **avoided** as it is neurotoxic; both it
and lactobacillus preparations are valueless.

Cholestyramine and **aluminium hydroxide
mixture** (section 1.1.1), bind unabsorbed bile salts
and provide symptomatic relief of diarrhoea following
ileal disease or resection, in bacterial colonisation of
the small bowel, and in post-vagotomy diarrhoea.

1.4.1 Adsorbents and bulk-forming drugs
Adsorbents such as kaolin are **not** recommended
for *acute diarrhoeas.* Bulk-forming drugs, such as
ispaghula, methylcellulose, and sterculia (see section 1.6.1) are useful in controlling faecal consistency in ileostomy and colostomy, and in controlling
diarrhoea associated with diverticular disease.

KAOLIN, LIGHT

Indications: diarrhoea but see notes above
Cautions: **interactions:** Appendix 1 (antacids and adsorbents)

Kaolin Mixture, BP
(Kaolin Oral Suspension)
Oral suspension, light kaolin or light kaolin (natural) 20%, light magnesium carbonate 5%, sodium bicarbonate 5% in a suitable vehicle with a peppermint flavour.
Dose: 10–20 mL every 4 hours
Note. Kaolin-containing preparations on sale to the public include NHS *Kaopectate*® and *KLN*®

1.4.2   Antimotility drugs

In *acute diarrhoeas* antimotility drugs have a very limited role as adjuncts to fluid and electrolyte replacement (see section 9.2.1.2); they are **not** recommended for acute diarrhoeas in young children.

For comments on their role in *chronic diarrhoeas* see section 1.5.

CODEINE PHOSPHATE

Indications: see notes above
Cautions; Contra-indications; Side-effects: see section 4.7.2; not for use in conditions where inhibition of peristalsis should be avoided, where abdominal distension develops, or in acute diarrhoeal conditions such as acute ulcerative colitis or antibiotic-associated colitis; not recommended for children; tolerance and dependence may occur with prolonged use; **interactions:** Appendix 1 (opioid analgesics)
Dose: see under Preparations

PoM **Codeine Phosphate** (Non-proprietary)
Tablets, codeine phosphate 15 mg, net price 20 = 35p; 30 mg, 20 = 39p; 60 mg, 20 = 97p. Label: 2
Dose: 30 mg 3–4 times daily (range 15–60 mg); CHILD not recommended
Note. Travellers needing to take codeine phosphate tablets abroad may require a doctor's letter explaining why they are necessary.

PoM **Diarrest**® (Galen)
Liquid, yellow, codeine phosphate 5 mg, dicyclomine hydrochloride 2.5 mg, potassium chloride 40 mg, sodium chloride 50 mg, sodium citrate 50 mg/5 mL. For diarrhoea, vomiting, and cramp. Net price 200 mL = £3.34
Dose: 20 mL 4 times daily with water; CHILD 4–5 years 5 mL, 6–9 years 10 mL, 10–13 years 15 mL but see cautions and notes above

NHS **Kaodene**® (Knoll)
Suspension, codeine phosphate 5 mg, light kaolin 1.5 g/5 mL. Net price 250 mL = £1.06
Dose: 20 mL 3–4 times daily; CHILD under 5 years not recommended, over 5 years 10 mL but see cautions and notes above

CO-PHENOTROPE

A mixture of diphenoxylate hydrochloride and atropine sulphate in the mass proportions 100 parts to 1 part respectively
Indications: adjunct to rehydration in acute diarrhoea (but see notes above); chronic mild ulcerative colitis

Cautions; Contra-indications; Side-effects: see under Codeine Phosphate; young children are particularly susceptible to **overdosage** and symptoms may be delayed and observation is needed for at least 48 hours after ingestion; presence of subclinical doses of atropine may give rise to atropine side-effects in susceptible individuals or in overdosage; **interactions:** Appendix 1 (opioid analgesics)

PoM **Lomotil**® (Searle)
Tablets, co-phenotrope 2.5/0.025 (diphenoxylate hydrochloride 2.5 mg, atropine sulphate 25 micrograms). Net price 20 = £1.57
Dose: initially 4 tablets, followed by 2 tablets every 6 hours until diarrhoea controlled; CHILD under 4 years not recommended, 4–8 years 1 tablet 3 times daily, 9–13 years 1 tablet 4 times daily, 13–16 years 2 tablets 3 times daily, but see also notes above
Note. Co-phenotrope 2.5/0.025 tablets are also available from Mepra-pharm (*Diarphen*®) and Norgine (*Tropergen*®)

LOPERAMIDE HYDROCHLORIDE

Indications: adjunct to rehydration in acute diarrhoea in adults and children over 4 years (but see notes above); chronic diarrhoea in adults only
Cautions: see under Codeine Phosphate (except dependence)
Contra-indications: see under Codeine Phosphate
Side-effects: abdominal cramps and skin reactions, including urticaria reported; paralytic ileus and abdominal bloating also reported
Dose: acute diarrhoea, 4 mg initially followed by 2 mg after each loose stool for up to 5 days; usual dose 6–8 mg daily; max. 16 mg daily; CHILD under 4 years not recommended, 4–8 years 1 mg 3–4 times daily for up to *3 days only,* 9–12 years 2 mg 4 times daily for up to 5 days
Chronic diarrhoea in adults, initially, 4–8 mg daily in divided doses, subsequently adjusted according to response and given in 2 divided doses for maintenance; max. 16 mg daily

PoM ¹ **Loperamide** (Non-proprietary)
Capsules, loperamide hydrochloride 2 mg. Net price 30 = £1.55
Available from Berk (*Diocaps*®), Cox, Generics, Hillcross, Norgine (*LoperaGen*®), Norton, Tillomed (*Norimode*®), Unichem
1. Loperamide can be sold to the public, for adults and children over 12 years, provided it is licensed and labelled for the treatment of acute diarrhoea; proprietary brands include NHS *Arret*® capsules, *Boots Diareze*® capsules, *Diasorb*® capsules, NHS *Diocalm Ultra*® capsules and NHS *Imodium*® (8- and 12-cap packs), *Imodium*® liquid and *Normaloe*® tablets are on sale to the public

PoM **Imodium**® (Janssen-Cilag)
Capsules, green/grey, loperamide hydrochloride 2 mg. Net price 30 = £2.21
Syrup, red, sugar-free, loperamide hydrochloride 1 mg/5 mL. Net price 100 mL = £1.90

MORPHINE

Indications: see notes above

Cautions; Contra-indications; Side-effects: see notes above and under Codeine Phosphate, sedation and the risk of dependence are greater

Kaolin and Morphine Mixture, BP

(Kaolin and Morphine Oral Suspension)

Oral suspension, light kaolin or light kaolin (natural) 20%, sodium bicarbonate 5%, and chloroform and morphine tincture 4% in a suitable vehicle. Contains anhydrous morphine 550–800 micrograms/10 mL.

Dose: 10 mL every 4 hours in water

1.5   Treatment of chronic diarrhoeas

Once tumours are ruled out individual complaints need specific treatment including dietary manipulation as well as drug treatment and the maintenance of a liberal fluid intake.

IRRITABLE BOWEL SYNDROME

Irritable bowel syndrome can present with pain, constipation, or diarrhoea, all of which may benefit from a high-fibre diet, with bran or with other agents which increase stool bulk (section 1.6.1). In some patients there may be important psychological aggravating factors which respond to reassurance. Antimotility drugs such as loperamide (section 1.4.2) may relieve diarrhoea and antispasmodic drugs (section 1.2) may relieve pain. Opioids with a central action such as codeine are better avoided because of the risk of dependence.

MALABSORPTION SYNDROMES

Individual conditions need specific management and also general nutritional consideration. Thus coeliac disease (gluten enteropathy) usually needs a gluten-free diet (Appendix 7) and pancreatic insufficiency needs pancreatin supplements (section 1.9.4).

ULCERATIVE COLITIS

For *acute attacks* of ulcerative colitis topical **corticosteroid** treatment such as budesonide or prednisolone enemas or prednisolone suppositories for localised rectal disease will induce remission; foam preparations are especially useful where patients have difficulty retaining liquid enemas. More extensive disease requires oral corticosteroid treatment and severe extensive or fulminant disease needs hospital admission and intravenous corticosteroid administration.

Sulphasalazine (sulfasalazine) a chemical combination of sulphapyridine and 5-aminosalicylic acid ('5-ASA') is useful in mild symptomatic disease requiring oral treatment; it is also available as suppositories for rectal disease. Activity resides in the 5-aminosalicylic acid moiety; sulphapyridine

acts only as a carrier to the colonic site of action (but it still causes side-effects). Newer aminosalicylates include **mesalazine** (5-aminosalicylic acid itself), **balsalazide** (a prodrug of 5-aminosalicylic acid), and **olsalazine** (a dimer of 5-aminosalicylic acid that cleaves in the lower bowel). Sulphonamide-related side-effects of sulphasalazine are avoided, but 5-aminosalicylate alone can still cause a range of adverse effects including blood disorders and lupoid phenomenon also seen with sulphasalazine. Olsalazine may also be particularly prone to cause watery diarrhoea. Some manufacturers of sulphasalazine and mesalazine recommend renal function tests, but evidence of practical value is unsatisfactory.

Sulphasalazine, mesalazine, and olsalazine all have value in preventing relapse and choice is related in part to their different side-effects. Corticosteroids are unsuitable for *maintenance treatment* because of side-effects. In resistant cases **azathioprine** (section 8.2.1), 2 mg/kg daily, given under close supervision may be helpful [unlicensed indication].

Laxatives are required to facilitate bowel movement when proctitis is present but a high-fibre diet and bulk-forming drugs such as **methylcellulose** are more useful in adjusting faecal consistency (section 1.6.1).

Antimotility drugs such as codeine and loperamide should not be used in severe colitis as they can precipitate paralytic ileus and megacolon. They have limited value in mild disease, but treatment of the inflammation is more logical. For similar reasons antispasmodics should **not** be used in ulcerative colitis.

General nutritional care and appropriate supplements are essential.

CROHN'S DISEASE

Treatment of Crohn's disease (particularly of colonic disease) is similar to that for ulcerative colitis. In small bowel disease the **aminosalicylates** may have marginal value. Symptoms and inflammation associated with disease exacerbation are suppressed by **oral corticosteroids** such as prednisolone; modified-release budesonide is also effective and causes fewer systemic side-effects. **Metronidazole** may be beneficial possibly through its antibacterial activity. Other antibacterials should be given if specifically indicated and for managing bacterial overgrowth in the small bowel.

General nutritional care and appropriate supplements are essential.

ANTIBIOTIC-ASSOCIATED COLITIS

Antibiotic-associated colitis (pseudomembranous colitis) is caused by colonisation of the colon with *Clostridium difficile* which may follow antibiotic therapy. It is usually of acute onset, but may run a chronic course; it is a particular hazard of clindamycin but few antibiotics are free of this side-effect. Oral **vancomycin** (see section 5.1.7) or **metronidazole** (see section 5.1.11) are used as specific treatment; vancomycin may be preferred for very sick patients.

DIVERTICULAR DISEASE

Diverticular disease is treated with a high-fibre diet, **bran supplements**, and **bulk-forming drugs**. **Antispasmodics** may provide symptomatic relief when colic is a problem (section 1.2). **Antibiotics** are used only when the diverticula in the intestinal wall become infected (specialist referral). **Antimotility** drugs which slow intestinal motility, e.g. codeine, diphenoxylate, and loperamide could possibly exacerbate the symptoms of diverticular disease and are **contra-indicated**.

AMINOSALICYLATES

> **Blood disorders**
> It is recommended that patients receiving aminosalicylates should be advised to report any unexplained bleeding, bruising, purpura, sore throat, fever or malaise that occurs during treatment. A blood count should be performed and the drug stopped immediately if there is suspicion of a blood dyscrasia.

BALSALAZIDE DISODIUM

Indications: induction of remission of ulcerative colitis

Cautions: asthma, liver disease, renal impairment (avoid if moderate or severe), pregnancy and breast-feeding

Contra-indications: salicylate hypersensitivity
BLOOD DISORDERS. See recommendation above

Side-effects: abdominal pain, diarrhoea, nausea, vomiting, headache; rarely, exacerbation of colitis, acute pancreatitis, hepatitis, blood dyscrasias

Dose: 2.25 g 3 times daily until remission occurs or for up to max. 12 weeks

▼ PoM **Colazide®** (Astra)
Capsules, red/maroon, balsalazide disodium 750 mg. Net price 130-cap pack = £39.00. Label: 21, 25, counselling, blood disorder symptoms (see recommendation above)

MESALAZINE

Indications: induction and maintenance of remission in ulcerative colitis; see also under preparations

Cautions: pregnancy and breast-feeding
BLOOD DISORDERS. See recommendation above

Contra-indications: salicylate hypersensitivity; renal impairment (nephrotoxic)

Side-effects: nausea, diarrhoea, and abdominal pain; headache; exacerbation of symptoms of colitis; rarely reversible pancreatitis, hepatitis, interstitial nephritis, nephrotic syndrome, rash, urticaria; leucopenia, neutropenia, thrombocytopenia and aplastic anaemia reported; myocarditis,

lupus phenomenon, fibrosing alveolitis also reported
Dose: see under preparations, below
> *Note.* The delivery characteristics of enteric-coated mesalazine preparations may vary; these preparations should not be considered interchangable

PoM **Asacol®** (SK&F)
Tablets, red, e/c, mesalazine 400 mg, net price 90-tab pack = £32.69, 120-tab pack = £43.58. Label: 5, 25, counselling, blood disorder symptoms (see recommendation above)
> *Dose:* ulcerative colitis, acute attack, 6 tablets daily in divided doses; maintenance of ulcerative colitis and Crohn's ileo-colitis, 3–6 tablets daily in divided doses; CHILD not recommended
> *Note.* Preparations that lower stool pH (e.g. lactulose) may prevent release of mesalazine

Foam enema, mesalazine 1 g/metered application. Net price 14 g (14 applications) with disposable applicators and plastic bags = £39.60. Counselling, blood disorder symptoms (see recommendation above)
> *Dose:* acute attack affecting the rectosigmoid region, 1 metered application (mesalazine 1 g) into the rectum daily for 4–6 weeks; acute attack affecting the descending colon, 2 metered applications (mesalazine 2 g) daily for 4–6 weeks; CHILD not recommended

Suppositories, mesalazine 250 mg, net price 20-suppos pack = £7.15; 500 mg, 10 = £7.15. Counselling, blood disorder symptoms (see recommendation above)
> *Dose:* 3–6 suppositories of 250 mg (max. 3 suppositories of 500 mg) daily in divided doses, with last dose at bedtime; CHILD not recommended

PoM **Coltec® EC** (Berk)
Tablets, brown, e/c, mesalazine 400 mg. Net price 120-tab pack = £42.00. Label: 5, 25, counselling, blood disorder symptoms (see recommendation above)
Mesalazine tablets also available from APS
> *Dose:* ulcerative colitis, acute attack, 6 tablets daily in divided doses; maintenance, 3–6 tablets daily in divided doses; CHILD not recommended
> *Note.* Preparations that lower stool pH (e.g. lactulose) may prevent release of mesalazine

PoM **Pentasa®** (Ferring)
Slow Release tablets, m/r, both scored, mesalazine 250 mg, net price 200-tab pack = £32.28; 500 mg (grey), 100-tab pack = £32.28. Counselling, administration, see dose, blood disorder symptoms (see recommendation above)
> *Dose:* acute attack, up to 4 g daily in 2–3 divided doses; maintenance, 1.5 g daily in 2–3 divided doses; tablets may be dispersed in water, but should not be chewed; CHILD under 15 years not recommended

Retention enema, mesalazine 1 g in 100-mL pack. Net price 7 enemas = £19.45. Counselling, blood disorder symptoms (see recommendation above)
> *Dose:* 1 enema at bedtime; CHILD not recommended

Suppositories, mesalazine 1 g. Net price 28-suppos pack = £44.68. Counselling, blood disorder symptoms (see recommendation above)
> *Dose:* ulcerative proctitis, acute attack, 1 suppository daily for 2–4 weeks; maintenance, 1 suppository daily; CHILD under 15 years not recommended

---

PoM **Salofalk®** (Thames)

Tablets, e/c, yellow, mesalazine 250 mg. Net price 100-tab pack = £18.41. Label: 5, 25, counselling, blood disorder symptoms (see recommendation above)

Dose: acute attack, 6 tablets daily in 3 divided doses; maintenance 3–6 tablets daily in divided doses; CHILD not recommended

Suppositories, mesalazine 500 mg. Net price 30-suppos pack = £20.45. Counselling, blood disorder symptoms (see recommendations above)

Dose: acute attack, 1–2 suppositories 2–3 times daily adjusted according to response; CHILD not recommended

Enema, mesalazine 2 g in 59-mL pack. Net price 7 enemas = £40.53. Counselling, blood disorder symptoms (see recommendations above)

Dose: acute attack *or* maintenance, 1 enema daily at bedtime; CHILD not recommended

OLSALAZINE SODIUM

Indications: induction and maintenance of remission in ulcerative colitis

Cautions: pregnancy and breast-feeding

BLOOD DISORDERS. See CSM recommendation above

Contra-indications: salicylate hypersensitivity; renal impairment

Side-effects: watery diarrhoea, abdominal cramps, headache, nausea, dyspepsia, arthralgia, and rash; rarely reversible pancreatitis

Dose: acute attack, 1 g daily in divided doses after meals increased if necessary over 1 week to max. 3 g daily (max. single dose 1 g)

Maintenance, 500 mg twice daily after meals

PoM **Dipentum®** (Pharmacia & Upjohn)

Capsules, brown, olsalazine sodium 250 mg. Net price 112-cap pack = £28.71. Label: 21, counselling, blood disorder symptoms (see recommendation above)

Tablets, yellow, scored, olsalazine sodium 500 mg. Net price 60-tab pack = £30.76. Label: 21, counselling, blood disorder symptoms (see recommendation above)

SULPHASALAZINE

(Sulfasalazine)

Indications: induction and maintenance of remission in ulcerative colitis; active Crohn's disease; rheumatoid arthritis, see section 10.1.3

Cautions: history of allergy; hepatic and renal disease; G6PD deficiency; slow acetylator status; risk of haematological and hepatic toxicity (differential white cell, red cell and platelet counts initially and at monthly intervals for first 3 months, liver function tests at monthly intervals for first 3 months; upper gastro-intestinal side-effects common over 4 g daily; pregnancy and breast-feeding (see Appendixes 4 and 5); porphyria (see section 9.8.2)

BLOOD DISORDERS. See recommendation above

Contra-indications: salicylate and sulphonamide hypersensitivity; CHILD under 2 years of age

Side-effects: nausea, vomiting, epigastric discomfort, headache, rashes; *occasionally:* fever, minor haematological abnormalities such as Heinz-body anaemia, reversible neutropenia, folate deficiency; reversible oligospermia; *rarely:* pancreatitis, hepatitis, exacerbation of colitis, thrombocytopenia, agranulocytosis, aplastic anaemia, Stevens–Johnson syndrome, neurotoxicity, photosensitisation, lupus erythematosus-like syndrome, and fibrosing alveolitis; proteinuria, crystalluria, haematuria, and nephrotic syndrome; urine may be coloured orange; some soft contact lenses may be stained

Dose: by *mouth*, acute attack 1–2 g 4 times daily (but see **cautions**) until remission occurs (if necessary corticosteroids may also be given), reducing to a maintenance dose of 500 mg 4 times daily; CHILD over 2 years, acute attack 40–60 mg/kg daily, maintenance dose 20–30 mg/kg daily

By *rectum*, in suppositories, alone or in conjunction with oral treatment 0.5–1 g morning and night after a bowel movement. As an enema, 3 g at night, retained for at least 1 hour

PoM **Sulphasalazine** (Non-proprietary)

Tablets, sulphasalazine 500 mg. Net price 100 = £6.99. Label: 14, counselling, blood disorder symptoms (see recommendation above), contact lenses may be stained

Available from APS, Berk, Cox, Lagap

Tablets, e/c, sulphasalazine 500 mg. Net price 112-tab pack = £12.11. Label: 5, 14, 25, counselling, blood disorder symptoms (see recommendation above), contact lenses may be stained

Available from Cox (*Sulazine EC®*)

PoM **Salazopyrin®** (Pharmacia & Upjohn)

Tablets, yellow, scored, sulphasalazine 500 mg. Net price 112-tab pack = £8.10. Label: 14, counselling, blood disorder symptoms (see recommendation above), contact lenses may be stained

EN-Tabs® (= tablets e/c), yellow, f/c, sulphasalazine 500 mg. Net price 112-tab pack = £12.11. Label: 5, 14, 21, 25, counselling, blood disorder symptoms (see recommendation above), contact lenses may be stained

Suspension, yellow, sulphasalazine 250 mg/5 mL. Net price 500 mL = £16.44. Label: 14, counselling, blood disorder symptoms (see recommendation above), contact lenses may be stained

Suppositories, yellow, sulphasalazine 500 mg. Net price 10 = £2.88. Label: 14, counselling, blood disorder symptoms (see recommendation above), contact lenses may be stained

Retention enema, sulphasalazine 3 g in 100-mL single-dose disposable packs fitted with a nozzle. Net price 7 × 100 mL = £12.43. Label: 14, counselling, blood disorder symptoms (see recommendation above), contact lenses may be stained

---

ANION-EXCHANGE RESINS

CHOLESTYRAMINE
(Colestyramine)

Indications: diarrhoea associated with Crohn's disease, ileal resection, vagotomy, diabetic vagal neuropathy, and radiation; pruritus in liver disease, and hypercholesterolaemia, see section 2.12

Cautions; Contra-indications; Side-effects: see section 2.12

Dose: diarrhoea, after initial introduction over 3–4 week period, 12–24 g daily mixed with water (or other suitable liquid), in single or up to 4 divided doses, subsequently adjusted as required; max. 36 g daily

CHILD 6–12 years, see product information

COUNSELLING. Other drugs should be taken at least 1 hour before or 4–6 hours after cholestyramine to reduce possible interference with absorption

Preparations
Section 2.12

CORTICOSTEROIDS

BUDESONIDE

Indications: see under preparations

Cautions; Contra-indications; Side-effects: see section 6.3.2

Dose: see under preparations

PoM **Entocort®** (Astra)

CR Capsules, e/c, m/r, grey/pink, budesonide 3 mg. Net price 100-cap pack = £90.00. Label: 5, 10 steroid card, 22, 25

Note. Dispense in original container (contains desiccant)

Dose: mild to moderate Crohn's disease affecting the ileum or ascending colon, 9 mg once daily in the morning before breakfast for up to 8 weeks; reduce dose for the last 2–4 weeks of treatment. See also section 6.3.2

CHILD not recommended

Enema, budesonide 2 mg/100 mL when dispersible tablet reconstituted in isotonic saline vehicle. Net price pack of 7 dispersible tablets and bottles of vehicle = £30.00

Dose: ulcerative colitis involving rectal and recto-sigmoid disease, 1 enema at bedtime for 4 weeks; CHILD not recommended

HYDROCORTISONE

Indications: ulcerative colitis, proctitis, proctosigmoiditis

Cautions; Contra-indications; Side-effects: systemic absorption may occur, section 6.3.2; local irritation may also occur; prolonged use should be avoided; avoid use of enemas and rectal foams in obstruction, bowel perforation, and extensive fistulas; contra-indicated in untreated infection

Dose: rectal, see under Preparations

PoM **Colifoam®** (Stafford-Miller)

Foam in aerosol pack, hydrocortisone acetate 10%. Net price 20.8 g (14 applications) with applicator = £7.07

Dose: initially 1 metered application (125 mg hydrocortisone acetate) inserted into the rectum once or twice daily for 2–3 weeks, then once on alternate days

---

PREDNISOLONE

Indications: ulcerative colitis, and Crohn's disease; other indications, see section 6.3.2, see also preparations

Cautions; Contra-indications; Side-effects: see under Hydrocortisone and section 6.3.2

Dose: by mouth, initial dose 20–40 mg daily, in single or divided doses, until remission occurs, followed by reducing doses

By rectum, see under preparations

Oral preparations, section 6.3.2

Rectal preparations

PoM **Predenema®** (Pharmax)

Retention enema, prednisolone 20 mg (as sodium metasulphobenzoate) in 100-mL single-dose disposable pack. Net price 1 (standard tube) = 80p, 1 (long tube) = £1.35

Dose: ulcerative colitis, initially 1 enema at bedtime for 2–4 weeks, continued if good response; CHILD not recommended

PoM **Predfoam®** (Pharmax)

Foam in aerosol pack, prednisolone 20 mg (as metasulphobenzoate sodium)/metered application. Net price 25 g (14 applications) with disposable applicators = £7.06

Dose: proctitis and distal ulcerative colitis, 1 metered application (containing 20 mg prednisolone) inserted into the rectum once or twice daily for 2 weeks, continued for further 2 weeks if good response; CHILD not recommended

PoM **Predsol®** (Evans)

Retention enema, prednisolone 20 mg (as sodium phosphate) in 100-mL single-dose disposable packs fitted with a nozzle. Net price 7 = £5.24

Dose: rectal and rectosigmoidal ulcerative colitis and Crohn's disease, initially 1 enema at bedtime for 2–4 weeks, continued if good response; CHILD not recommended

Suppositories, prednisolone 5 mg (as sodium phosphate). Net price 10 = £1.00

Dose: ADULT and CHILD proctitis and rectal complications of Crohn's disease, 1 suppository inserted night and morning after a bowel movement

---

CROMOGLYCATE

Allergy with classical symptoms of vomiting, colic and diarrhoea caused by specific foods such as shellfish should be managed by strict avoidance. The condition should be distinguished from symptoms of occasional food intolerance in those with irritable bowel syndrome. **Sodium cromoglycate** may be helpful as an adjunct to dietary avoidance.

SODIUM CROMOGLYCATE

(Sodium cromoglicate)

Indications: food allergy (in conjunction with dietary restriction); asthma, section 3.3; allergic conjunctivitis, section 11.4.2; allergic rhinitis, section 12.2.1

Side-effects: occasional nausea, rashes, and joint pain

Dose: 200 mg 4 times daily before meals; CHILD 2–14 years 100 mg; capsules may be swallowed whole or the contents dissolved in hot water and diluted with cold water before taking. May be increased if necessary after 2–3 weeks to a max. of 40 mg/kg daily and then reduced according to the response

PoM **Nalcrom**® (Fisons)

Capsules, sodium cromoglycate 100 mg. Net price 100 = £35.00. Label: 22, counselling, see dose above

---

1.6 Laxatives

1.6.1	Bulk-forming laxatives
1.6.2	Stimulant laxatives
1.6.3	Faecal softeners
1.6.4	Osmotic laxatives
1.6.5	Bowel cleansing solutions

Before prescribing laxatives it is important to be sure that the patient *is* constipated and that the constipation is *not* secondary to an underlying undiagnosed complaint.

It is also important for those who complain of constipation to understand that bowel habit can vary considerably in frequency without doing harm. Some people tend to consider themselves constipated if they do not have a bowel movement each day. A useful definition of constipation is the passage of hard stools less frequently than the patient's own normal pattern and this can be explained to the patient.

Misconceptions about bowel habits have led to excessive laxative use. Abuse may lead to hypokalaemia and an atonic non-functioning colon.

Thus, laxatives should generally be **avoided** except where straining will exacerbate a condition (such as angina) or increase the risk of rectal bleeding as in haemorrhoids. Laxatives are also of value in *drug-induced constipation*, for the expulsion of *parasites* after anthelmintic treatment, and to clear the alimentary tract before *surgery and radiological procedures.* Prolonged treatment of constipation is seldom necessary except occasionally in the elderly.

CHILDREN. The use of laxatives in children should be discouraged unless prescribed by a doctor. Infrequent defaecation may be normal in breast-fed babies or in response to poor intake of fluid or fibre. Delays of greater than 3 days between stools may increase the likelihood of pain on passing hard stools leading to anal fissure, anal spasm and eventually to a learned response to avoid defaecation.

If increased fluid and fibre intake is insufficient, an osmotic laxative such as lactulose or a bulk-forming laxative such as methylcellulose may be effective; methylcellulose is given in a dose of 0.5–1 g twice daily for a child over 7 years [unlicensed use]—an appropriate formulation for a younger child is not readily available. If there is evidence of minor faecal retention, the addition of a stimulant laxative such as senna may overcome withholding but may lead to colic or, in the presence of faecal impaction in the rectum, an increase of faecal overflow. Referral to hospital may be needed unless the child evacuates the impacted mass spontaneously. In hospital, enemas or suppositories may clear the mass but their use is frequently distressing for the child and may lead to a persistence of withholding. Enemas may be administered under heavy sedation in hospital where a bowel cleansing solution (section 1.6.5) may be tried. In severe cases or where the child is afraid, a manual evacuation under anaesthetic may be appropriate.

Long-term use of stimulant laxatives such as senna or sodium picosulphate is essential to prevent recurrence of the faecal impaction. Parents should be encouraged to use them regularly for many months; intermittent use may provoke a series of relapses.

> The laxatives that follow have been divided into 5 main groups (sections 1.6.1–1.6.5). This simple classification disguises the fact that some laxatives have a complex action.

1.6.1 Bulk-forming laxatives

Bulk-forming laxatives relieve constipation by increasing faecal mass which stimulates peristalsis; the full effect may take some days to develop and patients should be told this.

Bulk-forming laxatives are of particular value in those with small hard stools, but should not be required unless fibre cannot be increased in the diet. A balanced diet, including adequate fluid intake and fibre is of value in preventing constipation.

Bulk-forming laxatives are useful in the management of patients with *colostomy, ileostomy, haemorrhoids, anal fissure, chronic diarrhoea associated with diverticular disease, irritable bowel syndrome,* and as adjuncts in *ulcerative colitis* (section 1.5). Adequate fluid intake must be maintained to avoid intestinal obstruction. Unprocessed wheat **bran**, taken with food or fruit juice, is a most effective bulk-forming preparation. Finely ground bran, though more palatable, has poorer water-retaining properties, but can be taken as bran bread or biscuits in appropriately increased quantities. Oat bran is also used.

Methylcellulose, ispaghula, and **sterculia** are useful in patients who cannot tolerate bran. Methylcellulose also acts as a faecal softener.

BRAN

Indications: see notes above

Cautions; Contra-indications; Side-effects: see under Ispaghula Husk. Avoid in gluten enteropathies and coeliac disease

Dose: see preparation below

COUNSELLING. Preparations that swell in contact with liquid should always be carefully swallowed with water and should not be taken immediately before going to bed

Trifyba® (Sanofi Winthrop)

Powder, brown, wheat fibre 80%. Net price 56 sachets containing 3.5 g = £3.28. Counselling, see below

Note. Contains gluten

Dose: 1 sachet 2–3 times daily added to food; CHILD (but see section 1.6) half to one sachet 1–2 times daily added to food

COUNSELLING. At least one glass of water or other liquid should be drunk with the meal

ISPAGHULA HUSK

Indications: see notes above; hypercholesterolaemia, section 2.12

Cautions: adequate fluid intake should be maintained to avoid intestinal obstruction—it may be necessary to supervise elderly or debilitated patients or those with intestinal narrowing or decreased motility

Contra-indications: difficulty in swallowing, intestinal obstruction, colonic atony, faecal impaction

Side-effects: flatulence, abdominal distension, gastro-intestinal obstruction or impaction; hypersensitivity reported

Dose: see preparations below

COUNSELLING. Preparations that swell in contact with liquid should always be carefully swallowed with water and should not be taken immediately before going to bed

Fybogel® (R&C)

Granules, buff, effervescent, sugar- and gluten-free, ispaghula husk 3.5 g/sachet (low Na⁺). Net price 60 sachets (plain, lemon, or orange flavoured) = £4.24. Label: 13, counselling, see above

Note. Contains aspartame 50 mg/sachet (see section 9.4.1)

Dose: 1 sachet in water twice daily preferably after meals; CHILD (but see section 1.6) 6–12 years ½–1 level 5-mL spoonful (children under 6 years on doctor's advice only)

Konsyl® (Eastern)

Powder, gluten-free, ispaghula husk (micronised), *Konsyl Sugar Free* (6 g/sachet), net price 30-sachet pack = £3.99; *Konsyl Dex* (3.4 g/sachet with glucose 8 g), 60-sachet pack = £3.99; *Konsyl Orange* (3.4 g/sachet), 60-sachet pack = £3.99. Label 13, counselling, see above

Dose: 1 sachet in water 1–3 times daily before or after meals; CHILD (but see section 1.6) over 6 years, ½ adult dose or less (children under 6 years on doctor's advice only)

Diarrhoea (section 1.4.1), 1 sachet in water 3 times daily

Important. Each sachet of *Konsyl Sugar Free* contains almost twice as much ispaghula husk as *Konsyl Dex* or *Konsyl Orange*

Isogel® (Pfizer Consumer)

Granules, brown, sugar- and gluten-free, ispaghula husk 90%. Net price 300 g = £2.94. Label: 13, counselling, see above

Dose: constipation, 2 teaspoonfuls in water once or twice daily, preferably at mealtimes; CHILD (but see section 1.6) 1 teaspoonful

Diarrhoea (section 1.4.1), 1 teaspoonful 3 times daily

Regulan® (Procter & Gamble)

Powder, beige, sugar- and gluten-free, ispaghula husk 3.4 g/5.85-g sachet (orange or lemon/lime flavour). Net price 30 sachets = £2.12. Label: 13, counselling, see above

Note. Contains aspartame (see section 9.4.1)

Dose: 1 sachet in 150 mL water 1–3 times daily; CHILD (but see section 1.6) 6–12 years 2.5–5 mL

METHYLCELLULOSE

Indications: see notes above; obesity, see section 4.5.1

Cautions; Contra-indications; Side-effects: see under Ispaghula Husk

Dose: see preparations below

COUNSELLING. Preparations that swell in contact with liquid should always be carefully swallowed with water and should not be taken immediately before going to bed

Celevac® (Monmouth)

Tablets, pink, scored, methylcellulose '450' 500 mg. Net price 112-tab pack = £2.69. Counselling, see above and dose

Dose: 3–6 tablets twice daily. In constipation the dose should be taken with at least 300 mL of water. In diarrhoea, ileostomy, and colostomy control, minimise liquid intake for 30 minutes before and after the dose

STERCULIA

Indications: see notes above

Cautions; Contra-indications; Side-effects: see under Ispaghula Husk

COUNSELLING. Preparations that swell in contact with liquid should always be carefully swallowed with water and should not be taken immediately before going to bed

Normacol® (Norgine)

Granules, coated, gluten-free, sterculia 62%. Net price 500 g = £5.53; 60 × 7-g sachets = £4.65. Label: 25, 27, counselling, see above

Dose: 1–2 heaped 5-mL spoonfuls, or the contents of 1–2 sachets, washed down without chewing with plenty of liquid once or twice daily after meals; CHILD (but see section 1.6) 6–12 years half adult dose

Normacol Plus® (Norgine)

Granules, brown, coated, gluten-free, sterculia 62%, frangula (standardised) 8%. Net price 500 g = £5.92; 60 × 7 g sachets = £4.98. Label: 25, 27, counselling, see above

Dose: constipation and after haemorrhoidectomy, 1–2 heaped 5-mL spoonfuls or the contents of 1–2 sachets washed down without chewing with plenty of liquid once or twice daily after meals

---

1.6.2   Stimulant laxatives

The recognised stimulant laxatives include **bisacodyl** and members of the **anthraquinone** group, e.g. senna. **Docusate** sodium probably acts both as a stimulant and as a softening agent. **Danthron** (dantron) has limited indications (see below) because *rodent* studies indicate potential carcinogenic risk. Powerful stimulants such as **cascara** and **castor oil** are obsolete.

Stimulant laxatives increase intestinal motility and often cause abdominal cramp. They should not be used in intestinal obstruction, and prolonged use can precipitate the onset of an atonic non-functioning colon and hypokalaemia. See section 1.6 for the use of stimulant laxatives in children.

Glycerol suppositories act as a rectal stimulant by virtue of the mildly irritant action of glycerol.

Soft soap is a more severe irritant; the use of soft soap enema should be **avoided**, especially in pregnancy, as it may inflame the colonic mucosa.

The **parasympathomimetics** bethanechol, distigmine, neostigmine, and pyridostigmine (see section 7.4.1 and section 10.2.1) enhance parasympathetic activity in the gut and increase intestinal motility. They are rarely used for their gastro-intestinal effects. Organic obstruction of the gut must first be excluded and they should not be used shortly after bowel anastomosis.

Oxyphenisatin is indicated for diagnostic procedures or surgery only, since it causes hepatitis in chronic use.

BISACODYL

Indications: see under Dose; tablets act in 10–12 hours; suppositories act in 20–60 minutes

Cautions; Contra-indications; Side-effects: see notes on stimulant laxatives; tablets, griping; suppositories, local irritation

Dose: by mouth for constipation, 5–10 mg at night; occasionally necessary to increase to 15–20 mg; CHILD (but see section 1.6) under 10 years 5 mg

By rectum in suppositories for constipation, 10 mg in the morning; CHILD (but see section 1.6) under 10 years 5 mg

Before radiological procedures and surgery, 10 mg by mouth at bedtime for 2 days before examination and, if necessary, a 10-mg suppository 1 hour before examination; CHILD half adult dose

Bisacodyl (Non-proprietary)
Tablets, e/c, bisacodyl 5 mg. Net price 20 = 24p. Label: 5, 25
Suppositories, bisacodyl 10 mg. Net price 12 = 86p
Paediatric suppositories, bisacodyl 5 mg. Net price 5 = 81p
Note. The brand name NHS Dulco-lax® (Windsor) is used for bisacodyl tablets, net price 10-tab pack = 56p; suppositories (10 mg), 10 = £1.39; paediatric suppositories (5 mg), 5 = 81p
The brand name Dulco-lax® Liquid is used for sodium picosulphate elixir

DANTHRON
(Dantron)
Indications: only for: constipation in geriatric practice; prophylaxis and treatment of analgesic-induced constipation in terminally ill patients of all ages; constipation in cardiac failure and coronary thrombosis (conditions in which bowel movement must be free of strain); acts within 6–12 hours

Cautions; Contra-indications; Side-effects: see notes on stimulant laxatives; urine may be coloured red; avoid prolonged contact with skin (as in incontinent patients) since irritation and excoriation may occur; avoid in pregnancy and breast-feeding; *rodent* studies indicate potential carcinogenic risk

Dose: see under preparations

With poloxamer '188' (as co-danthramer)
Note. Co-danthramer suspension 5 mL = one co-danthramer capsule, **but** strong co-danthramer suspension 5 mL = two strong co-danthramer capsules
PoM **Co-danthramer** (Non-proprietary)
Capsules, co-danthramer 25/200 (danthron 25 mg, poloxamer '188' 200 mg). Net price 60-cap pack = £12.86. Label: 14 (urine red)
Dose: 1–2 capsules at bedtime; CHILD 1 capsule at bedtime (restricted indications, see notes above)
Available from Napp
Strong capsules, co-danthramer 37.5/500 (danthron 37.5 mg, poloxamer '188' 500 mg). Net price 60-cap pack = £15.55. Label: 14 (urine red)
Dose: 1–2 capsules at bedtime (restricted indications, see notes above); CHILD under 12 years not recommended
Available from Napp
Suspension, co-danthramer 25/200 in 5 mL (danthron 25 mg, poloxamer '188' 200 mg/5 mL). Net price 300 mL = £11.26, 1 litre = £37.53. Label: 14 (urine red)
Dose: 5–10 mL at night; CHILD 2.5–5 mL (restricted indications, see notes above)
Available from Galen (Ailax®), Hillcross, Napp (NHS Codalax®)
Strong suspension, co-danthramer 75/1000 in 5 mL (danthron 75 mg, poloxamer '188' 1 g/5 mL). Net price 300 mL = £30.12, 1 litre = £100.40. Label: 14 (urine red)
Dose: 5 mL at night (restricted indications, see notes above); CHILD under 12 years not recommended
Available from Galen (Ailax® Forte) and Napp (NHS Codalax Forte®)

With docusate sodium (as co-danthrusate)
PoM **Co-danthrusate** (Non-proprietary)
Capsules, co-danthrusate 50/60 (danthron 50 mg, docusate sodium 60 mg). Net price 63-cap pack = £13.46. Label: 14 (urine red)
Dose: 1–3 capsules, usually at night; CHILD 6–12 years 1 capsule (restricted indications, see notes above)
Available from Evans (NHS Normax®), Galen (Capsuvac®), Hillcross
Suspension, yellow, co-danthrusate 50/60 (danthron 50 mg, docusate sodium 60 mg/5 mL). Net price 200 mL = £6.40. Label: 14 (urine red)
Dose: 5–15 mL at night; CHILD 6–12 years 5 mL at night (restricted indications, see notes above)
Available from Evans (Normax®)

DOCUSATE SODIUM
(Dioctyl Sodium Sulphosuccinate)

Indications: constipation (oral preparations act within 1–2 days); adjunct in abdominal radiological procedures

Cautions; Contra-indications; Side-effects: see notes on stimulant laxatives; do not give with liquid paraffin; rectal preparations not indicated if haemorrhoids or anal fissure

Dose: by mouth, chronic constipation, up to 500 mg daily in divided doses
With barium meal, 400 mg

Dioctyl® (Schwarz)
Capsules, yellow/white, docusate sodium 100 mg. Net price 100-cap pack = £4.65

Rectal preparations
Fletchers' Enemette® (Pharmax)
Enema, docusate sodium 90 mg, glycerol 3.78 g/5 mL with macrogol and sorbic acid. Net price 5-mL unit = 32p
Dose: ADULT and CHILD (but see section 1.6) over 3 years, 5-mL unit when required
Norgalax Micro-enema® (Norgine)
Enema, docusate sodium 120 mg in 10-g single-dose disposable packs. Net price 10-g unit = 64p
Dose: ADULT and CHILD (but see section 1.6) over 12 years, 10-g unit

GLYCEROL
(Glycerin)
Indications: constipation
Dose: see below

Glycerol Suppositories, BP
(Glycerin Suppositories)
Suppositories, gelatin 140 mg, glycerol 700 mg, purified water to 1 g. Net price 12 = 50p (infant), 51p (child), 55p (adult)
Dose: 1 suppository moistened with water before use. The usual sizes are for *infants* small (1-g mould), *children* medium (2-g mould), *adults* large (4-g mould)

OXYPHENISATIN
(Oxyphenisatine)
Indications: see under Dose
Cautions; Contra-indications; Side-effects: see notes on stimulant laxatives; avoid repeated use owing to liver toxicity; **important:** consider general warnings relating to bowel cleansing solutions on p. 53

Veripaque® (Sanofi Winthrop)
Enema, powder for reconstitution, oxyphenisatin 50 mg in 3 g. Net price 1 vial = £2.03
Dose: by rectum before diagnostic procedures or surgery, oxyphenisatin 50 mg dissolved in 2 litres of water given over 5–8 minutes
Adjuvant to barium enema, oxyphenisatin 50 mg mixed thoroughly with 2 litres of barium sulphate enema

SENNA
Indications: constipation; acts in 8–12 hours
Cautions; Contra-indications; Side-effects: see notes on stimulant laxatives

Senna Tablets, total sennosides (calculated as sennoside B) 7.5 mg. Net price 20 = 30p
Dose: 2–4 tablets, usually at night; initial dose should be low then gradually increased; CHILD (but see section 1.6) over 6 years, half adult dose (on doctor's advice only)
Note. The brand name NHS Senokot® (see below) is used for Senna tablets; for those on sale to the public lower dose recommended
Manevac® (Galen)
Granules, coated, senna fruit 12.4%, ispaghula 54.2%. Net price 400 g = £5.76, 56 × 4-g sachets = £3.80. Label: 25, 27, counselling, see Ispaghula Husk
Dose: 1–2 level 5-mL spoonfuls (or sachets) with water or warm drink after supper and, if necessary, before breakfast *or* every 6 hours in resistant cases for 1–3 days; CHILD (but see section 1.6) 5–12 years 1 level 5-mL spoonful (or sachet) daily
Note. One level 5-mL spoonful is equivalent to one 4-g sachet
COUNSELLING. Preparations that swell in contact with liquid should always be carefully swallowed with water and should not be taken immediately before going to bed
Senokot® (R&C)
NHS *Tablets,* see above
Granules, brown, total sennosides (calculated as sennoside B) 15 mg/5 mL or 5.5 mg/g (one 5-mL spoonful = 2.7 g). Net price 100 g = £2.64
Dose: 5–10 mL, usually at bedtime; CHILD (but see section 1.6) over 6 years 2.5–5 mL in the morning
Note. Lower dose on packs on sale to the public
Syrup, brown, total sennosides (calculated as sennoside B) 7.5 mg/5 mL. Net price 100 mL pack = £1.98
Dose: 10–20 mL, usually at bedtime; CHILD (but see section 1.6) 2–6 years 2.5–5 mL in the morning (doctor's advice only), over 6 years 5–10 mL
Note. Lower dose on packs on sale to the public

SODIUM PICOSULPHATE
(Sodium Picosulfate)
Indications: constipation; bowel evacuation before abdominal radiological procedures, endoscopy, and surgery (section 1.6.5)
Cautions; Contra-indications; Side-effects: see notes on stimulant laxatives
Dose: see below

Sodium Picosulphate Elixir, sodium picosulphate 5 mg/5 mL. Acts within 10–14 hours. Net price 100 mL = £1.85
Dose: 5–15 mL at night; CHILD (but see section 1.6) 2–5 years 2.5 mL, 5–10 years 2.5–5 mL
Note. The brand names NHS Laxoberal® and Dulco-lax® Liquid (both Windsor) are used for sodium picosulphate elixir 5 mg/5 mL
The brand name Dulco-lax® is also used for bisacodyl tablets and suppositories

Before radiography, endoscopy or surgery
See section 1.6.5

OTHER STIMULANT LAXATIVES

Unstandardised preparations of cascara, frangula, rhubarb, and senna should be **avoided** as their laxative action is unpredictable. Aloes, colocynth, and jalap should be **avoided** as they have a drastic purgative action.

Phenolphthalein can cause rashes. It may colour alkaline urine pink.

Stimulant laxative preparations on sale to the public (not prescribable on the NHS) together with their significant ingredients:
Agarol® (agar, liquid paraffin, phenolphthalein), **Alophen**® (aloin, phenolphthalein)
Beechams Pills® (aloin), **Bonomint**® (phenolphthalein), **Boots Compound Laxative**® (fig, senna), **Boots Senna Tablets**® (senna), **Brooklax**® (phenolphthalein)
Califig® (fig, senna), **Calsalettes**® (aloin), **Carters Little Pills**® (aloin, phenolphthalein)
Delax® (liquid paraffin, phenolphthalein)
Ex-lax Senna® (senna)
Fam-lax® (phenolphthalein, rhubarb)
Juno Junipah Salts® (juniper berry oil, sodium bicarbonate, sodium phosphate, sodium sulphate), **Juno Junipah Tablets**® (juniper berry oil, phenolphthalein, sodium chloride, sodium phosphate, sodium sulphate)
Kest® (magnesium sulphate, phenolphthalein)
Nylax® (bisacodyl, phenolphthalein, senna)
Potter's Cleansing Herb® (aloes, cascara, senna)
Reguletts® (phenolphthalein), **Rhuaka**® (cascara, rhubarb, senna)
Senlax® (senna), **Sure-Lax**® (phenolphthalein)

1.6.3   Faecal softeners
Liquid paraffin, the classical lubricant, has disadvantages (see below). Bulk laxatives (section 1.6.1) and non ionic surfactant 'wetting' agents e.g. docusate sodium (section 1.6.2) also have softening properties. Such drugs are useful for oral administration in the management of haemorrhoids and anal fissure; glycerol suppositories (section 1.6.2) are useful for rectal use.

Enemas containing **arachis oil** (ground-nut oil, peanut oil) lubricate and soften impacted faeces and promote a bowel movement.

ARACHIS OIL
Indications: see notes above
Dose: see below

Fletchers' Arachis Oil Retention Enema®
(Pharmax)
Enema, arachis (peanut) oil in 130-mL single-dose disposable packs. Net price 130 mL = £1.07
Dose: to soften impacted faeces, 130 mL; the enema should be warmed before use; CHILD (but see section 1.6) under 3 years not recommended; over 3 years reduce adult dose in proportion to body-weight (medical supervision only)

LIQUID PARAFFIN
Indications: constipation
Cautions: CSM recommends avoid prolonged use, and has contra-indicated in children less than 3 years of age
Side-effects: anal seepage of paraffin and consequent anal irritation after prolonged use, granulomatous reactions caused by absorption of small quantities of liquid paraffin (especially from the emulsion), lipoid pneu-monia, and interference with the absorption of fat-soluble vitamins
Dose: see under preparation

Liquid Paraffin Oral Emulsion, BP
Oral emulsion, liquid paraffin 5 mL, vanillin 5 mg, chloroform 0.025 mL, benzoic acid solution 0.2 mL, methylcellulose-20 200 mg, saccharin sodium 500 micrograms, water to 10 mL
Dose: 10–30 mL at night when required
COUNSELLING. Should not be taken immediately before going to bed

With phenolphthalein, see Other Stimulant Laxatives

1.6.4   Osmotic laxatives
These act by retaining fluid in the bowel by osmosis or by changing the pattern of water distribution in the faeces.

Saline purgatives such as **magnesium hydroxide** are commonly abused but are satisfactory for occasional use; adequate fluid intake should be maintained. **Magnesium salts** are useful where rapid bowel evacuation is required. **Sodium salts** should be avoided as they may give rise to sodium and water retention in susceptible individuals. **Phosphate enemas** are useful in bowel clearance before radiology, endoscopy, and surgery.

Lactulose is a semi-synthetic disaccharide which is not absorbed from the gastro-intestinal tract. It produces an osmotic diarrhoea of low faecal pH, and discourages the proliferation of ammonia-producing organisms. It is therefore useful in the treatment of *hepatic encephalopathy*. **Lactitol** is a similar disaccharide.

LACTITOL
Indications; Contra-indications; Side-effects: see under Lactulose
Dose: constipation, initially 20 g daily in a single dose with morning or evening meal, subsequently adjusted to produce one stool daily (dose of 10 g daily may be sufficient); CHILD (but see section 1.6) 1–6 years 2.5–5 g, 6–12 years 5–10 g, 12–16 years 10–20 g daily, subsequently adjusted to produce one stool daily
Hepatic encephalopathy, 500–700 mg/kg daily in 3 divided doses with meals, subsequently adjusted to produce 2 soft stools daily
By nasogastric administration, as a 40% solution (200 g/500 mL), 1–2 mL/kg body-weight daily
COUNSELLING. Powder should be mixed with food or liquid and one to two glasses of liquid should be drunk with the meal

Lactitol (Non-proprietary)
Powder, lactitol 10 g/sachet. Net price 10-sachet pack = £1.00. Counselling, see above
Available from Novartis Consumer Health

LACTULOSE
Indications: constipation (may take up to 48 hours to act), hepatic encephalopathy (portal systemic encephalopathy)

Contra-indications: galactosaemia, intestinal obstruction

Side-effects: flatulence, cramps, and abdominal discomfort

Dose: see under preparations below

COUNSELLING. Powder can be placed on tongue and washed down with water or other liquid *or* sprinkled on food *or* mixed with water or other liquid before swallowing

Lactulose (Non-proprietary)
Solution, lactulose 3.1–3.7 g/5 mL with other ketoses. Net price 200-mL pack = £1.05

Dose: constipation, initially 15 mL twice daily, adjusted according to patient's needs; CHILD (but see section 1.6) under 1 year 2.5 mL, 1–5 years 5 mL, 5–10 years 10 mL twice daily

Hepatic encephalopathy, 30–50 mL 3 times daily, subsequently adjusted to produce 2–3 soft stools daily

Available from APS, Ashbourne (Osmolax®), Berk (Laxose®), Cox, CP, Galen (Lactugal®), Norton, Sandoz (Regulose®), Solvay (NHS Duphalac®)

Note. A proprietary brand of lactulose 3.3 g/5 mL (Regulose®) is on sale to the public

Powder, lactulose 10 g/sachet, with other ketoses. Net price 30-sachet pack = £3.00. Counselling, see above

Dose: constipation, 10 g twice daily, adjusted according to patient's needs; CHILD (but see section 1.6) 5–10 years 5 g twice daily, under 5 years lactulose solution recommended

Hepatic encephalopathy, 20–30 g 3 times daily, subsequently adjusted to produce 2–3 soft stools daily

Available from Solvay (Lactulose Dry, Duphalac Dry®)

MACROGOLS
(Polyethylene glycols)

Indications; Dose: see under preparation below

Cautions: pregnancy and breast-feeding

Contra-indications: intestinal perforation or obstruction, paralytic ileus, severe inflammatory conditions of the intestinal tract (such as Crohn's disease, ulcerative colitis, and toxic megacolon)

Side-effects: abdominal distension and pain, nausea

Movicol® (Norgine)
Oral powder, macrogol '3350' (polyethylene glycol '3350') 13.125 g, sodium bicarbonate 178.5 mg, sodium chloride 350.7 mg, potassium chloride 46.6 mg/sachet. Net price 20-sachet pack = £9.85. Label: 13

Dose: chronic constipation, 2–3 sachets daily in divided doses; each sachet dissolved in 125 mL water and drunk immediately usually for max. 2 weeks, course repeated if required; ELDERLY initially 1 sachet daily; CHILD not recommended

MAGNESIUM SALTS
Indications; Dose: see under preparations

Cautions: renal impairment (risk of magnesium accumulation); hepatic impairment (see Appendix 2); elderly and debilitated; see also notes above; **interactions:** Appendix 1 (magnesium salts)

Contra-indications: acute gastro-intestinal conditions

Side-effects: colic

Magnesium hydroxide
Magnesium Hydroxide Mixture, BP
(Cream of Magnesia)
Aqueous suspension containing about 8% hydrated magnesium oxide. Do not store in cold place

Dose: constipation, 25–50 mL when required

Magnesium hydroxide with liquid paraffin
Liquid Paraffin and Magnesium Hydroxide Emulsion, BP
Oral emulsion, 25% liquid paraffin in aqueous suspension containing 6% hydrated magnesium oxide

Dose: constipation, 5–20 mL when required

Note. Liquid paraffin and magnesium hydroxide preparations on sale to the public include: NHS Cremaffin® and NHS Milpar®

Magnesium sulphate
Magnesium Sulphate. Label: 13, 23
Dose: rapid bowel evacuation (acts in 2–4 hours) 5–10 g in a tumblerful of water preferably before breakfast

Note. Magnesium sulphate is on sale to the public as Epsom Salts; NHS Andrews Liver Salts® (citric acid, magnesium sulphate, sodium bicarbonate) is also on sale to the public

Bowel evacuation before radiography and surgery
Section 1.6.5

PHOSPHATES (RECTAL)
Indications: rectal use in constipation; bowel evacuation before abdominal radiological procedures, endoscopy, and surgery

Cautions: elderly and debilitated; see also notes above

Contra-indications: acute gastro-intestinal conditions

Side-effects: local irritation

Dose: see below

Carbalax® (Pharmax)
Suppositories, sodium acid phosphate 1.69 g (as anhydrous salt) in an effervescent basis. Net price 12 = £2.24

Dose: constipation, 1 suppository, inserted 30 minutes before evacuation is required; moisten with water before use; CHILD, not recommended

Fleet® Ready-to-use Enema (De Witt)
Enema, sodium acid phosphate 21.4 g, sodium phosphate 9.4 g/118 mL. Net price single-dose pack (standard tube) = 46p

Dose: ADULT and CHILD (but see section 1.6) over 12 years, 118 mL; CHILD 3–12 years, on doctor's advice only (under 3 years not recommended)

Fletchers' Phosphate Enema® (Pharmax)
Enema, sodium acid phosphate 12.8 g, sodium phosphate 10.24 g, purified water, freshly boiled and cooled, to 128 mL (corresponds to Phosphates Enema Formula B). Net price 128 mL with standard tube = 46p, with long rectal tube = 64p

Dose: 128 mL; CHILD (but see section 1.6) over 3 years, reduced according to body weight (under 3 years not recommended)

SODIUM CITRATE (RECTAL)

Indications: rectal use in constipation
Cautions: elderly and debilitated; see also notes above
Contra-indications: acute gastro-intestinal conditions
Dose: see below

Fleet® Micro-enema (De Witt)

Enema, sodium citrate 450 mg, sodium lauryl sulphoacetate 45 mg, together with glycerol, sorbitol, propylene glycol, and carbomer, in 5-mL single-dose disposable packs with nozzle. Net price 5 mL = 45p

Dose: ADULT and CHILD over 3 years, 5 mL (but see section 1.6)

Micolette Micro-enema® (Dexcel)

Enema, sodium citrate 450 mg, sodium lauryl sulphoacetate 45 mg, glycerol 625 mg, together with citric acid, potassium sorbate, and sorbitol in a viscous solution, in 5-mL single-dose disposable packs with nozzle. Net price 5 mL = 32p

Dose: ADULT and CHILD over 3 years, 5–10 mL (but see section 1.6)

Micralax Micro-enema® (Evans)

Enema, sodium citrate 450 mg, sodium alkylsulphoacetate 45 mg, sorbic acid 5 mg, together with glycerol and sorbitol in a viscous solution in 5-mL single-dose disposable packs with nozzle. Net price 5 mL = 45p

Dose: ADULT and CHILD over 3 years, 5 mL (but see section 1.6)

Relaxit Micro-enema® (Crawford)

Enema, sodium citrate 450 mg, sodium lauryl sulphate 75 mg, sorbic acid 5 mg, together with glycerol and sorbitol in a viscous solution in 5-mL single-dose disposable packs with nozzle. Net price 5 mL = 31p

Dose: ADULT and CHILD (but see section 1.6) 5 mL (insert only half nozzle length in child under 3 years)

1.6.5 Bowel cleansing solutions

Bowel cleansing solutions are used before colonic surgery, colonoscopy, or radiological examination to ensure the bowel is free of solid contents. They are **not** treatments for constipation.

BOWEL CLEANSING SOLUTIONS

Indications: see above
Cautions: pregnancy; renal impairment; heart disease; ulcerative colitis; diabetes mellitus; reflux oesophagitis; impaired gag reflex; unconscious or semiconscious or possibility of regurgitation or aspiration
Contra-indications: gastro-intestinal obstruction, gastric retention, gastro-intestinal ulceration, perforated bowel, congestive cardiac failure; toxic colitis, toxic megacolon or ileus
Side-effects: nausea and bloating; less frequently abdominal cramps (usually transient—reduced by taking more slowly); vomiting

Citramag® (Bioglan)

Powder, effervescent, providing when dissolved in water magnesium citrate 17.7 g/sachet. Net price 10-sachet pack = £12.55. Label 10, patient information leaflet, 13, counselling, see below

Dose: bowel evacuation before radiological examination and surgery, 1 sachet dissolved in 200 mL water and taken at 8 a.m. on day before procedure; CHILD 5–9 years one-third adult dose; over 10 years one-half adult dose

COUNSELLING. The patient information leaflet advises that hot water is needed to make the solution and provides guidance on reconstitution; it also mentions need for high fluid, low residue diet beforehand (according to hospital advice), and explains that only clear fluids can be taken after Citramag® until procedure completed

Fleet Phospho-soda® (De Witt)

Oral solution, sugar-free, sodium dihydrogen phosphate dihydrate 24.4 g, disodium phosphate dodecahydrate 10.8 g/45 mL. Net price 2×45-mL bottles = £4.79. Label: 10 patient information leaflet, counselling

Dose:
First dose, in the morning (7 a.m.) on the day before the procedure, 45 mL diluted with half a glass (120 mL) of cool water, followed by one full glass (240 mL) of cool water

At mid-day, follow with at least 3 full glasses (720 mL) of water or clear liquids

Second dose, in the evening (7 p.m.) on the day before the procedure, 45 mL diluted with half a glass (120 mL) of cool water, followed by one full glass (240 mL) of cool water

Additional clear liquids may be taken until midnight if necessary

CHILD not recommended

Note. No solid foods may be taken for breakfast, lunch or evening meal on the day of taking the preparation

Klean-Prep® (Norgine)

Oral powder, macrogol '3350' (polyethylene glycol '3350') 59 g, anhydrous sodium sulphate 5.685 g, sodium bicarbonate 1.685 g, sodium chloride 1.465 g, potassium chloride 743 mg/sachet. Contains aspartame (see section 9.4.1). Net price 4 sachets = £8.39. Label: 10 patient information leaflet, counselling

Four sachets when reconstituted with water to 4 litres provides an iso-osmotic solution for bowel cleansing before surgery, colonoscopy or radiological procedures

Dose:, 250 mL (1 tumblerful) of reconstituted solution every 10–15 minutes, or by nasogastric tube 20–30 mL/minute, until 4 litres have been consumed or watery stools are free of solid matter; CHILD not recommended

The solution from all 4 sachets should be drunk within 4–6 hours (250 mL drunk rapidly every 10–15 minutes); flavouring such as clear fruit cordials may be added if required; to facilitate gastric emptying domperidone or metoclopramide may be given 30 minutes before starting.

Alternatively the administration may be divided into two, e.g. taking the solutions from 2 sachets on the evening before examination and the remaining 2 on the morning of the examination

After reconstitution the solution should be kept in a refrigerator and discarded if unused after 24 hours

Note. Contra-indicated in patients under 20 kg body-weight; allergic reactions reported

Picolax® (Nordic)

Oral powder, sugar-free, sodium picosulphate 10 mg/sachet, with magnesium citrate (for bowel evacuation before radiological procedure, endoscopy, and surgery). Net price 2 sachets = 59p. Label: 10, patient information leaflet, 13, counselling, see below

Dose: ADULT and CHILD over 9 years, 1 sachet in water in morning (before 8 a.m.) and a second in afternoon (between 2 and 4 p.m.) of day preceding procedure; CHILD 1–2 years quarter sachet morning and afternoon, 2–4 years half sachet morning and afternoon, 4–9 years 1 sachet morning and half sachet afternoon

Acts within 3 hours of first dose

Note. Low residue diet recomended for 2 days before procedure and copious intake of water or other clear fluids recommended during treatment

COUNSELLING. Patients should be warned that heat is generated on addition to water; for this reason the powder should be added initially to 30 mL (2 tablespoonfuls) of water; after 5 minutes (when reaction complete) the solution should be further diluted to 150 mL (about a tumblerful)

1.7   Preparations for haemorrhoids

1.7.1 Soothing haemorrhoidal preparations
1.7.2 Compound haemorrhoidal preparations with corticosteroids
1.7.3 Rectal sclerosants

Anal and perianal pruritus, soreness, and excoriation are best treated by application of bland ointments and suppositories (section 1.7.1). These conditions occur commonly in patients suffering from haemorrhoids, fistulas, and proctitis. Careful local toilet with attention to any minor faecal soiling, adjustment of the diet to avoid hard stools, the use of bulk-forming materials such as bran (section 1.6.1) and a high residue diet are helpful. In proctitis these measures may supplement treatment with corticosteroids or sulphasalazine (see section 1.5).

When necessary topical preparations containing **local anaesthetics** (section 1.7.1) or **corticosteroids** (section 1.7.2) are used provided perianal thrush has been excluded. Perianal thrush is best treated with **nystatin** by mouth and by local application (see sections 5.2, 7.2.2, and 13.10.2).

1.7.1   Soothing haemorrhoidal preparations

Soothing preparations containing mild astringents such as bismuth subgallate, zinc oxide, and hamamelis may give symptomatic relief in haemorrhoids. Many proprietary preparations also contain lubricants, vasoconstrictors, or mild antiseptics.

Local anaesthetics are used to relieve pain associated with *haemorrhoids*, and *pruritus ani* but good evidence is lacking. Lignocaine ointment (see section 15.2) is used before emptying the bowel to relieve pain associated with *anal fissure*. Alternative local anaesthetics include amethocaine, cinchocaine, and pramoxine, but they are more irritant. Local anaesthetic ointments can be absorbed through the rectal mucosa therefore excessive application should be **avoided**, particularly in infants and children. They should be used for short periods only (no longer than a few days) since they may cause sensitisation of the anal skin.

Soothing haemorrhoidal preparations on sale to the public together with their significant ingredients include:

Anacal® (heparinoid, laureth '9'), **Anodesyn**® (allantoin, lignocaine), **Anusol**® **cream** (bismuth oxide, Peru balsam, zinc oxide), **Anusol**® **ointment** and **suppositories** (bismuth oxide, bismuth subgallate, Peru balsam, zinc oxide)
Boots Haemorrhoid Ointment® (lignocaine, zinc oxide), **Boots Suppositories for Haemorrhoids**® (benzyl alcohol, glycol monosalicylate, methyl salicylate, zinc oxide)
Germoloids® (lignocaine, zinc oxide)
Hemocane® (benzoic acid, bismuth oxide, cinnamic acid, lignocaine, zinc oxide)
Lanacane® **cream** (benzocaine, chlorothymol, resorcinol)
Nupercainal® (cinchocaine)
Preparation H® (shark liver oil, yeast cell extract)

1.7.2   Compound haemorrhoidal preparations with corticosteroids

Corticosteroids are often combined with local anaesthetics and soothing agents in preparations for haemorrhoids. They are suitable for occasional short-term use after exclusion of infections, such as herpes simplex; see section 13.4 for general comments on topical corticosteroids and section 1.7.1 for comment on local anaesthetics.

PoM **Anugesic-HC**® (P-D)

Cream, benzyl benzoate 1.2%, bismuth oxide 0.875%, hydrocortisone acetate 0.5%, Peru balsam 1.85%, pramoxine hydrochloride 1%, zinc oxide 12.35%. Net price 30 g (with rectal nozzle) = £3.09

Apply night and morning and after a bowel movement; do not use for longer than 7 days; CHILD not recommended

Suppositories, buff, benzyl benzoate 33 mg, bismuth oxide 24 mg, bismuth subgallate 59 mg, hydrocortisone acetate 5 mg, Peru balsam 49 mg, pramoxine hydrochloride 27 mg, zinc oxide 296 mg. Net price 12 = £2.24

Insert 1 suppository night and morning and after a bowel movement; do not use for longer than 7 days; CHILD not recommended

PoM **Anusol-HC**® (P-D)

Ointment, benzyl benzoate 1.25%, bismuth oxide 0.875%, bismuth subgallate 2.25%, hydrocortisone acetate 0.25%, Peru balsam 1.875%, zinc oxide 10.75%. Net price 30 g (with rectal nozzle) = £2.90

Apply night and morning and after a bowel movement; do not use for longer than 7 days; CHILD not recommended

Note. A proprietary brand (Anusol Plus HC® ointment) is on sale to the public

Suppositories, benzyl benzoate 33 mg, bismuth oxide 24 mg, bismuth subgallate 59 mg, hydrocortisone acetate 10 mg, Peru balsam 49 mg, zinc oxide 296 mg. Net price 12 = £2.24

Additives: include tartrazine lake

Insert 1 suppository night and morning and after a bowel movement; do not use for longer than 7 days; CHILD not recommended

Note. A proprietary brand (Anusol Plus HC® suppositories) is on sale to the public

PoM **Betnovate**® (GlaxoWellcome)

Rectal ointment, betamethasone valerate 0.05%, lignocaine hydrochloride 2.5%, phenylephrine hydrochloride 0.1%. Net price 30 g (with applicator) = £1.50

Apply 2–3 times daily until inflammation subsides then once daily, externally or by rectum; do not use for longer than 7 days; CHILD under 1 year not recommended

Perinal® (Dermal)

Spray application, hydrocortisone 0.2%, lignocaine hydrochloride 1%. Net price 30-mL pack = £6.87

Spray twice over the affected area up to 3 times daily; do not use for longer than 1–2 weeks; CHILD under 14 years not recommended

Proctocream HC® (Stafford-Miller)

Cream, hydrocortisone acetate 1%, pramoxine hydrochloride 1%. Net price 15 g (with applicator) = £2.24

ADULT over 18 years, apply morning and night after a bowel movement, externally or by rectum; do not use for longer than 7 days

PoM **Proctofoam HC**® (Stafford-Miller)

Foam in aerosol pack, hydrocortisone acetate 1%, pramoxine hydrochloride 1%. Net price 21.2-g pack (approx. 40 applications) with applicator = £4.71

Dose: haemorrhoids and proctitis, 1 applicatorful (4–6 mg hydrocortisone acetate, 4–6 mg pramoxine hydrochloride) by rectum 2–3 times daily and after a bowel movement (max. 4 times daily); do not use for longer than 7 days; CHILD not recommended

PoM **Proctosedyl**® (Hoechst Marion Roussel)

Ointment, cinchocaine (dibucaine) hydrochloride 0.5%, hydrocortisone 0.5%. Net price 30 g = £6.48 (with cannula)

Apply morning and night and after a bowel movement, externally or by rectum; do not use for longer than 7 days

Suppositories, cinchocaine (dibucaine) hydrochloride 5 mg, hydrocortisone 5 mg. Net price 12 = £2.93

Insert 1 suppository night and morning and after a bowel movement; do not use for longer than 7 days

PoM **Scheriproct**® (Schering Health)

Ointment, cinchocaine (dibucaine) hydrochloride 0.5%, prednisolone hexanoate 0.19%. Net price 30 g = £4.41

Apply twice daily for 5–7 days (3–4 times daily on 1st day if necessary), then once daily for a few days after symptoms have cleared

Suppositories, cinchocaine (dibucaine) hydrochloride 1 mg, prednisolone hexanoate 1.3 mg. Net price 12 = £2.08

Insert 1 suppository daily after a bowel movement, for 5–7 days (in severe cases initially 2–3 times daily)

PoM **Ultraproct**® (Schering Health)

Ointment, cinchocaine (dibucaine) hydrochloride 0.5%, fluocortolone hexanoate 0.095%, fluocortolone pivalate 0.092%. Net price 30 g (with rectal nozzle) = £4.57

Apply twice daily for 5–7 days (3–4 times daily on 1st day if necessary), then once daily for few days after symptoms have cleared

Suppositories, cinchocaine (dibucaine) hydrochloride 1 mg, fluocortolone hexanoate 630 micrograms, fluocortolone pivalate 610 micrograms. Net price 12 = £2.15

Insert 1 suppository daily after a bowel movement, for 5–7 days (in severe cases initially 2–3 times daily) then 1 suppository every other day for 1 week

PoM **Uniroid-HC**® (Unigreg)

Ointment, cinchocaine (dibucaine) hydrochloride 0.5%, hydrocortisone 0.5%. Net price 30 g (with applicator) = £4.43

Apply twice daily and after a bowel movement, externally or by rectum; do not use for longer than 7 days; CHILD under 12 years not recommended

Suppositories, cinchocaine (dibucaine) hydrochloride 5 mg, hydrocortisone 5 mg. Net price 12 = £2.00

Insert 1 suppository twice daily and after a bowel movement; do not use for longer than 7 days; CHILD under 12 years not recommended

PoM **Xyloproct**® (Astra)

Ointment (water-miscible), aluminium acetate 3.5%, hydrocortisone acetate 0.275%, lignocaine 5%, zinc oxide 18%. Net price 30 g (with applicator) = £3.39

Apply several times daily; short-term use only

Suppositories, aluminium acetate 50 mg, hydrocortisone acetate 5 mg, lignocaine 60 mg, zinc oxide 400 mg. Net price 10 = £1.59

Insert 1 suppository at night and after a bowel movement; short-term use only

1.7.3   Rectal sclerosants

Oily phenol injection is used to inject haemorrhoids particularly when unprolapsed.

PHENOL

Indications: see notes above

Side-effects: irritation, tissue necrosis

PoM **Oily Phenol Injection, BP**, phenol 5% in a suitable fixed oil. Net price 5-mL amp = £4.03

Dose: 2–3 mL into the submucosal layer at the base of the pile; several injections may be given at different sites, max. total injected 10 mL at any one time

Available from Evans

1.8   Stoma care

Prescribing for patients with stoma calls for special care. The following is a brief account of some of the main points to be borne in mind.

Enteric-coated and *modified-release* preparations are **unsuitable**, particularly in patients with ileostomies, as there may not be sufficient release of the active ingredient.

Laxatives. Enemas and washouts should **not** be prescribed for patients with ileostomies as they may cause rapid and severe dehydration.

Colostomy patients may suffer from constipation and whenever possible should be treated by increasing fluid intake or dietary fibre. **Bulk-forming drugs** (section 1.6.1) should be tried. If they are insufficient, as small a dose as possible of senna (section 1.6.2) should be used.

Antidiarrhoeals. Drugs such as **loperamide, codeine phosphate**, or **co-phenotrope** (diphenoxylate with atropine) are effective. Bulk-forming drugs (section 1.6.1) may be tried but it is often difficult to adjust the dose appropriately.

Antibiotics should **not** be given for an episode of acute diarrhoea.

Antacids. The tendency to diarrhoea from magnesium salts or constipation from aluminium salts may be increased in these patients.

Diuretics should be used with caution in patients with ileostomies as they may become excessively dehydrated and potassium depletion may easily occur. It is usually advisable to use a **potassium-sparing** diuretic (see section 2.2.3).

Digoxin. Patients with a stoma are particularly susceptible to hypokalaemia if on digoxin therapy and potassium supplements or a potassium-sparing diuretic may be advisable (for comment see section 9.2.1.1).

Potassium supplements. Liquid formulations are preferred to modified-release formulations (see above).

Analgesics. Opioid analgesics (see section 4.7.2) may cause troublesome constipation in colostomy patients. When a non-opioid analgesic is required **paracetamol** is usually suitable but anti-inflammatory analgesics may cause gastric irritation and bleeding.

Iron preparations may cause loose stools and sore skin in these patients. If this is troublesome and if iron is definitely indicated an intramuscular iron preparation (see section 9.1.1.2) should be used. Modified-release preparations should be **avoided** for the reasons given above.

Patients are usually given advice about the use of *cleansing agents, protective creams, lotions, deodorants,* or *sealants* whilst in hospital, either by the surgeon or by the health authority stoma care nurses. Voluntary organisations offer help and support to patients with stoma.

For details of **stoma appliances and associated products,** see Appendix 8.

1.9   Drugs affecting intestinal secretions

1.9.1   Drugs acting on the gall bladder
1.9.2   Drugs which increase gastric acidity
1.9.3   Aprotinin
1.9.4   Pancreatin

1.9.1   Drugs acting on the gall bladder

The use of laproscopic cholecystectomy and of endoscopic biliary techniques has limited the place of the bile acids **chenodeoxycholic acid** and **ursodeoxycholic acid** in gallstone disease. They are suitable for patients not treatable by other means who have mild symptoms, unimpaired gall bladder function, and small or medium sized radiolucent stones; they are not suitable for radio-opaque stones, which are unlikely to be dissolved. Patients should be given appropriate dietary advice (including avoidance of excessive cholesterol and calories) and should preferably be supervised in hospital because radiological monitoring is required. Long-term prophylaxis may be needed after complete dis-

solution of the gallstones has been confirmed (preferably with cholecystograms and ultrasound on two separate occasions) as gallstones may recur in up to 25% of patients within one year of stopping treatment.

Ursodeoxycholic acid is also used in primary biliary cirrhosis; it has also been tried in primary sclerosing cholangitis [unlicensed indication].

CHENODEOXYCHOLIC ACID

Indications: see notes above

Cautions: see notes above

Contra-indications: radio-opaque stones, pregnancy (see Appendix 4; non-hormonal contraceptive measures should be taken in women of childbearing age), non-functioning gall bladders, chronic liver disease, peptic ulceration, inflammatory diseases and other conditions of the small intestine and colon which interfere with entero-hepatic circulation of bile salts

Side-effects: diarrhoea particularly initially with high dosage (reduce dose for few days), pruritus, minor hepatic abnormalities and transient rise in serum transaminases

Dose: 10–15 mg/kg daily as a single dose at bedtime *or* in divided doses for 3–24 months, depending on size of stone; treatment is continued for at least 3 months after stones dissolve

PoM **Chendol 125®** (CP)

Capsules, orange/white, chenodeoxycholic acid 125 mg. Net price 224-cap pack = £47.50

PoM **Chenofalk®** (Thames)

Capsules, chenodeoxycholic acid 250 mg. Net price 60 = £25.20

With ursodeoxycholic acid

PoM **Combidol®** (CP)

Tablets, f/c, chenodeoxycholic acid 125 mg, ursodeoxycholic acid 125 mg. Net price 60-tab pack = £40.00

Dose: 3 tablets (patients greater than 120% of ideal body weight, 6 tablets) daily as a single dose at bedtime or in divided doses; treatment continued for approx. 3 months after stones dissolve; CHILD not recommended

URSODEOXYCHOLIC ACID

Indications: see notes above, under Dose and under preparations

Cautions: see notes above

Contra-indications: see under Chenodeoxycholic Acid; although chenodeoxycholic acid is contra-indicated in chronic liver disease, ursodeoxycholic acid preparations may be used in primary biliary cirrhosis

Side-effects: see under Chenodeoxycholic Acid; diarrhoea occurs rarely; liver changes have not been reported

Dose: dissolution of gallstones, 8–12 mg/kg daily as a single dose at bedtime *or* in two divided doses, for up to 2 years; treatment is continued for 3–4 months after stones dissolve

Primary biliary cirrhosis, see under *Ursofalk®*

PoM **Destolit**® (Hoechst Marion Roussel)
Tablets, scored, ursodeoxycholic acid 150 mg. Net price 60 = £18.92. Label: 21
PoM **Urdox**® (CP)
Tablets, f/c, ursodeoxycholic acid 300 mg, net price 60-tab pack = £30.24. Label: 21
PoM **Ursofalk**® (Thames)
Capsules, ursodeoxycholic acid 250 mg. Net price 60 = £34.65. Label: 21
Dose: primary biliary cirrhosis, 10–15 mg/kg daily in 2–4 divided doses
Dissolution of gallstones, see Dose, above
PoM **Ursogal**® (Galen)
Tablets, scored, ursodeoxycholic acid 150 mg, net price 60-cap pack = £18.92. Label: 21
Capsules, ursodeoxycholic acid 250 mg, net price 60-tab pack = £31.50. Label: 21

With chenodeoxycholic acid
See under Chenodcoxycholic acid

OTHER PREPARATIONS FOR BILIARY DISORDERS

A **terpene** mixture (Rowachol®) raises biliary cholesterol solubility. It is not considered to be a useful adjunct.
PoM **Rowachol**® (Rowa)
Capsules, green, e/c, borneol 5 mg, camphene 5 mg, cineole 2 mg, menthol 32 mg, menthone 6 mg, pinene 17 mg in olive oil. Net price 50-cap pack = £7.35. Label: 22
Dose: 1–2 capsules 3 times daily before food (but see notes above)
Interactions: Appendix 1 (*Rowachol*®)

1.9.2   Drugs which increase gastric acidity

Muripsin®, which contained glutamic acid hydrochloride, was formerly used in achlorhydria and hypochlorhydria but was of uncertain value. It has now been discontinued.

1.9.3   Aprotinin

Section 2.11.

1.9.4   Pancreatin

Supplements of pancreatin are given by mouth to compensate for reduced or absent exocrine secretion in cystic fibrosis, and following pancreatectomy, total gastrectomy, or chronic pancreatitis. They assist the digestion of starch, fat, and protein.

Pancreatin is inactivated by gastric acid therefore pancreatin preparations are best taken with food (or immediately before or after food). Gastric acid secretion may be reduced by giving cimetidine or ranitidine an hour beforehand (section 1.3). Concurrent use of antacids also reduces gastric acidity. The newer enteric-coated preparations such as *Creon*®, *Nutrizym GR*®, and *Pancrease*® deliver a higher enzyme concentration in the duodenum (provided the granules are swallowed whole without chewing). Higher-strength versions are now also available (**important:** CSM advice on p. 58).

Since pancreatin is also inactivated by heat, excessive heat should be avoided if preparations are mixed with liquids or food; the resulting mixtures should not be kept for more than one hour.

Dosage is adjusted according to size, number, and consistency of stools, so that the patient thrives; extra allowance may be needed if snacks are taken between meals.

Pancreatin can irritate the perioral skin and buccal mucosa if retained in the mouth, and excessive doses can cause perianal irritation. The most frequent side-effects are gastro-intestinal including nausea, vomiting, and abdominal discomfort; hyperuricaemia and hyperuricosuria have been associated with very high doses. Hypersensitivity reactions occur occasionally and may affect those handling the powder.

PANCREATIN

Note. The pancreatin preparations which follow are all of porcine origin
Indications; Cautions; Side-effects: see above and (for higher-strength preparations) see below

Creon® (Solvay)
Capsules, brown/yellow, enclosing buff-coloured e/c granules of pancreatin, providing: protease 210 units, lipase 8000 units, amylase 9000 units. Net price 100 = £13.33. Counselling, see dose
Dose: ADULT and CHILD initially 1–2 capsules with meals either taken whole or contents mixed with fluid or soft food (then swallowed immediately without chewing); higher doses may be required according to response
Granules, brown, e/c, pancreatin, providing: protease 1 125 units, lipase 20 000 units, amylase 22 500 units/sachet. Net price 40-sachet pack = £13.33. Counselling, see dose
Dose: ADULT and CHILD initially 1 sachet with meals either washed down or sprinkled on soft food (then swallowed immediately without chewing); higher doses may be required according to response
Note. One sachet of Creon granules contains the equivalent of 2½ Creon capsules
Creon® **10 000** (Solvay)
Capsules, brown/clear, enclosing buff-coloured e/c granules of pancreatin, providing: protease 600 units, lipase 10 000 units, amylase 8000 units. Net price 100-cap pack = £16.66. Counselling, see dose
Dose: ADULT and CHILD initially 1–2 capsules with meals either taken whole or contents mixed with fluid or soft food (then swallowed immediately without chewing)
Nutrizym GR® (Merck)
Capsules, green/orange, enclosing e/c pellets of pancreatin, providing minimum of: protease 650 units, lipase 10 000 units, amylase 10 000 units. Net price 100 = £13.15. Counselling, see dose
Dose: ADULT and CHILD 1–2 capsules with meals swallowed whole or contents sprinkled on soft food (then swallowed immediately without chewing); higher doses may be required according to response
Nutrizym 10® (Merck)
Capsules, red/yellow, enclosing e/c minitablets of pancreatin providing minimum of: protease 500 units, lipase 10 000 units, amylase 9000 units. Net price 100 = £13.15. Counselling, see dose
Dose: ADULT and CHILD 1–2 capsules with meals and 1 capsule with snacks, swallowed whole or contents taken with water or sprinkled on soft food (then swallowed immediately without chewing); higher doses may be required according to response

Pancrease® (Janssen-Cilag)

Capsules, enclosing e/c beads of pancrelipase USP, providing minimum of: protease 330 units, lipase 5000 units, amylase 2900 units. Net price 100 = £17.07. Counselling, see dose

Dose: ADULT and CHILD 1–2 (occasionally 3) capsules during each meal and 1 capsule with snacks swallowed whole or contents sprinkled on liquid or soft food (then swallowed immediately without chewing); higher doses may be required according to response

Pancrex® (Paines & Byrne)

Granules, pancreatin, providing minimum of: protease 300 units, lipase 5000 units, amylase 4000 units/g. Net price 300 g = £20.39. Label: 25, counselling, see dose

Dose: ADULT and CHILD 5–10 g just before meals washed down or mixed with liquid

Pancrex V® (Paines & Byrne)

Capsules, pancreatin, providing minimum of: protease 430 units, lipase 8000 units, amylase 9000 units. Net price 300-cap pack = £15.80. Counselling, see dose

Dose: ADULT and CHILD over 1 year 2–6 capsules with meals, swallowed whole or sprinkled on food; CHILD up to 1 year 1–2 capsules mixed with feeds

Capsules '125', pancreatin, providing minimum of: protease 160 units, lipase 2950 units, amylase 3300 units. Net price 300-cap pack = £9.72. Counselling, see dose

Dose: NEONATE 1–2 capsules with feeds

Tablets, e/c, s/c, pancreatin, providing minimum of: protease 110 units, lipase 1900 units, amylase 1700 units. Net price 300-tab pack = £4.51. Label: 5, 25, counselling, see dose

Dose: ADULT and CHILD 5–15 tablets before meals

Tablets forte, e/c, s/c, pancreatin, providing minimum of: protease 330 units, lipase 5600 units, amylase 5000 units. Net price 300-tab pack = £13.74. Label: 5, 25, counselling, see dose

Dose: ADULT and CHILD 6–10 tablets before meals

Powder, pancreatin, providing minimum of: protease 1400 units, lipase 25 000 units, amylase 30 000 units/g. Net price 300 g = £24.28. Counselling, see dose

Dose: ADULT and CHILD 0.5–2 g with meals washed down or mixed with liquid; NEONATE 250–500 mg with each feed

Higher-strength preparations

The **CSM** has advised of data associating the high-strength pancreatin preparations Nutrizym 22® and Pancreatin HL® with the development of large bowel strictures (fibrosing colonopathy) in children with cystic fibrosis aged between 2 and 13 years. There was only minimal use of Panzytrat® 25 000 during the study period but an identical preparation has been implicated in Denmark. No association was found with Creon® 25 000. The following was recommended:

—Pancrease HL®, Nutrizym 22®, Panzytrat® 25 000 [now discontinued] should not be used in children aged 15 years or less with cystic fibrosis;

—the total dose of pancreatic enzyme supplements used in patients with cystic fibrosis should not usually exceed 10 000 units of lipase per kg bodyweight daily;

—if a patient on any pancreatin preparation develops new abdominal symptoms (or any change in existing abdominal symptoms) the patient should be reviewed to exclude the possibility of colonic damage.

Possible risk factors are gender (boys at greater risk than girls), more severe cystic fibrosis, and concomitant use of laxatives. The peak age for developing fibrosing colonopathy is between 2 and 8 years.

COUNSELLING. It is important to ensure adequate hydration at all times in patients receiving higher-strength pancreatin preparations.

▼ PoM **Creon® 25 000** (Solvay)

Capsules, orange/yellow, enclosing brown-coloured e/c pellets of pancreatin, providing: protease (total) 1000 units, lipase 25 000 units, amylase 18 000 units. Net price 50-cap pack = £19.50. Counselling, see above and under dose

Dose: ADULT and CHILD initially 1 capsule with meals either taken whole or contents mixed with fluid or soft food (then swallowed immediately without chewing)

▼ PoM **Nutrizym 22®** (Merck)

Capsules, red/yellow, enclosing e/c minitablets of pancreatin, providing minimum of: protease 1100 units, lipase 22 000 units, amylase 19 800 units. Net price 100-cap pack = £30.30. Counselling, see above and under dose

Dose: 1–2 capsules with meals and 1 capsule with snacks, swallowed whole or contents taken with water or sprinkled on soft food (then swallowed immediately without chewing)

CHILD under 15 years not recommended

▼ PoM **Pancrease HL®** (Janssen-Cilag)

Capsules, enclosing light brown e/c minitablets of pancreatin, providing minimum of: protease 1250 units, lipase 25 000 units, amylase 22 500 units. Net price 100 = £36.18. Counselling, see above and under dose

Dose: 1–2 capsules during each meal and 1 capsule with snacks swallowed whole or contents sprinkled on liquid or soft food (then swallowed immediately without chewing)

CHILD under 15 years not recommended

2: Drugs used in the treatment of diseases of the
CARDIOVASCULAR SYSTEM

In this chapter, drug treatment is discussed under the following headings:

2.1   Positive inotropic drugs
2.2   Diuretics
2.3   Anti-arrhythmic drugs
2.4   Beta-adrenoceptor blocking drugs
2.5   Drugs affecting the renin-angiotensin system and some other antihypertensive drugs
2.6   Nitrates, calcium-channel blockers, and potassium-channel activators
2.7   Sympathomimetics
2.8   Anticoagulants and Protamine
2.9   Antiplatelet drugs
2.10   Myocardial infarction and fibrinolysis
2.11   Antifibrinolytic drugs and haemostatics
2.12   Lipid-regulating drugs
2.13   Local sclerosants

2.1   Positive inotropic drugs

2.1.1   Cardiac glycosides
2.1.2   Phosphodiesterase inhibitors

Positive inotropic drugs increase the force of contraction of the myocardium, for sympathomimetics with inotropic activity see section 2.7.1.

2.1.1   Cardiac glycosides

The principal actions of the cardiac glycosides are an increase in the force of myocardial contraction and a reduction in the conductivity within the atrioventricular node. They are most useful in the treatment of *supraventricular tachycardias*, especially for controlling ventricular response in atrial fibrillation. *Heart failure* may also be improved, even in patients in sinus rhythm, because of changes in the availability of intracellular calcium; this action is relatively unimportant, however, compared with the effects that can be achieved with diuretics and ACE inhibitors (see section 2.5.5). Except when needed to maintain satisfactory rhythm, cardiac glycosides can sometimes be withdrawn from patients with heart failure that is well controlled, without clinical deterioration. In the elderly who may be particularly susceptible to digitalis toxicity, cardiac glycosides should be used with special care in the management of heart failure without atrial fibrillation.

Loss of appetite, nausea, and vomiting are common toxic effects; sinus bradycardia, atrioventricular block, ventricular extrasystoles, and sometimes ventricular tachycardia or atrial tachycardia with block also occur—especially in the presence of underlying conducting system defects or myocardial disease. These unwanted effects depend both on the plasma concentrations of the drugs and on the sensitivity of the conducting system or myocardium, which is often increased in heart disease.

Thus, no one plasma concentration can indicate toxicity reliably but the likelihood increases progressively through the range 1.5 to 3 micrograms/litre for digoxin; higher steady-state concentrations must certainly be avoided. Measurements of plasma concentration are not necessary, however, unless problems occur during maintenance treatment. Hypokalaemia predisposes to toxicity, therefore diuretics used with digoxin should either be potassium sparing or should be given with potassium supplements.

Renal function is the most important determinant of digoxin dosage, whereas elimination of digitoxin depends on metabolism by the liver. Toxicity can often be managed by discontinuing therapy and correcting hypokalaemia if appropriate; serious manifestations require urgent specialist management. Digoxin-specific antibody fragments are available for reversal of life-threatening overdosage (see next page).

Digoxin is the glycoside most commonly used. In patients with *mild failure* a loading dose is not required, and a satisfactory plasma concentration can be achieved over a period of about a week, using a dose of 125 to 250 micrograms twice a day which may then be reduced having special regard to renal function. Because it has a long half-life maintenance doses need only be given once daily (but higher doses may be divided to avoid nausea). For management of *atrial fibrillation* the maintenance dose can usually be governed by ventricular response which should not be allowed to fall below 60 beats per minute except in special and recognised circumstances, e.g. with the concomitant administration of beta-blockers.

When *rapid control* is needed, digoxin may be given intravenously in a digitalising dose of 0.75 to 1 mg, preferably as an infusion (suggested volume 50 mL) over two or more hours (too rapid a rate of administration is associated with nausea and risk of arrhythmias); this is followed by normal maintenance therapy. The intramuscular route is not recommended.

Digitoxin has a long half-life and maintenance doses need only be given once daily or on alternate days.

CHILDREN. The dose is based on body-weight; they require a relatively larger dose of digoxin than adults.

DIGOXIN

Indications: heart failure, supraventricular arrhythmias (particularly atrial fibrillation)
Cautions: recent infarction; sick sinus syndrome; thyroid disease; reduce dose in the elderly and in renal impairment; avoid hypokalaemia; avoid rapid intravenous administration (nausea and risk of arrhythmias); pregnancy (see also Appendix 4); **interactions:** Appendix 1 (cardiac glycosides)

Contra-indications: intermittent complete heart block, second degree AV block; supraventricular arrhythmias caused by Wolff-Parkinson-White syndrome; hypertrophic obstructive cardiomyopathy (unless concomitant atrial fibrillation and heart failure — but with caution)

Side-effects: usually associated with excessive dosage, include: anorexia, nausea, vomiting, diarrhoea, abdominal pain; visual disturbances, headache, fatigue, drowsiness, confusion, delirium, hallucinations; arrhythmias, heart block; see also notes above

Dose: by mouth, rapid digitalisation, 1–1.5 mg in divided doses over 24 hours; less urgent digitalisation, 250–500 micrograms daily (higher dose may be divided)

Maintenance, 62.5–500 micrograms daily (higher dose may be divided) according to renal function and, in atrial fibrillation, on heart-rate response; usual range, 125–250 micrograms daily (lower dose may be appropriate in elderly)

Emergency loading dose *by intravenous infusion,* total dose of 0.5–1 mg given in divided doses with approx. half of the total dose given over 10–20 minutes (see also Cautions), followed by further fractions of the total dose (also given over 10–20 minutes) at intervals of 4–8 hours according to response (see notes above for an alternative regimen)

Note. The above doses may need to be reduced if digoxin (or another cardiac glycoside) has been given in the preceding 2 weeks. For plasma concentration monitoring blood should ideally be taken at least 6 hours after a dose

PoM **Digoxin** (Non-proprietary)

Tablets, digoxin 62.5 micrograms, net price 20 = 16p; 125 micrograms, 20 = 19p; 250 micrograms, 20 = 21p

Injection, digoxin 250 micrograms/mL, see Lanoxin®

Paediatric injection, digoxin 100 micrograms/mL (hosp. only, available from BCM Specials)

PoM **Lanoxin®** (GlaxoWellcome)

Tablets, digoxin 125 micrograms, net price 20 = 32p; 250 micrograms (scored), 20 = 32p

Injection, digoxin 250 micrograms/mL. Net price 2-mL amp = 65p

PoM **Lanoxin-PG®** (GlaxoWellcome)

Tablets, blue, digoxin 62.5 micrograms. Net price 20 = 32p

Elixir, yellow, digoxin 50 micrograms/mL. Do not dilute, measure with pipette. Net price 60 mL = £5.23. Counselling, use of pipette

DIGITOXIN

Indications: heart failure, supraventricular arrhythmias (particularly atrial fibrillation)

Cautions; Contra-indications; Side-effects: see under Digoxin

Dose: maintenance, 100 micrograms daily *or* on alternate days; may be increased to 200 micrograms daily if necessary

PoM **Digitoxin** (Non-proprietary)

Tablets, digitoxin 100 micrograms, net price 20 = £2.83

DIGOXIN-SPECIFIC ANTIBODY

Digoxin-specific antibody fragments are indicated for the treatment of known or strongly suspected digoxin or digitoxin overdosage, when measures beyond the withdrawal of the cardiac glycoside and correction of any electrolyte abnormality are felt to be necessary (see also notes above).

PoM **Digibind®** (GlaxoWellcome)

Injection, powder for preparation of infusion, digoxin-specific antibody fragments (F(ab)) 38 mg. Net price per vial = £87.44 (hosp. and poisons centres only)

Dose: see product literature

2.1.2   Phosphodiesterase inhibitors

Enoximone and **milrinone** are selective phosphodiesterase inhibitors which exert most of their effect on the myocardium. Sustained haemodynamic benefit has been observed after administration, but there is no evidence of any beneficial effect on survival.

ENOXIMONE

Indications: congestive heart failure where cardiac output reduced and filling pressures increased

Cautions: heart failure associated with hypertrophic cardiomyopathy, stenotic or obstructive valvular disease or other outlet obstruction; monitor blood pressure, heart rate, ECG, central venous pressure, fluid and electrolyte status, platelet count, hepatic enzymes; reduce dose in renal impairment; avoid extravasation; pregnancy and breast-feeding

Side-effects: ectopic beats; less frequently ventricular tachycardia or supraventricular arrhythmias (more likely in patients with pre-existing arrhythmias); hypotension; also headache, insomnia, nausea and vomiting, diarrhoea; occasionally, chills, oliguria, fever, urinary retention; upper and lower limb pain

Dose: by slow intravenous injection (rate not exceeding 12.5 mg/minute), diluted before use, initially 0.5–1 mg/kg, then 500 micrograms/kg every 30 minutes until satisfactory response or total of 3 mg/kg given; maintenance, initial dose of up to 3 mg/kg may be repeated every 3–6 hours as required

By intravenous infusion, initially 90 micrograms/kg/minute over 10–30 minutes, followed by continuous or intermittent infusion of 5–20 micrograms/kg/minute

Total dose over 24 hours should not normally exceed 24 mg/kg

PoM **Perfan®** (Hoechst Marion Roussel)

Injection, enoximone 5 mg/mL. For dilution before use. Net price 20-mL amp = £15.02

Note. Plastic apparatus should be used; crystal formation if glass used

---

MILRINONE

Indications: short-term treatment of severe congestive heart failure unresponsive to conventional maintenance therapy (not immediately after myocardial infarction); acute heart failure, including low output states, following heart surgery

Cautions; Side-effects: see under Enoximone; also correct hypokalaemia, monitor renal function, chest pain reported

Dose: by intravenous injection over 10 minutes, diluted before use, 50 micrograms/kg followed by *intravenous infusion* at a rate of 375–750 nanograms/kg/minute, usually for up to 12 hours following surgery or for 48–72 hours in congestive heart failure; max. daily dose 1.13 mg/kg

PoM **Primacor**® (Sanofi Winthrop)
Injection, milrinone (as lactate) 1 mg/mL. For dilution before use. Net price 10-mL amp = £17.39

2.2   Diuretics

2.2.1	Thiazides and related diuretics
2.2.2	Loop diuretics
2.2.3	Potassium-sparing diuretics
2.2.4	Potassium-sparing diuretics with other diuretics
2.2.5	Osmotic diuretics
2.2.6	Mercurial diuretics
2.2.7	Carbonic anhydrase inhibitors
2.2.8	Diuretics with potassium

Thiazides (section 2.2.1) are used to relieve oedema due to *heart failure* and, in lower doses, to reduce *blood pressure.*

Loop diuretics (section 2.2.2) are used in pulmonary oedema due to *left ventricular failure* and in patients with *longstanding heart failure* who no longer respond to thiazides.

Combination diuretic therapy may be effective in patients with *oedema resistant to treatment with one diuretic.* For example, a loop diuretic may be combined with a potassium-sparing diuretic (section 2.2.3) or with a thiazide or related diuretic (section 2.2.1). Vigorous diuresis, particularly with loop diuretics, may cause acute hypotension; rapid reduction of plasma volume should be avoided.

The combination of a thiazide with a potassium-sparing diuretic is of value in *less severe heart failure* when hypokalaemia is difficult to counter or when any degree of hypokalaemia should be avoided, as in patients with a continuing tendency to life-threatening ventricular arrhythmias.

ELDERLY. Diuretics are overprescribed in old age and the elderly are particularly susceptible to many of their side-effects. Lower initial doses should be used, and subsequently adjusted according to renal function. Diuretics should not be used on a long-term basis to treat simple gravitational oedema (which will usually respond to increased movement, raising the legs, and support stockings).

POTASSIUM LOSS. Hypokalaemia may occur with both thiazide and loop diuretics; the risk of hypokalaemia depends more on duration of action than on potency and is thus greater with thiazides than with loop diuretics.

Hypokalaemia is dangerous in severe coronary artery disease and in patients also being treated with cardiac glycosides. Often the use of potassium-sparing diuretics (section 2.2.3) avoids the need to take potassium supplements.

In hepatic failure hypokalaemia caused by diuretics can precipitate encephalopathy, particularly in alcoholic cirrhosis; diuretics may also increase the risk of hypomagnesaemia in alcoholic cirrhosis, leading to arrhythmias.

Potassium supplements are seldom necessary when thiazides are used in the routine treatment of hypertension. For further comment see section 9.2.1.1.

2.2.1   Thiazides and related diuretics

Thiazides and related compounds are moderately potent diuretics; they inhibit sodium reabsorption at the beginning of the distal convoluted tubule. They act within 1 to 2 hours of oral administration and most have a duration of action of 12 to 24 hours; they are usually administered early in the day so that the diuresis does not interfere with sleep.

In the management of *hypertension* a low dose of a thiazide, e.g. bendrofluazide 2.5 mg daily, produces a maximal or near-maximal blood pressure lowering effect, with very little biochemical disturbance. Higher doses cause more marked changes in plasma potassium, uric acid, glucose, and lipids, with no advantage in blood pressure control, and should not be used. Optimum doses for the control of *heart failure* may be larger, and long-term effects are of less importance.

Bendrofluazide (bendroflumethiazide) is widely used for mild or moderate heart failure when the patient is not desperately ill and severe pulmonary oedema is not present. It is also used for hypertension—alone in the treatment of mild hypertension or with other drugs in more severe hypertension.

Chlorthalidone (chlortalidone), a thiazide-related compound, has a longer duration of action than the thiazides and may be given on alternate days to control oedema. It is also useful if acute retention is liable to be precipitated by a more rapid diuresis or if patients dislike the altered pattern of micturition promoted by other diuretics.

Other thiazides and related diuretics (including benzthiazide, chlorothiazide, clopamide, cyclopenthiazide, hydrochlorothiazide, hydroflumethiazide, mefruside and polythiazide) do not offer any significant advantage over those mentioned above, and newer ones are more expensive than the longer-established thiazides.

Metolazone is particularly effective when combined with a loop diuretic (even in renal failure); profound diuresis may occur therefore the patient should be monitored carefully.

Cautionary label wordings, see inside back cover   Prices are **net**, see p.1

Xipamide resembles chlorthalidone structurally, and is more potent than the other thiazides.

Indapamide is also chemically related to chlorthalidone. It is claimed to lower blood pressure with less metabolic disturbance, particularly less aggravation of diabetes mellitus.

BENDROFLUAZIDE
(Bendroflumethiazide)

Indications: oedema, hypertension (see also notes above)

Cautions: may cause hypokalaemia, aggravates diabetes and gout; may exacerbate systemic lupus erythematosus; elderly (see notes above); pregnancy (see also Appendix 4) and breast-feeding; hepatic and renal impairment (avoid if severe, see Appendixes 2 and 3); see also notes above; porphyria (see section 9.8.2); **interactions:** Appendix 1 (diuretics)

Contra-indications: refractory hypokalaemia, hyponatraemia, hypercalcaemia; severe renal and hepatic impairment; symptomatic hyperuricaemia; Addison's disease

Side-effects: postural hypotension and mild gastro-intestinal effects; impotence (reversible on withdrawal of treatment); hypokalaemia (see also notes above), hypomagnesaemia, hyponatraemia, hypercalcaemia, hypochloraemic alkalosis, hyperuricaemia, gout, hyperglycaemia, and increases in plasma cholesterol concentration; less commonly rashes, photosensitivity; blood disorders (including neutropenia and thrombocytopenia—when given in late pregnancy neonatal thrombocytopenia has been reported); pancreatitis, intrahepatic cholestasis, and hypersensitivity reactions (including pneumonitis, pulmonary oedema, severe skin reactions) also reported

Dose: oedema, initially 5–10 mg in the morning, daily *or* on alternate days; maintenance 5–10 mg 1–3 times weekly

Hypertension, 2.5 mg in the morning; higher doses rarely necessary (see notes above)

PoM **Bendrofluazide** (Non-proprietary)
Tablets, bendrofluazide 2.5 mg, net price 20 = 12p; 5 mg, 20 = 11p
Available from APS, Ashbourne (Neo-Bendromax®), Berk (Berkozide®), Cox, Goldshield (Neo-NaClex®, 5 mg only), Hillcross, Knoll (Aprinox®), Norton

CHLOROTHIAZIDE

Indications: oedema, hypertension (see also notes above)

Cautions; Contra-indications; Side-effects: see under Bendrofluazide

Dose: oedema, usually 0.25–1 g daily in 1–2 divided doses; maintenance dose may be given daily, on alternate days, or less frequently; max. 1 g daily

Hypertension, initially 250 mg daily; max. 500 mg daily in single or divided doses (but see also notes above)

PoM **Saluric**® (MSD)
Tablets, scored, chlorothiazide 500 mg. Net price 20 = 46p

CHLORTHALIDONE
(Chlortalidone)

Indications: oedema, hypertension (see also notes above); diabetes insipidus (see section 6.5.2)

Cautions; Contra-indications; Side-effects: see under Bendrofluazide

Dose: oedema, initially 50 mg in the morning *or* 100–200 mg on alternate days, reduced for maintenance if possible

Hypertension, 25 mg, increased to 50 mg if necessary, in the morning (see also notes above)

PoM **Hygroton**® (Novartis)
Tablets, yellow, scored, chlorthalidone 50 mg, net price 28-tab pack = £1.37

CYCLOPENTHIAZIDE

Indications: oedema, hypertension (see also notes above)

Cautions; Contra-indications; Side-effects: see under Bendrofluazide

Dose: oedema, 250–500 micrograms daily in the morning; in heart failure may be increased to 1 mg daily (reduce to lowest effective dose for maintenance)

Hypertension, initially 250 micrograms daily in the morning, increased if necessary to 500 micrograms daily (see also notes above)

PoM **Navidrex**® (Novartis)
Tablets, scored, cyclopenthiazide 500 micrograms. Net price 28-tab pack = 50p
Additives: include gluten

HYDROCHLOROTHIAZIDE

Indications: oedema, hypertension (see also notes above)

Cautions; Contra-indications; Side-effects: see under Bendrofluazide

Dose: oedema, initially 25–50 mg daily, reduced for maintenance if possible; severe oedema in patients unable to tolerate loop diuretics, initially 75 mg daily

Hypertension, 25 mg daily, increased to 50 mg daily if necessary (see also notes above)

ELDERLY. In some patients (especially the elderly) an initial dose of 12.5 mg daily may be sufficient

PoM **HydroSaluric**® (MSD)
Tablets, both scored, hydrochlorothiazide 25 mg, net price 20 = 29p; 50 mg, 20 = 54p

HYDROFLUMETHIAZIDE

Indications: oedema, hypertension (see also notes above)

Cautions; Contra-indications; Side-effects: see under Bendrofluazide

Dose: oedema, initially 50–200 mg in the morning; maintenance 25–50 mg on alternate days

Hypertension, 25–50 mg daily (see also notes above)

PoM **Hydrenox**® (Knoll)
Tablets, hydroflumethiazide 50 mg. Net price 20 = 44p

INDAPAMIDE

Indications: essential hypertension

Cautions: renal impairment (stop if deterioration); monitor plasma potassium and urate concentrations in elderly, hyperaldosteronism, gout, or with concomitant cardiac glycosides; hyperparathyroidism (discontinue if hypercalcaemia); pregnancy and breast-feeding; **interactions:** Appendix 1 (diuretics)

Contra-indications: recent cerebrovascular accident, severe hepatic impairment

Side-effects: hypokalaemia, headache, dizziness, fatigue, muscular cramps, nausea, anorexia, diarrhoea, constipation, dyspepsia, rashes (erythema multiforme, epidermal necrolysis reported); rarely postural hypotension, palpitations, increase in liver enzymes, blood disorders (including thrombocytopenia), hyponatraemia, metabolic alkalosis, hyperglycaemia, increased plasma urate concentrations, paraesthesia, photosensitivity, impotence, renal impairment, reversible acute myopia; diuresis with doses above 2.5 mg daily

Dose: 2.5 mg in the morning

PoM Indapamide (Non-proprietary)

Tablets, s/c, indapamide 2.5 mg. Net price 60-tab pack = £5.41

Available from APS, Ashbourne (Nindaxa 2.5®), Bartholomew Rhodes, Cox, Hillcross, Norton, Opus (Opumide®), Trinity (Natramid®)

PoM Natrilix® (Servier)

Tablets, f/c, indapamide 2.5 mg. Net price 30-tab pack = £3.89, 60-tab pack = £7.63

Modified release

PoM Natrilix SR® (Servier)

Tablets, m/r, indapamide 1.5 mg. Net price 30-tab pack = £4.47. Label: 25

Dose: hypertension, 1 tablet daily, preferably in the morning

MEFRUSIDE

Indications: oedema, hypertension (see also notes above)

Cautions; Contra-indications; Side-effects: see under Bendrofluazide

Dose: initially 25–50 mg in the morning, increased to 75–100 mg for oedema; maintenance 25 mg daily *or* on alternate days (see also notes above)

PoM Baycaron® (Bayer)

Tablets, scored, mefruside 25 mg. Net price 20 = £1.41

METOLAZONE

Indications: oedema, hypertension (see also notes above)

Cautions; Contra-indications; Side-effects: see under Bendrofluazide; also profound diuresis on concomitant administration with frusemide (monitor patient carefully)

Dose: oedema, 5–10 mg in the morning, increased if necessary to 20 mg daily in resistant oedema, max. 80 mg daily

Hypertension, initially 5 mg in the morning; maintenance 5 mg on alternate days

PoM Metenix 5® (Hoechst Marion Roussel)

Tablets, blue, metolazone 5 mg. Net price 100-tab pack = £8.53

Note. The low dose formulation of metolazone (Xuret®) has been discontinued

POLYTHIAZIDE

Indications: oedema, hypertension (see also notes above)

Cautions; Contra-indications; Side-effects: see under Bendrofluazide

Dose: usually 1–4 mg daily; in hypertension 500 micrograms daily may be adequate

PoM Nephril® (Pfizer)

Tablets, scored, polythiazide 1 mg. Net price 28-tab pack = 79p

XIPAMIDE

Indications: oedema, hypertension (see also notes above)

Cautions; Contra-indications: see under Bendrofluazide

Side-effects: gastro-intestinal disturbances; mild dizziness; hypokalaemia, more rarely other electrolyte disturbances such as hyponatraemia

Dose: oedema, initially 40 mg in the morning, increased to 80 mg in resistant cases; maintenance 20 mg in the morning

Hypertension, 20 mg in the morning

PoM Diurexan® (ASTA Medica)

Tablets, scored, xipamide 20 mg. Net price 14-tab pack = £2.19

2.2.2   Loop diuretics

Loop diuretics are used in pulmonary oedema due to left ventricular failure; intravenous administration produces relief of breathlessness and reduces pre-load sooner than would be expected from the time of onset of diuresis. They are also used in patients with longstanding heart failure. Diuretic-resistant oedema (except oedema due to peripheral venous stasis or calcium-channel blockers) can be treated with a loop diuretic combined with a thiazide or related diuretic (e.g. bendrofluazide 5–10 mg daily or metolazone 5–20 mg daily).

Loop diuretics inhibit resorption from the ascending loop of Henle in the renal tubule and are powerful diuretics. Hypokalaemia may develop, and care is needed to avoid hypotension. If there is an enlarged prostate, urinary retention may occur; this is less likely if small doses and less potent diuretics are used initially.

Frusemide (furosemide) and **bumetanide** are similar in activity; both act within 1 hour of oral administration and diuresis is complete within 6 hours so that, if necessary, they can be given twice in one day without interfering with sleep. Following intravenous administration they have a peak effect within 30 minutes. The diuresis associated with these drugs is dose related. In patients with impaired renal function very large doses may occasionally be needed; in such doses both drugs can cause deafness and bumetanide can cause myalgia.

Ethacrynic acid (etacrynic acid) may also be given by injection when urgent diuresis is required; deafness may occur in renal failure. Ethacrynic acid is now rarely used.

Torasemide has properties similar to those of frusemide and bumetanide, and is indicated for oedema and for hypertension.

FRUSEMIDE
(Furosemide)

Indications: oedema, oliguria due to renal failure

Cautions: pregnancy (see also Appendix 4) and breast-feeding; may cause hypokalaemia and hyponatraemia; aggravates diabetes mellitus and gout; liver failure, prostatic enlargement; porphyria (see section 9.8.2); **interactions:** Appendix 1 (diuretics)

Contra-indications: precomatose states associated with liver cirrhosis; renal failure with anuria

Side-effects: hyponatraemia, hypokalaemia, and hypomagnesaemia (see also section 2.2), hypochloraemic alkalosis, increased calcium excretion, hypotension; less commonly nausea, gastro-intestinal disturbances, hyperuricaemia and gout; hyperglycaemia (less common than with thiazides); temporary increase in plasma cholesterol and triglyceride concentrations; rarely rashes, photosensitivity and bone marrow depression (withdraw treatment), pancreatitis (with large parenteral doses), tinnitus and deafness (usually with large parenteral doses and rapid administration and in renal impairment)

Dose: by mouth, oedema, initially 40 mg in the morning; maintenance 20 mg daily *or* 40 mg on alternate days, increased in resistant oedema to 80 mg daily; CHILD 1–3 mg/kg daily

Oliguria, initially 250 mg daily; if necessary larger doses, increasing in steps of 250 mg, may be given every 4–6 hours to a max. of a single dose of 2 g (rarely used)

By intramuscular injection or slow intravenous injection (rate not exceeding 4 mg/minute), initially 20–50 mg; CHILD 0.5–1.5 mg/kg to a max. daily dose of 20 mg

By intravenous infusion (by syringe pump if necessary), in oliguria, initially 250 mg over 1 hour (rate not exceeding 4 mg/minute); if satisfactory urine output not obtained in the subsequent hour further 500 mg over 2 hours, then if no satisfactory response within subsequent hour, further 1 g over 4 hours, if no response obtained dialysis probably required; effective dose (up to 1 g) can be repeated every 24 hours

PoM Frusemide (Non-proprietary)

Tablets, frusemide 20 mg, net price 20 = 31p; 40 mg, 20 = 22p; 500 mg, 20 = £6.78
Various strengths available from APS, Ashbourne (Froop®), Berk (Dryptal®), Cox, CP (including Rusyde®), Hillcross, Norton

Oral solutions, sugar-free, frusemide 1 mg/mL available as Lasix® paediatric liquid; frusemide 4 mg, 8 mg, and 10 mg/mL available from Rosemont (special order)

Injection, frusemide 10 mg/mL, net price 2-mL amp = 25p
Available from Antigen, Evans, Phoenix (all also 5-mL amp)

PoM Lasix® (Hoechst Marion Roussel)

Tablets, all scored, frusemide 20 mg, net price 28-tab pack = 82p; 40 mg, 28-tab pack = £1.18; 500 mg (yellow), 20 = £11.44

Paediatric liquid, sugar-free, frusemide 1 mg/mL when reconstituted with purified water, freshly boiled and cooled, net price 150 mL = £1.10

Injection, frusemide 10 mg/mL, net price 2-mL amp = 25p
Note. Large volume frusemide injections available from Antigen, IMS (Min-I-Jet®)

BUMETANIDE

Indications: oedema, oliguria due to renal failure

Cautions; Contra-indications: see under Frusemide (but has been used in porphyria, see section 9.8.2)

Side-effects: see under Frusemide; also myalgia (see notes above)

Dose: by mouth, 1 mg in the morning, repeated after 6–8 hours if necessary; severe cases, increased up to 5 mg or more daily
ELDERLY, 500 micrograms daily may be sufficient

By intravenous injection, 1–2 mg, repeated after 20 minutes; when *intramuscular injection* considered necessary, 1 mg initially then adjusted according to response

By intravenous infusion, 2–5 mg over 30–60 minutes

PoM Bumetanide (Non-proprietary)

Tablets, bumetanide 1 mg, net price 28-tab pack = £1.71; 5 mg, 28-tab pack = £10.93
Available from CP, Hillcross

PoM Burinex® (Leo)

Tablets, both scored, bumetanide 1 mg, net price 28-tab pack = £1.72; 5 mg, 20 = £7.81

Liquid, green, sugar-free, bumetanide 1 mg/5 mL. Net price 150 mL = £3.32

Injection, bumetanide 500 micrograms/mL. Net price 2-mL amp = 40p; 4-mL amp = 69p; 10-mL amp = £1.46

ETHACRYNIC ACID
(Etacrynic Acid)

Indications: oedema where urgent diuresis essential

Cautions; Contra-indications; Side-effects: see under Frusemide and notes above; also contra-indicated in breast-feeding; gastro-intestinal disturbances more severe; also pain on injection

Dose: by slow intravenous injection or infusion, 50 mg, increased to 100 mg if necessary

PoM Edecrin® (MSD)

Injection, powder for reconstitution, ethacrynic acid (as sodium salt). Net price 50-mg vial = £1.26

TORASEMIDE

Indications: oedema, hypertension

Cautions; Contra-indications; Side-effects: see under Frusemide; avoid in pregnancy and breast-feeding

Dose: oedema, 5 mg once daily, preferably in the morning, increased if required to 20 mg once daily; usual max. 40 mg daily

Hypertension, 2.5 mg daily, increased if necessary to 5 mg once daily

PoM **Torem**® (Boehringer Mannheim)
Tablets, torasemide 2.5 mg, net price 28-tab pack = £4.25; 5 mg (scored), 28-tab pack = £6.23; 10 mg (scored), 28-tab pack = £9.16

2.2.3 Potassium-sparing diuretics

Amiloride and **triamterene** on their own are weak diuretics. They cause retention of potassium and are therefore used as a more effective alternative to giving potassium supplements with thiazide or loop diuretics. (See section 2.2.4 for compound preparations with thiazides or loop diuretics.)

Spironolactone is also a potassium-sparing diuretic, and potentiates thiazide or loop diuretics by antagonising aldosterone. It is of value in the treatment of the oedema of cirrhosis of the liver and is effective in oedema of heart failure, particularly when congestion has caused hepatic engorgement.

Spironolactone is also used in primary hyperaldosteronism (Conn's syndrome).

Potassium canrenoate has similar uses to spironolactone, but can be given parenterally. It is metabolised to canrenone, which is also a metabolite of spironolactone.

Potassium supplements must **not** be given with potassium-sparing diuretics. It is also important to bear in mind that administration of a potassium-sparing diuretic to a patient receiving an ACE inhibitor can cause severe hyperkalaemia.

AMILORIDE HYDROCHLORIDE

Indications: oedema, potassium conservation with thiazide and loop diuretics
Cautions: pregnancy and breast-feeding; monitor in renal impairment (avoid if moderate to severe, see also Appendix 3); diabetes mellitus; elderly; **interactions:** Appendix 1 (diuretics)
Contra-indications: hyperkalaemia, renal failure
Side-effects: include gastro-intestinal disturbances, dry mouth, rashes, confusion, postural hypotension, hyperkalaemia, hyponatraemia
Dose: used alone, initially 10 mg daily *or* 5 mg twice daily, adjusted according to response; max. 20 mg daily

With other diuretics, congestive heart failure and hypertension, initially 5–10 mg daily; cirrhosis with ascites, initially 5 mg daily

PoM **Amiloride** (Non-proprietary)
Tablets, amiloride hydrochloride 5 mg, net price 20 = 39p
Available from APS, Ashbourne (Amilospare®), Berk (Berkamil®), Cox, CP, Hillcross, Norton
Oral solution, sugar-free, amiloride hydrochloride 5 mg/5 mL, net price 125 mL = £31.50
Available from Rosemont (Amilamont®)

Compound preparations with thiazide or loop diuretics, see section 2.2.4

TRIAMTERENE

Indications: oedema, potassium conservation with thiazide and loop diuretics
Cautions; Contra-indications: see under Amiloride Hydrochloride; may cause blue fluorescence of urine
Side-effects: include gastro-intestinal disturbances, dry mouth, rashes; slight decrease in blood pressure, hyperkalaemia, hyponatraemia; photosensitivity and blood disorders also reported; triamterene found in kidney stones
Dose: initially 150–250 mg daily, reducing to alternate days after 1 week; taken in divided doses after breakfast and lunch; lower initial dose when given with other diuretics
COUNSELLING. Urine may look slightly blue in some lights

PoM **Dytac**® (Pharmark)
Capsules, maroon, triamterene 50 mg. Net price 30-cap pack = £13.96. Label: 14 (see above), 21

Compound preparations with thiazides or loop diuretics, see section 2.2.4

ALDOSTERONE ANTAGONISTS

POTASSIUM CANRENOATE

Indications: oedema associated with secondary hyperaldosteronism, liver failure, chronic decompensated heart disease
Cautions; Contra-indications; Side-effects: see under Spironolactone; nausea and vomiting may occur, particularly after high doses; pain and irritation at injection site
Dose: by slow intravenous injection or intravenous infusion, 200–400 mg daily (exceptionally 800 mg)

PoM **Spiroctan-M**® (Boehringer Mannheim)
Injection, potassium canrenoate 20 mg/mL. Net price 10-mL amp = 71p

SPIRONOLACTONE

Indications: oedema and ascites in cirrhosis of the liver, malignant ascites, nephrotic syndrome, congestive heart failure; primary hyperaldosteronism
Cautions: potential human metabolic products carcinogenic in *rodents*; elderly; hepatic impairment; renal impairment (avoid if moderate to severe); monitor electrolytes (discontinue if hyperkalaemia occurs); porphyria (see section 9.8.2); **interactions:** Appendix 1 (diuretics)
Contra-indications: hyperkalaemia, hyponatraemia, severe renal impairment; pregnancy and breast-feeding; Addison's disease
Side-effects: gastro-intestinal disturbances; impotence, gynaecomastia; menstrual irregularities; lethargy, headache, confusion; rashes; hyperkalaemia (see also Cautions); hyponatraemia; hepatotoxicity, osteomalacia, and blood disorders reported
Dose: 100–200 mg daily, increased to 400 mg if required; CHILD initially 3 mg/kg daily in divided doses

---

Cautionary label wordings, see inside back cover

Prices are **net**, see p.1

PoM **Spironolactone** (Non-proprietary)

Tablets, spironolactone 25 mg, net price 20 = 73p; 50 mg, 20 = £1.97; 100 mg, 20 = £2.33

Available from APS, Ashbourne (Spirospare®), Berk (Spirolone®), Cox, Hillcross, Lagap (Laractone®), Norton

Oral suspensions, sugar-free, spironolactone 5 mg/ 5 ml, 10 mg/5 ml, 25 mg/5 ml, 50 mg/5 ml and 100 mg/5 mL available from Rosemont (special order)

PoM **Aldactone®** (Searle)

Tablets, all f/c, spironolactone 25 mg (buff), net price 100-tab pack = £9.88; 50 mg (off-white), 100-tab pack = £19.76; 100 mg (buff), 28-tab pack = £11.07

PoM **Spiroctan®** (Boehringer Mannheim)

Tablets, both s/c, spironolactone 25 mg (blue), net price 100-tab pack = £7.22; 50 mg (green), 100-tab pack = £13.85

Capsules, green, spironolactone 100 mg. Net price 28-cap pack = £7.56

Compound preparations with thiazides or loop diuretics, see section 2.2.4

2.2.4 Potassium-sparing diuretics with other diuretics

Although it is preferable to prescribe thiazides (section 2.2.1) and potassium-sparing diuretics (section 2.2.3) separately, the use of fixed combinations may be justified if compliance is a problem. Potassium-sparing diuretics are not usually necessary in the routine treatment of hypertension, unless hypokalaemia develops. For **interactions**, see Appendix 1 (diuretics).

Amiloride with thiazides

PoM **Co-amilozide** (Non-proprietary)

Tablets, co-amilozide 2.5/25 (amiloride hydrochloride 2.5 mg, hydrochlorothiazide 25 mg). Net price 28-tab pack = £1.94

Available from CP, Du Pont (Moduret 25®), Lagap

Dose: hypertension, oedema, 1–4 tablets, increased if necessary to a max. of 8, daily

Tablets, co-amilozide 5/50 (amiloride hydrochloride 5 mg, hydrochlorothiazide 50 mg). Net price 20 = 73p

Available from APS, Ashbourne (Amilmaxco 5/50®), Baker Norton (Amil-Co®), Berk (Delvas®), Cox, CP, Du Pont (Moduretic®), Hillcross, Lagap, Lennon, Norton, Opus (Zida-Co®)

Dose: hypertension, oedema, 1–2 tablets, increased if necessary to max. of 4, daily

Oral solution, co-amilozide 5/50 (amiloride hydrochloride 5 mg, hydrochlorothiazide 50 mg)/5 mL. Net price 200 mL = £4.61

Available from Du Pont (Moduretic®)

Dose: as for co-amilozide 5 /50 tablets above (5 mL = 1 tablet)

PoM **Navispare®** (Novartis)

Tablets, f/c, orange, amiloride hydrochloride 2.5 mg, cyclopenthiazide 250 micrograms. Net price 28-tab pack = £2.06

Additives: include gluten

Dose: hypertension, 1–2 tablets in the morning

Amiloride with loop diuretics

PoM **Co-amilofruse** (Non-proprietary)

Tablets, co-amilofruse 2.5/20 (amiloride hydrochloride 2.5 mg, frusemide 20 mg). Net price 28-tab pack = £3.00, 56-tab pack = £6.21

Available from CP (Aridil®), Hillcross, Rhône-Poulenc Rorer (Frumil LS®)

Dose: oedema, 1 tablet in the morning

Tablets, co-amilofruse 5/40 (amiloride hydrochloride 5 mg, frusemide 40 mg). Net price 28-tab pack = £2.74

Available from Baker Norton (Fru-Co®), Cox, CP, Hillcross, Hoechst Marion Roussel (Lasoride®), Lagap, Rhône-Poulenc Rorer (Frumil®)

Dose: oedema, 1–2 tablets in the morning

Tablets, co-amilofruse 10/80 (amiloride hydrochloride 10 mg, frusemide 80 mg). Net price 28-tab pack = £7.10, 56-tab pack = £14.11

Available from CP (Aridil®), Rhône-Poulenc Rorer (Frumil Forte®)

Dose: oedema, 1 tablet in the morning

PoM **Burinex A®** (Leo)

Tablets, ivory, scored, amiloride hydrochloride 5 mg, bumetanide 1 mg. Net price 28-tab pack = £3.20

Dose: oedema, 1–2 tablets daily

Triamterene with thiazides

COUNSELLING. Urine may look slightly blue in some lights

PoM **Dyazide®** (SK&F)

Tablets, peach, scored, co-triamterzide 50/25 (triamterene 50 mg, hydrochlorothiazide 25 mg). Net price 30-tab pack = £2.41. Label: 14 (see above), 21

Dose: hypertension, 1 tablet daily after breakfast; oedema, 2 tablets daily (1 after breakfast and 1 after midday meal) increased to 3 daily if necessary (2 after breakfast and 1 after midday meal); usual maintenance, 1 daily or 2 on alternate days; max. 4 daily

Note. Tablets containing co-triamterzide 50/25 (triamterene 50 mg and hydrochlorothiazide 25 mg) are also available from Ashbourne (TriamaxCo®), Baker Norton (Triam-Co®)

PoM **Dytide®** (Pharmark)

Capsules, clear/maroon, triamterene 50 mg, benzthiazide 25 mg. Net price 30-cap pack = £13.96. Label: 14 (see above), 21

Dose: oedema, initially 3 capsules daily (2 after breakfast and 1 after midday meal) for 1 week then 1 or 2 on alternate days

PoM **Kalspare®** (Dominion)

Tablets, orange, f/c, scored, triamterene 50 mg, chlorthalidone 50 mg. Net price 28-tab pack = £3.19. Label: 14 (see above), 21

Dose: hypertension, oedema, 1–2 tablets in the morning

Triamterene with loop diuretics

COUNSELLING. Urine may look slightly blue in some lights

PoM **Frusene®** (Orion)

Tablets, yellow, scored, triamterene 50 mg, frusemide 40 mg. Net price 56-tab pack = £5.94. Label: 14 (see above), 21

Dose: oedema, ½–2 tablets daily in the morning

Spironolactone with thiazides

PoM **Co-flumactone** (Non-proprietary)

Tablets, co-flumactone 25/25 (hydroflumethiazide 25 mg, spironolactone 25 mg). Net price 100-tab pack = £22.83

Available from Baker Norton (Spiro-Co®), Searle (Aldactide 25®)

Dose: congestive heart failure, initially 4 tablets daily; range 1–8 daily

Tablets, co-flumactone 50/50 (hydroflumethiazide 50 mg, spironolactone 50 mg). Net price 28-tab pack = £8.92

Available from Baker Norton (Spiro-Co 50®), Searle (Aldactide 50®)

Dose: congestive heart failure, initially 2 tablets daily; range 1–4 daily

Spironolactone with loop diuretics

PoM **Lasilactone**® (Hoechst Marion Roussel)

Capsules, blue/white, spironolactone 50 mg, frusemide 20 mg. Net price 28-cap pack = £4.91

Dose: resistant oedema, 1–4 capsules daily

2.2.5 Osmotic diuretics

Osmotic diuretics are rarely used in heart failure as they may acutely expand the blood volume. **Mannitol** is used in cerebral oedema—a typical dose is 1 g/kg as a 20% solution given by rapid intravenous infusion.

MANNITOL

Indications: see notes above; glaucoma (section 11.6)

Cautions: extravasation causes inflammation and thrombophlebitis

Contra-indications: congestive cardiac failure, pulmonary oedema

Side-effects: chills, fever

Dose: by intravenous infusion, diuresis, 50–200 g over 24 hours, preceded by a test dose of 200 mg/kg by slow intravenous injection

Cerebral oedema, see notes above

PoM **Mannitol** (Non-proprietary)

Intravenous infusion, mannitol 10% and 20%

Available from Baxter

2.2.6 Mercurial diuretics

Mercurial diuretics are effective but are now almost never used because of their nephrotoxicity.

2.2.7 Carbonic anhydrase inhibitors

The carbonic anhydrase inhibitor **acetazolamide** is a weak diuretic and is little used for its diuretic effect. It is used for prophylaxis against mountain sickness [unlicensed indication] but is not a substitute for acclimatisation.

Acetazolamide and eye drops of dorzolamide inhibit the formation of aqueous humour and are used in glaucoma (section 11.6)

2.2.8 Diuretics with potassium

Many patients on diuretics do not need potassium supplements (section 9.2.1.1). For many of those who do, the amount of potassium in combined preparations may not be enough, and for this reason their use is to be discouraged.

Diuretics with potassium and potassium-sparing diuretics should **not** usually be given together.

COUNSELLING. Modified-release potassium tablets should be swallowed whole with plenty of fluid during meals while sitting or standing

PoM **Burinex K**® (Leo)

Tablets, bumetanide 500 micrograms, potassium 7.7 mmol for modified release. Net price 20 = 85p. Label: 25, 27, counselling, see above

PoM **Diumide-K Continus**® (ASTA Medica)

Tablets, f/c, white/orange, frusemide 40 mg, potassium 8 mmol for modified release. Net price 30-tab pack = £3.13. Label: 25, 27, counselling, see above

PoM **Lasikal**® (Hoechst Marion Roussel)

Tablets, white/yellow, f/c, frusemide 20 mg, potassium 10 mmol for modified release. Net price 100-tab pack = £5.31. Label: 25, 27, counselling, see above

PoM **Neo-NaClex-K**® (Goldshield)

Tablets, pink/white, f/c, bendrofluazide 2.5 mg, potassium 8.4 mmol for modified release. Net price 20 = £1.47. Label: 25, 27, counselling, see above

2.3 Anti-arrhythmic drugs

2.3.1   Management of arrhythmias

2.3.2   Drugs for arrhythmias

2.3.1 Management of arrhythmias

Management of an arrhythmia, apart from the treatment of associated heart failure, requires precise diagnosis of the type of arrhythmia, and electrocardiography is essential.

ECTOPIC BEATS. If spontaneous with a normal heart, these rarely require treatment beyond reassurance. If they are particularly troublesome, beta-blockers are sometimes effective and may be safer than other suppressant drugs.

ATRIAL FIBRILLATION. The ventricular rate can usually be controlled with digoxin. If adequate control at rest or during exercise cannot be achieved readily, a beta-blocker or verapamil may be added if ventricular function is adequate. In some cases other classes of drugs may be appropriate. Anticoagulants are indicated especially in valvular or myocardial disease, and in the elderly; younger patients with lone atrial fibrillation in the absence of heart disease probably do not require anticoagulation. Aspirin is less effective than warfarin at preventing emboli but may be appropriate if there are no other risk factors for stroke. Doses of aspirin within the range 75–300 mg daily are used.

ATRIAL FLUTTER. The ventricular rate can often be controlled with digoxin. Reversion to sinus rhythm (if indicated) is best achieved by appropriately synchronised d.c. shock, rather than by drug therapy. If the arrhythmia is long-standing a period of treatment with anticoagulants should be considered before cardioversion to avoid the complication of emboli.

PAROXYSMAL SUPRAVENTRICULAR TACHYCARDIA. In most patients this remits spontaneously or can be returned to sinus rhythm by reflex vagal stimulation with respiratory manoeuvres, prompt squatting, or pressure over one carotid sinus (**important**: pressure over carotid sinus should be restricted to monitored patients—it can be dangerous in recent ischaemia, digitalis toxicity, or the elderly).

If vagal stimulation fails, intravenous administration of adenosine is usually the treatment of choice; digitalisation or intravenous administration of a beta-blocker may also be effective. Intravenous administration of verapamil is useful for patients without myocardial or valvular disease (**important:** never in patients recently treated with beta-blockers, see p. 101). For arrhythmias that are poorly tolerated, synchronised d.c. shock usually provides rapid relief.

In cases of paroxysmal supraventricular tachycardia with block, digitalis toxicity should be suspected. In addition to stopping administration of the cardiac glycoside and giving potassium supplements, intravenous administration of a beta-blocker may be useful. Specific digoxin antibody is available if the toxicity is considered life-threatening (section 2.1.1).

ARRHYTHMIAS AFTER MYOCARDIAL INFARCTION. In patients with a paroxysmal tachycardia or rapid irregularity of the pulse it is best not to administer an antiarrhythmic until an ECG record has been obtained. If the condition of the patient is such that death due to the arrhythmia seems possible lignocaine should be given intravenously (see p. 73). Bradycardia, particularly if complicated by hypotension, should be treated with atropine sulphate, given intravenously in a dose of 0.3 to 1 mg. If the initial dose is effective it may be repeated if necessary.

VENTRICULAR TACHYCARDIA. Drug treatment is used both for the treatment of ventricular tachycardia and for prophylaxis of recurrent attacks that merit suppression. Ventricular tachycardia requires treatment most commonly in the acute stage of myocardial infarction, but the likelihood of this and other life-threatening arrhythmias diminishes sharply over the first 24 hours after the attack, especially in patients without heart failure or shock. Lignocaine is the preferred drug for emergency use. Other drugs are best administered under specialist supervision. Very rapid ventricular tachycardia causes profound circulatory collapse and should be treated urgently with d.c. shock.

Torsades de pointes is a special form of ventricular tachycardia which tends to occur in the presence of a long QT interval (usually drug induced, but hypokalaemia, severe bradycardia, and genetic predisposition may also be implicated). The episodes are usually self-limiting, but are frequently recurrent and may cause impairment (or loss) of consciousness. If not controlled, the arrhythmia may progress to ventricular fibrillation. Intravenous infusion of magnesium sulphate (section 9.5.1.3) is usually effective. Anti-arrhythmics (including lignocaine) may further prolong the QT interval, thus worsening the condition.

2.3.2   Drugs for arrhythmias

Anti-arrhythmic drugs can be classified clinically into those that act on supraventricular arrhythmias (e.g. verapamil), those that act on both supraventricular and ventricular arrhythmias (e.g. disopyramide), and those that act on ventricular arrhythmias (e.g. lignocaine).

They can also be classified according to their effects on the electrical behaviour of myocardial cells during activity:

Class Ia, b, c: membrane stabilising drugs (e.g. quinidine, lignocaine, flecainide respectively)
Class II: beta-blockers
Class III: amiodarone, bretylium, and sotalol (also Class II)
Class IV: calcium-channel blockers (includes verapamil but not the nifedipine group)

This latter classification (the Vaughan Williams classification) is of less clinical significance.

CAUTIONS. The negative inotropic effects of anti-arrhythmic drugs tend to be additive therefore special care should be taken if two or more are used, especially in impaired myocardial function. Most or all drugs that are effective in countering arrhythmias can also provoke them in some circumstances; moreover, hypokalaemia enhances the arrhythmogenic (pro-arrhythmic) effect of many drugs.

SUPRAVENTRICULAR ARRHYTHMIAS

Adenosine is usually the treatment of choice for terminating paroxysmal supraventricular tachycardia. As it has a very short duration of action (half-life only about 8 to 10 seconds, but prolonged in those taking dipyridamole), most side-effects are short lived. Unlike verapamil, adenosine may be used after a beta-blocker. Verapamil may be preferable to adenosine in asthma.

Oral administration of a **cardiac glycoside** (such as digoxin, section 2.1.1) is the treatment of choice in slowing ventricular response in cases of atrial fibrillation and atrial flutter. Intravenous digoxin, preferably infused slowly, is occasionally required if the ventricular rate needs rapid control.

Verapamil (section 2.6.2) is usually effective for supraventricular tachycardias. An initial intravenous dose (**important**: serious beta-blocker interaction hazard, see p. 101) may be followed by oral treatment; hypotension may occur with larger doses. It should not be used for tachyarrhythmias where the QRS complex is wide (i.e. broad complex) unless a supraventricular origin has been established beyond reasonable doubt. It is also contra-indicated in atrial fibrillation with pre-excitation (e.g.Wolff-Parkinson-White syndrome). It should not be used in children with arrhythmias without specialist advice; some supraventricular arrhythmias in childhood can be accelerated by verapamil with dangerous consequences.

Drugs for both supraventricular and ventricular arrhythmias include **amiodarone**, **beta-blockers**, **disopyramide**, **flecainide**, **procainamide**, **propafenone** and **quinidine**, see below under Supraventricular and Ventricular Arrhythmias.

ADENOSINE

Indications: rapid reversion to sinus rhythm of paroxysmal supraventricular tachycardias, including those associated with accessory pathways (e.g. Wolff-Parkinson-White syndrome); aid to diagnosis of broad or narrow complex supraventricular tachycardias

Cautions: atrial fibrillation or flutter with accessory pathway (conduction down anomalous pathway may increase); heart transplant (see below); **interactions:** Appendix 1 (adenosine)

Contra-indications: second- or third-degree AV block and sick sinus syndrome (unless pacemaker fitted); asthma

Side-effects: include transient facial flush, chest pain, dyspnoea, bronchospasm, choking sensation, nausea, light-headedness; severe bradycardia reported (requiring temporary pacing); ECG may show transient rhythm disturbances

Dose: by rapid intravenous injection into central or large peripheral vein, 3 mg over 2 seconds with cardiac monitoring; if necessary followed by 6 mg after 1–2 minutes, and then by 12 mg after a further 1–2 minutes; increments should not be given if high level AV block develops at any particular dose

Note. 3-mg dose ineffective in a number of patients, therefore higher initial dose sometimes used but patients with *heart transplant* are **very sensitive** to effects of adenosine, and should **not** receive higher initial dose. Also if essential to give with dipyridamole reduce initial dose to 0.5–1 mg.

PoM **Adenocor®** (Sanofi Winthrop)
Injection, adenosine 3 mg/mL in physiological saline. Net price 2-mL vial = £4.05 (hosp. only)
Note. Intravenous infusion of adenosine (Adenoscan®, Sanofi Winthrop) may be used in conjunction with radionuclide myocardial perfusion imaging in patients who cannot exercise adequately or for whom exercise is inappropriate—consult product literature

SUPRAVENTRICULAR AND VENTRICULAR ARRHYTHMIAS

Amiodarone is used in the treatment of tachycardia associated with the Wolff-Parkinson-White syndrome. It may only be used for the treatment of other arrhythmias when other drugs are ineffective or contra-indicated and should be initiated only under hospital or specialist supervision. These include paroxysmal supraventricular, nodal and

ventricular tachycardias, atrial fibrillation and flutter, and ventricular fibrillation. It may be given by intravenous infusion as well as by mouth, and has the advantage of causing little or no myocardial depression. Unlike oral amiodarone, intravenous amiodarone may act relatively rapidly.

Amiodarone has a very long half-life (extending to several weeks) and only needs to be given once daily (but high doses may cause nausea unless divided). Many weeks or months may be required to achieve steady-state plasma concentrations; this is particularly important when interactions with amiodarone are considered (see also Appendix 1).

Most patients taking amiodarone develop corneal microdeposits (reversible on withdrawal of treatment); these rarely interfere with vision, but drivers may be dazzled by headlights at night. Because of the possibility of phototoxic reactions, patients should be advised to shield the skin from light and to use a wide-spectrum sunscreen such as RoC Total Sunblock® (section 13.8.1) to protect against both long ultraviolet and visible light.

Amiodarone contains iodine and can cause disorders of thyroid function; both hypothyroidism and hyperthyroidism may occur. Clinical assessment is unreliable, and laboratory tests should be performed every 6 months. Thyroxine (T4) may be raised in the absence of hyperthyroidism; therefore tri-iodothyronine (T3), T4, and thyroid-stimulating hormone (thyrotrophin, TSH) should all be measured. A raised T3 and T4 with a very low or undetectable TSH concentration suggests the development of thyrotoxicosis. The thyrotoxicosis may be very refractory, and amiodarone should usually be withdrawn at least temporarily to help achieve control; treatment with carbimazole may be required. Hypothyroidism can be treated with replacement therapy without withdrawing amiodarone if it is essential.

Pneumonitis should always be suspected if new or progressive shortness of breath or cough develops in a patient taking amiodarone. Fresh neurological symptoms should raise the possibility of peripheral neuropathy.

Amiodarone is also associated with hepatotoxicity and treatment should be discontinued if severe liver function abnormalities or clinical signs of liver disease develop.

Beta-blockers act as anti-arrhythmic drugs principally by attenuating the effects of the sympathetic system on automaticity and conductivity within the heart, for details see section 2.4. For special reference to the role of **sotalol** in ventricular arrhythmias, see also p. 75

Disopyramide may be given by intravenous injection to control arrhythmias after myocardial infarction (including those not responding to lignocaine), but it impairs cardiac contractility. Oral administration of disopyramide is useful but it has an antimuscarinic effect which limits its use in patients with glaucoma or prostatic hypertrophy.

Flecainide belongs to the same general class as lignocaine. It may be of value for serious symptomatic ventricular arrhythmias. It may also be indicated for junctional re-entry tachycardias.

Preliminary results with paroxysmal atrial fibrillation are promising. As with quinidine it may precipitate serious arrhythmias in a small minority of patients (including those with otherwise normal hearts).

Procainamide can be given by intravenous injection to control ventricular arrhythmias, but prolonged oral use can cause a syndrome resembling systemic lupus erythematosus.

Propafenone is used for the prophylaxis and treatment of ventricular arrhythmias and also for some supraventricular arrhythmias. It has complex mechanisms of action, including weak beta-blocking activity (therefore great caution is needed in obstructive airways disease—contra-indicated if severe).

Quinidine may be effective in suppressing supraventricular and ventricular arrhythmias. It may itself precipitate rhythm disorders, and is best used on specialist advice; it can cause hypersensitivity reactions and gastro-intestinal upsets.

Drugs for supraventricular arrhythmias include **adenosine, cardiac glycosides** and **verapamil**, see above under Supraventricular Arrhythmias. Drugs for ventricular arrhythmias include **bretylium, lignocaine, mexiletine, moracizine**, and **phenytoin**, see below under Ventricular Arrhythmias.

AMIODARONE HYDROCHLORIDE

Indications: see notes above (should be initiated in hospital or under specialist supervision)

Cautions: liver-function and thyroid-function tests required before treatment and then every 6 months (see notes above for tests of thyroid function); chest x-ray required before treatment; heart failure; renal impairment; elderly; severe bradycardia and conduction disturbances in excessive dosage; intravenous use may cause moderate and transient fall in blood pressure (circulatory collapse precipitated by rapid administration or overdosage); porphyria (section 9.8.2); **interactions:** Appendix 1 (amiodarone)

Contra-indications: sinus bradycardia, sino-atrial heart block; unless pacemaker fitted avoid in severe conduction disturbances or sinus node disease; thyroid dysfunction; pregnancy and breast-feeding (see also Appendixes 4 and 5); iodine sensitivity; avoid *intravenous use* in severe respiratory failure, circulatory collapse, severe arterial hypotension

Side-effects: reversible corneal microdeposits (sometimes with night glare), rarely impaired vision due to optic neuritis; peripheral neuropathy and myopathy (usually reversible on withdrawal); bradycardia and conduction disturbances (see Cautions); phototoxicity and rarely persistent slate-grey skin discoloration (see also notes); hypothyroidism, hyperthyroidism, diffuse pulmonary alveolitis, pneumonitis, and fibrosis; raised serum transaminases (may require dose reduction or withdrawal if accompanied by acute liver disorders); jaundice, hepatitis and cirrhosis reported; rarely nausea, vomiting, metallic taste, tremor, nightmares, vertigo, headache, sleeplessness,

fatigue, alopecia, paraesthesia, benign raised intracranial pressure, impotence, epididymo-orchitis; ataxia, rashes (including exfoliative dermatitis), hypersensitivity including vasculitis, renal involvement and thrombocytopenia; haemolytic or aplastic anaemia; anaphylaxis on rapid injection, also bronchospasm or apnoea in respiratory failure

Dose: by mouth, 200 mg 3 times daily for 1 week reduced to 200 mg twice daily for a further week; maintenance, usually 200 mg daily or the minimum required to control the arrhythmia

By intravenous infusion via caval catheter, 5 mg/kg over 20–120 minutes with ECG monitoring; max. 1.2 g in 24 hours

PoM Amiodarone Hydrochloride (Non-proprietary)

Tablets, amiodarone hydrochloride 100 mg, net price 28-tab pack = £4.18; 200 mg, 28-tab pack = £6.44. Label: 11

Available from APS, Cox, Generics, Hillcross, Norton

PoM Cordarone X® (Sanofi Winthrop)

Tablets, both scored, amiodarone hydrochloride 100 mg, net price 28-tab pack = £5.00; 200 mg, 28-tab pack = £8.19. Label: 11

Injection, amiodarone hydrochloride 50 mg/mL. Net price 3-mL amp = £1.50. For dilution and use as an infusion

---

DISOPYRAMIDE

Indications: ventricular arrhythmias, especially after myocardial infarction; supraventricular arrhythmias

Cautions: discontinue if hypotension, hypoglycaemia, ventricular, tachycardia, ventricular fibrillation or torsades de pointes develop; atrial flutter or tachycardia with partial block, bundle branch block, heart failure (avoid if severe); prostatic enlargement; glaucoma; hepatic and renal impairment (see Appendixes 2 and 3); pregnancy and breast-feeding (see Appendixes 4 and 5); **interactions:** Appendix 1 (disopyramide)

Contra-indications: second- and third-degree heart block and sinus node dysfunction (unless pacemaker fitted); cardiogenic shock; severe uncompensated heart failure

Side-effects: ventricular tachycardia, ventricular fibrillation or torsades de pointes (usually associated with prolongation of QRS complex or QT interval—see Cautions above), myocardial depression, hypotension, AV block; antimuscarinic effects include dry mouth, blurred vision, urinary retention; gastro-intestinal irritation; psychosis, cholestatic jaundice, hypoglycaemia also reported (see Cautions above)

Dose: by mouth, 300–800 mg daily in divided doses

By slow intravenous injection, 2 mg/kg over at least 5 minutes to a max. of 150 mg, with ECG monitoring, followed immediately *either* by 200 mg *by mouth,* then 200 mg every 8 hours for 24 hours *or* 400 micrograms/kg/hour *by intravenous infusion;* max. 300 mg in first hour and 800 mg daily

---

PoM **Disopyramide** (Non-proprietary)

Capsules, disopyramide (as phosphate) 100 mg, net price 20 = £1.73; 150 mg, 20 = £2.57

Available from APS, Hillcross, Lagap (100 mg), Norton (100 mg)

PoM **Rythmodan®** (Hoechst Marion Roussel)

Capsules, disopyramide 100 mg (green/beige), net price 84-cap pack = £7.53; 150 mg, 84-cap pack = £10.99

Injection, disopyramide (as phosphate) 10 mg/mL, net price 5-mL amp = 68p

Modified release

PoM **Dirythmin SA®** (Astra)

Durules® (= tablets, m/r), f/c, disopyramide (as phosphate) 150 mg. Net price 20 = £2.47. Label: 25

Dose: 300 mg every 12 hours; max. 750 mg daily

PoM **Rythmodan Retard®** (Hoechst Marion Roussel)

Tablets, m/r, scored, f/c, disopyramide (as phosphate) 250 mg. Net price 56-tab pack = £16.24. Label: 25

Dose: 250–375 mg every 12 hours

FLECAINIDE ACETATE

Indications: (should be initiated in hospital)

Tablets and injection: AV nodal reciprocating tachycardia, arrhythmias associated with Wolff-Parkinson-White syndrome and similar conditions with accessory pathways, paroxysmal atrial fibrillation in patients with disabling symptoms (arrhythmias of recent onset will respond more readily)

Tablets only: symptomatic sustained ventricular tachycardia, premature ventricular contractions and/or non-sustained ventricular tachycardia causing disabling symptoms in patients resistant to or intolerant of other therapy

Injection only: ventricular tachyarrhythmias resistant to other treatment

Cautions: patients with pacemakers (especially those who may be pacemaker dependent because stimulation threshold may rise appreciably); avoid in sinus node dysfunction, atrial conduction defects, second-degree or greater AV block, bundle branch block or distal block unless pacing rescue available; atrial fibrillation following heart surgery; elderly (see Dose); hepatic and renal impairment (see Appendixes 2 and 3); pregnancy (toxicity in *animal* studies) and breast-feeding; **interactions:** Appendix 1 (flecainide)

Contra-indications: heart failure; history of myocardial infarction and either asymptomatic ventricular ectopics or asymptomatic non-sustained ventricular tachycardia; long-standing atrial fibrillation where no attempt has been made to convert to sinus rhythm; haemodynamically significant valvular heart disease

Side-effects: dizziness, visual disturbances (corneal deposits reported); arrhythmogenic (pro-arrhythmic) effect; rarely nausea and vomiting, photosensitivity; reversible increases in liver enzymes, jaundice; ataxia, peripheral neuropathy, pulmonary fibrosis, pneumonitis also reported

Dose: by mouth, ventricular arrhythmias, 100 mg twice daily; max. 400 mg daily (usually reserved for rapid control or in heavily built patients), reduced after 3–5 days if possible

Supraventricular arrhythmias, 50 mg twice daily, increased if required to max. 300 mg daily

ELDERLY. Rate of elimination may be reduced—care on dose adjustment

By slow intravenous injection, 2 mg/kg over 10–30 minutes, max. 150 mg, with ECG monitoring; followed if required by *infusion* at a rate of 1.5 mg/kg/hour for 1 hour, subsequently reduced to 100–250 micrograms/kg/hour for up to 24 hours; max. cumulative dose in first 24 hours, 600 mg; transfer to *oral* treatment, as above

PoM **Tambocor®** (3M)

Tablets, flecainide acetate 50 mg, net price 60-tab pack = £16.28; 100 mg (scored), 60-tab pack = £23.26

Injection, flecainide acetate 10 mg/mL. Net price 15-mL amp = £4.95

PROCAINAMIDE HYDROCHLORIDE

Indications: ventricular arrhythmias, especially after myocardial infarction; atrial tachycardia

Cautions: elderly; hepatic and renal impairment, asthma, myasthenia gravis; pregnancy; **interactions:** Appendix 1 (procainamide)

Contra-indications: heart block, heart failure, hypotension; systemic lupus erythematosus; not indicated for torsades de pointes (can exacerbate); breast-feeding

Side-effects: nausea, diarrhoea, rashes, fever, myocardial depression, heart failure, lupus erythematosus-like syndrome, agranulocytosis after prolonged treatment; psychosis and angioedema also reported

Dose: by mouth, ventricular arrhythmias, up to 50 mg/kg daily in divided doses, preferably controlled by measurement of plasma concentration (dosage intervals can range from 3–6 hours); atrial arrhythmias, higher doses may be required

By slow intravenous injection, rate not exceeding 50 mg/minute, 100 mg with ECG monitoring, repeated at 5-minute intervals until arrhythmia controlled; max. 1 g

By intravenous infusion, 500–600 mg over 25–30 minutes with ECG monitoring, followed by maintenance at rate of 2–6 mg/minute, then if necessary oral treatment as above, starting 3–4 hours after infusion

PoM **Pronestyl®** (Squibb)

Tablets, scored, procainamide hydrochloride 250 mg. Net price 100-tab pack = £4.70

Injection, procainamide hydrochloride 100 mg/mL. Net price 10-mL vial = £1.90

PROPAFENONE HYDROCHLORIDE

Indications: ventricular arrhythmias; paroxysmal supraventricular tachyarrhythmias which include paroxysmal atrial flutter or fibrillation and paroxysmal re-entrant tachycardias involving the AV node or accessory pathway, where standard therapy ineffective or contra-indicated

Cautions: heart failure; hepatic and renal impairment; elderly; pacemaker patients; pregnancy and breast-feeding (see Appendixes 4 and 5); great caution in obstructive airways disease owing to beta-blocking activity (contra-indicated if severe); **interactions:** Appendix 1 (propafenone)

Contra-indications: uncontrolled congestive heart failure, cardiogenic shock (except arrhythmia induced), severe bradycardia, uncontrolled electrolyte disturbances, severe obstructive pulmonary disease, marked hypotension; myasthenia gravis; unless adequately paced avoid in sinus node dysfunction, atrial conduction defects, second degree or greater AV block, bundle branch block or distal block

Side-effects: constipation, blurred vision, dry mouth (due to antimuscarinic action); dizziness, nausea and vomiting, fatigue, bitter taste, diarrhoea, headache, and allergic skin reactions reported; postural hypotension, particularly in elderly; bradycardia, sino-atrial, atrioventricular, or intraventricular blocks; arrhythmogenic (proarrhythmic) effect; rarely hypersensitivity reactions (cholestasis, blood disorders, lupus syndrome), seizures; myoclonus also reported

Dose: 70 kg and over, initially 150 mg 3 times daily after food under direct hospital supervision with ECG monitoring and blood pressure control (if QRS interval prolonged by more than 20%, reduce dose or discontinue until ECG returns to normal limits); may be increased at intervals of at least 3 days to 300 mg twice daily and, if necessary, to max. 300 mg 3 times daily; under 70 kg, reduce dose

ELDERLY may respond to lower doses

PoM **Arythmol**® (Knoll)
Tablets, both f/c, propafenone hydrochloride 150 mg, net price 90-tab pack = £19.48; 300 mg (scored), 60-tab pack = £19.48. Label: 21, 25

QUINIDINE

Indications: suppression of supraventricular tachycardias and ventricular arrhythmias (see notes above)

Cautions: 200-mg test dose to detect hypersensitivity reactions; **interactions:** Appendix 1 (quinidine)

Contra-indications: heart block

Side-effects: see under Procainamide Hydrochloride; also ventricular arrhythmias, thrombocytopenia, haemolytic anaemia; rarely granulomatous hepatitis; also cinchonism (see Quinine, section 5.4.1)

Dose: by mouth, quinidine sulphate 200–400 mg 3–4 times daily

Note. Quinidine sulphate 200 mg ≡ quinidine bisulphate 250 mg

PoM **Quinidine Sulphate** (Non-proprietary)
Tablets, quinidine sulphate 200 mg; 300 mg
Note. May be difficult to obtain

Modified release
PoM **Kinidin Durules**® (Astra)
Tablets, m/r, f/c, quinidine bisulphate 250 mg. Net price 100-tab pack = £11.05. Label: 25
Dose: 500 mg every 12 hours, adjusted as required

VENTRICULAR ARRHYTHMIAS

Bretylium is only used as an anti-arrhythmic drug in resuscitation. It is given both intramuscularly and intravenously but can cause severe hypotension, particularly after intravenous administration; nausea and vomiting can occur with either route. The intravenous route should only be used in emergency when there is doubt about absorption because of inadequate circulation.

Lignocaine (lidocaine) is relatively safe when used by slow intravenous injection and should be considered first for emergency use. Though effective in suppressing ventricular tachycardia and reducing the risk of ventricular fibrillation following myocardial infarction, it has not been shown to reduce mortality when used prophylactically in this condition. In patients with cardiac or hepatic failure doses may need to be reduced to avoid convulsions, depression of the central nervous system, or depression of the cardiovascular system.

Mexiletine may be given as a slow intravenous injection if lignocaine is ineffective; it has a similar action. Adverse cardiovascular and central nervous system effects may limit the dose tolerated; nausea and vomiting may prevent an effective dose being given by mouth.

Moracizine is a newer drug for the prophylaxis and treatment of serious and life-threatening ventricular arrhythmias. In common with other anti-arrhythmic drugs it may aggravate arrhythmias and exacerbate congestive heart failure.

Phenytoin (section 4.8.2) by slow intravenous injection was formerly used in ventricular arrhythmias particularly those caused by cardiac glycosides, but this use is now obsolete.

Tocainide was used for life-threatening symptomatic ventricular tachyarrhythmias associated with severely compromised left ventricular function in patients who did not respond to other therapy or for whom other therapy was contra-indicated; it is no longer available.

Drugs for both supraventricular and ventricular arrhythmias include **amiodarone**, **beta-blockers**, **disopyramide**, **flecainide**, **procainamide**, **propafenone** and **quinidine**, see above under Supraventricular and Ventricular Arrhythmias.

BRETYLIUM TOSYLATE
(Bretylium Tosilate)

Indications: ventricular arrhythmias resistant to other treatment

Cautions: do not give noradrenaline or other sympathomimetic amines; may exacerbate ventricular arrhythmias due to cardiac glycosides; **interactions:** Appendix 1 (adrenergic neurone blockers)

Contra-indications: phaeochromocytoma

Side-effects: hypotension, nausea and vomiting; tissue necrosis reported after intramuscular injection (rotate sites)

Dose: by slow intravenous injection, 5–10 mg/kg over 8–10 minutes (preferably 15–30 minutes) with blood pressure and ECG monitoring; may be repeated after 1–2 hours to a total dosage of 30 mg/kg (intravenous dose being diluted to 10 mg/mL in glucose 5% or sodium chloride intravenous infusion)
Maintenance 5–10 mg/kg *by intramuscular injection, by intravenous infusion* (over 15–30 minutes) every 6–8 hours, *or* 1–2 mg/minute *by continuous intravenous infusion*

PoM **Bretylate®** (GlaxoWellcome)
Injection, bretylium tosylate 50 mg/mL. Net price 10-mL amp = £19.81
PoM **Min-I-Jet® Bretylium Tosylate** (IMS)
Injection, bretylium tosylate 50 mg/mL. Net price 10-mL disposable syringe = £19.75

LIGNOCAINE HYDROCHLORIDE
(Lidocaine Hydrochloride)
Indications: ventricular arrhythmias, especially after myocardial infarction
Cautions: lower doses in congestive cardiac failure, in hepatic failure, and following cardiac surgery; elderly; **interactions:** Appendix 1 (lignocaine)
Contra-indications: sino-atrial disorders, all grades of atrioventricular block, severe myocardial depression; porphyria (see section 9.8.2)
Side-effects: dizziness, paraesthesia, or drowsiness (particularly if injection too rapid); other CNS effects include confusion, respiratory depression and convulsions; hypotension and bradycardia (may lead to cardiac arrest); hypersensitivity reported
Dose: by intravenous injection, in patients without gross circulatory impairment, 100 mg as a bolus over a few minutes (50 mg in lighter patients or those whose circulation is severely impaired), followed immediately by *infusion* of 4 mg/minute for 30 minutes, 2 mg/minute for 2 hours, then 1 mg/minute; reduce concentration further if infusion continued beyond 24 hours (ECG monitoring and specialist advice for infusion)
IMPORTANT. Following intravenous injection lignocaine has a short duration of action (lasting for 15–20 minutes). If an *intravenous infusion* is not immediately available the initial *intravenous injection* of 50–100 mg can be repeated if necessary once or twice at intervals of not less than 10 minutes

PoM **Lignocaine in Glucose Infusion** (Non-proprietary)
Infusion, lignocaine hydrochloride 0.1% (1 mg/mL) and 0.2% (2 mg/mL) in glucose intravenous infusion 5%. 500-mL containers
Available from Baxter
PoM **Min-I-Jet® Lignocaine** (IMS)
Injection, lignocaine hydrochloride 1% (10 mg/mL), net price 10-mL disposable syringe = £3.39; 2% (20 mg/mL), 5-mL disposable syringe = £3.07

PoM **Xylocard®** (Astra)
Injection 100 mg, lignocaine hydrochloride (anhydrous) 20 mg/mL. Net price 5-mL syringe = £1.61

MEXILETINE HYDROCHLORIDE
Indications: ventricular arrhythmias, especially after myocardial infarction
Cautions: hepatic impairment; close monitoring on initiation of therapy (including ECG, blood pressure, etc.); **interactions:** Appendix 1 (mexiletine)
Contra-indications: bradycardia, cardiogenic shock; high degree AV block (unless pacemaker fitted)
Side-effects: nausea, vomiting, constipation; bradycardia, hypotension, atrial fibrillation, palpitations, conduction defects, exacerbation of arrhythmias, torsades de pointes; drowsiness, confusion, convulsions, psychiatric disorders, dysarthria, ataxia, paraesthesia, nystagmus, tremor; jaundice, hepatitis, and blood disorders reported; see also notes above
Dose: by mouth, initial dose 400 mg (may be increased to 600 mg if opioid analgesics also given), followed after 2 hours by 200–250 mg 3–4 times daily
By intravenous injection, 100–250 mg at a rate of 25 mg/minute with ECG monitoring followed by *infusion* of 250 mg as a 0.1% solution over 1 hour, 125 mg/hour for 2 hours, then 500 micrograms/minute

PoM **Mexitil®** (Boehringer Ingelheim)
Capsules, mexiletine hydrochloride 50 mg (purple/red), net price 100-cap pack = £4.95; 200 mg (red), 100-cap pack = £11.87
Injection, mexiletine hydrochloride 25 mg/mL. Net price 10-mL amp = £1.49

Modified release
PoM **Mexitil PL®** (Boehringer Ingelheim)
Perlongets® (= capsules, m/r, each enclosing 5 miniature tablets), turquoise/scarlet, mexiletine hydrochloride 360 mg. Net price 60-cap pack = £12.71. Label: 25
Dose: 1 capsule twice daily

MORACIZINE HYDROCHLORIDE
Indications: ventricular arrhythmias in patients with underlying cardiac disease and history of ventricular fibrillation or sustained ventricular tachycardia, or of symptomatic non-sustained ventricular tachycardia, or of disabling symptoms due to premature ventricular contraction
Cautions: sick sinus syndrome; pre-existing conduction abnormalities; congestive heart failure; hepatic and renal impairment; pregnancy and breast-feeding; **interactions:** Appendix 1 (moracizine)
Contra-indications: second-degree or greater AV block (unless paced); cardiogenic shock

---

Side-effects: include gastro-intestinal disturbances; dizziness, headache, fatigue, palpitations, dyspnoea; arrhythmogenic (pro-arrhythmic effect); chest pain; congestive heart failure; reversible increases in liver enzymes, jaundice; thrombocytopenia

Dose: (initiated in hospital) usually 600–900 mg daily in 3 divided doses, adjusted by steps of 150 mg daily at intervals of 3 days; max. recommended daily dose 900 mg; rapid control, initially 400–500 mg, then 200 mg every 8 hours

Note. Patients well controlled on 3 divided doses daily may be given same total daily dosage in 2 divided doses (every 12 hours)

▼ PoM **Ethmozine**® (Monmouth)
Tablets, all f/c, moracizine hydrochloride 200 mg, net price 100-tab pack = £47.93; 250 mg, 100-tab pack = £59.36; 300 mg, 100-tab pack = £71.60

2.4   Beta-adrenoceptor blocking drugs

Beta-adrenoceptor blocking drugs (beta-blockers) block the beta-adrenoreceptors in the heart, peripheral vasculature, bronchi, pancreas, and liver.

Many beta-blockers are now available and in general they are all equally effective. There are, however, differences between them which may affect choice in treating particular diseases or individual patients; esmolol and sotalol are used for the management of arrhythmia only (see below).

Intrinsic sympathomimetic activity (ISA, partial agonist activity) represents the capacity of beta-blockers to stimulate as well as to block adrenergic receptors. **Oxprenolol**, **pindolol**, **acebutolol** and **celiprolol** have intrinsic sympathomimetic activity; they tend to cause less bradycardia than the other beta-blockers and may also cause less coldness of the extremities.

Some beta-blockers are *lipid soluble* and some are *water soluble*. **Atenolol**, **celiprolol**, **nadolol**, and **sotalol** are the most water-soluble; they are less likely to enter the brain, and may therefore cause less sleep disturbance and nightmares. Water-soluble beta-blockers are excreted by the kidneys; they accumulate in renal impairment and dosage reduction is therefore often necessary.

Beta-blockers with a *relatively short duration of action* have to be given two or three times daily. Many of these are, however, available in modified-release formulations so that administration once daily is adequate for hypertension. For angina twice-daily treatment may sometimes be needed even with a modified-release formulation. Some beta-blockers such as atenolol, betaxolol, bisoprolol, carvedilol, celiprolol, and nadolol have an intrinsically longer duration of action and need to be given only once daily.

All beta-blockers *slow the heart* and may induce myocardial depression and precipitate heart failure. They should not therefore be given to patients who have incipient cardiac failure or those with second- or third-degree AV block; they may, however, be used with caution in patients whose heart failure is well controlled. **Sotalol** may prolong the QT interval, and has occasionally caused life-threatening ventricular arrhythmias (**important:** particular care should be taken to avoid hypokalaemia in patients taking sotalol).

Labetalol, **celiprolol**, and **carvedilol** are beta-blockers which have in addition an arteriolar vasodilating action, by diverse mechanisms, and thus lower peripheral resistance. There is no evidence that these drugs have important advantages over other beta-blockers in the treatment of hypertension.

Beta-blockers may *precipitate asthma* and this effect can be dangerous; they should be **avoided** in patients with a history of asthma or chronic obstructive airways disease (unless no alternative treatment is available, when a cardioselective one should be used with extreme caution and under specialist supervision). Some, such as **atenolol**, **betaxolol**, **bisoprolol**, **metoprolol**, and (to a lesser extent) **acebutolol**, have less effect on the beta$_2$ (bronchial) receptors and are, therefore, relatively *cardioselective*, but they are **not** *cardiospecific*. They have a lesser effect on airways resistance but are **not** free of this side-effect.

Beta-blockers are also associated with *fatigue*, *coldness of the extremities* (may be less common with those with ISA, see above), and *sleep disturbances with nightmares* (may be less common with the water-soluble ones, see above).

Beta-blockers can lead to a small deterioration of *glucose tolerance* in diabetics; they also interfere with metabolic and autonomic responses to hypoglycaemia. Their use is not contra-indicated in diabetics, but cardioselective beta-blockers (see above) may be preferable and they should be avoided altogether in those with frequent episodes of hypoglycaemia.

HYPERTENSION. Beta-blockers are effective *antihypertensives* but their mode of action is not understood; they reduce cardiac output, alter baroceptor reflex sensitivity, and block peripheral adrenoceptors. Some beta-blockers depress plasma renin secretion. It is possible that a central effect may also explain their mode of action. Blood pressure can usually be controlled with relatively few side-effects. In general the dose of beta-blocker does not have to be as high as originally thought. The maximum dose of **oxprenolol** and **propranolol** necessary is probably 320 mg daily. **Atenolol** can usually be given in a dose of 50 mg daily and it is no longer considered necessary to increase to 100 mg.

Combined thiazide and beta-blocker preparations may help compliance but combined preparations should only be used when blood pressure is not adequately controlled by a thiazide or a beta-blocker alone. Beta-blockers reduce, but do not abolish, the tendency for diuretics to cause hypokalaemia.

Beta-blockers can be used to control the pulse rate in patients with *phaeochromocytoma*. However, they should never be used alone as beta-blockade without concurrent alpha-blockade may lead to a hypertensive crisis. For this reason phenoxybenzamine should always be used together with the beta-blocker.

ANGINA. By reducing cardiac work beta-blockers improve exercise tolerance and relieve symptoms in patients with *angina* (for further details on the management of stable angina see section 2.6). As with hypertension there is no good evidence of the superiority of any one drug, although occasionally a patient will respond better to one beta-blocker than to another. There is some evidence that sudden withdrawal may cause an exacerbation of angina therefore gradual reduction of dose is preferable when beta-blockers are to be stopped. There is a risk of precipitating heart failure when beta-blockers and verapamil are used together in established ischaemic heart disease (**important**: see p. 101).

MYOCARDIAL INFARCTION. For advice on the management of myocardial infarction see section 2.10.1.

Several studies have shown that some beta-blockers can reduce the recurrence rate of *myocardial infarction*. However, pre-existing heart failure, hypotension, bradyarrhythmias, and obstructive airways disease render beta-blockers unsuitable in some patients following a myocardial infarction. **Atenolol** and **metoprolol** may reduce early mortality after intravenous and subsequent oral administration in the acute phase, while **acebutolol**, **metoprolol**, **propranolol**, and **timolol** have protective value when started in the early convalescent phase. The evidence relating to other beta-blockers is less convincing; some have not been tested in trials of secondary protection. It is also not known whether the protective effect of beta-blockers continues after two years; it is possible that sudden cessation may cause a rebound worsening of myocardial ischaemia.

ARRHYTHMIAS. Beta-blockers act as *anti-arrhythmic drugs* principally by attenuating the effects of the sympathetic system on automaticity and conductivity within the heart. They may be used in conjunction with digoxin to control the ventricular response in atrial fibrillation, especially in patients with thyrotoxicosis. Beta-blockers are also useful in the management of supraventricular tachycardias, and are used to control those following myocardial infarction, see above.

Esmolol is a relatively cardioselective beta-blocker with a very short duration of action, used intravenously for the short-term treatment of supraventricular arrhythmias, sinus tachycardia, or hypertension, particularly in the peri-operative period. It may also be used in other situations, such as acute myocardial infarction, where sustained beta blockade might be hazardous.

Sotalol, a non-cardioselective beta-blocker with additional class III anti-arrhythmic activity, is used for prophylaxis in paroxysmal supraventricular arrhythmias. It also suppresses ventricular ectopic beats and non-sustained ventricular tachycardia. It has been shown to be more effective than lignocaine in the termination of sustained spontaneous ventricular tachycardia due to coronary disease or cardiomyopathy. However, it may induce torsades de pointes in susceptible patients.

THYROTOXICOSIS. Beta-blockers are used in pre-operative preparation for thyroidectomy. Administration of propranolol can reverse clinical symptoms of *thyrotoxicosis* within 4 days. Routine tests of increased thyroid function remain unaltered. The thyroid gland is rendered less vascular thus making surgery easier (see section 6.2.2).

OTHER USES. Beta-blockers have been used to alleviate some symptoms of *anxiety*; probably patients with palpitations, tremor, and tachycardia respond best (see also sections 4.1.2 and 4.9.3). Beta-blockers are also used in the *prophylaxis of migraine* (see section 4.7.4.2). Betaxolol, carteolol, levobunolol, metipranolol and timolol are used topically in *glaucoma* (see section 11.6).

PROPRANOLOL HYDROCHLORIDE

Indications: see under Dose

Cautions: pregnancy and breast-feeding (see also Appendixes 4 and 5); avoid abrupt withdrawal in angina; reduce oral dose of propranolol in liver disease; liver function deteriorates in portal hypertension; reduce initial dose in renal impairment; diabetes; myasthenia gravis; history of hypersensitivity—may increase sensitivity to allergens and result in more serious hypersensitivity response, also may reduce response to adrenaline (see also section 3.4.3); see also notes above; **interactions:** Appendix 1 (beta-blockers), **important:** verapamil interaction, see also p. 101

Contra-indications: asthma or history of obstructive airways disease (**important:** see Bronchospasm below), uncontrolled heart failure, Prinzmetal's angina, marked bradycardia, hypotension, sick sinus syndrome, second or third degree AV block, cardiogenic shock; phaeochromocytoma (apart from specific use with alpha-blockers, see also notes above)

BRONCHOSPASM. The CSM has advised that beta-blockers, including those considered to be cardioselective, should not be given to patients with a history of asthma or bronchospasm. However, in these patients there are very rare situations where there is no alternative to the use of a beta-blocker, when a cardioselective one is given with extreme caution and under specialist supervision

Side-effects: bradycardia, heart failure, hypotension, conduction disorders, bronchospasm, peripheral vasoconstriction, gastro-intestinal disturbances, fatigue, sleep disturbances; rare reports of rashes and dry eyes (reversible on withdrawal), exacerbation of psoriasis; see also notes above; **overdosage:** see Emergency Treatment of Poisoning, p. 22

Dose: by mouth, hypertension, initially 80 mg twice daily, increased at weekly intervals as required; maintenance 160–320 mg daily

Portal hypertension, initially 40 mg twice daily, increased to 80 mg twice daily according to heart-rate; max. 160 mg twice daily

Phaeochromocytoma (only with an alpha-blocker), 60 mg daily for 3 days before surgery *or* 30 mg daily in patients unsuitable for surgery

Angina, initially 40 mg 2–3 times daily; maintenance 120–240 mg daily

Arrhythmias, hypertrophic obstructive cardio-myopathy, anxiety tachycardia, and thyrotoxicosis (adjunct), 10–40 mg 3–4 times daily

Anxiety with symptoms such as palpitations, sweating, tremor, 40 mg twice daily, increased to 3 times daily if necessary

Prophylaxis after myocardial infarction, 40 mg 4 times daily for 2–3 days, then 80 mg twice daily, beginning 5 to 21 days after infarction

Migraine prophylaxis and essential tremor, initially 40 mg 2–3 times daily; maintenance 80–160 mg daily

By intravenous injection, arrhythmias and thyrotoxic crisis, 1 mg over 1 minute; if necessary repeat at 2-minute intervals; max. 10 mg (5 mg in anaesthesia)

Note. Excessive bradycardia can be countered with intravenous injection of atropine sulphate 0.6–2.4 mg in divided doses of 600 micrograms; for **overdosage** see Emergency Treatment of Poisoning, p. 22

PoM **Propranolol** (Non-proprietary)

Tablets, propranolol hydrochloride 10 mg, net price 20 = 5p; 40 mg, 20 = 7p; 80 mg, 20 = 20p 160 mg, 20 = 31p. Label: 8

Available from APS (Apsolol®), Ashbourne (Propanix®), Berk (Berkolol®), Cox, CP (Cardinol®), DDSA (Angilol®), Hillcross

Oral solution (syrup), propranolol hydrochloride 5 mg/5 mL, 10 mg/5 mL, 40 mg/5 ml, 50 mg/5 ml and 80 mg/5 mL available from Rosemont (special order)

PoM **Inderal®** (Zeneca)

Tablets, all pink, f/c, propranolol hydrochloride 10 mg, net price 100-tab pack = 89p; 40 mg, 100-tab pack = £2.40; 80 mg, 60-tab pack = £2.35. Label: 8

Injection, propranolol hydrochloride 1 mg/mL, net price 1-mL amp = 21p

Modified release

PoM **Half-Inderal LA®** (Zeneca)

Capsules, m/r, lavender/pink, propranolol hydrochloride 80 mg. Net price 28-cap pack = £5.40. Label: 8, 25

Note. Modified-release capsules containing propranolol hydrochloride 80 mg also available from APS, Tillomed (Half Beta Prograne®)

PoM **Inderal-LA®** (Zeneca)

Capsules, m/r, lavender/pink, propranolol hydrochloride 160 mg. Net price 28-cap pack = £6.67. Label: 8, 25

Note. Modified-release capsules containing propranolol hydrochloride 160 mg also available from APS, Ashbourne (Propanix SR®), Hillcross, Lagap (Bedranol SR®), Opus (Lopranol LA®), Tillomed (Beta Prograne®), Trinity (Probeta LA®)

With diuretic

PoM **Inderetic®** (Zeneca)

Capsules, propranolol hydrochloride 80 mg, bendrofluazide 2.5 mg. Net price 60-cap pack = £5.85. Label: 8

Dose: hypertension, 1 capsule twice daily

PoM **Inderex®** (Zeneca)

Capsules, pink/grey, propranolol hydrochloride 160 mg (m/r), bendrofluazide 5 mg. Net price 28-cap pack = £7.45. Label: 8, 25

Dose: hypertension, 1 capsule daily

ACEBUTOLOL

Indications: see under Dose

Cautions; Contra-indications; Side-effects: see under Propranolol Hydrochloride

Dose: hypertension, initially 400 mg once daily *or* 200 mg twice daily, increased after 2 weeks to 400 mg twice daily if necessary

Angina, initially 400 mg once daily *or* 200 mg twice daily; 300 mg 3 times daily in severe angina; up to 1.2 g daily has been used

Arrhythmias, 0.4–1.2 g daily in 2–3 divided doses

PoM **Sectral®** (Rhône-Poulenc Rorer)

Capsules, acebutolol (as hydrochloride) 100 mg (buff/white), net price 84-cap pack = £8.43; 200 mg (buff/pink), 56-cap pack = £10.80. Label: 8

Tablets, f/c, acebutolol 400 mg (as hydrochloride). Net price 28-tab pack = £10.48. Label: 8

With diuretic

PoM **Secadrex®** (Rhône-Poulenc Rorer)

Tablets, f/c, acebutolol 200 mg (as hydrochloride), hydrochlorothiazide 12.5 mg. Net price 28-tab pack = £9.90. Label: 8

Dose: hypertension, 1 tablet daily, increased to 2 daily as a single dose if necessary

ATENOLOL

Indications: see under Dose

Cautions; Contra-indications; Side-effects: see under Propranolol Hydrochloride; reduce dose in renal impairment (25-mg tablets available)

Dose: by mouth,

Hypertension, 50 mg daily (higher doses no longer considered necessary)

Angina, 100 mg daily in 1 or 2 doses

Arrhythmias, 50–100 mg daily

By intravenous injection, arrhythmias, 2.5 mg at a rate of 1 mg/minute, repeated at 5-minute intervals to a max. of 10 mg

Note. Excessive bradycardia can be countered with intravenous injection of atropine sulphate 0.6–2.4 mg in divided doses of 600 micrograms; for **overdosage** see Emergency Treatment of Poisoning, p. 22

By intravenous infusion, arrhythmias, 150 micrograms/kg over 20 minutes, repeated every 12 hours if required

Early intervention within 12 hours of infarction, 5–10 mg *by slow intravenous injection*, then *by mouth* 50 mg after 15 minutes, 50 mg after 12 hours, then 100 mg daily

PoM **Atenolol** (Non-proprietary)

Tablets, atenolol 25 mg, net price 28-tab pack = £1.96; 50 mg, 28-tab pack = £1.06; 100 mg, 28-tab pack = £1.48. Label: 8

Various strengths available from Antigen, APS, Ashbourne (Atenix®), Berk (Antipressan®), Cox, CP (Totamol®), Hillcross, Lagap, Norton, Tillomed

PoM **Tenormin®** (Stuart)

'25' tablets, f/c, atenolol 25 mg. Net price 28-tab pack = £4.62. Label: 8

LS tablets, orange, f/c, scored, atenolol 50 mg. Net price 28-tab pack = £5.35. Label: 8

Tablets, orange, f/c, scored, atenolol 100 mg. Net price 28-tab pack = £6.81. Label: 8

Syrup, sugar-free, atenolol 25 mg/5mL. Net price 300 mL = £8.14. Label: 8

Injection, atenolol 500 micrograms/mL. Net price 10-mL amp = £1.00 (hosp. only)

With diuretic

PoM **Co-tenidone** (Non-proprietary)

Tablets, co-tenidone 50/12.5 (atenolol 50 mg, chlorthalidone 12.5 mg), net price 28-tab pack = £3.63; co-tenidone 100/25 (atenolol 100 mg, chlorthalidone 25 mg), 28-tab pack = £5.02. Label: 8

Available from APS, Ashbourne (AtenixCo®), Berk (Tenchlor®), Bioglan, Cox, CP (Totaretic®), Hillcross, Norton

Dose: hypertension, 1 tablet daily (but see also under Dose above)

PoM **Kalten®** (Stuart)

Capsules, red/ivory, atenolol 50 mg, co-amilozide 2.5/25 (anhydrous amiloride hydrochloride 2.5 mg, hydrochlorothiazide 25 mg). Net price 28-cap pack = £8.39. Label: 8

Dose: hypertension, 1 capsule daily

PoM **Tenben®** (Galen)

Capsules, pink/red, atenolol 25 mg, bendroflu-azide 1.25 mg. Net price 56-cap pack = £4.95. Label: 8

Dose: hypertension, 1–2 capsules daily

PoM **Tenoret 50®** (Stuart)

Tablets, brown, f/c, co-tenidone 50/12.5 (atenolol 50 mg, chlorthalidone 12.5 mg). Net price 28-tab pack = £5.70. Label: 8

Dose: hypertension, 1 tablet daily

PoM **Tenoretic®** (Stuart)

Tablets, brown, f/c, co-tenidone 100/25 (atenolol 100 mg, chlorthalidone 25 mg). Net price 28-tab pack = £8.12. Label: 8

Dose: hypertension, 1 tablet daily (but see also under Dose above)

With calcium-channel blocker

Note. Only indicated when calcium-channel blocker or beta-blocker alone proves inadequate

PoM **Beta-Adalat®** (Bayer)

Capsules, reddish-brown, atenolol 50 mg, nife-dipine 20 mg (m/r). Net price 28-cap pack = £10.90. Label: 8, 25

Dose: hypertension, 1 capsule daily, increased if necessary to twice daily; elderly, 1 daily

Angina, 1 capsule twice daily

PoM **Tenif®** (Stuart)

Capsules, reddish-brown, atenolol 50 mg, nife-dipine 20 mg (m/r). Net price 28-cap pack = £10.63. Label: 8, 25

Dose: hypertension, 1 capsule daily, increased if necessary to twice daily; elderly, 1 daily

Angina, 1 capsule twice daily

BETAXOLOL HYDROCHLORIDE

Indications: hypertension; glaucoma (section 11.6)

Cautions; Contra-indications; Side-effects: see under Propranolol Hydrochloride

Dose: 20 mg daily (elderly patients 10 mg), increased to 40 mg if required

PoM **Kerlone®** (Lorex)

Tablets, f/c, scored, betaxolol hydrochloride 20 mg. Net price 28-tab pack = £7.51. Label: 8

BISOPROLOL FUMARATE

Indications: hypertension, angina

Cautions; Contra-indications; Side-effects: see under Propranolol Hydrochloride; reduce dose in hepatic and renal impairment

Dose: usual dose 10 mg daily (5 mg may be adequate in some patients); max. recommended dose 20 mg daily

PoM **Emcor®** (Merck)

LS Tablets, yellow, f/c, scored, bisoprolol fumarate 5 mg. Net price 28-tab pack = £8.56. Label: 8

Tablets, orange, f/c, scored, bisoprolol fumarate 10 mg. Net price 28-tab pack = £9.61. Label: 8

PoM **Monocor®** (Lederle)

Tablets, both f/c, bisoprolol fumarate 5 mg (pink), net price 28-tab pack = £8.56; 10 mg, 28-tab pack £9.61. Label: 8

With diuretic

PoM **Monozide 10®** (Lederle)

Tablets, f/c, bisoprolol fumarate 10 mg, hydro-chlorothiazide 6.25 mg. Net price 28-tab pack = £11.20. Label: 8

Dose: hypertension, 1 tablet daily

CARVEDILOL

Indications: hypertension, angina

Cautions; Contra-indications: as for Propranolol Hydrochloride; also hepatic impairment

Side-effects: postural hypotension, dizziness, headache, fatigue, gastro-intestinal disturbances, bradycardia; occasionally diminished peripheral circulation, peripheral oedema and painful extremities, dry mouth, dry eyes, eye irritation or disturbed vision, impotence, disturbances of micturition, influenza-like symptoms; rarely angina, A-V block, exacerbation of intermittent claudication or Raynaud's phenomenon; allergic skin reactions, exacerbation of psoriasis, nasal stuffiness, wheezing, depressed mood, sleep disturbances, paraesthesia, heart failure, changes in liver enzymes, thrombocytopenia, leucopenia also reported

Dose: hypertension, initially 12.5 mg daily, increased after 2 days to usual dose of 25 mg once daily; if necessary may be further increased at intervals of at least 2 weeks to max. 50 mg daily in single or divided doses; ELDERLY initial dose of 12.5 mg may provide satisfactory control

Angina, initially 12.5 mg twice daily, increased after 2 days to 25 mg twice daily

PoM **Eucardic®** (Boehringer Mannheim)

Tablets, both scored, carvedilol 12.5 mg (peach), net price 28-tab pack = £9.56, 56-tab pack = £19.12; 25 mg, 28-tab pack = £11.95, 56-tab pack = £23.90. Label: 8

CELIPROLOL HYDROCHLORIDE

Indications: mild to moderate hypertension

Cautions; Contra-indications: as for Propranolol Hydrochloride; also avoid in severe renal impairment

Side-effects: headache, dizziness, fatigue, nausea and somnolence; also bradycardia, bronchospasm

Dose: 200 mg once daily in the morning, increased to 400 mg once daily if necessary

PoM **Celectol®** (Rhône-Poulenc Rorer)

Tablets, both f/c, scored, celiprolol hydrochloride 200 mg (yellow), net price 28-tab pack = £9.08; 400 mg, 28-tab pack = £18.01. Label: 8, 22

ESMOLOL HYDROCHLORIDE

Indications: short-term treatment of supraventricular arrhythmias (including atrial fibrillation, atrial flutter, sinus tachycardia); tachycardia and hypertension in peri-operative period

Cautions; Contra-indications; Side-effects: see under Propranolol Hydrochloride

Dose: by intravenous infusion, usually within range 50–200 micrograms/kg/minute (consult product literature for details of dose titration)

PoM **Brevibloc®** (Sanofi Winthrop)

Injection, esmolol hydrochloride 10 mg/mL, net price 10-mL vial = £5.90

Injection concentrate, esmolol hydrochloride 250 mg/mL (for dilution before infusion), 10-mL amp = £65.90

LABETALOL HYDROCHLORIDE

Indications: hypertension (including hypertension in pregnancy, hypertension with angina, and hypertension following acute myocardial infarction); hypertensive crisis (but see section 2.5); controlled hypotension in anaesthesia

Cautions; Contra-indications: as for Propranolol Hydrochloride; interferes with laboratory tests for catecholamines; liver damage (see below)

LIVER DAMAGE. Severe hepatocellular damage reported after both short-term and long-term treatment. Appropriate laboratory testing needed at first symptom of liver dysfunction and if laboratory evidence of damage (or if jaundice) labetalol should be stopped and not restarted

Side-effects: postural hypotension (avoid upright position during and for 3 hours after intravenous administration), tiredness, weakness, headache, rashes, scalp tingling, difficulty in micturition, epigastric pain, nausea, vomiting; liver damage (see above); rarely lichenoid rash

Dose: by mouth, initially 100 mg (50 mg in elderly) twice daily with food, increased at intervals of 14 days to usual dose of 200 mg twice daily; up to 800 mg daily in 2 divided doses (3–4 divided doses if higher); max. 2.4 g daily

By intravenous injection, 50 mg over at least 1 minute, repeated after 5 minutes if necessary; max. 200 mg

Note. Excessive bradycardia can be countered with intravenous injection of atropine sulphate 0.6–2.4 mg in divided doses of 600 micrograms; for **overdosage** see Emergency Treatment of Poisoning, p. 22

By intravenous infusion, 2 mg/minute; usual range 50–200 mg, higher doses in phaeochromocytoma

Hypertension of pregnancy, 20 mg/hour, doubled every 30 minutes; usual max. 160 mg/hour

Hypertension following infarction, 15 mg/hour, gradually increased to max. 120 mg/hour

PoM **Labetalol Hydrochloride** (Non-proprietary)

Tablets, all f/c, labetalol hydrochloride 100 mg, net price 20 = £1.50; 200 mg, 20 = £2.36; 400 mg, 20 = £3.66. Label: 8, 21

Available from APS, Cox, Hillcross, Norton

PoM **Trandate®** (Evans)

Tablets, all orange, f/c, labetalol hydrochloride 50 mg, net price 56-tab pack. £5.05; 100 mg, 56-tab pack = £5.56; 200 mg, 56-tab pack = £9.02; 400 mg, 50-tab pack = £11.21. Label: 8, 21

Injection, labetalol hydrochloride 5 mg/mL. Net price 20-mL amp = £2.83

METOPROLOL TARTRATE

Indications: see under Dose

Cautions; Contra-indications; Side-effects: see under Propranolol Hydrochloride; reduce dose in hepatic impairment

Dose: by mouth, hypertension, initially 100 mg daily, maintenance 100–200 mg daily in 1–2 doses

Angina, 50–100 mg 2–3 times daily

Arrhythmias, usually 50 mg 2–3 times daily; up to 300 mg daily in divided doses if necessary

Migraine prophylaxis, 100–200 mg daily in divided doses

Thyrotoxicosis (adjunct), 50 mg 4 times daily

By intravenous injection, arrhythmias, up to 5 mg at rate 1–2 mg/minute, repeated after 5 minutes if necessary, total dose 10–15 mg

Note. Excessive bradycardia can be countered with intravenous injection of atropine sulphate 0.6–2.4 mg in divided doses of 600 micrograms; for **overdosage** see Emergency Treatment of Poisoning, p. 22

In surgery, 2–4 mg *by slow intravenous injection* at induction or to control arrhythmias developing during anaesthesia; 2-mg doses may be repeated to a max. of 10 mg

Early intervention within 12 hours of infarction, 5 mg *by intravenous injection* every 2 minutes to a max. of 15 mg, followed after 15 minutes by 50 mg *by mouth* every 6 hours for 48 hours; maintenance 200 mg daily in divided doses

PoM **Metoprolol Tartrate** (Non-proprietary)

Tablets, metoprolol tartrate 50 mg, net price 20 = 67p; 100 mg, 20 = £1.23. Label: 8

Available from APS, Ashbourne (Mepranix®), Berk (Arbralene®), Cox, Hillcross, Norton

PoM **Betaloc®** (Astra)

Tablets, both scored, metoprolol tartrate 50 mg, net price 100-tab pack = £3.30; 100 mg, 100-tab pack = £6.13. Label: 8

Injection, metoprolol tartrate 1 mg/mL. Net price 5-mL amp = 44p

PoM **Lopresor**® (Novartis)

Tablets, both f/c, scored, metoprolol tartrate 50 mg (pink), net price 56-tab pack = £5.13; 100 mg (blue), 56-tab pack = £9.54. Label: 8

Modified release
PoM **Betaloc-SA**® (Astra)

Durules® (= tablets, m/r), metoprolol tartrate 200 mg. Net price 28-tab pack = £4.56. Label: 8, 25

Dose: hypertension, angina, 200–400 mg daily; migraine prophylaxis, 200 mg daily

PoM **Lopresor SR**® (Novartis)

Tablets, m/r, yellow, f/c, metoprolol tartrate 200 mg. Net price 28-tab pack = £8.98. Label: 8, 25

Dose: hypertension, 200 mg daily; angina, 200-400 mg daily; migraine prophylaxis, 200 mg daily

With diuretic
PoM **Co-Betaloc**® (Astra)

Tablets, scored, metoprolol tartrate 100 mg, hydrochlorothiazide 12.5 mg. Net price 28-tab pack = £4.66. Label: 8

Dose: hypertension, 1–3 tablets daily in single or divided doses

PoM **Co-Betaloc SA**® (Astra)

Tablets, yellow, f/c, metoprolol tartrate (m/r) 200 mg, hydrochlorothiazide 25 mg. Net price 28-tab pack = £5.74. Label: 8, 25

Dose: hypertension, 1 tablet daily

NADOLOL

Indications: see under Dose

Cautions; Contra-indications; Side-effects: see under Propranolol Hydrochloride; reduce dose in renal impairment

Dose: hypertension, 80 mg daily, increased at weekly intervals if required; max. 240 mg daily
Angina, 40 mg daily, increased at weekly intervals if required; usual max. 160 mg daily
Arrhythmias, initially 40 mg daily, increased to 160 mg if required; reduce to 40 mg if bradycardia occurs
Migraine prophylaxis, initially 40 mg daily, increased by 40 mg at weekly intervals; usual maintenance dose 80–160 mg daily
Thyrotoxicosis (adjunct), 80–160 mg daily

PoM **Corgard**® (Sanofi Winthrop)

Tablets, both blue, nadolol 40 mg, net price 28-tab pack = £3.76; 80 mg, 28-tab pack = £5.45. Label: 8

With diuretic
PoM **Corgaretic 40**® (Sanofi Winthrop)

Tablets, scored, nadolol 40 mg, bendrofluazide 5 mg. Net price 28-tab pack = £5.92. Label: 8
Dose: hypertension, 1–2 tablets daily

PoM **Corgaretic 80**® (Sanofi Winthrop)

Tablets, scored, nadolol 80 mg, bendrofluazide 5 mg. Net price 28-tab pack = £8.47. Label: 8
Dose: hypertension, 1–2 tablets daily

OXPRENOLOL HYDROCHLORIDE

Indications: see under Dose

Cautions; Contra-indications; Side-effects: see under Propranolol Hydrochloride

Dose: hypertension, 80–160 mg daily in 2–3 divided doses, increased as required at 1–2 week intervals; max. 480 mg daily
Angina, 40–160 mg 3 times daily
Arrhythmias, initially 20–40 mg 3 times daily, increased as necessary
Anxiety symptoms (short-term use), initially 40 mg twice daily, increased if necessary to 160 mg daily in divided doses

PoM **Oxprenolol** (Non-proprietary)

Tablets, all coated, oxprenolol hydrochloride 20 mg, net price 20 = 39p; 40 mg, 20 = 53p; 80 mg, 20 = 84p; 160 mg, 20 = £1.27. Label: 8

Available from APS (80-mg tablets contain tartrazine), Cox, Hillcross, Norton

PoM **Trasicor**® (Novartis)

Tablets, all f/c, oxprenolol hydrochloride 20 mg (contain gluten), net price 100-tab pack = £2.31; 40 mg (contain gluten), 56-tab pack = £2.59; 80 mg (yellow), 56-tab pack = £5.17. Label: 8

Modified release
PoM **Slow-Trasicor**® (Novartis)

Tablets, m/r, f/c, oxprenolol hydrochloride 160 mg. Net price 28-tab pack = £6.08. Label: 8, 25

Dose: hypertension, angina, initially 160 mg daily in the morning; if necessary may be increased to max. 480 mg daily in 1–2 divided doses

Note. Modified-release tablets containing oxprenolol hydrochloride 160 mg also available from Norton

With diuretic
PoM **Trasidrex**® (Novartis)

Tablets, red, s/c, co-prenozide 160/0.25 (oxprenolol hydrochloride 160 mg (m/r), cyclopenthiazide 250 micrograms). Net price 28-tab pack = £7.40. Label: 8, 25

Dose: hypertension, 1 tablet daily, increased if necessary to 2 daily as a single dose

PINDOLOL

Indications: see under Dose

Cautions; Contra-indications; Side-effects: see under Propranolol Hydrochloride; reduce dose in renal impairment

Dose: hypertension, initially 5 mg 2–3 times daily *or* 15 mg once daily, increased as required at weekly intervals; usual maintenance 15–30 mg daily; max. 45 mg daily
Angina, 2.5–5 mg up to 3 times daily

PoM **Visken**® (Novartis)

Tablets, both scored, pindolol 5 mg, net price 100-tab pack = £7.27; 15 mg, 30-tab pack = £6.54. Label: 8

With diuretic

PoM **Viskaldix®** (Novartis)

Tablets, scored, pindolol 10 mg, clopamide 5 mg. Net price 28-tab pack = £5.58. Label: 8

Dose: hypertension, 1 tablet daily in the morning, increased if necessary to 2 daily; max. 3 daily

SOTALOL HYDROCHLORIDE

Indications:

Tablets and injection: life-threatening arrhythmias including ventricular tachyarrhythmias, symptomatic non-sustained ventricular tachyarrhythmias

Tablets only: prophylaxis of paroxysmal atrial tachycardia or fibrillation, paroxysmal AV re-entrant tachycardias (both nodal and involving accessory pathways), paroxysmal supraventricular tachycardia after cardiac surgery, maintenance of sinus rhythm following cardioversion of atrial fibrillation or flutter

Injection only: electrophysiological study of inducible ventricular and supraventricular arrhythmias; temporary substitution for tablets

CSM advice. The use of sotalol should be limited to the treatment of ventricular arrhythmias or prophylaxis of supraventricular arrhythmias (see above). It should no longer be used for angina, hypertension, thyrotoxicosis or for secondary prevention after myocardial infarction; when stopping sotalol for these indications, the dose should be reduced gradually

Cautions: see under Propranolol Hydrochloride; reduce dose in renal impairment (avoid if severe); correct hypokalaemia, hypomagnesaemia, or other electrolyte disturbances; severe or prolonged diarrhoea; **interactions:** Appendix 1 (beta-blockers), **important:** verapamil interaction see also p. 101

Contra-indications: see under Propranolol Hydrochloride; congenital or acquired long QT syndrome; torsades de pointes; renal failure

Side-effects: see under Propranolol Hydrochloride; arrhythmogenic (pro-arrhythmic) effect (torsades de pointes—increased risk in women)

Dose: by mouth with ECG monitoring and measurement of corrected QT interval, arrhythmias, initially 80 mg daily in 1–2 divided doses increased gradually at intervals of 2–3 days to usual dose of 160–320 mg daily in 2 divided doses; higher doses of 480–640 mg daily for life-threatening ventricular arrhythmias under specialist supervision

By intravenous injection over 10 minutes, acute arrhythmias, 20–120 mg with ECG monitoring, repeated if necessary with 6-hour intervals between injections

Diagnostic use, see product literature

Note. Excessive bradycardia can be countered with intravenous injection of atropine sulphate 0.6–2.4 mg in divided doses of 600 micrograms; for **overdosage** see Emergency Treatment of Poisoning, p. 22

PoM **Sotalol** (Non-proprietary)

Tablets, both scored, sotalol hydrochloride 80 mg, net price 28-tab pack = £1.64; 160 mg, 28-tab pack = £6.89. Label: 8

Available from Generics, Hillcross

PoM **Beta-Cardone®** (Evans)

Tablets, all scored, sotalol hydrochloride 40 mg (green), net price 100-tab pack = £3.96; 80 mg (pink), 100-tab pack = £5.87; 200 mg, 30-tab pack = £4.15. Label: 8

PoM **Sotacor®** (Bristol-Myers)

Tablets, sotalol hydrochloride 80 mg, net price 28-tab pack = £3.49; 160 mg, 28-tab pack = £6.89. Label: 8

Injection, sotalol hydrochloride 10 mg/mL. Net price 4-mL amp = £1.76

TIMOLOL MALEATE

Indications: see under Dose

Cautions; Contra-indications; Side-effects: see under Propranolol Hydrochloride

Dose: hypertension, initially 5 mg twice daily *or* 10 mg once daily; gradually increased if necessary to max. 60 mg daily (given in divided doses above 20 mg daily)

Angina, initially 5 mg 2–3 times daily, usual maintenance 35–45 mg daily (range 15–45 mg daily)

Prophylaxis after infarction, initially 5 mg twice daily, increased after 2 days to 10 mg twice daily, starting 7 to 28 days after infarction

Migraine prophylaxis, 10–20 mg once daily

Glaucoma, see section 11.6

PoM **Betim®** (Leo)

Tablets, scored, timolol maleate 10 mg. Net price 100-tab pack = £8.55. Label: 8

PoM **Blocadren®** (MSD)

Tablets, blue, scored, timolol maleate 10 mg. Net price 100-tab pack = £8.55. Label: 8

With diuretic

PoM **Moducren®** (Morson)

Tablets, blue, scored, timolol maleate 10 mg, co-amilozide 2.5/25 (amiloride hydrochloride 2.5 mg, hydrochlorothiazide 25 mg). Net price 28-tab pack = £8.00. Label: 8

Dose: hypertension, 1–2 tablets daily as a single dose

PoM **Prestim®** (Leo)

Tablets, scored, timolol maleate 10 mg, bendrofluazide 2.5 mg. Net price 100-tab pack = £14.32. Label: 8

Dose: hypertension, 1–2 tablets daily; max. 4 daily

2.5   Drugs affecting the renin-angiotensin system and some other antihypertensive drugs

Antihypertensive therapy has improved the outlook for patients with high blood pressure by decreasing the frequency of stroke, heart failure, and renal failure: treatment also reduces the incidence of coronary events.

All patients should be given advice on non-pharmacological measures to reduce high blood pressure, including achieving ideal body weight, avoiding high alcohol intake, limiting sodium intake, and taking regular exercise. Cigarette smoking has a powerful adverse effect on cardiovascular risk in hypertensive subjects, and the importance of stopping should be emphasised.

Response to drug treatment for hypertension may be affected by the patient's ethnic background; the response to beta-blockers and to ACE inhibitors may be reduced in Afro-Caribbean subjects.

The recommendations of the British Hypertension Society are that specific antihypertensive treatment is indicated:

Where the initial blood pressure is systolic ≥ 200 mmHg or diastolic ≥ 110 mmHg, **treat** if these values are confirmed on 3 separate occasions over 1-2 weeks (**important:** if very severe or in presence of associated conditions such as heart failure, immediate treatment needed—see also below);

Where the initial blood pressure is systolic 160–199 mmHg or diastolic 90–109 mmHg (or when higher initial values fall to this range) take one of the following courses of action:

• if vascular complications or end-organ damage (e.g. left ventricular hypertrophy, renal impairment) or diabetes present, treat if systolic ≥ 160 mmHg or diastolic ≥ 90 mmHg confirmed on at least 3 separate occasions;

• if no vascular complications, no end-organ damage and no diabetes repeat blood pressure measurements at monthly intervals for 3–6 months and **treat** if the average value during this period is systolic ≥ 160 mmHg or diastolic ≥ 100 mmHg;

• if the average value is systolic <160 mmHg and diastolic 90–99 mmHg treatment may be withheld but continue to monitor; however **consider treatment** if sustained in this range in older patients (over 60 years), and in those with a particularly high risk of cardiovascular complications (e.g. strong family history).

The usual aim should be to reduce the systolic pressure to below 160 mmHg and the diastolic pressure to below 90 mmHg.

Malignant (or accelerated) hypertension or very severe hypertension (diastolic blood pressure > 140 mmHg) requires urgent treatment in hospital but is not an indication for parenteral antihypertensive therapy. Normally treatment should be by mouth with a beta-blocker (atenolol or labetalol) or a calcium-channel blocker (nifedipine). Within the first 24 hours the diastolic blood pressure should be reduced to 100–110 mmHg. Over the next two or three days blood pressure should be normalised by using beta-blockers, calcium-channel blockers, diuretics, vasodilators, or angiotensin-converting enzyme inhibitors. Very rapid falls in blood pressure can cause reduced cerebral perfusion leading to cerebral infarction and blindness, a reduction in renal perfusion causing a deterioration in renal function, and myocardial ischaemia. Parenteral antihypertensive drugs are, therefore, hardly ever necessary. (On the rare occasions when a parenteral antihypertensive is necessary, sodium nitroprusside by infusion is the drug of choice.)

In moderate to severe hypertension (diastolic blood pressure > 110 mmHg) or in patients with vascular complications, drugs are best added 'stepwise' until control has been achieved; an attempt can then be made to 'step down' treatment under supervision. In uncomplicated mild hypertension (diastolic blood pressure < 110 mmHg), drugs may be substituted rather than added. Whenever the blood pressure is consistently well below the target level it is reasonable to try stepping down treatment cautiously, by gradually decreasing the dose or number of drugs, under close supervision. In some patients, usually those with mild hypertension and no end organ damage, it may even be possible to withdraw treatment completely; any subsequent rise in blood pressure may be delayed for several months, therefore blood pressure should be monitored indefinitely.

The strategy for reducing blood pressure is probably best as follows:

1. Non-drug treatment—obesity, high alcohol intake, high salt intake, and lack of regular exercise, may elevate blood pressure and these should be corrected.

2. Diuretic therapy. The optimum dose of a thiazide (section 2.2.1) used to treat hypertension is the lowest possible dose; higher doses do not have a major additional antihypertensive effect, but do cause more metabolic side-effects. Potassium supplements or potassium-sparing diuretics are usually not necessary in the routine treatment of hypertension, but plasma potassium concentration should be checked 3 to 4 weeks after starting treatment.

3. Beta-adrenoceptor blocking drugs (section 2.4) are used with a thiazide where they are not effective alone.

4(a). ACE inhibitors (section 2.5.5.1) may cause a precipitate drop in blood pressure especially in patients with heart failure or those receiving diuretic therapy; they should be given in low initial doses and where possible diuretic therapy should be omitted for a few days before starting.

4(b). Calcium-channel blockers have antihypertensive efficacy broadly similar to that of thiazides or beta-blockers. Their safety during long-term treatment is less well established; they should therefore be considered for hypertension only when thiazides and beta-blockers are contra-indicated, not tolerated, or fail to control blood pressure (and should usually be avoided in heart failure). There are **important** differences between calcium-channel blockers (see section 2.6.2).

5. *Other drugs*—vasodilators (hydralazine, minoxidil), alpha-blockers (prazosin, terazosin, doxazosin), and centrally acting drugs (methyldopa, moxonidine) are generally reserved for patients whose blood pressure is not controlled by, or who have contra-indications to, the drugs already mentioned.

SYSTOLIC HYPERTENSION. Isolated systolic hypertension (systolic blood pressure > 160 mmHg, diastolic < 90 mmHg) is associated with an increased risk of stroke and coronary events, particularly in those over 60 years. Systolic blood pressure averaging 160 mmHg or higher over 3 to 6 months (despite appropriate non-drug treatment) should be lowered in those over 60 years, even if diastolic hypertension is absent. The regimen proven effective is a low dose of a thiazide, with addition of a beta-blocker when necessary. Patients with severe postural hypotension should not receive blood pressure lowering drugs.

Isolated systolic hypertension is uncommon in younger patients but by extrapolation it seems reasonable to recommend that a threshold pressure of 160 mmHg should also be an indication for treatment.

HYPERTENSION IN PREGNANCY. It is important to control blood pressure in pregnancy. High blood pressure may be due to pre-existing essential hypertension or to pre-eclampsia. Oral methyldopa is safe in pregnancy. Beta-blockers are effective and safe in the third trimester but may cause intra-uterine growth retardation when used earlier in pregnancy. Modified-release preparations of nifedipine are also used for hypertension in pregnancy. Hydralazine by intravenous injection can be used to control hypertensive crises. For use of magnesium sulphate in eclampsia, see section 9.5.1.3.

HYPERTENSION IN THE ELDERLY. Antihypertensive therapy reduces the incidence of cardiovascular complications substantially in elderly hypertensive subjects. The benefit is evident up to at least 85 years of age, and it is probably inappropriate to apply a strict age limit when coming to a decision on drug therapy. Elderly subjects who have a good outlook for longevity from other points of view should have their blood pressure lowered if they are hypertensive. The criteria for treatment are diastolic blood pressure averaging 90 mmHg or higher *or* systolic averaging 160 mmHg or higher over 3 to 6 months observation (despite appropriate non-drug treatment). A low dose of a thiazide is the clear drug of first choice, with addition of a beta-blocker when necessary.

2.5.1 Vasodilator antihypertensive drugs

These are potent drugs, especially when used in combination with a beta-blocker and a thiazide. **Important:** for a warning on the hazards of a very rapid fall in blood pressure, see section 2.5.

Diazoxide is used by intravenous injection in hypertensive emergencies.

Hydralazine given by mouth is a useful adjunct to other treatment, but when used alone causes tachycardia and fluid retention. Side-effects can be few if the dose is kept below 100 mg daily, but systemic lupus erythematosus should be suspected if there is unexplained weight loss, arthritis, or any other unexplained ill health.

Sodium nitroprusside is given by intravenous infusion to control severe hypertensive crises.

Minoxidil should be reserved for the treatment of severe hypertension resistant to other drugs. Vasodilatation is accompanied by increased cardiac output and tachycardia and the patients develop fluid retention. For this reason a beta-blocker and a diuretic (usually frusemide, in high dosage) are mandatory. Hypertrichosis is troublesome and renders this drug unsuitable for women.

Prazosin, doxazosin, and terazosin (section 2.5.4) have alpha-blocking and vasodilator properties.

DIAZOXIDE

Indications: acute treatment of severe hypertension associated with renal disease (but see section 2.5); hypoglycaemia, see section 6.1.4

Cautions: ischaemic heart disease, pregnancy, labour, impaired renal function; **interactions:** Appendix 1 (diazoxide)

Side-effects: tachycardia, hyperglycaemia, sodium and water retention

Dose: by rapid intravenous injection (less than 30 seconds), 1–3 mg/kg to max. single dose of 150 mg (see below); may be repeated after 5–15 minutes if required

Note. Single doses of 300 mg have been associated with angina and with myocardial and cerebral infarction

PoM **Eudemine**® (Link)
Injection, diazoxide 15 mg/mL. Net price 20-mL amp = £18.90

HYDRALAZINE HYDROCHLORIDE

Indications: moderate to severe hypertension, with beta-blocker and thiazide; hypertensive crisis (but see section 2.5)

Cautions: reduce initial dose in renal impairment; coronary artery disease (may provoke angina, avoid after myocardial infarction until stabilised), cerebrovascular disease; over-rapid blood pressure reduction is occasionally encountered even with low parenteral doses; pregnancy (see also Appendix 4), breast-feeding; **interactions:** Appendix 1 (hydralazine)

Contra-indications: idiopathic systemic lupus erythematosus, severe tachycardia, high output heart failure, myocardial insufficiency due to mechanical obstruction, cor pulmonale, dissecting aortic aneurysm; porphyria (see section 9.8.2)

Side-effects: tachycardia, fluid retention, nausea, and vomiting; headache; systemic lupus erythematosus-like syndrome after long-term therapy with over 100 mg daily (or less in women) (see also notes above); rarely rashes, fever, changes in blood count, peripheral neuritis; blood disorders reported (including haemolytic anaemia)

Dose: by mouth, 25 mg twice daily, increased to a max. of 50 mg twice daily (see notes above)

By slow intravenous injection, 5–10 mg over 20 minutes; may be repeated after 20–30 minutes (see Cautions)

By intravenous infusion, initially 200–300 micrograms/minute; maintenance usually 50–150 micrograms/minute

PoM **Hydralazine** (Non-proprietary)
Tablets, hydralazine hydrochloride 25 mg, net price 20 = 33p; 50 mg, 20 = 64p

PoM **Apresoline®** (Novartis)
Tablets, yellow, s/c, hydralazine hydrochloride 25 mg, net price 84-tab pack = £1.65
Additives: include gluten
Injection, powder for reconstitution, hydralazine hydrochloride. Net price 20-mg amp = 35p

MINOXIDIL

Indications: severe hypertension, in addition to a diuretic and a beta-blocker

Cautions: see notes above; angina; after myocardial infarction (until stabilised); lower doses in dialysis patients; pregnancy; porphyria (see section 9.8.2); **interactions:** Appendix 1 (minoxidil)

Contra-indications: phaeochromocytoma

Side-effects: sodium and water retention; weight gain; peripheral oedema, tachycardia, hypertrichosis; reversible rise in creatinine and blood urea nitrogen; occasionally, gastro-intestinal disturbances, breast tenderness, rashes

Dose: initially 5 mg (elderly, 2.5 mg) daily, in 1–2 doses, increased by 5–10 mg every 3 or more days; max. usually 50 mg daily

PoM **Loniten®** (Pharmacia & Upjohn)
Tablets, all scored, minoxidil 2.5 mg, net price 100-tab pack = £12.34; 5 mg, 100-tab pack = £21.98; 10 mg, 100-tab pack = £42.62

SODIUM NITROPRUSSIDE

Indications: hypertensive crisis (but see section 2.5); controlled hypotension in anaesthesia; acute or chronic heart failure

Cautions: hypothyroidism, renal impairment, hyponatraemia, ischaemic heart disease, impaired cerebral circulation, elderly; hypothermia; monitor blood pressure and blood-cyanide concentration and if treatment exceeds 3 days, also blood-thiocyanate concentration; avoid sudden withdrawal—terminate infusion over 15–30 minutes; pregnancy and breast-feeding; **interactions:** Appendix 1 (nitroprusside).

Contra-indications: severe hepatic impairment; severe vitamin B_{12} deficiency; Leber's optic atrophy; compensatory hypertension

Side-effects: associated with over rapid reduction in blood pressure (reduce infusion rate): headache, dizziness, nausea, retching, abdominal pain, perspiration, palpitations, apprehension, retrosternal discomfort; occasionally reduced platelet count, acute transient phlebitis

CYANIDE. Side-effects caused by excessive plasma concentration of the cyanide metabolite include tachycardia, sweating, hyperventilation, arrhythmias, marked metabolic acidosis (discontinue and give antidote, see p. 24)

Dose: hypertensive crisis, *by intravenous infusion,* initially 0.5–1.5 micrograms/kg/minute, then adjusted by increments of 0.5 micrograms/kg/minute every 5 minutes within range 0.5–8 micrograms/kg/minute (lower doses in patients already receiving other anti-

hypertensives); stop if marked response not obtained with max. dose in 10 minutes

Note. Lower initial dose of 0.3 micrograms/kg/minute has been used

Maintenance of blood pressure at 30–40% lower than pretreatment diastolic blood pressure, 20–400 micrograms/minute (lower doses for patients being treated with other antihypertensives)

Controlled hypotension in surgery, *by intravenous infusion,* max. 1.5 micrograms/kg/minute

Heart failure, *by intravenous infusion,* initially 10–15 micrograms/minute, increased every 5–10 minutes as necessary; usual range 10–200 micrograms/minute normally for max. 3 days

PoM **Sodium Nitroprusside** (Non-proprietary)
Intravenous solution, sodium nitroprusside 10 mg/mL. For dilution and use as an infusion. 5-mL vial available from Faulding DBL

2.5.2   Centrally acting antihypertensive drugs

This group includes **methyldopa**, which has the advantage of being safe in asthmatics, in heart failure, and in pregnancy. Side-effects are minimised if the daily dose is kept below 1 g.

Clonidine has the disadvantage that sudden withdrawal may cause a hypertensive crisis. Reserpine and rauwolfia are no longer used in Britain.

Moxonidine, a centrally acting drug, has been introduced recently for mild to moderate essential hypertension. It may have a role when thiazides, beta-blockers, ACE inhibitors and calcium-channel blockers are not appropriate or have failed to control blood pressure.

CLONIDINE HYDROCHLORIDE

Indications: hypertension (for use in migraine, see section 4.7.4.2)

Cautions: must be withdrawn gradually to avoid hypertensive crisis; Raynaud's syndrome or other occlusive peripheral vascular disease; history of depression; avoid in porphyria (see section 9.8.2); **interactions:** Appendix 1 (clonidine)

DRIVING. Drowsiness may affect performance of skilled tasks (e.g. driving); effects of alcohol may be enhanced

Side-effects: dry mouth, sedation, depression, fluid retention, bradycardia, Raynaud's phenomenon, headache, dizziness, euphoria, nocturnal unrest, rash, nausea, constipation, rarely impotence

Dose: by mouth, 50–100 micrograms 3 times daily, increased every second or third day; max. daily dose usually 1.2 mg

By slow intravenous injection, 150–300 micrograms; max. 750 micrograms in 24 hours

PoM **Catapres®** (Boehringer Ingelheim)
Tablets, both scored, clonidine hydrochloride 100 micrograms, net price 100-tab pack = £7.00; 300 micrograms, 100-tab pack = £16.30. Label: 3, 8

Injection, clonidine hydrochloride 150 micrograms/mL. Net price 1-mL amp = 29p

PoM **Dixarit®** (migraine), see section 4.7.4.2

Modified release
PoM **Catapres® Perlongets** (Boehringer Ingelheim)
Capsules, m/r, red/yellow, clonidine hydrochloride 250 micrograms. Net price 56-cap pack = £13.89. Label: 3, 8, 25

Dose: usually 1 capsule in the evening; 2–3 capsules daily (1 morning and 1–2 evening) if necessary

METHYLDOPA

Indications: hypertension, in conjunction with diuretic; hypertensive crisis when immediate effect not necessary

Cautions: positive direct Coombs' test in up to 20% of patients (may affect blood cross-matching); interference with laboratory tests; reduce initial dose in renal impairment; blood counts and liver-function tests advised; history of depression; **interactions:** Appendix 1 (methyldopa)

DRIVING. Drowsiness may affect performance of skilled tasks (e.g. driving); effects of alcohol may be enhanced

Contra-indications: depression, active liver disease, phaeochromocytoma; porphyria (see section 9.8.2)

Side-effects: dry mouth, sedation, depression, drowsiness, diarrhoea, fluid retention, failure of ejaculation, liver damage, haemolytic anaemia, lupus erythematosus-like syndrome, parkinsonism, rashes, nasal stuffiness

Dose: by mouth, 250 mg 2–3 times daily, gradually increased at intervals of 2 or more days; max. daily dose 3 g; ELDERLY 125 mg twice daily initially, gradually increased; max. daily dose 2 g (see also notes above)

By intravenous infusion, methyldopate hydrochloride 250–500 mg, repeated after 6 hours if required

PoM **Methyldopa** (Non-proprietary)

Tablets, coated, methyldopa (anhydrous) 125 mg, net price 20 = 43p; 250 mg, 20 = 61p; 500 mg, 20 = £1.22. Label: 3, 8

Available from APS, Berk (Dopamet®), Cox, CP, Hillcross, Norton

PoM **Aldomet**® (MSD)

Tablets, all yellow, f/c, methyldopa (anhydrous) 125 mg, net price 20 = 34p; 250 mg, 20 = 63p; 500 mg, 20 = £1.27. Label: 3, 8

Suspension, methyldopa 250 mg/5mL. Net price 200 mL = £3.96. Label: 3, 8

Injection, methyldopate hydrochloride 50 mg/mL. Net price 5-mL amp = £2.31

MOXONIDINE

Indications: mild to moderate essential hypertension

Cautions: renal impairment (see Appendix 3); avoid abrupt withdrawal (if concomitant treatment with beta-blocker has to be stopped, discontinue beta-blocker first, then moxonidine after few days); **interactions:** see Appendix 1 (moxonidine)

Contra-indications: history of angioedema; conduction disorders (sick sinus syndrome, sinoatrial block, second- or third-degree AV block); bradycardia; life-threatening arrhythmia; severe heart failure; severe coronary artery disease, unstable angina; severe liver disease or renal impairment; also on theoretical grounds: Raynaud's syndrome, intermittent claudication, epilepsy, depression, Parkinson's disease, glaucoma; pregnancy and breast-feeding

Side-effects: dry mouth; headache, fatigue, sedation, dizziness, nausea, sleep disturbance, vasodilatation

Dose: 200 micrograms once daily in the morning, increased if necessary after 3 weeks to 400 micrograms daily in 1–2 divided doses; max. 600 micrograms daily in 2 divided doses

▼ PoM **Physiotens**® (Solvay)

Tablets, f/c, moxonidine 200 micrograms (pink), net price 28-tab pack = £10.45; 400 micrograms (red), 28-tab pack = £14.26. Label: 3

2.5.3   Adrenergic neurone blocking drugs

These drugs prevent the release of noradrenaline from postganglionic adrenergic neurones. Guanethidine also depletes the nerve endings of noradrenaline. These drugs do not control supine blood pressure and may cause postural hypotension. For this reason they have largely fallen from use, but may be necessary with other therapy in resistant hypertension.

GUANETHIDINE MONOSULPHATE

Indications: hypertensive crisis (but see section 2.5)

Cautions: postural hypotension may cause falls in elderly; coronary or cerebral arteriosclerosis, asthma, history of peptic ulceration; pregnancy; **interactions:** Appendix 1 (adrenergic neurone blockers)

Contra-indications: phaeochromocytoma, renal impairment (Appendix 3), heart failure

Side-effects: postural hypotension, failure of ejaculation, fluid retention, nasal congestion, headache, diarrhoea, drowsiness

Dose: by intramuscular injection, 10–20 mg, repeated after 3 hours if required

PoM **Ismelin**® (Novartis)

Injection, guanethidine monosulphate 10 mg/mL. Net price 1-mL amp = 23p

BETHANIDINE SULPHATE

(Betanidine Sulphate)

Indications: hypertension

Cautions; Contra-indications; Side-effects: see under Guanethidine Monosulphate (except diarrhoea)

Dose: 10 mg (elderly 5 mg) 3 times daily after food, increased by 5 mg at intervals; max. daily dose 200 mg

PoM **Bendogen**® (Lagap)

Tablets, scored, bethanidine sulphate 10 mg, net price 100-tab pack = £15.14. Label: 21

DEBRISOQUINE

Indications: hypertension

Cautions; Contra-indications; Side-effects: see under Guanethidine Monosulphate (except diarrhoea)

Dose: 10 mg 1–2 times daily, increased by 10 mg every 3 days; usual range 20–60 mg daily (120 mg or higher in severe hypertension)

PoM ¹**Debrisoquine** (Cambridge)

Tablets, scored, debrisoquine (as sulphate) 10 mg, net price 100-tab pack = £14.74
1. Former brand name Declinax®

2.5.4   Alpha-adrenoceptor blocking drugs

Prazosin has post-synaptic alpha-blocking and vasodilator properties and rarely causes tachycardia. It may, however, cause a rapid reduction in blood pressure after the first dose and should be introduced with caution. **Doxazosin** and **terazosin** have properties similar to those of prazosin.

Indoramin is also an effective alpha-blocker but has many side-effects.

Alpha-blockers may be used with other antihypertensive drugs in the treatment of hypertension.

PROSTATIC HYPERPLASIA. Alfuzosin, doxazosin, indoramin, prazosin, tamsulosin and terazosin are indicated for benign prostatic hyperplasia (see section 7.4.1).

DOXAZOSIN

Indications: hypertension; benign prostatic hyperplasia (section 7.4.1)
Cautions: care with initial dose (postural hypotension); hepatic impairment (Appendix 2); pregnancy and breast-feeding (Appendixes 4 and 5); **interactions:** Appendix 1 (alpha-blockers)
Side-effects: postural hypotension (rarely associated with fainting); dizziness, vertigo, headache, fatigue, asthenia, oedema, somnolence, nausea, rhinitis, urinary incontinence and isolated cases of priapism reported
Dose: hypertension, 1 mg daily, increased after 1–2 weeks to 2 mg once daily, and thereafter to 4 mg once daily if necessary; max. 16 mg daily
Benign prostatic hyperplasia, see section 7.4.1

PoM **Cardura**® (Invicta)
Tablets, doxazosin (as mesylate) 1 mg, net price 28-tab pack = £10.56; 2 mg, 28-tab pack = £14.08; 4 mg, 28-tab pack = £17.60

INDORAMIN

Indications: hypertension; benign prostatic hyperplasia, see section 7.4.1
Cautions: avoid alcohol (enhances rate and extent of absorption); control incipient heart failure with diuretics and digoxin; hepatic or renal impairment; elderly patients; Parkinson's disease; epilepsy (convulsions in *animal* studies); history of depression; **interactions:** Appendix 1 (alpha-blockers)
DRIVING. Drowsiness may affect performance of skilled tasks (e.g. driving); effects of alcohol may be enhanced
Contra-indications: established heart failure; patients receiving MAOIs
Side-effects: sedation; also dizziness, depression, failure of ejaculation, dry mouth, nasal congestion, extrapyramidal effects, weight gain
Dose: hypertension, initially 25 mg twice daily, increased by 25–50 mg daily at intervals of 2 weeks; max. daily dose 200 mg in 2–3 divided doses
Benign prostatic hyperplasia, see section 7.4.1

PoM **Baratol**® (Monmouth)
Tablets, both f/c, indoramin (as hydrochloride) 25 mg (blue), net price 84-tab pack = £19.32; 50 mg (green, scored), 84-tab pack = £34.26. Label: 2

Prostatic hyperplasia
PoM **Doralese**®: see section 7.4.1

PRAZOSIN HYDROCHLORIDE

Indications: see under Dose
Cautions: first dose may cause collapse due to hypotension (therefore should be taken on retiring to bed); elderly; reduce initial dose in renal impairment; pregnancy and breast-feeding; **interactions:** Appendix 1 (alpha-blockers)
Contra-indications: not recommended for congestive heart failure due to mechanical obstruction (e.g. aortic stenosis)
Side-effects: postural hypotension, drowsiness, weakness, dizziness, headache, lack of energy, nausea, palpitations; urinary frequency, incontinence and priapism reported
Dose: hypertension, 500 micrograms 2–3 times daily, the initial dose on retiring to bed at night (to avoid collapse, see Cautions); increased to 1 mg 2–3 times daily after 3–7 days; further increased if necessary to max. 20 mg daily
Congestive heart failure, 500 micrograms 2–4 times daily (initial dose at bedtime, see above), increasing to 4 mg daily in divided doses; maintenance 4–20 mg daily (but rarely used)
Raynaud's syndrome, initially 500 micrograms twice daily (initial dose at bedtime, see above); maintenance 1–2 mg twice daily
Benign prostatic hyperplasia, see section 7.4.1

PoM **Prazosin** (Non-proprietary)
Tablets, prazosin hydrochloride 500 micrograms, net price 100-tab pack = £3.96; 1 mg, 100-tab pack = £4.96; 2 mg, 100-tab pack = £6.74; 5 mg, 100-tab pack = £14.60. Label: 3, counselling, see dose above
Available from APS, Ashbourne (Alphavase®), Cox, Hillcross, Norton
PoM **Hypovase**® (Invicta)
Tablets, prazosin hydrochloride 500 micrograms, net price 56-tab pack = £2.09; 1 mg (orange, scored), 56-tab pack = £2.69; 2 mg (scored), 56-tab pack = £3.66; starter pack of 8 × 500-microgram tabs with 32 × 1-mg tabs = £2.52. Label: 3, counselling, see dose above
Note. Hypovase® (Benign Prostatic Hypertrophy), see section 7.4.1

TERAZOSIN

Indications: mild to moderate hypertension; benign prostatic hyperplasia (section 7.4.1)
Cautions: first dose may cause collapse due to hypotension (within 30–90 minutes, therefore should be taken on retiring to bed) (may also occur with rapid dose increase); **interactions:** Appendix 1 (alpha-blockers)

Side-effects: dizziness, lack of energy, peripheral oedema; urinary frequency and priapism reported
Dose: hypertension, 1 mg at bedtime (compliance with bedtime dose important, see Cautions); dose doubled after 7 days if necessary; usual maintenance dose 2–10 mg once daily; more than 20 mg daily rarely improves efficacy
Benign prostatic hyperplasia, see section 7.4.1

PoM **Hytrin**® (Abbott)
Tablets, terazosin (as hydrochloride) 2 mg (yellow), net price 28-tab pack = £12.55; 5 mg (tan), 28-tab pack = £18.89; 10 mg (blue), 28-tab pack = £26.59; starter pack of 7 × 1-mg tabs with 21 × 2-mg tabs = £13.00. Label: 3, counselling, see dose above
Note. Hytrin BPH® (for benign prostatic hyperplasia), see section 7.4.1

PHAEOCHROMOCYTOMA

Phenoxybenzamine is a powerful alpha-blocker with many side-effects. It is used with a beta-blocker in the short-term management of severe hypertensive episodes associated with phaeochromocytoma; it is also used in the management of severe shock unresponsive to conventional therapy.

Phentolamine is a short-acting alpha-blocker used rarely as a suppression test for phaeochromocytoma.

PHENOXYBENZAMINE HYDROCHLORIDE
Indications: hypertensive episodes in phaeochromocytoma, see also above
Cautions: elderly; congestive heart failure; severe heart disease (see also Contra-indications); cerebrovascular disease (avoid if history of cerebrovascular accident); renal impairment; carcinogenic in *animals*; pregnancy; avoid in porphyria (see section 9.8.2); avoid infusion in hypovolaemia; avoid extravasation (irritant to tissues)
Contra-indications: history of cerebrovascular accident; during recovery period after myocardial infarction (usually 3–4 weeks)
Side-effects: postural hypotension with dizziness and marked compensatory tachycardia, lassitude, nasal congestion, miosis, inhibition of ejaculation; rarely gastro-intestinal disturbances; decreased sweating and dry mouth after intravenous infusion; idiosyncratic profound hypotension within few minutes of starting infusion
Dose: see under preparations

PoM **Phenoxybenzamine** (Goldshield)
Injection concentrate, phenoxybenzamine hydrochloride 50 mg/mL. To be diluted before use. Net price 3 × 2-mL amp = £43.88 (hosp. only)
Dose: by intravenous infusion (preferably through large vein), phaeochromocytoma and adjunct in severe shock, 1 mg/kg daily in 200 mL physiological saline over at least 2 hours; do not repeat within 24 hours (intensive care facilities needed)
CAUTION. Owing to risk of contact sensitisation doctors, nurses, and other health workers should avoid contamination of hands

PoM **Dibenyline**® (Goldshield)
Capsules, red/white, phenoxybenzamine hydrochloride 10 mg. Net price 30-cap pack = £21.68
Dose, phaeochromocytoma, 10 mg daily, increased by 10 mg daily; usual dose 1–2 mg/kg daily in 2 divided doses

PHENTOLAMINE MESYLATE
(Phentolamine mesilate)
Indications: hypertensive episodes due to phaeochromocytoma e.g. during surgery; diagnosis of phaeochromocytoma
Cautions: monitor blood pressure (avoid in hypotension), heart rate; renal impairment; gastritis, peptic ulcer; elderly; **interactions:** Appendix 1 (alpha-blockers)
ASTHMA. Presence of sulphites in ampoules may (especially in patients with asthma) lead to hypersensitivity (with bronchospasm and shock)
Contra-indications: hypotension; history of myocardial infarction; coronary insufficiency, angina, or other evidence of coronary artery disease
Side-effects: postural hypotension, tachycardia, dizziness; nausea and vomiting, diarrhoea, nasal congestion; also acute or prolonged hypotension, angina, chest pain, arrhythmias
Dose: hypertensive episodes, *by intravenous injection*, 2–5 mg repeated if necessary
Diagnosis of phaeochromocytoma, consult product literature

PoM **Rogitine**® (Novartis)
Injection, phentolamine mesylate 10 mg/mL. Net price 1-mL amp = 27p

2.5.5 Drugs affecting the renin-angiotensin system

2.5.5.1 Angiotensin-converting enzyme inhibitors
2.5.5.2 Angiotensin-II receptor antagonists

2.5.5.1 ANGIOTENSIN-CONVERTING ENZYME INHIBITORS

Angiotensin-converting enzyme inhibitors (ACE inhibitors) inhibit the conversion of angiotensin I to angiotensin II. They are effective and generally well tolerated.

HYPERTENSION. ACE inhibitors should be considered for hypertension when thiazides and beta-blockers are contra-indicated, not tolerated, or fail to control blood pressure; they are particularly indicated for hypertension in insulin-dependent diabetics with nephropathy (see also section 6.1.5), and possibly for hypertension in all diabetics. ACE inhibitors may cause very rapid falls of blood pressure in some patients. Therefore where possible any diuretic therapy should be stopped for a few days before initiating therapy and the first dose should preferably be given at bedtime (see Cautions).

DIABETIC NEPHROPATHY. For comment on the role of ACE inhibitors in the management of diabetic nephropathy, see section 6.1.5.

HEART FAILURE. ACE inhibitors have a valuable role in all grades of heart failure, combined when appropriate with diuretic and digoxin treatment. They improve prognosis substantially, and in this respect are superior to regimens such as modified-release nitrates with hydralazine. ACE inhibitor treatment is indicated in any patient with heart failure who has no contra-indications. To avoid dangerous hyperkalaemia, any potassium-sparing diuretic should be omitted from the diuretic regimen before introducing an ACE inhibitor, changing to the loop diuretic alone; potassium supplements should also be discontinued. Profound first-dose hypotension may occur when ACE inhibitors are introduced to patients with heart failure who are already taking a high dose of a loop diuretic (e.g. frusemide 80 mg daily or higher). Temporary withdrawal of the loop diuretic reduces the risk, but may cause severe rebound pulmonary oedema. The ACE inhibitor should therefore be started at very low dosage (e.g. captopril 6.25 mg), with the patient recumbent and under close medical supervision, and with facilities to treat profound hypotension. In these circumstances and in other special risk groups (see below) the patient should be admitted to hospital for initiation.

MYOCARDIAL INFARCTION. ACE inhibitors are used in the immediate and long-term management of patients who have had a myocardial infarction, see section 2.10.1.

INITIATION IN HOSPITAL. ACE inhibitor therapy for heart failure should be initiated under close medical supervision (in hospital in severe heart failure). Initiation in hospital is also recommended for patients with mild to moderate heart failure:

receiving multiple or high-dose diuretic therapy (e.g. more than 80 mg of frusemide daily or its equivalent);

with hypovolaemia;

with hyponatraemia (plasma-sodium concentration below 130 mmol/litre);

with pre-existing hypotension (systolic blood pressure below 90 mmHg);

with unstable heart failure;

with renal impairment (plasma-creatinine concentration above 150 micromol/litre);

receiving high-dose vasodilator therapy;

aged 70 years or more.

RENAL EFFECTS. In patients with severe bilateral renal artery stenosis (or severe stenosis of the artery supplying a single functioning kidney), ACE inhibitors reduce or abolish glomerular filtration and are likely to cause severe and progressive renal failure. They are thus contra-indicated in patients known to have these forms of critical renovascular disease.

ACE inhibitor treatment is unlikely to have an adverse effect on overall renal function in patients with severe unilateral renal artery stenosis and a normal contralateral kidney, but glomerular filtration is likely to be reduced (or even abolished) in the affected kidney and the long-term consequences are unknown.

In general, ACE inhibitors are therefore best avoided in patients with known or suspected renovascular disease, unless the blood pressure cannot be controlled by other drugs. If they are used in these circumstances renal function needs to be monitored.

ACE inhibitors should also be used with particular caution in patients who may have undiagnosed and clinically silent renovascular disease. This includes patients with peripheral vascular disease or with severe generalised atherosclerosis.

Renal function and electrolytes should be checked before starting ACE inhibitors and monitored during treatment (more frequently if features mentioned above present). Although ACE inhibitors now have a specialised role in some forms of renal disease they also occasionally cause impairment of renal function which may progress and become severe in other circumstances (at particular risk are the elderly).

Concomitant treatment with NSAIDs increases the risk of renal damage, and potassium-sparing diuretics (or potassium-containing salt substitutes) increase the risk of hyperkalaemia.

CAUTIONS. ACE inhibitors should be used with caution in patients receiving diuretics (**important:** see Concomitant diuretics, below); first doses may cause hypotension especially in patients taking diuretics, on a low-sodium diet, on dialysis, dehydrated or with heart failure (see above). They should also be used with caution in peripheral vascular disease or generalised atherosclerosis owing to risk of clinically silent renovascular disease (see also above). Renal function should be monitored before and during treatment, and the dose reduced in renal impairment (see also above and Appendix 3). The risk of agranulocytosis is possibly increased in collagen vascular disease (blood counts recommended). Use ACE inhibitors with caution in breast-feeding (see Appendix 5). **Interactions:** Appendix 1 (ACE inhibitors)

ANAPHYLACTOID REACTIONS. To prevent anaphylactoid reactions, ACE inhibitors should be avoided during dialysis with high-flux polyacrylonitrile membranes and during low-density lipoprotein apheresis with dextran sulphate; they should also be withheld before desensitisation with wasp or bee venom

Concomitant diuretics. ACE inhibitors can cause very rapid falls of blood pressure in volume-depleted patients. Therefore, if possible, any diuretic should be discontinued, or the dose reduced significantly, 2–3 days before initiation of an ACE inhibitor; as usual the first dose of the ACE inhibitor should preferably be given at bedtime. Diuretic therapy may be resumed if necessary after a few weeks. If diuretic therapy cannot be stopped, medical supervision is recommended for at least 2 hours after administration of the first dose of the ACE inhibitor or until the blood pressure has stabilised.

CONTRA-INDICATIONS ACE inhibitors are contra-indicated in patients with hypersensitivity to ACE inhibitors (including angioedema) and in known or suspected renovascular disease (see also above), aortic stenosis or outflow tract obstruction. ACE inhibitors should not be used in pregnancy (Appendix 4).

SIDE-EFFECTS. ACE inhibitors can cause profound hypotension (see Cautions) and renal impairment (see Renal effects above). They may also cause angioedema (onset may be delayed), rash (which may be associated with pruritus and urticaria), persistent dry cough, pancreatitis and upper respiratory-tract symptoms such as sinusitis, rhinitis and sore throat. Gastro-intestinal effects reported with ACE inhibitors include nausea, vomiting, dyspepsia, diarrhoea and constipation. Altered liver function tests, cholestatic jaundice and hepatitis have been reported. Blood dyscrasias including thrombocytopenia, leucopenia, neutropenia and haemolytic anaemia have also been reported. Other reported side-effects include headache, dizziness, fatigue, malaise, taste disturbance, paraesthesia and bronchospasm.

SYMPTOM COMPLEX. A symptom complex has been reported for some ACE inhibitors and may include fever, serositis, vasculitis, myalgia, arthralgia, positive antinuclear antibody, raised erythrocyte sedimentation rate, eosinophilia, leucocytosis; rash, photosensitivity or other skin reactions may occur.

COMBINATION PRODUCTS. A number of products incorporating an ACE inhibitor with a thiazide diuretic are now available for the treatment of hypertension. Use of these combination products should be reserved for patients whose blood pressure has not responded to a thiazide diuretic or an ACE inhibitor alone.

A product combining an ACE inhibitor with a calcium-channel blocker is also available for the management of hypertension. Use of this combination is rarely justified; the range of adverse effects may be increased considerably. The combination product should be considered only for those patients who have been stabilised on the individual components in the same proportions.

CAPTOPRIL

Indications: mild to moderate essential hypertension alone or with thiazide therapy and severe hypertension resistant to other treatment; congestive heart failure (adjunct); following myocardial infarction, see dose; diabetic nephropathy (microalbuminuria greater than 30 mg/day) in insulin-dependent diabetes

Cautions: see notes above

Contra-indications: see notes above; porphyria (section 9.8.2)

Side-effects: see notes above; tachycardia, serum sickness, weight loss, stomatitis, maculopapular rash, photosensitivity, flushing and acidosis

Dose: hypertension, used alone, initially 12.5 mg twice daily; if used in addition to diuretic (see notes above), or in elderly, initially 6.25 mg twice daily (first dose at bedtime); usual maintenance dose 25 mg twice daily; max. 50 mg twice daily (rarely 3 times daily in severe hypertension)
Heart failure (adjunct), initially 6.25–12.5 mg under close medical supervision (see notes above); usual maintenance dose 25 mg 2–3 times daily; usual max. 150 mg daily

Prophylaxis after infarction in clinically stable patients with asymptomatic or symptomatic left ventricular dysfunction (radionuclide ventriculography or echocardiography undertaken before initiation), initially 6.25 mg, starting as early as 3 days after infarction, then increased over several weeks to 150 mg daily (if tolerated) in divided doses
Diabetic nephropathy, 75–100 mg daily in divided doses; if further blood pressure reduction required, other antihypertensives may be used in conjunction with captopril; in severe renal impairment, initially 12.5 mg twice daily (if concomitant diuretic therapy required, loop diuretic rather than thiazide should be chosen)

PoM **Captopril** (Non-proprietary)
Tablets, captopril 12.5 mg, net price 56-tab pack = £4.64, 100-tab pack = £6.10; 25 mg, 56-tab pack = £5.63; 50 mg, 56-tab pack = £9.51
Available from Berk (Kaplon®), Cox, CP, Ethical Generics Ltd, Galen, Generics, Genus, Hillcross, Lagap, Sterwin

PoM **Capoten®** (Squibb)
Tablets, captopril 12.5 mg (scored), net price 56-tab pack = £10.56; 25 mg, 56-tab pack = £12.03, 84-tab pack = £18.05; 50 mg (scored), 56-tab pack = £20.50, 84-tab pack = £30.75 (also available as Acepril®)

With diuretic
Note. For mild to moderate hypertension in patients stabilised on the individual components in the same proportions
PoM **Capozide®** (Squibb)
LS tablets, scored, captopril 25 mg, hydrochlorothiazide 12.5 mg. Net price 28-tab pack = £11.25
Tablets, scored, captopril 50 mg, hydrochlorothiazide 25 mg. Net price 28-tab pack = £14.14 (also available as Acezide®)

CILAZAPRIL

Indications: essential and renovascular hypertension; congestive heart failure (adjunct)

Cautions: see notes above

Contra-indications: see notes above; ascites

Side-effects: see notes above; dyspnoea and bronchitis

Dose: hypertension, initially 1–1.25 mg once daily (initial dose reduced in those receiving a diuretic, in the elderly, in renal impairment and in severe hepatic impairment—consult product literature); usual maintenance dose 2.5–5 mg once daily; max. 5 mg daily
Renovascular hypertension (see notes above), initially 250–500 micrograms once daily, then adjusted according to response
Heart failure (adjunct), initially 500 micrograms once daily under close medical supervision (see notes above), increased to 1 mg once daily; usual maintenance dose 1–2.5 mg daily; max. 5 mg daily

PoM **Vascace®** (Roche)

Tablets, all f/c, cilazapril 250 micrograms (pink), net price 28-tab pack = £3.87; 500 micrograms (white), 28-tab pack = £4.10; 1 mg (yellow), 28-tab pack = £6.76; 2.5 mg (pink), 28-tab pack = £8.60; 5 mg (brown), 28-tab pack = £14.95

ENALAPRIL MALEATE

Indications: essential and renovascular hypertension; congestive heart failure (adjunct); prevention of symptomatic heart failure and prevention of coronary ischaemic events in patients with left ventricular dysfunction

Cautions: see notes above

Contra-indications: see notes above; porphyria (section 9.8.2)

Side-effects: see notes above; also palpitations, arrhythmias, angina, chest pain, syncope, cerebrovascular accident, myocardial infarction; anorexia, ileus, stomatitis, hepatic failure; dermatological side-effects including erythema multiforme, Stevens-Johnson syndrome, toxic epidermal necrolysis, exfoliative dermatitis and pemphigus; confusion, depression, nervousness, asthenia, drowsiness, insomnia, blurred vision, tinnitus, sweating, flushing, impotence, alopecia, dyspnoea, asthma, pulmonary infiltrates and muscle cramps

Dose: hypertension, used alone, initially 5 mg once daily; if used in addition to diuretic (see notes above), in elderly patients, or in renal impairment, initially 2.5 mg daily; usual maintenance dose 10–20 mg once daily; in severe hypertension may be increased to max. 40 mg once daily

Heart failure (adjunct), asymptomatic left ventricular dysfunction, initially 2.5 mg daily under close medical supervision (see notes above); usual maintenance dose 20 mg daily in 1–2 divided doses

PoM **Innovace®** (MSD)

Tablets, enalapril maleate 2.5 mg, net price 28-tab pack = £5.60; 5 mg (scored), 28-tab pack = £7.86; 10 mg (red), 28-tab pack = £11.03; 20 mg (peach), 28-tab pack = £13.10

Wafers (*Innovace Melt®*), enalapril maleate 2.5 mg, net price 30-wafer pack = £5.60; 5 mg, 30-wafer pack = £7.86; 10 mg, 30-wafer pack = £11.03; 20 mg, 30-wafer pack = £13.10. Label: 10 patient information leaflet

Note. Innovace Melt® wafers should be placed on the tongue and allowed to dissolve; contain aspartame (section 9.4.1) equivalent to phenylalanine 1.4 mg/2.5 mg enalapril maleate

With diuretic

Note. For mild to moderate hypertension in patients stabilised on the individual components in the same proportions

PoM **Innozide®** (MSD)

Tablets, yellow, scored, enalapril maleate 20 mg, hydrochlorothiazide 12.5 mg. Net price 28-tab pack = £14.56

FOSINOPRIL

Indications: hypertension; congestive heart failure (adjunct)

Cautions: see notes above

Contra-indications: see notes above

Side-effects: see notes above; chest pain and musculoskeletal pain

Dose: hypertension, initially 10 mg daily, increased if necessary after 4 weeks; usual dose range 10–40 mg (doses over 40 mg not shown to increase efficacy); if used in addition to diuretic see notes above

Heart failure (adjunct), initially 10 mg daily under close medical supervision (see notes above); if initial dose well tolerated, may be increased to up to 40 mg once daily

PoM **Staril®** (Squibb)

Tablets, fosinopril sodium 10 mg, net price 28-tab pack = £12.04; 20 mg, 28-tab pack = £13.00

LISINOPRIL

Indications: essential and renovascular hypertension; congestive heart failure (adjunct); following myocardial infarction in haemodynamically stable patients

Cautions: see notes above

Contra-indications: see notes above; porphyria (section 9.8.2)

Side-effects: see notes above; tachycardia, cerebrovascular accident, myocardial infarction; dry mouth, confusion, mood changes, asthenia, sweating, impotence and alopecia

Dose: hypertension, initially 2.5 mg daily; usual maintenance dose 10–20 mg daily; max. 40 mg daily; if used in addition to diuretic see notes above

Heart failure (adjunct), initially 2.5 mg daily under close medical supervision (see notes above); usual maintenance dose 5–20 mg daily

Prophylaxis after myocardial infarction, systolic blood pressure >120 mmHg, 5 mg within 24 hours, followed by further 5 mg 24 hours later, then 10 mg after a further 24 hours, and continuing with 10 mg once daily for 6 weeks (or continued if heart failure); systolic blood pressure 100-120 mmHg, initially 2.5 mg, increasing to maintenance dose of 5 mg once daily

Note. Should not be started after myocardial infarction if systolic blood pressure <100 mmHg; temporarily reduce maintenance dose to 5 mg and if necessary 2.5 mg daily if systolic blood pressure ≤ 100 mmHg during treatment; withdraw if prolonged hypotension occurs (systolic blood pressure < 90 mmHg for more than 1 hour)

PoM **Carace®** (Du Pont)

Tablets, lisinopril 2.5 mg (blue), net price 28-tab pack = £7.64; 5 mg (pink, scored), 28-tab pack = £9.58; 10 mg (yellow, scored), 28-tab pack = £11.83; 20 mg (orange, scored), 28-tab pack = £13.38

PoM **Zestril®** (Zeneca)

Tablets, lisinopril (as dihydrate) 2.5 mg, net price 28-tab pack = £7.64; 5 mg (pink, scored), 28-tab pack = £9.58; 10 mg (pink), 28-tab pack = £11.83; 20 mg (red), 28-tab pack = £13.38

With diuretic

Note. For mild to moderate hypertension in patients stabilised on the individual components in the same proportions

PoM **Carace Plus**® (Du Pont)

Carace 10 Plus tablets, blue, lisinopril 10 mg, hydrochlorothiazide 12.5 mg. Net price 28-tab pack = £11.83

Carace 20 Plus tablets, yellow, scored, lisinopril 20 mg, hydrochlorothiazide 12.5 mg. Net price 28-tab pack = £13.38

PoM **Zestoretic**® (Zeneca)

Zestoretic 10 tablets, peach, lisinopril (as dihydrate) 10 mg, hydrochlorothiazide 12.5 mg. Net price 28-tab pack = £11.83

Zestoretic 20 tablets, lisinopril (as dihydrate) 20 mg, hydrochlorothiazide 12.5 mg. Net price 28-tab pack = £13.38

MOEXIPRIL HYDROCHLORIDE

Indications: essential hypertension

Cautions: see notes above

Contra-indications: see notes above

Side-effects: see notes above; arrhythmias, angina, chest pain, syncope, cerebrovascular accident, myocardial infarction; appetite and weight changes; dry mouth, photosensitivity, flushing, nervousness, mood changes, anxiety, drowsiness, sleep disturbance, tinnitus, influenza-like syndrome, sweating and dyspnoea

Dose: used alone, initially 7.5 mg once daily; if used in addition to diuretic (see notes above), with nifedipine, in elderly, in renal or hepatic impairment, initially 3.75 mg once daily; usual range 15–30 mg once daily; doses above 30 mg daily not shown to increase efficacy

▼ PoM **Perdix**® (Schwarz)

Tablets, f/c, both pink, scored, moexipril hydrochloride 7.5 mg, net price 28-tab pack = £8.50; 15 mg, 28-tab pack = £9.80

PERINDOPRIL

Indications: essential and renovascular hypertension; congestive heart failure (adjunct)

Cautions: see notes above

Contra-indications: see notes above

Side-effects: see notes above; asthenia, flushing, mood and sleep disturbances

Dose: hypertension, initially 2 mg daily; usual maintenance dose 4 mg once daily; max. 8 mg daily; if used in addition to diuretic see notes above

Heart failure (adjunct), initial dose 2 mg in the morning under close medical supervision (see notes above); usual maintenance 4 mg daily

PoM **Coversyl**® (Servier)

Tablets, perindopril erbumine (= tert-butylamine) 2 mg, net price 30-tab pack = £9.45; 4 mg (scored), 30-tab pack = £13.65. Label: 22

QUINAPRIL

Indications: essential hypertension; congestive heart failure (adjunct)

Cautions: see notes above

Contra-indications: see notes above

Side-effects: see notes above; asthenia, chest pain, oedema, flatulence, nervousness, depression, insomnia, blurred vision, impotence, back pain and myalgia

Dose: hypertension, initially 10 mg once daily; with a diuretic, in elderly, or in renal impairment initially 2.5 mg daily; usual maintenance dose 20–40 mg daily in single or 2 divided doses; up to 80 mg daily has been given

Heart failure (adjunct), initial dose 2.5 mg under close medical supervision (see notes above); usual maintenance 10–20 mg daily in single or 2 divided doses; up to 40 mg daily has been given

PoM **Accupro**® (P-D)

Tablets, all brown, f/c, quinapril 5 mg, net price 28-tab pack = £10.30; 10 mg, 28-tab pack = £10.07; 20 mg, 28-tab pack = £9.79; 40 mg, 28-tab pack = £9.75

With diuretic

Note. For hypertension in patients stabilised on the individual components in the same proportions

PoM **Accuretic**® (P-D)

Tablets, pink, f/c, scored, quinapril 10 mg, hydrochlorothiazide 12.5 mg. Net price 28-tab pack = £9.79

RAMIPRIL

Indications: mild to moderate hypertension; congestive heart failure (adjunct); following myocardial infarction in patients with clinical evidence of heart failure

Cautions: see notes above

Contra-indications: see notes above

Side-effects: see notes above; arrhythmias, angina, chest pain, syncope, cerebrovascular accident, myocardial infarction, loss of appetite, stomatitis, dry mouth, skin reactions including erythema multiforme and pemphigoid exanthema; precipitation or exacerbation of Raynaud's syndrome; conjunctivitis, onycholitis, confusion, nervousness, depression, anxiety, impotence, decreased libido, alopecia, bronchitis and muscle cramps

Dose: hypertension, initially 1.25 mg daily, increased at intervals of 1–2 weeks; usual range 2.5–5 mg once daily; max. 10 mg daily; if used in addition to diuretic see notes above

Heart failure (adjunct), initially 1.25 mg once daily under close medical supervision (see notes above), increased if necessary at intervals of 1–2 weeks; max. 10 mg daily (daily doses of 2.5 mg or more may be taken in 1–2 divided doses)

Prophylaxis after myocardial infarction (started in hospital 3 to 10 days after infarction), initially 2.5 mg twice daily, increased after 2 days to 5 mg twice daily; maintenance 2.5–5 mg twice daily

Note. If initial 2.5-mg dose not tolerated, give 1.25 mg twice daily for 2 days before increasing to 2.5 mg twice daily, then 5 mg twice daily; withdraw if 2.5 mg twice daily not tolerated

PoM **Tritace**® (Hoechst Marion Roussel)
Capsules, ramipril 1.25 mg (yellow/white), net price 28-cap pack = £5.30; 2.5 mg (orange/white), 28-cap pack = £7.51; 5 mg (red/white), 28-cap pack = £9.55

TRANDOLAPRIL
Indications: mild to moderate hypertension; following myocardial infarction in patients with left ventricular dysfunction
Cautions: see notes above
Contra-indications: see notes above
Side-effects: see notes above; tachycardia, arrhythmias, angina, transient ischaemic attacks, cerebral haemorrhage, myocardial infarction; ileus, dry mouth; skin reactions including Stevens-Johnson syndrome, toxic epidermal necrolysis, psoriasis-like efflorescence; asthenia, alopecia, dyspnoea and bronchitis
Dose: hypertension, initially 500 micrograms once daily, increased at intervals of 2–4 weeks; usual range 1–2 mg once daily; max. 4 mg daily; if used in addition to diuretic see notes above
Prophylaxis after myocardial infarction (starting as early as 3 days after infarction), initially 500 micrograms daily, gradually increased to max. 4 mg once daily
Note. If symptomatic hypotension develops during titration, do not increase dose further; if possible, reduce dose of any adjunctive treatment and if this is not effective or feasible, reduce dose of trandolapril

PoM **Gopten**® (Knoll)
Capsules, trandolapril 500 micrograms (red/yellow), net price 14-cap pack = £4.09; 1 mg (red/orange), 28-cap pack = £10.33; 2 mg (red/red), 28-cap pack = £12.28
PoM **Odrik**® (Hoechst Marion Roussel)
Capsules, trandolapril 500 micrograms (red/yellow), net price 28-cap pack = £8.19; 1 mg (red/orange), 28-cap pack = £10.34; 2 mg (red/red), 28-cap pack = £12.29

With calcium-channel blocker
Note. For hypertension in patients stabilised on the individual components in the same proportions but combination with calcium-channel blocker rarely justified. For cautions, contra-indications and side-effects of verapamil, see section 2.6.2
PoM **Tarka**® (Knoll)
Capsules, pink, trandolapril 2 mg, verapamil hydrochloride 180 mg (m/r). Net price 28 cap-pack = £16.23. Label: 25

2.5.5.2 ANGIOTENSIN-II RECEPTOR ANTAGONISTS

Losartan and **valsartan** are specific angiotensin-II receptor antagonists with properties similar to those of the ACE inhibitors; **candesartan** and **irbesartan** have been introduced recently. However, unlike ACE inhibitors, they do not inhibit the breakdown of bradykinin and other kinins, and thus do not appear to cause the persistent dry cough which commonly complicates ACE inhibitor therapy. They are therefore a useful alternative for patients who have to discontinue an ACE inhibitor because of persistent cough. Beyond this their role in the management of hypertension remains to be established.

CAUTIONS. Angiotensin-II receptor antagonists should be used with caution in renal artery stenosis (see also Renal Effects, p. 87). Monitoring of plasma potassium is advised, particularly in the elderly and in patients with renal impairment; lower initial doses may be appropriate in these patients. **Interactions:** Appendix 1 (as for ACE inhibitors).

CONTRA-INDICATIONS. Angiotensin-II receptor antagonists, like the ACE inhibitors, should be avoided in pregnancy (see also Appendix 4).

SIDE-EFFECTS. Side-effects are usually mild. Symptomatic hypotension may occur, particularly in patients with intravascular volume depletion (e.g. those taking high-dose diuretics). Hyperkalaemia occurs occasionally; angioedema has also been reported with some angiotensin-II receptor antagonists.

CANDESARTAN CILEXETIL
Indications: hypertension (see also notes above)
Cautions: see notes above; hepatic and renal impairment (Appendixes 2 and 3), aortic and mitral valve stenosis
Contra-indications: see notes above; breast-feeding (Appendix 5), severe hepatic impairment and cholestasis
Side-effects: see notes above; also upper respiratory tract and influenza-like symptoms including rhinitis and pharyngitis; altered liver function tests, back pain, peripheral oedema and nausea have also been reported
Dose: initially 4 mg (2 mg in hepatic and renal impairment) once daily adjusted according to response; usual maintenance dose 8 mg once daily; max. 16 mg once daily

▼ PoM **Amias**® (Astra, Takeda)
Tablets, candesartan cilexetil 2 mg, net price 7-tab pack = £3.00; 4 mg (scored), 7-tab pack = £3.35, 28-tab pack = £13.40; 8 mg (orange, scored), 28-tab pack = £15.75; 16 mg (scored), 28-tab pack = £19.10

IRBESARTAN
Indications: hypertension (see also notes above)
Cautions: see notes above; also aortic and mitral valve stenosis
Contra-indications: see notes above; breast-feeding (Appendix 5)
Side-effects: see notes above; flushing, increase in plasma concentration of creatine kinase reported
Dose: 150 mg once daily, increased if necessary to 300 mg once daily (in haemodialysis or in elderly over 75 years, initial dose of 75 mg once daily may be used)

▼ PoM **Aprovel**® (Bristol-Myers)
Tablets, irbesartan 75 mg, net price 28-tab pack = £15.50; 150 mg, 28-tab pack = £17.22; 300 mg, 28-tab pack = £23.26

LOSARTAN POTASSIUM
Indications: hypertension (see also notes above)
Cautions: see notes above; hepatic and renal impairment (Appendixes 2 and 3)
Contra-indications: see notes above; breast-feeding (Appendix 5)
Side-effects: see notes above; dizziness, taste disturbance, rarely, altered liver function tests
Dose: usually 50 mg once daily (elderly over 75 years, moderate to severe renal impairment, intravascular volume depletion, initially 25 mg once daily); if necessary increased after several weeks to 100 mg once daily

▼ PoM **Cozaar**® (MSD)
Tablets, both f/c, losartan potassium 25 mg (Half Strength), net price 7-tab pack = £4.31; 50 mg (scored), 28-tab pack = £17.23

With diuretic
Note. For hypertension in patients stabilised on the individual components in the same proportions
▼ PoM **Cozaar-Comp**® (MSD)
Tablets, f/c, yellow, losartan potassium 50 mg, hydrochlorothiazide 12.5 mg. Net price 28-tab pack = £17.23

VALSARTAN
Indications: hypertension (see also notes above)
Cautions: see notes above; mild to moderate hepatic impairment (Appendix 2) and renal impairment (Appendix 3)
Contra-indications: see notes above; severe hepatic impairment (Appendix 2), cirrhosis, biliary obstruction, breast-feeding (Appendix 5)
Side-effects: see notes above; fatigue, rarely epistaxis; neutropenia reported
Dose: usually 80 mg once daily (elderly over 75 years, mild to moderate hepatic impairment, moderate to severe renal impairment, intravascular volume depletion, initially 40 mg once daily); if necessary increased after at least 4 weeks to 160 mg daily (80 mg daily in hepatic impairment)

▼ PoM **Diovan**® (Novartis)
Capsules, valsartan 40 mg (grey), net price 7-cap pack = £3.35; 80 mg (grey/pink), 7-cap pack = £3.94 (hosp. only), 28-cap pack = £15.75; 160 mg (dark grey/pink), 7-cap pack = £4.92 (hosp. only), 28-cap pack = £19.69

2.5.6   Ganglion-blocking drugs

TRIMETAPHAN CAMSYLATE
(Trimetaphan Camsilate)
Indications: controlled hypotension in surgery
Cautions: hepatic or renal impairment, diabetes mellitus, elderly, cerebral or coronary vascular disease, adrenal insufficiency, Addison's disease, CNS degenerative disease

Contra-indications: severe arteriosclerosis, severe cardiac disease, pyloric stenosis, pregnancy
Side-effects: tachycardia and respiratory depression (particularly with muscle relaxants); constipation, increased intra-ocular pressure, pupillary dilatation
Dose: by intravenous infusion, 3–4 mg/minute initially, then adjusted according to response

PoM **Trimetaphan Camsylate** (Cambridge)
Injection, trimetaphan camsylate 50 mg/mL. Net price 5-mL amp = £11.62. For dilution and use as an infusion

2.5.7   Tyrosine hydroxylase inhibitors
Metirosine inhibits the enzyme tyrosine hydroxylase, and hence the synthesis of catecholamines. It is used in the pre-operative management of phaeochromocytoma, and long term in patients unsuitable for surgery; an alpha-adrenoceptor blocking drug (e.g. phenoxybenzamine, section 2.5.4) may also be required. Metirosine should **not** be used to treat essential hypertension.

METIROSINE
Indications: see notes above
Cautions: maintain high fluid intake and adequate blood volume; may impair ability to drive or operate machinery; **interactions:** Appendix 1 (metirosine)
Side-effects: sedation; extrapyramidal symptoms; diarrhoea (may be severe); hypersensitivity reactions
Dose: initially 250 mg 4 times daily, increased to max. of 4 g daily in divided doses; doses of 2–3 g daily should be given for 5–7 days before surgery

PoM **Demser**® (MSD)
Capsules, blue, metirosine 250 mg (hosp. only). Label: 2

2.6   Nitrates, calcium-channel blockers, and potassium-channel activators

2.6.1   Nitrates
2.6.2   Calcium-channel blockers
2.6.3   Potassium-channel activators
2.6.4   Peripheral and cerebral vasodilators

Nitrates, calcium-channel blockers and potassium-channel activators have a vasodilating effect. Vasodilators are known to act in heart failure either by: arteriolar dilatation which reduces both peripheral vascular resistance and left ventricular pressure at systole and results in improved cardiac output, *or* venous dilatation which results in dilatation of capacitance vessels, increase of venous pooling, and diminution of venous return to the heart (decreasing left ventricular end-diastolic pressure).

MANAGEMENT OF STABLE ANGINA. Acute attacks of stable angina should be managed with sublingual

---

glyceryl trinitrate. If attacks occur more than twice a week, regular drug therapy is required and should be introduced in a stepwise manner according to response. Aspirin should be given to patients with angina; a dose of 75–150 mg daily is suitable. Revascularisation procedures may also be appropriate.

Patients with mild or moderate stable angina who do not have left ventricular dysfunction, may be managed effectively with sublingual glyceryl trinitrate and regular administration of a beta-blocker (section 2.4). If necessary a dihydropyridine calcium-channel blocker (section 2.6.2) and then a long-acting nitrate (section 2.6.1) may be added. For those without left ventricular dysfunction and in whom beta-blockers are inappropriate, diltiazem or verapamil may be given (section 2.6.2) and a long-acting nitrate (section 2.6.1) may be added if symptom control is not adequate. For those intolerant of standard treatment, or where standard treatment has failed, nicorandil may be tried.

For patients with left ventricular dysfunction a long-acting nitrate (section 2.6.1) should be used and a long-acting dihydropyridine calcium-channel blocker (section 2.6.2) may be added if necessary.

A statin (section 2.12) should be considered for those with an elevated plasma-cholesterol concentration.

2.6.1   Nitrates

Nitrates have a useful role in *angina* (for details on the management of stable angina, see section 2.6). Although they are potent coronary vasodilators, their principal benefit follows from a reduction in venous return which reduces left ventricular work. Unwanted effects such as flushing, headache, and postural hypotension may limit therapy, especially when angina is severe or when patients are unusually sensitive to the effects of nitrates.

Sublingual **glyceryl trinitrate** is one of the most effective drugs for providing rapid symptomatic relief of angina, but its effect lasts only for 20 to 30 minutes; the 300-microgram tablet is often appropriate when glyceryl trinitrate is first used. Duration of action may be prolonged by *modified-release* preparations. The *aerosol spray* provides an alternative method of rapid relief of symptoms for those who find difficulty in dissolving sublingual preparations. The *percutaneous* preparations may be useful in the prophylaxis of angina for patients who suffer attacks at rest, especially at night.

Isosorbide dinitrate is active *sublingually* and is a more stable preparation for those who only require nitrates infrequently. It is also effective by mouth for prophylaxis; although the effect is slower in onset, it may persist for several hours. Duration of action of up to 12 hours is claimed for *modified-release* preparations. The activity of isosorbide dinitrate may depend on the production of active metabolites, the most important of which is isosorbide mononitrate. **Isosorbide mononitrate** itself is also available for angina prophylaxis, though the advantages over isosorbide dinitrate have not yet been firmly established.

Glyceryl trinitrate or isosorbide dinitrate may be tried by *intravenous injection* when the sublingual form is ineffective in patients with chest pain due to myocardial infarction or severe ischaemia. Intravenous injections are also useful in the treatment of acute left ventricular failure.

TOLERANCE. Many patients on long-acting or transdermal nitrates rapidly develop tolerance (with reduced therapeutic effects). Reduction of blood-nitrate concentrations to low levels for 4 to 8 hours each day usually maintains effectiveness in such patients. If tolerance is suspected during the use of transdermal patches they should be left off for several consecutive hours in each 24 hours; in the case of modified-release tablets of isosorbide dinitrate (and conventional formulations of isosorbide mononitrate), the second of the two daily doses can be given after about 8 hours rather than after 12 hours. Conventional formulations of isosorbide mononitrate should not usually be given more than twice daily unless small doses are used; modified-release formulations of isosorbide mononitrate should only be given once daily.

GLYCERYL TRINITRATE
Indications: prophylaxis and treatment of angina; left ventricular failure
Cautions: severe hepatic or renal impairment; hypothyroidism, malnutrition, or hypothermia; recent history of myocardial infarction, metal-containing transdermal systems should be removed before cardioversion or diathermy; tolerance (see notes above); **interactions:** Appendix 1 (glyceryl trinitrate)
Contra-indications: hypersensitivity to nitrates; hypotensive conditions and hypovolaemia; hypertrophic obstructive cardiomyopathy, aortic stenosis, cardiac tamponade, constrictive pericarditis, mitral stenosis; marked anaemia, head trauma, cerebral haemorrhage, closed-angle glaucoma
Side-effects: throbbing headache, flushing, dizziness, postural hypotension, tachycardia (but paradoxical bradycardia has occurred)
INJECTION. Specific side-effects following injection (particularly if given too rapidly) include severe hypotension, nausea and retching, diaphoresis, apprehension, restlessness, muscle twitching, retrosternal discomfort, palpitations, abdominal pain, syncope; prolonged administration has been associated with methaemoglobinaemia
Dose: *sublingually*, 0.3–1 mg, repeated as required
By mouth, see under Preparations
By intravenous infusion, 10–200 micrograms/minute

Short-acting tablets and sprays
Glyceryl Trinitrate (Non-proprietary)
Sublingual tablets, glyceryl trinitrate 300 micrograms, net price 100 = £2.84; 500 micrograms, 100 = 75p; 600 micrograms, 100 = £1.72. Label: 16
Note. Glyceryl trinitrate tablets should be supplied in glass containers of not more than 100 tablets, closed with a foil-lined cap, and containing no cotton wool wadding; they should be discarded after 8 weeks in use

---

Cautionary label wordings, see inside back cover   Prices are **net**, see p.1

Coro-Nitro Pump Spray® (Boehringer Mannheim)

Aerosol spray, glyceryl trinitrate 400 micrograms/metered dose. Net price 200-dose unit = £3.28

Dose: treatment or prophylaxis of angina, spray 1–2 doses under tongue and then close mouth

Glytrin Spray® (Sterwin)

Aerosol spray, glyceryl trinitrate 400 micrograms/metered dose. Net price 200-dose unit = £3.65

Dose: treatment or prophylaxis of angina, spray 1–2 doses under tongue and then close mouth

Caution: flammable

GTN 300 mcg (Martindale)

Sublingual tablets, glyceryl trinitrate 300 micrograms. Net price 100 = £2.84. Label: 16

Nitrolingual Pumpspray® (Lipha)

Aerosol spray, glyceryl trinitrate 400 micrograms/metered dose. Net price 200-dose unit = £4.10

Dose: treatment or prophylaxis of angina, spray 1–2 doses under tongue and then close mouth

Nitromin® (Dominion)

Aerosol spray, glyceryl trinitrate 400 micrograms/metered dose. Net price 180-dose unit = £2.92

Dose: treatment or prophylaxis of angina, spray 1–2 doses under tongue and then close mouth

Longer-acting tablets

Suscard® (Pharmax)

Buccal tablets, m/r, glyceryl trinitrate 1 mg, net price 20 = £1.96; 2 mg, 20 = £2.84; 3 mg, 20 = £4.10; 5 mg, 20 = £5.58. Counselling, see administration below

Dose: treatment of angina, 2 mg as required (1 mg in sensitive patients), increased to 3 mg if necessary; prophylaxis 1–3 mg 3 times daily; 5 mg in severe angina

Unstable angina (adjunct), up to 5 mg with ECG monitoring

Congestive heart failure, 5 mg 3 times daily, increased to 10 mg 3 times daily in severe cases

Acute heart failure, 5 mg repeated until symptoms abate

ADMINISTRATION: Tablets have rapid onset of effect; they are placed between upper lip and gum, and left to dissolve; vary site to reduce risk of dental caries

Sustac® (Pharmax)

Tablets, m/r, all pink, glyceryl trinitrate 2.6 mg, net price 20 = £1.19; 6.4 mg, 20 = £1.72; 10 mg, 20 = £2.39. Label: 25

Dose: prophylaxis of angina, 2.6–12.8 mg 3 times daily or 10 mg 2-3 times daily

Parenteral preparations

Note. Glass or polyethylene apparatus is preferable; loss of potency will occur if PVC is used

PoM **Glyceryl Trinitrate** (Non-proprietary)

Injection, glyceryl trinitrate 5 mg/mL. To be diluted before use. Net price 5-mL amp = £6.49; 10-mL amp = £12.98

Available from Faulding DBL

PoM **Nitrocine®** (Schwarz)

Injection, glyceryl trinitrate 1 mg/mL. To be diluted before use or given undiluted with syringe pump. Net price 10-mL amp = £8.27; 50-mL bottle = £19.38

PoM **Nitronal®** (Lipha)

Injection, glyceryl trinitrate 1 mg/mL. To be diluted before use or given undiluted with syringe pump. Net price 5-mL vial = £2.16; 50-mL vial = £17.64

Transdermal preparations

Deponit® (Schwarz)

Patches, self-adhesive, transparent, glyceryl trinitrate, *'5' patch* (releasing approx. 5 mg/24 hours when in contact with skin), net price 28 = £17.97; *'10' patch* (releasing approx. 10 mg/24 hours), 28 = £19.78

ADMINISTRATION: prophylaxis of angina, apply one '5' or one '10' patch to lateral chest wall, upper arm, or shoulder; replace every 24 hours, siting replacement patch on different area; see also notes above

Minitran® (Bayer)

Patches, self-adhesive, transparent, glyceryl trinitrate, *'5' patch* (releasing approx. 5 mg/24 hours when in contact with skin), net price 30 = £13.08; *'10' patch* (releasing approx. 10 mg/24 hours), 30 = £14.49; *'15' patch* (releasing approx. 15 mg/24 hours), 30 = £15.98

ADMINISTRATION: prophylaxis of angina, apply one '5' patch to chest or upper arm; replace every 24 hours, siting replacement patch on different area; adjust dose according to response; see also notes above

Maintenance of venous patency ('5' patch only), see literature

Nitro-Dur® (Schering-Plough)

Patches, self-adhesive, buff, glyceryl trinitrate, *'0.1 mg/h' patch* (releasing approx. 2.5 mg/24 hours when in contact with skin), net price 28 = £11.85; *'0.2 mg/h' patch* (releasing approx. 5 mg/24 hours), 28 = £13.15; *'0.4 mg/h' patch* (releasing approx. 10 mg/24 hours), 28 = £14.56; *'0.6 mg/h' patch* (releasing approx. 15 mg/24 hours), 28 = £16.02

ADMINISTRATION: prophylaxis of angina, apply one '0.2 mg/h' patch to chest or outer upper arm; replace every 24 hours, siting replacement patch on different area: adjust dose according to response; see also notes above

Percutol® (Dominion)

Ointment, glyceryl trinitrate 2%. Net price 60 g = £9.55. Counselling, see administration below

Additives: include wool fat

ADMINISTRATION: prophylaxis of angina, usual dose 1–2 inches of ointment measured on to *Applirule®*, and applied (usually to chest, abdomen, or thigh) without rubbing in and secured with surgical tape, every 3–4 hours as required; to determine dose, ½ inch on first day then increased by ½ inch/day until headache occurs, then reduced by ½ inch

Note. 1 inch of ointment contains glyceryl trinitrate 16.64 mg

Transiderm-Nitro® (Novartis)

Patches, self-adhesive, pink, glyceryl trinitrate, *'5' patch* (releasing approx. 5 mg/24 hours when in contact with skin), net price 28 = £17.71; *'10' patch* (releasing approx. 10 mg/24 hours), 28 = £19.47

ADMINISTRATION: prophylaxis of angina, apply one '5' or one '10' patch to lateral chest wall; replace every 24 hours, siting replacement patch on different area; max. two '10' patches daily; see also notes above

Prophylaxis of phlebitis and extravasation ('5' patch only), see product literature

ISOSORBIDE DINITRATE

Indications: prophylaxis and treatment of angina; left ventricular failure

Cautions; Contra-indications; Side-effects: see under Glyceryl Trinitrate

Dose: sublingually, 5–10 mg
By mouth, daily in divided doses, angina 30–120 mg, left ventricular failure 40–160 mg, up to 240 mg if required
By intravenous infusion, 2–10 mg/hour; higher doses up to 20 mg/hour may be required

Short-acting tablets and sprays
Isosorbide Dinitrate (Non-proprietary)
Tablets, isosorbide dinitrate 10 mg, net price 20 = 16p; 20 mg, 20 = 35p
Available from APS, Berk (Jeridin®), Cox, Hillcross, Norton
Isordil® (Monmouth)
Tablets (sublingual), pink, isosorbide dinitrate 5 mg. Net price 100-tab pack = £1.43. Label: 26
Tablets, both scored, isosorbide dinitrate 10 mg, net price 112-tab pack = £1.62; 30 mg, 112-tab pack = £3.86
Sorbichew® (Stuart)
Tablets (chewable), green, scored, isosorbide dinitrate 5 mg. Net price 100-tab pack = £1.51. Label: 24
Sorbitrate® (Stuart)
Tablets, both scored, isosorbide dinitrate 10 mg (yellow), net price 100-tab pack = £1.51; 20 mg (blue), 100-tab pack = £2.10

Modified-release preparations
Cedocard Retard® (Pharmacia & Upjohn)
Retard-20 tablets, m/r, yellow, scored, isosorbide dinitrate 20 mg. Net price 60-tab pack = £5.71. Label: 25
Dose: prophylaxis of angina, 1 tablet every 12 hours
Retard-40 tablets, m/r, orange-red, scored, isosorbide dinitrate 40 mg. Net price 60-tab pack = £11.09. Label: 25
Dose: prophylaxis of angina, 1–2 tablets every 12 hours
Isoket Retard® (Schwarz)
Retard-20 tablets, m/r, yellow, scored, isosorbide dinitrate 20 mg. Net price 50-tab pack = £3.24. Label: 25
Retard-40 tablets, m/r, orange, scored, isosorbide dinitrate 40 mg. Net price 50-tab pack = £7.99. Label: 25
Dose: prophylaxis of angina, 20–40 mg every 12 hours
Isordil Tembids® (Monmouth)
Capsules, m/r, blue/clear, isosorbide dinitrate 40 mg. Net price 56-cap pack = £8.70. Label: 25
Dose: prophylaxis of angina, 1 capsule 2–3 times daily
Sorbid SA® (Stuart)
Sorbid-20 SA capsules, m/r, red/yellow, isosorbide dinitrate 20 mg. Net price 56-cap pack = £3.50. Label: 25
Dose: prophylaxis of angina, 1–2 capsules twice daily
Sorbid-40 SA capsules, m/r, red/clear, isosorbide dinitrate 40 mg. Net price 56-cap pack = £5.00. Label: 25
Dose: prophylaxis of angina, 1–2 capsules twice daily

Parenteral preparations
PoM **Isoket**® (Schwarz)
Injection 0.05%, isosorbide dinitrate 500 micrograms/mL. To be diluted before use or given undiluted with syringe pump. Net price 50-mL bottle = £10.06

Injection 0.1%, isosorbide dinitrate 1 mg/mL. To be diluted before use. Net price 10-mL amp = £3.79; 50-mL bottle = £18.81; 100-mL bottle = £25.98
Note. Glass or polyethylene infusion apparatus is preferable; loss of potency if PVC used

Transdermal preparations
Isocard® (Eastern)
Transdermal spray, isosorbide dinitrate, 30 mg/metered dose. Net price 65-dose unit = £17.50. Label: 10 patient information leaflet, counselling, administration
Dose: prophylaxis of angina, initially (in those not previously receiving nitrates) 1 spray daily for 3 days, increased if necessary to 2 sprays daily for 3 days and then to 2 sprays twice daily; usual dose, 1–2 sprays in the morning and at night if necessary
COUNSELLING. Apply to clean dry skin on the chest wall holding can vertically. Spray each dose onto the chest from a distance of about 20 cm and then rub in gently; avoid contact with eyes; do not inhale
Caution: flammable

ISOSORBIDE MONONITRATE
Indications: prophylaxis of angina; adjunct in congestive heart failure
Cautions; Contra-indications; Side-effects: see under Glyceryl Trinitrate
Dose: initially 20 mg 2–3 times daily *or* 40 mg twice daily (10 mg twice daily in those who have not previously received nitrates); up to 120 mg daily in divided doses if required

Isosorbide Mononitrate (Non-proprietary)
Tablets, isosorbide mononitrate 10 mg, net price 20 = 38p; 20 mg, 20 = 42p; 40 mg, 20 = £1.40. Label: 25
Various strengths available from APS, Ashbourne (Isib®), Berk (Dynamin®), Cox, Dominion, Hillcross, Lagap, Lennon, Norton, Opus (Angeze®)
Elantan® (Schwarz)
Elantan 10 tablets, scored, isosorbide mononitrate 10 mg. Net price 50 = £2.83. Label: 25
PoM *Elantan 20 tablets*, scored, isosorbide mononitrate 20 mg. Net price 50 = £4.11. Label: 25
PoM *Elantan 40 tablets*, scored, isosorbide mononitrate 40 mg. Net price 50 = £7.07. Label: 25
Ismo® (Boehringer Mannheim)
Ismo 10 tablets, isosorbide mononitrate 10 mg. Net price 60-tab pack = £3.39. Label: 25
Ismo 20 tablets, isosorbide mononitrate 20 mg. Net price 60-tab pack = £4.97. Label: 25
Ismo 40 tablets, isosorbide mononitrate 40 mg. Net price 60-tab pack = £8.17. Label: 25
Isotrate® (Bioglan)
Tablets, isosorbide mononitrate 20 mg. Net price 60-tab pack = £7.09. Label: 25
Monit® (Lorex)
LS Tablets, isosorbide mononitrate 10 mg. Net price 56-tab pack = £3.37. Label: 25
Tablets, scored, isosorbide mononitrate 20 mg. Net price 56-tab pack = £4.30. Label: 25

Mono-Cedocard® (Pharmacia & Upjohn)

Mono-Cedocard 10 tablets, orange, scored, isosorbide mononitrate 10 mg. Net price 60-tab pack = £3.68. Label: 25

Mono-Cedocard 20 tablets, scored, isosorbide mononitrate 20 mg. Net price 100-tab pack = £6.83. Label: 25

Mono-Cedocard 40 tablets, scored, isosorbide mononitrate 40 mg. Net price 60-tab pack = £9.12. Label: 25

Modified release

Elantan LA® (Schwarz)

Elantan LA 25 capsules, m/r, brown/white, enclosing white micropellets, isosorbide mononitrate 25 mg. Net price 28-cap pack = £7.00. Label: 25

Dose: prophylaxis of angina, 1 capsule in the morning, increased if necessary to 2 capsules

Elantan LA 50 capsules, m/r, brown/pink, enclosing white micropellets, isosorbide mononitrate 50 mg. Net price 28-cap pack = £11.30. Label: 25

Dose: prophylaxis of angina, 1 capsule daily in the morning, increased if necessary to 2 capsules

PoM **Imdur®** (Astra)

Durules® (= tablets m/r), yellow, f/c, scored, isosorbide mononitrate 60 mg. Net price 28-tab pack = £11.14. Label: 25

Dose: prophylaxis of angina, 1 tablet in the morning (half a tablet if headache occurs), increased to 2 tablets if required

Isib 60XL® (Ashbourne)

Tablets, m/r, scored, ivory, isosorbide mononitrate 60 mg. Net price 28-tab pack = £10.02. Label: 25

Dose: prophylaxis of angina, 1 tablet in the morning (half a tablet for 2–4 days if headache occurs), increased if necessary to 2 tablets

Note. Also available as Isotard 60XL® (Bartholomew Rhodes, Hillcross)

Ismo Retard® (Boehringer Mannheim)

Tablets, m/r, s/c, isosorbide mononitrate 40 mg. Net price 28-tab pack = £10.24. Label: 25

Dose: prophylaxis of angina, 1 tablet daily in morning

¹**MCR-50®** (Pharmacia & Upjohn)

Capsules, m/r, containing white micropellets, isosorbide mononitrate 50 mg. Net price 28-cap pack = £11.02. Label: 25

Dose: prophylaxis of angina, 1 capsule in morning, increased to 2 capsules if required

1. Full product name Mono Cedocard Retard-50®

Modisal XL® (Lagap)

Tablets, m/r, ivory, isosorbide mononitrate 60 mg. Net price 28-tab pack = £11.14. Label: 25

Dose: prophylaxis of angina, 1 tablet daily in the morning (half a tablet for first 2–4 days to minimise possibility of headache), increased if necessary to 2 tablets once daily

Monit SR® (Lorex)

Tablets, m/r, s/c, isosorbide mononitrate 40 mg. Net price 28-tab pack = £10.24. Label: 25

Dose: prophylaxis of angina, 1 tablet daily in morning

Monomax SR® (Trinity)

Capsules, m/r, isosorbide mononitrate 40 mg, net price 28-cap pack = £8.70; 60 mg, 28-cap pack = £9.46. Label: 25

Dose: prophylaxis of angina, 40 mg once daily, increased if necessary to 60 mg daily

Note. Also available as Angeze SR® (Opus)

Monosorb XL 60® (Dexcel)

Tablets, m/r, f/c, isosorbide mononitrate 60 mg. Net price 28-tab pack = £11.14. Label: 25

Dose: prophylaxis of angina, 1 tablet daily in the morning (half a tablet for first 2–4 days to minimise possibility of headache) increased if necessary to 2 tablets

PENTAERYTHRITOL TETRANITRATE
(Pentaerithrityl Tetranitrate)

Indications: prophylaxis of angina

Cautions; Contra-indications; Side-effects: see under Glyceryl Trinitrate

Mycardol® (Sanofi Winthrop)

Tablets, scored, pentaerythritol tetranitrate 30 mg. Net price 168-tab pack = £8.05. Label: 22

Dose: 2 tablets 3–4 times daily

2.6.2   Calcium-channel blockers

Calcium-channel blockers (less correctly called 'calcium-antagonists') interfere with the inward displacement of calcium ions through the slow channels of active cell membranes. They influence the myocardial cells, the cells within the specialised conducting system of the heart, and the cells of vascular smooth muscle. Thus, myocardial contractility may be reduced, the formation and propagation of electrical impulses within the heart may be depressed, and coronary or systemic vascular tone may be diminished. They should usually be **avoided** in *heart failure* because they may further depress cardiac function and cause clinically significant deterioration.

Calcium-channel blockers differ in their predilection for the various possible sites of action therefore their therapeutic effects are disparate, with much greater variation than those of beta-blockers. There are important differences between verapamil and the dihydropyridine calcium-channel blockers, such as nifedipine, nicardipine and isradipine.

Verapamil is used for the treatment of *angina* (section 2.6), *hypertension*, and *arrhythmias* (section 2.3.2). It reduces cardiac output, slows the heart rate, and may impair atrioventricular conduction. It may precipitate heart failure, exacerbate conduction disorders, and cause hypotension at high doses and should **not** be used with beta-blockers (see p. 101). Constipation is the most common side-effect.

Nifedipine relaxes vascular smooth muscle and dilates coronary and peripheral arteries. It has more influence on vessels and less on the myocardium than does verapamil, and unlike verapamil has no anti-arrhythmic activity. It rarely precipitates heart failure because any negative inotropic effect is offset by a reduction in left ventricular work. Short-acting formulations of nifedipine are not recommended for long-term management of hypertension; their use may be associated with large variations in blood pressure, reducing their potential to prevent complications. **Nicardipine** has similar effects to those of nifedipine and may produce less reduction of myocardial contractility. **Amlodipine** and **felodipine** also resemble nifedipine and nicardipine in their effects and do not reduce myocardial contractility. They have a longer duration of action and can be given once daily. Nifedipine, nicardipine, amlodipine, and felodipine are used for the treatment of angina (section 2.6) or hypertension. All are valuable in forms of *angina associated with coronary vasospasm*. Side-effects associated with vasodilatation such as flushing and headache (which become less obtrusive after a few days), and ankle swelling (which may respond only partially to diuretics) are common.

Isradipine, **lacidipine** and **nisoldipine** have similar effects to those of nifedipine and nicardipine; isradipine and lacidipine are only indicated for *hypertension* whereas nisoldipine is indicated for angina and hypertension.

Nimodipine is related to nifedipine but the smooth muscle relaxant effect preferentially acts on cerebral arteries. Its use is confined to prevention of *vascular spasm following subarachnoid haemorrhage*.

Diltiazem is effective in most forms of *angina* (section 2.6); the longer-acting formulation is also used for *hypertension*. It may be used in patients for whom beta-blockers are contra-indicated or ineffective. It has a less negative inotropic effect than verapamil and significant myocardial depression occurs rarely. Nevertheless because of the risk of bradycardia it should be used with caution in association with beta-blockers.

UNSTABLE ANGINA. Calcium-channel blockers do not reduce the risk of myocardial infarction in unstable angina. Their use should be reserved for patients resistant to treatment with beta-blockers, nitrates, and anticoagulation with aspirin and intravenous heparin.

WITHDRAWAL. There is some evidence that sudden withdrawal of calcium-channel blockers may be associated with an exacerbation of angina.

AMLODIPINE BESYLATE
(Amlodipine Besilate)
Indications: hypertension, prophylaxis of angina
Cautions: hepatic impairment; **interactions:** Appendix 1 (calcium-channel blockers)
Contra-indications: cardiogenic shock, unstable angina, significant aortic stenosis; pregnancy and breast-feeding
Side-effects: headache, oedema, fatigue, nausea, flushing, dizziness, gum hyperplasia; erythema multiforme reported
Dose: hypertension or angina, initially 5 mg once daily; max. 10 mg once daily

PoM **Istin**® (Pfizer)
Tablets, amlodipine (as besylate) 5 mg. Net price 28-tab pack = £11.85; 10 mg, 28-tab pack = £17.70

DILTIAZEM HYDROCHLORIDE
Indications: prophylaxis and treatment of angina; hypertension
Cautions: reduce dose in hepatic and renal impairment; heart failure or significantly impaired left ventricular function, mild bradycardia (avoid if severe), first degree AV block, or prolonged PR interval; **interactions:** Appendix 1 (calcium-channel blockers)
Contra-indications: severe bradycardia, left ventricular failure, second- or third-degree AV block (unless pacemaker fitted), sick sinus syndrome; pregnancy and breast-feeding (see Appendixes 4 and 5)
Side-effects: bradycardia, sino-atrial block, AV block, dizziness, hypotension, malaise, asthenia, headache, hot flushes, gastro-intestinal disturbances, oedema (notably of ankles); rarely rashes (erythema multiforme reported); altered liver function tests; hepatitis and depression reported
Dose: angina, 60 mg 3 times daily (elderly initially twice daily); increased if necessary to 360 mg daily
Longer-acting formulations, see under preparations below

Standard formulations
Note. These formulations are licensed as generics and there is no requirement for brand name dispensing. Although their means of formulation has called for the strict designation 'modified-release' their duration of action corresponds to that of tablets requiring administration 3 times daily

PoM **Diltiazem** (Non-proprietary)
Tablets, m/r (but see note above), diltiazem hydrochloride 60 mg. Net price 100 = £7.39. Label: 25
Available from APS, Ashbourne (Angiozem®), Berk (Calazem®), Cox, Hillcross, Lagap, Norton, Thames (Britiazim®)

PoM **Adizem-60**® (Napp)
Tablets, m/r (but see note above), f/c, diltiazem hydrochloride 60 mg. Net price 100-tab pack = £15.38. Label: 25

PoM **Tildiem**® (Lorex)
Tablets, m/r (but see note above), off-white, diltiazem hydrochloride 60 mg. Net price 90-tab pack = £10.35. Label: 25

Longer-acting formulations
Note. To avoid confusion between these different formulations of diltiazem, prescribers should specify the brand to be dispensed

PoM **Adizem-SR**® (Napp)
Capsules, m/r, diltiazem hydrochloride 90 mg (white), net price 56-cap pack = £11.06; 120 mg (brown/white), 56-cap pack = £12.29; 180 mg (brown/white), 56-cap pack = £18.43. Label: 25
Tablets, m/r, f/c, scored, diltiazem hydrochloride 120 mg. Net price 56-tab pack = £18.14. Label: 25
Dose: mild to moderate hypertension, usually 120 mg twice daily (dose form not appropriate for initial dose titration)
Angina, initially 90 mg twice daily (elderly, dose form not appropriate for initial dose titration); increased to 180 mg twice daily if required

---

PoM **Adizem-XL®** (Napp)

Capsules, m/r, diltiazem hydrochloride 120 mg (pink/blue), net price 28-cap pack = £10.72; 180 mg (dark pink/blue), 28-cap pack = £12.16; 240 mg (red/blue), 28-cap pack = £13.51; 300 mg (maroon/blue), 28-cap pack = £10.72. Label: 25

Dose: angina and mild to moderate hypertension, initially 240 mg once daily, increased if necessary to 300 mg once daily; in elderly and in hepatic or renal impairment, initially 120 mg daily

PoM **Angitil SR®** (Trinity)

Capsules, m/r, diltiazem hydrochloride 90 mg (white), net price 56-cap pack = £8.85; 120 mg (brown), 56-cap pack = £9.83; 180 mg (brown), 56-cap pack = £14.74. Label: 25

Dose: angina and mild to moderate hypertension, initially 90 mg twice daily (elderly and in hepatic and renal impairment, dose form not appropriate for initial dose titration); increased if necessary to 120 mg or 180 mg twice daily

PoM **Calcicard CR®** (Norton)

Tablets, m/r, both f/c, diltiazem hydrochloride 90 mg, net price 56-tab pack = £8.85; 120 mg, 56-tab pack = £9.83. Label: 25

Dose: mild to moderate hypertension, initially 90 mg or 120 mg twice daily; up to 360 mg daily may be required: ELDERLY and in hepatic and renal impairment, initially 120 mg once daily; up to 240 mg daily may be required Angina, initially 90 mg or 120 mg twice daily; up to 480 mg daily in divided doses may be required; ELDERLY and in hepatic and renal impairment, dose form not appropriate for initial dose titration; up to 240 mg daily may be required

PoM **Dilzem SR®** (Elan)

Capsules, m/r, all beige, diltiazem hydrochloride 60 mg, net price 56-cap pack = £7.56; 90 mg, 56-cap pack = £10.21; 120 mg, 56-cap pack = £11.34. Label: 25

Dose: angina and mild to moderate hypertension, initially 90 mg twice daily (elderly 60 mg twice daily); up to 180 mg twice daily may be required

PoM **Dilzem XL®** (Elan)

Capsules, m/r, diltiazem hydrochloride 120 mg, net price 28-cap pack = £7.56; 180 mg, 28-cap pack = £10.36; 240 mg, 28-cap pack = £10.64. Label: 25

Dose: angina and mild to moderate hypertension, initially 180 mg once daily (elderly and in hepatic and renal impairment, 120 mg once daily); if necessary may be increased to 360 mg once daily

PoM **Slozem®** (Lipha)

Capsules, m/r, diltiazem hydrochloride 120 mg (pink/clear), net price 28-cap pack = £7.00; 180 mg (pink/clear), 28-cap pack = £9.24; 240 mg (red/clear), 28-cap pack = £9.80. Label: 25

Dose: angina and mild to moderate hypertension, initially 240 mg once daily (elderly and in hepatic and renal impairment, 120 mg once daily); if necessary may be increased to 360 mg once daily

PoM **Tildiem LA®** (Lorex)

Capsules, m/r, diltiazem hydrochloride 200 mg (pink/grey, containing white pellets), net price 28-cap pack = £11.61; 300 mg (white/yellow, containing white pellets), 28-cap pack = £12.80. Label: 25

Dose: angina and mild to moderate hypertension, initially 300 mg once daily before or with food, increased to 400 mg daily, and if necessary to 500 mg daily; ELD-ERLY and in hepatic or renal impairment, initially 200 mg daily, increased if necessary to 300 mg daily

PoM **Tildiem Retard®** (Lorex)

Tablets, m/r, diltiazem hydrochloride 90 mg, net price 56-tab pack = £11.06; 120 mg, 56-tab pack = £12.29. Label: 25

COUNSELLING. Tablet membrane may pass through gastro-intestinal tract unchanged, but being porous has no effect on efficacy

Dose: mild to moderate hypertension, initially 90 mg or 120 mg twice daily (elderly once daily); up to 360 mg daily may be required (elderly up to 240 mg daily) Angina, initially 90 mg or 120 mg twice daily (elderly, dose form not appropriate for initial dose titration); up to 480 mg daily in divided doses may be required (elderly up to 240 mg daily)

PoM **Viazem XL®** (Du Pont)

Capsules, m/r, diltiazem hydrochloride 120 mg (lavender), net price 28-cap pack = £10.50; 180 mg (white/blue-green), 28-cap pack = £10.94; 240 mg (blue-green/lavender), 28-cap pack = £12.16; 300 mg (white/lavender), 28-cap pack = £9.65; 360 mg (blue-green), 28-cap pack = £21.00. Label: 25

Dose: mild to moderate hypertension, titrate to usual maintenance dose of 300 mg once daily, adjusted according to response

ELDERLY and in hepatic or renal impairment, initially 120 mg once daily, adjusted according to response

PoM **Zemtard 300 XL®** (Bartholomew Rhodes)

Capsules, m/r, blue/white, diltiazem hydrochloride 300 mg. Net price 28-cap pack = £11.21. Label: 25

Dose: angina and mild to moderate hypertension, 180–300 mg once daily, increased if necessary to 360 mg once daily in hypertension and to 480 mg once daily in angina (only 300 mg dose form available)

ELDERLY and in hepatic or renal impairment, initially 120 mg once daily (dose form not appropriate for initial dose titration)

FELODIPINE

Indications: hypertension, prophylaxis of angina

Cautions: withdraw if ischaemic pain occurs or existing pain worsens shortly after initiating treatment or if cardiogenic shock develops; severe left ventricular dysfunction; hepatic impairment; breast-feeding; avoid grapefruit juice (may affect metabolism); **interactions:** Appendix 1 (calcium-channel blockers)

Contra-indications: pregnancy; unstable angina; significant aortic stenosis; within 1 month of myocardial infarction

Side-effects: flushing, headache, palpitations, dizziness, fatigue, gravitational oedema, rash and pruritus, gum hyperplasia

Dose: hypertension, initially 5 mg (elderly 2.5 mg) daily in the morning; usual maintenance 5–10 mg once daily; doses above 20 mg daily rarely needed

Angina, initially 5 mg daily in the morning, increased if necessary to 10 mg once daily

PoM **Plendil®** (Astra)

Tablets, m/r, f/c, felodipine 2.5 mg, net price 28-tab pack = £6.09; 5 mg, 28-tab pack = £8.12; 10 mg, 28-tab pack = £10.92. Label: 25

ISRADIPINE

Indications: hypertension

Cautions: tight aortic stenosis; sick sinus syndrome (if pacemaker not fitted); reduce dose in hepatic or renal impairment; pregnancy (may prolong labour); avoid grapefruit juice (may affect metabolism); **interactions:** Appendix 1 (calcium-channel blockers)

Side-effects: headache, flushing, dizziness, tachycardia and palpitations, localised peripheral oedema; hypotension uncommon; rarely weight gain, fatigue, abdominal discomfort, rashes

Dose: 2.5 mg twice daily (1.25 mg twice daily in elderly, hepatic or renal impairment); increased if necessary after 3–4 weeks to 5 mg twice daily (exceptionally up to 10 mg twice daily); maintenance 2.5 or 5 mg once daily may be sufficient

PoM **Prescal**® (Novartis)
Tablets, yellow, scored, isradipine 2.5 mg. Net price 56-tab pack = £12.53

LACIDIPINE

Indications: hypertension

Cautions: cardiac conduction abnormalities; poor cardiac reserve; hepatic impairment; withdraw if ischaemic pain occurs shortly after initiating treatment or if cardiogenic shock develops; avoid grapefruit juice (may affect metabolism); **interactions:** Appendix 1 (calcium-channel blockers)

Contra-indications: aortic stenosis; pregnancy and breast-feeding; avoid within 1 month of myocardial infarction

Side-effects: headache, flushing, oedema, dizziness, palpitations; also asthenia, rash (including pruritus and erythema), gastro-intestinal disturbances, gum hyperplasia, muscle cramps, polyuria, chest pain (see Cautions); mood disturbances

Dose: initially 2 mg as a single daily dose, preferably in the morning; increased after 3–4 weeks to 4 mg daily, then if necessary to 6 mg daily

PoM **Motens**® (Boehringer Ingelheim)
Tablets, both f/c, lacidipine 2 mg, net price 28-tab pack = £10.23; 4 mg (scored), 28-tab pack = £15.30

MIBEFRADIL

Indications: hypertension, prophylaxis of angina

Cautions: hepatic impairment (Appendix 2), severe aortic stenosis, mild heart failure, bradycardia (avoid if severe); **interactions:** Appendix 1 (calcium-channel blockers)

Contra-indications: sick sinus syndrome, second or third degree AV block (unless pacemaker fitted), moderate or severe heart failure, avoid within one month of myocardial infarction, unstable angina, severe hepatic impairment (Appendix 2), pregnancy (Appendix 4) and breast-feeding (Appendix 5)

Side-effects: peripheral oedema, fatigue, dizziness, bradycardia, AV block; thrombocytopenia and angioedema reported

Dose: initially 50 mg once daily, increased to 100 mg once daily if necessary

▼ PoM **Posicor**® (Roche)
Tablets, f/c, scored, mibefradil (as dihydrochloride) 50 mg, net price 28-tab pack = £11.26; 100 mg (pink), 28-tab pack = £16.82

NICARDIPINE HYDROCHLORIDE

Indications: prophylaxis of angina; mild to moderate hypertension

Cautions: withdraw if ischaemic pain occurs or existing pain worsens within 30 minutes of initiating treatment or increasing dose; congestive heart failure or significantly impaired left ventricular function; elderly; hepatic or renal impairment; avoid grapefruit juice (may affect metabolism); **interactions:** Appendix 1 (calcium-channel blockers)

Contra-indications: cardiogenic shock; advanced aortic stenosis; unstable or acute attacks of angina; pregnancy and breast-feeding; avoid within 1 month of myocardial infarction

Side-effects: dizziness, headache, peripheral oedema, flushing, palpitations, nausea; also gastro-intestinal disturbances, drowsiness, insomnia, tinnitus, hypotension, rashes, dyspnoea, paraesthesia, frequency of micturition; thrombocytopenia, depression and impotence reported

Dose: initially 20 mg 3 times daily, increased, after at least three days, to 30 mg 3 times daily (usual range 60–120 mg daily); patients with hypertension controlled on 20–30 mg 3 times daily can be given 30–40 mg twice daily

PoM **Cardene**® (Yamanouchi)
Capsules, nicardipine hydrochloride 20 mg (blue/white), net price 56-cap pack = £8.95; 30 mg (blue/pale blue), 56-cap pack = £10.39

Modified release
PoM **Cardene SR**® (Yamanouchi)
Capsules, m/r, nicardipine hydrochloride 30 mg, net price 56-cap pack = £10.33; 45 mg (blue), 56-cap pack = £14.35. Label: 25
Dose: mild to moderate hypertension, initially 30 mg twice daily; usual effective dose 45 mg twice daily (range 30–60 mg twice daily)

NIFEDIPINE

Indications: prophylaxis and treatment of angina; hypertension; Raynaud's phenomenon

Cautions: withdraw if ischaemic pain occurs or existing pain worsens shortly after initiating treatment; poor cardiac reserve; heart failure or significantly impaired left ventricular function (heart failure deterioration observed); severe hypotension; reduce dose in hepatic impairment; diabetes mellitus; may inhibit labour; breast-feeding (see Appendix 5); avoid grapefruit juice (may affect metabolism); **interactions:** Appendix 1 (calcium-channel blockers)

Contra-indications: cardiogenic shock; advanced aortic stenosis; pregnancy (toxicity in *animal* studies); porphyria (see section 9.8.2)

Side-effects: headache, flushing, dizziness, lethargy; tachycardia, palpitations: also gravitational oedema, rash (erythema multiforme reported), nausea, increased frequency of micturition, eye pain, gum hyperplasia; depression reported; telangiectasia reported

Dose: see preparations below

PoM **Adalat**® (Bayer)

Capsules, both orange, nifedipine 5 mg, net price 20 = £1.42; 10 mg, 20 = £1.80. Label: 21, counselling, see dose

Dose: angina and Raynaud's phenomenon, initially 10 mg (elderly and hepatic impairment, 5 mg) 3 times daily with or after food; usual maintenance 5–20 mg 3 times daily; for immediate effect in angina bite into capsule and swallow liquid
Hypertension, not recommended therefore no dose stated

Note. Nifedipine capsules also available from APS, Ashbourne (Angiopine®), Berk (Calanif®), Cox, CP, Hillcross, Norton

Modified release

Note. To avoid confusion between these different formulations of nifedipine, prescribers should specify the brand to be dispensed

PoM **Adalat**® **LA** (Bayer)

LA 30 tablets, m/r, pink, nifedipine 30 mg. Net price 28-tab pack = £10.36. Label: 25

LA 60 tablets, m/r, pink, nifedipine 60 mg. Net price 28-tab pack = £15.40. Label: 25

COUNSELLING. Tablet membrane may pass through gastro-intestinal tract unchanged, but being porous has no effect on efficacy
Dose: mild to moderate hypertension and angina prophylaxis, 30 mg once daily, increased if necessary; max. 90 mg once daily
Caution: dose form not appropriate for use in hepatic impairment or where there is a history of oesophageal or gastro-intestinal obstruction, decreased lumen diameter of the gastro-intestinal tract, or inflammatory bowel disease (including Crohn's disease)

PoM **Adalat**® **Retard** (Bayer)

Retard 10 tablets, m/r, pink, nifedipine 10 mg. Net price 56-tab pack = £8.66. Label: 21, 25

Retard 20 tablets, m/r, pink, nifedipine 20 mg. Net price 56-tab pack = £10.81. Label: 21, 25

Dose: hypertension and angina prophylaxis, 20 mg twice daily with or after food (initial titration 10 mg twice daily); usual maintenance 10–40 mg twice daily

PoM **Adipine**® **MR** (Trinity)

Tablets, m/r, nifedipine 10 mg (apricot), net price 56-tab pack = £6.93; 20 mg (pink), 56-tab pack = £8.65. Label: 21, 25

Dose: hypertension and angina prophylaxis, 20 mg twice daily after food (initial titration 10 mg twice daily); max. 40 mg twice daily
Note. Also available as Nimodrel MR® (Opus)

PoM **Cardilate MR**® (Norton)

Tablets, m/r, nifedipine 10 mg (pink), net price 56-tab pack = £6.93; 20 mg (brown), net price 100-tab pack = £15.44. Label: 25

Dose: hypertension and angina prophylaxis, 20 mg twice daily (initial titration 10 mg twice daily); max. 80 mg daily
Note. Also available as Angiopine MR® (Ashbourne)

PoM **Coracten**® (Evans)

Capsules, m/r, nifedipine 10 mg (grey/pink, enclosing yellow pellets), net price 60-cap pack = £7.15; 20 mg (pink/brown, enclosing yellow pellets), 60-cap pack = £9.97. Label: 25

Dose: hypertension and angina prophylaxis, one 20-mg capsule every 12 hours, adjusted within range 10–40 mg every 12 hours

PoM **Hypolar**® **Retard 20** (Lagap)

Tablets, m/r, red, f/c, nifedipine 20 mg. Net price 56-tab pack = £12.81. Label: 25

Dose: hypertension and angina prophylaxis, 20 mg twice daily, increased if necessary to 40 mg twice daily

PoM **Nifedotard 20 MR**® (Bartholomew Rhodes)

Tablets, m/r, red, nifedipine 20 mg. Net price 56-tab pack = £10.62. Label: 25

Dose: hypertension and angina prophylaxis, 20 mg twice daily, increased if necessary to 40 mg twice daily (dose form not appropriate for initial dose titration in hepatic impairment)

PoM **Nifelease**® (Lennon)

Tablets, m/r, scored, pink, nifedipine 20 mg. Net price 100-tab pack = £18.99. Label: 25

Dose: hypertension and angina prophylaxis, 20 mg twice daily, increased if necessary to 40 mg twice daily

PoM **Nifensar XL**® (Rhône-Poulenc Rorer)

Tablets, m/r, yellow, nifedipine 20 mg. Net price 28-tab pack = £7.37. Label: 21, 25

Dose: mild to moderate hypertension, initially 40 mg once daily (initially 20 mg in elderly not previously treated with nifedipine, or in renal impairment); usual maintenance dose 20–40 mg daily; max. 100 mg daily
Note. May be temporarily unavailable

PoM **Tensipine MR**® (Ethical Generics Ltd)

Tablets, m/r, both pink, nifedipine 10 mg, net price 56-tab pack = £7.62; 20 mg, 56-tab pack = £9.51. Label: 21, 25

Dose: hypertension and angina prophylaxis, initially 10 mg twice daily adjusted according to response to 40 mg twice daily

PoM **Unipine XL**® (Ethical Generics Ltd)

Tablets, m/r, red, f/c, nifedipine 30 mg. Net price 28-tab pack = £10.08. Label: 22, 25

Dose: mild to moderate hypertension, 30 mg once daily, preferably in the morning, increased if necessary to 60 mg once daily

With atenolol
Section 2.4

NIMODIPINE

Indications: prevention and treatment of ischaemic neurological deficits following subarachnoid haemorrhage

Cautions: cerebral oedema or severely raised intracranial pressure; avoid concomitant administration of nimodipine tablets and infusion, other calcium-channel blockers, or beta-blockers; impaired renal function or nephrotoxic drugs; pregnancy; avoid grapefruit juice (may affect metabolism); **interactions:** Appendix 1 (calcium-channel blockers)

Side-effects: hypotension, variation in heart-rate, flushing, headache, gastro-intestinal disorders, nausea, and feeling of warmth; thrombocytopenia and ileus reported; transient increase in liver enzymes after intravenous administration

Dose: prevention, *by mouth*, 60 mg every 4 hours (total daily dose 360 mg), starting within 4 days of subarachnoid haemorrhage and continued for 21 days

Treatment, *by intravenous infusion* via central catheter, 1 mg/hour initially, increased after 2 hours to 2 mg/hour, providing no severe decrease in blood pressure; patients with unstable blood pressure or weighing less than 70 kg, 500 micrograms/hour initially or less if necessary; treatment should start as soon as possible and should continue for at least 5 days (max. 14 days); in the event of surgical intervention during treatment continue for at least 5 days after

PoM Nimotop® (Bayer)

Tablets, yellow, f/c, nimodipine 30 mg. Net price 100-tab pack = £38.85

Intravenous infusion, nimodipine 200 micrograms/mL; also contains ethanol 20% and macrogol '400' 17%. Net price 50-mL vial (with polyethylene infusion catheter) = £13.24; 250-mL bottle = £66.20

Note. Polyethylene or polypropylene apparatus should be used; PVC should be avoided

NISOLDIPINE

Indications: prophylaxis of angina, mild to moderate hypertension

Cautions: elderly; hypotension; avoid grapefruit juice (may affect metabolism); **interactions:** Appendix 1 (calcium-channel blockers)

Contra-indications: cardiogenic shock, aortic stenosis; hepatic impairment (dose form not appropriate); pregnancy and breast-feeding

Side-effects: gravitational oedema, headache, flushing, tachycardia, palpitations; dizziness, gastro-intestinal disturbances (including nausea, constipation); less frequently paraesthesia, hypotension, weakness, dyspnoea, allergic skin reactions, frequency of micturition, liver enzyme disturbances

Dose: initially 10 mg daily, preferably before breakfast; if necessary increase at intervals of at least 1 week (usual maintenance in angina 20–40 mg once daily); max. 40 mg daily

▼ **PoM Syscor MR®** (Bayer)

Tablets, m/r, all f/c, yellow, nisoldipine 10 mg, net price 28-tab pack = £9.80; 20 mg, 28-tab pack = £13.72; 30 mg, 28-tab pack = £17.64. Label: 22, 25

VERAPAMIL HYDROCHLORIDE

Indications: see under Dose and preparations

Cautions: first-degree AV block; acute phase of myocardial infarction (avoid if bradycardia, hypotension, left ventricular failure); patients taking beta-blockers (**important:** see below); reduce dose in hepatic impairment; children, specialist advice only (see section 2.3.2); pregnancy and

breast-feeding; avoid grapefruit juice (may affect metabolism); **interactions:** Appendix 1 (calcium-channel blockers)

VERAPAMIL AND BETA-BLOCKERS. Verapamil should not be injected into patients recently treated with beta-blockers because of the risk of hypotension and asystole. It has been suggested that when verapamil injection has been given first, an interval of 30 minutes before giving a beta-blocker is sufficient but this too is open to doubt.

It may even be hazardous to give verapamil and a beta-blocker together by mouth (should only be contemplated if myocardial function well preserved).

Contra-indications: hypotension, bradycardia, second- and third-degree AV block, sick sinus syndrome, cardiogenic shock, sino-atrial block; history of heart failure or significantly impaired left ventricular function, even if controlled by therapy; atrial flutter or fibrillation complicating Wolff-Parkinson-White syndrome; porphyria (see section 9.8.2)

Side-effects: constipation; less commonly nausea, vomiting, flushing, headache, dizziness, fatigue, ankle oedema; rarely reversible impairment of liver function, allergic reactions (erythema, pruritus, urticaria, Stevens-Johnson syndrome); myalgia, arthralgia, paraesthesia, erythromelalgia; increased prolactin concentration; rarely gynaecomastia and gingival hyperplasia after long-term treatment; after intravenous administration or high doses, hypotension, bradycardia, heart block, and asystole

Dose. by mouth, supraventricular arrhythmias (but see also Contra-indications), 40–120 mg 3 times daily

Angina, 80–120 mg 3 times daily

Hypertension, 240–480 mg daily in 2–3 divided doses

By slow intravenous injection over 2 minutes (3 minutes in elderly), 5–10 mg (preferably with ECG monitoring); in paroxysmal tachyarrhythmias a further 5 mg after 5–10 minutes if required

PoM Verapamil (Non-proprietary)

Tablets, coated, verapamil hydrochloride 40 mg, net price 20 = 18p; 80 mg, 20 = 33p; 120 mg, 20 = 58p; 160 mg, 20 = 92p

Various strengths available from APS, Berk (Berkatens®), Cox, Hillcross, Lagap, Norton

Oral solution, sugar-free, verapamil hydrochloride 40 mg/5 mL available from Rosemont (special order)

PoM Cordilox® (Baker Norton)

Tablets, all yellow, f/c, verapamil hydrochloride 40 mg, net price 100-tab pack = £4.57; 80 mg, 100-tab pack = £9.15; 120 mg, 100-tab pack = £13.70; 160 mg, 56-tab pack = £12.77

Injection, verapamil hydrochloride 2.5 mg/mL, net price 2-mL amp = £1.11

PoM Securon® (Knoll)

Tablets, f/c, verapamil hydrochloride 40 mg, net price 100 = £4.57; 80 mg (scored), 100 = £9.14; 120 mg (scored), 60-tab pack = £7.67

Injection, verapamil hydrochloride 2.5 mg/mL. Net price 2-mL amp = £1.08

Modified release
PoM Half Securon SR® (Knoll)
Tablets, m/r, f/c, verapamil hydrochloride 120 mg.
Net price 28-tab pack = £6.82. Label: 25
Dose: see Securon SR®

PoM Securon SR® (Knoll)
Tablets, m/r, pale green, f/c, scored, verapamil
hydrochloride 240 mg. Net price 28-tab pack =
£10.64. Label: 25
Dose: hypertension, 240 mg daily (new patients initially
120 mg), increased if necessary to max. 480 mg daily
(doses above 240 mg daily as 2 divided doses)
Angina, 240 mg twice daily (may sometimes be reduced
to once daily)
Prophylaxis after myocardial infarction where beta-
blockers not appropriate (started at least 1 week after
infarction), 360 mg daily in divided doses, given as
240 mg in the morning and 120 mg in the evening *or*
120 mg 3 times daily

PoM Univer® (Rhône-Poulenc Rorer)
Capsules, m/r, verapamil hydrochloride 120 mg
(yellow/dark blue), net price 28-cap pack = £6.83;
180 mg (yellow), 56-cap pack = £16.50; 240 mg
(yellow/dark blue), 28-cap pack = £11.13. Label:
25
Dose: hypertension, 240 mg daily, max. 480 mg daily
(new patients, initial dose 120 mg); angina, 360 mg
daily, max. 480 mg daily

PoM Verapress MR® (Dexcel)
Tablets, m/r, pale green, f/c, verapamil hydrochloride 240 mg. Net price 28-tab pack = £10.64.
Label: 25
Dose: hypertension, 1 tablet daily, increased to twice
daily if necessary; angina, 1 tablet twice daily (may
sometimes be reduced to once daily)

2.6.3   Potassium-channel activators

Nicorandil is a member of a new class of drugs
termed potassium-channel activators. It has both
arterial and venous vasodilating properties and is
indicated for the prevention and long-term treatment of angina. Its place in therapy is currently
uncertain.

NICORANDIL
Indications: prophylaxis and treatment of angina
Cautions: hypovolaemia; low systolic blood pressure; acute pulmonary oedema; acute myocardial
infarction with acute left ventricular failure and
low filling pressures; pregnancy and breast-feeding; **interactions:** Appendix 1 (nicorandil)
DRIVING. Patients should be warned not to drive or operate machinery until it is established that their performance is unimpaired
Contra-indications: cardiogenic shock; left ventricular failure with low filling pressures; hypotension
Side-effects: headache (especially on initiation,
usually transitory); cutaneous vasodilatation with
flushing; nausea, vomiting, dizziness, weakness
also reported; at high dosage, reduction in blood
pressure and/or increase in heart rate
Dose: initially 10 mg twice daily (if susceptible to
headache 5 mg twice daily); usual dose 10–20 mg
twice daily; up to 30 mg twice daily may be used

▼ PoM Ikorel® (Rhône-Poulenc Rorer)
Tablets, both scored, nicorandil 10 mg, net price
60-tab pack = £11.66; 20 mg, 60-tab pack =
£19.88

2.6.4   Peripheral and cerebral vasodilators

2.6.4.1 Peripheral vasodilators and related drugs
2.6.4.2 Cerebral vasodilators

2.6.4.1 PERIPHERAL VASODILATORS AND RELATED DRUGS

Most serious peripheral disorders, such as *intermittent claudication*, are now known to be due to
occlusion of vessels, either by spasm or sclerotic
plaques; use of vasodilators may increase blood
flow at rest, but the few controlled studies carried
out have shown little improvement in walking distance. Rest pain is rarely affected.

Management of *Raynaud's syndrome* includes
avoidance of exposure to cold and stopping
smoking. More severe symptoms may require
vasodilator treatment, which is most often successful in primary Raynaud's syndrome. Nifedipine
(section 2.6.2), prazosin (section 2.5.4) and thymoxamine (moxisylyte) have all been shown to be
beneficial; cinnarizine, naftidrofuryl, nicotinic acid
derivatives, and oxpentifylline (pentoxifylline) are
not established as being effective.

Vasodilator therapy is not established as being
effective for *chilblains* (section 13.14).

CINNARIZINE
Indications: peripheral vascular disease, Raynaud's
syndrome
Cautions; Side-effects: see section 4.6
Dose: initially, 75 mg 3 times daily; maintenance, 75 mg
2–3 times daily

Stugeron Forte® (Janssen-Cilag)
Capsules, orange/ivory, cinnarizine 75 mg. Net price 100-
cap pack = £7.85. Label: 25
Stugeron®: see section 4.6

NAFTIDROFURYL OXALATE
Indications: see under Dose
Side-effects: nausea, epigastric pain, rash, hepatitis,
hepatic failure
Dose: peripheral vascular disease, 100–200 mg 3 times
daily; cerebral vascular disease, 100 mg 3 times daily

PoM Naftidrofuryl (Non-proprietary)
Capsules, naftidrofuryl oxalate 100 mg. Net price 84-cap
pack = £7.90. Label: 25, 27
Available from Berk (*Stimlor®*)
PoM Praxilene® (Lipha)
Capsules, pink, naftidrofuryl oxalate 100 mg. Net price
84-cap pack = £8.60. Label: 25, 27

NICOTINIC ACID DERIVATIVES
Indications: peripheral vascular disease (for hyperlipidaemia, see section 2.12)
Side-effects: flushing, dizziness, nausea, vomiting, hypotension (more frequent with nicotinic acid than derivatives); occasional diabetogenic effect reported with
nicotinic acid and nicotinyl alcohol; rarely associated
with nodular changes to liver (monitor on prolonged
high dosage)

Hexopal® (Sanofi Winthrop)
Tablets, scored, inositol nicotinate 500 mg. Net price 20 = £4.07
Dose: 1 g 3 times daily, increased to 4 g daily if required
Tablets forte, scored, inositol nicotinate 750 mg. Net price 112-tab pack = £34.02
Dose: 1.5 g twice daily
Suspension, sugar-free, inositol nicotinate 1 g/5 mL. Net price 300 mL = £20.85
Dose: as for tablets (above)

Ronicol® (Tillomed)
Tablets, scored, nicotinyl alcohol 25 mg (as tartrate). Net price 100-tab pack = £5.55
Dose: 25–50 mg 4 times daily
Timespan® (= tablets m/r), red, s/c, nicotinyl alcohol 150 mg (as tartrate). Net price 100-tab pack = £23.70. Label: 25
Dose: 150–300 mg twice daily

OXPENTIFYLLINE
(Pentoxifylline)
Indications: peripheral vascular disease
Cautions: hypotension, coronary artery disease; renal impairment, severe hepatic impairment; avoid in porphyria (section 9.8.2); **interactions:** Appendix 1 (oxpentifylline)
Contra-indications: cerebral haemorrhage, extensive retinal haemorrhage, acute myocardial infarction; pregnancy and breast-feeding
Side-effects: gastro-intestinal disturbances, dizziness, agitation, sleep disturbances, headache; rarely flushing, tachycardia, angina, hypotension, thrombocytopenia, intrahepatic cholestasis, hypersensitivity reactions including rash, pruritus and bronchospasm
Dose: 400 mg 2–3 times daily

PoM **Trental®** (Hoechst Marion Roussel)
Tablets, m/r, pink, s/c, oxpentifylline 400 mg. Net price 90-tab pack = £15.11. Label: 21, 25

THYMOXAMINE
(Moxisylyte)
Indications: primary Raynaud's syndrome (short-term treatment); erectile dysfunction (section 7.4.5)
Cautions: diabetes mellitus
Contra-indications: active liver disease
Side-effects: nausea, diarrhoea, flushing, headache, dizziness; hepatic reactions including cholestatic jaundice and hepatitis reported to CSM
Dose: initially 40 mg 4 times daily, increased to 80 mg 4 times daily if poor initial response; discontinue after 2 weeks if no response

PoM **Opilon®** (P-D)
Tablets, yellow, f/c, thymoxamine 40 mg (as hydrochloride). Net price 112-tab pack = £26.13. Label: 21

OTHER PREPARATION USED IN PERIPHERAL VASCULAR DISEASE

Rutosides (oxerutins, *Paroven®*) are not vasodilators and are not generally regarded as effective preparations as capillary sealants or for the treatment of cramps; side-effects include headache, flushing, rashes, mild gastro-intestinal disturbances.

Paroven® (Novartis Consumer Health)
Capsules, yellow, oxerutins 250 mg. Net price 120-cap pack = £13.67
Dose: relief of symptoms of oedema associated with chronic venous insufficiency, 500 mg twice daily

2.6.4.2 CEREBRAL VASODILATORS

These drugs are claimed to improve mental function. Some improvements in performance of psychological tests have been reported but the drugs have not been shown clinically to be of much benefit in dementia.

CO-DERGOCRINE MESYLATE
A mixture in equal proportions of dihydroergocornine mesylate, dihydroergocristine mesylate, and (in the ratio 2 : 1) α- and β-dihydroergocryptine mesylates
Indications: adjunct in elderly patients with mild to moderate dementia
Cautions: severe bradycardia
Side-effects: gastro-intestinal disturbances, flushing, headache, rash, nasal congestion; dizziness and postural hypotension in hypertensive patients
Dose: 1.5 mg 3 times daily before meals *or* 4.5 mg once daily before a meal

PoM **Hydergine®** (Novartis)
Tablets, co-dergocrine mesylate 1.5 mg (scored), net price 100-tab pack = £10.78; 4.5 mg, 28-tab pack = £10.78. Label: 22

2.7   Sympathomimetics

2.7.1   Inotropic sympathomimetics
2.7.2   Vasoconstrictor sympathomimetics
2.7.3   Cardiopulmonary resuscitation

The properties of sympathomimetics vary according to whether they act on alpha or on beta adrenergic receptors. Adrenaline (section 2.7.3) acts on both alpha and beta receptors and increases both heart rate and contractility (beta$_1$ effects); it can cause peripheral vasodilation (a beta$_2$ effect) or vasoconstriction (an alpha effect).

2.7.1   Inotropic sympathomimetics

The cardiac stimulants **dobutamine** and **dopamine** act on beta$_1$ receptors in cardiac muscle, and increase contractility with little effect on rate; they are used in cardiogenic shock. Dosage of dopamine is critical since although low doses induce vasodilatation and increase renal perfusion, higher doses (more than 5 micrograms per kg per minute) lead to vasoconstriction and may exacerbate heart failure.

Xamoterol also acts on beta$_1$ receptors but being a partial agonist it provokes only a modest stimulatory response at rest. **Important:** restricted to **mild heart failure only**, owing to deterioration in patients with moderate to severe heart failure, see p. 104.

Dopexamine acts on beta$_2$ receptors in cardiac muscle to produce its positive inotropic effect; and on peripheral dopamine receptors to increase renal perfusion; it is reported not to induce vasoconstriction.

Isoprenaline is less selective and increases both heart rate and contractility; it may prevent Stokes-Adams attacks, but insertion of a pacemaker is preferable. It is now only used as a short-term emergency treatment of heart block or severe bradycardia.

Arbutamine (GenESA®, manufactured by Gensia) which is used in the GenESA® system for pharmacological stress testing, simulates the effects of physical exercise on the heart, and thus provides an alternative in patients unable to perform exercise tests adequately.

DOBUTAMINE

Indications: inotropic support in infarction, cardiac surgery, cardiomyopathies, septic shock, and cardiogenic shock

Cautions: severe hypotension complicating cardiogenic shock; **interactions:** Appendix 1 (sympathomimetics)

Side-effects: tachycardia and marked increase in systolic blood pressure indicate overdosage

Dose: by intravenous infusion, 2.5–10 micrograms/kg/minute, adjusted according to response

PoM **Dobutrex®** (Lilly)

Strong sterile solution, dobutamine (as hydrochloride) 12.5 mg/mL. For dilution and use as an intravenous infusion. Net price 20-mL vial = £8.35

Note. Strong sterile solution containing dobutamine (as hydrochloride) 12.5 mg/mL also available in 20-mL amps from Faulding DBL, Phoenix

PoM **Posiject®** (Boehringer Ingelheim)

Strong sterile solution, dobutamine (as hydrochloride) 50 mg/mL. For dilution and use as an intravenous infusion. Net price 5-mL amp = £5.50

DOPAMINE HYDROCHLORIDE

Indications: cardiogenic shock in infarction or cardiac surgery

Cautions: correct hypovolaemia; low dose in shock due to acute myocardial infarction—see notes above; **interactions:** Appendix 1 (sympathomimetics)

Contra-indications: tachyarrhythmia, phaeochromocytoma

Side-effects: nausea and vomiting, peripheral vasoconstriction, hypotension, hypertension, tachycardia

Dose: by intravenous infusion, 2–5 micrograms/kg/minute initially (see notes above)

PoM **Dopamine Hydrochloride** (Nonproprietary)

Strong sterile solution, dopamine hydrochloride 40 mg/mL; 160 mg/mL, 5-mL amps. For dilution and use as an intravenous infusion
Available from Antigen, Faulding DBL

PoM **Dopamine Hydrochloride in Dextrose (Glucose) Injection** (Abbott)

Intravenous infusion, dopamine hydrochloride 1.6 mg/mL in glucose 5% intravenous infusion, net price 250-mL container (400 mg) = £11.69; 3.2 mg/mL, 250-mL container (800 mg) = £22.93 (both hosp. only)

PoM **Select-A-Jet® Dopamine** (IMS)

Strong sterile solution, dopamine hydrochloride 40 mg/mL. Net price 5-mL vial = £4.14; 10-mL vial = £6.65; 20-mL vial = £11.86. For dilution and use as an intravenous infusion

DOPEXAMINE HYDROCHLORIDE

Indications: inotropic support and vasodilator in exacerbations of chronic heart failure and in heart failure associated with cardiac surgery

Cautions: myocardial infarction, recent angina, hypokalaemia, hyperglycaemia; correct hypovolaemia before starting, monitor blood pressure, pulse, plasma potassium, blood glucose; avoid abrupt withdrawal; **interactions:** Appendix 1 (sympathomimetics)

Contra-indications: left ventricular outlet obstruction such as hypertrophic cardiomyopathy or aortic stenosis; phaeochromocytoma, thrombocytopenia

Side-effects: tachycardia, other arrhythmias; also reported: nausea, vomiting, anginal pain, tremor, headache

Dose: by intravenous infusion into central or large peripheral vein, 500 nanograms/kg/minute, may be increased to 1 microgram/kg/minute and further increased up to 6 micrograms/kg/minute in increments of 0.5–1 microgram/kg/minute at intervals of not less than 15 minutes

PoM **Dopacard®** (Speywood)

Strong sterile solution, dopexamine hydrochloride 10 mg/mL (1%). For dilution and use as an intravenous infusion. Net price 5-mL amp = £21.00

Note. Contact with metal in infusion apparatus should be minimised

ISOPRENALINE HYDROCHLORIDE

Indications: heart block, severe bradycardia

Cautions: ischaemic heart disease, diabetes mellitus, hyperthyroidism; **interactions:** Appendix 1 (sympathomimetics)

Side-effects: tachycardia, arrhythmias, hypotension, sweating, tremor, headache

Dose: by intravenous infusion, 0.5–10 micrograms/minute

PoM **Min-I-Jet® Isoprenaline** (IMS)

Injection, isoprenaline hydrochloride 20 micrograms/mL. Net price 10-mL disposable syringe = £4.05

PoM **Saventrine IV®** (Pharmax)

Strong sterile solution, isoprenaline hydrochloride 1 mg/mL. For dilution and use as an intravenous infusion. Net price 2-mL amp = 44p

XAMOTEROL

Indications: chronic mild heart failure (in patients not breathless at rest but limited by symptoms on exertion)

Cautions: withdraw if heart failure deteriorates; cardiac outflow obstruction, arrhythmias (maintain concurrent digoxin in atrial fibrillation), obstructive airways disease (withdraw if worsening, and reverse bronchospasm with inhaled bronchodilator such as salbutamol), reduce dose in renal impairment; pregnancy (toxicity in *animal* studies); **interactions**: Appendix 1 (xamoterol)

Contra-indications: moderate to severe heart failure; breast-feeding

HEART FAILURE. Patients in whom xamoterol is contra-indicated are those:

who are short of breath or fatigued at rest or limited on minimal exercise;

with resting tachycardia (>90 beats per minute) or hypotension (systolic BP <100 mmHg);

with peripheral oedema, raised jugular venous pressure, enlarged liver, or third heart sound;

with (or with history of) acute pulmonary oedema;

who require treatment with frusemide in dose in excess of 40 mg daily (or equivalent);

who require ACE inhibitor treatment

Side-effects: gastro-intestinal disturbances, headache, dizziness, bronchospasm, hypotension; also reported: chest pain, palpitations, muscle cramp, rashes

Dose: 200 mg daily for 1 week, then 200 mg twice daily

IMPORTANT. Treatment should be started in hospital after full assessment of severity of heart failure by exercise test

PoM **Corwin®** (Stuart)

Tablets, yellow, f/c, xamoterol (as fumarate) 200 mg. Net price 56-tab pack = £25.94

2.7.2 Vasoconstrictor sympathomimetics

Vasoconstrictor sympathomimetics raise blood pressure transiently by acting on alpha-adrenergic receptors to constrict peripheral vessels. They are sometimes used as an emergency method of elevating blood pressure, notably in spinal anaesthesia.

The danger of vasoconstrictors is that although they raise blood pressure they do so at the expense of perfusion of vital organs such as the kidney. Further, in many patients with shock the peripheral resistance is already high, and to raise it further is unhelpful. Thus the use of vasoconstrictors in the treatment of shock is to be generally **deprecated**. The use of plasma substitutes, or of inotropic agents such as dopamine or dobutamine (section 2.7.1) is more appropriate. Treatment of the underlying condition is obviously important.

Spinal and epidural anaesthesia may result in sympathetic block with resultant hypotension. Management may include intravenous fluids (which are usually given prophylactically), oxygen, elevation of the legs, and injection of a pressor drug such as ephedrine or methoxamine. As well as constricting peripheral vessels **ephedrine** also accelerates the heart rate (by acting on beta receptors). Use is made of this dual action of ephedrine to manage associated bradycardia (although intravenous injection of atropine sulphate 400 to 600 micrograms may also be required if bradycardia persists). When

the hypotension occurs in association with tachycardia the pure alpha-adrenergic stimulant action of **methoxamine** is more appropriate.

EPHEDRINE HYDROCHLORIDE

Indications: see under Dose

Cautions: hyperthyroidism, diabetes mellitus, ischaemic heart disease, hypertension, elderly; may cause acute retention in prostatic hypertrophy; **interactions:** Appendix 1 (sympathomimetics)

Side-effects: tachycardia, anxiety, restlessness, insomnia; also tremor, arrhythmias, dry mouth, cold extremities; acute retention in prostatic hypertrophy

Dose: reversal of hypotension from spinal or epidural anaesthesia, *by slow intravenous injection* of a solution containing ephedrine hydrochloride 3 mg/mL, 3–6 mg (max. 9 mg) repeated every 3–4 minutes to max. 30 mg

PoM **Ephedrine Hydrochloride** (Non-proprietary)

Injection, ephedrine hydrochloride 30 mg/mL. For dilution before intravenous administration. 1-mL amp [unlicensed]

METARAMINOL

Indications: acute hypotension (see notes above)

Cautions; Contra-indications; Side-effects: see under Noradrenaline Acid Tartrate; metaraminol has a longer duration of action than noradrenaline, see also warning below; also tachycardia; fatal ventricular arrhythmia reported in Laennec's cirrhosis

HYPERTENSIVE RESPONSE. Since metaraminol has a longer duration of action than noradrenaline, an excessive vasopressor response may cause a prolonged rise in blood pressure

Dose: by intravenous infusion, 15–100 mg in 500 mL, adjusted according to response

PoM **Aramine®** (MSD)

Injection, metaraminol 10 mg (as tartrate)/mL. Net price 1-mL amp = 57p

METHOXAMINE HYDROCHLORIDE

Indications: acute hypotension (see notes above)

Cautions; Contra-indications; Side-effects: see under Noradrenaline Acid Tartrate; methoxamine has a longer duration of action than noradrenaline, see also warning below

HYPERTENSIVE RESPONSE. Since methoxamine has a longer duration of action than noradrenaline, an excessive vasopressor response may cause a prolonged rise in blood pressure

Dose: by intramuscular injection, 5–20 mg

By slow intravenous injection, 5–10 mg (rate 1 mg/minute)

PoM **Vasoxine®** (GlaxoWellcome)

Injection, methoxamine hydrochloride 20 mg/mL. Net price 1-mL amp = 52p

NORADRENALINE ACID TARTRATE
(Norepinephrine Bitartrate)
Indications: see preparations
Cautions: coronary, mesenteric, or peripheral vascular thrombosis; following myocardial infarction, Prinzmetal's variant angina, thyroid disease, diabetes mellitus; hypoxia or hypercapnia; appropriate blood volume replacement required; elderly; extravasation at injection site may cause necrosis; **interactions:** Appendix 1 (sympathomimetics)
Contra-indications: hypertension (monitor blood pressure and rate of flow frequently), pregnancy
Side-effects: hypertension, headache, bradycardia, arrhythmias, peripheral ischaemia
Dose: see under preparations

PoM **Levophed®** (Sanofi Winthrop)
Strong sterile solution, noradrenaline acid tartrate 2 mg/mL (equivalent to noradrenaline base 1 mg/mL). For dilution and use as an intravenous infusion. Net price 2-mL amp = £1.01; 4-mL amp = £1.50; 20-mL amp = £6.35
  Dose: acute hypotension, *by intravenous infusion,* via central venous catheter, of a solution containing noradrenaline acid tartrate 80 micrograms/mL (equivalent to noradrenaline base 40 micrograms/mL) at an initial rate of 0.16–0.33 mL/minute, adjusted according to response

PoM **Levophed Special®** (Sanofi Winthrop)
Injection, noradrenaline acid tartrate 200 micrograms/mL (equivalent to noradrenaline base 100 micrograms/mL). Net price 2-mL amp = 98p
  Dose: cardiac arrest, *by rapid intravenous or intracardiac injection,* 0.5 to 0.75 mL of a solution containing noradrenaline acid tartrate 200 micrograms/mL (equivalent to noradrenaline base 100 micrograms/mL)

PHENYLEPHRINE HYDROCHLORIDE
Indications: acute hypotension (see notes above)
Cautions; Contra-indications; Side-effects: see under Noradrenaline Acid Tartrate; phenylephrine has a longer duration of action than noradrenaline, see also warning below; since phenylephrine induces tachycardia or reflex bradycardia it should be avoided in severe hyperthyroidism and used with caution in severe coronary disease
HYPERTENSIVE RESPONSE. Since phenylephrine has a longer duration of action than noradrenaline, an excessive vasopressor response may cause a prolonged rise in blood pressure
Dose: by subcutaneous or intramuscular injection, 2–5 mg, followed if necessary by further doses of 1–10 mg
By slow intravenous injection, 100–500 micrograms repeated as necessary after at least 15 minutes
By intravenous infusion, initial rate up to 180 micrograms/minute reduced to 30–60 micrograms/minute according to response

PoM **Phenylephrine** (Knoll)
Injection, phenylephrine hydrochloride 10 mg/mL (1%). Net price 1-mL amp = £2.40

2.7.3   Cardiopulmonary resuscitation

In *cardiac arrest* **adrenaline** (epinephrine) 1 in 10 000 (1 mg per 10 mL) is recommended in a dose of 10 mL by central intravenous injection. The procedure for cardiopulmonary resuscitation is given in the algorithm (see p. 107) which reflects the recommendations of the European Resuscitation Council and the Resuscitation Council (UK). Other drugs used in cardiopulmonary resuscitation include **atropine** (section 15.1.3) and **calcium** (section 9.5.1.1).

For *acute anaphylaxis* see section 3.4.3.

ADRENALINE
(Epinephrine)
Indications; Dose: see notes above
Cautions: ischaemic heart disease, diabetes mellitus, hyperthyroidism, hypertension; **interactions:** Appendix 1 (sympathomimetics)
Side-effects: anxiety, tremor, tachycardia, headache, cold extremities; in overdosage arrhythmias, cerebral haemorrhage, pulmonary oedema

PoM **Adrenaline Injection, 1 in 10 000** (Non-proprietary)
Injection, adrenaline (as acid tartrate) 100 micrograms/mL. 10-mL amp.
  Available from Martindale (special order); also from Aurum (10-mL prefilled syringe), IMS (Min-I-Jet® Adrenaline 3- and 10-mL disposable syringes)
  Note. Adrenaline Injection BP is 1 in 1000 (adrenaline 1 mg/mL, as acid tartrate), see section 3.4.3

2.8   Anticoagulants and protamine

> 2.8.1   Parenteral anticoagulants
> 2.8.2   Oral anticoagulants
> 2.8.3   Protamine sulphate

The main use of anticoagulants is to prevent thrombus formation or extension of an existing thrombus in the slower-moving venous side of the circulation, where the thrombus consists of a fibrin web enmeshed with platelets and red cells. They are therefore widely used in the prevention and treatment of *deep-vein thrombosis* in the legs.

Anticoagulants are of less use in preventing thrombus formation in arteries, for in faster-flowing vessels thrombi are composed mainly of platelets with little fibrin. They are used to prevent thrombi forming on *prosthetic heart valves.*

2.8.1   Parenteral anticoagulants

HEPARIN

Heparin initiates anticoagulation rapidly but has a short duration of action. It is now often referred to as being **standard** or **unfractionated heparin** to distinguish it from the **low molecular weight heparins** (see p. 109), which have a longer duration of action.

Adult Advanced Life Support

1997 guidelines for use in the UK

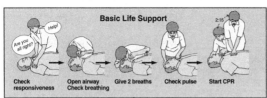

Basic Life Support 2:15

Check responsiveness — Open airway / Check breathing — Give 2 breaths — Check pulse — Start CPR

Call for help

Fill in local emergency no.

Fetch
1. Defibrillator
2. Oxygen & Airway Adjuncts
3. Resuscitation kit

Precordial thump
if appropriate

Attach defibrillator-monitor

Assess rhythm

± check pulse

VF / VT

Non VF / VT

Defibrillate x 3 as necessary

CPR 1 min

CPR up to 3 min

DURING CPR
if not already:

- **Check:** electrode/paddle positions & contact
- **Attempt/verify:** ETT / IV Access
- **Give epinephrine (adrenaline) every 3 min**
- **Correct reversible causes**
- **Consider:** buffers / antiarrhythmics / atropine / pacing

Potentially reversible causes:
Hypoxia
Hypovolaemia
Hyper/hypokalaemia & metabolic disorders
Hypothermia
Tension pneumothorax
Tamponade
Toxic/therapeutic disturbances
Thromboembolic/mechanical obstruction

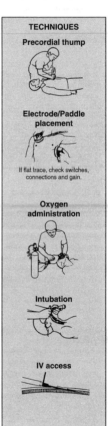

TECHNIQUES

Precordial thump

Electrode/Paddle placement

If flat trace, check switches, connections and gain.

Oxygen administration

Intubation

IV access

© Design and illustrations, Laerdal 1997

Resuscitation Council (UK)

These guidelines are based on the ILCOR advisory statement and are being assessed on behalf of the ERC

European Resuscitation Council

TREATMENT. For the initial treatment of *deep-vein thrombosis and pulmonary embolism* heparin is given as an *intravenous loading dose,* followed by *continuous intravenous infusion* (using an infusion pump) or by *intermittent subcutaneous injection*; the use of *intermittent intravenous injection* is no longer recommended. An oral anticoagulant (usually warfarin, section 2.8.2) is started at the same time as the heparin (which needs to be continued for at least 3 days, until the oral anticoagulant has taken effect). Laboratory monitoring is essential—preferably on a daily basis, determination of the APTT (activated partial thromboplastin time) being the most widely used technique. Heparin is also used in regimens for the management of *myocardial infarction* (see also section 2.10.1), the management of *unstable angina*, and the management of *acute peripheral arterial occlusion.*

PROPHYLAXIS. In patients undergoing *general surgery*, low-dose heparin by subcutaneous injection is widely advocated to *prevent postoperative deep-vein thrombosis and pulmonary embolism* in 'high risk' patients (i.e. those with obesity, malignant disease, history of deep-vein thrombosis or pulmonary embolism, patients over 40 years, or those with an established thrombophilic disorder or who are undergoing large or complicated surgical procedures); laboratory monitoring is not required with this *standard prophylactic regimen.*

To combat the increased risk in *major orthopaedic surgery* an *adjusted dose regimen* may be used (with monitoring) or *low molecular weight heparin* (see p. 109) may be selected.

EXTRACORPOREAL CIRCUITS. Heparin is also used in the maintenance of extracorporeal circuits in *cardiopulmonary bypass* and *haemodialysis.*

HAEMORRHAGE. If haemorrhage occurs it is usually sufficient to withdraw heparin, but if rapid reversal of the effects of heparin is required, protamine sulphate (section 2.8.3) is a specific antidote (but only partially reverses the effects of low molecular weight heparins).

HEPARIN

Indications: see under Dose

Cautions: hepatic and renal impairment (avoid if severe); pregnancy; **interactions:** Appendix 1 (heparin)

THROMBOCYTOPENIA. Clinically important thrombocytopenia is immune-mediated, and does not usually develop until after 6 to 10 days; it may be complicated by thrombosis. The CSM has recommended platelet counts for patients receiving heparin for longer than 5 days (and that heparin should be stopped immediately in those who develop thrombocytopenia). Patients requiring continued anticoagulation should preferably be given a heparinoid such as danaparoid; alternatives include low molecular weight heparins (but cross reactivity may occur), warfarin, or epoprostenol

Contra-indications: haemophilia and other haemorrhagic disorders, thrombocytopenia, peptic ulcer, recent cerebral haemorrhage, severe hypertension, severe liver disease (including oeso-

phageal varices), renal failure, after major trauma or recent surgery (especially to eye or nervous system), hypersensitivity to heparin

Side-effects: haemorrhage (see notes above), skin necrosis, thrombocytopenia (see Cautions), hypersensitivity reactions (including urticaria, angioedema, and anaphylaxis); osteoporosis after prolonged use (and rarely alopecia)

Dose:

Treatment of deep-vein thrombosis and pulmonary embolism, *by intravenous injection,* loading dose of 5000 units (10 000 units in severe pulmonary embolism) followed by continuous *infusion* of 1000–2000 units/hour *or* by *subcutaneous injection* of 15 000 units every 12 hours (laboratory monitoring essential—preferably on a daily basis)

SMALL ADULT OR CHILD, lower loading dose *then,* 15–25 units/kg/hour *by intravenous infusion, or* 250 units/kg every 12 hours by *subcutaneous injection*

Unstable angina, acute peripheral arterial occlusion, as intravenous regimen for deep-vein thrombosis and pulmonary embolism, above

Prophylaxis in orthopaedic surgery, see notes above

Prophylaxis in general surgery (see notes above), *by subcutaneous injection,* 5000 units 2 hours before surgery, then every 8–12 hours for 7 days or until patient is ambulant (monitoring not needed); during pregnancy (with monitoring), 5000–10 000 units every 12 hours (**important:** not intended to cover prevention of prosthetic heart valve thrombosis in pregnancy which calls for separate specialist management)

MYOCARDIAL INFARCTION. For the prevention of *coronary re-occlusion after thrombolysis* heparin is used in a variety of regimens according to locally agreed protocols

For the prevention of *mural thrombosis* heparin is considered effective when given by *subcutaneous injection* of 12 500 units every 12 hours for at least 10 days

Note. Doses above reflect the guidelines of the British Society for Haematology; for doses of the low molecular weight heparins, see p. 109

PoM **Heparin Injection** (heparin sodium)
1000 units/mL, net price 1-mL amp = 18p; 5-mL amp = 54p; 5-mL vial = 46p
5000 units/mL, net price 1-mL amp = 36p; 5-mL amp = 95p; 5-mL vial = 92p
25 000 units/mL, net price 1-mL amp = 97p; 5-mL vial = £3.84

PoM **Calciparine®** (Sanofi Winthrop)
Injection (subcutaneous only), heparin calcium 25 000 units/mL. Net price 0.2-mL syringe = 68p; 0.5-mL syringe = £1.46; 0.8-mL syringe = £1.76

PoM **Minihep®** (Leo)
Injection (subcutaneous only), heparin sodium 25 000 units/mL. Net price 0.2-mL amp = 41p

PoM **Minihep Calcium®** (Leo)
Injection (subcutaneous only), heparin calcium 25 000 units/mL. Net price 0.2-mL amp = 44p

PoM **Monoparin®** (CP)

Injection, heparin sodium (mucous) 1000 units/
mL, net price 1-mL amp = 18p; 5-mL amp = 54p;
10-mL amp = 72p; 20-mL = £1.38; 5000 units/
mL, 1-mL amp = 36p; 5-mL amp = 95p; 25 000
units/mL, 0.2-mL amp = 44p, 1-mL amp = 97p

PoM **Monoparin Calcium®** (CP)

Injection, heparin calcium 25 000 units/mL. Net
price 0.2-mL amp = 47p

PoM **Multiparin®** (CP)

Injection, heparin sodium (mucous) 1000 units/
mL, net price 5-mL vial = 46p; 5000 units/mL, 5-
mL vial = 92p; 25 000 units/mL, 5-mL vial =
£3.84

PoM **Pump-Hep®** (Leo)

Injection, heparin sodium (mucous) 1000 units/
mL. Net price 5-mL amp = 39p; 10-mL amp =
64p; 20-mL amp = 95p

PoM **Unihep®** (Leo)

Injection, heparin sodium (mucous) 1000 units/
mL, net price 1-mL amp = 13p; 5000 units/mL, 1-
mL amp = 27p; 10 000 units/mL, 1-mL amp =
44p; 25 000 units/mL, 1-mL amp = £1.04

PoM **Uniparin Calcium®** (CP)

Injection (subcutaneous only), heparin calcium
25 000 units/mL. Net price 0.5-mL syringe =
£1.50

PoM **Uniparin Forte®** (CP)

Injection (subcutaneous only), heparin sodium
25 000 units/mL. Net price 0.4-mL syringe =
£1.53

LOW MOLECULAR WEIGHT HEPARINS

There is evidence that the low molecular weight
heparins, **certoparin**, **dalteparin**, **enoxaparin**, and
tinzaparin, are as effective and as safe as unfractionated heparin in the prevention of venous
thrombo-embolism; in orthopaedic practice they are
probably more effective. They have a longer duration of action than unfractionated heparin; *once-
daily subcutaneous* dosage means that they are convenient to use. The standard prophylactic regimen
does not require monitoring.

Some low molecular weight heparins are also
used in the treatment of deep-vein thrombosis,
unstable coronary artery disease and for the prevention of clotting in extracorporeal circuits.

HAEMORRHAGE. See under Heparin.

CERTOPARIN

Indications: see notes above and under preparations

Cautions; Contra-indications; Side-effects: see
under Heparin

PoM **Alphaparin®** (Alpha)

Injection, certoparin sodium 3000 units/0.3-mL
syringe, net price 1 syringe = £3.00; 3000 units/
0.5-mL amp = £2.75

Dose: prophylaxis of deep-vein thrombosis, *by subcutaneous injection*, 3000 units 1–2 hours before surgery,
then 3000 units every 24 hours for 7–10 days (or until
the patient is mobile)

DALTEPARIN SODIUM

Indications: see notes above and under preparations

Cautions; Contra-indications; Side-effects: see
under Heparin

PoM **Fragmin®** (Pharmacia & Upjohn)

Injection (single-dose syringe), dalteparin sodium
12 500 units/mL, net price 0.2-mL (2500-unit)
syringe = £1.95; 25 000 units/mL, 0.2-mL (5000-
unit) syringe = £2.96

Dose: prophylaxis of deep-vein thrombosis, *by subcutaneous injection*, moderate risk, 2500 units 1–2 hours
before surgery then 2500 units every 24 hours for 5–7
days or longer; high risk, 2500 units 1–2 hours before
surgery, then 2500 units 8–12 hours later (*or* 5000 units
on the evening before surgery, then 5000 units on the
following evening), then 5000 units every 24 hours for
5–7 days or longer (5 weeks in hip replacement)

Injection (for subcutaneous or intravenous use),
dalteparin sodium 2500 units/mL, net price 4-mL
(10 000-unit) amp = £5.36; 10 000 units/mL, 1-
mL (10 000-unit) amp = £5.36; 25 000 units/mL,
4-mL (100 000-unit) vial = £50.95

Dose: treatment of deep-vein thrombosis, *by subcutaneous injection*, 200 units/kg (max. 18 000 units) as a single daily dose (*or* 100 units/kg twice daily if increased
risk of haemorrhage) with oral anticoagulant treatment
until prothrombin complex concentration in therapeutic
range (usually for at least 5 days)

Note. For monitoring, blood should be taken 3–4 hours
after a dose (recommended plasma concentration of
anti-Factor Xa 0.5–1 unit/mL), monitoring not required
for once-daily treatment regimen and not generally necessary for twice-daily regimen

Unstable coronary artery disease, *by subcutaneous
injection*, 120 units/kg every 12 hours (max. 10 000 units
twice daily) for 5–8 days

Prevention of clotting in extracorporeal circuits, consult
product literature

ENOXAPARIN

Indications: see notes above and under preparations

Cautions; Contra-indications; Side-effects: see
under Heparin

PoM **Clexane®** (Rhône-Poulenc Rorer)

Injection, enoxaparin 100 mg/mL. Net price 0.2-
mL syringe (20 mg, 2000 units) = £3.55; 0.4-mL
syringe (40 mg, 4000 units) = £4.73; 0.6-mL
syringe (60 mg, 6000 units) = £5.35; 0.8-mL
syringe (80 mg, 8000 units) = £6.08; 1-mL
syringe (100 mg, 10 000 units) = £7.53

Dose: prophylaxis of deep-vein thrombosis, *by subcutaneous injection*, moderate risk, 20 mg (2000 units)
approx. 2 hours before surgery then 20 mg (2000 units)
every 24 hours for 7–10 days; *high risk*, 40 mg
(4000 units) 12 hours before surgery then 40 mg
(4000 units) every 24 hours for 7–10 days

Treatment of deep-vein thrombosis, *by subcutaneous
injection*, 1 mg/kg (100 units/kg) every 12 hours, usually
for at least 5 days (and until adequate oral anticoagulation established)

Prevention of clotting in extracorporeal circuits, consult
product literature

TINZAPARIN

Indications: see notes above and under preparations

Cautions: severe hepatic and renal impairment (Appendixes 2 and 3); pregnancy; **interactions:** Appendix 1 (heparin)

ASTHMA. Presence of sulphites in ampoules may (especially in patients with asthma) lead to hypersensitivity (with bronchospasm and shock)

Contra-indications: see under Heparin

Side-effects: see under Heparin

PoM **Innohep**® (Leo)

Injection, tinzaparin 3500 units/0.3-mL syringe, net price 1 syringe = £3.12; 5000 units/0.5-mL ampoule, 1 amp = £2.97

Dose: prophylaxis of deep-vein thrombosis, *by subcutaneous injection,* general surgery, 3500 units 2 hours before surgery, then 3500 units every 24 hours for 7–10 days; orthopaedic surgery (high risk), 50 units/kg 2 hours before surgery, then 50 units/kg every 24 hours for 7–10 days

▼*Injection,* tinzaparin sodium 20 000 units/mL, net price 0.5-mL (10 000-unit) syringe = £10.11, 0.7-mL (14 000-unit) syringe = £14.15, 0.9-mL (18 000-unit) syringe = £18.19, 2-mL (40 000-unit) vial = £38.50

Dose: treatment of deep-vein thrombosis and pulmonary embolism, *by subcutaneous injection,* 175 units/kg once daily for at least 6 days (and until adequate oral anticoagulation established)

Note. This treatment regimen does not require monitoring

Injection, tinzaparin sodium 1000 units/mL, net price 5-mL amp = £4.20

Dose: for prevention of clotting in extracorporeal circuits, consult product literature

---

HEPARINOIDS

Danaparoid is a heparinoid used for prophylaxis of deep-vein thrombosis in patients undergoing general or orthopaedic surgery. Providing there is no evidence of cross-reactivity, it also has a role in patients who develop thrombocytopenia in association with heparin [unlicensed indication].

DANAPAROID SODIUM

Indications: prophylaxis of deep vein thrombosis in general and orthopaedic surgery

Cautions: hepatic and renal impairment (avoid if severe); pregnancy and breast-feeding

ASTHMA. Presence of sulphite in ampoules may (especially in patients with asthma) lead to hypersensitivity (with bronchospasm and shock)

Contra-indications: see under Heparin; cross-reactivity to heparin-induced thrombocytopenia

Side-effects: haemorrhage (see notes above); thrombocytopenia (may be cross-reactivity with heparin); hypersensitivity reactions (including rash); liver enzyme changes; osteoporosis with excessive dosage; bruising or pain at injection site

Dose: by subcutaneous injection, 750 units 1–4 hours before surgery, then twice daily for 7–10 days

Note. If patient cannot be operated on immediately (e.g. after hip fracture), twice daily administration may be initiated, providing the last pre-operative dose is given not later than 1 hour before surgery

PoM **Organan**® (Durbin)

Injection, danaparoid sodium 1250 units/mL, net price 0.6-mL amp (750 units) = £15.00

HEPARIN FLUSHES

For maintaining catheter patency sodium chloride injection 0.9% is as effective as heparin flushes for up to 48 hours, and is therefore recommended for cannulas intended to be in place for 48 hours or less. Heparin flushes are recommended for cannulas intended to be in place for longer than 48 hours.

PoM **Canusal**® (CP)

Solution, heparin sodium 100 units/mL. Net price 2-mL amp = 29p. To maintain patency of catheters, cannulas, etc., 200 units flushed through every 4 hours or as required. Not for therapeutic use

PoM **Hep-Flush**® (Leo)

Solution, heparin sodium 100 units/mL. Net price 2-mL amp = 25p; 10-mL vial = £1.27. To maintain patency of catheters, cannulas, etc., 200 units flushed through every 4–8 hours. Not for therapeutic use

PoM **Heplok**® (Leo)

Solution, heparin sodium 10 units/mL. Net price 5-mL amp = 29p. To maintain patency of catheters, cannulas, etc., 10–50 units flushed through every 4 hours. Not for therapeutic use

PoM **Hepsal**® (CP)

Solution, heparin sodium 10 units/mL. Net price 5-mL amp = 25p (glass), 30p (polypropylene). To maintain patency of catheters, cannulas, etc., 50 units flushed through every 4 hours or as required. Not for therapeutic use

---

EPOPROSTENOL

Epoprostenol (prostacyclin) can be given to inhibit platelet aggregation during renal dialysis either alone or with heparin. Since its half-life is only about 3 minutes it must be given by continuous intravenous infusion. It is a potent vasodilator and therefore its side-effects include flushing, headache, and hypotension.

EPOPROSTENOL

Indications: see notes above

Cautions: anticoagulant monitoring required when given with heparin

Side-effects: see notes above; also bradycardia, pallor, sweating with higher doses

Dose: see product literature

PoM **Flolan**® (GlaxoWellcome)

Infusion, powder for reconstitution, epoprostenol (as sodium salt). Net price 500-microgram vial (with diluent) = £103.86

2.8.2   Oral anticoagulants

Oral anticoagulants antagonise the effects of vitamin K, and take at least 48 to 72 hours for the anticoagulant effect to develop fully; if an immediate effect is required, heparin must be given concomitantly.

USES. The main indication for oral anticoagulant therapy is *deep-vein thrombosis.* Patients with *pulmonary embolism* should also be treated, as should those with *atrial fibrillation who are at risk of embolisation* (see also section 2.3.1), and those

---

with *prosthetic heart valves* (to prevent emboli developing on the valves); antiplatelet drugs may also be useful in these patients.

Oral anticoagulants should not be used in cerebral thrombosis or peripheral arterial occlusion, but may be of value in patients with *transient brain ischaemic attacks* whether due to carotid or vertebrobasilar arterial disease; if these patients also have severe hypertension anticoagulants are contra-indicated, and antiplatelet drugs are an alternative (section 2.9).

Warfarin is the drug of choice; **nicoumalone** (acenocoumarol) and **phenindione** are seldom used.

DOSE. Whenever possible, the base-line prothrombin time should be determined before the initial dose is given.

The usual adult induction dose of warfarin is 10 mg[1] daily for 2 days (higher doses no longer recommended). The subsequent maintenance dose depends upon the prothrombin time (reported as INR); the currently recommended therapeutic ranges are:

INR 2–2.5 for prophylaxis of deep-vein thrombosis including surgery on high-risk patients;

INR 2–3 for prophylaxis in hip surgery and fractured femur operations, for treatment of deep-vein thrombosis, pulmonary embolism, systemic embolism, prevention of venous thrombo-embolism in myocardial infarction, mitral stenosis with embolism, transient ischaemic attacks, atrial fibrillation, and tissue prosthetic heart valves;

INR 3–4.5 for recurrent deep-vein thrombosis and pulmonary embolism, arterial disease including myocardial infarction, and mechanical prosthetic heart valves.

It is essential that the INR be determined:

daily or on alternate days in early days of treatment, *then* at longer intervals (depending on response[2]) *then* up to every 8 weeks

The daily maintenance dose of warfarin is usually 3 to 9 mg (taken at the **same time** each day).

HAEMORRHAGE. The main adverse effect of all oral anticoagulants is haemorrhage. Omission of dosage with checking of the INR is essential. The following recommendations of the British Society for Haematology are based on the result of the INR and the clinical state:

Life-threatening haemorrhage—immediately give phytomenadione (vitamin K_1) 5 mg by slow intravenous injection and a concentrate of factors II, IX, X (with factor VII concentrate if available). If no concentrate is available, fresh frozen plasma should be infused (approximately 1 litre for an adult) but this may not be as effective

Less severe haemorrhage e.g. haematuria and epistaxis—withhold warfarin for one or more days and consider giving phytomenadione (vitamin K_1) 0.5–2 mg[3] by slow intravenous injection

INR 4.5–7 without haemorrhage—withhold warfarin for 1 or 2 days then review

INR > 7 without haemorrhage—withhold warfarin and consider giving phytomenadione (vitamin K_1) 500 micrograms by slow intravenous injection

Unexpected bleeding at therapeutic levels[4]—investigate possibility of underlying cause e.g. unsuspected renal or alimentary tract pathology

PREGNANCY. Oral anticoagulants are teratogenic and should not be given in the first trimester of pregnancy. Women at risk of pregnancy should be warned of this danger since stopping warfarin before the sixth week of gestation may largely avoid the risk of fetal abnormality. Oral anticoagulants cross the placenta with risk of placental or fetal haemorrhage, especially during the last few weeks of pregnancy and at delivery. Therefore, if at all possible, oral anticoagulants should be avoided in pregnancy, especially in the first and third trimesters. Difficult decisions may have to be made, particularly in women with prosthetic heart valves or with a history of recurrent venous thrombosis or pulmonary embolism.

TREATMENT BOOKLETS. Anticoagulant treatment booklets should be issued to patients, and are available for distribution to local healthcare professionals from Health Authorities and also from:

England:
The Stationary Office
Broadway
Chadderton
Oldham
Lancs OL9 6QH

Scotland:
The Stationary Office
21, South Gyle Crescent
Edinburgh EH12 9EB

Northern Ireland Office
Central Services Agency
27 Adelaide St
Belfast BT2 8FH

These booklets include advice for patients on anticoagulant treatment.

1. Less than 10 mg if base-line prothrombin time prolonged, if liver-function tests abnormal, or if patient in cardiac failure, on parenteral feeding, less than average body weight, or over 80 years of age.
2. Change in patient's clinical condition, particularly associated with liver disease, intercurrent illness, or drug administration, necessitates more frequent testing. See also **interactions**, Appendix 1 (warfarin). Major changes in diet (especially involving salads and vegetables) and in alcohol consumption may also affect warfarin control.
3. Usually 1 mg adequate and should be given if INR greater than desired; higher doses will prevent oral anticoagulants from acting for several days or even weeks.
4. Should always be investigated regardless of INR since even if patients over-anticoagulated bleeding generally has an additional underlying cause.

WARFARIN SODIUM

Indications: prophylaxis of embolisation in rheumatic heart disease and atrial fibrillation; prophylaxis after insertion of prosthetic heart valve; prophylaxis and treatment of venous thrombosis and pulmonary embolism; transient ischaemic attacks

Cautions: hepatic or renal disease, recent surgery; **interactions:** Appendix 1 (warfarin)

Contra-indications: pregnancy (see notes above), peptic ulcer, severe hypertension, bacterial endocarditis

Side-effects: haemorrhage—see notes above for British Society for Haematology recommendations; other side-effects reported include hypersensitivity, rash, alopecia, diarrhoea, unexplained drop in haematocrit, 'purple toes', skin necrosis, jaundice, hepatic dysfunction; also nausea, vomiting, and pancreatitis

Dose: see notes above

PoM **Warfarin** (Non-proprietary)
Tablets, all scored, warfarin sodium 1 mg (brown), net price 20 = 51p; 3 mg (blue), 20 = 57p; 5 mg (pink), 20 = 86p. Label: 10 anticoagulant card
Available from APS, Cox, Goldshield (Marevan®), Hillcross, Lagap, Norton

NICOUMALONE
(Acenocoumarol)

Indications; Cautions; Contra-indications; Side-effects: see under Warfarin Sodium; avoid breast-feeding

Dose: 8–12 mg on 1st day; 4–8 mg on 2nd day; maintenance dose usually 1–8 mg daily

PoM **Sinthrome®** (Novartis)
Tablets, nicoumalone 1 mg. Net price 20 = 49p.
Label: 10 anticoagulant card

PHENINDIONE

Indications: prophylaxis of embolisation in rheumatic heart disease and atrial fibrillation; prophylaxis after insertion of prosthetic heart valve; prophylaxis and treatment of venous thrombosis and pulmonary embolism

Cautions; Contra-indications; Side-effects: see under Warfarin Sodium; also hypersensitivity reactions including rashes, fever, leucopenia, agranulocytosis, diarrhoea, renal and hepatic damage; urine coloured pink; avoid breast-feeding; **interactions:** Appendix 1 (phenindione)

Dose: 200 mg on 1st day; 100 mg on 2nd day; maintenance dose usually 50–150 mg daily

PoM **Dindevan®** (Goldshield)
Tablets, phenindione 10 mg, net price 20 = £1.36; 25 mg (green), 20 = £1.90; 50 mg, 20 = £2.42.
Label: 10 anticoagulant card, 14 (urine pink)

2.8.3   Protamine sulphate

Although protamine sulphate is used to counteract overdosage with heparin, if used in excess it has an anticoagulant effect.

PROTAMINE SULPHATE
(Protamine Sulfate)

Indications; Cautions: see above; also if increased risk of allergic reaction to protamine (includes previous treatment with protamine insulin, allergy to fish, men who are infertile or who have had a vasectomy)

Side-effects: flushing, hypotension, bradycardia, dyspnoea

Dose: *by intravenous injection* over approx. 10 minutes, 1 mg neutralises 100 units heparin (mucous) or 80 units heparin (lung) when given within 15 minutes of heparin; if longer time, less protamine required as heparin rapidly excreted; max. 50 mg

PoM **Protamine Sulphate** (Non-proprietary)
Injection, protamine sulphate 10 mg/mL. Net price 5-mL amp = 98p
Available from Evans, Knoll
PoM **Prosulf®** (CP)
Injection, protamine sulphate 10 mg/mL. Net price 5-mL amp = 96p (glass), £1.20 (polypropylene)

2.9   Antiplatelet drugs

By decreasing platelet aggregation, these drugs may inhibit thrombus formation on the arterial side of the circulation, where thrombi are formed by platelet aggregation and anticoagulants have little effect.

Encouraging results have been obtained using **aspirin** 75–300 mg daily for the *secondary* prevention of thrombotic cerebrovascular or cardiovascular disease. Aspirin 150–300 mg daily is used to reduce mortality after myocardial infarction (section 2.10.1). Low doses of aspirin (such as 75 or 100 mg daily) are also given following bypass surgery. For details on the use of aspirin in atrial fibrillation see section 2.3.1 and for stable angina see section 2.6.

Dipyridamole is used by mouth as an adjunct to oral anticoagulation for prophylaxis of thromboembolism associated with prosthetic heart valves.

Abciximab (ReoPro®, Lilly) is a monoclonal antibody which inhibits platelet aggregation and thrombus formation. It is indicated for use by experienced physicians as an adjunct to heparin and aspirin for the prevention of ischaemic complications in high-risk patients undergoing percutaneous transluminal coronary angioplasty. Abciximab should be used once only.

For use of epoprostenol, see section 2.8.1.

ASPIRIN (antiplatelet)
(Acetylsalicylic Acid)

Indications: prophylaxis of cerebrovascular disease or myocardial infarction (see section 2.10.1 and notes above)

Cautions: asthma; uncontrolled hypertension; pregnancy (but see Appendix 4); **interactions:** Appendix 1 (aspirin)

Contra-indications: children under 12 years and in breast-feeding (Reye's syndrome, section 4.7.1); active peptic ulceration; haemophilia and other bleeding disorders

Side-effects: bronchospasm; gastro-intestinal haemorrhage (occasionally major), also other haemorrhage (e.g. subconjunctival)

Dose: see notes above

Aspirin (Non-proprietary)
Dispersible tablets, aspirin 75 mg, net price 20 = 5p; 300 mg, see section 4.7.1. Label: 13, 21, 32

Angettes 75® (Bristol-Myers)
Tablets, aspirin 75 mg. Net price 56-tab pack = £1.88. Label: 32

Caprin® (Sinclair)
Tablets, e/c, pink, aspirin 75 mg, net price 56-tab pack = £3.08; 300 mg, see section 4.7.1. Label: 5, 25, 32

Disprin CV® (R&C)
Tablets, both m/r, aspirin 100 mg, net price 28-tab pack = £1.68; 300 mg, 28-tab pack = £1.99. Label: 25, 32

Nu-Seals® **Aspirin** (Lilly)
Tablets, e/c, aspirin 75 mg, net price 56-tab pack = £3.09; 300 mg, see section 4.7.1. Label: 5, 25, 32
Note. Tablets may be chewed at diagnosis for rapid absorption
Aspirin enteric-coated tablets also available from Ashbourne (*postMI 75EC*®)

DIPYRIDAMOLE

Indications: see notes above and under preparations
Cautions: rapidly worsening angina, aortic stenosis, recent myocardial infarction, heart failure; may exacerbate migraine; hypotension; **interactions:** Appendix 1 (dipyridamole)
Side-effects: gastro-intestinal effects, dizziness, myalgia, throbbing headache, hypotension, hot flushes and tachycardia; rarely worsening symptoms of coronary heart disease, hypersensitivity reactions such as rash and urticaria, increased bleeding during or after surgery
Dose: by mouth, 300–600 mg daily in 3–4 divided doses before food
Modified-release preparations, see under preparation below
By intravenous injection, diagnostic only, consult product literature

PoM **Dipyridamole** (Non-proprietary)
Tablets, coated, dipyridamole 25 mg, net price 20 = 37p; 100 mg, 20 = £1.14. Label: 22
Available from APS, Ashbourne (Cerebrovase®), Berk (Modaplate®), Cox, Hillcross, Lagap (100 mg), Norton
Oral suspension, dipyridamole 50 mg/5 ml. Available from Rosemont (sugar-free, special order)

PoM **Persantin**® (Boehringer Ingelheim)
Tablets, both s/c, dipyridamole 25 mg (orange), net price 84-tab pack = £1.78; 100 mg, 84-tab pack = £4.95. Label: 22
Injection, dipyridamole 5 mg/mL. Net price 2-mL amp = 11p

Modified release
PoM **Persantin**® **Retard** (Boehringer Ingelheim)
Capsules, m/r, red/orange containing yellow pellets, dipyridamole 200 mg. Net price 60-cap pack = £9.75. Label: 21, 25
Dose: secondary prevention of ischaemic stroke and transient ischaemic attacks (used alone or with aspirin), adjunct to oral anticoagulation for prophylaxis of thromboembolism associated with prosthetic heart valves, 200 mg twice daily preferably with food
Note. Dispense in original container (pack contains a desiccant) and discard any capsules remaining 6 weeks after opening

2.10 Myocardial infarction and fibrinolysis

2.10.1 Management of myocardial infarction
2.10.2 Fibrinolytic drugs

2.10.1 Management of myocardial infarction

Local guidelines for the management of myocardial infarction should be followed where they exist

These notes give an overview of the initial and long-term management of myocardial infarction. The aims of management are to provide supportive care and pain relief, to promote revascularisation and to reduce mortality. Oxygen, diamorphine and nitrates provide initial support and pain relief; thrombolytics and aspirin promote revascularisation; long-term use of aspirin, beta-blockers, ACE inhibitors and statins help to reduce mortality further.

INITIAL MANAGEMENT. **Oxygen** (section 3.6) should be administered unless the patient has severe chronic obstructive airways disease.

The pain (and anxiety) of myocardial infarction is managed with slow intravenous injection of **diamorphine** (section 4.7.2); an antiemetic such as metoclopramide (or, if left ventricular function is not compromised, cyclizine) by intravenous injection should also be given (section 4.6).

Aspirin (chewed or dispersed in water) is given for its antiplatelet effect (section 2.9); a dose of 150–300 mg is suitable. If aspirin is given prior to arrival at hospital, a note saying that it has been given should be sent with the patient.

Thrombolytic drugs (alteplase, anistreplase, reteplase or streptokinase, section 2.10.2) are given to patients without contra-indications who present within 12 hours of a myocardial infarction; use after 12 hours requires specialist advice. **Streptokinase** remains the drug of choice although antibodies appear after 4 days and streptokinase or anistreplase should not therefore be used again after this time.

Nitrates (section 2.6.1) are used to relieve ischaemic pain. If sublingual glyceryl trinitrate is not effective, intravenous glyceryl trinitrate or isosorbide dinitrate is given.

Early intravenous administration of some **beta-blockers** (section 2.4) has been shown to be of benefit and patients without contra-indications should receive **atenolol** by intravenous injection at a dose of 5 mg over 5 minutes, repeated after 10–15 minutes; **metoprolol** by intravenous injection is an alternative.

ACE inhibitors (section 2.5.5.1) are also of benefit to patients who have no contra-indications; in normotensive patients treatment with an ACE inhibitor can be started within 24 hours of the myocardial infarction and continued for at least 5–6 weeks (see below for long-term treatment).

LONG-TERM MANAGEMENT. **Aspirin** (section 2.9) should be given to all patients, unless contra-indicated, at a dose of 75–150 mg daily.

Beta-blockers (section 2.4) should be given to all patients in whom they are not contra-indicated and continued for 2–3 years. Acebutolol, metoprolol, propranolol and timolol are suitable.

Although other calcium-channel blockers (section 2.6.2) have no place in routine management, **verapamil** may be useful in patients in whom beta-blockers are inappropriate.

ACE inhibitors (section 2.5.5.1) are recommended for any patient with evidence of left ventricular dysfunction.

Nitrates (section 2.6.1) are used for patients with angina.

Statins are beneficial in preventing recurrent coronary events, particularly for patients at high risk because of other factors (section 2.12).

2.10.2   Fibrinolytic drugs

Fibrinolytic drugs act as thrombolytics by activating plasminogen to form plasmin, which degrades fibrin and so breaks up thrombi.

Streptokinase is used in the treatment of *life-threatening venous thrombosis*, and in *pulmonary embolism*, but treatment must be started rapidly.

Urokinase is currently used for *thrombolysis in the eye* and in *arteriovenous shunts*. It has the advantage of being non-immunogenic.

The value of thrombolytic drugs for the treatment of *myocardial infarction* has been established (section 2.10.1). **Streptokinase, alteplase,** and **anistreplase** have all been shown to reduce mortality; **reteplase** has been licensed recently for acute myocardial infarction. Thrombolytic drugs are indicated for any patient with acute myocardial infarction for whom the benefit is believed to outweigh the risk of treatment. Trials have shown that the benefit is greatest in those with ECG changes that include ST segment elevation and in those with anterior infarction. Patients should not be excluded on account of age alone because mortality in this group is high and the percentage reduction in mortality is the same as in younger patients.

CAUTIONS. Risk of bleeding including that from venepuncture or invasive procedures, any external chest compression, pregnancy (see Appendix 4), abdominal aneurysm or conditions in which thrombolysis might give rise to embolic complications such as enlarged left atrium with atrial fibrillation (risk of dissolution of clot and subsequent embolisation), diabetic retinopathy, recent or concurrent anticoagulant therapy.

CONTRA-INDICATIONS. Recent haemorrhage, trauma, or surgery (including dental extraction), coagulation defects, bleeding diatheses, aortic dissection, coma, history of cerebrovascular disease especially recent events or with any residual disability, recent symptoms of possible peptic ulceration, heavy vaginal bleeding, severe hypertension, pulmonary disease with cavitation, acute pancreatitis, severe liver disease, oesophageal varices; also

in the case of streptokinase or anistreplase, previous allergic reactions to either drug.

Prolonged persistence of antibodies to streptokinase and anistreplase may reduce the effectiveness of subsequent treatment, therefore neither drug should be repeated beyond 4 days of first administration.

SIDE-EFFECTS. Side-effects of thrombolytics are mainly nausea and vomiting and bleeding. Back pain has been reported. Bleeding is usually limited to the site of injection, but intracerebral haemorrhage or bleeding from other sites may occur. Serious bleeding calls for discontinuation of the thrombolytic and may require administration of coagulation factors and antifibrinolytic drugs (aprotinin or tranexamic acid). Streptokinase and anistreplase may cause allergic reactions (including rash, flushing and uveitis) and anaphylaxis has been reported (for details of management see Allergic Emergencies, section 3.4.3). Guillain-Barré syndrome has been reported rarely after streptokinase treatment.

ALTEPLASE

(rt-PA, tissue-type plasminogen activator)

Indications: acute myocardial infarction (see notes above); pulmonary embolism

Cautions; Contra-indications; Side-effects: see notes above

Dose:

Myocardial infarction, accelerated regimen (initiated within 6 hours), 15 mg by *intravenous injection*, followed by *intravenous infusion* of 50 mg over 30 minutes, then 35 mg over 60 minutes (total dose 100 mg over 90 minutes); lower doses in patients less than 65 kg

Myocardial infarction, initiated within 6–12 hours, 10 mg by *intravenous injection*, followed by *intravenous infusion* of 50 mg over 60 minutes, then 4 *infusions* each of 10 mg over 30 minutes (total dose 100 mg over 3 hours; max. 1.5 mg/kg in patients less than 65 kg)

Pulmonary embolism, 10 mg by *intravenous injection* over 1–2 minutes followed by *intravenous infusion* of 90 mg over 2 hours; max. 1.5 mg/kg in patients less than 65 kg

PoM **Actilyse®** (Boehringer Ingelheim)

Injection, powder for reconstitution, alteplase 10 mg (5.8 million units)/vial, net price per vial (with diluent and transfer device) = £150.00; 20 mg (11.6 million units)/vial (with diluent and transfer device) = £200.00; 50 mg (29 million units)/vial, pack of 2 vials (with diluent, transfer device, and infusion bag) = £750.00

ANISTREPLASE

(APSAC)

Indications: acute myocardial infarction (see notes above)

Cautions; Contra-indications; Side-effects: see notes above

Dose: by intravenous injection, 30 units over 4–5 minutes; treatment should be initiated as soon as possible and preferably within 6 hours

PoM **Eminase®** (Monmouth)
Injection, powder for reconstitution, anistreplase. Net price 30-unit vial = £495.00 (also available in injection pack with 5-mL amp water for injections and disposable syringe and needle)

RETEPLASE
Indications: acute myocardial infarction (see also section 2.10.1)
Cautions; Contra-indications; Side-effects: see notes above
Dose: by intravenous injection, 10 units over not more than 2 minutes, followed after 30 minutes by a further 10 units

▼ PoM **Rapilysin®** (Boehringer Mannheim)
Injection, powder for reconstitution, reteplase 10 units (1.16 g)/vial, net price pack of 2 vials (with 2 prefilled syringes of diluent and transfer device) = £750.00

STREPTOKINASE
Indications: deep-vein thrombosis, pulmonary embolism, acute arterial thromboembolism, thrombosed arteriovenous shunts; acute myocardial infarction (section 2.10.1); topical use, see section 13.11.7
Cautions; Contra-indications; Side-effects: see notes above
Dose: by intravenous infusion, 250 000 units over 30 minutes, then 100 000 units every hour for up to 24–72 hours according to condition (see product literature)
Myocardial infarction, 1 500 000 units over 60 minutes

PoM **Kabikinase®** (Pharmacia & Upjohn)
Injection, powder for reconstitution, streptokinase; net price 250 000-unit vial = £15.00; 750 000-unit vial = £40.00; 1.5 million-unit vial = £85.00
PoM **Streptase®** (Hoechst Marion Roussel)
Injection, powder for reconstitution, streptokinase; net price 250 000-unit vial = £17.11; 750 000-unit vial = £44.86; 1.5 million-unit vial = £89.72 (hosp. only)

UROKINASE
Indications: thrombosed arteriovenous shunts and intravenous cannulas; thrombolysis in the eye; deep-vein thrombosis, pulmonary embolism, peripheral vascular occlusion
Cautions; Contra-indications; Side-effects: see notes above
Dose: by instillation into arteriovenous shunt, 5000–25 500 International units in 2–3 mL sodium chloride injection 0.9%
By intravenous infusion 4400 International units/kg over 10 minutes, then 4400 units/kg/hour for

12 hours in pulmonary embolism or 12–24 hours in deep-vein thrombosis; for bolus injection for pulmonary embolism consult product literature
Peripheral vascular occlusion, consult product literature
Intra-ocular administration, 5000 International units in 2 mL sodium chloride injection 0.9%

PoM **Urokinase** (Non-proprietary)
Injection, powder for reconstitution, urokinase; net price 5000 International unit vial = £9.75; 25 000 International unit vial = £27.79; 100 000 International unit vial = £60.00
Available from Leo, Serono (Ukidan®)

2.11   Antifibrinolytic drugs and haemostatics
Fibrin dissolution can be impaired by the administration of **tranexamic acid**, which inhibits plasminogen activation and fibrinolysis. It may be useful when haemorrhage cannot be staunched (e.g. in prostatectomy and dental extraction in haemophilia) and can be particularly useful in menorrhagia. Tranexamic acid may also be used in hereditary angioedema and in thrombolytic overdose.

Desmopressin (see section 6.5.2) is used in the management of mild to moderate haemophilia.

Aprotinin is a proteolytic enzyme inhibitor acting on plasmin and kallidinogenase (kallikrein). It is indicated for patients at high risk of major blood loss during and after open heart surgery with extracorporeal circulation and for patients in whom optimal blood conservation during open heart surgery is an absolute priority; it is also indicated for the treatment of life-threatening haemorrhage due to hyperplasminaemia (occasionally observed during the mobilisation and dissection of malignant tumours, in acute promyelocytic leukaemia, and following thrombolytic therapy).

Ethamsylate (etamsylate) reduces capillary bleeding in the presence of a normal number of platelets. It does not act by fibrin stabilisation, but probably by correcting abnormal platelet adhesion.

APROTININ
Indications: see notes above
Side-effects: occasionally hypersensitivity reactions and localised thrombophlebitis
Dose: by slow intravenous injection or infusion
Open heart surgery, loading dose, 2 000 000 units (200 mL) after induction of anaesthesia and before sternotomy—initial 50 000 units (5 mL) *by slow intravenous injection* over several minutes (to detect allergy), remainder *by intravenous infusion* over 20 minutes; maintenance dose, *by intravenous infusion* 500 000 units (50 mL) every hour until end of operation (or early postoperative period in septic endocarditis); pump prime, 2 000 000 units (200 mL) in priming volume of extracorporeal circuit; in septic endocarditis 3 000 000 units (300 mL) added to pump prime
Hyperplasminaemia, *by slow intravenous injection or by infusion* initially, 500 000 units (50 mL) to 1 000 000 units (100 mL) at max. rate 10 mL/min; followed if necessary by 200 000 units (20 mL) every hour until bleeding stops

PoM **Trasylol®** (Bayer)
Injection, aprotinin 10000 kallikrein inactivator units/
mL. Net price 50-mL vial = £20.53
Note. Aprotinin injection containing 10000 kallikrein
inactivator units/mL also available from Paines & Byrne

ETHAMSYLATE
(Etamsylate)
Indications: see under preparations
Contra-indications: porphyria (see section 9.8.2)
Side-effects: nausea, headache, rashes
Dose: see below

PoM **Dicynene®** (Delandale)
Tablets, scored, ethamsylate 500 mg, net price
100-tab pack = £22.13
Dose: short-term treatment of blood loss in menorrhagia, 500 mg 4 times daily during menstruation
Injection, ethamsylate 125 mg/mL. Net price 2-mL
amp = 82p
Dose: prophylaxis and treatment of periventricular
haemorrhage in low birth-weight infants, by intramuscular or intravenous injection, 12.5 mg/kg every 6 hours
IMPORTANT. The ampoules currently available contain a
total of 250 mg in 2 mL volume therefore **small fraction
only** required for neonatal use

TRANEXAMIC ACID
Indications: see notes above
Cautions: reduce dose in renal impairment; massive haematuria (avoid if risk of ureteric obstruction); regular eye examinations and liver function
tests in long-term treatment of hereditary angioedema
Note. Requirement for regular eye examinations during
long-term treatment is based on unsatisfactory evidence
Contra-indications: thromboembolic disease
Side-effects: nausea, vomiting, diarrhoea (reduce
dose); giddiness on rapid intravenous injection
Dose: by mouth, local fibrinolysis, 15–25 mg/kg
2–3 times daily
Menorrhagia (initiated when heavy bleeding has
started), 1–1.5 g 3–4 times daily for 3–4 days
By slow intravenous injection, local fibrinolysis,
0.5–1 g 3 times daily

PoM **Cyklokapron®** (Pharmacia & Upjohn)
Tablets, f/c, scored, tranexamic acid 500 mg. Net
price 60-tab pack = £14.97
Syrup, tranexamic acid 500 mg/5 mL. Net price
300 mL = £15.60
Injection, tranexamic acid 100 mg/mL. Net price
5-mL amp = £1.35

BLOOD PRODUCTS

FACTOR VIIa (RECOMBINANT)
Recombinant factor VIIa is used in patients with
inhibitors to factors VIII and IX
Available from Novo Nordisk (▼*NovoSeven®*)

FACTOR VIII FRACTION, DRIED
(Human Antihaemophilic Fraction, Dried)
Dried factor VIII fraction is prepared from human plasma
by a suitable fractionation technique
Indications: control of haemorrhage in haemophilia A
Cautions: intravascular haemolysis after large or
frequently repeated doses in patients with blood
groups A, B, or AB—less likely with high
potency concentrates
Side-effects: allergic reactions including chills,
fever; hyperfibrinogenaemia occurred after massive doses with earlier products but less likely
since fibrinogen content has now been substantially reduced
Available from Alpha (*Alphanate®*), Armour
(*Monoclate-P®*), BPL (*Replenate®*, *8Y®*), SNBTS
(*Liberate®*, High Potency Factor VIII Concentrate)
Note. Preparation of recombinant human antihaemophilic factor VIII (octocog alfa) available from Bayer
(*Kogenate®*), Baxter Hyland (*Recombinate®*)

FACTOR VIII INHIBITOR BYPASSING FRACTION
Preparations with factor VIII inhibitor bypassing activity
are prepared from human plasma
Human Factor VIII Inhibitor Bypassing Fraction
(*FEIBA*, Immuno) is used in patients with factor
VIII inhibitors
Note. A porcine preparation of antihaemophilic factor
for patients with inhibitors to human factor VIII is avail-
able from Speywood (*Hyate C®*)

FACTOR IX FRACTION, DRIED
Dried factor IX fraction is prepared from human plasma
by a suitable fractionation technique; it may also contain
clotting factors II, VII, and X.
Indications: congenital factor IX deficiency
(haemophilia B)
Cautions: risk of thrombosis—principally with
former low purity products
Contra-indications: disseminated intravascular
coagulation
Side-effects: allergic reactions, including chills,
fever
Available from Alpha (*AlphaNine®*), Armour
(*Mononine®*), BPL (Dried Factor IX Fraction,
Heat-Treated; *Replenine®*), SNBTS (Human Factor IX Concentrate, Heat Treated; *HT Defix®*)

FRESH FROZEN PLASMA
Fresh frozen plasma is prepared from the supernatant liquid obtained by centrifugation of one donation of whole
blood
Indications: to replace coagulation factors or other
plasma proteins where their concentration or
functional activity is critically reduced, e.g. to
reverse warfarin effect
Cautions: avoid in circulatory overload; need for
compatibility
Side-effects: allergic reactions including chills,
fever, bronchospasm; adult respiratory distress
syndrome
Available from Regional Blood Transfusion Services and BPL

2.12   Lipid-regulating drugs

There are a number of common conditions, some familial, in which there are very high plasma concentrations of cholesterol, or triglycerides, or both. There is evidence that therapy which lowers low density lipoprotein (LDL) cholesterol and raises high density lipoprotein (HDL) cholesterol reduces the progression of coronary atherosclerosis and may even induce regression. There is also evidence that lowering LDL-cholesterol by 25 to 35% is effective in both the primary and secondary prevention of clinical manifestations of coronary heart disease.

Lipid-regulating drugs are indicated in patients with coronary heart disease or with severe hyperlipidaemia inadequately controlled by a modified fat diet. Treatment should also be considered in those at high risk of developing coronary heart disease on account of multiple risk factors (including smoking, hypertension, diabetes mellitus, and a family history of premature coronary heart disease). Any drug therapy must be combined with strict adherence to diet, maintenance of near-ideal body weight and, if appropriate, reduction of blood pressure and cessation of smoking.

Statins are drugs of first choice for treating hypercholesterolaemia, fibrates for hypertriglyceridaemia and statins or fibrates can be used, either alone or together, to treat mixed hyperlipidaemia.

Severe hyperlipidaemia often requires combinations of lipid-regulating drugs such as an anion-exchange resin with a fibrate, a statin, or nicotinic acid. Combinations of a statin with nicotinic acid or a fibrate carry an increased risk of side-effects (including rhabdomyolysis) and should be used with caution.

> **Muscle effects.** The CSM has advised that rhabdomyolysis associated with lipid-regulating drugs such as the fibrates and statins appears to be rare (approx. 1 case in every 100 000 treatment years) but may be increased in those with renal impairment and possibly in those with hypothyroidism. Concomitant treatment with cyclosporin may increase plasma-statin concentrations and the risk of muscle toxicity; concomitant treatment with a fibrate and a statin may also be associated with an increased risk of serious muscle toxicity.

ANION-EXCHANGE RESINS

Cholestyramine (colestyramine) and **colestipol** are anion-exchange resins used in the management of hypercholesterolaemia. They act by binding bile acids, preventing their reabsorption; this promotes hepatic conversion of cholesterol into bile acids; the resultant increased LDL-receptor activity of liver cells increases the breakdown of LDL-cholesterol. Thus both compounds effectively reduce LDL-cholesterol but can aggravate hypertriglyceridaemia.

CAUTIONS. Anion-exchange resins interfere with the absorption of fat-soluble vitamins; supplements of vitamins A, D and K may be required when treatment is prolonged. **Interactions:** Appendix 1 (cholestyramine and colestipol).

SIDE-EFFECTS. As cholestyramine and colestipol are not absorbed, gastro-intestinal side-effects predominate. Constipation is common, but diarrhoea has occurred, as have nausea, vomiting, and gastro-intestinal discomfort. An increased bleeding tendency has been reported due to hypoprothrombinaemia associated with vitamin K deficiency.

COUNSELLING. Other drugs should be taken at least 1 hour before or 4–6 hours after cholestyramine or colestipol to reduce possible interference with absorption.

CHOLESTYRAMINE
(Colestyramine)

Indications: hyperlipidaemias, particularly type IIa, in patients who have not responded adequately to diet and other appropriate measures; primary prevention of coronary heart disease in men aged 35–59 years with primary hypercholesterolaemia who have not responded to diet and other appropriate measures; pruritus associated with partial biliary obstruction and primary biliary cirrhosis; diarrhoeal disorders, see section 1.5

Cautions: see notes above; pregnancy and breast-feeding

Contra-indications: complete biliary obstruction (not likely to be effective)

Side-effects: see notes above; hyperchloraemic acidosis reported on prolonged use

Dose: lipid reduction (after initial introduction over 3–4 weeks) 12–24 g daily in water (or other suitable liquid) in single or up to 4 divided doses; up to 36 g daily if necessary

Pruritus, 4–8 g daily in water (or other suitable liquid)

Diarrhoeal disorders, see section 1.5

CHILD 6–12 years, see product literature

PoM **Cholestyramine** (Non-proprietary)

Powder, cholestyramine (anhydrous) 4 g/sachet, net price 180-sachet pack = £50.55. Label: 13, counselling, avoid other drugs at same time (see notes above)

Available from Dominion

PoM **Questran®** (Bristol-Myers)

Powder, orange, cholestyramine (anhydrous) 4 g/sachet. Net price 60-sachet pack = £21.06, 180-sachet pack = £63.19. Label: 13, counselling, avoid other drugs at same time (see notes above)

PoM **Questran Light®** (Bristol-Myers)

Powder, orange, cholestyramine (anhydrous) 4 g/sachet, with aspartame. Net price 60-sachet pack = £22.11, 180-sachet pack = £66.34. Label: 13, counselling, avoid other drugs at same time (see notes above)

COLESTIPOL HYDROCHLORIDE

Indications: hyperlipidaemias, particularly type IIa, in patients who have not responded adequately to diet and other appropriate measures

Cautions: see notes above; pregnancy

Side-effects: see notes above

Dose: 5 g 1–2 times daily in liquid increased if necessary at intervals of 1–2 months to max. of 30 g daily (in single or 2 divided doses)

PoM **Colestid**® (Pharmacia & Upjohn)
Granules, yellow, colestipol hydrochloride 5 g/ sachet. Net price 30 sachets = £12.54. Label: 13, counselling, avoid other drugs at same time (see notes above)
Colestid Orange, granules, yellow/orange, colestipol hydrochloride 5 g/sachet, with aspartame. Net price 30 sachets = £12.54. Label: 13, counselling, avoid other drugs at same time (see notes above)

CLOFIBRATE GROUP

Clofibrate, bezafibrate, ciprofibrate, fenofibrate, and **gemfibrozil** can be regarded as broad-spectrum lipid-modulating agents in that although their main action is to decrease serum triglycerides they also tend to reduce LDL-cholesterol and to raise HDL-cholesterol.

All can cause a myositis-like syndrome (see also CSM advice above), especially in patients with impaired renal function. In addition, clofibrate predisposes to gallstones by increasing biliary cholesterol excretion; it is therefore only indicated in patients who have had a cholecystectomy.

BEZAFIBRATE

Indications: hyperlipidaemias of types IIa, IIb, III, IV and V in patients who have not responded adequately to diet and other appropriate measures

Cautions: renal impairment (avoid if severe—see also under Myotoxicity below); **interactions:** Appendix 1 (clofibrate group)

MYOTOXICITY. Special care needed in patients with renal disease, as progressive increases in serum creatinine concentration or failure to follow dosage guidelines may result in myotoxicity (rhabdomyolysis)

Contra-indications: severe renal or hepatic impairment, hypoalbuminaemia, primary biliary cirrhosis, gall bladder disease, nephrotic syndrome, pregnancy and breast-feeding

Side-effects: gastro-intestinal (e.g. nausea, anorexia, gastric pain), pruritus, urticaria, impotence; also headache, dizziness, vertigo, fatigue, hair loss; myotoxicity (with myasthenia or myalgia)—special risk in renal impairment (see Cautions)

Dose: see preparations below

PoM **Bezalip**® (Boehringer Mannheim)
Tablets, f/c, bezafibrate 200 mg. Net price 100-tab pack = £10.30. Label: 21
Dose: 200 mg 3 times daily with or after food
PoM **Bezalip-Mono**® (Boehringer Mannheim)
Tablets, m/r, f/c, bezafibrate 400 mg. Net price 28-tab pack = £8.50. Label: 21, 25
Dose: 1 tablet daily after food (dose form not appropriate in renal impairment)

CIPROFIBRATE

Indications: hyperlipidaemias of types IIa, IIb, III, and IV in patients who have not responded adequately to diet

Cautions; Contra-indications; Side-effects: see under Bezafibrate

Dose: 100 mg daily

PoM **Modalim**® (Sanofi Winthrop)
Tablets, scored, ciprofibrate 100 mg. Net price 28-tab pack = £13.38

CLOFIBRATE

Indications: hyperlipidaemias of types IIb, III, IV and V in patients who have not responded adequately to diet and other appropriate measures (but see also notes above)

Cautions; Contra-indications: see under Bezafibrate and notes above

Side-effects: see under Bezafibrate; also cholesterol cholelithiasis

Dose: over 65 kg, 2 g daily (50–65 kg, 1.5 g daily) in 2 or 3 divided doses

PoM **Atromid-S**® (Zeneca)
Capsules, red, clofibrate 500 mg. Net price 100-cap pack = £4.08. Label: 21

FENOFIBRATE

Indications: hyperlipidaemias of types IIa, IIb, III, IV, and V in patients who have not responded adequately to diet and other appropriate measures

Cautions: see under Bezafibrate; renal impairment (Appendix 3)

Contra-indications: severe renal or hepatic impairment, existing gall bladder disease; pregnancy and breast-feeding

Side-effects: see under Bezafibrate

Dose: see preparations below

PoM **Lipantil**® (Fournier)
Lipantil® *Micro 67 capsules,* yellow, fenofibrate (micronised) 67 mg. Net price 90-cap pack = £24.40. Label: 21
Dose: initially 3 capsules daily in divided doses; usual range 2–4 capsules daily; CHILD 1 capsule/20 kg daily
Lipantil® *Micro 200 capsules,* orange, fenofibrate (micronised) 200 mg. Net price 30-cap pack = £24.40. Label: 21
Dose: initially 1 capsule daily (dose form not appropriate for children or in renal impairment)
Note. For an equivalent therapeutic effect, 100 mg previously available non-micronised fenofibrate ≡ 67 mg micronised fenofibrate

---

GEMFIBROZIL

Indications: hyperlipidaemias of types IIa, IIb, III, IV and V in patients who have not responded adequately to diet and other appropriate measures; primary prevention of coronary heart disease in men aged 40–55 years with hyperlipidaemias that have not responded to diet and other appropriate measures

---

Cautions: lipid profile, blood counts, and liver-function tests before initiating long-term treatment; renal impairment; **interactions:** Appendix 1 (clofibrate group)

Contra-indications: alcoholism, hepatic impairment, gallstones; pregnancy and breast-feeding

Side-effects: gastro-intestinal disturbances; also rash, dermatitis, pruritus, urticaria, impotence, headache, dizziness, blurred vision, cholestatic jaundice, angioedema, laryngeal oedema, atrial fibrillation, pancreatitis, myasthenia, myopathy, rhabdomyolysis, painful extremities, myalgia accompanied by increases in creatine kinase

Dose: 1.2 g daily, usually in 2 divided doses; range 0.9–1.5 g daily

PoM **Gemfibrozil** (Non-proprietary)
Capsules, gemfibrozil 300 mg, net price 112-cap pack = £21.56
Available from Berk (*Emfib*®)
Tablets, gemfibrozil 600 mg, net price 30-tab pack = £15.88
Available from Norton
PoM **Lopid**® (P-D)
'300' capsules, white/maroon, gemfibrozil 300 mg. Net price 112-cap pack = £29.64
'600' tablets, f/c, gemfibrozil 600 mg. Net price 56-tab pack = £29.64

ISPAGHULA

Ispaghula husk, a form of soluble fibre, can be used as an adjunct to a lipid-lowering diet in patients with mild to moderate hypercholesterolaemia. It probably acts by reducing reabsorption of bile acids; plasma triglycerides remain unchanged.

ISPAGHULA

Indications: primary hypercholesterolaemia in patients with cholesterol concentration of 6.5–7.8 mmol/litre who have not responded adequately to dietary control; constipation, see section 1.6.1

Cautions: maintain adequate fluid intake; diabetes mellitus

Contra-indications: intestinal obstruction, faecal impaction, colonic atony

Side-effects: flatulence, abdominal bloating, particularly on starting treatment (if necessary, reduce dosage to once daily for few days); gastro-intestinal obstruction or impaction

Dose: see under preparation below

Fybozest Orange® (R&C)
Granules, effervescent, sugar-free, ispaghula husk. Net price 265-g tub (with measure) = £6.43. Label: 13, counselling, see below
Note. Contains aspartame 50 mg/3.5-g dose (section 9.4.1) also, sodium 0.4 mmol/3.5-g dose and potassium 0.7 mmol/3.5-g dose
Dose: 3.5 g (1 measure) in at least 150 mL water twice daily; for earlier onset of cholesterol reduction (under medical supervision only), initially 5.25 g (1½ measures) twice daily for 2–3 months
COUNSELLING. Preparations that swell in contact with liquid should always be carefully swallowed with water and should not be taken immediately before going to bed

---

STATINS

The statins (**atorvastatin**, **cerivastatin**, **fluvastatin**, **pravastatin** and **simvastatin**) competitively inhibit 3-hydroxy-3-methylglutaryl coenzyme A (HMG CoA) reductase, an enzyme involved in cholesterol synthesis, especially in the liver. They are more effective than anion-exchange resins in lowering LDL-cholesterol but less effective than the clofibrate group in reducing triglycerides and raising HDL-cholesterol.

There is evidence that statins produce important reductions in coronary events, in all cardiovascular events, and in total mortality in patients aged up to 70 years with coronary heart disease (history of angina or acute myocardial infarction) and with plasma cholesterol of 5.5 mmol/litre or greater. In patients who have had a myocardial infarction, treatment may be appropriate when the total plasma cholesterol concentration is as low as 4.8 mmol/litre. They also have a role in primary prevention of coronary heart disease in some patients with hypercholesterolaemia and increased risk of coronary events.

CAUTIONS. Statins should be used with caution in those with a history of liver disease or with a high alcohol intake (use should be avoided in active liver disease). Liver-function tests should be carried out before and during treatment. Treatment should be discontinued if serum transaminase concentrations rise to, and persist at, three times the upper limit of normal. Patients should be advised to report unexplained muscle pain (see Muscle Effects below). **Interactions:** Appendix 1 (statins).

CONTRA-INDICATIONS. Statins are contra-indicated in those with active liver disease and in pregnancy (adequate contraception should be ensured during and for one month after treatment) and breast-feeding (see Appendixes 4 and 5).

SIDE-EFFECTS. Reversible myositis is a rare but significant side-effect of the statins (see also Muscle Effects, p. 117 and below). The statins also cause headache, altered liver-function tests and gastro-intestinal effects including abdominal pain, nausea and vomiting.

MUSCLE EFFECTS. Myalgia, myositis and myopathy have been reported with the statins; if the creatine kinase concentration is markedly elevated (> 10 times upper limit of normal), and myopathy is suspected or diagnosed, treatment should be discontinued. There is an increased incidence of myopathy if the statins are given with a fibrate, with lipid-lowering doses of nicotinic acid, or with immunosuppressants such as cyclosporin; close monitoring of liver function and if, symptomatic, of creatine kinase is required in patients receiving these drugs. Rhabdomyolysis with acute renal impairment secondary to myoglobinuria has also been reported

COUNSELLING. Advise patient to report promptly unexplained muscle pain, tenderness, weakness.

ATORVASTATIN

Indications: primary hypercholesterolaemia, heterozygous familial hypercholesterolaemia, homozygous familial hypercholesterolaemia or combined (mixed) hyperlipidaemia in patients who have not responded adequately to diet and other appropriate measures

Cautions: see notes above

Contra-indications: see notes above

Side-effects: see notes above; also insomnia, angioedema, anorexia, alopecia, impotence, chest pain, hypoglycaemia and hyperglycaemia reported

Dose: primary hypercholesterolaemia and combined hyperlipidaemia, usually 10 mg once daily Familial hypercholesterolaemia, initially 10 mg daily, increased at intervals of 4 weeks to 40 mg once daily; if necessary, further increased to max. 80 mg once daily (or combined with anion-exchange resin in heterozygous familial hypercholesterolaemia)

▼ PoM **Lipitor®** (P-D)

Tablets, all f/c, atorvastatin (as calcium trihydrate) 10 mg, net price 28-tab pack = £18.88; 20 mg, 28-tab pack = £30.60; 40 mg 28-tab pack = £47.04. Counselling, muscle effects, see notes above

CERIVASTATIN

Indications: primary hypercholesterolaemia (types IIa and IIb) in patients who have not responded adequately to dietary control

Cautions: see notes above; renal impairment

Contra-indications: see notes above

Side-effects: see notes above; also insomnia, influenza-like syndrome, arthralgia, back pain

Dose: initially 100 micrograms once daily in the evening, increased by increments of 100 micrograms at intervals of not less than 4 weeks to max. 300 micrograms once daily (200 micrograms daily in moderate to severe renal impairment)

▼ PoM **Lipobay®** (Bayer)

Tablets, all f/c, cerivastatin 100 micrograms (yellow), net price 28-tab pack = £12.95; 200 micrograms (light yellow-brown), net price 28-tab pack = £17.35; 300 micrograms (yellow-brown), net price 28-tab pack = £18.20. Counselling, muscle effects, see notes above

FLUVASTATIN

Indications: primary hypercholesterolaemia (hyperlipidaemia type IIa) in patients with cholesterol concentration of 6.5 mmol/litre or greater who have not responded adequately to dietary control; adjunct to diet in retarding progression of coronary atherosclerosis in primary hypercholesterolaemia and concomitant coronary heart disease

Cautions: see notes above

Contra-indications: see notes above; also severe renal impairment

Side-effects: see notes above; also insomnia

Dose: initially 20 mg daily in the evening; usual range 20–40 mg daily in the evening, adjusted at intervals of 4 weeks; up to 40 mg twice daily may be required

▼ PoM **Lescol®** (Novartis)

Capsules, fluvastatin (as sodium salt) 20 mg (brown/yellow), net price 28-cap pack = £14.90; 40 mg (brown/orange), 28-cap pack = £15.90, 56-cap pack = £29.80. Counselling, muscle effects, see notes above

PRAVASTATIN

Indications: primary hypercholesterolaemia (hyperlipidaemia type IIa), in patients with cholesterol concentration of 6.5 mmol/litre or greater who have not responded adequately to dietary control; adjunct to diet to slow progressive course of coronary atherosclerosis and reduce incidence of clinical cardiac events in patients with hypercholesterolaemia and documented atherosclerotic coronary artery disease; adjunct to diet in hypercholesterolaemia without clinically evident coronary heart disease

Cautions: see notes above

Contra-indications: see notes above

Side-effects: see notes above; also rash, chest pain, fatigue

Dose: usual range 10–40 mg once daily at night, adjusted at intervals of not less than 4 weeks

PoM **Lipostat®** (Squibb)

Tablets, all yellow, pravastatin sodium 10 mg, net price 28-tab pack = £16.18; 20 mg, 28-tab pack = £31.09; 40 mg, 28-tab pack = £46.48. Counselling, muscle effects, see notes above

SIMVASTATIN

Indications: primary hypercholesterolaemia (hyperlipidaemia type IIa) in patients who have not responded adequately to diet and other appropriate measures; to reduce incidence of clinical coronary events and slow progression of coronary atherosclerosis in patients with coronary heart disease and cholesterol concentration of 5.5 mmol/litre or greater

Cautions: see notes above

Contra-indications: see notes above; also porphyria (see section 9.8.2)

Side-effects: see notes above; also rash, alopecia, anaemia, dizziness, depression, paraesthesia, peripheral neuropathy, hepatitis, jaundice, pancreatitis; hypersensitivity syndrome (including angioedema) reported rarely

Dose: hypercholesterolaemia, 10 mg daily at night, adjusted at intervals of not less than 4 weeks; usual range 10–40 mg once daily at night
Coronary heart disease, initially 20 mg once daily at night

PoM **Zocor**® (MSD)

Tablets, all f/c, simvastatin 10 mg (peach), net price 28-tab pack = £18.29; 20 mg (tan), 28-tab pack = £31.09; 40 mg (red), 28-tab pack = £47.04. Counselling, muscle effects, see notes above

NICOTINIC ACID GROUP

The value of **nicotinic acid** is limited by its side-effects, especially vasodilatation. In doses of 1.5 to 3 g daily it lowers both cholesterol and triglyceride concentrations by inhibiting synthesis; it also increases HDL-cholesterol. **Acipimox** seems to have fewer side-effects but may be less effective in its lipid-modulating capabilities.

ACIPIMOX

Indications: hyperlipidaemias of types IIa, IIb, and IV in patients who have not responded adequately to diet and other appropriate measures
Cautions: renal impairment
Contra-indications: peptic ulcer; pregnancy
Side-effects: vasodilatation, flushing, itching, rashes, erythema; occasionally, heartburn, epigastric pain, nausea, diarrhoea, headache, malaise
Dose: usually 500–750 mg daily in divided doses

PoM **Olbetam**® (Pharmacia & Upjohn)
Capsules, brown/pink, acipimox 250 mg. Net price 90-cap pack = £38.61. Label: 21

NICOTINIC ACID

Indications: see notes above
Cautions: diabetes mellitus, gout, liver disease, peptic ulcer; **interactions:** Appendix 1 (nicotinic acid)
Contra-indications: pregnancy, breast-feeding
Side-effects: flushing, dizziness, headache, palpitations, pruritus (prostaglandin-mediated symptoms can be reduced by low initial doses taken with meals, or by taking aspirin 75 mg 30 minutes before the dose); nausea, vomiting; rarely impaired liver function and rashes
Dose: initially 100–200 mg 3 times daily (see above), gradually increased over 2–4 weeks to 1–2 g 3 times daily

PoM **¹Nicotinic Acid Tablets,** nicotinic acid 50 mg, net price 100 = £9.26. Label: 21
1. If max. daily dose exceeds 600 mg or if intended for treatment of hyperlipidaemia

FISH OILS

A fish-oil preparation (Maxepa®), rich in omega-3 marine triglycerides, is useful in the treatment of severe hypertriglyceridaemia; however, it can sometimes aggravate hypercholesterolaemia.

OMEGA-3 MARINE TRIGLYCERIDES

Indications: reduction of plasma triglycerides in patients with severe hypertriglyceridaemia judged to be at special risk of ischaemic heart disease or pancreatitis, in conjunction with dietary and other methods (see notes above)
Side-effects: occasional nausea and belching
Dose: see under preparations below

Maxepa® (Seven Seas)
Capsules, 1 g (approx. 1.1 mL) concentrated fish oils containing, as percentage of total fatty acid composition, eicosapentaenoic acid 18%, docosahexaenoic acid 12%. Vitamin A content less than 100 units/g, vitamin D content less than 10 units/g. Net price 200-cap pack = £28.57. Label: 21
Dose: 5 capsules twice daily with food
Liquid, golden-coloured, concentrated fish oils containing, as percentage of total fatty acid composition, eicosapentaenoic acid 18% w/w, docosahexaenoic acid 12% w/w. Vitamin A content less than 100 units/g, vitamin D content less than 10 units/g. Net price 150 mL = £21.43. Label: 21
Dose: 5 mL twice daily with food

2.13 Local sclerosants

Ethanolamine oleate and sodium tetradecyl sulphate are used in sclerotherapy of varicose veins, and phenol is used in haemorrhoids (see section 1.7.3).

ETHANOLAMINE OLEATE
(Monoethanolamine Oleate)

Indications: sclerotherapy of varicose veins
Cautions: extravasation may cause necrosis of tissues
Contra-indications: inability to walk, acute phlebitis, oral contraceptive use, obese legs
Side-effects: allergic reactions (including anaphylaxis)

PoM **Ethanolamine Oleate Injection,** ethanolamine oleate 5%. Net price 5-mL amp = £1.97
Available from Evans
Dose: by slow injection into empty isolated segment of vein, 2–5 mL divided between 3–4 sites; repeated at weekly intervals

SODIUM TETRADECYL SULPHATE

Indications: sclerotherapy of varicose veins
Cautions; Contra-indications; Side-effects: see under Ethanolamine Oleate

PoM **Fibro-Vein**® (STD Pharmaceutical)
Injection, sodium tetradecyl sulphate 0.2%, net price 5-mL amp = £2.20; 0.5%, 2-mL amp = £1.35; 1%, 2-mL amp = £1.46; 3%, 2-mL amp = £1.64, 5-mL vial = £3.15
Dose: by slow injection into empty isolated segment of vein, 0.1–1 mL according to site and condition being treated (consult product literature)

3: Drugs used in the treatment of diseases of the
RESPIRATORY SYSTEM

In this chapter, drug treatment is described under the following headings:

The initial treatment of exacerbations of chronic bronchitis and bacterial pneumonia is indicated in section 5.1 (table 1) and the treatment of tuberculosis is discussed in section 5.1.9.

3.1 Bronchodilators

3.1.1 Adrenoceptor stimulants
(Sympathomimetics)

3.1.1.1 Selective beta$_2$-adrenoceptor stimulants
3.1.1.2 Other adrenoceptor stimulants

The selective beta$_2$-adrenoceptor stimulants (selective beta$_2$-stimulants, selective beta$_2$-agonists) (section 3.1.1.1) such as salbutamol or terbutaline (preferably given by aerosol inhalation) are the safest and most effective beta-stimulants for asthma. They are recommended over the less selective beta-adrenoceptor stimulants such as orciprenaline (section 3.1.1.2), which should be avoided whenever possible.

Adrenaline (which has both alpha- and beta-adrenoceptor stimulant properties) is used in the emergency management of allergic and anaphylactic reactions (section 3.4.3).

3.1.1.1 SELECTIVE BETA$_2$-ADRENOCEPTOR STIMULANTS

Most mild to moderate symptoms of asthma respond rapidly to aerosol administration of a selective short-acting beta$_2$-adrenoceptor stimulant such as salbutamol or terbutaline. If beta$_2$-adrenoceptor stimulant inhalation is needed more than once daily prophylactic treatment should be considered, using a stepped approach as outlined on p. 124. However in more severe exacerbations a short course of an oral corticosteroid may be necessary to bring the asthma under control (section 3.2). Treatment of patients with acute severe asthma or airways obstruction (see also below) is safer in hospital where oxygen and resuscitation facilities are immediately available (see also Acute Severe Asthma table, p. 125).

Patients with chronic bronchitis and emphysema are often described as having irreversible airways obstruction, but they usually respond partially to the beta$_2$-adrenoceptor stimulant drugs or to the antimuscarinic drugs ipratropium or oxitropium (section 3.1.2).

There are some differences among the various selective beta$_2$-adrenoceptor stimulant drugs. **Salbutamol** and **terbutaline** are available in the widest range of formulations. **Fenoterol** may be less beta$_2$-selective than salbutamol.

Salmeterol and **eformoterol** are longer-acting beta$_2$-adrenoceptor stimulants which are administered by inhalation on a twice-daily basis. They are not suitable for the relief of an acute attack. Salmeterol or eformoterol should be added to existing corticosteroid therapy and **not** replace it. Salmeterol and eformoterol can be useful in nocturnal asthma.

REGULAR TREATMENT. Short-acting beta$_2$-adrenoceptor stimulants should not be prescribed on a regular basis in patients with mild or moderate asthma since several studies show that regular treatment provides no clinical benefit (compared with placebo). In contrast, the longer acting beta$_2$-adrenoceptor stimulants, salmeterol and eformoterol when taken regularly have shown clear benefit compared to placebo and to regular treatment with short-acting beta$_2$-adrenoceptor stimulants.

Chronic Asthma table, see p. 124
Acute Severe Asthma table, see p. 125

INHALATION. Administration by inhalation delivers the drug directly to the bronchi and is therefore effective in smaller doses; inhalation is preferred to administration by tablets or oral liquid because it provides relief more rapidly and causes fewer side-effects (such as tremor and nervous tension).

Pressurised (aerosol) inhalation (using a metered dose inhaler) is an effective and convenient method of administration for mild to moderate airways obstruction. The duration of action of an aerosol inhalation depends on the drug that it contains and the dose administered. With recommended doses salbutamol, terbutaline and fenoterol will usually last for 3 to 5 hours, and salmeterol and eformoterol for around 12 hours

CFC-FREE INHALERS. Chloroflurocarbon (CFC) propellants in pressurised aerosol inhalers are being replaced by hydrofluroalkane (HFA) propellants. Patients receiving CFC-free inhalers should be reassured about the efficacy of the new inhalers and counselled that the aerosol may feel and taste different; any difficulty with the new inhaler should be discussed with the doctor or pharmacist.

CSM advice. The CSM has requested doctors to report any adverse reaction to the new HFA-containing inhalers and to include the brand name of the inhaler on the yellow card.

Patients should be given careful instruction on the use of their pressurised (aerosol) inhalers and it is important to check that they continue to use them correctly as inadequate technique may be mistaken for drug failure. In particular, it should be emphasised that they must inhale slowly and hold their breath for 10 seconds after inhalation. Most patients can be successfully taught to use pressurised (aerosol) inhalers but some patients, particularly the elderly, the arthritic, and small children experience difficulty using them; some patients are unable to synchronise their breathing with the administration of aerosol. For such patients a variety of *breath-actuated aerosol inhalers* and *spacing devices* (section 3.1.5) is now available. Alternatively *dry powder inhalers*, activated by the patient's inspiration, are of value; some occasionally cause coughing.

The **dose** in terms of the number of inhalations at one time, the frequency, and the maximum number of inhalations allowed in 24 hours should be **stated explicitly** to the patient. High doses of beta$_2$-stimulants can be dangerous in some patients. Excessive use is usually an indication of **inadequately treated** asthma and should be treated with preventative medication such as an inhaled corticosteroid. Patients should be advised to seek medical advice when they fail to obtain their usual degree of symptomatic relief as this usually indicates a worsening of the asthma and may require alternative medication (see Chronic Asthma table, p. 124).

Respirator (or *nebuliser*) *solutions* of salbutamol and terbutaline are used for the treatment of acute asthma both in hospital and in general practice. They are administered over a period of 5–10 minutes from a nebuliser, usually driven by oxygen in hospital. An electric compressor is most suitable for domiciliary use but these are costly and not currently prescribable under the NHS. Patients with a severe attack of asthma should have oxygen if possible during nebulisation since beta$_2$-adrenoceptor stimulants can cause an increase in arterial hypoxaemia. For patients with chronic bronchitis and hypercapnia, however, oxygen can be dangerous, and the nebuliser should be driven by air. The dose prescribed by nebuliser is substantially higher than that prescribed by metered dose inhaler. Patients should therefore be warned that it is dangerous to exceed the stated dose and that if they fail to respond to the usual dose of their respirator solution they should call for help. See also guidelines in section 3.1.5.

ORAL. *Oral preparations* are available for patients who cannot manage the inhaled route. They are sometimes used for children, although the inhaled route is better and most children can use one or other of the inhalation devices available. Oral preparations have a slower onset and a slightly more prolonged action than the aerosol inhalers. The longer-acting preparations may be of value in patients with nocturnal asthma as an alternative to the modified-release theophylline preparations (section 3.1.3).

PARENTERAL. *Intravenous* and occasionally *subcutaneous* injections of salbutamol and terbutaline are given for severe bronchospasm. Although some patients with chronic asthma are treated with a beta$_2$-adrenoceptor stimulant by subcutaneous injection on a regular basis, the evidence of benefit is uncertain and it may be difficult to withdraw such treatment once started; patients supplied with either adrenaline injection or a selective beta$_2$-adrenoceptor stimulant injection for severe attacks should be advised to attend hospital immediately after using the injection for further assessment.

CHILDREN. Selective beta$_2$-adrenoceptor stimulants are useful even in children under the age of 18 months. They are most effective by the *inhaled route*, but an inhalation device may be needed (with the technique carefully checked). They may also be administered as tablets or oral liquids although administration by inhalation is preferred. In severe attacks *nebulisation* using a selective beta$_2$-adrenoceptor stimulant or ipratropium is advisable (see also Asthma tables, pp. 124–5).

PREGNANCY AND BREAST-FEEDING. It is particularly important that asthma should be well controlled during pregnancy; where this is achieved asthma has no important effects on pregnancy, labour, or the fetus.

Inhalation has particular advantages as a means of drug administration during pregnancy because the therapeutic action can be achieved without the need for plasma drug concentrations liable to have a pharmacological effect on the fetus.

Severe exacerbations of asthma can have an adverse effect on pregnancy and should be treated promptly with conventional therapy, including oral or parenteral administration of corticosteroids and nebulisation of a selective beta$_2$-adrenoceptor stimulant; prednisolone is the preferred corticosteroid for oral administration since placental transfer is slower than with some others.

Although theophylline has been given without adverse effects during pregnancy or breast-feeding there have been occasional reports of toxicity in the fetus and neonate.

Chronic Asthma table, see p. 124
Acute Severe Asthma table, see p. 125

Start at **step most appropriate** to initial severity; **'rescue'** course of prednisolone at **any time** or **any step**

Chronic asthma: **adults** and **schoolchildren**

Step 1: occasional relief bronchodilators

Inhaled short-acting beta$_2$ stimulant as required (up to once daily)

Note. Move to step 2 if needed more than once daily (or night-time symptoms); check compliance, inhaler technique

Step 2: regular inhaled preventer therapy

Inhaled short-acting beta$_2$ stimulant as required
  plus
Either regular standard-dose[1] inhaled corticosteroid
Or regular cromoglycate or nedocromil (but change to inhaled corticosteroid if control not achieved)

Note. Higher dose of inhaled corticosteroid may be required to gain initial control; some individuals benefit from doubling for short period to cover an exacerbation

Step 3: high-dose inhaled corticosteroids *or* standard-dose inhaled corticosteroids + long-acting inhaled beta$_2$ stimulant

Inhaled short-acting beta$_2$ stimulant as required
  plus
Either regular high-dose[2] inhaled corticosteroid
Or regular standard-dose[1] inhaled corticosteroid *plus* regular inhaled long-acting beta$_2$ stimulant (salmeterol 50 micrograms twice daily *or* in those over 18 years, eformoterol 12 micrograms twice daily)

Note. In few who have problems with high-dose inhaled corticosteroid use standard-dose inhaled corticosteroid with *either* inhaled long-acting beta$_2$ stimulant option *or* regular modified-release oral theophylline *or* try regular cromoglycate or nedocromil

Step 4: high-dose inhaled corticosteroids + regular bronchodilators

Inhaled short-acting beta$_2$ stimulant as required
  with
Regular high-dose[2] inhaled corticosteroid
  plus sequential therapeutic trial of one or more of
    Inhaled long-acting beta$_2$ stimulant
    Modified-release oral theophylline
    Inhaled ipratropium or, in adults, oxitropium
    Modified-release oral beta$_2$ stimulant
    High-dose inhaled bronchodilators
    Cromoglycate or nedocromil

Step 5: regular corticosteroid tablets

Inhaled short-acting beta$_2$ stimulant as required
  with
Regular high-dose[2] inhaled corticosteroid *and* one or more long-acting bronchodilators (see step 4)
  plus
Regular prednisolone tablets (as single daily dose)

Note. In addition to regular prednisolone, continue high-dose inhaled corticosteroid (in exceptional cases may exceed licensed doses); these patients should normally be referred to an asthma clinic

Stepping down

Review treatment every 3–6 months; if control achieved stepwise reduction may be possible; if treatment started recently at step 4 or 5 (or contained corticosteroid tablets) reduction may take place after short interval; in other patients a 1–3 month or longer period of stability needed before slow stepwise reduction is undertaken

1. Standard-dose inhaled corticosteroids are beclomethasone dipropionate or budesonide 100–400 micrograms twice daily *or* fluticasone propionate 50–200 micrograms twice daily
2. High-dose inhaled corticosteroids are beclomethasone dipropionate or budesonide 0.8–2 mg daily (in divided doses) *or* fluticasone propionate 0.4–1 mg daily (in divided doses); use a large-volume spacer

Chronic asthma: **children under 5 years**

Step 1: occasional relief bronchodilators

Short-acting beta$_2$ stimulant as required (not more than once daily)

Note. Whenever possible inhaled (less effective and more side-effects when given by mouth); check compliance, technique and that inhaler device is appropriate

Step 2: regular inhaled preventer therapy

Inhaled short-acting beta$_2$ stimulant as required
  plus
Either regular inhaled cromoglycate (powder or metereddose inhaler via large-volume spacer)
Or regular inhaled corticosteroid in standard paediatric dose[3]
    Consider for stabilisation
    5-day course of soluble prednisolone tablets[5] *or* temporary doubling of dose of inhaled corticosteroid

Note. Try cromoglycate for 4–6 weeks. For inhaled corticosteroids assess effect on symptoms after 1 month and adjust doses; if control not adequate consider doubling dose of inhaled corticosteroid for 1 month (alternatively give 5-day course of soluble prednisolone tablets or consider introducing other treatments before increasing dose of inhaled corticosteroid for long periods)

Step 3: increased-dose inhaled corticosteroids

Inhaled short-acting beta$_2$ stimulant as required
  plus
Regular inhaled corticosteroid in high paediatric dose[4]
    Consider
    Short course of soluble prednisolone tablets[5]
    Regular inhaled long-acting beta$_2$ stimulant *or* regular modified-release oral theophylline

Note. Long-acting beta$_2$ stimulant should probably be reserved for supplementing treatment in child already receiving cromoglycate or a corticosteroid; modified-release oral theophylline may be helpful (particularly for nocturnal symptoms), but has appreciable side-effects in up to one-third of children (plasma- or salivary-concentration monitoring recommended)

Step 4: high-dose inhaled corticosteroid + regular bronchodilators

Inhaled short-acting beta$_2$ stimulant as required
  with
Regular inhaled corticosteroid in high dose (beclomethasone dipropionate or budesonide up to 2 mg daily *via* large-volume spacer)
    Consider (as in step 3)
    Short course of soluble prednisolone[5]
    Regular inhaled long-acting beta$_2$ stimulant
    Regular modified-release oral theophylline
    Also nebulised beta$_2$ stimulant

Stepping down

Regularly review need for treatment

3. Standard paediatric dose of inhaled corticosteroid is beclomethasone dipropionate or budesonide up to 400 micrograms daily (in divided doses) *or* fluticasone propionate up to 200 micrograms daily (in divided doses); initial dose according to age, weight and severity of asthma; use a large-volume spacer
4. High paediatric dose of inhaled corticosteroid is beclomethasone dipropionate or budesonide up to 800 micrograms daily (in divided doses) *or* fluticasone propionate up to 500 micrograms daily (in divided doses); use a large-volume spacer
5. Doses of prednisolone tablets are child under 1 year 1–2 mg/kg daily, 1–5 years 20 mg daily; rescue courses usually for 1–3 days

Based on tables in: British Thoracic Society and others. The British Guidelines on Asthma Management. *Thorax* 1997; **52** (suppl): S1–S21. Reproduced with permission of BMJ Specialist Journals

MANAGEMENT OF ACUTE SEVERE ASTHMA IN GENERAL PRACTICE

Uncontrolled asthma in adults
— Speech normal
— Pulse <110 beats/minute
— Respiration <25 breaths/minute
— Peak flow >50% of predicted or best
Treat at home but response to treatment **must** be assessed before doctor leaves
Treatment:
Nebulised salbutamol 5 mg or nebulised terbutaline 10 mg
Monitor response 15–30 minutes after nebulisation
If peak flow 50–75% of predicted or best give:
Oral prednisolone 30–60 mg
and step up usual treatment
Alternatively if peak flow >75% of predicted or best:
Step up usual treatment
Follow up
Monitor symptoms and peak flow
Set up self management plan
Review in surgery within 48 hours
Modify treatment at review according to guidelines for chronic asthma (see opposite page)

Important: regard each emergency consultation as being for acute severe asthma until shown otherwise.

Important: failure to respond adequately at any time requires immediate referral to hospital.

Acute episodes or exacerbations of asthma in young children in primary care
Mild/moderate episode in young children
— short-acting beta₂ stimulant from metered dose inhaler via large-volume spacer (and face mask in very young), up to 10 puffs (1 puff every 15–30 seconds); alternatively give by nebuliser every 3–4 hours
— if favourable response (respiratory rate reduced, reduced use of accessory muscles, improved 'behaviour' pattern), repeat inhaled beta₂ stimulant every 3–4 hours; consider doubling dose of inhaled corticosteroids

Acute severe asthma in adults
— Cannot complete sentences
— Pulse ≥110 beats/minute
— Respiration ≥25 breaths/minute
— Peak flow ≤50% of predicted or best
Seriously consider hospital admission if more than one of above features present
Treatment:
Oxygen 40–60% if available
Nebulised salbutamol 5 mg or nebulised terbutaline 10 mg
Oral prednisolone 30–60 mg or i/v hydrocortisone 200 mg
Monitor response 15–30 minutes after nebulisation
If any signs of acute asthma persist:
Arrange hospital admission
While awaiting ambulance repeat nebulised beta₂ stimulant and give with nebulised ipratropium 500 micrograms
or give subcutaneous terbutaline (or salbutamol)
or give slow intravenous aminophylline 250 mg
(important: not if taking an oral theophylline)
Alternatively if symptoms have improved, respiration and pulse settling, and peak flow >50% of predicted or best:
Step up usual treatment and continue prednisolone
Follow up
Monitor symptoms and peak flow
Set up self management plan
Review in surgery within 24 hours
Modify treatment at review (see opposite page)

Signs of acute asthma in children
Acute severe asthma:
— too breathless to talk
— too breathless to feed
— respiration >50 breaths/minute (≤40/minute in children over 5 years)
— pulse >140 beats/minute (≥120 beats/minute in children over 5 years)
— in younger children, use of accessory muscles of breathing
— in older children, peak flow ≤50% of predicted or best

— if beta₂ stimulant still required every 3–4 hours after 12 hours, start short course of oral prednisolone for 1–3 days (under 1 year 1–2 mg/kg daily; 1–5 years 20 mg daily)
— if unresponsive or relapse within 3–4 hours:
— immediately refer to hospital
— increase frequency of beta₂ stimulant (give as frequently as needed)
— start oral prednisolone
— give high-flow oxygen via face mask

Life-threatening asthma in adults
— Silent chest
— Cyanosis
— Bradycardia or exhaustion
— Peak flow <33% of predicted or best
Arrange IMMEDIATE hospital admission
Treatment:
Oral prednisolone 30–60 mg or i/v hydrocortisone 200 mg (immediately)
Oxygen-driven nebuliser in ambulance
Nebulised[1] beta₂ stimulant with nebulised ipratropium or subcutaneous terbutaline (or salbutamol)
or slow intravenous aminophylline 250 mg (important: not if taking an oral theophylline)
STAY WITH PATIENT UNTIL AMBULANCE ARRIVES

1. If no nebuliser available give 2 puffs of beta₂ stimulant using large-volume spacer and repeat 10–20 times

Important: do not give bolus aminophylline to patient already taking an oral theophylline.

Important: patients with severe or life-threatening attacks may not be distressed and may not have all these abnormalities; the presence of any should alert doctor.

Life-threatening features:
— cyanosis, silent chest, or poor respiratory effort
— fatigue or exhaustion
— agitation or reduced level of consciousness
— in older children, peak flow <33% of predicted or best

ACUTE SEVERE ASTHMA

Severe asthma can be fatal and **must** be treated promptly and energetically. It is characterised by persistent dyspnoea poorly relieved by broncho-dilators, exhaustion, a high pulse rate (usually over 110/minute), and a very low peak expiratory flow. The respiration is so shallow that wheezing may be absent. Such patients should be given oxygen (if available) and a large dose of a **corticosteroid** (see section 6.3.2)—for adults prednisolone 30–60 mg by mouth *or* hydrocortisone 200 mg (preferably as sodium succinate) intravenously, children predniso-lone 1–2 mg/kg (max. 40 mg) by mouth *or* hydro-cortisone 100 mg (preferably as sodium succinate) intravenously; if the patient experiences vomiting, the parenteral route may be preferred for the first dose. They should also be given **salbutamol** or **ter-butaline** by nebuliser with oxygen if available. For a table outlining the management of acute severe asthma, see p. 125.

If there is little response the following additional treatment should be considered: **ipratropium** by nebuliser (section 3.1.2), **aminophylline** by slow intravenous injection if the patient has not already been receiving theophylline (section 3.1.3), or administer the beta$_2$-selective adrenoceptor stimu-lant by the intravenous route.

Further treatment of these patients is safer in hos-pital where resuscitation facilities are immediately available. Treatment should **never** be delayed for investigations, patients should **never** be sedated, and the possibility of a pneumothorax should also be remembered.

If the patient deteriorates despite appropriate pharmacological treatment, intermittent positive pressure ventilation may be needed temporarily.

Chronic Asthma table, see p. 124
Acute Severe Asthma table, see p. 125

SALBUTAMOL

Indications: asthma and other conditions associ-ated with reversible airways obstruction; prema-ture labour (section 7.1.3)

Cautions: hyperthyroidism, myocardial insuffi-ciency, arrhythmias, susceptibility to QT-interval prolongation, hypertension, pregnancy and breast-feeding (but appropriate to use, see notes above); diabetes—especially intravenous admin-istration to diabetics (monitor blood glucose; ketoacidosis reported); see also notes above; **interactions:** Appendix 1 (sympathomimetics, beta$_2$)

HYPOKALAEMIA. The CSM has advised that potentially serious hypokalaemia may result from beta$_2$-adreno-ceptor stimulant therapy. Particular caution is required in severe asthma, as this effect may be potentiated by concomitant treatment with theophylline and its deriva-tives, corticosteroids, and diuretics, and by hypoxia. Plasma-potassium concentrations should therefore be monitored in severe asthma.

Side-effects: fine tremor (usually hands), nervous tension, headache, peripheral vasodilatation, pal-pitations, tachycardia (seldom troublesome when given by aerosol inhalation); rarely muscle cramps; hypokalaemia after high doses (for **CSM** advice see under Cautions above); hypersensi-tivity reactions including paradoxical broncho-spasm, urticaria, and angioedema reported; slight pain on intramuscular injection

Dose: by mouth, 4 mg (elderly and sensitive patients initially 2 mg) 3–4 times daily; max. sin-gle dose 8 mg (but unlikely to provide much extra benefit or to be tolerated); CHILD under 2 years 100 micrograms/kg 4 times daily; 2–6 years 1–2 mg 3–4 times daily, 6–12 years 2 mg

By subcutaneous or intramuscular injection, 500 micrograms, repeated every 4 hours if neces-sary

By slow intravenous injection, 250 micrograms, repeated if necessary

By intravenous infusion, initially 5 micrograms/minute, adjusted according to response and heart-rate usually in range 3–20 micrograms/minute, or more if necessary

By aerosol inhalation, 100–200 micrograms (1–2 puffs); for persistent symptoms up to 3–4 times daily (but see also Chronic Asthma table); CHILD 100 micrograms (1 puff), increased to 200 micrograms (2 puffs) if necessary

Prophylaxis in exercise-induced bronchospasm, 200 micrograms (2 puffs); CHILD 100 micrograms (1 puff)

By inhalation of powder (Rotacaps®, Ventodisks®; for *Accuhaler®* dose see under preparation), 200–400 micrograms; for persistent symptoms up to 3–4 times daily (but see also Chronic Asthma table); CHILD 200 micrograms

Prophylaxis in exercise-induced bronchospasm (*powder*), 400 micrograms; CHILD 200 micrograms

Note. Bioavailability appears to be lower, so recom-mended doses for dry powder inhalers are twice those in a metered inhaler

By inhalation of nebulised solution, chronic bron-chospasm unresponsive to conventional therapy and severe acute asthma, ADULT and CHILD over 18 months 2.5 mg, repeated up to 4 times daily; may be increased to 5 mg if necessary, but medi-cal assessment should be considered since alter-native therapy may be indicated; CHILD under 18 months, clinical efficacy uncertain (transient hypoxaemia may occur—consider supplemental oxygen)

Oral

PoM **Salbutamol** (Non-proprietary)

Tablets, salbutamol (as sulphate) 2 mg, net price 20 = 28p; 4 mg, 20 = 27p

Available from APS, Berk (Asmaven®), Cox, Hillcross, Norton

Oral solution, salbutamol (as sulphate) 2 mg/5 mL. Net price 150 mL = 71p

Available from Lagap (sugar-free)

PoM **Ventolin®** (A&H)

Syrup, sugar-free, salbutamol (as sulphate) 2 mg/5 mL. Net price 150 mL = 71p

PoM **Volmax**® (DF)

Tablets, m/r, salbutamol (as sulphate) 4 mg, net price 56-tab pack = £10.55; 8 mg, 56-tab pack = £12.66. Label: 25

Dose: 8 mg twice daily; CHILD 3–12 years 4 mg twice daily

Parenteral

PoM **Ventolin**® (A&H)

Injection, salbutamol (as sulphate) 50 micrograms/mL, net price 5-mL amp = 57p; 500 micrograms/mL, 1-mL amp = 43p

Solution for intravenous infusion, salbutamol (as sulphate) 1 mg/mL. Dilute before use. Net price 5-mL amp = £3.08

Inhalation

COUNSELLING. Advise patients not to exceed prescribed dose and to follow manufacturer's directions; if a previously effective dose of inhaled salbutamol fails to provide at least 3 hours relief, a doctor's advice should be obtained as soon as possible

PoM **Salbutamol** (Non-proprietary)

Aerosol inhalation, salbutamol 100 micrograms/metered inhalation, net price 200-dose unit = £1.80. Counselling, dose

Available from A&H (*Ventolin*®), APS, Ashbourne (*Maxivent*®), Berk (*Asmaven*®), Cox, Norton

Note. Vortex-based aerosol inhalers releasing salbutamol 100 micrograms/metered inhalation also available from Evans (*Asmasal Spacehaler*®)

Additives: include CFC propellants

PoM **Aerolin**® **Autohaler** (3M)

Aerosol inhalation, salbutamol (as sulphate) 100 micrograms/metered inhalation. Net price 200-dose breath-actuated unit = £10.51; also 100-dose unit = £5.50 (hosp. only). Counselling, dose

Additives: include CFC propellants

▼ PoM **Airomir**® (3M)

Aerosol inhalation, salbutamol (as sulphate) 100 micrograms/metered inhalation. Net price 200-dose unit = £2.06. Counselling, dose

Additives: include HFA-134a (a non-CFC propellant), alcohol

Note. Can only be supplied against a generic prescription when prescription has been written for 'salbutamol sulphate inhaler', 'salbutamol sulphate inhaler CFC free', or 'salbutamol inhaler CFC free'

PoM **Steri-Neb Salamol**® (Baker Norton)

Nebuliser solution, salbutamol (as sulphate) 0.1% (1 mg/mL), net price 20 × 2.5 mL (2.5 mg) = £3.06; 0.2% (2 mg/mL), 20 × 2.5 mL (5 mg) = £6.14. May be diluted with sterile sodium chloride 0.9% if administration time in excess of 10 minutes is required

PoM **Ventodisks**® (A&H)

Dry powder for inhalation, disks containing 8 blisters of salbutamol (as sulphate) 200 micrograms/blister, net price 14 disks with *Diskhaler*® device = £7.11; 5-disk refill = £2.53 (hosp. only), 14-disk refill = £6.54; 400 micrograms/blister, 14 disks with *Diskhaler*® device = £12.02; 5-disk refill = £4.30 (hosp. only), 14-disk refill = £11.45. Counselling, dose

PoM **Ventolin**® (A&H)

Accuhaler® (dry powder for inhalation), disk containing 60 blisters of salbutamol (as sulphate)

200 micrograms/blister with *Accuhaler*® device, net price = £5.00. Counselling, dose

Dose: by inhalation of powder, 200 micrograms; for persistant symptoms up to 4 times daily (but see also Chronic Asthma table); CHILD 200 micrograms

Prophylaxis in allergen- or exercise-induced bronchospasm, 200 micrograms

Aerosol inhalation, salbutamol 100 micrograms/metered inhalation. Net price 80-dose unit = £1.16 (hosp. only), 200-dose unit = £2.30. Counselling, dose

Additives: include CFC propellants

Easi-Breathe® *aerosol inhalation*, salbutamol 100 micrograms/metered inhalation, net price 200-dose breath-actuated unit = £6.30. Counselling, dose

Additives: include CFC propellants

Nebules® (for use with nebuliser), salbutamol (as sulphate) 0.1% (1 mg/mL), net price 2.5 mL (2.5 mg) = 19p; 0.2% (2 mg/mL), 2.5 mL (5 mg) = 38p. May be diluted with sterile sodium chloride 0.9% if administration time in excess of 10 minutes is required

Respirator solution (for use with a nebuliser or ventilator), salbutamol (as sulphate) 0.5% (5 mg/mL). Net price 20 mL = £2.71 (hosp. only). May be diluted with sterile sodium chloride 0.9%

Rotacaps® (dry powder for inhalation; for use with *Ventolin Rotahaler*®), salbutamol (as sulphate), 200 micrograms (light-blue/clear), net price 112-cap pack = £5.92; 400 micrograms (dark-blue/clear), 112-cap pack = £10.01. Counselling, dose

Compound preparations

For some **compound preparations** containing salbutamol, see section 3.1.4

Inhaler devices

Section 3.1.5

TERBUTALINE SULPHATE

Indications; Cautions; Side-effects: see under Salbutamol; premature labour (section 7.1.3)

Dose: by mouth, initially 2.5 mg 3 times daily for 1–2 weeks, then up to 5 mg 3 times daily

CHILD 75 micrograms/kg 3 times daily; 7–15 years 2.5 mg 2–3 times daily

By subcutaneous, intramuscular, or slow intravenous injection, 250–500 micrograms up to 4 times daily; CHILD 2–15 years 10 micrograms/kg to a max. of 300 micrograms

By continuous intravenous infusion as a solution containing 3–5 micrograms/mL, 1.5–5 micrograms/minute for 8–10 hours; reduce dose for children

By aerosol inhalation, adults and children 250–500 micrograms (1–2 puffs); for persistent symptoms up to 3–4 times daily (but see also Chronic Asthma table)

By inhalation of powder (*Turbohaler*®), 500 micrograms (1 inhalation); for persistent symptoms up to 4 times daily (but see also Chronic Asthma table)

By inhalation of nebulised solution, 5–10 mg 2–4 times daily; additional doses may be necessary in severe acute asthma; CHILD, up to 3 years 2 mg, 3–6 years 3 mg; 6–8 years 4 mg, over 8 years 5 mg, 2–4 times daily

Oral and parenteral

PoM **Bricanyl**® (Astra)

Tablets, scored, terbutaline sulphate 5 mg. Net price 20 = 74p

Syrup, sugar-free, terbutaline sulphate 1.5 mg/ 5 mL. Net price 300 mL = £2.36

Injection, terbutaline sulphate 500 micrograms/ mL. Net price 1-mL amp = 27p; 5-mL amp = £1.27

PoM **Bricanyl SA**® (Astra)

Tablets, m/r, terbutaline sulphate 7.5 mg. Net price 20 = £1.55. Label: 25

Dose: 7.5 mg twice daily

PoM **Monovent**® (Lagap)

Syrup, terbutaline sulphate 1.5 mg/5 mL. Net price 300 mL = £2.25

Inhalation

COUNSELLING. Advise patients not to exceed prescribed dose and to follow manufacturer's directions; if a previously effective dose of inhaled terbutaline fails to provide at least 3 hours relief, a doctor's advice should be obtained as soon as possible; little sensation associated with use of *Turbohaler*®

PoM **Bricanyl**® (Astra)

Aerosol inhalation, terbutaline sulphate 250 micrograms/metered inhalation. Net price 400-dose unit = £5.31; 400-dose unit with *Spacer* device (collapsible extended mouthpiece) = £7.21; 400-dose refill canister for use with *Nebuhaler* or *Spacer* inhaler = £5.21. Counselling, dose

Additives: include CFC propellants

Turbohaler® (= dry powder inhaler), terbutaline sulphate 500 micrograms/inhalation. Net price 100-dose unit = £7.96. Counselling, dose

Respules® (= single-dose units for nebulisation), terbutaline sulphate 2.5 mg/mL. Net price 20 × 2-mL units = £3.67

Respirator solution (for use with a nebuliser or ventilator), terbutaline sulphate 10 mg/mL. Net price 10 mL = £1.32. Before use dilute with sterile sodium chloride 0.9%

Inhaler devices
Section 3.1.5

BAMBUTEROL HYDROCHLORIDE

Note. Bambuterol is a pro-drug of terbutaline

Indications: asthma and other conditions associated with reversible airways obstruction

Cautions; Side-effects: see under Salbutamol; reduce dose in renal impairment; avoid in cirrhosis, severe hepatic impairment; manufacturer advises avoid in pregnancy

Dose: 20 mg once daily at bedtime if patient has previously tolerated beta$_2$-adrenoceptor stimulants; other patients, initially 10 mg once daily at bedtime, increased if necessary after 1–2 weeks to 20 mg once daily; CHILD not recommended

PoM **Bambec**® (Astra)

Tablets, both scored, bambuterol hydrochloride 10 mg, net price 7-tab pack = £2.50, 28-tab pack = £10.95; 20 mg, 28-tab pack = £13.14

EFORMOTEROL FUMARATE

(Formoterol Fumarate)

Indications: reversible airways obstruction (including nocturnal asthma and prevention of exercise-induced bronchospasm) in patients requiring long-term regular bronchodilator therapy, who should normally also be receiving regular and adequate doses of inhaled anti-inflammatory drugs (e.g. corticosteroids and/or sodium cromoglycate) or oral corticosteroids; see also Chronic Asthma table, p. 124

Note. Eformoterol is not for immediate relief of acute attacks and existing corticosteroid therapy should not be reduced or withdrawn

Cautions: see under Salbutamol and notes above; severe liver cirrhosis; pregnancy (Appendix 4 and notes above); avoid in breast-feeding

Side-effects: see under Salbutamol; oropharyngeal irritation, conjunctival irritation and eyelid oedema, taste disturbances, rash, insomnia, nausea and pruritus also reported; **important:** potential for paradoxical bronchospasm (calling for discontinuation and alternative therapy)

Dose: see under preparations below

▼ PoM **Foradil**® (Novartis)

Dry powder for inhalation, eformoterol fumarate 12 micrograms/capsule, net price 56-dose unit (with inhaler device) = £24.00, 14-dose unit (with inhaler device) = £6.00 (hosp. only). Counselling, dose

Dose: by inhalation of powder, 12 micrograms twice daily, increased to 24 micrograms twice daily in more severe airways obstruction; CHILD under 18 years not recommended

COUNSELLING. Advise patients that eformoterol should **not** be used for relief of acute attacks, not to exceed prescribed dose, and to follow manufacturer's directions; if a previously effective dose of inhaled eformoterol fails to provide adequate relief, a doctor's advice should be obtained as soon as possible

▼ PoM **Oxis**® (Astra)

Turbohaler® (= dry powder inhaler), eformoterol fumarate 6 micrograms/inhalation, net price 60-dose unit = £24.80; 12 micrograms/inhalation, 60-dose unit = £24.80. Counselling, dose

Dose: by inhalation of powder, 6–12 micrograms once or twice daily, increased to 24 micrograms twice daily in more severe airways obstruction; CHILD under 12 years not recommended

COUNSELLING. Advise patients that eformoterol should **not** be used for relief of acute attacks, not to exceed prescribed dose, and to follow manufacturer's directions; if a previously effective dose of inhaled eformoterol fails to provide adequate relief, a doctor's advice should be obtained as soon as possible; little sensation associated with use of *Turbohaler*®

FENOTEROL HYDROBROMIDE

Indications: reversible airways obstruction

Cautions; Side-effects: see under Salbutamol

Dose: by aerosol inhalation, 200 micrograms (2 puffs *Berotec '100'*) 1–3 times daily, and see also *Berotec '200'* below (but see also Chronic Asthma table); CHILD 6–12 years 100 micrograms (1 puff *Berotec '100'*)

Persistent bronchospasm not adequately controlled by *Berotec '100'*, by aerosol inhalation, 200–400 micrograms (1–2 puffs *Berotec '200'*) 1–3 times daily; not more than 400 micrograms (2 puffs *Berotec '200'*) every 6 hours; max. 1.6 mg daily (**important:** see also Chronic asthma table); CHILD under 16 years, not recommended

PoM **Berotec®** (Boehringer Ingelheim)
'100' aerosol inhalation, fenoterol hydrobromide 100 micrograms/metered inhalation. Net price 200-dose unit = £2.36. Counselling, dose
Additives: include CFC propellants
'200' aerosol inhalation, fenoterol hydrobromide 200 micrograms/metered inhalation. Net price 200-dose unit = £2.78. Counselling, dose
Additives: include CFC propellants
Note. Only for persistent bronchospasm inadequately controlled by *Berotec '100'*
COUNSELLING. Advise patients not to exceed prescribed dose and to follow manufacturer's directions; if a previously effective dose of inhaled fenoterol fails to provide at least 3 hours relief, a doctor's advice should be obtained as soon as possible

Compound preparations
For some **compound preparations** containing fenoterol, see section 3.1.4

REPROTEROL HYDROCHLORIDE
Indications: reversible airways obstruction
Cautions; Side-effects: see under Salbutamol
Dose: by aerosol inhalation, 0.5–1 mg (1–2 puffs); persistent symptoms, up to 3 times daily (but see also Chronic Asthma table); CHILD 6–12 years 500 micrograms (1 puff)

PoM **Bronchodil®** (ASTA Medica)
Aerosol inhalation, reproterol hydrochloride 500 micrograms/metered inhalation. Net price 400-dose unit = £7.34. Counselling, dose
Additives: include CFC propellants
COUNSELLING. Advise patients not to exceed prescribed dose and to follow manufacturer's directions; if a previously effective dose of inhaled reproterol fails to provide at least 3 hours relief, a doctor's advice should be obtained as soon as possible

SALMETEROL
Indications: reversible airways obstruction (including nocturnal asthma and prevention of exercise-induced bronchospasm) in patients requiring long-term regular bronchodilator therapy, who should normally also be receiving regular and adequate doses of inhaled anti-inflammatory drugs (e.g. corticosteroids and/or, in children, sodium cromoglycate) or oral corticosteroids; see also Chronic Asthma table, p. 124
Note. CSM has emphasised that salmeterol is not for immediate relief of acute attacks and that existing

corticosteroid therapy should not be reduced or withdrawn
Cautions; Side-effects: see under Salbutamol and notes above; **important**: significant incidence of paradoxical bronchospasm, which may be clinically important in severe or deteriorating asthma
Dose: by inhalation, 50 micrograms (2 puffs or 1 blister) twice daily; up to 100 micrograms (4 puffs or 2 blisters) twice daily in more severe airways obstruction; CHILD under 4 years not recommended, over 4 years, 50 micrograms (2 puffs or 1 blister) twice daily

PoM **Serevent®** (A&H)
Accuhaler® (dry powder for inhalation), disk containing 60 blisters of salmeterol (as xinafoate (= hydroxynaphthoate)) 50 micrograms/blister with *Accuhaler®* device, net price = £29.97. Counselling, dose
Aerosol inhalation, salmeterol (as xinafoate (= hydroxynaphthoate)) 25 micrograms/metered inhalation, net price 60-dose unit = £14.30 (hosp. only), 120-dose unit = £28.60. Counselling, dose
Additives: include CFC propellants
Diskhaler® (dry powder for inhalation), disks containing 4 blisters of salmeterol (as xinafoate (= hydroxynaphthoate)) 50 micrograms/blister, net price 14 disks with *Diskhaler®* device = £29.97, 5-disk refill = £9.99 (hosp. only), 14-disk refill = £29.40. Counselling, dose
COUNSELLING. Advise patients that salmeterol should **not** be used for relief of acute attacks, not to exceed prescribed dose, and to follow manufacturer's directions; if a previously effective dose of inhaled salmeterol fails to provide adequate relief, a doctor's advice should be obtained as soon as possible

TULOBUTEROL HYDROCHLORIDE
Indications: reversible airways obstruction
Cautions: see under Salbutamol; also mild renal impairment (avoid if severe); pregnancy (manufacturer states not yet established)
Contra-indications: moderate to severe renal impairment; acute liver failure, chronic liver disease
Side-effects: see under Salbutamol
Dose: 2 mg twice daily; increased if necessary to 2 mg 3 times daily; CHILD 6–10 years 0.5–1 mg twice daily; over 10 years, 1–2 mg twice daily

PoM **Respacal®** (UCB Pharma)
Tablets, f/c, scored, tulobuterol hydrochloride 2 mg. Net price 60-tab pack = £12.54
Syrup, sugar-free, tulobuterol hydrochloride 1 mg/5 mL. Net price 150 mL = £4.48

3.1.1.2 OTHER ADRENOCEPTOR STIMULANTS

These preparations (including the partially selective orciprenaline) are now regarded as less suitable and less safe for use as bronchodilators than the selective beta₂-adrenoceptor stimulants, as they are more likely to cause arrhythmias and other side-effects. They should be avoided whenever possible.

Adrenaline injection (1 in 1000) is used in the emergency treatment of acute allergic and anaphylactic reactions (section 3.4.3).

EPHEDRINE HYDROCHLORIDE

Indications: reversible airways obstruction, but see notes above

Cautions: hyperthyroidism, diabetes mellitus, ischaemic heart disease, hypertension, renal impairment, elderly; may cause acute retention in prostatic hypertrophy; interaction with MAOIs a disadvantage; **interactions:** Appendix 1 (sympathomimetics)

Side-effects: tachycardia, anxiety, restlessness, insomnia common; also tremor, arrhythmias, dry mouth, cold extremities

Dose: 3 times daily, 15–60 mg; CHILD 3 times daily, up to 1 year 7.5 mg, 1–5 years 15 mg, 6–12 years 30 mg (not recommended, see above)

PoM ¹ **Ephedrine Hydrochloride** (Non-proprietary)
Tablets, ephedrine hydrochloride 15 mg, net price 28 = £1.40; 30 mg, 28 = £1.46; 60 mg, 20 = £1.22
Elixir, ephedrine hydrochloride 15 mg/5 mL in a suitable flavoured vehicle, containing alcohol 12%. Net price 100 mL = 83p
1. For exemptions see *Medicines, Ethics and Practice,* No. 19, London, Pharmaceutical Press, 1998 (and subsequent editions as available)
For a list of **cough and decongestant preparations on sale to the public,** including those containing ephedrine, see section 3.9.2

ORCIPRENALINE SULPHATE

Indications: reversible airways obstruction, but see notes above

Cautions; Side-effects: see under Salbutamol (section 3.1.1.1) and note above; **interactions:** Appendix 1 (sympathomimetics)

Dose: by mouth, 20 mg 4 times daily; CHILD up to 1 year 5–10 mg 3 times daily, 1–3 years 5–10 mg 4 times daily, 3–12 years 40–60 mg daily in divided doses (but not recommended, see notes above)

By aerosol inhalation, 750–1500 micrograms (1–2 puffs) repeated if necessary after not less than 30 minutes to a max. of 9 mg (12 puffs) daily; CHILD up to 6 years 750 micrograms (1 puff) up to 4 times daily, 6–12 years 750–1500 micrograms (1–2 puffs) up to 4 times daily (but not recommended, see notes above)

PoM **Alupent**® (Boehringer Ingelheim)
Tablets, scored, orciprenaline sulphate 20 mg. Net price 100-tab pack = £3.80
Syrup, sugar-free, orciprenaline sulphate 10 mg/5 mL. Net price 300 mL = £2.51
Aerosol inhalation, orciprenaline sulphate 750 micrograms/metered inhalation. Net price 300-dose vial with mouthpiece = £3.22; refill vial = £2.66. Counselling, dose
Additives: include CFC propellants
COUNSELLING. Advise patients not to exceed prescribed dose and to follow manufacturer's directions; if a previously effective dose of inhaled orciprenaline fails to provide at least 3 hours relief, a doctor's advice should be obtained as soon as possible

3.1.2   Antimuscarinic bronchodilators

Ipratropium or **oxitropium** may be used by inhalation in the management of chronic asthma in patients who already require high-dose inhaled corticosteroids (see Chronic Asthma table, p. 124). Ipratropium by nebulisation may be added to other standard treatment in life-threatening asthma or where acute asthma fails to improve with standard therapy (see Acute Severe Asthma table, p. 125).

Antimuscarinic bronchodilators have traditionally been regarded as more effective in relieving bronchoconstriction associated with chronic bronchitis in patients who fail to respond to the selective beta$_2$-adrenoceptor stimulants (section 3.1.1.1). The aerosol inhalation of ipratropium has a maximum effect 30–60 minutes after use; its duration of action is 3 to 6 hours and bronchodilation can usually be maintained with treatment three times a day. **Oxitropium** has a similar action to that of ipratropium.

IPRATROPIUM BROMIDE

Indications: reversible airways obstruction, particularly in chronic bronchitis

Cautions: glaucoma (standard doses unlikely to be harmful but see also under nebuliser, below); prostatic hypertrophy; pregnancy

Side-effects: dry mouth occasionally reported; rarely urinary retention, constipation

Dose: see below

PoM **Ipratropium Bromide** (Non-proprietary)
Nebuliser solution, ipratropium bromide 0.025% (250 micrograms/mL), net price 20 × 1-mL (250 micrograms) unit-dose vials (preservative-free) = £5.71, 60 × 1-mL = £16.78; 20 × 2-mL (500 micrograms) = £6.65, 60 × 2-mL = £19.52. If dilution is necessary use only sterile sodium chloride 0.9%
Dose (and cautions relating to paradoxical bronchospasm and glaucoma): see under Atrovent® *Nebuliser Solution* below
Available from Bartholomew Rhodes

PoM **Atrovent**® (Boehringer Ingelheim)
COUNSELLING. Advise patient not to exceed prescribed dose and to follow manufacturer's directions
Aerocaps® (dry powder for inhalation; for use with *Atrovent Aerohaler*®), green, ipratropium bromide 40 micrograms. Net price pack of 100 caps with *Aerohaler*® = £14.53; 100 caps = £10.53. Counselling, dose
Dose: by inhalation of powder, 40 micrograms (1 *Aerocap*®) 3–4 times daily (may be doubled in less responsive patients); CHILD under 12 years, not recommended
Note. one *Atrovent Aerocap*® is equivalent to 2 puffs of *Atrovent*® metered aerosol inhalation *or* 1 puff of *Atrovent Forte*® metered aerosol inhalation
Aerosol inhalation, ipratropium bromide 20 micrograms/metered inhalation. Net price 200-dose unit = £4.21. Counselling, dose
Additives: include CFC propellants
Dose: by aerosol inhalation, 20–40 micrograms (1–2 puffs), in early treatment up to 80 micrograms (4 puffs) at a time, 3–4 times daily; CHILD up to 6 years 20 micrograms (1 puff) 3 times daily, 6–12 years 20–40 micrograms (1–2 puffs) 3 times daily
Autohaler® (= breath-actuated aerosol inhalation), ipratropium bromide 20 micrograms/metered inhalation. Net price 200-dose unit = £10.43. Counselling, dose
Additives: include CFC propellants
Dose: by aerosol inhalation, 20–40 micrograms (1–2 puffs), in early treatment up to 80 micrograms (4 puffs) at a time, 3–4 times daily; CHILD up to 6 years 20 micrograms (1 puff) 3 times daily, 6–12 years 20–40 micrograms (1–2 puffs) 3 times daily

---

Forte aerosol inhalation, ipratropium bromide 40 micrograms/metered inhalation. Net price 200-dose unit = £6.22. Counselling, dose

Additives: include CFC propellants

Dose: by aerosol inhalation 40 micrograms (1 puff), in early treatment 80 micrograms (2 puffs), 3–4 times daily; CHILD 6–12 years 40 micrograms (1 puff) 3 times daily

Nebuliser solution, isotonic, ipratropium bromide 250 micrograms/mL (0.025%); net price 20 × 1-mL unit-dose vials (preservative-free) = £6.82; 20 × 2-mL vials = £8.00. If dilution is necessary use only sterile sodium chloride solution 0.9%

Dose: reversible airways obstruction, *by inhalation of nebulised solution*, 100–500 micrograms (0.4–2 mL of a 0.025% solution) up to 4 times daily; CHILD 3–14 years 100–500 micrograms up to 3 times daily. Dilution of solution is adjusted according to equipment and length of administration. Because paradoxical bronchospasm has occurred, *first dose* should be inhaled under medical supervision

GLAUCOMA. *Acute angle closure glaucoma* has been reported in patients given nebulised ipratropium, particularly when used in association with nebulised salbutamol. Special caution is needed and care should be taken to **avoid** escape from mask to patient's eyes

PoM **Steri-Neb Ipratropium®** (Baker Norton)

Nebuliser solution unit, ipratropium bromide 0.025% (250 micrograms/mL), net price 20 × 1-mL (250 micrograms) unit-dose vials (preservative-free) = £6.14; 20 × 2-mL (500 micrograms) = £7.20. If dilution is necessary use only sterile sodium chloride 0.9%

Dose (and cautions relating to paradoxical broncho spasm and glaucoma): see under *Atrovent®* *Nebuliser Solution* above

For some **compound preparations** containing ipratropium, see section 3.1.4

OXITROPIUM BROMIDE

Indications: reversible airways obstruction, particularly in chronic bronchitis

Cautions; Side-effects: see under Ipratropium Bromide; rarely blurring of vision

Dose: by aerosol inhalation, 200 micrograms (2 puffs) 2–3 times daily; CHILD not recommended

PoM **Oxivent®** (Boehringer Ingelheim)

Aerosol inhalation, oxitropium bromide 100 micrograms/metered inhalation. Net price 200-dose unit = £8.36. Counselling, dose

Additives: include CFC propellants

Autohaler® (= breath-actuated aerosol inhalation), oxitropium bromide 100 micrograms/metered inhalation. Net price 200-dose unit = £19.65. Counselling, dose

Additives: include CFC propellants

COUNSELLING. Advise patient not to exceed prescribed dose and to follow manufacturer's directions

3.1.3 Theophylline

Theophylline is a bronchodilator used for reversible airways obstruction. It may have an additive effect when used in conjunction with small doses of beta$_2$-adrenoceptor stimulants; the combination may increase the risk of side-effects, including hypokalaemia (for CSM advice see p. 126).

Theophylline is metabolised in the liver; there is considerable variation in its half-life particularly in smokers, in patients with hepatic impairment or heart failure, or if certain drugs are taken concurrently. The half-life is *increased* in heart failure, cirrhosis, viral infections, in the elderly, and by drugs such as cimetidine, ciprofloxacin, erythromycin, fluvoxamine, and oral contraceptives. The half-life is *decreased* in smokers and in heavy drinkers, and by drugs such as phenytoin, carbamazepine, rifampicin, and barbiturates. For other interactions of theophylline see Appendix 1.

These differences in half-life are important because theophylline has a narrow margin between the therapeutic and toxic dose. In most subjects plasma theophylline concentrations of between 10 and 20 mg/litre are required for satisfactory bronchodilation. However, adverse effects can occur within this range and both the frequency and severity increase at concentrations above 20 mg/litre.

Theophylline modified-release preparations are usually able to produce adequate plasma concentrations for up to 12 hours. When given as a single dose at night they have a useful role in controlling *nocturnal asthma* and *early morning wheezing*. The use of *rapid-release* oral theophylline preparations has declined because of the high incidence of side-effects associated with rapid absorption.

Theophylline is given by injection as **aminophylline**, a mixture of theophylline with ethylenediamine, which is 20 times more soluble than theophylline alone. Aminophylline must be given by **very slow** intravenous injection (over at least 20 minutes); it is too irritant for intramuscular use.

Intravenous aminophylline has a role in the treatment of severe attacks of asthma that do not respond rapidly to a nebulised beta$_2$-adrenoceptor stimulant (see also Acute Severe Asthma table, p. 125). Measurement of plasma theophylline concentrations may be helpful, and is **essential** if aminophylline is to be given to patients who have been taking oral theophylline preparations, as serious side-effects such as convulsions and arrhythmias can occasionally occur before the appearance of other symptoms of toxicity.

Aminophylline injection was formerly also used in the treatment of left ventricular failure but has been superseded for this purpose by diuretics (section 2.2.1 and section 2.2.2) and the opioid analgesics (section 4.7.2). However, it may have a role in patients with heart failure who are also suffering from asthma and bronchitis, where opioids are contra-indicated, though care is needed in those with increased myocardial excitability.

Aminophylline was formerly available for rectal administration as suppositories but these caused proctitis and the response was unpredictable; there was a particular risk of toxicity in children.

THEOPHYLLINE

Indications: reversible airways obstruction, acute severe asthma; for guidelines see also Asthma tables (pp. 124–5)

Cautions: cardiac disease, hypertension, hyperthyroidism, peptic ulcer, hepatic impairment (reduce dose), epilepsy, pregnancy and breast-feeding, elderly, fever; **CSM** advice on hypokalaemia risk, p. 126; avoid in porphyria (see section 9.8.2); **interactions:** Appendix 1 (theophylline) and notes above

Side-effects: tachycardia, palpitations, nausea, gastro-intestinal disturbances, headache, insomnia, arrhythmias, and convulsions especially if given rapidly by intravenous injection; **overdosage:** see Emergency Treatment of Poisoning, p. 24

Dose: see below

Note. Plasma theophylline concentration for optimum response 10–20 mg/litre (55–110 micromol/litre); narrow margin between therapeutic and toxic dose, see also notes above

Nuelin® (3M)

Tablets, scored, theophylline 125 mg. Net price 90-tab pack = £3.44. Label: 21

Dose: 125 mg 3–4 times daily after food, increased to 250 mg if required; CHILD 7–12 years 62.5–125 mg 3–4 times daily

Liquid, brown, theophylline hydrate (as sodium glycinate) 60 mg/5 mL. Net price 300 mL = £3.07. Label: 21

Dose: 120–240 mg 3–4 times daily after food; CHILD 2–6 years 60–90 mg, 7–12 years 90–120 mg, 3–4 times daily

Modified release

Note. The Council of the Royal Pharmaceutical Society of Great Britain advises pharmacists that if a general practitioner prescribes a modified-release, oral theophylline preparation without specifying a brand name, the pharmacist should contact the prescriber and agree the brand to be dispensed. Additionally, it is essential that a patient discharged from hospital should be maintained on the brand on which that patient was stabilised as an in-patient.

Lasma® (Pharmax)

Tablets, m/r, scored, theophylline 300 mg. Net price 20 = £1.89. Label: 25

Dose: 300 mg every 12 hours (increased after 1 week to 450 mg every 12 hours in patients over 70 kg); adjust dose by 150-mg increments as required

Total daily dose may be given as single dose at night when nocturnal symptoms predominate (daytime symptoms then controlled with inhaled bronchodilators)

Nuelin SA® (3M)

SA tablets, m/r, theophylline 175 mg. Net price 60-tab pack = £3.59. Label: 25

Dose: 175–350 mg every 12 hours; CHILD over 6 years 175 mg every 12 hours

SA 250 tablets, m/r, scored, theophylline 250 mg. Net price 60-tab pack = £5.03. Label: 25

Dose: 250–500 mg every 12 hours; CHILD over 6 years 125–250 mg every 12 hours

Slo-Phyllin® (Lipha)

Capsules, all m/r, theophylline 60 mg (white/clear, enclosing white pellets), net price 56-cap pack = £1.92; 125 mg (brown/clear, enclosing white pellets), 56-cap pack = £2.42; 250 mg (blue/clear, enclosing white pellets), 56-cap pack = £3.02. Label: 25 *or* counselling, see below

Dose: 250–500 mg every 12 hours; CHILD, every 12 hours, 2–6 years 60–120 mg, 7–12 years 125–250 mg

COUNSELLING. Swallow whole with fluid *or* swallow enclosed granules with soft food (e.g. yoghurt)

Theo-Dur® (Astra)

Tablets, m/r, both scored, theophylline 200 mg, net price 20 = £1.21; 300 mg, 20 = £1.75. Label: 25

Dose: 300 mg every 12 hours, adjust dose by 100–150-mg steps as required; CHILD up to 35 kg 100 mg, over 35 kg 200 mg, every 12 hours

For nocturnal asthma, total daily requirement may be given as single evening dose

Uniphyllin Continus® (Napp)

Tablets, m/r, all scored, theophylline 200 mg, net price 56-tab pack = £4.05; 300 mg, 56-tab pack = £6.17; 400 mg, 56-tab pack = £7.32. Label: 25

Dose: 200 mg every 12 hours increased after 1 week to 300 mg every 12 hours; over 70 kg 200–300 mg every 12 hours increased after 1 week to 400 mg every 12 hours

May be appropriate to give larger evening or morning dose to achieve optimum therapeutic effect when symptoms most severe; in patients whose night- or daytime symptoms persist despite other therapy, who are not currently receiving theophylline, total daily requirement may be added as single evening or morning dose

CHILD over 7 years, 9 mg/kg twice daily; some children with chronic asthma may require 10–16 mg/kg every 12 hours

For a list of **cough and decongestant preparations on sale to the public**, including those containing theophylline, see section 3.9.2

AMINOPHYLLINE

Note. Aminophylline is a stable mixture or combination of theophylline and ethylenediamine; the ethylenediamine confers greater solubility in water

Indications: reversible airways obstruction, acute severe asthma

Cautions; Side-effects: see under Theophylline; also allergy to ethylenediamine can cause urticaria, erythema, and exfoliative dermatitis

Dose: see under preparations, below

Note. Plasma theophylline concentration for optimum response 10–20 mg/litre (55–110 micromol/litre); narrow margin between therapeutic and toxic dose, see also notes above

Aminophylline (Non-proprietary)

Tablets, aminophylline 100 mg, net price 20 = 71p. Label: 21

Dose: by mouth, 100–300 mg, 3–4 times daily, after food

℞oM *Injection,* aminophylline 25 mg/mL, net price 10-mL amp = 61p

Available from Antigen, Evans, IMS (Min-I-Jet®), Phoenix

Dose: deteriorating acute severe asthma **not** previously treated with theophylline, *by slow intravenous injection* over at least 20 minutes, 250–500 mg (5 mg/kg), then as for acute severe asthma; CHILD 5 mg/kg, then as for acute severe asthma

Acute severe asthma, *by intravenous infusion,* 500 micrograms/kg/hour, adjusted according to plasma-theophylline concentration; CHILD 6 months–9 years 1 mg/kg/hour, 10–16 years 800 micrograms/kg/hour, adjusted according to plasma-theophylline concentration

Note. Patients taking oral theophylline or aminophylline should not normally receive intravenous aminophylline unless plasma-theophylline concentration is available to guide dosage

---

Modified release
See advice on p. 132
Pecram® (Novartis Consumer Health)
Tablets, m/r, yellow, aminophylline hydrate 225 mg. Net price 60 = £3.29. Label: 25
Dose: 1 tablet twice daily initially, increased if necessary to 2 tablets twice daily (steady-state concentrations usually reached after 3–4 days); CHILD not recommended
Phyllocontin Continus® (Napp)
Tablets, m/r, yellow, f/c, aminophylline hydrate 225 mg. Net price 56-tab pack = £3.29. Label: 25
Dose: 1 tablet twice daily initially, increased after 1 week to 2 tablets twice daily
Forte tablets, m/r, yellow, f/c, aminophylline hydrate 350 mg. Net price 56-tab pack = £5.46. Label: 25
Note. Forte tablets are for smokers and other patients with decreased theophylline half-life (see notes above)
Paediatric tablets, m/r, peach, aminophylline hydrate 100 mg. Net price 56-tab pack = £2.12. Label: 25
Dose: CHILD over 3 years, 6 mg/kg twice daily initially, increased after 1 week to 12 mg/kg twice daily; some children with chronic asthma may require 13–20 mg/kg every 12 hours
Note. Modified-release tablets containing aminophylline 225 mg and 350 mg also available from Ashbourne (Amnivent®), Norton (Norphyllin® SR)

3.1.4 Compound bronchodilator preparations

Most compound bronchodilator preparations have no place in the management of patients with airways obstruction.

In general, patients are best treated with single-ingredient preparations, such as a selective beta$_2$-adrenoceptor stimulant (section 3.1.1.1) or ipratropium bromide (section 3.1.2), so that the dose of each drug can be adjusted. This flexibility is lost with combinations, although those in which both components are effective may occasionally have a role when compliance is a problem.

For **cautions, contra-indications** and **side-effects** see under individual monographs.

PoM **Combivent®** (Boehringer Ingelheim)
Aerosol inhalation, ipratropium bromide 20 micrograms, salbutamol (as sulphate) 100 micrograms/metered inhalation. Net price 200-dose unit = £6.45. Counselling, dose
Additives: include CFC propellants
Dose: 2 puffs 4 times daily; CHILD under 12 years not recommended
Nebuliser solution, isotonic, ipratropium bromide 500 micrograms, salbutamol (as sulphate) 2.5 mg/2.5-mL vial, net price 60 unit-dose vials (preservative-free) = £33.00
Dose: by inhalation of nebulised solution, 1 vial 3–4 times daily; CHILD under 12 years not recommended
GLAUCOMA. In addition to other potential side-effects acute angle glaucoma has been reported with nebulised ipratropium—for details, see p. 131
PoM **Duovent®** (Boehringer Ingelheim)
Aerosol inhalation, fenoterol hydrobromide 100 micrograms, ipratropium bromide 40 micrograms/metered inhalation. Net price 200-dose unit with mouthpiece = £6.48 (extension tube also available). Counselling, dose
Additives: include CFC propellants
Dose: 1–2 puffs 3–4 times daily; CHILD over 6 years 1 puff 3 times daily

Autohaler® (= breath-actuated aerosol inhalation), fenoterol hydrobromide 100 micrograms, ipratropium bromide 40 micrograms/metered inhalation. Net price 200-dose unit = £12.73. Counselling, dose
Additives: include CFC propellants
Dose: 1–2 puffs 3–4 times daily; CHILD over 6 years 1 puff 3 times daily
Nebuliser solution, isotonic, fenoterol hydrobromide 1.25 mg, ipratropium bromide 500 micrograms/4-mL vial, net price 20 unit-dose vials = £11.00
Dose: acute severe asthma or acute exacerbation of chronic asthma, by inhalation of nebulised solution, 1 vial (4 mL); may be repeated up to max. 4 vials in 24 hours; CHILD under 14 years, not recommended
GLAUCOMA. In addition to other potential side-effects acute angle-closure glaucoma has been reported with nebulised ipratropium—for details, see p. 131

Preparations on sale to the public
For **compound bronchodilator preparations** on sale to the public, see p. 153

3.1.5 Peak flow meters, inhaler devices and nebulisers

PEAK FLOW METERS

Measurement of peak flow is particularly helpful for patients who are 'poor perceivers' and hence slow to detect deterioration in their asthma, and for those with moderate or severe asthma. Patients must be given clear guidelines as to the action they should take if their peak flow falls below a certain level. Patients can be encouraged to adjust some of their own treatment (within specified limits) according to changes in peak flow rate.

Ferraris Pocketpeak® (Ferraris)
Peak flow meter, standard (90–710 litres/minute), net price = £6.42, low range (40–370 litres/minute) = £6.42, replacement mouthpiece = 38p (for adult or child)
Mini-Wright® (Clement Clarke)
Peak flow meter, standard (60 to 800 litres/minute), net price = £6.74, low range (30 to 400 litres/minute) = £6.78, replacement mouthpiece = 38p (for adult or child)
Vitalograph® (Vitalograph)
Peak flow meter, standard (50 to 750 litres/minute), now called *Asmaplan®*, net price = £6.65, low range (25 to 280 litres/minute) = £6.65, replacement mouthpiece = 40p (for adult or child)

INHALER DEVICES

A variety of *spacing devices* is now available for use with *pressurised (aerosol) inhalers* (metered dose inhalers). By providing a space between inhaler and mouth, they reduce the velocity of the aerosol and subsequent impaction on the oropharynx; in addition they allow more time for evaporation of the propellant so that a larger proportion of the particles can be inhaled and deposited in the lungs; also co-ordination of inspiration with actuation of the aerosol is less important. The size of the spacer is important and the larger spacing devices with a one-way valve (*Nebuhaler®, Volumatic®*) are the most effective. Spacing devices are particularly useful for patients with poor inhalation technique, for children, for patients requiring higher doses, for nocturnal asthma, and for patients prone to develop candidiasis with inhaled corticosteroids.

Alternatively *dry powder inhalers*, activated by the patient's inspiration, are of value; some occasionally cause coughing.

USE AND CARE OF LARGE-VOLUME SPACER DEVICES. Patients should inhale from the spacer devices as soon as possible after actuation since the drug aerosol is very short-lived; single-dose actuation is recommended. The device is cleansed once a week by washing, rinsing and then allowing to dry in air (wiping should be avoided since any electrostatic charge may affect drug delivery). Spacer devices should be replaced every 6–12 months.

AeroChamber® (3M)
Spacer device, medium-volume device. For use with *Airomir®* inhaler, net price standard device (blue) = £4.28, with mask (blue) = £16.36; child device (yellow) with mask = £14.36; infant device (orange) with mask = £14.36

NHS **Babyhaler®** (A&H)
Spacer device for paediatric use with *Becotide-50®* and *Ventolin®* inhalers. Net price = £11.34

NHS **E-Z Spacer®** (Vitalograph) ·
Spacer device, large-volume, collapsible device. For use with pressurised (aerosol) inhalers, price (direct from manufacturer) = £22.50

NHS **Haleraid®** (GlaxoWellcome)
Device to place over standard inhalers as aid to operation by patients with impaired strength in hands (e.g. with arthritis). Available as Haleraid-120 for 120-dose inhalers and Haleraid-200 for 200-dose inhalers. Net price = £1.38

Nebuhaler® (Astra)
Spacer inhaler, large-volume device. For use with *Bricanyl®* and *Pulmicort®* refill canisters, net price = £4.28; with paediatric mask = £4.28

Rotahaler® (A&H)
Breath-actuated device for use with *Rotacaps®*. Available as *Becotide Rotahaler®*, *Ventolin Rotahaler®*, and *Ventide Rotahaler®*. Net price = 78p

Spinhaler® (Fisons)
Breath-actuated device for use with *Intal Spincaps®*. Net price = £1.89

Volumatic® (A&H)
Spacer inhaler, large-volume device. For use with *Becloforte®*, *Becotide®*, *Flixotide®*, *Serevent®*, *Ventide®*, and *Ventolin®* inhalers, net price = £2.75; with paediatric mask = £2.75

NEBULISERS

Nebulisers convert a solution of a drug into an aerosol for inhalation. They are used to deliver higher doses of drug to the airways than is usual with standard inhalers. The main indications for use of a nebuliser are:

To deliver a beta-adrenoceptor stimulant or ipratropium to a patient with an *acute exacerbation* of asthma or of chronic airway obstruction

To deliver a beta-adrenoceptor stimulant or ipratropium on a *regular basis* to a patient with severe asthma or reversible airways obstruction who has been shown to benefit from regular treatment with higher doses

To deliver *prophylactic medication* such as cromoglycate or a corticosteroid to a patient unable to use other inhalational devices (particularly a young child)

To deliver an antibiotic (such as colistin) to a patient with chronic purulent infection (as in cystic fibrosis or bronchiectasis)

To deliver pentamidine for the prophylaxis and treatment of pneumocystis pneumonia to a patient with AIDS.

In England and Wales nebulisers and compressors are not available on the NHS (but they are free of VAT); some nebulisers (but not compressors) are available on form GP10A in Scotland (for details consult Scottish Drug Tariff).

The proportion of a nebuliser solution that reaches the lungs depends on the type of nebuliser and although it can be as high as 30% it is more frequently close to 10% and sometimes below 10%. The remaining solution is left in the nebuliser as residual volume or it is deposited in the mouthpiece and tubing. The extent to which the nebulised solution is deposited in the airways or alveoli depends on particle size. Particles with a mass median diameter of 1–5 microns are deposited in the airways and are therefore appropriate for asthma whereas a particle size of 1–2 microns is needed for alveolar deposition of pentamidine to combat pneumocystis infection. The type of nebuliser is therefore chosen according to the deposition required and according to the viscosity of the solution (antibiotic solutions usually being more viscous).

Some jet nebulisers are able to increase drug output during inspiration and hence increase efficiency.

The patient should be aware that the dose of a bronchodilator given by nebulisation is usually **much higher** than that from an aerosol inhaler; see below for British Thoracic Society guidelines.

The British Thoracic Society has advised that nebulised bronchodilators may be given to patients with chronic persistent asthma or those with sudden catastrophic severe asthma (brittle asthma). In chronic asthma, nebulised bronchodilators should only be used to relieve persistent daily wheeze (see Chronic Asthma table p. 124). The British Thoracic Society has further recommended that the use of nebulisers in chronic persistent asthma should only be considered:

After a review of the diagnosis

If the airflow obstruction is significantly reversible by bronchodilators without unacceptable side-effects

After the patient has been using the usual hand-held inhaler correctly

After a larger dose of bronchodilator from a hand-held inhaler (with a spacer if necessary) has been tried for at least 2 weeks

If the patient is complying with the prescribed dose and frequency of anti-inflammatory treatment including regular use of high-dose inhaled corticosteroid

Before prescribing, a home trial should preferably be undertaken to monitor peak flow for up to 2

---

weeks on standard treatment and up to 2 weeks on nebulised treatment. If prescribed patients must:

Have clear instructions from doctor, specialist nurse or pharmacist on the use of the nebuliser and on peak-flow monitoring

Be instructed not to treat acute attacks at home without also seeking help

Receive an education program

Have regular follow up including peak-flow monitoring and be seen by doctor, specialist nurse or physiotherapist

Jet nebulisers

Jet nebulisers utilise the Venturi principle for nebulisation; they are more widely used than ultrasonic nebulisers. Most jet nebulisers require an optimum gas flow rate of 6–8 litres/minute and in hospital can be driven by piped air or oxygen. Domiciliary oxygen cylinders do not provide an adequate flow rate therefore for domiciliary use an electrical compressor is used.

For patients with *chronic bronchitis and hypercapnia*, oxygen can be dangerous and the nebuliser should be driven by air (see also p. 123).

Important: the Department of Health has reminded users of the need to use the correct grade of tubing when connecting a nebuliser to a medical gas supply or compressor.

NHS Medix All Nebuliser® (Medix)

Jet nebuliser, disposable; for use with bronchodilators, antimuscarinics, corticosteroids, and antibiotics, replacement recommended every 2–3 months if used 4 times a day. Compatible with **NHS AC 2000 Hi Flo®**, **NHS World Traveller Hi Flo®**, and **NHS Econoneb®**. Net price 5 = £7.50

NHS Medix Antibiotic Circuit® (Medix)

Jet nebuliser, closed-system; for use with antibiotics and other respiratory drugs. Compatible with **NHS AC 2000 Hi Flo®**, **NHS Econoneb®**, and **NHS Turboneb®**. Net price 1 = £7.30

NHS Medix System® (Medix)

Jet nebuliser, consisting of mouthpiece, tubing, and nebuliser chamber. Net price 1 = £2.80; mask kits with tubing and nebuliser chamber also available, net price 1 (adult) = £2.90; 1 (child) = £2.90

NHS Pari LC Plus Filter® (Pari)

Jet nebuliser, closed system, non-disposable, for hospital or home use with low flow compressors; supplied with filter/valve set. Compatible with **NHS Pari TurboBoy®** and **NHS Pari JuniorBoy®** compressors. Net price 1 = £19.90, replacement filters 100 = £33.30

NHS Pari LC Plus® (Pari)

Jet nebuliser, non-disposable, for hospital or home use with low flow compressors; for use with bronchodilators, antibiotics, and corticosteroids, replacement recommended yearly if used 4 times a day. Compatible with **NHS Pari TurboBoy®**, **NHS Pari JuniorBoy®** and **NHS Pari WalkBoy®** compressors. Net price 1 = £13.90

NHS Pari Baby® (Pari)

Jet nebuliser, non-disposable, for hospital or home use with low flow compressors; for use with bronchodilators, antibiotics and corticosteroids, replacement recommended yearly if used 4 times a day. Compatible with **NHS Pari TurboBoy®**, **NHS Pari JuniorBoy®**, **NHS Pari WalkBoy®** compressors. Available separately for children aged less than 1 year, 1–4 years or 4–7 years. Net price 1 (with connection hose) = £25.00

NHS Sidestream Durable® (Medic-Aid)

Jet nebuliser, non-disposable, for home use; for use with bronchodilators; yearly replacement recommended if 4 six-minute treatments used per day. Compatible with **NHS CR50®**, **NHS Freeway Lite®** and **NHS Porta-Neb 50®** (depending on nebulising solution). Net price 10 pack = £94.50; patient pack with **NHS CR50®** compressor = £98.50. **NHS Disposable Sidestream®** nebuliser also available

Note. This has been developed to replace the **NHS System 22 Acorn®**

NHS Ventstream® (Medic-Aid)

Jet nebuliser, closed-system, for use with low flow compressors, compatible with **NHS CR50®**, **NHS Porta-Neb 50®**, and **NHS Freeway Lite®** compressors; for use with antibiotics, bronchodilators, and corticosteroids, replacement recommended yearly if used 3 times a day. Net price 1 with filter = £27.00; 10-pack with filter = £250.00; 1 without filter = £23.00; 10-pack without filter = £215.00; patient pack with **NHS CR 50®** compressor = £119.95

Home compressors with nebulisers

NHS AC 2000 HI FLO® (Medix)

Portable, home use, containing 1 **NHS Jet Nebuliser®** set with mouthpiece, 1 adult or 1 child mask, 1 spare inlet filter, filter spanner. Mains operated. Nebulises bronchodilators and antibiotics. Net price 1 = £99.00; carrying case available

NHS Aquilon® (Henleys)

Portable, home use, with 1 adult or 1 child mask and tubing. Mains operated; for use with bronchodilators, corticosteroids and antibiotics. Net price = £81.00

NHS Econoneb® (Medix)

Home, clinic and hospital use, used with 1 **NHS Jet Nebuliser®** set with mouthpiece, 1 adult or 1 child mask, 1 spare inlet filter, filter spanner. Compatible with all types of jet nebuliser sets and also the **NHS Micro Cirrus®** nebuliser (recommended for alveolar deposition). Nebulises bronchodilators, corticosteroids, and antibiotics. Mains operated. Net price 1 = £90.00

NHS Freeway Lite® (Medic-Aid)

Portable, containing 1 **NHS Sidestream Durable®** reusable nebuliser, 1 adult or 1 child mask, 1 mouthpiece, 1 Coiled Duratube®, 2 filters. Net price 1 = £149.00 with carrying case. **NHS Freeway Lite Luxury®** contains additional battery. Net price 1 = £198.00

Also compatible with **NHS Ventstream®** closed system nebuliser

NHS M-Flo® (Medix)

Portable, home use, containing 1 **NHS Jet Nebuliser®** set with mouthpiece, spare inlet filter, filter spanner. Mains operated. Nebulises bronchodilators and corticosteroids. Net price 1 = £85.00

NHS Medi-Neb® (Timesco)

Range of compressors all supplied with adult and child mask, vapourising chamber, and PVC tubing, including: **NHS Medi-Neb Elite®**, *home use*. Mains operated. Net price 1 = £84.95. **NHS Medi-Neb Companion®**, *portable*. Mains/car battery operated. Net price 1 = £104.95 (includes car battery adaptor and carrying case). **NHS Medi-Neb Companion Plus®**, *portable*. Mains/battery operated. Net price 1 = £144.95 (includes rechargeable battery, car battery adaptor, and carrying case). **NHS Medi-Neb Tempest®**, *home/hospital use*. Mains operated. Net price 1 = £94.95

All used for nebulising antibiotics and bronchodilators

NHS Pari TurboBoy® (Pari)

Portable, for hospital or home use, containing **NHS Pari LC Plus** with connection tube and mains cable. Filter replacement recommended every 12 months or 550 hours of use. Compatible with **NHS Pari LC Plus®**, **NHS Pari LC Plus Filter®**, and **NHS Pari Baby®** nebulisers. Net price = £109.00

NHS **Pari JuniorBoy**® (Pari)

Portable, for hospital or home use, containing NHS **Pari LC Plus** with connection tube and mains cable. Filter replacement recommended every 12 months or 550 hours of use. Compatible with NHS **Pari LC Plus**®, NHS **Pari LC Plus Filter**®, and NHS **Pari Baby**® nebulisers. Net price = £119.00

NHS **Pari WalkBoy**® (Pari)

Portable, containing 1 NHS **Pari LC Plus**® nebuliser with connection tube, mains cable, rechargeable battery and carrying bag. Compatible with NHS **Pari LC Plus**® and NHS **Pari Baby**® nebulisers. Net price 1 = £219.00; car cigarette lighter adapter = £63.00

NHS **Porta-Neb**® (Medic-Aid)

Portable, containing 1 NHS **Sidestream Durable**® reusable nebuliser, 1 angled flow-through mouthpiece, 1 adult or 1 child mask, 1 Duratube® supply tubing, 4 spare filters. Mains operated; for use with bronchodilators. Net price 1 = £109.50; carrying case available

Also compatible with NHS **Ventstream**® closed-system nebuliser; for use with antibiotics, bronchodilators, and corticosteroids

NHS **Pulmo-Aide**® (De Vilbiss)

Home, clinic use, containing disposable nebuliser set, mouthpiece, mask, mains lead, tubing, thumb-valve. For use with bronchodilators. Net price 1 = £99.50. NHS **Pulmo-Aide Escort**®, *portable*, containing disposable nebuliser set, transformer, rechargeable battery, AC to DC adapter charger, DC lead with car adapter, and carrying case. Net price 1 = £198.50. NHS **Pulmo-Aide AP50**®, *home, clinic, hospital use*. Net price 1 = £180.00, 1 with antipollution kit = £188.50. NHS **Pulmo-Aide Sunmist**®, *home, clinic use*, containing nebuliser set, mouthpiece, face mask, mains lead. Net price 1 = £84.25

NHS **SunMist**® (De Vilbiss)

Home, clinic and hospital use, with mouthpiece. Mains operated. Net price = £89.50. NHS **SunMist Plus**®, *home, clinic and hospital use*, with mouthpiece, higher flow rate. Mains operated. Net price = £107.50

NHS **Tourer**® (Henleys)

Portable, home use. Mains/car battery operated; for use with bronchodilators, corticosteroids and antibiotics. Net price = £118.50, rechargeable battery pack = £54.00

NHS **Ultima**® (Henleys)

Portable, home use. Rechargable or mains/car battery operated. Nebulises bronchodilators and corticosteroids. Net price = £184.00 (includes case)

NHS **World Traveller HI FLO**® (Medix)

Portable, containing 1 NHS **Jet Nebuliser**® set with mouthpiece, 1 adult or 1 child mask, 1 spare inlet filter, filter spanner. Battery/mains operated; rechargeable battery pack available. Nebulises bronchodilators, corticosteroids, and antibiotics. Net price 1 excluding battery = £135.00; 1 with battery = £180.00; carrying case available

Compressors

NHS **System 22 CR50**® (Medic-Aid)

Home, clinic and hospital use. Mains operated. Net price 1 = £89.50. Also compatible with NHS **Ventstream**®, and NHS **Sidestream Durable**®

NHS **System 22 CR60**® (Medic-Aid)

Hospital use, high flow compressor. Mains operated. Net price = £199.90. Also compatible with NHS **System 22 Antibiotic Tee**® for nebulisation of high viscosity drugs such as antibiotics

NHS **Turboneb**® (Medix)

Hospital use, high flow compressor. Mains operated. Net price 1 = £115.00. Also compatible with NHS **Medix Antibiotic Circuit**® for nebulisation of respiratory drugs in particular viscous antibiotics

Ultrasonic nebulisers

Ultrasonic nebulisers produce an aerosol by ultrasonic vibration of the drug solution and therefore do not require a gas flow

NHS **AeroSonic**® (De Vilbiss)

Portable, containing 1 controlling unit, chamber assembly, carrying case, AC to DC adapter/charger, DC lead, 1 mouthpiece with check valve and adapter. Net price 1 = £250.00

NHS **Omron U1 MicroAir**® (Hutchings)

Portable. Battery operated/mains adaptor. Net price 1 = £325.00

NHS **Omron NE U07**® (Hutchings)

Portable. Mains operated or rechargeable battery pack. Net price = £166.00 (mains version), £253.00 (rechargeable version)

NHS **Sonix 2000**® (Medix)

Portable, delivery rate adjustable to suit user. Supplied with carrying case and DC lead. Mains/car battery operated; rechargeable battery pack available. Net price 1 excluding battery = £150.00, 1 with battery = £215.00

NHS **Ultra Neb 2000**® (De Vilbiss)

Hospital, clinic and home use, delivery rate adjustable. Supplied with stand. Net price = £1125.50

NEBULISER DILUENT

Nebulisation may be carried out using an undiluted nebuliser solution or it may require dilution beforehand. The usual diluent is sodium chloride 0.9% (physiological saline).

PoM **Steri-Neb Saline**® (Baker Norton)

Solution, sodium chloride 0.9% in single-dose units of 2.5 mL. Net price 20 = £3.66

3.2   Corticosteroids

Corticosteroids are effective in *asthma*; they reduce bronchial mucosal inflammation (and hence reduce oedema and secretion of mucus into the airway).

Corticosteroids are usually of no benefit in patients with *chronic bronchitis* and *emphysema*; some patients with asthma, however, may be clinically indistinguishable from those with chronic bronchitis except that they will respond to a trial course of corticosteroids.

INHALATION. Inhaled corticosteroids are recommended for prophylactic treatment of asthma when patients are using a beta$_2$-stimulant more than once daily (see Chronic Asthma table). They have many fewer side-effects than those associated with systemic administration (section 6.3.2), but nevertheless these need to be borne in mind, including the potential of higher inhaled doses to adrenal suppression and to have effects on bone metabolism (for further details see below). The growth retardation in children associated with oral corticosteroid therapy does not appear to be a significant problem with recommended doses of inhaled therapy although it is wise to monitor linear growth.

Corticosteroid *aerosol inhalations* must be used regularly to obtain maximum benefit; alleviation of symptoms usually occurs 3 to 7 days after initiation. **Beclomethasone** (beclometasone) **dipropionate**, **budesonide** and **fluticasone propionate** appear to be equally effective; fluticasone achieves the same effect as the other two with half the dose (when given by an equivalent delivery system). If a

---

beta$_2$-adrenoceptor stimulant is to be used at the same time as an inhaled corticosteroid it should be used first to help increase the penetration of the inhaled corticosteroid.

Patients who have been taking long-term oral corticosteroids can often be transferred to an inhaled corticosteroid but the transfer must be done slowly, with gradual reduction in dose of oral corticosteroid, and at a time when the asthma is well controlled.

High-dose aerosol inhalations are available for patients who only have a partial response to standard inhalers. The maximum doses for high-dose corticosteroid inhalations are associated with some adrenal suppression (section 6.3.2), therefore patients on high doses should be given a 'steroid card' and may need corticosteroid cover during an episode of stress (e.g. an operation). Systemic therapy may also be necessary during episodes of infection or increased bronchoconstriction where higher doses are needed and access of inhaled drug to small airways may be reduced; patients may need a reserve supply of tablets.

Inhaled corticosteroids have considerably fewer systemic effects than oral corticosteroids, but adverse effects have been reported including a small increased risk of glaucoma with prolonged high doses of inhaled corticosteroids; cataracts have also been reported with inhaled corticosteroids. Effects on bone metabolism can be detected following inhalation of higher doses of beclomethasone, budesonide and fluticasone. Although there is no firm evidence that this may lead to increased osteoporosis in the future, it is sensible to ensure that the dose of inhaled corticosteroid is no higher than necessary to keep a patient's asthma under good control. The dose may therefore be reduced cautiously when the asthma has been well controlled for a few weeks as long as the patient knows that it is necessary to reinstate it should the asthma deteriorate or the peak flow rate fall.

Corticosteroids are preferably inhaled from aerosol inhalers using large-volume 'spacer devices' (section 3.1.5) particularly if high doses are required. Spacer devices increase airway deposition and reduce oropharyngeal deposition, resulting in a marked reduction in the incidence of candidiasis. *Dry powder inhalers* are actuated by the patient's inhalation and are particularly useful for patients who are unable to use the aerosol inhalers.

Budesonide is available as a suspension for nebulisation (*Pulmicort Respules*®).

ORAL. *Acute attacks* of asthma should be treated with short courses of oral corticosteroids starting with a high dose, e.g. prednisolone 30 to 60 mg (30 to 40 mg usually adequate) daily for a few days, gradually reducing once the attack has been controlled. Patients whose asthma has deteriorated rapidly usually respond quickly to corticosteroids, which can then be tailed down over a few days; more gradual reduction is necessary in those whose asthma has deteriorated gradually. For use of corticosteroids in the emergency treatment of *acute severe asthma* see table on p. 125.

In *chronic continuing asthma*, when the response to other anti-asthma drugs has been relatively small, continued administration of oral corticosteroids may be necessary; in such cases high doses of inhaled corticosteroids should be continued so that oral requirements are reduced to a minimum. Oral corticosteroids should normally be taken as a single dose in the morning to reduce the disturbance to circadian cortisol secretion. Dosage should always be titrated to the lowest dose which controls symptoms. Regular peak flow measurements often help both patient and doctor to adjust the dose optimally. Prednisolone is available as tablets of 1 mg as well as 5 mg, and the smaller tablets may conveniently be used to adjust the maintenance dosage to the minimum necessary.

Alternate-day administration has not been very successful in the management of asthma in adults as they tend to deteriorate during the second 24 hours. If an attempt is made to introduce this, pulmonary function should be monitored carefully over the 48 hours.

PARENTERAL. For the use of hydrocortisone injection in the emergency treatment of acute severe asthma, see Acute Severe Asthma table, p. 125.

BECLOMETHASONE DIPROPIONATE
(Beclometasone Dipropionate)

Indications: prophylaxis of asthma especially if not fully controlled by bronchodilators or cromoglycate

Cautions: see notes above; also active or quiescent tuberculosis; may need to reinstate systemic therapy during periods of stress or when airways obstruction or mucus prevent drug access to smaller airways

PARADOXICAL BRONCHOSPASM. The potential for paradoxical bronchospasm (calling for discontinuation and alternative therapy) should be borne in mind—if mild it may be prevented by inhalation of a beta$_2$-adrenoceptor stimulant (or by transfer from an aerosol inhalation to a dry powder inhalation)

Side-effects: see notes above; also hoarseness and candidiasis of mouth or throat (usually only with large doses); rarely rash

CANDIDIASIS. Candidiasis can be reduced by using spacer, see notes above, and responds to antifungal lozenges (section 12.3.2) without discontinuation of therapy—rinsing the mouth with water (or cleaning child's teeth) after inhalation of a dose may also be helpful

Dose: Standard dose inhalers

By aerosol inhalation, 200 micrograms twice daily *or* 100 micrograms 3–4 times daily (in more severe cases initially 600–800 micrograms daily); CHILD 50–100 micrograms 2–4 times daily

By inhalation of powder, 200 micrograms 3–4 times daily *or* 400 micrograms twice daily; CHILD 100 micrograms 2–4 times daily *or* 200 micrograms twice daily

High dose inhalers

By aerosol inhalation, 500 micrograms twice daily *or* 250 micrograms 4 times daily; if necessary may be increased to 500 micrograms 4 times daily; CHILD not recommended

By inhalation of powder, 400 micrograms twice daily; if necessary may be increased to 800 micrograms twice daily; CHILD not recommended

---

Standard-dose inhalers

PoM **Beclomethasone** (Non-proprietary)

Aerosol inhalation, beclomethasone dipropionate 50 micrograms/metered inhalation, net price 200-dose unit = £4.34; 100 micrograms/metered inhalation, 200-dose unit = £8.24. Label: 8, counselling, dose

Available from Baker Norton (*Beclazone®*), Generics and 3M (*Filair®*); vortex-based aerosol inhalers releasing beclomethasone dipropionate 50 micrograms/metered inhalation and 100 micrograms/metered inhalation available from Evans (*Asmabec Spacehaler®*)

Additives: include CFC propellants

PoM **AeroBec®** (3M)

AeroBec 50 Autohaler® (breath-actuated aerosol inhalation), beclomethasone dipropionate 50 micrograms/metered inhalation, net price 200-dose unit = £11.00. Label: 8, counselling, dose

Additives: include CFC propellants

AeroBec 100 Autohaler® (breath-actuated aerosol inhalation), beclomethasone dipropionate 100 micrograms/metered inhalation, net price 200-dose unit = £13.50. Label: 8, counselling, dose

Additives: include CFC propellants

PoM **Becodisks®** (A&H)

Dry powder for inhalation, disks containing 8 blisters of beclomethasone dipropionate 100 micrograms/blister, net price 14 disks with *Diskhaler®* device = £10.99, 5-disk refill = £3.93 (hosp. only), 14-disk refill = £10.42; 200 micrograms/blister, 14 disks with *Diskhaler®* device = £20.90, 5-disk refill = £7.46 (hosp. only), 14-disk refill = £20.33; 400 micrograms/blister, 7 disks with *Diskhaler®* device = £20.90, 7-disk refill = £20.33. Label: 8, counselling, dose

PoM **Becotide®** (A&H)

Becotide-50 aerosol inhalation, beclomethasone dipropionate 50 micrograms/metered inhalation. Net price 80-dose unit = £2.00 (hosp. only), 200-dose unit = £5.43. Label: 8, counselling, dose

Becotide-100 aerosol inhalation, beclomethasone dipropionate 100 micrograms/metered inhalation. Net price 80-dose unit = £4.00 (hosp. only), 200-dose unit = £10.32. Label: 8, counselling, dose

Becotide-200 aerosol inhalation, beclomethasone dipropionate 200 micrograms/metered inhalation. Net price 200-dose unit = £19.61. Label: 8, counselling, dose, 10 steroid card

Note. Becotide-200 not indicated for children

Additives: all include CFC propellants

Easi-Breathe® aerosol inhalation, beclomethasone dipropionate 50 micrograms/metered inhalation, net price 200-dose breath-actuated unit = £4.34; 100 micrograms/metered inhalation, 200-dose breath-actuated unit = £8.24. Label: 8, counselling, dose

Additives: include CFC propellants

Rotacaps® (dry powder for inhalation; for use with *Becotide Rotahaler®*), beclomethasone dipropionate 100 micrograms (buff/clear), net price 112-cap pack = £8.47; 200 micrograms (brown/clear), 112-cap pack = £16.07; 400 micrograms (dark brown/clear), 112-cap pack = £30.54. Label: 8, counselling, dose

High-dose inhalers

Note. High-dose inhalers not indicated for children

PoM **Beclomethasone** (Non-proprietary)

Aerosol inhalation, beclomethasone dipropionate 250 micrograms/metered inhalation, net price 200-dose unit = £18.02. Label: 8, counselling, dose, 10 steroid card

Available from Baker Norton (*Beclazone®*), Generics and 3M (*Filair Forte®*); vortex-based aerosol inhalers releasing beclomethasone dipropionate 250 micrograms/metered inhalation available from Evans (*Asmabec Spacehaler®*)

Additives: include CFC propellants

PoM **AeroBec Forte®** (3M)

Aerosol inhalation, beclomethasone dipropionate 250 micrograms/metered inhalation, net price 200-inhalation breath-actuated unit (*Autohaler®*) = £25.10. Label: 8, counselling, dose, 10 steroid card

Additives: include CFC propellants

PoM **Becloforte®** (A&H)

Aerosol inhalation, beclomethasone dipropionate 250 micrograms/metered inhalation. Net price 80-dose unit = £9.24 (hosp. only), 200-dose unit = £23.10; 200-puff unit with spacer device (*Becloforte Integra®*) = £23.10; 200-dose refill for use with *Becloforte Integra®* = £18.02. Label: 8, counselling, dose, 10 steroid card

Additives: include CFC propellants

Easi-Breathe® aerosol inhalation, beclomethasone dipropionate 250 micrograms/metered inhalation, net price 200-dose breath-actuated unit = £18.02. Label: 8, counselling, dose, 10 steroid card

Additives: include CFC propellants

Dry powder for inhalation, disks containing 8 blisters of beclomethasone dipropionate 400 micrograms/blister, net price 14 disks with *Diskhaler®* device = £39.70; 14-disk refill = £39.13. Label: 8, counselling, dose, 10 steroid card

Compound preparations

(Not recommended)

PoM **Ventide®** (A&H)

Aerosol inhalation, beclomethasone dipropionate 50 micrograms, salbutamol 100 micrograms/metered inhalation. Net price 200-dose unit = £6.02. Label: 8, counselling, dose

Additives: include CFC propellants

Dose: maintenance, 2 puffs 3–4 times daily; CHILD 1–2 puffs 2–4 times daily

Paediatric Rotacaps® (dry powder for inhalation; for use with *Ventide Rotahaler®*), light grey/clear, beclomethasone dipropionate 100 micrograms, salbutamol (as sulphate) 200 micrograms. Net price 112-cap pack = £14.10. Label: 8, counselling, dose

Dose: by inhalation of powder, 1 *Paediatric Rotacap®* 2–4 times daily

Rotacaps® (dry powder for inhalation; for use with *Ventide Rotahaler®*), dark grey/clear, beclomethasone dipropionate 200 micrograms, salbutamol (as sulphate) 400 micrograms. Net price 112-cap pack = £25.57. Label: 8, counselling, dose

Dose: by inhalation of powder, 1 *Rotacap®* 3–4 times daily

Inhaler devices

See section 3.1.5

Chronic Asthma table, see p. 124
Acute Severe Asthma table, see p. 125

BUDESONIDE

Indications; Cautions; Side-effects: see under Beclomethasone Dipropionate
Dose: see preparations below

PoM **Pulmicort®** (Astra)

LS aerosol inhalation, budesonide 50 micrograms/metered inhalation. Net price 200-dose unit with standard or *Spacer* inhaler = £6.66; 200-dose refill for use with *Nebuhaler®* or *Spacer* inhaler = £4.54. Label: 8, counselling, dose

Additives: include CFC propellants

Aerosol inhalation, budesonide 200 micrograms/metered inhalation. Net price 200-dose unit with standard or *Spacer* inhaler = £19.00; 200-dose refill for use with *Nebuhaler®* or *Spacer* inhaler = £17.00; 100-dose unit with standard and *Spacer* inhaler = £7.96 (hosp. only). Label: 8, counselling, dose, 10 steroid card

Additives: include CFC propellants

Dose: by aerosol inhalation, 200 micrograms twice daily; may be reduced in well-controlled asthma to not less than 200 micrograms daily; in severe asthma dose may be increased to 1.6 mg daily; CHILD 50–400 micrograms twice daily; in severe asthma may be increased to 800 micrograms daily

Turbohaler® (= dry powder inhaler), budesonide 100 micrograms/inhalation, net price 200-dose unit = £18.50; 200 micrograms/inhalation, 100-dose unit = £18.50; 400 micrograms/inhalation, 50-dose unit = £18.50. Label: 8, counselling, dose, 10 steroid card

Note. Little sensation associated with use

Dose: by inhalation of powder, when starting treatment, during periods of severe asthma, and while reducing or discontinuing oral corticosteroids, 0.2–1.6 mg twice daily; patients already controlled on an inhaled corticosteroid administered twice daily may be transferred to once-daily dosing (each evening) at the same equivalent total daily dose (up to 800 micrograms once daily); CHILD 200–800 micrograms daily in divided doses (800 micrograms daily in severe asthma)

Respules® (= single-dose units for nebulisation), budesonide 250 micrograms/mL, net price 20 × 2-mL (500 micrograms) unit = £32.00; 500 micrograms/mL, 20 × 2-mL (1 mg) unit = £44.64. May be diluted up to 50% with sterile sodium chloride 0.9%. Label: 8, counselling, dose, 10 steroid card

Dose: by inhalation of nebulised suspension, when starting treatment, during periods of severe asthma, and while reducing or discontinuing oral corticosteroids, 1–2 mg twice daily (may be increased further in very severe asthma); CHILD 3 months–12 years, 0.5–1 mg twice daily

Maintenance, usually half above doses

Croup, 2 mg as a single dose (*or* as two 1-mg doses separated by 30 minutes)

Inhaler devices
Section 3.1.5

FLUTICASONE PROPIONATE

Indications; Cautions; Side-effects: see under Beclomethasone Dipropionate
Dose: see preparations below

PoM **Flixotide®** (A&H)

Accuhaler® (dry powder for inhalation), disk containing 60 blisters of fluticasone propionate 50 micrograms/blister with *Accuhaler®* device, net price = £8.23; 100 micrograms/blister with *Accuhaler®* device = £12.80; 250 micrograms/blister with *Accuhaler®* device = £24.23; 500 micrograms/blister with *Accuhaler®* device = £40.23. Label: 8, counselling, dose; 250- and 500-microgram strengths also label 10 steroid card

Note. Flixotide Accuhaler® 250 micrograms and 500 micrograms are not indicated for children

Dose: by inhalation of powder, ADULT and CHILD over 16 years, 100–250 micrograms twice daily, increased according to severity of asthma to 1 mg twice daily; CHILD under 4 years not recommended, 4–16 years, 50–100 micrograms twice daily adjusted as necessary

Aerosol inhalation, fluticasone propionate 25 micrograms/metered inhalation, net price 120-dose unit = £6.86; 50 micrograms/metered inhalation, 120-dose unit = £11.43; 125 micrograms/metered inhalation, 60-dose unit = £11.43 (hosp. only), 120-dose unit = £22.86; 250 micrograms/metered inhalation, 60 dose unit = £19.43 (hosp. only), 120-dose unit = £38.86. Label: 8, counselling, dose; 250-microgram strength also label 10 steroid card

Additives: include CFC propellants

Note. Flixotide® 125 micrograms and 250 micrograms inhalers not indicated for children

Dose: by aerosol inhalation, ADULT and CHILD over 16 years, 100–250 micrograms twice daily, increased according to severity of asthma to 1 mg twice daily; CHILD 4–16 years, 50–100 micrograms twice daily adjusted as necessary

Diskhaler® (dry powder for inhalation), fluticasone propionate
50 micrograms/blister, net price 14 disks of 4 blisters with *Diskhaler®* device = £8.23, 14-disk refill = £7.66;
100 micrograms/blister, 14 disks of 4 blisters with *Diskhaler®* device = £12.80, 14-disk refill = £12.23;
250 micrograms/blister, 14 disks of 4 blisters with *Diskhaler®* device = £24.23, 5-disk refill = £8.65 (hosp. only), 14-disk refill = £23.66;
500 micrograms/blister, 14 disks of 4 blisters with *Diskhaler®* device = £40.23, 5-disk refill = £14.37 (hosp. only), 14-disk refill = £39.66. Label: 8, counselling, dose; 250- and 500-microgram strengths also label 10 steroid card

Note. Flixotide Diskhaler® 250 micrograms and 500 micrograms are not indicated for children

Dose: by inhalation of powder, ADULT and CHILD over 16 years, 100–250 micrograms twice daily, increased according to severity of asthma to 1 mg twice daily; CHILD 4–16 years, 50–100 micrograms twice daily adjusted as necessary

3.3   Cromoglycate and related therapy

Regular inhalation of **sodium cromoglycate** (sodium cromoglicate) can reduce the incidence of attacks of asthma and allow dosage reduction of bronchodilators and oral corticosteroids. In general, prophylaxis with sodium cromoglycate is less effective in adults than prophylaxis with corticosteroid inhalations (see Chronic Asthma table, p. 124) but the fact that in the long term corticosteroid inhalations may be associated with more side-effects needs to be borne in mind. Children may respond better than adults although sodium cromoglycate appears not to be effective in children under the age of 4 years. Sodium cromoglycate is of no value in the treatment of acute attacks of asthma.

Sodium cromoglycate is of value in the prevention of exercise-induced asthma, a single dose being inhaled half-an-hour beforehand.

The mode of action of sodium cromoglycate is not completely understood. It may be of value in asthma with an allergic basis, but, in practice, it is difficult to predict who will benefit, therefore it is reasonable to try it for a period of 4 to 6 weeks. Dose frequency is adjusted according to response but is usually 3 to 4 times a day initially; this may subsequently be reduced.

If inhalation of the dry powder form of sodium cromoglycate causes bronchospasm a selective beta$_2$-adrenoceptor stimulant such as salbutamol or terbutaline should be inhaled a few minutes beforehand. The nebuliser solution is an alternative means of delivery for children who cannot manage the dry powder inhaler or the aerosol.

Nedocromil has a pharmacological action similar to that of sodium cromoglycate.

SODIUM CROMOGLYCATE
(Sodium Cromoglicate)

Indications: prophylaxis of asthma; food allergy, section 1.5

Side-effects: coughing, transient bronchospasm, and throat irritation due to inhalation of powder (see also notes above)

Dose: by aerosol inhalation, ADULT and CHILD, 10 mg (2 puffs) 4 times daily, increased in severe cases or during periods of risk to 6–8 times daily; additional doses may also be taken before exercise; maintenance 5 mg (1 puff) 4 times daily

By inhalation of powder (Spincaps®), ADULT and CHILD, 20 mg 4 times daily, increased in severe cases to 8 times daily

By inhalation of nebulised solution, ADULT and CHILD, 20 mg 4 times daily, increased in severe cases to 6 times daily

COUNSELLING. Regular use is necessary

PoM **Sodium Cromoglycate** (Non-proprietary)

Aerosol inhalation, sodium cromoglycate 5 mg/ metered inhalation. Net price 112-dose unit = £13.91. Label: 8

Available from Baker Norton (*Cromogen®*)
Additives: include CFC propellants

Nebuliser solution, sodium cromoglycate 10 mg/ mL. Net price 60 × 2-mL unit-dose vials = £12.87
Available from Baker Norton (*Steri-Neb Cromogen®*)

PoM **Cromogen Easi-Breathe®** (Baker Norton)

Aerosol inhalation, sodium cromoglycate 5 mg/ metered inhalation. Net price 112-dose breath-actuated unit = £13.91. Label: 8
Additives: include CFC propellants

PoM **Intal®** (Fisons)

Aerosol inhalation, sodium cromoglycate 5 mg/ metered inhalation. Net price 112-puff unit = £17.35; 2 × 112-puff unit with spacer device (*Syncroner®*) = £34.52; also available with large volume spacer inhaler (*Fisonair®*), complete unit = £20.05. Label: 8
Additives: include CFC propellants

Spincaps®, yellow/clear, sodium cromoglycate 20 mg. Net price 112-cap pack = £15.08. Label: 8

Spinhaler insufflator® (for use with Intal Spincaps). Net price = £1.89

Nebuliser solution, sodium cromoglycate 10 mg/ mL. Net price 2-mL amp = 31p. For use with power-operated nebuliser

Compound preparations

Note. The compound inhalation of sodium cromoglycate with a beta-adrenoceptor stimulant is not recommended as the inhalation is liable to be used inappropriately for relief of bronchospasm rather than for its prophylactic effect

PoM **Aerocrom®** (Fisons)

Aerosol inhalation, sodium cromoglycate 1 mg, salbutamol (as sulphate) 100 micrograms/metered inhalation, net price 200-puff unit = £18.02; 200-puff unit with spacer device (*Syncroner®*) = £18.02. Label: 8
Additives: include CFC propellants
Dose: by aerosol inhalation, 2 inhalations 4 times daily; CHILD, not recommended

NEDOCROMIL SODIUM

Indications: prophylaxis of asthma

Side-effects: see under Sodium Cromoglycate; also headache, nausea, vomiting, dyspepsia, abdominal pain (mild and transient); bitter taste (masked by mint flavour)

Dose: by aerosol inhalation, ADULT and CHILD over 6 years 4 mg (2 puffs) 4 times daily, when control achieved may be possible to reduce to twice daily

COUNSELLING. Regular use is necessary

PoM **Tilade®** (Fisons)

Aerosol inhalation, nedocromil sodium 2 mg/ metered inhalation. Net price 2 × 56-puff mint-flavoured units = £22.64; 2 × 112-puff unit with spacer device (*Syncroner®*) = £45.26. Label: 8
Additives: include CFC propellants

RELATED THERAPY

Antihistamines are of no value in the treatment of bronchial asthma. **Ketotifen** is an antihistamine with an action said to resemble that of sodium cromoglycate, but it has proved disappointing.

KETOTIFEN

Indications: see notes above

Cautions: previous anti-asthmatic treatment should be continued for a minimum of 2 weeks after initiation of ketotifen treatment; pregnancy and breast-feeding (see Appendixes 4 and 5); **interactions:** Appendix 1 (antihistamines)—also, manufacturer advises avoid with oral antidiabetics (fall in thrombocyte count reported)

DRIVING. Drowsiness may affect performance of skilled tasks (e.g. driving); effects of alcohol enhanced

Side-effects: drowsiness, dry mouth, slight dizziness; CNS stimulation, weight gain also reported

Dose: 1 mg twice daily with food increased if necessary to 2 mg twice daily; initial treatment in readily sedated patients 0.5–1 mg at night; CHILD over 2 years 1 mg twice daily

PoM **Zaditen**® (Novartis)

Capsules, ketotifen (as hydrogen fumarate) 1 mg. Net price 60-cap pack = £8.14. Label: 2, 8, 21

Tablets, scored, ketotifen (as hydrogen fumarate) 1 mg. Net price 60-tab pack = £8.14. Label: 2, 8, 21

Elixir, ketotifen (as hydrogen fumarate) 1 mg/5 mL. Net price 300 mL = £9.64. Label: 2, 8, 21

3.4 Antihistamines, hyposensitisation, and allergic emergencies

3.4.1   Antihistamines
3.4.2   Hyposensitisation
3.4.3   Allergic emergencies

3.4.1   Antihistamines

All antihistamines are of potential value in the treatment of nasal allergies, particularly seasonal allergic rhinitis (hay fever), and may be of some value in vasomotor rhinitis. They reduce rhinorrhoea and sneezing but are usually less effective for nasal congestion.

Oral antihistamines are also of some value in preventing urticaria and are used to treat urticarial rashes, pruritus, and insect bites and stings; they are also used in drug allergies. Injections of chlorpheniramine or promethazine are used as an adjunct to adrenaline in the emergency treatment of anaphylaxis and angioedema (section 3.4.3). For the use of antihistamines (including cinnarizine, cyclizine, dimenhydrinate, and promethazine theoclate) in nausea and vomiting, see section 4.6. Buclizine is included as an anti-emetic in a preparation for migraine (section 4.7.4.1). For reference to the use of antihistamines for occasional insomnia, see section 4.1.1.

Antihistamines differ in their duration of action and incidence of drowsiness and antimuscarinic effects. Many older antihistamines are relatively short acting but some (e.g. promethazine) act for up to 12 hours, while most of the newer non-sedating antihistamines are long acting.

All older antihistamines cause sedation but **dimenhydrinate**, **promethazine**, and **trimeprazine** (alimemazine) (section 4.6) may be more sedating whereas **chlorpheniramine** (chlorphen-

amine), **cyclizine** (section 4.6), and **mequitazine** may be less so. This sedating activity is sometimes used to alleviate the pruritus associated with some allergies. There is little evidence that any one of the older, 'sedating' antihistamines is superior to another and patients vary widely in their responses.

Non-sedating antihistamines such as **acrivastine**, **astemizole**, **cetirizine**, **loratadine**, and **terfenadine** cause less sedation and psychomotor impairment than the older antihistamines because they penetrate the blood brain barrier only to a slight extent (and for this reason do not alleviate pruritus of non-allergic origin). Astemizole has a relatively slow onset of action and is more appropriate for use on a regular basis than when symptoms occur. **Fexofenadine**, an active metabolite of terfenadine, has been introduced recently.

CAUTIONS and CONTRA-INDICATIONS. All antihistamines should be used with caution in epilepsy, prostatic hypertrophy, urinary retention, glaucoma, and hepatic disease (astemizole and terfenadine in particular should be **avoided** in significant impairment). Children and the elderly are more susceptible to side-effects. Many antihistamines should be avoided in porphyria although some (e.g. chlorpheniramine and cetirizine) are thought to be safe (section 9.8.2). **Interactions:** Appendix 1 (antihistamines); **important:** see also under *Astemizole* and *Terfenadine.*

SIDE-EFFECTS. Drowsiness is a significant side-effect with most of the older antihistamines (although paradoxical stimulation may occur rarely, especially in high dosage or in children and the elderly) but this side-effect may diminish after a few days of continued treatment; drowsiness is considerably less of a problem with the newer antihistamines (see also notes above). Other side-effects that are more common with the older antihistamines include headache, psychomotor impairment, and antimuscarinic effects such as urinary retention, dry mouth, blurred vision, and gastro-intestinal disturbances.

Other side-effects of antihistamines reported include palpitations and arrhythmias (**important:** see especially risks associated with *astemizole* and *terfenadine*, pp. 142 and 143), hypotension, hypersensitivity reactions (including bronchospasm, angioedema, and anaphylaxis), rashes and photosensitivity reactions, extrapyramidal effects, confusion, depression, sleep disturbances, tremor, convulsions, sweating, myalgia, paraesthesia, blood disorders, liver dysfunction, and hair loss.

NON-SEDATING ANTIHISTAMINES

DRIVING. Although drowsiness is rare, nevertheless patients should be advised that it can occur and may affect performance of skilled tasks (e.g. driving); excess alcohol should be avoided.

ACRIVASTINE

Indications: symptomatic relief of allergy such as hay fever, urticaria

Cautions: see notes above

Contra-indications: see notes above; avoid in renal impairment
Side-effects: see notes above; incidence of sedation and antimuscarinic effects low
Dose: 8 mg 3 times daily; CHILD under 12 years, not recommended; ELDERLY not recommended

PoM **Semprex**® (GlaxoWellcome)
Capsules, acrivastine 8 mg. Net price 84-cap pack = £5.04. Counselling, driving

ASTEMIZOLE

Indications: symptomatic relief of allergy such as hay fever, urticaria
Cautions: see notes above
Contra-indications: see notes above; pregnancy and breast-feeding (see below); **important:** see also Arrhythmias, below

PREGNANCY AND BREAST-FEEDING. Manufacturer advises avoid in pregnancy (toxicity at high doses in *animals*) and advises that women of childbearing potential should use contraception while taking astemizole and (owing to long half-life) for several weeks after stopping. Manufacturer also advises avoid in breast-feeding

ARRHYTHMIAS. Rare hazardous arrhythmias are associated with astemizole and terfenadine particularly in association with increased blood concentrations—these two antihistamines should *not* be taken concomitantly (and the long half-life of astemizole should be borne in mind).

Recommendations are: *not to exceed* recommended dose, *to avoid* in significant hepatic impairment, and *to avoid* concomitant administration of *ketoconazole, itraconazole and other imidazole antifungals* and of *erythromycin and clarithromycin, to avoid* if hypokalaemia (or other electrolyte imbalance) or prolonged QT interval known or suspected and *to avoid* concomitant administration of potentially arrhythmogenic drugs such as *anti-arrhythmics, antipsychotics, tricyclic antidepressants, quinine,* and of drugs liable to produce electrolyte imbalance such as *diuretics*.

If syncope occurs the antihistamine should be discontinued and patient evaluated for potential arrhythmias

Side-effects: see notes above; weight gain occurs infrequently; incidence of sedation and antimuscarinic effects low; **important:** ventricular arrhythmias (including torsades de pointes) have followed excessive dosage, for recommendations see also Arrhythmias above

Dose: 10 mg daily (must **not** be exceeded); CHILD under 6 years not recommended, 6–12 years 5 mg daily (must **not** be exceeded)

PoM ¹**Hismanal**® (Janssen-Cilag)
Tablets, scored, astemizole 10 mg. Net price 30-tab pack = £5.40. Counselling, driving
Suspension, sugar-free, astemizole 5 mg /5 mL. Net price 200 mL = £5.80. Counselling, driving
1. Tablets can be sold to the public for the treatment of hay fever in adults and children over 12 years (NHS *Hismanal*® 10-tab pack); another brand on sale to the public is NHS *Pollon-eze*®

CETIRIZINE HYDROCHLORIDE

Indications: symptomatic relief of allergy such as hay fever, urticaria
Cautions: see notes above; halve dose in renal impairment

Contra-indications: pregnancy and breast-feeding
Side-effects: see notes above; incidence of sedation and antimuscarinic effects low
Dose: ADULT and CHILD over 6 years, 10 mg daily *or* 5 mg twice daily; CHILD 2–6 years, hayfever, 5 mg daily *or* 2.5 mg twice daily

PoM ¹**Zirtek**® (UCB Pharma)
Tablets, f/c, scored, cetirizine hydrochloride 10 mg. Net price 30-tab pack = £8.73. Counselling, driving
Oral solution, sugar-free, cetirizine hydrochloride 5 mg/5 mL. Net price 200 mL = £14.95. Counselling, driving
1. Tablets can be sold to the public for adults and children over 12 years provided packs do not contain more than 10 days' supply (NHS *Zirtek 7*®)

FEXOFENADINE HYDROCHLORIDE

Indications: see under preparations below
Cautions: see notes above; pregnancy
Contra-indications: breast-feeding
Dose: see under preparations below

▼ PoM **Telfast 120**® (Hoechst Marion Roussel)
Tablets, f/c, peach, fexofenadine hydrochloride 120 mg. Net price 30-tab pack = £7.40. Counselling, driving
Dose: symptomatic relief of seasonal allergic rhinitis, 120 mg once daily; CHILD under 12 years, not recommended

▼ PoM **Telfast 180**® (Hoechst Marion Roussel)
Tablets, f/c, peach, fexofenadine hydrochloride 180 mg. Net price 30-tab pack = £9.63. Counselling, driving
Dose: symptomatic relief of chronic idiopathic urticaria, 180 mg once daily; CHILD under 12 years, not recommended

LORATADINE

Indications: symptomatic relief of allergy such as hay fever, urticaria
Cautions: see notes above
Contra-indications: see notes above; pregnancy (toxicity at high doses in *animals*) and breast-feeding (Appendix 5)
Side-effects: see notes above; incidence of sedation and antimuscarinic effects low
Dose: 10 mg daily; CHILD 2–12 years, under 30 kg 5 mg daily, over 30 kg 10 mg daily

PoM ¹**Clarityn**® (Schering-Plough)
Tablets, scored, loratadine 10 mg. Net price 30-tab pack = £7.57. Counselling, driving
Syrup, yellow, loratadine 5 mg/5 mL. Net price 100 mL = £7.57. Counselling, driving
1. Tablets and syrup can be sold to the public provided packs do not contain more than 10 days' supply (NHS *Clarityn Allergy*®); another brand on sale to the public is *Boots Hayfever Relief*®

TERFENADINE

Indications: symptomatic relief of allergy such as hay fever, urticaria
Cautions: see notes above: pregnancy and breast-feeding

Contra-indications: see notes above; avoid grapefruit juice (may inhibit metabolism of terfenadine); **important:** see also Arrhythmias, below

ARRHYTHMIAS. Rare hazardous arrhythmias are associated with astemizole and terfenadine particularly in association with increased blood concentrations—these two antihistamines should *not* be taken concomitantly (and the long half-life of astemizole should be borne in mind).

Recommendations are: *not to exceed* recommended dose, *to avoid* in significant hepatic impairment, and *to avoid* concomitant administration of ketoconazole, itraconazole and other imidazole antifungals, erythromycin and clarithromycin, mibefradil, fluvoxamine, nefazodone, protease inhibitors including indinavir, ritonavir, and saquinavir, and cisapride, *to avoid* if hypokalaemia (or other electrolyte imbalance) or prolonged QT interval known or suspected and *to avoid* concomitant administration of potentially arrhythmogenic drugs such as anti-arrhythmics, antipsychotics, tricyclic antidepressants and of drugs liable to produce electrolyte imbalance such as diuretics.

If syncope occurs the antihistamine should be discontinued and patient evaluated for potential arrhythmias

Side-effects: see notes above; incidence of sedation and antimuscarinic effects low; erythema multiforme and galactorrhoea reported; **important:** ventricular arrhythmias (including torsades de pointes) have followed excessive dosage, see also Arrhythmias above

Dose: hay fever, allergic rhinitis, 60 mg daily increased if necessary to 120 mg daily, in single or 2 divided doses;

Allergic skin conditions, 120 mg daily in single or 2 divided doses

CHILD (hay fever, allergic rhinitis or allergic skin conditions) 3–6 years 15 mg twice daily; 6–12 years 30 mg twice daily

PoM **Terfenadine** (Non-proprietary)
Tablets, terfenadine 60 mg, net price 60-tab pack = £3.38; 120 mg, 30-tab pack = £4.70. Counselling, driving
Available from APS, Berk (*Histafen*®), Ashbourne (*Terfinax*®), Cox, Hillcross, Norton

PoM **Triludan**® (Hoechst Marion Roussel)
Tablets, scored, terfenadine 60 mg. Net price 60-tab pack = £5.40. Counselling, driving
Forte tablets, terfenadine 120 mg. Net price 30-tab pack = £5.40. Counselling, driving
Suspension, sugar-free, terfenadine 30 mg/5 mL. Net price 200 mL = £4.13. Counselling, driving

---

SEDATING ANTIHISTAMINES

DRIVING. Drowsiness may affect performance of skilled tasks (e.g. driving); sedating effects enhanced by alcohol.

AZATADINE MALEATE

Indications: symptomatic relief of allergy such as hay fever, urticaria
Cautions: see notes above
Contra-indications: see notes above; pregnancy and breast-feeding
Side-effects: see notes above

Dose: 1 mg, increased if necessary to 2 mg, twice daily; CHILD under 1 year not recommended, 1–6 years 250 micrograms twice daily, 6–12 years 0.5–1 mg twice daily

Optimine® (Schering-Plough)
Tablets, scored, azatadine maleate 1 mg. Net price 56-tab pack = £2.80. Label: 2
Syrup, azatadine maleate 500 micrograms/5 mL. Net price 120 mL = £1.39. Label: 2

BROMPHENIRAMINE MALEATE

Indications: symptomatic relief of allergy such as hay fever, urticaria
Cautions: see notes above
Contra-indications: see notes above
Side-effects: see notes above

Dose: 4–8 mg 3–4 times daily; CHILD up to 3 years 0.4–1 mg/kg daily in 4 divided doses, 3–6 years 2 mg 3–4 times daily, 6–12 years 2–4 mg 3–4 times daily

Dimotane® (Wyeth)
Tablets, peach, scored, brompheniramine maleate 4 mg. Net price 20 = 59p. Label: 2
Elixir, yellow-green, brompheniramine maleate 2 mg/5 mL. Net price 100 mL = 71p. Label: 2

Dimotane LA® (Wyeth)
Tablets, m/r, peach, s/c, brompheniramine maleate 12 mg. Net price 20 = 89p. Label: 2, 25
Dose: 12–24 mg twice daily; CHILD 6–12 years 12 mg at bedtime, increased if necessary to 12 mg twice daily

For a list of **cough and decongestant preparations on sale to the public,** including those containing brompheniramine, see section 3.9.2.

CHLORPHENIRAMINE MALEATE
(Chlorphenamine Maleate)
Indications: symptomatic relief of allergy such as hay fever, urticaria; emergency treatment of anaphylactic reactions (section 3.4.3)
Cautions: see notes above; injections may be irritant
Contra-indications: see notes above
Side-effects: see notes above; exfoliative dermatitis and tinnitus reported; injections may cause transient hypotension or CNS stimulation
Dose: by mouth, 4 mg every 4–6 hours, max. 24 mg daily; CHILD under 1 year not recommended, 1–2 years 1 mg twice daily; 2–5 years 1 mg every 4–6 hours, max. 6 mg daily; 6–12 years 2 mg every 4–6 hours, max. 12 mg daily
By subcutaneous or intramuscular injection, 10–20 mg, repeated if required; max. 40 mg in 24 hours
By slow intravenous injection over 1 minute, 10–20 mg

Chlorpheniramine (Non-proprietary)
Tablets, chlorpheniramine maleate 4 mg, net price 20 = 7p. Label: 2
Available from Cox, Hillcross
PoM *Injection,* chlorpheniramine maleate 10 mg/mL, net price 1-mL amp = 50p
Available from Link (*Piriton*®)

Piriton® (Stafford-Miller)

Tablets, ivory, chlorpheniramine maleate 4 mg. Net price 20 = 19p. Label: 2

Syrup, chlorpheniramine maleate 2 mg/5 mL. Net price 150 mL = £1.62. Label: 2

Note. In addition to NHS *Piriton Allergy®*, proprietary brands of chlorpheniramine maleate tablets on sale to the public include *Calimal®*

For a list of **cough and decongestant preparations on sale to the public**, including those containing chlorpheniramine, see section 3.9.2

CLEMASTINE

Indications: symptomatic relief of allergy such as hay fever, urticaria

Cautions: see notes above; pregnancy and breast-feeding

Contra-indications: see notes above

Side-effects: see notes above

Dose: 1 mg twice daily, increased up to 6 mg daily if required; CHILD under 1 year not recommended, 1–3 years 250–500 micrograms twice daily; 3–6 years 500 micrograms twice daily; 6–12 years 0.5–1 mg twice daily

Tavegil® (Novartis)

Tablets, scored, clemastine (as hydrogen fumarate) 1 mg. Net price 60-tab pack = £2.46. Label: 2

Elixir, sugar-free, clemastine (as hydrogen fumarate) 500 micrograms/5 mL. Net price 150 mL = 96p. Label: 2

Note. In addition to *Tavegil®*, proprietary brands of clemastine hydrogen fumarate on sale to the public include NHS *Aller-eze®*; it is also on sale to the public combined with phenylpropanolamine (NHS *Aller-eze Plus®*)

CYPROHEPTADINE HYDROCHLORIDE

Indications: symptomatic relief of allergy such as hay fever, urticaria; migraine

Cautions: see notes above; pregnancy

Contra-indications: see notes above; breast-feeding

Side-effects: see notes above; may cause weight gain

Dose: allergy, usual dose 4 mg 3–4 times daily; usual range 4–20 mg daily, max. 32 mg daily; CHILD under 2 years not recommended, 2–6 years 2 mg 2–3 times daily, max. 12 mg daily; 7–14 years 4 mg 2–3 times daily, max. 16 mg daily

Migraine, 4 mg with a further 4 mg after 30 minutes if necessary; maintenance, 4 mg every 4–6 hours

Periactin® (MSD)

Tablets, scored, cyproheptadine hydrochloride 4 mg. Net price 30 = 86p. Label: 2

DIPHENHYDRAMINE HYDROCHLORIDE

Indications: see under Preparations

Cautions; Contra-indications; Side-effects: see notes above

Preparations

Proprietary brands of diphenhydramine hydrochloride on sale to the public to aid relief of temporary sleep disturbance in adults include *Medinex®* (diphenhydramine hydrochloride 10 mg/5 mL), NHS *Nytol®* (diphenhydramine hydrochloride tablets 25 mg and 50 mg), *Sleepia®* (diphenhydramine hydrochloride 50 mg), and *Panadol Night®* (diphenhydramine hydrochloride 25 mg and paracetamol 500 mg, for relief of temporary sleeplessness and night-time pain)

For a list of **cough and decongestant preparations on sale to the public**, including those containing diphenhydramine, see section 3.9.2

DIPHENYLPYRALINE HYDROCHLORIDE

Cautions; Contra-indications; Side-effects: see notes above

Preparations

For a list of **cough and decongestant preparations on sale to the public**, including those containing diphenylpyraline, see section 3.9.2

DOXYLAMINE

Cautions; Contra-indications; Side-effects: see notes above

Preparations

Ingredient of **cough and decongestant preparations** (section 3.9.2.) and of **compound analgesics** (section 4.7.1.) on sale to the public

HYDROXYZINE HYDROCHLORIDE

Indications: pruritus, anxiety (short-term)

Cautions: see notes above; renal impairment (Appendix 3)

Contra-indications: see notes above; pregnancy and breast-feeding

Side-effects: see notes above

Dose: pruritus, initially 25 mg at night increased if necessary to 25 mg 3–4 times daily; CHILD 6 months–6 years initially 5–15 mg daily increased if necessary to 50 mg daily in divided doses; over 6 years initially 15–25 mg daily increased if necessary to 50–100 mg daily in divided doses

Anxiety (adults only), 50–100 mg 4 times daily

PoM **Atarax®** (Pfizer)

Tablets, both s/c, hydroxyzine hydrochloride 10 mg (orange), net price 84-tab pack = £1.52; 25 mg (green), 28-tab pack = £1.02. Label: 2

PoM **Ucerax®** (UCB Pharma)

NHS *Tablets*, f/c, scored, hydroxyzine hydrochloride 25 mg, net price 25-tab pack = £1.73. Label: 2

Syrup, hydroxyzine hydrochloride 10 mg/5 mL. Net price 200-mL pack = £1.91. Label: 2

MEQUITAZINE

Indications: symptomatic relief of allergy such as hay fever, urticaria

Cautions: see notes above

Contra-indications: see notes above; pregnancy
Side-effects: see notes above
Dose: 5 mg twice daily; CHILD under 12 years, not recommended

PoM **Primalan**® (Rhône-Poulenc Rorer)
Tablets, mequitazine 5 mg. Net price 56-tab pack = £2.80. Label: 2

PHENINDAMINE TARTRATE

Indications: symptomatic relief of allergy such as hay fever, urticaria
Cautions: see notes above
Contra-indications: see notes above
Side-effects: see notes above; may cause mild CNS stimulation
Dose: 25–50 mg 1–3 times daily; CHILD over 10 years 25 mg 1–3 times daily

Thephorin® (Sinclair)
Tablets, s/c, phenindamine tartrate 25 mg. Net price 50-tab pack = £1.66. Label: 2

PHENIRAMINE MALEATE

Cautions; Contra-indications; Side-effects: see notes above

Preparations
For a list of **cough and decongestant preparations on sale to the public**, including those containing pheniramine, see section 3.9.2

PROMETHAZINE HYDROCHLORIDE

Indications: symptomatic relief of allergy such as hay fever, urticaria; emergency treatment of anaphylactic reactions (section 3.4.3)
For use in premedication, see section 15.1.4.1; sedation, see section 4.1.1; motion sickness see section 4.6
Cautions: see notes above; intramuscular injection may be painful
Contra-indications: see notes above
Side-effects: see notes above
Dose: by mouth, 25 mg at night increased to 25 mg twice daily if necessary *or* 10–20 mg 2–3 times daily; CHILD under 2 years not recommended, 2–5 years 5–15 mg daily in 1–2 divided doses, 5–10 years 10–25 mg daily in 1–2 divided doses
By deep intramuscular injection, 25–50 mg; max. 100 mg; CHILD 5–10 years 6.25–12.5 mg
By slow intravenous injection in emergencies, 25–50 mg as a solution containing 2.5 mg/mL in water for injections; max. 100 mg

Phenergan® (Rhône-Poulenc Rorer)
Tablets, both blue, f/c, promethazine hydrochloride 10 mg, net price 56-tab pack = £1.10; 25 mg, 56-tab pack = £1.64. Label: 2
Elixir, sugar-free, golden, promethazine hydrochloride 5 mg/5 mL. Net price 100 mL = £1.23. Label: 2

PoM *Injection*, promethazine hydrochloride 25 mg/mL. Net price 1-mL amp = 38p
Promethazine hydrochloride injection 25 mg/mL (1-mL and 2-mL ampoules) also available from Antigen
Note. Proprietary brands of promethazine hydrochloride on sale to the public include *Phenergan Nightime*® (promethazine hydrochloride tablets 25 mg, for occasional insomnia in adults), **NHS** *Sominex*® (promethazine hydrochloride tablets 20 mg, for occasional insomnia in adults) and *Q-Mazine*® (promethazine hydrochloride 5 mg/5 mL for urticaria and other skin conditions in children)

For a list of **cough and decongestant preparations on sale to the public**, including those containing promethazine, see section 3.9.2

TRIMEPRAZINE TARTRATE
(Alimemazine Tartrate)

Indications: urticaria and pruritus; premedication (section 15.1.4.1)
Cautions: see notes above; see also under Chlorpromazine Hydrochloride, section 4.2.1
Contra-indications: see notes above; pregnancy and breast-feeding; see also under Chlorpromazine Hydrochloride, section 4.2.1
Side-effects: see notes above; see also under Chlorpromazine Hydrochloride, section 4.2.1
Dose: 10 mg 2–3 times daily, in severe cases up to max. 100 mg daily has been used; ELDERLY 10 mg 1–2 times daily; CHILD under 2 years not recommended; over 2 years 2.5–5 mg 3–4 times daily

PoM **Vallergan**® (Rhône-Poulenc Rorer)
Tablets, blue, f/c, trimeprazine tartrate 10 mg. Net price 28-tab pack = £1.13. Label: 2
Syrup, straw-coloured, trimeprazine tartrate 7.5 mg/5 mL. Net price 100 mL = £1.29. Label: 2
Syrup forte, trimeprazine tartrate 30 mg/5 mL. Net price 100 mL = £2.66. Label: 2
Note. For use of Forte Syrup see section 15.1.4.1

TRIPROLIDINE HYDROCHLORIDE

Cautions; Contra-indications; Side-effects: see notes above

Preparations
For a list of **cough and decongestant preparations on sale to the public**, including those containing triprolidine, see section 3.9.2

3.4.2 Hyposensitisation

Except for wasp and bee sting allergy, specific hyposensitisation with allergen extract vaccines has usually shown little benefit in asthma. Hyposensitisation may be effective in allergic rhinitis if sensitisation to a particular allergen can be proven. However, the benefit of hyposensitisation needs to be balanced against the significant risk of anaphylaxis, particularly in patients with asthma (see CSM advice below).
Diagnostic skin tests are unreliable and can only be used in conjunction with a detailed history of allergen exposure.

CSM advice. After re-examination of the efficacy and safety of desensitising vaccines, the CSM has concluded that they should only be used for the following indications:

—Seasonal allergic hay fever (which has not responded to anti-allergy drugs) caused by pollens, using licensed products only—patients with *asthma* should not be treated with desensitising vaccines as they are more likely to develop severe adverse reactions.

—Hypersensitivity to wasp and bee venoms—since reactions can be life-threatening, *asthma* is not an absolute contra-indication. There is inadequate evidence of benefit from desensitisation to other allergens such as house dust, house dust mite, animal danders and foods and it is *not* recommended. Desensitising vaccines should be avoided in pregnant women, in children under five years old, and in those taking beta-blockers.

Recent experience indicates that bronchospasm usually develops within 1 hour and anaphylaxis within 30 minutes of injection. Therefore patients need to be monitored for 1 hour after injection. If symptoms or signs of hypersensitivity **develop** (e.g. rash, urticaria, bronchospasm, faintness), **even when mild**, the patient should be observed until these have **completely resolved**.

For details of the management of anaphylactic shock, see section 3.4.3.

BEE AND WASP ALLERGEN EXTRACTS

Each set usually contains vials for the administration of graded amounts to patients undergoing hyposensitisation. Maintenance sets containing vials at the highest strength are also available. Product literature must be consulted for details of allergens, vial strengths, and administration

Indications: hypersensitivity to wasp or bee venom (see notes above)

Cautions: see notes above including CSM advice; manufacturers recommend that patients should be warned not to eat a heavy meal before the injection

CSM advice. The CSM has advised that facilities for cardiopulmonary resuscitation must be immediately available and patients monitored closely for one hour after each injection, for full details see above.

Contra-indications: pregnancy, febrile conditions, inadequately controlled asthma

Side-effects: allergic reactions, especially in small children

Dose: by subcutaneous injection, see product literature

PoM **Pharmalgen**® (ALK)

Bee venom extract (*Apis mellifera*) or wasp venom extract (*Vespula* spp.). Net price initial treatment set = £62.59 (bee), £76.73 (wasp); maintenance treatment set = £72.82 (bee), £93.67 (wasp)

3.4.3   Allergic emergencies

Adrenaline (epinephrine) provides physiological reversal of the immediate symptoms (such as laryngeal oedema, bronchospasm, and hypotension) associated with hypersensitivity reactions such as *anaphylaxis* and *angioedema*. See below for full details of adrenaline administration and for adjunctive treatment.

ANAPHYLAXIS

Anaphylactic shock requires prompt energetic treatment of *laryngeal oedema, bronchospasm*, and *hypotension*. Atopic individuals are particularly susceptible. Insect bites are a recognised risk (in particular wasp and bee stings). Certain foods, including eggs, fish, cow's milk protein, peanuts, and nuts may also precipitate anaphylaxis. Medicinal products particularly associated with anaphylaxis include blood products, vaccines, hyposensitising (allergen) preparations, antibiotics, aspirin and other NSAIDs, iron injections, heparin, and neuromuscular blocking drugs. In the case of drugs, anaphylaxis is more likely after parenteral administration; resuscitation facilities must always be available for injections associated with special risk. Anaphylactic reactions may also be associated with *additives and excipients* in foods and medicines; some oils, such as arachis (peanut) oil, may be contaminated with allergenic proteins from their original source—it is wise to check the full formula of preparations which may contain allergenic fats or oils (including those for topical application, particularly if they are intended for use in the mouth or for application to the nasal mucosa).

First-line treatment includes securing the airway, restoration of blood pressure (laying the patient flat, raising the feet), and administration of **adrenaline** (epinephrine) injection. This is given **intramuscularly** in a dose of 0.5–1 mg (0.5–1 mL adrenaline injection 1 in 1000); a dose of 300 micrograms (0.3 mL adrenaline injection 1 in 1000) may be appropriate for *immediate self-administration*. The dose is repeated every 10 minutes, according to blood pressure and pulse, until improvement occurs [important: possible need for *intravenous route* using *dilute solution*, see below]. **Oxygen** administration is also of primary importance. An antihistamine (e.g. **chlorpheniramine**, given by slow intravenous injection in a dose of 10–20 mg, see p. 143) is a useful adjunctive treatment, given after adrenaline injection and continued for 24 to 48 hours to prevent relapse. In patients on non-cardioselective beta-blockers severe anaphylaxis may not respond to adrenaline injection, calling for addition of **salbutamol** by intravenous injection.

Continuing deterioration requires further treatment including intravenous fluids (see section 9.2.2), intravenous aminophylline (see p. 132) or a nebulised beta$_2$-adrenoceptor stimulant (such as salbutamol or terbutaline, see p. 126 and p. 127); in addition to oxygen, assisted respiration and possibly emergency tracheotomy may be necessary.

An intravenous corticosteroid e.g. **hydrocortisone** (as sodium succinate) in a dose of 100–300 mg is of secondary value in the initial management of anaphylactic shock as the onset of action is delayed for several hours, but should be given to prevent further deterioration in severely affected patients.

When a patient is so ill that there is doubt as to the adequacy of the circulation, the initial injection of adrenaline may need to be given as a *dilute solution by the intravenous route*, for details of cautions, dose and strength, see under Intravenous Adrenaline, below.

Some patients with severe allergy to insect stings or foods are encouraged to carry pre-filled adrenaline syringes (e.g. *EpiPen®*) for *self-administration* during periods of risk.

ANGIOEDEMA

Angioedema is dangerous if *laryngeal oedema* is present. In this circumstance adrenaline injection and oxygen should be given as described under Anaphylaxis (see above); antihistamines and corticosteroids should also be given (see again above). Tracheal intubation and other measures may be necessary.

The administration of C_1 esterase inhibitor (in fresh frozen plasma or in partially purified form) may terminate acute attacks of *hereditary angioedema*, but is not practical for long-term prophylaxis.

INTRAMUSCULAR (OR SUBCUTANEOUS) ADRENALINE

The *intramuscular route* is the *first choice route* for the administration of adrenaline in the management of anaphylactic shock. Adrenaline has a rapid onset of action after intramuscular administration and in the shocked patient its absorption from the intramuscular site may be faster and more reliable than from the subcutaneous site (the intravenous route should be reserved for extreme emergency when there is doubt as to the adequacy of the circulation, for details of cautions, dose and strength see under Intravenous Adrenaline, below).

Patients with severe allergy should ideally be instructed in the self-administration of adrenaline by intramuscular injection (for details see under Self-administration of Adrenaline, below).

Prompt injection of adrenaline is of paramount importance and the recommendations in the following table avoid the need for complex dosage calculations in children.

Volume of adrenaline injection **1 in 1000** (1 mg/mL) for **intramuscular** injection (or alternatively **subcutaneous** injection) in anaphylactic shock

Age	Volume of adrenaline 1 in 1000
Under 1 year	0.05 mL
1 year	0.1 mL
2 years	0.2 mL[1]
3–4 years	0.3 mL[1]
5 years	0.4 mL[1]
6–12 years	0.5 mL[1]
Adult	0.5–1 mL

These doses may be repeated every 10 minutes, according to blood pressure and pulse, until improvement occurs (may be repeated several times).

1. Suitable for robust children in these age groups; for underweight children use half these doses.

INTRAVENOUS ADRENALINE

Where the patient is severely ill and there is real doubt about adequacy of the circulation and absorption from the intramuscular injection site, adrenaline may be given by **slow** *intravenous injection* in a dose of 500 micrograms (5 mL of the dilute 1 in 10 000 adrenaline injection) given at a rate of 100 micrograms (1 mL of the dilute 1 in 10 000 adrenaline injection) per minute, *stopping when a response has been obtained*; children can be given a dose of 10 micrograms/kg (0.1 mL/kg of the dilute 1 in 10 000 adrenaline injection) by **slow** *intravenous injection* over several minutes. Constant vigilance is needed to ensure that the *correct strength* is used; anaphylactic shock kits need to make a *very clear distinction* between the 1 in 10 000 strength and the 1 in 1000 strength. It is also important that, where intramuscular injection might still succeed, time should not be wasted seeking intravenous access.

For reference to the use of the intravenous route for *cardiac resuscitation*, see section 2.7.3.

SELF-ADMINISTRATION OF ADRENALINE

Individuals who are at considerable risk of anaphylaxis need to carry adrenaline with them at all times and need to be *instructed in advance* how to inject it. In addition, the packs need to be labelled so that in the case of rapid collapse someone else is able to administer the adrenaline. It is important to ensure that an adequate supply is provided to treat symptoms until medical assistance is available.

Some patients may best be able to cope with a pre-assembled syringe fitted with a needle suitable for very rapid administration (if necessary by a bystander). *EpiPen®* consists of a fully assembled syringe and needle delivering a dose of 300 micrograms of adrenaline by *intramuscular injection*; a 150-microgram version (*EpiPen® Jr*) is also available for use in children. Other products for the immediate treatment of anaphylaxis are available but are not licensed for use in the UK. *Anapen® Adult* is a fully assembled device that delivers 300 micrograms of adrenaline *by intramuscular injection*; a 150-microgram version (*Anapen® Junior*) is also available. *Anapen®* is available on a named-patient basis from Allerayde. *Ana-Guard®* is a pre-filled syringe that delivers two 300-microgram doses of adrenaline *by subcutaneous or intramuscular injection*; it can be adjusted to administer smaller doses for children. *Ana-Kit®* includes a similar pre-filled adrenaline syringe, chewable tablets of chlorpheniramine maleate 2 mg, 2 sterile pads impregnated with 70% isopropyl alcohol, and a tourniquet. *Ana-Guard®* and *Ana-Kit®* are available on a named-patient basis from IDIS.

ADRENALINE
(Epinephrine)

Indications: emergency treatment of acute anaphylaxis; angioedema; cardiopulmonary resuscitation (section 2.7.3)

Cautions: hyperthyroidism, diabetes mellitus, ischaemic heart disease, hypertension, elderly patients

INTERACTIONS. Severe anaphylaxis in patients on non-cardioselective beta-blockers may not respond to adrenaline injection calling for intravenous injection of salbutamol (see p. 126). Patients on tricyclic antidepressants are considerably more susceptible to arrhythmias calling for a much reduced dose of adrenaline. Other **interactions**, see Appendix 1 (sympathomimetics).

Side-effects: anxiety, tremor, tachycardia, arrhythmias, cold extremities; also hypertension (risk of cerebral haemorrhage) and pulmonary oedema (on excessive dosage or extreme sensitivity); nausea, vomiting, sweating, weakness, and dizziness also reported

Dose: acute anaphylaxis, *by intramuscular (or subcutaneous) injection*, see notes and table above
Acute anaphylaxis when there is doubt as to the adequacy of the circulation, *by intravenous injection* (dilute, extreme caution), see notes above

IMPORTANT. Intravenous route should be used with **extreme care**, see notes above

Intramuscular or subcutaneous
PoM **Adrenaline Injection, BP, 1 in 1000** (Non-proprietary)
Injection, adrenaline (as acid tartrate) 1 mg/mL, net price 0.5-mL amp = 39p; 1-mL amp = 29p
Available from Antigen, BCM Specials, Evans, Hillcross, Martindale, Phoenix

PoM **Min-I-Jet® Adrenaline** (IMS)
Injection, adrenaline (as hydrochloride) 1 in 1000 (1 mg/mL). Net price 1 mL (with 25 gauge × 0.25 inch needle for subcutaneous injection) = £7.37, 1 mL (with 21 gauge × 1.5 inch needle for intramuscular injection) = £3.91 (both disposable syringes)

Intravenous
Extreme caution, see notes above
PoM **Adrenaline Injection, 1 in 10 000** (Non-proprietary)
Injection, adrenaline (as acid tartrate) 100 micrograms/mL. 10-mL amp.
Available from Martindale (special order); also from Aurum (10-mL prefilled syringe) and IMS (Min-I-Jet® Adrenaline 3- and 10-mL disposable syringes)

Intramuscular injection for self-administration
PoM **EpiPen®** (ALK)
EpiPen® Auto-injector 0.3 mg (delivering a single dose of adrenaline 300 micrograms), adrenaline 1 mg/mL (1 in 1000), net price 2-mL *Auto-injector* = £23.50
Note. 1.7 mL of the solution remains in the *Auto-injector* after use
Dose: by intramuscular injection, ADULT and CHILD over 30 kg, 300 micrograms repeated after 15 minutes as necessary

Epipen® Jr Auto-injector 0.15 mg (delivering a single dose of adrenaline 150 micrograms), adrenaline 500 micrograms/mL (1 in 2000), net price 2-mL *Auto-injector* = £23.50
Note. 1.7 mL of the solution remains in the *Auto-injector* after use
Dose: by intramuscular injection, CHILD 15–30 kg, 10 micrograms/kg repeated after 10 minutes as necessary

3.5 Respiratory stimulants and pulmonary surfactants

3.5.1   Respiratory stimulants
3.5.2   Pulmonary surfactants

3.5.1   Respiratory stimulants

Respiratory stimulants (analeptic drugs) have a limited place in the treatment of ventilatory failure in patients with chronic obstructive airways disease. They are effective only when given by intravenous injection or infusion and have a short duration of action. Their use has largely been replaced by ventilatory support including nasal intermittent positive pressure ventilation. However, occasionally when ventilatory support is contra-indicated and in patients with hypercapnic respiratory failure who are becoming drowsy or comatose, respiratory stimulants in the short term may arouse patients sufficiently to co-operate and clear their secretions.

Respiratory stimulants can also be harmful in respiratory failure since they stimulate non-respiratory as well as respiratory muscles. They should only be given under **expert supervision** in hospital and must be combined with active physiotherapy. There is at present no oral respiratory stimulant available for long-term use in chronic respiratory failure.

Doxapram (section 15.1.7) is given by continuous intravenous infusion. Frequent arterial blood gas studies and pH measurements are necessary during treatment to ensure the correct dosage (for full details see section 15.1.7).

Nikethamide (now discontinued by most suppliers) is not recommended because the effective doses are close to those causing toxic effects, especially convulsions.

3.5.2   Pulmonary surfactants

A number of pulmonary surfactants have recently been developed for the management of respiratory distress syndrome (hyaline membrane disease) in preterm infants.

BERACTANT

Indications: treatment of respiratory distress syndrome in preterm infants who are intubated and receiving mechanical ventilation, whose heart rate and arterial oxygenation are continuously monitored

Cautions: continuous monitoring required to avoid hyperoxaemia (due to rapid improvement in arterial oxygen concentration)

Side-effects: pulmonary haemorrhage reported

Dose: by endotracheal tube, phospholipid 100 mg/kg equivalent to a volume of 4 mL/kg, preferably within 8 hours of birth; may be repeated within 48 hours at intervals of at least 6 hours for up to 4 doses

PoM Survanta® (Abbott)
Suspension, beractant (bovine lung extract) providing phospholipid 25 mg/mL, with lipids and proteins, Net price 8-mL vial = £306.43

COLFOSCERIL PALMITATE

Indications: see under Beractant (also prophylaxis of respiratory distress syndrome)

Cautions: see under Beractant

Side-effects: may increase incidence of pulmonary haemorrhage; obstruction of endotracheal tube by mucous secretions

Dose: by endotracheal tube, treatment, 67.5 mg/kg; if still intubated, may be repeated after 12 hours; prophylaxis, first dose soon after birth, if still intubated may be repeated 12 and 24 hours later

PoM Exosurf Neonatal® (GlaxoWellcome)
Suspension, colfosceril palmitate 108 mg for reconstitution with 8 mL water for injections (when reconstituted, contains 67.5 mg/5 mL). Net price per vial (with endotracheal tube connectors) = £306.43

PORACTANT ALFA

Indications: treatment of respiratory distress syndrome or hyaline membrane disease in neonates over 700 g (also prophylaxis of respiratory distress syndrome)

Cautions: see under Beractant

Side-effects: transient depression of cerebro-electrical activity

Dose: by endotracheal tube, treatment, 100–200 mg/kg; further doses of 100 mg/kg may be repeated at 12-hour intervals if still intubated; prophylaxis, 100–200 mg/kg soon after birth (preferably within 15 minutes); further doses of 100 mg/kg may be repeated 6–12 hours after the first dose and again 12 hours later if still intubated; max. total dose 300–400 mg/kg

PoM Curosurf® (Serono)
Suspension, poractant alfa (porcine lung phospholipid fraction) 80 mg/mL. Net price 1.5-mL vial = £400.00; 3-mL vial = £800.00

PUMACTANT

Indications: see under Beractant (also prophylaxis of respiratory distress syndrome)

Cautions: see under Beractant

Side-effects: obstruction of endotracheal tube

Dose: by endotracheal tube, 100 mg as soon as possible after intubation; may be repeated after 1 hour and again at 24 hours if still intubated

PoM Alec® (Britannia)
Suspension, pumactant 100 mg (synthetic lung phospholipids) for reconstitution with 1.2 mL cold sterile sodium chloride 0.9%. Net price per vial (with syringe and catheter) = £150.00

3.6   Oxygen

Oxygen should be regarded as a drug. It is prescribed for hypoxaemic patients to increase alveolar oxygen tension and decrease the work of breathing necessary to maintain a given arterial oxygen tension. The concentration depends on the condition being treated; an inappropriate concentration may have serious or even lethal effects.

High concentration oxygen therapy, with concentrations of up to 60% for short periods, is safe in conditions such as pneumonia, pulmonary thromboembolism, and fibrosing alveolitis. In such conditions low arterial oxygen ($P_a O_2$) is usually associated with low or normal arterial carbon dioxide ($P_a CO_2$), therefore there is little risk of hypoventilation and carbon dioxide retention.

In acute severe asthma, the arterial carbon dioxide ($P_a CO_2$) is usually subnormal but as asthma deteriorates may rise steeply (particularly in children). These patients usually require high concentrations of oxygen and if the arterial carbon dioxide ($P_a CO_2$) remains high despite other treatment intermittent positive pressure ventilation needs to be considered urgently. Where facilities for blood gas measurements are not immediately available, for example while transferring the patient to hospital, 35% to 50% oxygen delivered through a conventional mask is recommended. Exceptionally, asthma is diagnosed in patients with a long history of chronic bronchitis and probable respiratory failure; in these patients a lower concentration (24% to 28%) may be needed to limit oxygen-induced reduction of respiratory drive.

Low concentration oxygen therapy (controlled oxygen therapy) is reserved for patients with ventilatory failure due to chronic obstructive airways disease or other causes. The concentration should not exceed 28% and in some patients a concentration above 24% may be excessive. The aim is to provide the patient with just enough oxygen to improve hypoxaemia without worsening pre-existing carbon dioxide retention and respiratory acidosis. Treatment should be initiated in hospital as repeated blood gas measurements are required to estimate the correct concentration.

DOMICILIARY OXYGEN. Oxygen should only be prescribed for patients in the home after careful evaluation in hospital by respiratory experts; it should never be prescribed on a placebo basis.

Patients should be **advised of the fire risks** when receiving oxygen therapy.

OXYGEN CYLINDERS

Oxygen is occasionally prescribed for intermittent use for episodes of hypoxaemia of short duration, for example asthma. It is important, however, that the patient does not rely on oxygen instead of obtaining medical help or taking more specific treatment.

Alternatively, intermittent oxygen may be prescribed for patients with advanced irreversible respiratory disorders to increase mobility and capacity for exercise and to ease discomfort, for example in chronic obstructive bronchitis, emphysema, widespread fibrosis, and primary or thromboembolic pulmonary hypertension. Appropriate patients may be prescribed portable equipment through the hospital service, refillable from cylinders in the home.

Under the NHS oxygen may be supplied by pharmacy contractors as cylinders. Oxygen flow can be adjusted as the cylinders are equipped with an oxygen flow meter with 'medium' (2 litres/minute) and 'high' (4 litres/minute) settings. The Health Authorities have lists of pharmacy contractors who provide domiciliary oxygen services.

Patients are supplied with either constant or variable performance masks. The *Intersurgical 010 28%* or *Ventimask Mk IV 28%* are constant performance masks and provide a nearly constant supply of oxygen (28%) over a wide range irrespective of the patient's breathing pattern. The variable performance masks include the *Intersurgical 005 Mask* and the *Venticaire Mask*; the concentration of oxygen supplied to the patient varies with the rate of flow of oxygen and with the patient's breathing pattern.

PORTABLE OXYGEN CYLINDERS. Portable oxygen sets are not prescribable on the NHS since the fitting is not compatible with the Drug Tariff oxygen equipment. However, Medigas and BOC supply a portable oxygen cylinder called a 'PD oxygen cylinder', which has the same bull-nose fitting as the normal domiciliary headsets (prescriptions must therefore specify 'PD oxygen cylinder'). The PD oxygen cylinder holds about 300 litres of oxygen which will last approximately 2 hours at a standard flow rate of 2 litres/minute.

OXYGEN CONCENTRATORS

Long-term administration of oxygen (at least 15 hours daily) may prolong survival in patients with severe chronic obstructive airways disease with cor pulmonale.

Department of Health guidelines suggest that this treatment should be provided for patients who fulfil the following criteria:

$P_aO_2 < 7.3kPa$; $P_aCO_2 > 6kPa$;

FEV$_1$ < 1.5 litre and FVC < 2 litre

The measurements should be stable on two occasions at least three weeks apart after the patient has received appropriate bronchodilator therapy.

Less information is available on long-term oxygen in patients with a similar degree of hypoxaemia and airflow obstruction but no hypercapnia; the Department of Health suggests that these patients should not be denied this form of treatment but the effects of long-term therapy have not yet been assessed completely.

Increased respiratory depression is seldom a problem in patients with stable respiratory failure treated with low concentrations of oxygen although it may occur during exacerbations; patients and relatives should be warned to call for medical help if drowsiness or confusion occur.

Oxygen concentrators are more economical for patients requiring oxygen for long periods, and in England and Wales are now prescribable on the NHS on a regional tendering basis (see below). A concentrator was formerly only provided for a patient who required oxygen for 15 hours a day but it has been found to be cost-effective to provide one for a patient requiring it for 8 hours a day (or 21 cylinders per month).

PRESCRIBING ARRANGEMENTS FOR OXYGEN CONCENTRATORS

Prescribe concentrator and accessories (face mask, nasal cannula, and humidifier) on form FP10. Specify amount of oxygen required (hours per day) and flow rate. If required, prescribe back-up oxygen set and cylinder at same time. Inform patient that the supplier will be in contact to make arrangements and that the prescription form is to be given to the person who installs the concentrator.

Inform supplier by telephone (see table below) that a concentrator has been prescribed. The supplier will send written confirmation of the order to the prescriber, the patient, and the Health Authority.

Follow the same procedure if a back-up oxygen set and cylinder are required later.

Health Authority regional group	Supplier
Eastern	De Vilbiss Health Care UK Ltd
North Western	*to order*:
London North	Dial 0800 020202
North Wales	
West Midlands	
London South (includes Kent, Surrey, and Sussex)	Omnicare Group Ltd *to order:* Dial 0500 823773
Central and South Wales	Oxygen Therapy Co Ltd *to order:* Dial 0800 373580
Northern	
South Western	
Yorkshire (South and West) and Humberside	

In **Scotland** refer the patient for assessment by a respiratory consultant. If the need for a concentrator is confirmed the consultant will arrange for the provision of a concentrator through the Common Services Agency.

3.7   Mucolytics

Mucolytics are often prescribed to facilitate expectoration by reducing sputum viscosity in chronic asthma and bronchitis. Few patients, however, have been shown to derive much benefit from them although they do render sputum less viscid. Steam inhalation with postural drainage, is good expectorant therapy in bronchiectasis and some chronic bronchitics.

For reference to the newly introduced dornase alfa, see below.

CARBOCISTEINE

Indications: reduction of sputum viscosity
Contra-indications: active peptic ulceration

                    Prices are **net**, see p. 1

Side-effects: occasional gastro-intestinal irritation, rashes

Dose: 750 mg 3 times daily initially, then 1.5 g daily in divided doses; CHILD 2–5 years 62.5–125 mg 4 times daily, 6–12 years 250 mg 3 times daily

NHS * PoM **Carbocisteine Capsules** (Non-proprietary)

Capsules, carbocisteine 375 mg. Net price 30-cap pack = £4.48

NHS * PoM **Carbocisteine Syrup** (Non-proprietary)

Oral liquid, carbocisteine 125 mg/5 mL, net price 300 mL = £4.91; 250 mg/5 mL, 300 mL = £6.28

* except, for patients under the age of 18 years and in whom any condition which, through damage or disease, affects the airways and has required a tracheostomy and endorsed 'SLS'

Note. The brand name NHS Mucodyne® (Rhône-Poulenc Rorer) is used for carbocisteine preparations; capsules and 250 mg/5 mL strength of syrup contain tartrazine

METHYL CYSTEINE HYDROCHLORIDE
(Mecysteine Hydrochloride)

Indications: reduction of sputum viscosity

Dose: 100–200 mg 3–4 times daily before meals reduced to 200 mg twice daily after 6 weeks; CHILD over 5 years 100 mg 3 times daily

Prophylaxis, 100–200 mg 2–3 times every other day during winter months

NHS **Visclair®** (Sinclair)

Tablets, yellow, s/c, e/c, methyl cysteine hydrochloride 100 mg. Net price 20 = £3.66. Label: 5, 22, 25

DORNASE ALFA

Dornase alfa is a genetically engineered version of a naturally occurring human enzyme which cleaves extracellular deoxyribonucleic acid (DNA). It is administered by inhalation using a jet nebuliser (section 3.1.5).

DORNASE ALFA
Phosphorylated glycosylated recombinant human deoxyribonuclease 1 (rhDNase)

Indications: management of cystic fibrosis patients with a forced vital capacity (FVC) of greater than 40% of predicted to improve pulmonary function

Cautions: pregnancy (Appendix 4)

Side-effects: pharyngitis, voice changes, chest pain; occasionally laryngitis, rashes, urticaria, conjunctivitis

Dose: by inhalation of nebulised solution (by jet nebuliser), 2500 units (2.5 mg) once daily (patients over 21 years may benefit from twice daily dosage); CHILD under 5 years not recommended

▼ PoM **Pulmozyme®** (Roche)

Nebuliser solution, dornase alfa 1000 units (1 mg)/mL. Net price 2.5-mL (2500 units) vial = £20.39

Note. For use undiluted with jet nebulisers only; ultrasonic nebulisers are unsuitable

3.8 Aromatic inhalations

Inhalations containing volatile substances such as eucalyptus oil are traditionally used and although the vapour may contain little of the additive it encourages deliberate inspiration of warm moist air which is often comforting in bronchitis; boiling water should not be used owing to the risk of scalding. Inhalations are also used for the relief of nasal obstruction in acute rhinitis or sinusitis.

CHILDREN. The use of strong aromatic decongestants (applied as rubs or to pillows) is not advised for infants under the age of 3 months. Mothers with young infants in whom nasal obstruction with mucus is a problem can readily be taught appropriate techniques of suction aspiration.

Benzoin Tincture, Compound, BP
(Friars' Balsam)

Tincture, balsamic acids approx. 4.5%. Label: 15

Directions for use: add one teaspoonful to a pint of hot, **not** boiling, water and inhale the vapour

Menthol and Eucalyptus Inhalation, BP 1980

Inhalation, racementhol or levomenthol 2 g, eucalyptus oil 10 mL, light magnesium carbonate 7 g, water to 100 mL

Directions for use: add one teaspoonful to a pint of hot, **not** boiling, water and inhale the vapour

NHS **Karvol®** (Crookes)

Inhalation capsules, levomenthol 35.55 mg, with chlorbutol, pine oils, terpineol, and thymol. Net price 10-cap pack = £1.14; 20-cap pack = £2.07

Inhalation solution, levomenthol 7.92 mg with chlorbutol, pine oils, terpineol, and thymol. Net price 12-mL dropper bottle = £1.56

Directions for use: inhale vapour from contents of 1 capsule *or* 6 drops of solution expressed into handkerchief or a pint of hot, **not** boiling, water; avoid in infants under 3 months

3.9 Cough preparations

3.9.1 Cough suppressants
3.9.2 Expectorant and demulcent cough preparations

3.9.1 Cough suppressants

The drawbacks of prescribing cough suppressants are rarely outweighed by the benefits of treatment and only occasionally are they useful, as, for example, if sleep is disturbed by a dry cough. Cough suppressants may cause sputum retention and this may be harmful in patients with chronic bronchitis and bronchiectasis.

Opioid cough suppressants such as codeine, dextromethorphan, and pholcodine are seldom sufficiently potent to be effective in severe cough; all tend to cause constipation.

Sedating antihistamines, such as diphenhydramine, are used as the cough suppressant component of many compound cough preparations on sale to the public; all tend to cause drowsiness which may reflect their main mode of action.

CHILDREN. The use of cough suppressants containing codeine or similar opioid analgesics is not generally recommended in children and should be avoided altogether in those under 1 year of age.

CODEINE PHOSPHATE

Indications: dry or painful cough
Cautions: asthma; hepatic and renal impairment; history of drug abuse; see also notes above and section 4.7.2; **interactions:** Appendix 1 (opioid analgesics)
Contra-indications: liver disease, ventilatory failure
Side-effects: constipation, respiratory depression in sensitive patients or if given large doses

PoM [1] **Codeine Linctus, BP**
Linctus, codeine phosphate 15 mg/5 mL. Net price 100 mL = 38p (diabetic, 68p)
Dose: 5–10 mL 3–4 times daily; CHILD 5–12 years, 2.5–5 mL
Available from APS, Cox, Galen (Galcodine®, sugar-free), Norton
Note. BP 1993 directs that when Diabetic Codeine Linctus is prescribed, Codeine Linctus formulated with a vehicle appropriate for administration to diabetics, whether or not labelled 'Diabetic Codeine Linctus', shall be dispensed or supplied
1. Can be sold to the public provided the maximum single dose does not exceed 5 mL
Codeine Linctus, Paediatric, BP
Linctus, codeine phosphate 3 mg/5 mL. Net price 100 mL = 20p
Dose: CHILD 1–5 years 5 mL 3–4 times daily
Available from Evans, Galen (Galcodine® Paediatric, sugar-free)
Note. BP 1993 directs that Paediatric Codeine Linctus may be prepared extemporaneously by diluting Codeine Linctus with a suitable vehicle in accordance with the manufacturer's instructions
For a list of **cough and decongestant preparations on sale to the public,** including those containing codeine, see section 3.9.2

PHOLCODINE

Indications: dry or painful cough
Cautions; Contra-indications; Side-effects: see under Codeine Phosphate

Pholcodine Linctus, BP
Linctus, pholcodine 5 mg/5 mL in a suitable flavoured vehicle, containing citric acid monohydrate 1%. Net price 100 mL = 25p
Dose: 5–10 mL 3–4 times daily; CHILD 5–12 years 2.5–5 mL
Available from APS, Boehringer Ingelheim (Pavacol-D®, sugar-free), Cox, Galen (Galenphol®, sugar-free), Norton
Pholcodine Linctus, Strong, BP
Linctus, pholcodine 10 mg/5 mL in a suitable flavoured vehicle, containing citric acid monohydrate 2%. Net price 100 mL = 36p
Dose: 5 mL 3–4 times daily
Available from APS (sugar-free), Cox, Norton

Galenphol® (Galen)
Paediatric linctus, orange, sugar-free, pholcodine 2 mg/5 mL. Net price 90-mL pack = £1.11
Dose: CHILD 1–5 years 5 mL 3 times daily; 6–12 years 5–10 mL
For a list of **cough and decongestant preparations on sale to the public,** including those containing pholcodine, see section 3.9.2

PALLIATIVE CARE

Diamorphine and methadone are available in linctuses to control distressing cough in terminal lung cancer although morphine is now preferred (see Palliative Care, p. 13). In other circumstances they are contra-indicated because they induce sputum retention and ventilatory failure as well as causing opioid dependence.

DIAMORPHINE HYDROCHLORIDE

Indications: cough in terminal disease
Cautions; Contra-indications; Side-effects: see notes in section 4.7.2; more potent than morphine
Dose: see below

CD Diamorphine Linctus, BPC 1973
Linctus, diamorphine hydrochloride 3 mg, oxymel 1.25 mL, glycerol 1.25 mL, compound tartrazine solution 0.06 mL, syrup to 5 mL. It should be recently prepared. Label: 2
Dose: 2.5–10 mL every 4 hours

METHADONE HYDROCHLORIDE

Indications: cough in terminal disease
Cautions; Contra-indications; Side-effects: see notes in section 4.7.2; longer-acting than morphine therefore effects may be cumulative
Dose: see below

CD Methadone Linctus
Linctus, methadone hydrochloride 2 mg/5 mL in a suitable vehicle with a tolu flavour. Label: 2
Dose: 2.5–5 mL every 4–6 hours, reduced to twice daily on prolonged use

MORPHINE HYDROCHLORIDE

Indications: cough in terminal disease (see also p. 13)
Cautions; Contra-indications; Side-effects: see notes in section 4.7.2
Dose: initially 5 mg every 4 hours

Preparations
See section 4.7.2

3.9.2   Expectorant and demulcent cough preparations

Expectorants are claimed to promote expulsion of bronchial secretions but there is no evidence that any drug can specifically facilitate expectoration. The assumption that sub-emetic doses of expectorants, such as ammonium chloride, ipecacuanha, and squill promote expectoration is a myth. However, a simple expectorant mixture may serve a useful placebo function and has the advantage of being inexpensive.

Demulcent cough preparations contain soothing substances such as syrup or glycerol and certainly some patients believe that such preparations relieve a dry irritating cough. Preparations such as **simple linctus** have the advantage of being harmless and inexpensive; **paediatric simple linctus** is particularly useful in children and sugar-free versions are available.

Compound cough preparations are on sale to the public; the rationale for some is dubious.

Ammonia and Ipecacuanha Mixture, BP

Mixture, ammonium bicarbonate 200 mg, liquorice liquid extract 0.5 mL, ipecacuanha tincture 0.3 mL, concentrated camphor water 0.1 mL, concentrated anise water 0.05 mL, double-strength chloroform water 5 mL, water to 10 mL. It should be recently prepared
Dose: 10–20 mL 3–4 times daily

Simple Linctus, BP

Linctus, citric acid monohydrate 2.5% in a suitable vehicle with an anise flavour. Net price 100 mL = 17p
Dose: 5 mL 3–4 times daily
A sugar-free version is available from Pinewood and various wholesalers.

Simple Linctus, Paediatric, BP

Linctus, citric acid monohydrate 0.625% in a suitable vehicle with an anise flavour. Net price 100 mL = 16p
Dose: CHILD, 5–10 mL 3–4 times daily
A sugar-free version is available from Pinewood and various wholesalers.

3.10 Systemic nasal decongestants

These preparations are of doubtful value but unlike the preparations for local application (see section 12.2.2) they do not give rise to rebound nasal congestion. They contain sympathomimetics, and should therefore be **avoided** in patients with hypertension, hyperthyroidism, coronary heart disease, or diabetes, and in patients taking monoamine-oxidase inhibitors; **interactions:** Appendix 1 (sympathomimetics). Many of the preparations also contain antihistamines which may cause drowsiness and affect ability to drive or operate machinery.

The main ingredients in systemic nasal decongestant preparations are shown in the list of cough and decongestant preparations on sale to the public.

PSEUDOEPHEDRINE HYDROCHLORIDE

Indications; Dose: see notes above and under preparations
Cautions; Side-effects: see under Ephedrine Hydrochloride (section 3.1.1.2)

Galpseud® (Galen)
Tablets, pseudoephedrine hydrochloride 60 mg. Net price 20 = 87p
Dose: 1 tablet 4 times daily
Linctus, orange, sugar-free, pseudoephedrine hydrochloride 30 mg/5 mL. Net price 140 mL = £1.70
Dose: 10 mL 3 times daily; CHILD 2–6 years 2.5 mL, 6–12 years 5 mL
Sudafed® (Warner Lambert)
Tablets, red, f/c, pseudoephedrine hydrochloride 60 mg. Net price 20 = £1.15
Dose: 1 tablet every 4–6 hours (up to 4 times daily)
Elixir, red, pseudoephedrine hydrochloride 30 mg/5 mL. Net price 100 mL = £1.23
Dose: 10 mL every 4–6 hours (up to 4 times daily); CHILD 2–5 years 2.5 mL, 6–12 years 5 mL

Systemic cough and decongestant preparations on sale to the public, together with their significant ingredients.
Important: in overdose contact **Poisons Information Services** (p. 18) for full details of the ingredients.

Actifed® (pseudoephedrine, triprolidine), **Actifed Compound Linctus®** (dextromethorphan, pseudoephedrine, triprolidine), **Actifed Expectorant®** (guaiphenesin, pseudoephedrine, triprolidine), **Actifed Junior Cough Relief®** (dextromethorphan, triprolidine), **Adult Meltus® Expectorant with Decongestant** (guaiphenesin, pseudoephedrine, menthol), **Advil Cold and Sinus®** (ibuprofen, pseudoephedrine), **Anidox Spansules®** (diphenylpyraline, phenylpropanolamine)

Baby Meltus® (dilute acetic acid), **Balm of Gilead Cough Mixture®** (Gilead extract, squill, lobelia), **Barum Cold Relief with Decongestant®** (paracetamol, phenylephrine), **Beechams All-In-One®** (guaiphenesin, paracetamol, phenylephrine), **Beechams Flu-Plus Caplets®** (paracetamol, phenylephrine), **Beechams Hot Lemon®**, **Hot Lemon and Honey®**, **Hot Blackcurrant®**, **Beechams Powders Capsules® with Decongestant** (paracetamol, phenylephrine), **Benylin Chesty Cough®** (ammonium chloride, diphenhydramine, menthol), **Benylin Children's Chesty Cough®** (guaiphenesin), **Benylin Children's Cough®** (diphenhydramine, menthol), **Benylin Children's Dry Cough®** (pholcodine), **Benylin Children's Night Cough®** (diphenhydramine), **Benylin with Codeine®** (codeine, diphenhydramine, menthol), **Benylin Cough and**

Congestion® (dextromethorphan, diphenhydramine, menthol, pseudoephedrine), **Benylin Dry Cough®** (dextromethorphan, diphenhydramine, menthol), **Benylin Four Flu®** (diphenhydramine, paracetamol, pseudoephedrine), **Benylin Non-drowsy for Chesty Coughs®** (guaiphenesin, menthol), **Benylin Non-drowsy for Dry Coughs®** (dextromethorphan), **Benylin Sugar-free for Children®** (diphenhydramine, menthol), **Benylin Day and Night Cold and Flu Relief®** (day tablets, paracetamol, phenylpropanolamine, night tablets, paracetamol, diphenhydramine), **Boots Bronchial Cough Mixture®** (ammonium carbonate, ammonium chloride, guaiphenesin), **Boots Catarrh Syrup for Children®** (diphenhydramine, pseudoephedrine), **Boots Catarrh Cough Syrup®** (codeine, creosote), **Boots Cold Capsules®** (diphenylpyraline, phenylpropanolamine), **Boots Cold and Influenza Mixture®** (squill, ammonium acetate), **Boots Cold Relief Tablets®** (paracetamol, phenylephrine), **Boots Cough Linctus for Children®** (ephedrine, ipecacuanha), **Boots Cough Relief for Children®** (diphenhydramine, pholcodine), **Boots Day Cold Comfort®** (paracetamol, pholcodine, pseudoephedrine), **Boots Day-time Cough Relief®** (pholcodine), **Boots Decongestant Tablets®** (pseudoephedrine), **Boots Night-Cold Comfort®** (diphenhydramine, paracetamol, pholcodine, pseudo-

---

ephedrine), **Boots Night-time Cough Relief**® (diphenhydramine, pholcodine), **Bronal**® (dextromethorphan), **Bronalin Decongestant Elixir**® (pseudoephedrine), **Bronalin Dry Cough**® (dextromethorphan, pseudoephedrine), **Bronalin Expectorant**® (ammonium chloride, diphenhydramine), **Bronalin Junior Linctus**® (diphenhydramine), **Buttercup Syrup Traditional**® (squill), **Buttercup Honey and Lemon**® and **Blackcurrant**® (ipecacuanha, menthol)

Cabdrivers® and **Cabdrivers Sugar-free**® (dextromethorphan, menthol), **Cabdrivers Junior**® (ephedrine), **CAM**® (ephedrine), **Catarrh-Ex**® (paracetamol, pseudoephedrine), **Coldrex Blackcurrant Powders**®, **Hot Lemon Powders**® and **Tablets**® (paracetamol, phenylephrine), **Contac 400**® (phenylpropanolamine, chlorpheniramine), **Contac CoughCaps**® (dextromethorphan), **Covonia**® (dextromethorphan, menthol), **Covonia for Children**® (dextromethorphan, menthol), **Cupal Baby Cough**® (dilute acetic acid)

Davenol® (carbinoxamine, ephedrine, pholcodine), **Day Nurse**®, **Day Nurse Hot**® (dextromethorphan, paracetamol, phenylpropanolamine), **Dimotane Elixir**®, **Tablets**® and **Dimotane LA**® (brompheniramine), **Dimotane Expectorant**® (brompheniramine, guaiphenesin, pseudoephedrine), **Dimotane Co**® and **Dimotane Co Paediatric**® (brompheniramine, codeine, pseudoephedrine),**Dimotane Plus**® and **Dimotane Plus Paediatric**® (brompheniramine, pseudoephedrine), **Dimotapp**®, **Dimotapp Paediatric**®, and **Dimotapp LA**® (brompheniramine, phenylephrine, phenylpropanolamine), **Do-Do Expectorant**® (guaiphenesin), **Do-Do Chesteze**® (ephedrine, theophylline), **Dristan Tablets**® (aspirin, chlorpheniramine, phenylephrine)

Ecdylin® (ammonium chloride, diphenhydramine), **ES Bronchial**® (ammonium bicarbonate, ipecacuanha, senna, squill), **Eskornade**® (diphenylpyraline, phenylpropanolamine), **Evacode**® (codeine), **Evaphol**® (pholcodine), **Expulin**® (chlorpheniramine, menthol, pholcodine, pseudoephedrine), **Expulin Chesty Cough**® (guaiphenisin, menthol), **Expulin Decongestant for Babies and Children**® (chlorpheniramine, ephedrine, menthol), **Expulin Dry**® (menthol, pholcodine), **Expulin Paediatric**® chlorpheniramine, menthol, pholcodine)

Famel Expectorant® (guaiphenesin), **Famel Original**® (codeine, creosote), **Fennings Little Healers**® (ipecacuanha), **Fisherman's Friend Honey Cough Syrup**® (cineole, menthol, squill), **Franol**® and **Franol Plus**® (both ephedrine, theophylline), **Franolyn Chesty**® (ephedrine, guaiphenesin, theophylline), **Franolyn Dry**® (dextromethorphan)

Galcodine® (codeine), **Galcodine Paediatric**® (codeine), **Galenphol**® (pholcodine), **Galenphol Paediatric**® (pholcodine), **Galenphol Strong**® (pholcodine), **Galloway's**® (ipecacuanha, squill), **Galpseud**® (pseudoephedrine), **Galpseud Plus**® (chlorpheniramine, pseudoephedrine), **Gee's Linctus**® (opium, squill, tolu), **Guanor Expectorant**® (ammonium chloride, diphenhydramine, menthol)

Haymine® (chlorpheniramine, ephedrine), **Hill's Balsam Adult Expectorant**® (ipecacuanha, pholcodine), **Hill's Balsam Cough Suppressant**® (pholcodine), **Histalix**® (ammonium chloride, diphenhydramine, menthol)

Jackson's All Fours® (guaiphenesin), **Junior Lemsip**® (paracetamol, phenylephrine), **Junior Meltus Dry Cough**® (dextromethorphan, pseudoephedrine), **Junior Meltus Expectorant**® (guaiphenesin), **Junior Mucron**® (ipecacuanha, phenylpropanolamine)

Lem-Plus Capsules® (paracetamol, phenylephrine), **Lemsip Lemcaps**®, **Lemsip Flu Strength**®, **Lemsip Lemon**® or **Blackcurrant**®, **Lemsip Junior**®,

Lemsip Menthol Extra® (all paracetamol, phenylephrine), **Lemsip Chesty Cough**® (guaiphenesin), **Lemsip Expectorant**® (ammonium chloride, diphenhydramine), **Lemsip Flu Strength Nightime**® (chlorpheniramine, dextromethorphan, paracetamol, phenylpropanolamine), **Lemsip Power +**® (ibuprofen, pseudoephedrine), **Liqufruta Honey and Lemon**®, **Blackcurrant**® (ipecacuanha, menthol), **Liqufruta Garlic**® (guaiphenesin)

Medised® (paracetamol, promethazine), **Melo**® (ipecacuanha), **Meltus Baby**® (dilute acetic acid), **Meltus Dry Cough**® (dextromethorphan, pseudoephedrine), **Meltus Expectorant**®, **Meltus Honey and Lemon**® (guaiphenesin), **Mu-Cron Tablets**® (paracetamol, phenylpropanolamine)

Night Nurse® (dextromethorphan, paracetamol, promethazine), **Nirolex**® (ephedrine, guaiphenesin, menthol), **Nirolex for Children**® (guaiphenesin), **Numark Cold Relief Capsules**® **With Decongestant** (paracetamol, phenylephrine), **Numark Cold Relief Powders**® (paracetamol), **Nurofen Cold and Flu**® (ibuprofen, pseudoephedrine), **Nurse Sykes Balsam**® (guaiphenesin)

Owbridges® (dilute acetic acid, guaiphenesin, ammonium acetate)

Pavacol D® (pholcodine), **Phensedyl Plus**® (promethazine, pholcodine, pseudoephedrine), **Procol**® (pseudoephedrine), **Pulmo Bailly**® (codeine, guaiacol)

Robitussin Chesty Cough® (guaiphenesin), **Robitussin Chesty Cough with Congestion**® (guaiphenesin, pseudoephedrine), **Robitussin Dry Cough**® (dextromethorphan), **Robitussin Junior Persistant Cough**® (dextromethorphan), **Robitussin Night-Time**® (brompheniramine, codeine, pseudoephedrine)

Secron® (ephedrine, vinegar of ipecacuanha), **Sinutab**® (paracetamol, phenylpropanolamine), **Sinutab Nightime**® (paracetamol, phenylpropanolamine, phenyltoloxamine), **SP Cold Relief Capsules**® (paracetamol, phenylephrine), **Sudafed**® (pseudoephedrine), **Sudafed Co**® (paracetamol, pseudoephedrine), **Sudafed Expectorant**® (guaiphenesin, pseudoephedrine), **Sudafed Linctus**® (dextromethorphan, pseudoephedrine), **Sudafed Plus**® (pseudoephedrine, triprolidine)

Tancolin® (dextromethorphan), **Terpoin**® (cineole, codeine, menthol), **Throaties Family Cough Linctus**® (ipecacuanha), **Tixylix Catarrh**® (diphenhydramine, menthol), **Tixylix Chesty Cough**® (guaiphenesin), **Tixylix Cough and Cold**® (chlorpheniramine, pholcodine, pseudoephedrine), **Tixylix Daytime**® (pholcodine), **Tixylix Night-time**® (pholcodine, promethazine), **Triogesic**® (paracetamol, phenylpropanolamine), **Triominic**® (pheniramine, phenylpropanolamine)

Uniflu with Gregovite C® (codeine, diphenhydramine, paracetamol, phenylephrine)

Venos for Dry Coughs®, **Venos Expectorant**® (guaiphenesin), **Venos Honey and Lemon**®, **Vicks Action**® (ibuprofen, pseudoephedrine), **Vicks Children's Vaposyrup Dry Cough**® (dextromethorphan), **Vicks Coldcare**® (paracetamol, dextromethorphan, phenylpropanolamine), **Vicks Expectorant Cough Syrup**® (guaiphenesin), **Vicks Medinite**® (dextromethorphan, doxylamine, ephedrine, paracetamol), **Vicks Original Formula**® (honey, menthol), **Vicks Vaposyrup Chesty Cough**® (guaiphenesin), **Vicks Vaposyrup Dry Cough**® (dextromethorphan), **Vicks Vaposyrup Chesty Coughs and Nasal Congestion**® (guaiphenesin, phenylpropanolamine), **Vicks Vaposyrup Dry Coughs and Nasal Congestion**® (dextromethorphan, phenylpropanolamine)

4: Drugs acting on the
CENTRAL NERVOUS SYSTEM

In this chapter, drug treatments are discussed under the following headings:

4.1 Hypnotics and anxiolytics

Most anxiolytics ('sedatives') will induce sleep when given at night and most hypnotics will sedate when given during the day. Prescribing of these drugs is widespread but dependence (both physical and psychological) and tolerance occurs. This may lead to difficulty in withdrawing the drug after the patient has been taking it regularly for more than a few weeks (see Dependence and Withdrawal, below). Hypnotics and anxiolytics should therefore, be reserved for short courses to alleviate acute conditions after causal factors have been established.

Benzodiazepines are the most commonly used anxiolytics and hypnotics; they act at benzodiazepine receptors which are associated with gamma-aminobutyric acid (GABA) receptors. Older drugs such as meprobamate and barbiturates (section 4.1.3) are **not** recommended—they have more side-effects and interactions than benzodiazepines and are much more dangerous in overdosage.

PARADOXICAL EFFECTS. A paradoxical increase in hostility and aggression may be reported by patients taking benzodiazepines. The effects range from talkativeness and excitement, to aggressive and antisocial acts. Adjustment of the dose (up or down) usually attenuates the impulses. Increased anxiety and perceptual disorders are other paradoxical effects. Increased hostility and aggression after barbiturates and alcohol usually indicates intoxication.

DRIVING. Hypnotics and anxiolytics may impair judgement and increase reaction time, and so affect ability to drive or operate machinery; they increase the effects of alcohol. Moreover, the hangover effects of a night dose may impair driving on the following day.

DEPENDENCE AND WITHDRAWAL. Withdrawal of a benzodiazepine should be gradual as abrupt withdrawal may produce confusion, toxic psychosis, convulsions, or a condition resembling delirium tremens. Abrupt withdrawal of an older drug, such as a barbiturate (section 4.1.3), may be even more likely to have serious effects.

The benzodiazepine withdrawal syndrome may not develop until up to 3 weeks after stopping a long-acting benzodiazepine, but may occur within a few hours in the case of a short-acting one. It is characterised by insomnia, anxiety, loss of appetite and body-weight, tremor, perspiration, tinnitus, and perceptual disturbances. These symptoms may be similar to the original complaint and encourage further prescribing; some symptoms may continue for weeks or months after stopping benzodiazepines entirely.

A benzodiazepine can be withdrawn in steps of about one-eighth (range one-tenth to one-quarter) of the daily dose every fortnight. A suggested withdrawal protocol for patients who have difficulty is as follows:

1. Transfer patient to equivalent daily dose of diazepam[1] preferably taken at night
2. Reduce diazepam dose in fortnightly steps of 2 or 2.5 mg; if withdrawal symptoms occur, maintain this dose until symptoms improve
3. Reduce dose further, if necessary in smaller fortnightly steps[2]; it is better to reduce too slowly rather than too quickly
4. Stop completely; time needed for withdrawal can vary from about 4 weeks to a year or more

Counselling may help; beta-blockers should **only** be tried if other measures fail; antidepressants should **only** be used if clinical depression present; **avoid** antipsychotics (which may aggravate withdrawal symptoms)

> **CSM advice**
> 1. Benzodiazepines are indicated for the short-term relief (two to four weeks only) of anxiety that is severe, disabling or subjecting the individual to unacceptable distress, occurring alone or in association with insomnia or short-term psychosomatic, organic or psychotic illness.
> 2. The use of benzodiazepines to treat short-term 'mild' anxiety is inappropriate and unsuitable.
> 3. Benzodiazepines should be used to treat insomnia only when it is severe, disabling, or subjecting the individual to extreme distress.

1. Approximate equivalent doses, diazepam 5 mg
   ≡ chlordiazepoxide 15 mg
   ≡ loprazolam 0.5–1 mg
   ≡ lorazepam 500 micrograms
   ≡ lormetazepam 0.5–1 mg
   ≡ nitrazepam 5 mg
   ≡ oxazepam 15 mg
   ≡ temazepam 10 mg
2. Steps may be adjusted according to initial dose and duration of treatment and can range from diazepam 500 micrograms (one-quarter of a 2-mg tablet) to 2.5 mg

4.1.1   Hypnotics

Before a hypnotic is prescribed the cause of the insomnia should be established and, where possible, underlying factors should be treated. However, it should be noted that some patients have unrealistic sleep expectations, and others understate their alcohol consumption which is often the cause of the insomnia.

Transient insomnia may occur in those who normally sleep well and may be due to extraneous factors such as noise, shift work, and jet lag. If a hypnotic is indicated one that is rapidly eliminated should be chosen, and only one or two doses should be given.

Short-term insomnia is usually related to an emotional problem or serious medical illness. It may last for a few weeks and may recur; a hypnotic can be useful but should not be given for more than three weeks (preferably only one week). Intermittent use is desirable with omission of some doses. A rapidly eliminated drug is generally appropriate.

Chronic insomnia is rarely benefited by hypnotics and is more often due to mild dependence caused by injudicious prescribing. Psychiatric disorders such as anxiety, depression, and abuse of drugs and alcohol are common causes. Sleep disturbance is very common in depressive illness and early wakening is often a useful pointer. The underlying psychiatric complaint should be treated, adapting the drug regimen to alleviate insomnia. For example, amitriptyline, prescribed for depression, will also help to promote sleep if it is taken at night. Other causes of insomnia include daytime cat-napping and physical causes such as pain, pruritus, and dyspnoea.

Hypnotics should **not** be prescribed indiscriminately and routine prescribing is undesirable. They should be reserved for short courses in the acutely distressed. Tolerance to their effects develops within 3 to 14 days of continuous use and long-term efficacy cannot be assured. A major drawback of long-term use is that withdrawal causes rebound insomnia and precipitates a withdrawal syndrome (section 4.1).

Where prolonged administration is unavoidable hypnotics should be discontinued as soon as feasible and the patient warned that sleep may be disturbed for a few days before normal rhythm is re-established; broken sleep with vivid dreams and increased REM (rapid eye movement) may persist for several weeks.

- CHILDREN. The prescribing of hypnotics to children, except for occasional use such as for night terrors and somnambulism (sleep-walking), is not justified.

ELDERLY. Hypnotics should be avoided in the elderly, who are at risk of becoming ataxic and confused and so liable to fall and injure themselves.

BENZODIAZEPINES

Benzodiazepines used as hypnotics include **nitrazepam**, **flunitrazepam**, and **flurazepam** which have a prolonged action and may give rise to residual effects on the following day; repeated doses tend to be cumulative.

Loprazolam, **lormetazepam**, and **temazepam** act for a shorter time and they have little or no hangover effect. Withdrawal phenomena however are more common with the short-acting benzodiazepines.

Benzodiazepine anxiolytics such as **diazepam** given as a single dose at night may also be used as hypnotics.

For general guidelines on benzodiazepine prescribing see section 4.1.2 and for benzodiazepine withdrawal see section 4.1.

NITRAZEPAM

Indications: insomnia (short-term use)

Cautions: respiratory disease, muscle weakness, history of drug or alcohol abuse, marked personality disorder, pregnancy and breast-feeding (Appendixes 4 and 5); reduce dose in elderly and debilitated, and in hepatic (avoid if severe) and renal impairment (Appendixes 2 and 3); avoid prolonged use (and abrupt withdrawal thereafter); porphyria (section 9.8.2); **interactions:** Appendix 1 (anxiolytics and hypnotics)

DRIVING. Drowsiness may persist the next day and affect performance of skilled tasks (e.g. driving); effects of alcohol enhanced

Contra-indications: respiratory depression; acute pulmonary insufficiency; severe hepatic impairment, myasthenia gravis, sleep apnoea syndrome; not for phobic or obsessional states and not for use alone to treat depression (or anxiety associated with depression) or chronic psychosis

Side-effects: drowsiness and lightheadedness the next day; confusion and ataxia (especially in the elderly); amnesia may occur; dependence; see also under Diazepam (section 4.1.2); **overdosage:** see Emergency Treatment of Poisoning, p. 23

Dose: 5–10 mg at bedtime; ELDERLY (or debilitated) 2.5–5 mg; CHILD not recommended

PoM **Nitrazepam** (Non-proprietary)

Tablets, nitrazepam 5 mg, net price 20 = 16p. Label: 19

Available from APS, Berk, Cox, CP, DDSA (NHS Remnos®), Norton, Roche (NHS Mogadon®), Unigreg (NHS Unisomnia®)

Oral suspension, nitrazepam 2.5 mg/5 mL. Net price 150 mL = £4.95. Label: 19

Available from Norgine (NHS Somnite®)

FLUNITRAZEPAM

Indications: insomnia (short-term use)

Cautions; Contra-indications; Side-effects: see under Nitrazepam

Dose: 0.5–1 mg at bedtime; max. 2 mg; ELDERLY (or debilitated) 500 micrograms (max. 1 mg); CHILD not recommended

NHS PoM **Rohypnol**® (Roche)

Tablets, purple, f/c, scored, flunitrazepam 1 mg. Net price 30-tab pack = £4.41. Label: 19

FLURAZEPAM

Indications: insomnia (short-term use)
Cautions; Contra-indications; Side-effects: see under Nitrazepam
Dose: 15–30 mg at bedtime; ELDERLY (or debilitated) 15 mg; CHILD not recommended

NHS PoM **Dalmane®** (Roche)
Capsules, flurazepam (as hydrochloride), 15 mg (grey/yellow), net price 30-cap pack = £2.92; 30 mg (black/grey), 30-cap pack = £3.75. Label: 19

LOPRAZOLAM

Indications: insomnia (short-term use)
Cautions; Contra-indications; Side-effects: see under Nitrazepam
Dose: 1 mg at bedtime, increased to 1.5 or 2 mg if required; ELDERLY (or debilitated) 0.5–1 mg; CHILD not recommended

PoM **Loprazolam** (Non-proprietary)
Tablets, loprazolam 1 mg (as mesylate). Net price 28-tab pack = £4.46. Label: 19
Available from Hoechst Marion Roussel (previously NHS Dormonoct®)

LORMETAZEPAM

Indications: insomnia (short-term use)
Cautions; Contra-indications; Side-effects: see under Nitrazepam; shorter acting
Dose: 0.5–1.5 mg at bedtime; ELDERLY (or debilitated) 500 micrograms; CHILD not recommended

PoM **Lormetazepam** (Non-proprietary)
Tablets, lormetazepam 500 micrograms, net price 20 = 53p; 1 mg, 20 = 96p. Label: 19
Available from APS, Cox, Norton, Wyeth

TEMAZEPAM

Indications: insomnia (short-term use); see also section 15.1.4.1 for peri-operative use
Cautions; Contra-indications; Side-effects: see under Nitrazepam; shorter acting
Dose: 10–20 mg at bedtime, exceptional circumstances 30–40 mg; ELDERLY (or debilitated) 10 mg at bedtime, exceptional circumstances 20 mg; CHILD not recommended

CD [1] **Temazepam** (Non-proprietary)
NHS *Gel-filled capsules* (soft gelatin), temazepam 10 mg, net price 20 = 37p; 15 mg, 20 = 62p; 20 mg, 20 = 60p; 30 mg, 20 = £1.24. Label: 19
Note. The name NHS Temazepam Gelthix® is used for some gel-filled capsules
WARNING. Gel-filled capsules may be particularly subject to abuse; gangrene has followed abuse by injection
Tablets, temazepam 10 mg, net price 20 = 67p; 20 mg, 20 = £1.13. Label: 19
Oral solution, temazepam 10 mg/5 mL, net price 300 mL = £9.95. Label: 19
Available from Generics (sugar-free), Genus, Hillcross (sugar-free), Lagap, Rosemont (sugar-free)
1. See p. 7 for prescribing requirements for temazepam

ZOLPIDEM AND ZOPICLONE

Zopiclone is a cyclopyrrolone and **zolpidem** is an imidazopyridine. Although neither are benzodiazepines both act on the same receptors (or receptor sub-types) as benzodiazepines. Both have a short duration of action with little or no hangover effect. As with other hypnotics they should not be used for long-term treatment.

ZOLPIDEM TARTRATE

Indications: insomnia (short-term use)
Cautions: depression, history of drug or alcohol abuse, hepatic impairment (reduce dose, avoid if severe); renal impairment; elderly; avoid prolonged use (and abrupt withdrawal thereafter); **interactions:** Appendix 1 (anxiolytics and hypnotics)
DRIVING. Drowsiness may persist the next day and affect performance of skilled tasks (e.g. driving); effects of alcohol enhanced
Contra-indications: obstructive sleep apnoea, acute pulmonary insufficiency, respiratory depression, myasthenia gravis, severe hepatic impairment, psychotic illness, pregnancy and breast-feeding
Side-effects: diarrhoea, nausea, vomiting, vertigo, dizziness, headache, daytime drowsiness, asthenia; dependence, memory disturbances, nightmares, nocturnal restlessness, depression, confusion, perceptual disturbances or diplopia, tremor, ataxia, falls reported
Dose: 10 mg at bedtime; ELDERLY (or debilitated) 5 mg; CHILD not recommended

PoM **Stilnoct®** (Lorex)
Tablets, both f/c, zolpidem tartrate 5 mg, net price 28-tab pack = £3.36; 10 mg, 28-tab pack = £6.72. Label: 19

ZOPICLONE

Indications: insomnia (short-term use)
Cautions: hepatic (avoid if severe) and renal impairment (Appendixes 2 and 3); elderly; history of drug abuse, psychiatric illness; avoid prolonged use (and abrupt withdrawal thereafter); **interactions:** Appendix 1 (anxiolytics and hypnotics)
DRIVING. Drowsiness may persist the next day and affect performance of skilled tasks (e.g. driving); effects of alcohol enhanced
Contra-indications: myasthenia gravis, respiratory failure, severe sleep apnoea syndrome, severe hepatic impairment; pregnancy and breast-feeding
Side-effects: bitter or metallic taste; gastro-intestinal disturbances including nausea and vomiting, dry mouth; irritability, confusion, depressed mood; drowsiness, dizziness, lightheadedness, and incoordination, headache; dependence; hypersensitivity reactions reported (including urticaria and rashes); hallucinations, nightmares, amnesia, and behavioural disturbances (including aggression) reported
Dose: 7.5 mg at bedtime; ELDERLY initially 3.75 mg at bedtime increased if necessary; CHILD not recommended

---

PoM **Zimovane®** (Rhône-Poulenc Rorer)
LS tablets, f/c, blue, zopiclone 3.75 mg. Net price
28-tab pack = £3.08. Label: 19
Tablets, f/c, zopiclone 7.5 mg. Net price 28-tab
pack = £4.48. Label: 19

CHLORAL AND DERIVATIVES

Chloral hydrate and derivatives were formerly popular
hypnotics for children (but the use of hypnotics in children
is not usually justified). There is no convincing evidence
that they are particularly useful in the elderly and their role
as hypnotics is now very limited. **Triclofos** causes fewer
gastro-intestinal disturbances than chloral hydrate.

CHLORAL HYDRATE
Indications: insomnia (short-term use)
Cautions: respiratory disease, history of drug or alcohol
abuse, marked personality disorder; reduce dose in elderly and debilitated; avoid prolonged use (and abrupt
withdrawal thereafter); avoid contact with skin and
mucous membranes; **interactions:** Appendix 1 (anxiolytics and hypnotics)
DRIVING. Drowsiness may persist the next day and
affect performance of skilled tasks (e.g. driving); effects
of alcohol enhanced
Contra-indications: cardiac disease, gastritis, hepatic or
renal impairment; pregnancy and breast-feeding; not
recommended in porphyria
Side-effects: gastric irritation (nausea and vomiting
reported), abdominal distention and flatulence; also
vertigo, ataxia, staggering gait, rashes, headache, light
headedness, malaise, ketonuria, excitement, nightmares,
delirium (especially in the elderly), eosinophilia, reduction in white cell count; dependence (may be associated
with gastritis and renal damage) on prolonged use
Dose: insomnia, 0.5–1 g (max. 2 g) with plenty of water
at bedtime; CHILD 30–50 mg/kg up to a max. single dose
of 1 g

PoM Chloral Mixture, BP
(Chloral Oral Solution)
Mixture, chloral hydrate 10% in a suitable vehicle.
Extemporaneous preparations should be recently pre-
pared according to the following formula: chloral
hydrate 1 g, syrup 2 mL, water to 10 mL. Net price
100 mL = 40p. Label: 19, 27
Dose: 5–20 mL; CHILD 1–5 years 2.5–5 mL, 6–12 years
5–10 mL, taken well diluted with water at bedtime
Important. This preparation differs from Chloral Syrup
BPC 1968 which contains 20% (1 g in 5 mL; dose: 2.5–
10 mL, taken well diluted with water at bedtime)
PoM Chloral Elixir, Paediatric, BP
(Chloral Oral Solution, Paediatric)
Elixir, chloral hydrate 4% in a suitable vehicle with a
blackcurrant flavour. Extemporaneous preparations
should be recently prepared according to the following
formula: chloral hydrate 200 mg, water 0.1 mL, blackcurrant syrup 1 mL, syrup to 5 mL. Net price 100 mL =
95p. Label: 1, 27
Dose: up to 1 year 5 mL, taken well diluted with water at
bedtime
PoM **Welldorm®** (S&N Hlth.)
Tablets, blue-purple, f/c, chloral betaine 707 mg
(≡ chloral hydrate 414 mg). Net price 30-tab pack =
£2.54. Label: 19, 27
Dose: 1–2 tablets with water or milk at bedtime, max. 5
tablets (2 g chloral hydrate) daily
Elixir, red, chloral hydrate 143 mg/5 mL. Net price 150-
mL pack = £2.15. Label: 19, 27
Dose: 15–45 mL (0.4–1.3 g chloral hydrate) with water
or milk, at bedtime, max. 70 mL (2 g chloral hydrate)
daily; CHILD 1–1.75 mL/kg (30–50 mg/kg chloral
hydrate), max. 35 mL (1 g chloral hydrate) daily

TRICLOFOS SODIUM
Indications: insomnia (short-term use)
Cautions; Contra-indications; Side-effects: see under
Chloral Hydrate; less gastric irritation
Dose: see under preparation below

PoM Triclofos Oral Solution, BP
(Triclofos Elixir)
Oral solution, triclofos sodium 500 mg/5 mL. Net price
100 mL = £2.74. Label: 19
Available from Norton
Dose: 10–20 mL (1–2 g triclofos sodium) at bedtime;
CHILD up to 1 year 25–30 mg/kg, 1–5 years 2.5–5 mL
(250–500 mg triclofos sodium), 6–12 years 5–10 mL
(0.5–1 g triclofos sodium)

CHLORMETHIAZOLE

Chlormethiazole (clomethiazole) may be a useful
hypnotic for elderly patients because of its freedom
from hangover but, as with all hypnotics, routine
administration is undesirable and dependence
occurs. It is indicated for use as a hypnotic only in
the elderly (and for *very short-term use* in younger
adults to attenuate alcohol withdrawal symptoms,
see section 4.10).

CHLORMETHIAZOLE
(Clomethiazole)
Indications: see under Dose; status epilepticus
(section 4.8.2); alcohol withdrawal (section 4.10);
sedation during regional anaesthesia (section
15.1.4.1); eclampsia, see product literature
Cautions: cardiac and respiratory disease (confusional state may indicate hypoxia); history of
drug abuse; marked personality disorder; excessive sedation may occur (particularly with higher
doses); hepatic impairment (especially if severe
since sedation can mask hepatic coma); renal
impairment; avoid prolonged use (and abrupt
withdrawal thereafter); see also section 4.10;
interactions: Appendix 1 (anxiolytics and hypnotics)
DRIVING. Drowsiness may persist the next day and
affect performance of skilled tasks (e.g. driving); effects
of alcohol enhanced
Contra-indications: acute pulmonary insufficiency; alcohol-dependent patients who continue
to drink
Side-effects: nasal congestion and irritation
(increased nasopharyngeal and bronchial secretions), conjunctival irritation, headache; rarely,
paradoxical excitement, confusion, dependence,
gastro-intestinal disturbances, rash, urticaria, bullous eruption, anaphylaxis, alterations in liver
enzymes; intravenous infusion, see section 4.10
Dose: by mouth, severe insomnia in the elderly
(short-term use), 1–2 capsules (or 5–10 mL
syrup) at bedtime; CHILD not recommended
Restlessness and agitation in the elderly, 1 capsule (or 5 mL syrup) 3 times daily
Note. For an equivalent therapeutic effect 1 capsule ≡
5 mL syrup

PoM **Heminevrin®** (Astra)
Capsules, grey-brown, chlormethiazole base
192 mg in an oily basis. Net price 60-cap pack =
£4.34. Label: 19

Syrup, sugar-free, chlormethiazole edisylate 250 mg/5 mL. Net price 300-mL pack = £3.63.
Label: 19
Intravenous infusion 0.8%, section 4.10

ANTIHISTAMINES

Some **antihistamines** such as diphenhydramine (section 3.4.1) and promethazine are on sale to the public for occasional insomnia; their prolonged duration of action may often lead to drowsiness the following day.

Promethazine is also popular for use in children, but the use of hypnotics in children is not usually justified.

PROMETHAZINE HYDROCHLORIDE

Indications: night sedation and insomnia (short-term use); other indications, see sections 3.4.1, 4.6, 15.1.4.1

Cautions; Contra-indications; Side-effects: section 3.4.1

Dose: by mouth, 25 mg at bedtime increased to 50 mg if necessary; CHILD under 2 years not recommended, 2–5 years 15–20 mg, 5–10 years 20–25 mg, at bedtime

Preparations: section 3.4.1

ALCOHOL

Alcohol is a poor hypnotic because its diuretic action interferes with sleep during the latter part of the night. With chronic use, alcohol disturbs sleep patterns and causes insomnia; **interactions.** Appendix 1 (alcohol).

4.1.2 Anxiolytics

Benzodiazepine anxiolytics can be effective in alleviating definite anxiety states and they are widely prescribed. Although there has been a tendency to prescribe these drugs to almost anyone with stress-related symptoms, unhappiness, or minor physical disease, their use in many situations is unjustified. In particular, they are not appropriate for treating depression, phobic or obsessional states, or chronic psychosis. In bereavement, psychological adjustment may be inhibited by benzodiazepines. In children anxiolytic treatment should be used only to relieve acute anxiety (and related insomnia) caused by fear (e.g. before surgery).

Anxiolytic treatment should be limited to the lowest possible dose for the shortest possible time (see CSM advice, section 4.1). Dependence is particularly likely in patients with a history of alcohol or drug abuse and in patients with marked personality disorders.

Anxiolytics, particularly the benzodiazepines, have been termed 'minor tranquillisers'. This term is misleading because not only do they differ markedly from the antipsychotic drugs ('major tranquillisers') but their use is by no means minor. Antipsychotics, in low doses, are also sometimes used in severe anxiety for their sedative action but long-term use should be avoided in view of a possible risk of tardive dyskinesia (section 4.2.1). The use of antihistamines (e.g. hydroxyzine, section 3.4.1) for their sedative effect in anxiety is not considered to be appropriate.

BENZODIAZEPINES

Benzodiazepines are indicated for the *short-term relief of severe anxiety* but long-term use should be avoided (see p. 155). Diazepam, alprazolam, bromazepam, chlordiazepoxide, clobazam, and clorazepate have a sustained action. Shorter-acting compounds such as **lorazepam** and **oxazepam** may be preferred in patients with hepatic impairment but they carry a greater risk of withdrawal symptoms.

Diazepam or lorazepam are very occasionally administered intravenously for the *control of panic attacks*. This route is the most rapid but the procedure is not without risk (section 4.8.2) and should be used only when alternative measures have failed. The intramuscular route has no advantage over the oral route.

For guidelines on benzodiazepine withdrawal, see p. 155.

DIAZEPAM

Indications: short-term use in anxiety or insomnia, adjunct in acute alcohol withdrawal; status epilepticus (section 4.8.2); febrile convulsions (section 4.8.3); muscle spasm (section 10.2.2); peri-operative use (section 15.1.4.1)

Cautions: respiratory disease, muscle weakness (special care in myasthenia gravis), history of drug or alcohol abuse, marked personality disorder, pregnancy and breast-feeding (Appendixes 4 and 5); reduce dose in elderly and debilitated, and in hepatic (avoid if severe) and renal impairment (Appendixes 2 and 3); avoid prolonged use (and abrupt withdrawal thereafter); special precautions for intravenous injection (section 4.8.2); porphyria (section 9.8.2); **interactions:** Appendix 1 (anxiolytics and hypnotics)

DRIVING. Drowsiness may affect performance of skilled tasks (e.g. driving); effects of alcohol enhanced

Contra-indications: respiratory depression; acute pulmonary insufficiency; severe hepatic impairment; not for phobic or obsessional states, not for chronic psychosis; should not be used alone in depression or in anxiety with depression

Side-effects: drowsiness and lightheadedness the next day; confusion and ataxia (especially in the elderly); amnesia may occur; dependence; paradoxical increase in aggression (see also section 4.1); *occasionally:* headache, vertigo, hypotension, salivation changes, gastro-intestinal disturbances, rashes, visual disturbances, changes in libido, urinary retention; blood disorders and jaundice reported; on intravenous injection, pain, thrombophlebitis, and rarely apnoea; **overdosage:** see Emergency Treatment of Poisoning, p. 23

Dose: by mouth, anxiety, 2 mg 3 times daily increased if necessary to 15–30 mg daily in divided doses; ELDERLY (or debilitated) half adult dose

Insomnia associated with anxiety, 5–15 mg at bedtime

CHILD night terrors and somnambulism, 1–5 mg at bedtime

Cautionary label wordings, see inside back cover

By intramuscular injection or slow intravenous injection (into a large vein, at a rate of not more than 5 mg/minute), for severe acute anxiety, control of acute panic attacks, and acute alcohol withdrawal, 10 mg, repeated if necessary after not less than 4 hours

Note. Only use intramuscular route when oral and intravenous routes not possible; special precautions for intravenous injection see section 4.8.2

By intravenous infusion—section 4.8.2

By rectum as rectal solution, for acute anxiety and agitation, 500 micrograms/kg repeated after 12 hours as required; ELDERLY 250 micrograms/kg; CHILD not recommended

CHILD febrile convulsions, see p. 220

By rectum as suppositories for anxiety when oral route not appropriate, 10–30 mg (higher dose divided); dose form not appropriate for less than 10 mg

PoM **Diazepam** (Non-proprietary)
Tablets, diazepam 2 mg, net price 20 = 7p; 5 mg, 20 = 8p; 10 mg, 20 = 15p. Label: *2 or 19*
Available from APS, Berk, Cox, DDSA (NHS Tensium®), Norton, Rima (NHS Rimapam®), Roche (NHS Valium®)
Oral solution, diazepam 2 mg/5 mL, net price 100 mL = £2.16. Label: *2 or 19*
Available from Cox, Lagap (NHS Dialar®), Roche (NHS Valium®)
NHS *Strong oral solution,* diazepam 5 mg/5 mL, net price 100-mL pack = £3.07. Label: *2 or 19*
Available from Lagap (NHS Dialar®)
Injection (solution), diazepam 5 mg/mL. Do not dilute (except for intravenous infusion). Net price 2-mL amp = 25p
Available from CP, Roche (Valium®), Phoenix
Injection (emulsion), diazepam 5 mg/mL. For intravenous injection or infusion. Net price 2-mL amp = 76p
Available from Dumex (Diazemuls®)
Rectal tubes (= rectal solution), diazepam 2 mg/mL, net price 1.25-mL (2.5-mg) tube = 90p, 2.5-mL (5-mg) tube = £1.27; 4 mg/mL, 2.5-mL (10-mg) tube = £1.62, 5-mL (20-mg) tube = £2.92
Available from CP (Diazepam Rectubes® 2.5 mg, 5 mg, 10 mg, 20 mg), Dumex (Stesolid® 5 mg, 10 mg), Lagap
Suppositories, diazepam 10 mg, net price 6 = £6.51. Label: *2 or 19*
Available from Sinclair (Valclair®)

ALPRAZOLAM

Indications: anxiety (short-term use)
Cautions; Contra-indications; Side-effects: see under Diazepam
Dose: 250–500 micrograms 3 times daily (elderly or debilitated 250 micrograms 2–3 times daily), increased if necessary to a total of 3 mg daily; CHILD not recommended

NHS PoM **Xanax®** (Pharmacia & Upjohn)
Tablets, both scored, alprazolam 250 micrograms, net price 60-tab pack = £2.75; 500 micrograms (pink), 60-tab pack = £5.27. Label: 2

BROMAZEPAM

Indications: anxiety (short-term use)
Cautions; Contra-indications; Side-effects: see under Diazepam
Dose: 3–18 mg daily in divided doses; ELDERLY (or debilitated) half adult dose; max. (in exceptional circumstances in hospitalised patients) 60 mg daily in divided doses; CHILD not recommended

NHS PoM **Lexotan®** (Roche)
Tablets, both scored, bromazepam 1.5 mg (lilac), net price 60-tab pack = £5.47; 3 mg (pink), 60-tab pack = £6.93. Label: 2

CHLORDIAZEPOXIDE

Indications: anxiety (short-term use); adjunct in acute alcohol withdrawal (section 4.10)
Cautions; Contra-indications; Side-effects: see under Diazepam
Dose: anxiety, 10 mg 3 times daily increased if necessary to 60–100 mg daily in divided doses; ELDERLY (or debilitated) half adult dose; CHILD not recommended

Note. The doses stated above refer equally to chlordiazepoxide and to its hydrochloride

PoM **Chlordiazepoxide Capsules,** chlordiazepoxide hydrochloride 5 mg, net price 20 = 27p; 10 mg, 20 = 29p.
Various strengths available from APS, Cox, DDSA (NHS Tropium®), Hillcross, Lagap, Roche (NHS Librium®)
PoM **Chlordiazepoxide Hydrochloride Tablets,** chlordiazepoxide hydrochloride 5 mg, net price 20 = 26p; 10 mg, 20 = 32p; 25 mg, 20 = 70p. Label: 2

CLORAZEPATE DIPOTASSIUM

Indications: anxiety (short-term use)
Cautions; Contra-indications; Side-effects: see under Diazepam
Dose: 7.5–22.5 mg daily in 2–3 divided doses *or* a single dose of 15 mg at bedtime; ELDERLY (or debilitated) half adult dose; CHILD not recommended

NHS PoM **Tranxene®** (Boehringer Ingelheim)
Capsules, clorazepate dipotassium 7.5 mg (maroon/grey), net price 20-cap pack = £2.66; 15 mg (pink/grey), 20-cap pack = £2.78. Label: *2 or 19*

LORAZEPAM

Indications: short-term use in anxiety or insomnia; status epilepticus (section 4.8.2); peri-operative (section 15.1.4.1)
Cautions; Contra-indications; Side-effects: see under Diazepam; short acting
Dose: by mouth, anxiety, 1–4 mg daily in divided doses; ELDERLY (or debilitated) half adult dose
Insomnia associated with anxiety, 1–2 mg at bedtime; CHILD not recommended
By intramuscular or slow intravenous injection (into a large vein), acute panic attacks, 25–30 micrograms/kg, repeated every 6 hours if necessary; CHILD not recommended
Note. Only use intramuscular route when oral and intravenous routes not possible

---

PoM **Lorazepam** (Non-proprietary)

Tablets, lorazepam 1 mg, net price 20 = 24p; 2.5 mg, 20 = 36p. Label: 2 *or* 19

Available from APS, Cox, CP, Lagap, Norton, Wyeth (NHS Ativan®)

Injection, lorazepam 4 mg/mL. Net price 1-mL amp = 40p

For intramuscular injection it should be diluted with an equal volume of water for injections or physiological saline (but only use when oral and intravenous routes not possible)

Available from Wyeth (Ativan®)

OXAZEPAM

Indications: anxiety (short-term use)

Cautions; Contra-indications; Side-effects: see under Diazepam; short acting

Dose: anxiety, 15–30 mg (elderly or debilitated 10–20 mg) 3–4 times daily; CHILD not recommended

Insomnia associated with anxiety, 15–25 mg (max. 50 mg) at bedtime; CHILD not recommended

PoM **Oxazepam** (Non-proprietary)

Tablets, oxazepam 10 mg, net price 20 = 23p; 15 mg, 20 = 24p; 30 mg, 20 = 32p. Label: 2

Available from most generic manufacturers

BUSPIRONE

Buspirone is thought to act at specific serotonin (5HT$_{1A}$) receptors. Response to treatment may take up to 2 weeks. It does not alleviate the symptoms of benzodiazepine withdrawal. Therefore a patient taking a benzodiazepine still needs to have the benzodiazepine withdrawn gradually; it is advisable to do this before starting buspirone. The dependence and abuse liability of buspirone has not yet been established.

BUSPIRONE HYDROCHLORIDE

Indications: anxiety (short-term use)

Cautions: does not alleviate benzodiazepine withdrawal (see notes above); history of hepatic or renal impairment; **interactions:** Appendix 1 (anxiolytics and hypnotics)

DRIVING. May affect performance of skilled tasks (e.g. driving); effects of alcohol may be enhanced

Contra-indications: epilepsy, severe hepatic or renal impairment, pregnancy and breast-feeding

Side-effects: nausea, dizziness, headache, nervousness, lightheadedness, excitement; rarely tachycardia, palpitations, chest pain, drowsiness, confusion, dry mouth, fatigue, and sweating

Dose: initially 5 mg 2–3 times daily, increased as necessary every 2–3 days; usual range 15–30 mg daily in divided doses; max. 45 mg daily; CHILD not recommended

PoM **Buspar®** (Bristol-Myers)

Tablets, buspirone hydrochloride 5 mg, net price 126-tab pack = £39.31; 10 mg, 100-tab pack = £46.80. Counselling, driving

BETA-BLOCKERS

Beta-blockers (e.g. propranolol, oxprenolol) (see section 2.4) do not affect psychological symptoms, such as worry, tension, and fear, but they do reduce autonomic symptoms, such as palpitations and tremor; they do not reduce non-autonomic symptoms, such as muscle tension. Beta-blockers are therefore indicated for patients with predominantly somatic symptoms; this, in turn, may prevent the onset of worry and fear. Patients with predominantly psychological symptoms may obtain no benefit.

MEPROBAMATE

Meprobamate is **less effective** than the benzodiazepines, more hazardous in overdosage, and can also induce dependence. It is **not** recommended.

MEPROBAMATE

Indications: short-term use in anxiety, but see notes above

Cautions: respiratory disease, muscle weakness, epilepsy (may induce seizures), history of drug or alcohol abuse, marked personality disorder, pregnancy; elderly and debilitated; hepatic and renal impairment; avoid prolonged use, abrupt withdrawal may precipitate convulsions; **interactions:** Appendix 1 (anxiolytics and hypnotics)

DRIVING. Drowsiness may affect performance of skilled tasks (e.g. driving); effects of alcohol enhanced

Contra-indications: acute pulmonary insufficiency; respiratory depression; porphyria (section 9.8.2); breast-feeding

Side-effects: see under Diazepam, but the incidence is greater and drowsiness is the most common side-effect. Also gastro-intestinal disturbances, hypotension, paraesthesia, weakness, CNS effects which include headache, paradoxical excitement, disturbances of vision; rarely agranulocytosis and rashes

Dose: 400 mg 3–4 times daily; elderly patients half adult dose or less; CHILD not recommended

CD **Meprobamate** (Non-proprietary)

Tablets, scored, meprobamate 400 mg. Net price 84-tab pack = £3.60. Label: 2

CD **Equagesic®**

Section 4.7.1

4.1.3 Barbiturates

The intermediate-acting **barbiturates** only have a place in the treatment of severe intractable insomnia in patients **already taking** barbiturates; they should be **avoided** in the elderly. The long-acting barbiturates, phenobarbitone and methylphenobarbitone, are still sometimes of value in epilepsy (section 4.8.1) but their use as sedatives is unjustified. The very short-acting barbiturates, methohexitone and thiopentone, are used in anaesthesia (section 15.1.1).

IMPORTANT. Barbiturates should **not** be prescribed as a hypnotic other than for patients who are **already** receiving them and who are suffering from severe intractable insomnia.

BARBITURATES

Indications: severe intractable insomnia in patients already taking barbiturates; see also notes above

Cautions: avoid use where possible; dependence and tolerance readily occur; abrupt withdrawal may precipitate a serious withdrawal syndrome (rebound insomnia, anxiety, tremor, dizziness, nausea, convulsions, delirium, and death); repeated doses are cumulative and may lead to excessive sedation; caution in respiratory disease, renal disease, hepatic impairment; **interactions:** Appendix 1 (barbiturates and primidone)

DRIVING. Drowsiness may persist the next day and affect performance of skilled tasks (e.g. driving); effects of alcohol enhanced

Contra-indications: insomnia caused by pain; porphyria (see section 9.8.2), pregnancy, breast-feeding; avoid in children, young adults, elderly and debilitated patients, also patients with a history of drug or alcohol abuse

Side-effects: include hangover with drowsiness, dizziness, ataxia, respiratory depression, hypersensitivity reactions, headache, particularly in elderly; paradoxical excitement and confusion occasionally precede sleep; **overdosage:** see Emergency Treatment of Poisoning, p. 23

Dose: see under preparations below

CD Amytal® (Flynn)

Tablets, amylobarbitone (amobarbital) 50 mg, net price 20 = £1.84. Label: 19

Dose: 100–200 mg at bedtime (**important:** but see also contra-indications)

CD Sodium Amytal® (Flynn)

Capsules, both blue, amylobarbitone (amobarbital) sodium 60 mg, net price 20 = £3.43; 200 mg, 20 = £6.75. Label: 19

Dose: 60–200 mg at bedtime (**important:** but see also contra-indications)

Injection, powder for reconstitution, amylobarbitone (amobarbital) sodium. Net price 500-mg vial = £28.83. For specialised use in procedures in **expert epilepsy centres only**

Dose: by deep intramuscular injection into large muscle, preferably gluteal, (max. 5 mL at any one site) or by slow intravenous injection (max. 50 mg/minute), 0.25–1 g; max. single dose, intramuscular 500 mg, intravenous 1 g

CD Soneryl® (Concord)

Tablets, pink, scored, butobarbitone (butobarbital) 100 mg. Net price 56-tab pack = £10.65. Label: 19

Dose: 100–200 mg at bedtime (**important:** but see also contra-indications)

Preparations containing quinalbarbitone (secobarbital)

Note. Quinalbarbitone (secobarbital) has been transferred from schedule 3 to schedule 2 of the Misuse of Drugs Regulations 1985; receipt and supply must therefore be recorded in the CD register.

CD Seconal Sodium® (Flynn)

Capsules, both orange, quinalbarbitone (secobarbital) sodium 50 mg, net price 20 = £5.30; 100 mg, 20 = £6.96. Label: 19

Dose: 100 mg at bedtime (**important:** but see also contra-indications)

CD Tuinal® (Flynn)

Capsules, orange/blue, a mixture of amylobarbitone (amobarbital) sodium 50 mg, quinalbarbitone (secobarbital) sodium 50 mg. Net price 20 = £3.88. Label: 19

Dose: 1–2 capsules at bedtime (**important:** but see also contra-indications)

Note. Prescriptions need only specify 'Tuinal capsules'

4.2   Drugs used in psychoses and related disorders

4.2.1   Antipsychotic drugs
4.2.2   Antipsychotic depot injections
4.2.3   Antimanic drugs

Advice of Royal College of Psychiatrists on doses above BNF upper limit

Unless otherwise stated, doses in the BNF are licensed doses—any higher dose is therefore **unlicensed** (for an explanation of the significance of this, see p. 2).

1. Consider alternative approaches including adjuvant therapy and newer or atypical neuroleptics such as clozapine.
2. Bear in mind risk factors, including obesity—particular caution is indicated in older patients especially those over 70.
3. Consider potential for drug interactions—see **interactions:** Appendix 1 (antipsychotics).
4. Carry out ECG to exclude untoward abnormalities such as prolonged QT interval; repeat ECG periodically and reduce dose if prolonged QT interval or other adverse abnormality develops.
5. Increase dose slowly and not more often than once weekly.
6. Carry out regular pulse, blood pressure, and temperature checks; ensure that patient maintains adequate fluid intake.
7. Consider high-dose therapy to be for limited period and review regularly; abandon if no improvement after 3 months (return to standard dosage).

Important: When prescribing an antipsychotic for administration on an emergency basis, the intramuscular dose should be **lower** than the corresponding oral dose (owing to absence of first-pass effect), particularly if the patient is very active (increased blood flow to muscle considerably increases the rate of absorption). The prescription should specify the dose for **each route** and should **not** imply that the same dose can be given by mouth or by intramuscular injection. The dose of antipsychotic for emergency use should be reviewed at least **daily**.

4.2.1   Antipsychotic drugs

Antipsychotic drugs are also known as 'neuroleptics' and (misleadingly) as 'major tranquillisers'. Antipsychotic drugs generally tranquillise without impairing consciousness and without causing paradoxical excitement but they should not be regarded merely as tranquillisers. For conditions such as schizophrenia the tranquillising effect is of secondary importance.

In the short term they are used to quieten disturbed patients whatever the underlying psychopathology, which may be brain damage, mania, toxic delirium, agitated depression, or acute behavioural disturbance.

They are used to alleviate severe anxiety but this too should be a short-term measure. Some antipsychotic drugs (e.g. chlorpromazine, thioridazine, flupenthixol) also have an antidepressant effect while others may exacerbate depression (e.g. fluphenazine, pimozide, pipothiazine).

SCHIZOPHRENIA. Antipsychotic drugs relieve florid psychotic symptoms such as thought disorder, hallucinations, and delusions, and prevent relapse.

Although they are usually less effective in apathetic withdrawn patients, they sometimes appear to have an activating influence. For example, chlorpromazine may restore an acutely ill schizophrenic, who was previously withdrawn or even mute and akinetic, to normal activity and social behaviour. Patients with acute schizophrenia generally respond better than those with chronic symptoms.

Long-term treatment of a patient with a definite diagnosis of schizophrenia may be necessary even after the first episode of illness in order to prevent the manifest illness from becoming chronic. Withdrawal of drug treatment requires careful surveillance because the patient who appears well on medication may suffer a disastrous relapse if treatment is withdrawn inappropriately. In addition the need for continuation of treatment may not become immediately evident because relapse is often delayed for several weeks after cessation of treatment.

Antipsychotic drugs are considered to act by interfering with dopaminergic transmission in the brain by blocking dopamine receptors, which may give rise to the extrapyramidal effects described below, and also to hyperprolactinaemia. Antipsychotic drugs also affect cholinergic, alpha-adrenergic, histaminergic, and serotonergic receptors.

SIDE-EFFECTS. Extrapyramidal symptoms are the most troublesome. They are caused most frequently by the piperazine phenothiazines (fluphenazine, perphenazine, prochlorperazine, and trifluoperazine), the butyrophenones (benperidol, droperidol and haloperidol), and the depot preparations. They are easy to recognise but cannot be accurately predicted because they depend partly on the dose and partly on the type of drug, and on patient susceptibility. They consist of *parkinsonian symptoms* (including tremor) which may occur gradually, *dystonia* (abnormal face and body movements) which may appear after only a few doses, *akathisia* (restlessness) which may resemble an exacerbation of the condition being treated, and *tardive dyskinesia* (which usually takes longer to develop).

Parkinsonian symptoms remit if the drug is withdrawn and may be suppressed by the administration of **antimuscarinic** drugs (section 4.9.2). Routine administration of such drugs is **not** justified as not all patients are affected and because tardive dyskinesia may be unmasked or worsened by them. Furthermore, these drugs are sometimes abused for their mood-altering effects. Tardive dyskinesia is of particular concern because it may be irreversible on withdrawing therapy and treatment may be ineffective. It occurs fairly frequently in patients (especially the elderly) on long-term therapy and with high dosage, and the treatment of such patients must be carefully and regularly reviewed. Tardive dyskinesia may also occur occasionally after short-term treatment with low dosage.

Hypotension and *interference with temperature regulation* are dose-related side-effects and are liable to cause dangerous falls and hypothermia in the elderly; very serious consideration should be given before prescribing these drugs for patients over 70 years of age.

Neuroleptic malignant syndrome (hyperthermia, fluctuating level of consciousness, muscular rigidity and autonomic dysfunction with pallor, tachycardia, labile blood pressure, sweating, and urinary incontinence) is a rare but potentially fatal side-effect of some drugs. Drugs for which it has been reported in the UK include haloperidol, chlorpromazine, and flupenthixol decanoate. Discontinuation of drug therapy is essential as there is no proven effective treatment but bromocriptine and dantrolene have been used. The syndrome, which usually lasts for 5–10 days after drug discontinuation, may be unduly prolonged if depot preparations have been used.

Overdosage: see Emergency Treatment of Poisoning, p. 23.

CLASSIFICATION OF ANTIPSYCHOTICS. The **phenothiazine** derivatives can be divided into 3 main groups.

Group 1: chlorpromazine, methotrimeprazine, and promazine, generally characterised by pronounced sedative effects and moderate antimuscarinic and extrapyramidal side-effects.

Group 2: pericyazine, pipothiazine, and thioridazine, generally characterised by moderate sedative effects, marked antimuscarinic effects, but fewer extrapyramidal side-effects than groups 1 or 3.

Group 3: fluphenazine, perphenazine, prochlorperazine, and trifluoperazine, generally characterised by fewer sedative effects, fewer antimuscarinic effects, but more pronounced extrapyramidal side-effects than groups 1 and 2.

Drugs of other chemical groups tend to resemble the phenothiazines of *group 3*. They include the **butyrophenones** (benperidol, droperidol, and haloperidol); **diphenylbutylpiperidines** (pimozide); **thioxanthenes** (flupenthixol and zuclopenthixol), **substituted benzamides** (sulpiride); **oxypertine**; and **loxapine**.

For details of the newer antipsychotic drugs amisulpride, clozapine, olanzapine, quetiapine, risperidone, and sertindole, see under Atypical Antipsychotics below.

CHOICE. As indicated above, the various drugs differ somewhat in predominant actions and side-effects. Selection is influenced by the degree of sedation required and the patient's susceptibility to extrapyramidal side-effects. However, the differences between antipsychotic drugs are less important than the great variability in patient response; moreover, tolerance to these secondary effects usually develops. The newer antipsychotics may be appropriate in refractory cases or if extrapyramidal side-effects are a particular concern, see under Atypical Antipsychotics, below.

Prescribing of more than one antipsychotic at the same time is **not** recommended; it may constitute a hazard and there is no significant evidence that side-effects are minimised.

Chlorpromazine is widely used. It has a marked sedating effect and is useful for treating violent patients without causing stupor. Agitated states in the elderly can be controlled without confusion, a dose of 10 to 25 mg once or twice daily usually being adequate.

Flupenthixol and **pimozide** (see CSM advice p. 168) are less sedating than chlorpromazine.

Sulpiride in high doses controls florid positive symptoms, but in lower doses it has an alerting effect on apathetic withdrawn schizophrenics.

Fluphenazine, haloperidol, and **trifluoperazine** are also of value but their use is limited by the high incidence of extrapyramidal symptoms. Haloperidol may be preferred for the rapid control of hyperactive psychotic states. It is less hypotensive than chlorpromazine and is therefore also popular for agitation in the elderly, despite the high incidence of extrapyramidal side-effects.

Thioridazine was formerly popular for treating the elderly as there is a reduced incidence of extrapyramidal symptoms. However, there is a high incidence of antimuscarinic effects and possibly an increased risk of cardiotoxicity.

Promazine is not sufficiently active by mouth to be used as an antipsychotic drug.

Loxapine causes relatively little sedation; in overdosage it has a high potential for serious neurological and cardiac toxicity.

OTHER USES. Nausea and vomiting (section 4.6), choreas, motor tics (section 4.9.3), and intractable hiccup (see under Chlorpromazine Hydrochloride and under Haloperidol). **Benperidol** is used in deviant antisocial sexual behaviour but its value is not established.

Equivalent doses of oral antipsychotics
These equivalences are intended **only** as an approximate guide; individual dosage instructions should **also** be checked; patients should be carefully monitored after **any** change in medication

Antipsychotic	Daily dose
Chlorpromazine	100 mg
Clozapine	50 mg[1]
Haloperidol	2–3 mg[2]
Loxapine	10–20 mg
Pimozide	2 mg[3]
Risperidone	0.5–1 mg
Sulpiride	200 mg
Thioridazine	100 mg
Trifluoperazine	5 mg

1. The prescribing of clozapine needs to comply with the Clozaril Patient Monitoring Service, see p. 171
2. In specialist psychiatric units where very high doses are required the equivalent dose of haloperidol might be up to 10 mg
3. See also the CSM warning concerning pimozide dose, p. 168

IMPORTANT. These equivalences must **not** be extrapolated beyond the max. dose for the drug.

WITHDRAWAL. Withdrawal of antipsychotic drugs after long-term therapy should always be gradual and closely monitored to avoid the risk of acute withdrawal syndromes or rapid relapse.

DOSAGE. After an initial period of stabilisation, in most patients, the long half-life of antipsychotic drugs allows the total daily oral dose to be given as a single dose. For the advice of The Royal College of Psychiatrists on doses above the BNF upper limit, see p. 162.

CHLORPROMAZINE HYDROCHLORIDE

WARNING. Owing to the risk of contact sensitisation, pharmacists, nurses, and other health workers should avoid direct contact with chlorpromazine; tablets should not be crushed and solutions should be handled with care

Indications: see under Dose; antiemetic (in terminal illness), section 4.6; peri-operative use, see section 15.1.4.1

Cautions: cardiovascular and cerebrovascular disease, respiratory disease, parkinsonism, epilepsy (possibly avoid), acute infections, pregnancy, breast-feeding, renal and hepatic impairment (avoid if severe), history of jaundice, leucopenia (blood counts if unexplained infection or fever); hypothyroidism, myasthenia gravis, prostatic hypertrophy, angle-closure glaucoma; caution in elderly particularly in very hot or very cold weather; avoid abrupt withdrawal; patients should remain supine and the blood pressure monitored for 30 minutes after intramuscular injection; **interactions:** Appendix 1 (antipsychotics)

DRIVING. Drowsiness may affect performance of skilled tasks (e.g. driving); effects of alcohol enhanced

Contra-indications: coma caused by CNS depressants; bone-marrow depression; avoid in phaeochromocytoma

Side-effects: extrapyramidal symptoms (reversed by dose reduction or antimuscarinic drugs) and, on prolonged administration, occasionally tardive dyskinesia; hypothermia (occasionally pyrexia), drowsiness, apathy, pallor, nightmares, insomnia, depression, and, more rarely, agitation, EEG changes, convulsions; nasal congestion; antimuscarinic symptoms such as dry mouth, constipation, difficulty with micturition, and blurred vision; cardiovascular symptoms such as hypotension, tachycardia, and arrhythmias; ECG changes; respiratory depression; endocrine effects such as menstrual disturbances, galactorrhoea, gynaecomastia, impotence, and weight gain; sensitivity reactions such as agranulocytosis, leucopenia, leucocytosis, and haemolytic anaemia, photosensitisation (more common with chlorpromazine than with other antipsychotics), contact sensitisation and rashes, jaundice (including cholestatic) and alterations in liver function; neuroleptic malignant syndrome; lupus erythematosus-like syndrome reported; with prolonged high dosage, corneal and lens opacities and purplish pigmentation of the skin, cornea, conjunctiva, and retina; intramuscular injection may be painful, cause hypotension and tachycardia (see Cautions), and give rise to nodule formation; **overdosage:** see Emergency Treatment of Poisoning, p. 23

Dose: by mouth,

Schizophrenia and other psychoses, mania, short-term adjunctive management of severe anxiety, psychomotor agitation, excitement, and violent or dangerously impulsive behaviour initially 25 mg 3 times daily (*or* 75 mg at night), adjusted according to response, to usual maintenance dose of 75–300 mg daily (but up to 1 g daily may be required in psychoses); ELDERLY (or debilitated) third to half adult dose; CHILD (childhood schizophrenia and autism) 1–5 years 500 micrograms/kg every 4–6 hours (max. 40 mg daily); 6–12 years third to half adult dose (max. 75 mg daily)

Intractable hiccup, 25–50 mg 3–4 times daily

By deep intramuscular injection, (for relief of acute symptoms but see also Cautions and Side-effects), 25–50 mg every 6–8 hours; CHILD, 1–5 years 500 micrograms/kg every 6–8 hours (max. 40 mg daily); 6–12 years 500 micrograms/kg every 6–8 hours (max. 75 mg daily)

Induction of hypothermia (to prevent shivering), *by deep intramuscular injection,* 25–50 mg every 6–8 hours; CHILD 1–12 years, initially 0.5–1 mg/kg, followed by maintenance 500 micrograms/kg every 4–6 hours

By rectum in suppositories as chlorpromazine base 100 mg every 6–8 hours [unlicensed]

Note. For equivalent therapeutic effect 100 mg chlorpromazine base given *rectally* as a suppository ≡ 20–25 mg chlorpromazine hydrochloride *by intramuscular injection* ≡ 40–50 mg of chlorpromazine base or hydrochloride *by mouth*

PoM Chlorpromazine (Non-proprietary)

Tablets, coated, chlorpromazine hydrochloride 10 mg, net price 20 = 14p; 25 mg, 20 = 15p; 50 mg, 20 = 27p; 100 mg, 20 = 31p. Label: 2, 11

Available from Antigen, APS, DDSA (Chloractil®), Hillcross, Norton

Oral solution, chlorpromazine hydrochloride 25 mg/5 mL, net price 100 mL = 58p, 100 mg/5 mL, 100 mL = £1.41. Label: 2, 11

Available from Hillcross, Rosemont

Injection, chlorpromazine hydrochloride 25 mg/mL, net price 1-mL amp = 32p; 2-mL amp = 37p

Available from Antigen

Suppositories, chlorpromazine 100 mg. Label: 2, 11

'Special order' [unlicensed] product; contact Martindale or regional hospital manufacturing unit

PoM Largactil® (Rhône-Poulenc Rorer)

Tablets, all off-white, f/c, chlorpromazine hydrochloride 10 mg. Net price 56-tab pack = 39p; 25 mg, 56-tab pack = 54p; 50 mg, 56-tab pack = £1.13; 100 mg, 56-tab pack = £2.10. Label: 2, 11

Syrup, brown, chlorpromazine hydrochloride 25 mg/5 mL. Net price 100-mL pack = 61p. Label: 2, 11

Suspension forte, orange, sugar-free, chlorpromazine hydrochloride 100 mg (as embonate)/5 mL. Net price 100-mL pack = £1.41. Label: 2, 11

Injection, chlorpromazine hydrochloride 25 mg/mL. Net price 2-mL amp = 37p

BENPERIDOL

Indications: control of deviant antisocial sexual behaviour (but see notes above)

Cautions; Contra-indications; Side-effects: see under Haloperidol

Dose: 0.25–1.5 mg daily in divided doses, adjusted according to the response; ELDERLY (or debilitated) initially half adult dose; CHILD not recommended

PoM Anquil® (Janssen-Cilag)

Tablets, benperidol 250 micrograms. Net price 100-tab pack = £26.13. Label: 2

DROPERIDOL

Indications: see under Dose

Cautions; Contra-indications; Side-effects: see under Haloperidol

Dose: by mouth, tranquillisation and emergency control in mania, 5–20 mg repeated every 4–8 hours if necessary (elderly, initially half adult dose); CHILD, 0.5–1 mg daily

By intramuscular injection, up to 10 mg repeated every 4–6 hours if necessary (elderly, initially half adult dose); CHILD, 0.5–1 mg daily

By intravenous injection, 5–15 mg repeated every 4–6 hours if necessary (elderly, initially half adult dose)

Cancer chemotherapy-induced nausea and vomiting, *by intramuscular or intravenous injection,* 1–10 mg 30 minutes before starting therapy, followed by *continuous intravenous infusion* of 1–3 mg/hour or 1–5 mg *by intramuscular or intravenous injection* every 1–6 hours as necessary; CHILD *by intramuscular or intravenous injection,* 20–75 micrograms/kg

Premedication, *by intramuscular injection,* up to 10 mg 60 minutes before operation; CHILD 200–500 micrograms/kg

Neuroleptanalgesia, *by intravenous injection,* 5–15 mg at induction with an opioid analgesic; CHILD 200–300 micrograms/kg

PoM Droleptan® (Janssen-Cilag)

Tablets, yellow, scored, droperidol 10 mg. Net price 50-tab pack = £12.30. Label: 2

Oral liquid, sugar-free, droperidol 1 mg/mL. Net price 100-mL pack (with graduated cap) = £4.47; 500-mL pack = £21.25. Label: 2

Injection, droperidol 5 mg/mL. Net price 2-mL amp = 90p

FLUPENTHIXOL

(Flupentixol)

Indications: schizophrenia and other psychoses, particularly with apathy and withdrawal but not mania or psychomotor hyperactivity; depression, section 4.3.4

Cautions; Contra-indications; Side-effects: see under Chlorpromazine Hydrochloride but less sedating; extrapyramidal symptoms more frequent (25% of patients); avoid in senile confusional states, excitable and overactive patients; porphyria (see section 9.8.2)

Dose: psychosis, initially 3–9 mg twice daily adjusted according to the response; max. 18 mg daily; ELDERLY (or debilitated) initially quarter to half adult dose; CHILD not recommended

Depression, see section 4.3.4

PoM **Depixol®** (Lundbeck)

Tablets, yellow, s/c, flupenthixol 3 mg (as dihydrochloride). Net price 20 = £2.85. Label: 2

Depot injection (flupenthixol decanoate): section 4.2.2

PoM **Fluanxol®** (depression), see section 4.3.4

FLUPHENAZINE HYDROCHLORIDE

Indications: see under Dose

Cautions; Contra-indications; Side-effects: see under Chlorpromazine Hydrochloride, but less sedating and fewer antimuscarinic or hypotensive symptoms; extrapyramidal symptoms, particularly dystonic reactions and akathisia, are more frequent; avoid in depression

Dose: schizophrenia and other psychoses, mania, initially 2.5–10 mg daily in 2–3 divided doses, adjusted according to response to 20 mg daily; doses above 20 mg daily (10 mg in elderly) only with special caution; CHILD not recommended

Short-term adjunctive management of severe anxiety, psychomotor agitation, excitement, and violent or dangerously impulsive behaviour, initially 1 mg twice daily, increased as necessary to 2 mg twice daily; CHILD not recommended

PoM **Moditen®** (Sanofi Winthrop)

Tablets, all s/c, fluphenazine hydrochloride 1 mg (pink), net price 20 = £1.06; 2.5 mg (yellow), 20 = £1.33; 5 mg, 20 = £1.77. Label: 2

Depot injections (fluphenazine decanoate): section 4.2.2

HALOPERIDOL

Indications: see under Dose; motor tics, section 4.9.3

Cautions; Contra-indications; Side-effects: see under Chlorpromazine Hydrochloride but less sedating, and fewer antimuscarinic or hypotensive symptoms; pigmentation and photosensitivity reactions rare. Extrapyramidal symptoms, particularly dystonic reactions and akathisia are more frequent especially in thyrotoxic patients. Rarely weight loss. Avoid in basal ganglia disease

Dose: by mouth,

Schizophrenia and other psychoses, mania, short-term adjunctive management of psychomotor agitation, excitement, and violent or dangerously impulsive behaviour, initially 1.5–3 mg 2–3 times daily *or* 3–5 mg 2–3 times daily in severely affected or resistant patients; in resistant schizophrenia up to 100 mg (rarely 120 mg) daily may be needed; adjusted according to response to lowest effective maintenance dose (as low as 5–10 mg daily); ELDERLY (or debilitated) initially half adult dose; CHILD initially 25–50 micrograms/kg daily (in 2 divided doses) to a max. of 10 mg; adolescents up to 30 mg daily (exceptionally 60 mg)

Short-term adjunctive management of severe anxiety, adults 500 micrograms twice daily; CHILD not recommended

Intractable hiccup, 1.5 mg 3 times daily adjusted according to response; CHILD not recommended

By intramuscular injection, 2–10 mg, subsequent doses being given every 4–8 hours according to response (up to every hour if necessary) to total max. 60 mg; severely disturbed patients may require initial dose of up to 30 mg; CHILD not recommended

Nausea and vomiting, 0.5–2 mg

PoM **Haloperidol** (Non-proprietary)

Tablets, haloperidol 1.5 mg, net price 20 = 92p; 5 mg, 20 = £2.64; 10 mg, 20 = £5.00; 20 mg, 20 = £9.10. Label: 2

PoM **Dozic®** (Rosemont)

Oral liquid, sugar-free, haloperidol 1 mg/mL. Net price 100-mL pack = £7.65. Label: 2

PoM **Haldol®** (Janssen-Cilag)

Tablets, both scored, haloperidol 5 mg (blue), net price 20 = £1.65; 10 mg (yellow), 20 = £3.21. Label: 2

Oral liquid, sugar-free, haloperidol 2 mg/mL. Net price 100-mL pack (with pipette) = £5.08. Label: 2

Injection, haloperidol 5 mg/mL. Net price 1-mL amp = 33p; 2-mL amp = 62p

Depot injection (haloperidol decanoate): section 4.2.2

PoM **Serenace®** (Baker Norton)

Capsules, green, haloperidol 500 micrograms. Net price 20 = 65p. Label: 2

Tablets, haloperidol 1.5 mg, net price 20 = £1.16; 5 mg (pink), 20 = £3.27; 10 mg (pale pink), 20 = £5.87; 20 mg (dark pink), 20 = £10.58. Label: 2

Oral liquid, sugar-free, haloperidol 2 mg/mL. Net price 100-mL pack = £8.77. Label: 2

Injection, haloperidol 5 mg/mL, net price 1-mL amp = 59p; 10 mg/mL, 2-mL amp = £2.03

LOXAPINE

Indications: acute and chronic psychoses

Cautions; Contra-indications: see under Chlorpromazine Hydrochloride; porphyria (see section 9.8.2)

Side-effects: see under Chlorpromazine Hydrochloride; nausea and vomiting, weight gain or loss, dyspnoea, ptosis, hyperpyrexia, flushing and headache, paraesthesia, and polydipsia also reported

Dose: initially 20–50 mg daily in 2 divided doses, increased as necessary over 7–10 days to 60–100 mg daily (max. 250 mg) in 2–4 divided doses, then adjusted to usual maintenance dose of 20–100 mg daily; CHILD not recommended

PoM **Loxapac®** (Lederle)

Capsules, loxapine (as succinate) 10 mg (yellow/green), net price 100-cap pack = £9.52; 25 mg (light green/dark green), 100-cap pack = £19.05; 50 mg (blue/dark green), 100-cap pack = £34.27. Label: 2

METHOTRIMEPRAZINE
(Levomepromazine)

Indications: see under Dose

Cautions; Contra-indications; Side-effects: see under Chlorpromazine Hydrochloride but more sedating

ELDERLY. Risk of postural hypotension particularly in patients over 50 years—not recommended for ambulant patients over 50 years unless risk of hypotensive reaction has been assessed

Dose: by mouth, schizophrenia, initially 25–50 mg daily in divided doses increased as necessary; bedpatients initially 100–200 mg daily usually in 3 divided doses, increased if necessary to 1 g daily; ELDERLY, see Cautions

Adjunctive treatment in palliative care (including management of pain and associated restlessness, distress, or vomiting), 12.5–50 mg every 4–8 hours

By intramuscular injection or by intravenous injection (by intravenous injection after dilution with an equal volume of sodium chloride 0.9% injection), adjunct in palliative care, 12.5–25 mg (severe agitation up to 50 mg) every 6–8 hours if necessary

By continuous subcutaneous infusion, adjunct in palliative care (via syringe driver), 25–200 mg daily (over 24-hour period), diluted in a suitable volume of sodium chloride 0.9% injection; CHILD (experience limited), 0.35–3 mg/kg daily

PoM **Nozinan®** (Link)
Tablets, scored, methotrimeprazine maleate 25 mg. Net price 20 = £3.00. Label: 2
Injection, methotrimeprazine hydrochloride 25 mg/mL. Net price 1-mL amp = £1.75

OXYPERTINE

Indications: see under Dose

Cautions; Contra-indications; Side-effects: see under Chlorpromazine Hydrochloride, but extrapyramidal symptoms may occur less frequently. With low doses agitation and hyperactivity occur and with high doses sedation. Occasionally photophobia may occur

Dose: schizophrenia and other psychoses, mania, short-term adjunctive management of psychomotor agitation, excitement, and violent or dangerously impulsive behaviour, initially 80–120 mg daily in divided doses adjusted according to the response; max. 300 mg daily; CHILD not recommended

Short-term adjunctive management of severe anxiety, initially 10 mg 3–4 times daily preferably after food; max. 60 mg daily; CHILD not recommended

PoM **Oxypertine** (Sanofi Winthrop)
Capsules, oxypertine 10 mg. Net price 20 = £2.12. Label: 2
Tablets, scored, oxypertine 40 mg. Net price 20 = £6.64. Label: 2
Note. The brand name Integrin® was formerly used for oxypertine preparations

PERICYAZINE
(Periciazine)

Indications: see under Dose

Cautions; Contra-indications; Side-effects: see under Chlorpromazine Hydrochloride, but more sedating; hypotension commonly occurs when treatment initiated

Dose: schizophrenia and other psychoses, initially 75 mg daily in divided doses increased at weekly intervals by steps of 25 mg according to response; usual max. 300 mg daily (elderly initially 15–30 mg daily)

Short-term adjunctive management of severe anxiety, psychomotor agitation, and violent or dangerously impulsive behaviour, initially 15–30 mg (elderly 5–10 mg) daily divided into 2 doses, taking the larger dose at bedtime, adjusted according to response

CHILD (severe mental or behavioural disorders only), initially, 500 micrograms daily for 10-kg child, increased by 1 mg for each additional 5 kg to max. total daily dose of 10 mg; dose may be gradually increased according to response but maintenance should not exceed twice initial dose; INFANT under 1 year not recommended

PoM **Neulactil®** (JHC)
Tablets, all yellow, scored, pericyazine 2.5 mg, net price 84-tab pack = £8.05; 10 mg, 84-tab pack = £21.77. Label: 2
Syrup forte, brown, pericyazine 10 mg/5 mL. Net price 100-mL pack = £10.54. Label: 2

PERPHENAZINE

Indications: see under Dose; anti-emetic, section 4.6

Cautions; Contra-indications; Side-effects: see under Chlorpromazine Hydrochloride, but less sedating; extrapyramidal symptoms, especially dystonia, more frequent, particularly at high dosage; not indicated for agitation and restlessness in the elderly

Dose: schizophrenia and other psychoses, mania, short-term adjunctive management of severe anxiety, psychomotor agitation, excitement, and violent or dangerously impulsive behaviour, initially 4 mg 3 times daily adjusted according to the response; max. 24 mg daily; ELDERLY quarter to half adult dose (but see Cautions); CHILD under 14 years not recommended

PoM **Fentazin®** (Goldshield)
Tablets, both s/c, perphenazine 2 mg, net price 20 = £3.53; 4 mg, 20 = £4.19. Label: 2

PIMOZIDE

Indications: see under Dose

Cautions; Contra-indications; Side-effects: see under Chlorpromazine Hydrochloride, but less sedating; contra-indicated in breast-feeding; serious arrhythmias reported (contra-indicated if history of arrhythmias or pre-existing congenital QT prolongation); following reports of sudden unex-

---

plained death, the CSM recommends ECG before treatment in all patients, periodic ECGs at doses over 16 mg daily and review of need for pimozide if repolarisation changes or arrhythmias develop (close supervision and preferably dose reduction advised)—for additional CSM warnings see also below; concurrent cardioactive or antipsychotic drugs, or electrolyte disturbances (notably hypo-kalaemia) may predispose to cardiotoxicity

ADDITIONAL CSM WARNING. In addition to the advice above, the CSM now also recommends that patients on pimozide should have an annual ECG (if the QT interval is found to be prolonged treatment should be reviewed and either withdrawn or the dose reduced under close supervision) and that pimozide should **not** be given with other antipsychotic drugs (including depot prepara-tions), tricyclic antidepressants or other drugs known to prolong the QT interval, such as certain antimalarials, anti-arrhythmic drugs and certain antihistamines (terfen-adine, astemizole) and should **not** be given with drugs which cause electrolyte disturbances (especially diur-etics)

Dose: schizophrenia, initially 10 mg daily in acute conditions, adjusted according to response in increments of 2–4 mg at intervals of not less than 1 week; max. 20 mg daily; prevention of relapse, initially 2 mg daily (range 2–20 mg daily); ELD-ERLY half usual starting dose; CHILD not recom-mended

Monosymptomatic hypochondriacal psychosis, paranoid psychoses, initially 4 mg daily, adjusted according to response in increments of 2–4 mg at intervals of not less than 1 week; max. 16 mg daily; ELDERLY half usual starting dose; CHILD not recommended

Mania, hypomania, short-term adjunctive manage-ment of excitement and psychomotor agitation, initially 10 mg daily adjusted according to response in increments of 2–4 mg at intervals of not less than 1 week; max. 20 mg daily; ELDERLY half usual starting dose; CHILD not recommended

PoM **Orap®** (Janssen-Cilag)

Tablets, all scored, pimozide 2 mg, net price 20 = £3.17; 4 mg (green), 20 = £6.13; 10 mg, 20 = £11.76. Label: 2

PROCHLORPERAZINE

Indications: see under Dose; anti-emetic, section 4.6

Cautions; Contra-indications; Side-effects: see under Chlorpromazine Hydrochloride, but less sedating; extrapyramidal symptoms, particularly dystonic reactions, more frequent; avoid in chil-dren (but see section 4.6 for use as anti-emetic)

Dose: by mouth, schizophrenia and other psych-oses, mania, prochlorperazine maleate or mesy-late, 12.5 mg twice daily for 7 days adjusted at intervals of 4–7 days to usual dose of 75–100 mg daily according to response; CHILD not recom-mended

Short-term adjunctive management of severe anxiety, 15–20 mg daily in divided doses; max. 40 mg daily; CHILD not recommended

By deep intramuscular injection, psychoses, mania, prochlorperazine mesylate 12.5–25 mg 2–3 times daily; CHILD not recommended

By rectum in suppositories, psychoses, mania, the equivalent of prochlorperazine maleate 25 mg 2–3 times daily; CHILD not recommended

Preparations
Section 4.6

PROMAZINE HYDROCHLORIDE

Indications: see under Dose

Cautions; Contra-indications; Side-effects: see under Chlorpromazine Hydrochloride

Dose: by mouth, short-term adjunctive manage-ment of psychomotor agitation, 100–200 mg 4 times daily; CHILD not recommended

Agitation and restlessness in elderly, 25–50 mg 4 times daily

By intramuscular injection, short-term adjunctive management of psychomotor agitation, 50 mg (25 mg in elderly or debilitated), repeated if nec-essary after 6–8 hours; CHILD not recommended

PoM **Promazine** (Non-proprietary)

Tablets, coated, promazine hydrochloride 25 mg and 50 mg. Label: 2

Available from Biorex

Oral solution, promazine hydrochloride 25 mg/5 mL, net price 200 mL = £1.50; 50 mg/5 mL, 200 mL = £1.72. Label: 2

Available from Rosemont

Suspension, yellow, promazine hydrochloride (as embonate) 50 mg/5 mL. Net price 150-mL pack = £1.46. Label: 2

Note. Not recommended for children

Available from Genus

PoM **Sparine®** (Wyeth)

Injection, promazine hydrochloride 50 mg/mL. Net price 1-mL amp = 26p

---

SULPIRIDE

Indications: schizophrenia

Cautions; Contra-indications; Side-effects: see under Chlorpromazine Hydrochloride, but less sedating; structurally distinct from chlorprom-azine hence not associated with jaundice or skin reactions; porphyria (see section 9.8.2); avoid in breast-feeding; reduce dose (preferably avoid) in renal impairment

Dose: 200–400 mg twice daily; max. 800 mg daily in patients with predominantly negative symp-toms, and 2.4 g daily in patients with mainly posi-tive symptoms; ELDERLY, initially quarter to half adult dose; CHILD under 14 not recommended

PoM **Sulpiride** (Non-proprietary)

Tablets, sulpiride 200 mg. Net price 100-tab pack = £18.98. Label: 2

Available from Cox, Norton

PoM **Dolmatil®** (Lorex)

Tablets, both scored, sulpiride 200 mg, net price 100-tab pack = £19.50; 400 mg (f/c), 100-tab pack = £38.00. Label: 2

PoM **Sulparex®** (Bristol-Myers)
Tablets, scored, sulpiride 200 mg. Net price 100-tab pack = £20.03. Label: 2

PoM **Sulpitil®** (Pharmacia & Upjohn)
Tablets, scored, sulpiride 200 mg. Net price 28-tab pack = £5.61; 112-tab pack = £22.43. Label: 2

THIORIDAZINE

Indications: see under Dose
Cautions; Contra-indications; Side-effects: see under Chlorpromazine Hydrochloride, but less sedating and extrapyramidal symptoms and hypothermia rarely occur; more likely to induce hypotension and possibly increased risk of cardiotoxicity and prolongation of QT interval. Pigmentary retinopathy (with reduced visual acuity, brownish colouring of vision, and impaired night vision) occurs rarely with high doses—on prolonged use examinations for eye defects are required; sexual dysfunction, particularly retrograde ejaculation, may occur; porphyria (see section 9.8.2)
Dose: schizophrenia and other psychoses, mania, 150–600 mg daily (initially in divided doses); max. 800 mg daily (hospital patients only) for up to 4 weeks
Short-term adjunctive management of psychomotor agitation, excitement, violent or dangerously impulsive behaviour, 75–200 mg daily
Short-term adjunctive management of severe anxiety, and agitation and restlessness in the elderly, 30–100 mg daily
CHILD (severe mental or behavioural problems only) 1–5 years 1 mg/kg daily, 5–12 years 75–150 mg daily (in severe cases, up to 300 mg daily)

PoM **Thioridazine** (Non-proprietary)
Tablets, coated, thioridazine hydrochloride 25 mg, net price 20 = 34p; 50 mg, 20 = 69p; 100 mg, 20 = £1.31. Label: 2
Available from Cox, DDSA (Rideril®), Hillcross, Norton
Oral solution, thioridazine (as hydrochloride) 25 mg/5 mL. Net price 500-mL = £2.61. Label: 2
Available from Rosemont

PoM **Melleril®** (Novartis)
Tablets, all f/c, thioridazine hydrochloride 10 mg, net price 20 = 22p; 25 mg, 20 = 31p; 50 mg, 20 = 60p; 100 mg, 20 = £1.14. Label: 2
Suspension 25 mg/5 mL, thioridazine 25 mg/5 mL. Net price 500-mL = £2.98. Label: 2
Suspension 100 mg/5 mL, thioridazine 100 mg/5 mL. Net price 500-mL = £10.89. Label: 2
Note. These suspensions should not be diluted but the two preparations may be mixed with each other to provide intermediate doses
Syrup, orange, thioridazine (as hydrochloride) 25 mg/5 mL. Net price 300-mL pack = £2.28. Label: 2
Note. Also available as a generic from Hillcross

TRIFLUOPERAZINE

Indications: see under Dose; anti-emetic (section 4.6)
Cautions; Contra-indications; Side-effects: see under Chlorpromazine Hydrochloride but less sedating, and hypotension, hypothermia, and

antimuscarinic side-effects occur less frequently; extrapyramidal symptoms, particularly dystonic reactions and akathisia, are more frequent (particularly when the daily dose exceeds 6 mg); caution in children
Dose: by mouth (reduce initial doses in elderly by at least half)
Schizophrenia and other psychoses, short-term adjunctive management of psychomotor agitation, excitement, and violent or dangerously impulsive behaviour, initially 5 mg twice daily, *or* 10 mg daily in modified-release form, increased by 5 mg after 1 week, then at intervals of 3 days, according to the response; CHILD up to 12 years, initially up to 5 mg daily in divided doses, adjusted according to response, age, and body-weight
Short-term adjunctive management of severe anxiety, 2–4 mg daily in divided doses *or* 2–4 mg daily in modified-release form, increased if necessary to 6 mg daily; CHILD 3–5 years up to 1 mg daily, 6–12 years up to 4 mg daily

PoM **Trifluoperazine** (Non-proprietary)
Tablets, coated, trifluoperazine (as hydrochloride) 1 mg, net price 20 = 36p; 5 mg, 20 = 44p. Label: 2
Available from most generic manufacturers
Oral solution, trifluoperazine (as hydrochloride) 5 mg/5 mL. Net price 200-mL = £9.25. Label: 2
Available from Rosemont (sugar-free)

PoM **Stelazine®** (SK&F)
Tablets, both blue, f/c, trifluoperazine (as hydrochloride) 1 mg, net price 20 = 61p; 5 mg, 20 = 87p. Label: 2
Spansules® (– capsules m/r), all clear/yellow, enclosing dark blue, light blue, and white pellets, trifluoperazine (as hydrochloride) 2 mg, net price 60-cap pack = £3.97; 10 mg, 30-cap pack = £2.58; 15 mg, 30-cap pack = £3.89. Label: 2, 25
Syrup, yellow, sugar-free, trifluoperazine (as hydrochloride) 1 mg/5 mL. Net price 200-mL pack = £2.42. Label: 2

ZUCLOPENTHIXOL ACETATE

Indications: short-term management of acute psychosis, mania, or exacerbations of chronic psychosis
Cautions; Contra-indications; Side-effects: see under Chlorpromazine Hydrochloride; porphyria (see section 9.8.2); treatment duration should not exceed 2 weeks
Dose: by deep intramuscular injection into the gluteal muscle or lateral thigh, 50–150 mg (elderly 50–100 mg), if necessary repeated after 2–3 days (1 additional dose may be needed 1–2 days after the first injection); max. cumulative dose 400 mg per course and max. 4 injections; max. duration of treatment 2 weeks—if maintenance treatment necessary change to an oral antipsychotic 2–3 days after last injection, *or* to a longer acting antipsychotic depot injection given concomitantly with last injection of zuclopenthixol acetate; CHILD not recommended

PoM **Clopixol Acuphase®** (Lundbeck)

Injection (oily), zuclopenthixol acetate 50 mg/mL. Net price 1-mL amp = £4.95; 2-mL amp = £9.55

ZUCLOPENTHIXOL DIHYDROCHLORIDE

Indications: schizophrenia and other psychoses, particularly when associated with agitated, aggressive, or hostile behaviour

Cautions; Contra-indications; Side-effects: see under Chlorpromazine Hydrochloride; should not be used in apathetic or withdrawn states; porphyria (see section 9.8.2)

Dose: initially 20–30 mg daily in divided doses, increasing to a max. of 150 mg daily if necessary; usual maintenance dose 20–50 mg daily; ELDERLY (or debilitated) initially quarter to half adult dose; CHILD not recommended

PoM **Clopixol®** (Lundbeck)

Tablets, all f/c, zuclopenthixol (as dihydrochloride) 2 mg (pink), net price 20 = 61p; 10 mg (light brown), 20 = £1.65; 25 mg (brown), 20 = £3.30. Label: 2

Depot injection (zuclopenthixol decanoate): section 4.2.2

ATYPICAL ANTIPSYCHOTICS

The newer 'atypical antipsychotics' **amisulpride**, **clozapine**, **olanzapine**, **quetiapine**, **risperidone**, and **sertindole** may be effective in patients refractory to other treatment; extrapyramidal symptoms and prolactin elevation may be less frequent than with older antipsychotics.

Clozapine is indicated only for the treatment of schizophrenia in patients unresponsive to, or intolerant of, conventional antipsychotic drugs. It can cause agranulocytosis and its use is restricted to patients registered with the Clozaril Patient Monitoring Service (see under Clozapine, below).

Risperidone is indicated for psychoses in which both positive and negative symptoms are prominent.

Olanzapine, **sertindole**, and **quetiapine** have been introduced only recently and experience with their use is limited. Olanzapine is effective in maintaining clinical improvement in patients who have responded to initial treatment. Sertindole and quetiapine are indicated for the treatment of both positive and negative symptoms. Sertindole is associated with QT interval prolongation which may lead to serious ventricular arrhythmias; it should not be used with other drugs that prolong the QT interval. Quetiapine should also be used with caution in cardiovascular disease because it may prolong the QT interval; it is occasionally associated with neutropenia.

Amisulpride has been introduced recently; it is indicated for both positive and negative symptoms of schizophrenia.

CAUTIONS. Atypical antipsychotics should be used with caution in patients with cardiovascular disease, history of epilepsy, Parkinsons disease; **interactions:** Appendix 1 (antipsychotics)

DRIVING. Atypical antipsychotics may affect performance of skilled tasks (e.g. driving); effects of alcohol enhanced

SIDE-EFFECTS. Side-effects of the atypical antipsychotics include weight gain, dizziness, postural hypotension (especially during initial dose titration period) which may be associated with syncope or reflex tachycardia in some patients, extrapyramidal symptoms (which are usually mild and transient and respond to dose reduction or to antimuscarinic drugs), occasionally tardive dyskinesia on long-term administration; neuroleptic malignant syndrome has been reported rarely.

AMISULPRIDE

Indications: schizophrenia; see also notes above

Cautions: see notes above; renal impairment (Appendix 3), elderly (risk of hypotension or sedation); **interactions:** Appendix 1 (antipsychotics)

Contra-indications: pregnancy and breast-feeding, phaeochromocytoma, prolactin-dependent tumours

Side-effects: see notes above; insomnia, anxiety, agitation, drowsiness, gastro-intestinal disorders such as constipation, nausea, vomiting, and dry mouth, hyperprolactinaemia (with galactorrhoea, amenorrhoea, gynaecomastia, breast pain, sexual dysfunction), occasionally bradycardia, seizures; QT interval prolongation reported

Dose: acute psychotic episode, 400–800 mg daily in divided doses, adjusted according to response; max. 1.2 g daily

Predominently negative symptoms, 50–300 mg daily; CHILD under 15 years, not recommended

Note. Doses up to 300 mg may be administered once daily

▼ PoM **Solian®** (Lorex)

Tablets, scored, amisulpride 50 mg, net price 60-tab pack = £16.45, 90-tab pack = £24.69; 200 mg, net price 60-tab pack = £60.00, 90-tab pack = £90.00. Label: 2

CLOZAPINE

Indications: schizophrenia in patients unresponsive to, or intolerant of, conventional antipsychotic drugs

Cautions: see notes above; initiation must be in hospital in-patients; leucocyte and differential blood counts must be normal before starting treatment and must be monitored weekly for first 18 weeks then at least fortnightly—patients who have received clozapine for a year or more and have stable blood counts may have their blood monitoring reduced to every 4 weeks (monitoring must continue for 4 weeks after discontinuation); avoid drugs which depress leucopoiesis (Appendix 1) and taper off conventional neuroleptic

---

before starting; withdraw treatment permanently if leucocyte count falls below 3000/mm³ or absolute neutrophil count falls below 1500/mm³; patients should report any symptoms of infection immediately; mild to moderate renal impairment (Appendix 3); prostatic hypertrophy, angle-closure glaucoma; **interactions:** Appendix 1 (antipsychotics)

WITHDRAWAL. On planned withdrawal reduce dose gradually over 1–2 weeks to avoid risk of rebound psychosis. If abrupt withdrawal necessary observe patient carefully

Contra-indications: severe cardiac failure; hepatic impairment (Appendix 2), severe renal impairment (Appendix 3); history of drug-induced neutropenia or agranulocytosis; bone marrow disorders; alcoholic and toxic psychoses; history of circulatory collapse or paralytic ileus; drug intoxication; coma or severe CNS depression; uncontrolled epilepsy; pregnancy and breast-feeding

Side-effects: see notes above; neutropenia and potentially fatal agranulocytosis (**important:** see Cautions), fever (evaluate to rule out underlying infection or agranulocytosis), drowsiness, anxiety, agitation, confusion, fatigue, blurred vision, dry mouth, constipation, paralytic ileus, nausea and vomiting, dysphagia, headache, dizziness, hypersalivation, urinary incontinence and retention, priapism, abnormal temperature regulation, liver enzyme abnormalities (asymptomatic elevation occurs commonly during early stages of treatment), hepatitis, jaundice (discontinue immediately), rarely fulminant hepatic necrosis; arrhythmias, pericarditis, myocarditis, delirium; tachycardia, rarely circulatory collapse with cardiac and respiratory arrest (but hypertension also reported), acute pancreatitis; thromboembolism, hyperglycaemia, skin rash, elevated creatine kinase concentrations, interstitial nephritis also reported

Dose: (close medical supervision on initiation—risk of collapse due to hypotension) 12.5 mg once or twice on first day then 25–50 mg on second day then increased gradually (if well tolerated) in steps of 25–50 mg over 14–21 days to 300 mg daily in divided doses (larger dose at night, up to 200 mg daily may be taken as a single dose at bedtime); if necessary may be further increased in steps of 50–100 mg once (preferably) or twice weekly; usual antipsychotic dose 200–450 mg daily (max. 900 mg daily); subsequent adjustment to usual maintenance of 150–300 mg; CHILD not recommended

Note. Restarting after *interval of more than 2 days*, 12.5 mg once or twice on first day (but may be feasible to increase more quickly than on initiation)—unless previous respiratory or cardiac arrest with initial dosing in which case extreme caution

ELDERLY AND SPECIAL RISK GROUPS. In *elderly*, 12.5 mg once on first day—subsequent adjustments restricted to 25 mg daily; in *cardiovascular disease*, *hepatic* or *renal impairment* or if history of *epilepsy*, 12.5 mg on first day—subsequent adjustments slowly and in small steps (if epileptic seizures (see also Cautions), suspend for 24 hours and resume at lower dose)

PoM **Clozaril®** (Novartis)
Tablets, both yellow, clozapine 25 mg (scored), net price 28-tab pack = £12.52, 84-tab pack (hosp. only) = £37.54; 100 mg, 28-tab pack = £50.05, 84-tab pack (hosp. only) = £150.15. Label: 2, 10 patient information leaflet
Note. Patient, prescriber, and supplying pharmacist must be registered with the Clozaril Patient Monitoring Service—takes several days to do this

OLANZAPINE
Indications: schizophrenia
Cautions: see notes above; pregnancy, prostatic hypertrophy, paralytic ileus, hepatic impairment (Appendix 2), renal impairment (Appendix 3), low leucocyte or neutrophil count, bone marrow depression, hypereosinophilic disorders, myeloproliferative disease; concomitant administration of drugs that prolong QT interval (especially in elderly); **interactions:** Appendix 1 (antipsychotics)
Contra-indications: angle closure glaucoma; breast-feeding
Side-effects: see notes above; mild, transient antimuscarinic effects; drowsiness, increased appetite, peripheral oedema, hyperprolactinaemia (but clinical manifestations are rare), occasionally blood dyscrasias, transient asymptomatic elevations of liver enzymes, rarely photsensitivity and elevated creatine kinase concentrations
Dose: 10 mg daily adjusted to usual range of 5–20 mg daily; doses of 15 mg daily or greater only after reassessment
Note. When one or more factors present that might result in slower metabolism (e.g. female gender, elderly, non-smoker) consider lower initial dose and more gradual dose escalation

▼ PoM **Zyprexa®** (Lilly)
Tablets, f/c, olanzapine 5 mg, net price 28-tab pack = £52.73; 7.5 mg, 56-tab pack = £158.20; 10 mg, 28-tab pack = £105.47, 56-tab pack = £210.93. Label: 2

QUETIAPINE
Indications: schizophrenia, see also notes above
Cautions: see notes above; pregnancy, hepatic impairment (Appendix 2), renal impairment (Appendix 3), elderly, concomitant administration of drugs that prolong QT interval (especially in elderly), cerebrovascular disease; **interactions:** Appendix 1 (antipsychotics)
Contra-indications: breast-feeding
Side-effects: see notes above; drowsiness, dyspepsia, constipation, dry mouth, asymptomatic liver enzyme abnormalities, mild asthenia, rhinitis, tachycardia; anxiety, fever, myalgia, rash; leucopenia, neutropenia and occasionally, eosinophilia reported; elevated plasma-triglyceride and cholesterol concentrations, reduced plasma-thyroid hormone concentrations; possible QT interval prolongation
Dose: 25 mg twice daily on day 1, 50 mg twice daily on day 2, 100 mg twice daily on day 3, 150 mg twice daily on day 4, then adjusted according to response, usual range 300–450 mg daily in 2 divided doses; max. 750 mg daily; ELDERLY initially 25 mg daily, increased in steps of 25–50 mg daily

---

▼ PoM **Seroquel**® (Zeneca)
Tablets, f/c, quetiapine (as fumarate) 25 mg (peach), net price 60-tab pack = £28.20; 100 mg (yellow), 60-tab pack = £113.10, 90-tab pack = £169.65; 200 mg (white), 60-tab pack = £113.10, 90-tab pack = £169.65; starter pack of 6 × 25 mg with 2 × 100 mg = £6.59. Label: 2

RISPERIDONE

Indications: acute and chronic psychoses, see also notes above

Cautions: see notes above; pregnancy; hepatic impairment (Appendix 2), renal impairment (Appendix 3), concomitant administration of drugs that prolong QT interval; **interactions:** Appendix 1 (antipsychotics)

Contra-indications: breast-feeding

Side-effects: see notes above; insomnia, agitation, anxiety, headache, drowsiness, impaired concentration, fatigue, blurred vision, constipation, nausea and vomiting, dyspepsia, abdominal pain, hyperprolactinaemia (with galactorrhoea, menstrual disturbances, amenorrhoea, gynaecomastia), sexual dysfunction, priapism, urinary incontinence, liver enzyme abnormalities, tachycardia, hypertension, skin rash, rhinitis; neutropenia and thrombocytopenia have been reported; rarely, water intoxication with hyponatraemia, abnormal temperature regulation, seizures

Dose: 2 mg in 1–2 divided doses on first day *then* 4 mg in 1–2 divided doses on second day *then* 6 mg in 1–2 divided doses on third day (slower titration appropriate in some patients); usual range 4–8 mg daily; doses above 10 mg daily only if benefit considered to outweigh risk (max. 16 mg daily); ELDERLY (or in hepatic or renal impairment) initially 500 micrograms twice daily increased in steps of 500 micrograms twice daily to 1–2 mg twice daily; CHILD under 15 years not recommended

PoM **Risperdal**® (Janssen-Cilag, Organon)
Tablets, all f/c, scored, risperidone 1 mg (white), net price, 6-tab starter pack = £4.15, 20-tab pack = £13.45; 2 mg (orange), 60-tab pack = £79.56; 3 mg (yellow), 60-tab pack = £117.00; 4 mg (green), 60-tab pack = £154.44; 6 mg (yellow), 28-tab pack = £109.20. Label: 2
Liquid, risperidone 1 mg/mL, net price 100 mL = £65.00. Label: 2
Note. Liquid may be diluted with mineral water, orange juice or black coffee (should be used within 4 hours)

SERTINDOLE

Indications: schizophrenia, see also notes above

Cautions: see notes above; mild or moderate hepatic impairment (Appendix 2); diabetes; correct hypokalaemia or hypomagnesaemia before treatment; monitor ECG during treatment; monitor blood pressure during dose titration and early maintenance therapy (risk of postural hypotension); **interactions:** Appendix 1 (antipsychotics)

Contra-indications: see notes above; pregnancy and breast-feeding, severe hepatic impairment, QT interval prolongation (ECG required before treatment); concomitant administration of drugs which prolong QT interval or cause hypokalaemia (see interactions)

Side-effects: see notes above; prolonged QT interval, peripheral oedema, dry mouth, rhinitis, nasal congestion, dyspnoea, paraesthesia, abnormal ejaculation (decreased volume); rarely seizures, hyperglycaemia

Dose: initially 4 mg daily increased in steps of 4 mg at intervals of 4–5 days to usual maintenance of 12–20 mg as a single daily dose; max. 24 mg daily; ELDERLY and in hepatic impairment consider slower dose titration and lower maintenance dose

▼ PoM **Serdolect**® (Lundbeck)
Tablets, sertindole 4 mg, net price 30-tab pack = £36.63; 12 mg, 28-tab pack = £102.55; 16 mg, 28-tab pack = £102.55; 20 mg, 28-tab pack = £102.55

4.2.2   Antipsychotic depot injections

For maintenance therapy, long-acting depot injections of antipsychotic drugs are used because they are more convenient than oral preparations and ensure better patient compliance. However, they may give rise to a higher incidence of extrapyramidal reactions than oral preparations.

ADMINISTRATION. Depot antipsychotics are administered by deep intramuscular injection at intervals of 1 to 4 weeks. Patients should first be given a small test-dose as undesirable side-effects are prolonged. In general not more than 2–3 mL of oily injection should be administered at any one site; correct injection technique (including the use of z-track technique) and rotation of injection sites are essential. If the dose needs to be reduced to alleviate side-effects, it is important to recognise that the plasma-drug concentration may not fall for some time after reducing the dose, therefore it may be a month or longer before side-effects subside.

DOSAGE. Individual responses to neuroleptic drugs are very variable and to achieve optimum effect, dosage and dosage interval must be titrated according to the patient's response. For the advice of The Royal College of Psychiatrists on doses above the BNF upper limit, see p. 162

Equivalent doses of depot antipsychotics
These equivalences are intended **only** as an approximate guide; individual dosage instructions should **also** be checked; patients should be carefully monitored after **any** change in medication

Antipsychotic	Dose (mg)	Interval
Flupenthixol decanoate	40	2 weeks
Fluphenazine decanoate	25	2 weeks
Haloperidol (as decanoate)	100	4 weeks
Pipothiazine palmitate	50	4 weeks
Zuclopenthixol decanoate	200	2 weeks

IMPORTANT. These equivalences must **not** be extrapolated beyond the max. dose for the drug

CHOICE. There is no clear-cut division in the use of these drugs, but **zuclopenthixol** may be suitable for the treatment of agitated or aggressive patients whereas **flupenthixol** can cause over-excitement in such patients. The incidence of extrapyramidal reactions is similar for all these drugs.

CAUTIONS. Treatment requires careful monitoring for optimum effect; extrapyramidal symptoms occur frequently. When transferring from oral to depot therapy, dosage by mouth should be gradually phased out.

CONTRA-INDICATIONS. Do not use in children, confusional states, coma caused by CNS depressants, parkinsonism, intolerance to antipsychotics.

SIDE-EFFECTS. Pain may occur at injection site and occasionally erythema, swelling, and nodules. For side-effects of specific antipsychotics see under the relevant monograph.

FLUPENTHIXOL DECANOATE
(Flupentixol Decanoate)

Indications: maintenance in schizophrenia and other psychoses

Cautions; Contra-indications; Side-effects: see under Chlorpromazine Hydrochloride (section 4.2.1) and notes above, but it may have a mood elevating effect; extrapyramidal symptoms usually appear 1–3 days after administration and continue for about 5 days but may be delayed; an alternative antipsychotic may be necessary if symptoms such as aggression or agitation appear; porphyria (see section 9.8.2)

Dose: by deep intramuscular injection into the gluteal muscle, test dose 20 mg, then after at least 7 days 20–40 mg repeated at intervals of 2–4 weeks, adjusted according to response; max. 400 mg weekly; usual maintenance dose 50 mg every 4 weeks to 300 mg every 2 weeks; ELDERLY initially quarter to half adult dose; CHILD not recommended

PoM **Depixol®** (Lundbeck)
Injection (oily), flupenthixol decanoate 20 mg/mL. Net price 1-mL amp = £1.55; 2-mL amp = £2.60
PoM **Depixol Conc.®** (Lundbeck)
Injection (oily), flupenthixol decanoate 100 mg/ mL. Net price 0.5-mL amp = £3.49; 1-mL amp = £6.40
PoM **Depixol Low Volume®** (Lundbeck)
Injection (oily), flupenthixol decanoate 200 mg/ mL. Net price 1-mL amp = £19.98

FLUPHENAZINE DECANOATE

Indications: maintenance in schizophrenia and other psychoses

Cautions; Contra-indications; Side-effects: see under Chlorpromazine Hydrochloride (section 4.2.1) and notes above. Extrapyramidal symptoms usually appear a few hours after the dose has been administered and continue for about 2 days

but may be delayed. Contra-indicated in severely depressed states

Dose: by deep intramuscular injection into the gluteal muscle, test dose 12.5 mg (6.25 mg in elderly), then after 4–7 days 12.5–100 mg repeated at intervals of 14–35 days, adjusted according to response; CHILD not recommended

PoM **Modecate®** (Sanofi Winthrop)
Injection (oily), fluphenazine decanoate 25 mg/ mL. Net price 0.5-mL amp = £1.42; 1-mL amp = £2.46; 1-mL syringe = £2.72; 2-mL amp = £4.84; 2-mL syringe = £4.93; 10-mL vial = £23.45
Note. Contains sesame oil
Note. Fluphenazine decanoate injection also available from Antigen, Berk, Faulding DBL, Hillcross—at least some versions contain sesame oil
PoM **Modecate Concentrate®** (Sanofi Winthrop)
Injection (oily), fluphenazine decanoate 100 mg/ mL. Net price 0.5-mL amp = £4.87; 1-mL amp = £9.53
Note. Contains sesame oil
Note. Fluphenazine decanoate injection also available from Antigen, Berk, Faulding DBL, Hillcross—at least some versions contain sesame oil

---

HALOPERIDOL DECANOATE

Indications: maintenance in schizophrenia and other psychoses

Cautions; Contra-indications; Side-effects: see under Haloperidol (section 4.2.1) and notes above

Dose: by deep intramuscular injection into the gluteal muscle, haloperidol (as decanoate), initially 50 mg every 4 weeks, if necessary increasing after 2 weeks by 50-mg increments to 300 mg every 4 weeks; higher doses may be needed in some patients; ELDERLY, initially 12.5–25 mg every 4 weeks; CHILD not recommended

PoM **Haldol Decanoate®** (Janssen-Cilag)
Injection (oily), haloperidol (as decanoate) 50 mg/ mL, net price 1-mL amp = £4.35; 100 mg/mL, 1-mL amp = £5.77

PIPOTHIAZINE PALMITATE
(Pipotiazine Palmitate)

Indications: maintenance in schizophrenia and other psychoses

Cautions; Contra-indications; Side-effects: see under Chlorpromazine Hydrochloride (section 4.2.1) and notes above

Dose: by deep intramuscular injection into the gluteal muscle, test dose 25 mg, then a further 25–50 mg after 4–7 days, then adjusted according to response at intervals of 4 weeks; usual maintenance range 50–100 mg (max. 200 mg) every 4 weeks; ELDERLY initially 5–10 mg; CHILD not recommended

PoM **Piportil Depot®** (JHC)
Injection (oily), pipothiazine palmitate 50 mg/mL. Net price 1-mL amp = £11.85; 2-mL amp = £19.38

ZUCLOPENTHIXOL DECANOATE

Indications: maintenance in schizophrenia and
other psychoses, particularly with aggression and
agitation

Cautions; Contra-indications; Side-effects: see
under Chlorpromazine Hydrochloride (section
4.2.1) and notes above, but less sedating; porphyria (see section 9.8.2)

Dose: by deep intramuscular injection into the
gluteal muscle, test dose 100 mg, followed after
7–28 days by 100–200 mg or more, followed by
200–400 mg at intervals of 2–4 weeks, adjusted
according to response; max. 600 mg weekly;
CHILD not recommended

PoM **Clopixol**® (Lundbeck)
Injection (oily), zuclopenthixol decanoate 200 mg/
mL. Net price 1-mL amp = £3.23
PoM **Clopixol Conc.**® (Lundbeck)
Injection (oily), zuclopenthixol decanoate 500 mg/
mL. Net price 1-mL amp with needle = £7.61

4.2.3   Antimanic drugs

Drugs are used in mania both to control acute
attacks and also to prevent their recurrence.

BENZODIAZEPINES

Use of benzodiazepines (section 4.1) may be helpful in the initial stages of treatment until lithium
achieves its full effect; they should not be used for
long periods because of the risk of dependence.

ANTIPSYCHOTIC DRUGS

In an acute attack of mania, treatment with an antipsychotic drug (section 4.2.1) is usually required
because it may take a few days for lithium to exert
its antimanic effect. Lithium may be given concurrently with the antipsychotic drug, and treatment
with the antipsychotic gradually tailed off as lithium becomes effective. Alternatively, lithium therapy may be commenced once the patient's mood
has been stabilised with the antipsychotic. Haloperidol may be preferred for rapid control of acute
mania. However, high doses of haloperidol, fluphenazine, or flupenthixol may be hazardous when
used with lithium; irreversible toxic encephalopathy
has been reported.

LITHIUM

Lithium salts are used in the prophylaxis and treatment of mania, in the prophylaxis of manic-depressive illness (bipolar illness or bipolar depression)
and in the prophylaxis of recurrent depression (unipolar illness or unipolar depression). Lithium is
unsuitable for children.

The decision to give prophylactic lithium usually
requires *specialist advice*, and must be based on
careful consideration of the likelihood of recurrence
in the individual patient, and the benefit weighed
against the risks. In long-term use, therapeutic concentrations have been thought to cause histological
and functional changes in the kidney. The signifi-

cance of such changes is not clear but is of sufficient concern to discourage long-term use of
lithium unless it is definitely indicated. Patients
should therefore be maintained on lithium after 3–5
years only if, on assessment, benefit persists.

PLASMA CONCENTRATIONS. Lithium salts have a narrow therapeutic/toxic ratio and should therefore not
be prescribed unless facilities for monitoring
plasma-lithium concentrations are available. There
seem few if any reasons for preferring one or other
of the salts of lithium available. Doses are adjusted
to achieve plasma-lithium concentration of 0.4 to
1.0 mmol/litre (lower end of the range for maintenance therapy and elderly patients) on samples
taken 12 hours after the preceding dose. It is important to determine the optimum range for each individual patient.

Overdosage, usually with plasma-lithium concentration over 1.5 mmol/litre, may be fatal and toxic
effects include tremor, ataxia, dysarthria, nystagmus, renal impairment, and convulsions. If these
potentially hazardous signs occur, treatment should
be stopped, plasma-lithium concentrations redeter-
mined, and steps taken to reverse lithium toxicity.
In mild cases withdrawal of lithium and administration of generous amounts of sodium and fluid will
reverse the toxicity. Plasma-lithium concentration
in excess of 2.0 mmol/litre require emergency treatment as indicated under Emergency Treatment of
Poisoning, p. 23. When toxic concentrations are
reached there may be a delay of 1 or 2 days before
maximum toxicity occurs.

INTERACTIONS. Lithium toxicity is made worse by
sodium depletion, therefore concurrent use of diuretics (particularly thiazides) is hazardous and
should be avoided. For other **interactions** with lithium, see Appendix 1 (lithium).

WITHDRAWAL. There is no evidence of a lithium
withdrawal state nor of rebound psychosis on withdrawal. Nevertheless, to allay any concerns about
relapse, if possible lithium should be withdrawn
slowly over a period of weeks.

LITHIUM CARDS. A lithium treatment card available
from pharmacies tells patients how to take lithium
preparations, what to do if a dose is missed, and what
side-effects to expect. It also explains why regular
blood tests are important and warns that some medicines and illnesses can change plasma-lithium concentrations

Cards may be obtained from NPA Services, 38–42
St. Peter's St, St. Albans, Herts AL1 3NP.

LITHIUM CARBONATE

Indications: treatment and prophylaxis of mania,
manic-depressive illness, and recurrent depression (see also notes above); aggressive or self-
mutilating behaviour

Cautions: measure plasma concentrations regularly (every 3 months on stabilised regimens),

monitor thyroid function; maintain adequate sodium and fluid intake; avoid in renal impairment, cardiac disease, and conditions with sodium imbalance such as Addison's disease; reduction in dose or discontinuation may be necessary in diarrhoea, vomiting and intercurrent infection (especially when associated with profuse sweating); caution in pregnancy (Appendix 4), breast-feeding, elderly (reduce dose), diuretic treatment, myasthenia gravis; surgery (section 15.1); if possible avoid abrupt withdrawal (see notes above); **interactions:** Appendix 1 (lithium)

COUNSELLING. Patients should maintain an adequate fluid intake and should avoid dietary changes which might reduce or increase sodium intake; lithium treatment cards are available from pharmacies (see above)

Note. **Different preparations vary widely in bioavailability**; a change in the preparation used requires the same precautions as initiation of treatment

Side-effects: gastro-intestinal disturbances, fine tremor, polyuria and polydipsia; also weight gain and oedema (may respond to dose reduction). Signs of lithium intoxication are blurred vision, increasing gastro-intestinal disturbances (anorexia, vomiting, diarrhoea), muscle weakness, increasing CNS disturbances (mild drowsiness and sluggishness increasing to giddiness with ataxia, coarse tremor, lack of co-ordination, dysarthria), and require withdrawal of treatment. With severe **overdosage** (plasma-lithium concentrations above 2 mmol/litre) hyperreflexia and hyperextension of limbs, convulsions, toxic psychoses, syncope, oliguria, circulatory failure, coma, and occasionally, death. Goitre, raised antidiuretic hormone concentration, hypothyroidism, hypokalaemia, ECG changes, exacerbation of psoriasis, and kidney changes may also occur. See also Emergency Treatment of Poisoning, p. 23

Dose: see under preparations below, adjusted to achieve a plasma-lithium concentration of 0.4–1.0 mmol/litre 12 hours after a dose on the fourth to seventh day of treatment, then every week until dosage has remained constant for 4 weeks and every 3 months thereafter; doses are initially divided throughout the day, but once daily administration is preferred when plasma-lithium concentration stabilised

PoM **Camcolit®** (Norgine)

Camcolit 250® tablets, f/c, scored, lithium carbonate 250 mg (6.8 mmol Li⁺). Net price 20 = 58p. Label: 10 lithium card, counselling, see above

Camcolit 400® tablets, m/r, f/c, scored, lithium carbonate 400 mg (10.8 mmol Li⁺). Net price 20 = 77p. Label: 10 lithium card, 25, counselling, see above

Dose (plasma monitoring, see above):

Treatment, initially 1.5–2 g daily (elderly, 0.5–1 g daily); prophylaxis, initially 0.5–1.2 g daily (elderly, 0.5–1 g daily); CHILD not recommended

Camcolit 250® should be given in divided doses, whereas *Camcolit 400®* may be given in single or divided doses

Note. *Camcolit 400®* also available as *Lithonate®* (Berk)

PoM **Liskonum®** (SK&F)

Tablets, m/r, f/c, scored, lithium carbonate 450 mg (12.2 mmol Li⁺). Net price 60-tab pack = £2.82. Label: 10 lithium card, 25, counselling, see above

Dose (plasma monitoring, see above):

Treatment, initially 450–675 mg twice daily (elderly, initially 225 mg twice daily); prophylaxis, initially 450 mg twice daily (elderly, 225 mg twice daily); CHILD not recommended

PoM **Priadel®** (Delandale)

Tablets, both m/r, scored, lithium carbonate 200 mg (5.4 mmol Li⁺), net price 20 = 41p; 400 mg (10.8 mmol Li⁺), 20 = 68p. Label: 10 lithium card, 25, counselling, see above

Dose (plasma monitoring, see above):

Treatment and prophylaxis, initially 0.4 1.2 g daily as a single dose or in 2 divided doses (elderly or patients less than 50 kg, 400 mg daily); CHILD not recommended

Liquid, see under Lithium Citrate, below

LITHIUM CITRATE

Indications; Cautions; Side-effects: see under Lithium Carbonate and notes above

COUNSELLING. Patients should maintain an adequate fluid intake and should avoid dietary changes which might reduce or increase sodium intake; lithium treatment cards are available from pharmacies (see previous page)

Note. **Different preparations vary widely in bioavailability**; a change in the preparation used requires the same precautions as initiation of treatment

Dose: see under preparations below, adjusted to achieve plasma-lithium concentrations of 0.4–1.0 mmol/litre as described under Lithium Carbonate

PoM **Li-Liquid®** (Rosemont)

Oral solution, lithium citrate 509 mg/5 mL (5.4 mmol Li⁺/5 mL), yellow, net price 100-mL pack = £4.50, 100 × g/5 mL, (10 × mmol Li)/5 mL), orange, 100-mL pack = £8.60. Label: 10 lithium card, counselling, see above

Dose (plasma monitoring, see above):

Treatment and prophylaxis, initially 1.018–3.054 g daily in 2 divided doses (elderly or patients less than 50 kg, initially 509 mg twice daily); CHILD not recommended

PoM **Litarex®** (Dumex)

Tablets, m/r, lithium citrate 564 mg (6 mmol Li⁺). Net price 20 = 72p. Label: 10 lithium card, 25, counselling, see above

Dose (plasma monitoring, see above):

Treatment and prophylaxis, initially 564 mg twice daily; CHILD not recommended

PoM **Priadel®** (Delandale)

Tablets, see under Lithium Carbonate, above

Liquid, sugar-free, lithium citrate 520 mg/5 mL (approx. 5.4 mmol Li⁺/5 mL), net price 150-mL pack = £6.58, 300-mL pack = £13.16. Label: 10 lithium card, counselling, see above

Dose (plasma monitoring, see above):

Treatment and prophylaxis, initially 1.04–3.12 g daily in 2 divided doses (elderly or patients less than 50 kg, 520 mg twice daily); CHILD not recommended

CARBAMAZEPINE

Carbamazepine may be used for the prophylaxis of manic-depressive illness in patients unresponsive to lithium; it seems to be particularly effective in patients with rapid cycling manic-depressive illness (4 or more affective episodes per year).

CARBAMAZEPINE

Indications: prophylaxis of manic-depressive illness unresponsive to lithium; for use in epilepsy see section 4.8.1

Cautions; Contra-indications; Side-effects: see section 4.8.1

Dose: initially 400 mg daily in divided doses increased until symptoms controlled; usual range 400–600 mg daily; max. 1.6 g daily

Preparations

Section 4.8.1

4.3   Antidepressant drugs

4.3.1	Tricyclic and related antidepressant drugs
4.3.2	Monoamine-oxidase inhibitors (MAOIs)
4.3.3	SSRIs and related antidepressants
4.3.4	Other antidepressant drugs

Tricyclic and related antidepressants and the selective serotonin re-uptake inhibitors (SSRIs) and related antidepressants are preferred to the traditional MAOIs because they are more effective and do not show the dangerous interactions with some *foods* and have fewer of the dangerous interactions with *drugs* that are characteristic of the traditional MAOIs.

The choice between **older tricyclics** (e.g. amitriptyline) and **related drugs within the group** (e.g. maprotiline) depends mainly on the lower incidence of antimuscarinic side-effects associated with the related ones, such as less dry mouth and constipation; the related ones may also be associated with a lower risk of cardiotoxicity in overdosage; however, some have additional side-effects (for further details see section 4.3.1).

The **SSRIs** also have fewer antimuscarinic side-effects than the **older tricyclics** and they also seem to be less cardiotoxic in overdosage. Therefore, although not more effective, they may be preferred where there is a major risk of overdosage. The SSRIs do, however, have characteristic side-effects of their own. Hence, drowsiness, dry mouth and cardiotoxicity may be less of a problem, but gastro-intestinal side-effects such as nausea and vomiting may be more common.

See section 4.2.3 for references to the role of **lithium** and **carbamazepine** in depression or in manic depressive illness.

Where the depression is very severe **electroconvulsive therapy** may be indicated.

Prescribing more than one antidepressant at the same time is **not** recommended. It may constitute a hazard and there is no evidence that side-effects are minimised.

Compound preparations of an antidepressant and an anxiolytic are **not** recommended because the dosage of the individual components should be adjusted separately. Whereas antidepressants are given continuously over several months, anxiolytics are prescribed on a **short-term** basis.

It should be noted that although anxiety is often present in depressive illness and may be the presenting symptom, the use of antipsychotics or anxiolytics may mask the true diagnosis. They should therefore be used with caution (but are useful adjuncts in agitated depression).

CSM advice (hyponatraemia). Hyponatraemia (usually in the elderly and possibly due to inappropriate secretion of antidiuretic hormone) has been associated with all types of antidepressants and should be considered in all patients who develop drowsiness, confusion or convulsions while taking an antidepressant.

MANAGEMENT. The patient must be assessed frequently, especially in the early weeks of treatment, to detect any suicidal tendencies. Limited quantities of antidepressant drugs should be prescribed at any one time since antidepressant drugs and in particular tricyclic antidepressants are dangerous in overdosage. Some of the newer drugs seem less dangerous in overdose than the older tricyclics.

Treatment should be continued for 2 weeks before suppression of symptoms can be expected and thereafter should be maintained at the optimum level for at least 4–6 months after the depression has resolved. Treatment should not be withdrawn prematurely, otherwise symptoms are likely to recur. The natural history of depressive illness suggests that remission usually occurs after 3 months to a year or more. In recurrent depression, prophylactic maintenance therapy with an effective dose may need to be continued for several years.

In patients who do not respond to antidepressants, the diagnosis, dosage, compliance, and possible continuation of psychosocial or physical aggravating causes should all be carefully reviewed; other drug treatment may be successful.

WITHDRAWAL. Gastro-intestinal symptoms of nausea, vomiting, and anorexia, accompanied by headache, giddiness, 'chills', and insomnia, and sometimes by hypomania, panic-anxiety, and extreme motor restlessness may occur if an antidepressant (particularly an MAOI) is stopped suddenly after regular administration for 8 weeks or more. Reduction in dosage should preferably be carried out gradually over a period of about 4 weeks. SSRIs and in particular paroxetine have been associated with a specific withdrawal syndrome (section 4.3.3).

4.3.1   Tricyclic and related antidepressant drugs

This section covers tricyclic antidepressants and also 1-, 2-, and 4-ring structured drugs with broadly similar properties.

These drugs are most effective for treating moderate to severe *endogenous depression* associated with psychomotor and physiological changes such as loss of appetite and sleep disturbances; improvement in sleep is usually the first benefit of therapy. Since there may be an interval of 2 weeks before the antidepressant action takes place electroconvulsive treatment may be required in severe depression when delay is hazardous or intolerable.

Some tricyclic antidepressants are also effective in the management of *panic disorder.*

For reference to the role of some tricyclic antidepressants in some forms of *neuralgia,* see section 4.7.3, and in *nocturnal enuresis* in children, see section 7.4.2.

DOSAGE. About 10 to 20% of patients fail to respond to tricyclic and related antidepressant drugs and inadequate dosage may account for some of these failures. It is important to use doses that are sufficiently high for effective treatment but not so high as to cause toxic effects. Low doses should be used for initial treatment in the **elderly** (see under Side-effects, below).

In most patients the long half-life of tricyclic antidepressant drugs allows **once-daily** administration, usually at night; the use of modified-release preparations is therefore unnecessary.

CHOICE. Tricyclic and related antidepressant drugs can be roughly divided into those with additional sedative properties and those which are less so. Agitated and anxious patients tend to respond best to the sedative compounds whereas withdrawn and apathetic patients will often obtain most benefit from the less sedating ones. Those with **sedative** properties include amitriptyline, clomipramine, dothiepin (dosulepin), doxepin, maprotiline, mianserin, trazodone, and trimipramine. Those with **less sedative** properties include amoxapine, imipramine, lofepramine, nortriptyline, and viloxazine. Protriptyline has a **stimulant** action.

Imipramine and **amitriptyline** are well established and relatively safe and effective, but nevertheless have more marked antimuscarinic or cardiac side-effects than compounds such as **doxepin, mianserin, trazodone,** and **viloxazine**; this may be important in individual patients. Lofepramine also has a lower incidence of antimuscarinic and sedative side-effects and may be less dangerous in overdosage; it is, however, associated with hepatic toxicity. **Amoxapine** is related to the antipsychotic loxapine and its side-effects include tardive dyskinesia.

For a comparison of tricyclic and related antidepressants with SSRIs and related antidepressants and MAOIs, see section 4.3.

SIDE-EFFECTS. *Arrhythmias* and *heart block* occasionally follow the use of tricyclic antidepressants, particularly amitriptyline, and may be a factor in the sudden death of patients with cardiac disease. They are also sometimes associated with *convulsions* (and should be prescribed with special caution in epilepsy as they lower the convulsive threshold); maprotiline has particularly been associated with convulsions. *Hepatic* and *haematological* reactions may occur and have been particularly associated with mianserin.

Other side-effects of tricyclic and related antidepressants include *drowsiness, dry mouth, blurred vision, constipation,* and *urinary retention* (all attributed to antimuscarinic activity), and sweating. The patient should be encouraged to persist with treatment as some tolerance to these side-effects seems to develop. They are reduced if low doses are given initially and then gradually increased, but this must be balanced against the need to obtain a full therapeutic effect as soon as possible. Gradual introduction of treatment is particularly important in the elderly, who, because of the hypotensive effects of these drugs, are prone to attacks of *dizziness* or even *syncope.* Another side-effect to which the elderly are particularly susceptible is *hyponatraemia* (see CSM advice on p. 176).

Neuroleptic malignant syndrome (section 4.2.1) may, very rarely, arise in the course of antidepressant treatment.

Limited quantities of tricyclic antidepressants should be prescribed at any one time because they are dangerous in overdosage. For advice on **overdosage** see Emergency Treatment of Poisoning, p. 22.

WITHDRAWAL. If possible tricyclic and related antidepressants should be withdrawn slowly (see also section 4.3).

INTERACTIONS. A tricyclic or related antidepressant (or an SSRI or related antidepressant) should not be started until 2 weeks after stopping an MAOI. Conversely, an MAOI should not be started until at least a week after a tricyclic or related antidepressant (or an SSRI or related antidepressant) has been stopped (2 weeks in the case of paroxetine and sertraline and at least 5 weeks in the case of fluoxetine). For guidance relating to the reversible monoamine oxidase inhibitor, moclobemide, see p. 182. For other tricyclic antidepressant **interactions**, see Appendix 1 (antidepressants, tricyclic).

TRICYCLIC ANTIDEPRESSANTS

AMITRIPTYLINE HYDROCHLORIDE

Indications: depressive illness, particularly where sedation is required; nocturnal enuresis in children (section 7.4.2)

Cautions: cardiac disease (particularly with arrhythmias, see Contra-indications below), history of epilepsy, pregnancy and breast-feeding (Appendixes 4 and 5), elderly, hepatic impairment (avoid if severe), thyroid disease, phaeochromocytoma, history of mania, psychoses (may aggravate psychotic symptoms), angle-closure glaucoma, history of urinary retention, concurrent electroconvulsive therapy; avoid abrupt withdrawal; also caution in anaesthesia (increased risk of arrhythmias and hypotension, see surgery section 15.1); porphyria (section 9.8.2); see section 7.4.2 for additional nocturnal enuresis warnings; **interactions:** Appendix 1 (antidepressants, tricyclic)

DRIVING. Drowsiness may affect performance of skilled tasks (e.g. driving); effects of alcohol enhanced

Contra-indications: recent myocardial infarction, arrhythmias (particularly heart block), not indicated in manic phase, severe liver disease

---

Side-effects: dry mouth, sedation, blurred vision (disturbance of accommodation, increased intra-ocular pressure), constipation, nausea, difficulty with micturition; cardiovascular side-effects (such as ECG changes, arrhythmias, postural hypotension, tachycardia, syncope, particularly with high doses); sweating, tremor, rashes and hypersensitivity reactions (including urticaria, photosensitivity), behavioural disturbances (particularly children), hypomania or mania, confusion (particularly elderly), interference with sexual function, blood sugar changes; increased appetite and weight gain (occasionally weight loss); endocrine side-effects such as testicular enlargement, gynaecomastia, galactorrhoea; also convulsions (see also Cautions), movement disorders and dyskinesias, fever, agranulocytosis, leucopenia, eosinophilia, purpura, thrombocytopenia, hyponatraemia (may be due to inappropriate antidiuretic hormone secretion) see CSM advice, p. 176, abnormal liver function tests (jaundice); for a general outline of side-effects see also notes above; **overdosage:** see Emergency Treatment of Poisoning, p. 22

Dose: by mouth, depression, initially 75 mg (elderly and adolescents 30–75 mg) daily in divided doses *or* as a single dose at bedtime increased gradually as necessary to max. 150 mg; CHILD under 16 years not recommended for depression

Nocturnal enuresis, CHILD 7–10 years 10–20 mg, 11–16 years 25–50 mg at night; max. period of treatment (including gradual withdrawal) 3 months—full physical examination before further course

By intramuscular or intravenous injection, depression, 10–20 mg 4 times daily; CHILD under 16 years not recommended

PoM **Amitriptyline** (Non-proprietary)
Tablets, coated, amitriptyline hydrochloride 10 mg, net price 20 = 14p; 25 mg, 20 = 9p; 50 mg, 20 = 41p. Label: 2
Available from Antigen, APS, Berk (Domical®), Cox, DDSA (Elavil®)
Oral solution, amitriptyline (as hydrochloride) 25 mg/5 mL, net price 200-mL = £14.40; 50 mg/5 mL, 200-mL = £15.75. Label: 2
Available from Rosemont (sugar-free)
PoM **Lentizol®** (P-D)
Capsules, m/r, both enclosing white pellets, amitriptyline hydrochloride 25 mg (pink), net price 56-cap pack = £2.58; 50 mg (pink/red), 56-cap pack = £4.79. Label: 2, 25
PoM **Tryptizol®** (Morson)
Tablets, all f/c, amitriptyline hydrochloride 10 mg (blue), net price 30-tab pack = 20p; 25 mg (yellow), 30-tab pack = 13p; 50 mg (brown), 30-tab pack = 52p. Label: 2
Mixture, pink, sugar-free, amitriptyline 10 mg (as embonate)/5 mL. Net price 200-mL pack = £1.87. Label: 2
Injection, amitriptyline hydrochloride 10 mg/mL. Net price 10-mL vial = 54p

Compound preparations
Not recommended, see notes above.
PoM **Triptafen®** (Forley)
Tablets, pink, s/c, amitriptyline hydrochloride 25 mg, perphenazine 2 mg. Net price 20 = £4.05. Label: 2
PoM **Triptafen-M®** (Forley)
Tablets, pink, s/c, amitriptyline hydrochloride 10 mg, perphenazine 2 mg. Net price 20 = £3.60. Label: 2

AMOXAPINE
Indications: depressive illness
Cautions; Contra-indications; Side-effects: see under Amitriptyline Hydrochloride; tardive dyskinesia reported; menstrual irregularities, breast enlargement, and galactorrhoea reported in women
Dose: initially 100–150 mg daily in divided doses *or* as a single dose at bedtime increased as necessary to max. 300 mg daily; ELDERLY initially 25 mg twice daily increased as necessary after 5–7 days to max. 50 mg 3 times daily; CHILD under 16 years not recommended

PoM **Asendis®** (Lederle)
Tablets, amoxapine 25 mg, net price 100-tab pack = £10.89; 50 mg (orange, scored), 100-tab pack = £18.16; 100 mg (blue, scored), 100-tab pack = £30.27. Label: 2

CLOMIPRAMINE HYDROCHLORIDE
Indications: depressive illness, phobic and obsessional states; adjunctive treatment of cataplexy associated with narcolepsy
Cautions; Contra-indications; Side-effects: see under Amitriptyline Hydrochloride
Dose: by mouth, initially 10 mg daily, increased gradually as necessary to 30–150 mg daily in divided doses *or* as a single dose at bedtime; max. 250 mg daily; ELDERLY initially 10 mg daily increased to 30–50 mg daily; CHILD not recommended
Phobic and obsessional states, initially 25 mg daily (elderly 10 mg daily) increased over 2 weeks to 100–150 mg daily; CHILD not recommended
Adjunctive treatment of cataplexy associated with narcolepsy, initially 10 mg daily gradually increased until satisfactory response (range 10–75 mg daily)
By intramuscular injection, initially 25–50 mg daily, increased by 25 mg daily to 100–150 mg daily; CHILD not recommended
By intravenous infusion (careful monitoring) initially to assess tolerance, 25–50 mg, then increase by 25 mg daily to usual dose of 100 mg daily for 7–10 days—see product literature for details; CHILD not recommended

PoM **Clomipramine** (Non-proprietary)
Capsules, clomipramine hydrochloride 10 mg, net price 20 = 56p; 25 mg, 20 = £1.09; 50 mg, 20 = £2.11. Label: 2
Available from APS, Berk (Tranquax®), Cox, Generics, Hillcross, Norton

---

PoM **Anafranil**® (Novartis)

Capsules, clomipramine hydrochloride 10 mg (yellow/caramel), net price 84-cap pack = £3.23; 25 mg (orange/caramel), 84-cap pack = £6.35; 50 mg (grey/caramel), 56-cap pack = £8.06. Label: 2

Syrup, clomipramine hydrochloride 25 mg/5 mL. Net price 150-mL pack = £7.23. Label: 2

Injection, clomipramine hydrochloride 12.5 mg/ mL. Net price 2-mL amp = 47p

PoM **Anafranil SR**® (Novartis)

Tablets, m/r, grey-red, f/c, clomipramine hydrochloride 75 mg. Net price 28-tab pack = £8.83. Label: 2, 25

DOTHIEPIN HYDROCHLORIDE
(Dosulepin Hydrochloride)

Indications: depressive illness, particularly where sedation is required

Cautions; Contra-indications; Side-effects: see under Amitriptyline Hydrochloride

Dose: initially 75 mg (elderly 50–75 mg) daily in divided doses *or* as a single dose at bedtime, increased gradually as necessary to 150 mg daily (elderly 75 mg may be sufficient); up to 225 mg daily in some circumstances (e.g. hospital use); CHILD not recommended

PoM **Dothiepin** (Non-proprietary)

Capsules, dothiepin hydrochloride 25 mg, net price 20 = 78p. Label: 2
Available from APS, Ashbourne (Dothapax®), Berk (Prepadine®), Cox, Generics, Hillcross, Kent, Norton

Tablets, dothiepin hydrochloride 75 mg, net price 28-tab pack = £3.23. Label: 2
Available from APS, Ashbourne (Dothapax®), Berk (Prepadine®), Cox, Generics, Hillcross, Kent, Norton

PoM **Prothiaden**® (Knoll)

Capsules, red/brown, dothiepin hydrochloride 25 mg. Net price 20 = £1.00. Label: 2

Tablets, red, s/c, dothiepin hydrochloride 75 mg. Net price 28-tab pack = £4.00. Label: 2

DOXEPIN

Indications: depressive illness, particularly where sedation is required

Cautions; Contra-indications; Side-effects: see under Amitriptyline Hydrochloride; avoid in breast-feeding (see Appendix 5)

Dose: initially 75 mg daily in divided doses *or* as a single dose at bedtime, increased as necessary to max. 300 mg daily in 3 divided doses (up to 100 mg may be given as a single dose); ELDERLY initially 10–50 mg daily, range of 30–50 mg daily may be adequate; CHILD not recommended

PoM **Sinequan**® (Pfizer)

Capsules, doxepin (as hydrochloride) 10 mg (orange), net price 56-cap pack = £1.21; 25 mg (orange/blue), 28-cap pack = 87p; 50 mg (blue), 28-cap pack = £1.43; 75 mg (yellow/blue), 28-cap pack = £2.26. Label: 2

IMIPRAMINE HYDROCHLORIDE

Indications: depressive illness; nocturnal enuresis in children (see section 7.4.2)

Cautions; Contra-indications; Side-effects: see under Amitriptyline Hydrochloride, but less sedating

Dose: depression, initially up to 75 mg daily in divided doses increased gradually to 150–200 mg (up to 300 mg in hospital patients); up to 150 mg may be given as a single dose at bedtime; ELDERLY initially 10 mg daily, increased gradually to 30–50 mg daily; CHILD not recommended for depression

Nocturnal enuresis, CHILD 7 years 25 mg, 8–11 years 25–50 mg, over 11 years 50–75 mg at bedtime; max. period of treatment (including gradual withdrawal) 3 months—full physical examination before further course

PoM **Imipramine** (Non-proprietary)

Tablets, coated, imipramine hydrochloride 10 mg, net price 20 = 20p; 25 mg, 20 = 15p. Label: 2

PoM **Tofranil**® (Novartis)

Tablets, red-brown, s/c, imipramine hydrochloride 25 mg, net price 84-tab pack = £3.05. Label: 2

Syrup, imipramine hydrochloride 25 mg/5 mL. Net price 150-mL pack = £3.11. Label: 2

LOFEPRAMINE

Indications: depressive illness

Cautions; Contra-indications; Side-effects: see under Amitriptyline Hydrochloride, but less sedating; hepatic disorders reported; contra-indicated in hepatic and severe renal impairment

Dose: 140–210 mg daily in divided doses; ELDERLY may respond to lower doses; CHILD not recommended

PoM **Lofepramine** (Non-proprietary)

Tablets, lofepramine 70 mg (as hydrochloride). Net price 56-tab pack = £9.59. Label: 2
Available from Cox, Hillcross

Oral suspension, lofepramine 70 mg/5 mL (as hydrochloride). Net price 200 mL = £27.10. Label: 2
Available from Rosemont (Lomont®, sugar-free)

PoM **Gamanil**® (Merck)

Tablets, f/c, brown-violet, lofepramine 70 mg (as hydrochloride). Net price 56-tab pack = £9.84. Label: 2

NORTRIPTYLINE

Indications: depressive illness; nocturnal enuresis in children (section 7.4.2)

Cautions; Contra-indications; Side-effects: see under Amitriptyline Hydrochloride but less sedating

Dose: depression, low dose intially increased as necessary to 75–100 mg daily in divided doses *or* as a single dose; plasma concentration monitoring above 100 mg daily (max. 150 mg daily, in hospitalised patients); ADOLESCENT and ELDERLY 30–50 mg daily in divided doses; CHILD not recommended for depression

---

Nocturnal enuresis, CHILD 7 years 10 mg, 8–11 years 10–20 mg, over 11 years 25–35 mg, at night; max period of treatment (including gradual withdrawal) 3 months—full physical examination and ECG before further course

PoM **Allegron**® (Dista)
Tablets, nortriptyline (as hydrochloride) 10 mg, net price 20 = £2.39; 25 mg (orange, scored), 20 = £4.85. Label: 2

Compound preparations
Not recommended, see notes above.
PoM **Motipress**® (Sanofi Winthrop)
Tablets, yellow, s/c, fluphenazine hydrochloride 1.5 mg, nortriptyline 30 mg (as hydrochloride). Net price 28-tab pack = £2.83. Label: 2
PoM **Motival**® (Sanofi Winthrop)
Tablets, pink, s/c, fluphenazine hydrochloride 500 micrograms, nortriptyline 10 mg (as hydrochloride). Net price 20 = 69p. Label: 2

PROTRIPTYLINE HYDROCHLORIDE
Indications: depressive illness, particularly with apathy and withdrawal
Cautions; Contra-indications; Side-effects: see under Amitriptyline Hydrochloride but less sedating; anxiety, agitation, tachycardia, and hypotension more common; rashes associated with photosensitisation (avoid direct sunlight); daily dose above 20 mg in elderly (increased risk of cardiovascular side-effects)
Dose: initially 10 mg 3–4 times daily (elderly 5 mg 3 times daily initially), increased gradually up to 60 mg daily in divided doses according to response; if insomnia, last dose not after 4 p.m.; CHILD under 16 years not recommended

PoM **Concordin**® (MSD)
Tablets, both f/c, protriptyline hydrochloride 5 mg (pink), net price 30-tab pack = 66p; 10 mg, 30-tab pack = 98p. Label: 2, 11

TRIMIPRAMINE
Indications: depressive illness, particularly where sedation is required
Cautions; Contra-indications; Side-effects: see under Amitriptyline Hydrochloride
Dose: 50–75 mg daily as a single dose 2 hours before bedtime *or* as 25 mg midday and 50 mg evening, increased as necessary to max. of 300 mg daily for 4–6 weeks; ELDERLY 10–25 mg 3 times daily initially, half adult maintenance dose may be sufficient; CHILD not recommended

PoM **Surmontil**® (Rhône-Poulenc Rorer)
Capsules, green/white, trimipramine 50 mg (as maleate). Net price 28-cap pack = £5.71. Label: 2
Tablets, trimipramine (as maleate) 10 mg, net price 50-tab pack = £2.78; 25 mg, 50-tab pack = £4.62. Label: 2

RELATED ANTIDEPRESSANTS

MAPROTILINE HYDROCHLORIDE
Indications: depressive illness, particularly where sedation is required
Cautions; Contra-indications; Side-effects: see under Amitriptyline Hydrochloride, antimuscarinic effects may occur less frequently but rashes common and increased risk of convulsions at higher dosage; contra-indicated if history of epilepsy
Dose: initially 25–75 mg (elderly 30 mg) daily in 3 divided doses *or* as a single dose at bedtime, increased gradually as necessary to max. 150 mg daily; CHILD not recommended

PoM **Ludiomil**® (Novartis)
Tablets, all f/c, maprotiline hydrochloride 10 mg (pale yellow), net price 28-tab pack = 98p; 25 mg (greyish-red), 28-tab pack = £2.11; 50 mg (light orange), 28-tab pack = £4.18; 75 mg (brownish-orange), 28-tab pack = £6.21. Label: 2
Additives: include gluten

MIANSERIN HYDROCHLORIDE
Indications: depressive illness, particularly where sedation is required
Cautions; Contra-indications; Side-effects: see under Amitriptyline Hydrochloride; leucopenia, agranulocytosis and aplastic anaemia (particularly in the elderly); jaundice; arthritis, arthralgia; fewer and milder antimuscarinic and cardiovascular effects; **interactions:** Appendix 1 (mianserin)
BLOOD COUNTS. A full **blood count** is recommended every 4 weeks during the first 3 months of treatment; subsequent clinical monitoring should continue and treatment should be stopped and a full blood count obtained if *fever, sore throat, stomatitis*, or other signs of infection develop.
Dose: initially 30–40 mg (elderly 30 mg) daily in divided doses *or* as a single dose at bedtime, increased gradually as necessary; usual dose range 30–90 mg; CHILD not recommended

PoM **Mianserin** (Non-proprietary)
Tablets, mianserin hydrochloride 10 mg, net price 20 = 97p; 20 mg, 20 = £2.07; 30 mg, 20 = £2.89. Label: 2, 25
Available from Cox, Norton

MIRTAZAPINE
Indications: depressive illness
Cautions: epilepsy, hepatic or renal impairment, cardiac disorders, hypotension, history of urinary retention, angle-closure glaucoma, diabetes mellitus, psychoses (may aggravate psychotic symptoms), history of bipolar depression, avoid abrupt withdrawal; manufacturer advises avoid in pregnancy and in breast-feeding; **interactions:** Appendix 1 (mirtazapine)
BLOOD DISORDERS. Patients should be advised to report any fever, sore throat, stomatitis or other signs of infection that occur during treatment. A blood count should be performed and the drug stopped immediately if blood dyscrasia suspected

---

Abbreviations and symbols, see inside front cover

Side-effects: increased appetite and weight gain, sedation, less commonly elevated liver enzymes, jaundice (discontinue treatment); rarely oedema, postural hypotension, exanthema, tremor, myoclonus; reversible agranulocytosis (see Cautions above), leucopenia, granulocytosis

Dose: initially 15 mg daily at bedtime increased according to response up to 45 mg daily as a single dose at bedtime or in 2 divided doses; CHILD not recommended

▼ PoM **Zispin**® (Organon)
Tablets, scored, red/brown, mirtazapine 30 mg. Net price 28-tab pack = £24.00. Label: 2, 25

TRAZODONE HYDROCHLORIDE

Indications: depressive illness, particularly where sedation is required

Cautions; Contra-indications; Side-effects: see under Amitriptyline Hydrochloride but fewer antimuscarinic and cardiovascular effects; rarely priapism [discontinue immediately]; **interactions:** Appendix 1 (trazodone)

Dose: initially 150 mg (elderly 100 mg) daily in divided doses after food *or* as a single dose at bedtime; may be increased to 300 mg daily; hospital patients up to max. 600 mg daily in divided doses; CHILD not recommended

PoM **Molipaxin**® (Hoechst Marion Roussel)
Capsules, trazodone hydrochloride 50 mg (violet/green), net price 84-cap pack = £17.31; 100 mg (violet/fawn), 56-cap pack = £20.38. Label: 2, 21
Tablets, pink, f/c, trazodone hydrochloride 150 mg. Net price 28-tab pack = £11.62. Label: 2, 21
Liquid, sugar-free, trazodone hydrochloride 50 mg/5 mL. Net price 150-mL pack = £7.74. Label: 2, 21
CR tablets, m/r, blue, f/c, trazodone hydrochloride 150 mg. Net price 28-tab pack = £11.62. Label: 2, 21, 25
Dose: initially 1 tablet daily (elderly, dose form not appropriate for initial dose titration), increased if necessary to 2 tablets daily (up to 4 tablets daily in hospital patients); CHILD not recommended

---

VILOXAZINE HYDROCHLORIDE

Indications: depressive illness

Cautions; Contra-indications; Side-effects: see under Amitriptyline Hydrochloride, but less sedating and antimuscarinic and cardiovascular side-effects are fewer and milder; nausea and headache may occur; **interactions:** Appendix 1 (viloxazine)

Dose: 300 mg daily (preferably as 200 mg in the morning and 100 mg at midday), increased gradually as necessary; max. 400 mg daily; last dose not later than 6 p.m.; ELDERLY 100 mg daily initially, half adult maintenance dose may be sufficient; CHILD under 14 years not recommended

PoM **Vivalan**® (Zeneca)
Tablets, f/c, viloxazine 50 mg (as hydrochloride). Net price 20 = £1.23. Label: 2

4.3.2 Monoamine-oxidase inhibitors (MAOIs)

Monoamine-oxidase inhibitors are used much less frequently than tricyclic and related antidepressants, or SSRIs and related antidepressants because of the dangers of dietary and drug interactions and the fact that it is easier to prescribe MAOIs when tricyclic antidepressants have been unsuccessful than vice versa. **Tranylcypromine** is the most **hazardous** of the MAOIs because of its stimulant action. The drugs of choice are **phenelzine** or **isocarboxazid** which are less stimulant and therefore safer.

Phobic patients and depressed patients with atypical, hypochondriacal, or hysterical features are said to respond best to MAOIs. However, MAOIs should be tried in any patients who are refractory to treatment with other antidepressants as there is occasionally a dramatic response. Response to treatment may be delayed for 3 weeks or more and may take an additional 1 or 2 weeks to become maximal.

WITHDRAWAL. If possible MAOIs should be withdrawn slowly (see also section 4.3).

INTERACTIONS. MAOIs inhibit monoamine oxidase, thereby causing an accumulation of amine neurotransmitters. The metabolism of some amine drugs such as *indirect-acting sympathomimetics* (present in many cough and decongestant preparations, see section 3.10) is also inhibited and their pressor action may be potentiated; the pressor effect of tyramine (in some foods, such as cheese, pickled herring, broad bean pods, and *Bovril*®, *Oxo*®, *Marmite*® or any similar meat or yeast extract or fermented soya bean extract) may also be dangerously potentiated. These interactions may cause a dangerous rise in blood pressure. An early warning symptom may be a throbbing headache. Patients should be advised to eat only fresh foods and avoid food that is suspected of being stale or 'going off'. This is especially important with meat, fish, poultry or offal; game should be avoided. The danger of interaction persists for up to 2 weeks after treatment with MAOIs is discontinued. Patients should also avoid alcoholic drinks or de-alcoholised (low alcohol) drinks.

Other antidepressants should **not** be started for 2 weeks after treatment with MAOIs has been stopped. Some psychiatrists use selected tricyclics in conjunction with MAOIs but this is hazardous, indeed potentially lethal, except in experienced hands and there is no evidence that the combination is more effective than when either constituent is used alone. The combination of tranylcypromine with clomipramine is particularly **dangerous**.

Conversely, an MAOI should not be started until at least 1 week (phenelzine manufacturer specifies 2 weeks) after a *tricyclic or related antidepressant* or an *SSRI or related antidepressant* has been stopped (2 weeks in the case of paroxetine and sertraline, at least 5 weeks in the case of fluoxetine).

In addition, an MAOI should not be started for at least a week (phenelzine manufacturer specifies 2 weeks) after a previous MAOI has been stopped (then started at a reduced dose).

For other interactions with MAOIs including those with opioid analgesics (notably pethidine), see Appendix 1 (MAOIs). For guidance on interactions relating to the reversible monoamine oxidase inhibitor, moclobemide, see below.

PHENELZINE
Indications: depressive illness
Cautions: diabetes mellitus, cardiovascular disease, epilepsy, blood disorders, concurrent electroconvulsive therapy; elderly (great caution); monitor blood pressure to detect hypotensive responses (postural hypotension) and hypertensive responses (discontinue if palpitations or frequent headaches); if possible avoid abrupt withdrawal; severe hypertensive reactions to certain drugs and foods; avoid in agitated patients; porphyria (see section 9.8.2); pregnancy and breast-feeding; surgery (see section 15.1); **interactions:** Appendix 1 (MAOIs)
DRIVING. Drowsiness may affect performance of skilled tasks (e.g. driving)
Contra-indications: hepatic impairment or abnormal liver function tests (see Appendix 2), cerebrovascular disease, phaeochromocytoma; not indicated in manic phase
Side-effects: adverse effects commonly associated with phenelzine and other MAOIs include postural hypotension (especially in elderly) and dizziness; other side-effects include drowsiness, insomnia, headache, weakness and fatigue, dryness of mouth, constipation and other gastrointestinal disturbances, oedema, myoclonic movement, hyperreflexia, elevated liver enzymes; agitation and tremors, nervousness, euphoria, arrhythmias, blurred vision, nystagmus, difficulty in micturition, sweating, convulsions, rashes, purpura, leucopenia, sexual disturbances, and weight gain with inappropriate appetite may also occur; psychotic episodes with hypomanic behaviour, confusion, and hallucinations, may be induced in susceptible persons; jaundice has been reported and, on rare occasions, fatal progressive hepatocellular necrosis; paraesthesia, peripheral neuritis, peripheral neuropathy may be due to pyridoxine deficiency; for CSM advice on possible hyponatraemia, see p. 176 (hypernatraemia also reported)
Dose: 15 mg 3 times daily, increased if necessary to 4 times daily after 2 weeks (hospital patients, max. 30 mg 3 times daily), then reduced gradually to lowest possible maintenance dose (15 mg on alternate days may be adequate); CHILD not recommended

PoM **Nardil**® (P-D)
Tablets, orange, f/c, phenelzine 15 mg (as sulphate). Net price 20 = £1.33. Label: 3, 10 patient information leaflet

ISOCARBOXAZID
Indications: depressive illness
Cautions; Contra-indications; Side-effects: see under Phenelzine

Dose: initially up to 30 mg daily in single or divided doses increased after 4 weeks if necessary to max. 60 mg daily for up to 6 weeks under close supervision only; then reduced to usual maintenance dose 10–20 mg daily (but up to 40 mg daily may be required); CHILD not recommended

PoM **Isocarboxazid** (Cambridge)
Tablets, pink, scored, isocarboxazid 10 mg. Net price 50 = £11.96. Label: 3, 10 patient information leaflet
Note. The brand name Marplan® was formerly used for isocarboxazid preparations

TRANYLCYPROMINE
Indications: depressive illness
Cautions; Contra-indications: see under Phenelzine; also contra-indicated in hyperthyroidism
Side-effects: see under Phenelzine; insomnia if given in evening; hypertensive crises with throbbing headache requiring discontinuation of treatment occur more frequently than with other MAOIs; liver damage occurs less frequently than with phenelzine
Dose: initially 10 mg twice daily not later than 3 p.m., increasing the second daily dose to 20 mg after 1 week if necessary; doses above 30 mg daily under close supervision only; usual maintenance dose 10 mg daily; CHILD not recommended

PoM **Parnate**® (SK&F)
Tablets, red, s/c, tranylcypromine 10 mg (as sulphate). Net price 28-tab pack = £1.27. Label: 3, 10 patient information leaflet

Compound preparation
Not recommended, see section 4.3
PoM **Parstelin**® (SK&F)
Tablets, green, s/c, tranylcypromine 10 mg (as sulphate), trifluoperazine 1 mg (as hydrochloride). Net price 28-tab pack = £1.30. Label: 3, 10 patient information leaflet
Caution: contains MAOI

REVERSIBLE MAOIs

Moclobemide is indicated for major depression only; it is reported to act by reversible inhibition of monoamine oxidase type A (it is therefore termed a RIMA).

INTERACTIONS. Moclobemide is claimed to cause less potentiation of the pressor effect of tyramine than the traditional (irreversible) MAOIs, but patients should avoid consuming large amounts of tyramine-rich food (such as mature cheese, yeast extracts and fermented soya bean products).
The risk of drug interactions is also claimed to be less but patients still need to avoid sympathomimetics such as ephedrine, pseudoephedrine, and phenylpropanolamine. In addition, moclobemide should not be given with another antidepressant. Owing to its short duration of action no treatment-free period is required after it has been stopped but it should not be started until at least a week after a tricyclic or related antidepressant or an SSRI or

related antidepressant has been stopped (2 weeks in the case of paroxetine and sertraline, and at least 5 weeks in the case of fluoxetine), or for at least a week after an MAOI has been stopped. For other interactions, see Appendix 1 (moclobemide).

MOCLOBEMIDE

Indications: major depression

Cautions: avoid in agitated or excited patients (or give with sedative for up to 2–3 weeks), thyrotoxicosis, severe hepatic impairment, may provoke manic episodes in bipolar disorders, pregnancy and breast-feeding (patient information leaflet advises avoid); **interactions:** see notes above and Appendix 1 (moclobemide)

Contra-indications: acute confusional states, phaeochromocytoma

Side-effects: sleep disturbances, dizziness, nausea, headache, restlessness, agitation; confusional states reported; rarely raised liver enzymes; for CSM advice on possible hyponatraemia, see p. 176

Dose: initially 300 mg daily usually in divided doses after food, adjusted according to response; usual range 150–600 mg daily; CHILD not recommended

▼ PoM **Manerix**® (Roche)

Tablets, yellow, f/c, scored, moclobemide 150 mg, net price 30-tab pack = £10.50, 300 mg, 30 tab pack = £15.75. Label: 10 patient information leaflet, 21

4.3.3   SSRIs and related antidepressants

SSRIs

Citalopram, fluoxetine, fluvoxamine, paroxetine, and **sertraline** selectively inhibit the re-uptake of serotonin (5-hydroxytryptamine, 5-HT); they are termed selective serotonin re-uptake inhibitors (SSRIs) and appear to be effective antidepressants. They are less sedative than many of the tricyclic antidepressants, with few antimuscarinic effects and with low cardiotoxicity. They do not cause weight gain. Gastro-intestinal side-effects (diarrhoea, nausea and vomiting) are dose-related; headache, restlessness and anxiety may also occur. As with tricyclic antidepressants caution is necessary in epilepsy. For a general comment on the comparison between *tricyclic and related antidepressants* and the *SSRIs and related antidepressants,* see section 4.3.

WITHDRAWAL. If possible SSRIs should be withdrawn slowly (see also section 4.3 and under individual drugs). See next page for a CSM warning relating to paroxetine withdrawal.

INTERACTIONS. An SSRI or related antidepressant should not be started until 2 weeks after stopping an MAOI. Conversely, an MAOI should not be started

until at least a week after an SSRI or related antidepressant has been stopped (2 weeks in the case of paroxetine and sertraline, at least 5 weeks in the case of fluoxetine). For guidance relating to the reversible monoamine oxidase inhibitor, moclobemide, see above. For other SSRI antidepressant interactions, see Appendix 1 (antidepressants, SSRI).

FLUOXETINE

Indications: see under Dose

Cautions: see notes above; cardiac disease, epilepsy (avoid if poorly controlled, discontinue if convulsions develop), concurrent electroconvulsive therapy (prolonged seizures reported), history of mania, hepatic and renal impairment (see Appendixes 2 and 3), pregnancy and breast-feeding (see Appendixes 4 and 5); **interactions:** Appendix 1 (antidepressants, SSRI)

DRIVING. May impair performance of skilled tasks (e.g. driving)

Contra-indications: not indicated in manic phase

Side-effects: gastro-intestinal (fairly common—include nausea, vomiting, dyspepsia, abdominal pain, diarrhoea, constipation, anorexia with weight loss and possible changes in blood sugar); hypersensitivity reactions (**important:** see also below); also dry mouth, nervousness, anxiety, headache, insomnia, palpitations, tremor, confusion, dizziness, hypotension, hypomania or mania, drowsiness, asthenia, convulsions (see Cautions above), fever, sexual dysfunction, sweating; movement disorders and dyskinesias, neuroleptic malignant syndrome-like event; hyponatraemia (may be due to inappropriate antidiuretic hormone secretion), see CSM warning on p. 176; abnormal liver function tests reported; also reported (no causal relationship established): abnormal bleeding, aplastic anaemia, cerebrovascular accident, ecchymoses, eosinophilic pneumonia, gastro-intestinal haemorrhage, hyperprolactinaemia, haemolytic anaemia, pancreatitis, pancytopenia, suicidal ideation, thrombocytopenia, thrombocytopenic purpura, vaginal bleeding on withdrawal, violent behaviour; hair loss also reported

HYPERSENSITIVITY. Angioedema, urticaria, pruritus, and other allergic reactions including anaphylaxis have been reported (discontinue if rash occurs, may be warning of impending serious systemic reaction, possibly associated with vasculitis); pharyngitis and rarely pulmonary inflammation or fibrosis (with dyspnoea only warning sign) also reported; other possible hypersensitivity signs include arthralgia, myalgia

Dose: depressive illness, 20 mg daily; CHILD not recommended

Bulimia nervosa, 60 mg daily; CHILD not recommended

Obsessive-compulsive disorder, initially 20 mg daily, dose increase may be considered if no response after several weeks, but may be increased potential for side-effects; max. 60 mg daily; CHILD not recommended

LONG DURATION OF ACTION. Account should be taken of the long half-life of fluoxetine when adjusting dosage (or in overdosage)

PoM **Prozac**® (Dista)

Capsules, fluoxetine (as hydrochloride) 20 mg (green/yellow), net price 30-cap pack = £20.77, 98-cap pack = £67.85; 60 mg (yellow), 30-cap pack = £62.31. Counselling, driving

Liquid, fluoxetine (as hydrochloride) 20 mg/5 mL. Net price 70-mL pack = £19.39. Counselling, driving

CITALOPRAM

Indications: depressive illness, panic disorder

Cautions; Contra-indications; Side-effects: see notes above and under Fluoxetine

Dose: depressive illness, 20 mg daily as a single dose in the morning or evening increased if necessary to max. 60 mg daily (ELDERLY max 40 mg daily); CHILD not recommended

Panic disorder, initially 10 mg daily increased to 20 mg after 7 days, usual dose 20–30 mg daily; max. 60 mg daily (elderly max. 40 mg daily); CHILD not recommended

▼ PoM **Cipramil**® (Lundbeck, Du Pont)

Tablets, f/c, scored, citalopram (as hydrobromide) 20 mg. Net price 28-tab pack = £21.28. Counselling, driving

FLUVOXAMINE MALEATE

Indications: depressive illness, obsessive-compulsive disorder

Cautions; Contra-indications; Side-effects: see notes above and under Fluoxetine; avoid abrupt withdrawal; may cause decrease in heart rate; rarely increase in hepatic enzymes, usually with symptoms (discontinue treatment); galactorrhoea reported

CSM ADVICE. The CSM has advised that concomitant use of fluvoxamine and theophylline or aminophylline preparations should usually be avoided. Where this is not possible, patients taking this combination should have their theophylline dose halved and plasma theophylline levels monitored closely.

Dose: initially 100 mg daily increased if necessary to max. 300 mg daily (over 100 mg in divided doses); CHILD not recommended

Note. If no improvement in obsessive-compulsive disorder within 10 weeks, treatment should be reconsidered

PoM **Faverin**® (Solvay)

Tablets, f/c, scored, fluvoxamine maleate 50 mg, net price 60-tab pack = £19.00; 100 mg, 30-tab pack = £19.00. Counselling, driving

PAROXETINE

Indications: depressive illness, obsessive-compulsive disorder, panic disorder

Cautions; Contra-indications; Side-effects: see under Fluoxetine; consider gradual discontinuation by dose tapering or alternate day administration (dizziness, paraesthesia, anxiety, sleep disturbances, agitation, tremor, nausea, sweating

and confusion reported on abrupt discontinuation—see also CSM advice below)

IMPORTANT. During initial treatment of panic disorder, there is potential for worsening of panic symptomatology

CSM ADVICE. Extrapyramidal reactions (including orofacial dystonias) and withdrawal syndrome are reported to the CSM more commonly than with other SSRIs

Dose: depressive illness, usually 20 mg each morning, if necessary increased gradually in increments of 10 mg to max. 50 mg daily (elderly, 40 mg daily); CHILD not recommended

Obsessive-compulsive disorder, initially 20 mg each morning, if necessary increased gradually in weekly increments of 10 mg to usual dose 40 mg daily (max. 60 mg daily, max. in elderly 40 mg daily); CHILD not recommended

Panic disorder, initially 10 mg each morning, if necessary increased gradually in weekly increments of 10 mg to usual dose of 40 mg daily (max. 50 mg daily, max. in elderly 40 mg daily); CHILD not recommended

PoM **Seroxat**® (SmithKline Beecham)

Tablets, both f/c, scored, paroxetine (as hydrochloride) 20 mg, net price 30-tab pack = £20.77; 30 mg (blue), 30-tab pack = £31.16. Label: 21, counselling, driving

Liquid, orange, sugar-free, paroxetine (as hydrochloride) 10 mg/5 mL. Net price 150-mL pack = £20.77. Label: 21, counselling, driving

SERTRALINE

Indications: depressive illness

Cautions; Contra-indications; Side-effects: see notes above and under Fluoxetine; avoid abrupt withdrawal; asymptomatic elevation in serum transaminases diminishes on withdrawal; rarely erythema multiforme reported

Dose: initially 50 mg daily, increased if necessary by increments of 50 mg over several weeks to max. 200 mg daily, then reduced to usual maintenance of 50 mg daily; doses of 150 mg or greater should not be used for more than 8 weeks; CHILD not recommended

PoM **Lustral**® (Invicta)

Tablets, sertraline (as hydrochloride) 50 mg, net price 28-tab pack = £26.51; 100 mg, 28-tab pack = £39.77. Counselling, driving

RELATED ANTIDEPRESSANTS

Venlafaxine is a new antidepressant which potentiates neurotransmitter activity in the central nervous system, probably by inhibiting re-uptake of serotonin and noradrenaline.

Nefazodone is another new antidepressant. It inhibits re-uptake of serotonin and also selectively blocks serotonin receptors.

NEFAZODONE HYDROCHLORIDE

Indications: depressive illness

Cautions: epilepsy, concurrent electroconvulsive therapy (no studies), history of mania or hypomania, elderly (especially female), hepatic and renal

---

impairment (lower end of dose range), pregnancy; **interactions:** Appendix 1 (nefazodone)

DRIVING. May impair performance of skilled tasks (e.g. driving)

Contra-indications: breast-feeding

Side-effects: asthenia, dry mouth, nausea, somnolence, dizziness; less frequently, chills, fever, postural hypotension, constipation, lightheadedness, paraesthesia, confusion, ataxia, amblyopia and other minor visual disturbances; rarely syncope

Dose: initially 100 mg twice daily increased after 5–7 days to 200 mg twice daily, may be gradually increased if necessary to max. 300 mg twice daily (elderly usual max. 100–200 mg twice daily); ADOLESCENT and CHILD under 18 years not recommended

▼ PoM **Dutonin**® (Bristol-Myers)

Tablets, both scored, nefazodone hydrochloride 100 mg (white), net price 56-tab pack = £16.80; 200 mg (yellow), 56-tab pack = £16.80; starter pack consisting of 14 × 50 mg (pink) tablets, 14 × 100 mg tablets and 28 × 200 mg tablets = £16.80. Label: 3

VENLAFAXINE

Indications: depressive illness

Cautions: history of myocardial infarction or unstable heart disease, blood pressure monitoring may be advisable in patients taking more than 200 mg daily, history of epilepsy, hepatic or renal impairment (Appendixes 2 and 3), history of drug abuse, avoid abrupt withdrawal (if taken for more than 1 week withdraw over a few days, if taken for more than 6 weeks withdraw over at least 1 week); **interactions:** Appendix 1 (venlafaxine)

DRIVING. May affect performance of skilled tasks (e.g. driving)

SKIN REACTIONS. Patients should be advised to contact doctor if rash, urticaria or related allergic reaction develops

Contra-indications: severe hepatic or renal impairment; pregnancy and breast-feeding

Side-effects: nausea, headache, insomnia, somnolence, dry mouth, dizziness (and occasionally hypotension), constipation, asthenia, sweating, nervousness, convulsions (discontinue); other side-effects reported include anorexia, dyspepsia, abdominal pain, anxiety, sexual dysfunction, visual disturbances, vasodilatation, vomiting, tremor, abnormal dreams, paraesthesia, chills, hypertension (see Cautions), palpitations, weight changes, agitation, hypertonia, rash (see Cautions); hyponatraemia, reversible increase in liver enzymes, and alterations in serum cholesterol also reported

Dose: initially 75 mg daily in 2 divided doses increased if necessary after several weeks to 150 mg daily in 2 divided doses

Severely depressed or hospitalised patients, initially 150 mg daily in 2 divided doses increased if necessary in steps of up to 75 mg every 2–3 days to max. 375 mg daily then gradually reduced; ADOLESCENT and CHILD under 18 years not recommended

▼ PoM **Efexor**® (Wyeth)

Tablets, both peach, venlafaxine (as hydrochloride) 37.5 mg, net price 56-tab pack = £23.97; 50 mg, 42-tab pack = £23.97; 75 mg, 56-tab pack = £39.97. Label: 21, counselling, driving, skin reactions

▼ PoM **Efexor**® **XL** (Wyeth)

Capsules, m/r, venlafaxine (as hydrochloride) 75 mg (peach), net price 28-cap pack = £23.97, 150 mg (orange), 28-cap pack = £39.97. Label: 21, 25, counselling, driving, skin reactions

Dose: 75 mg daily as a single dose, increased if necessary after at least 2 weeks to 150 mg once daily; max. 225 mg once daily; ADOLESCENT and CHILD under 18 years not recommended

4.3.4 Other antidepressant drugs

FLUPENTHIXOL

The thioxanthene **flupenthixol** (*Fluanxol*®) has antidepressant properties, and low doses (1 to 3 mg daily) are given by mouth for this purpose. Flupenthixol is also used for the treatment of psychoses (section 4.2.1 and section 4.2.2)

FLUPENTHIXOL

(Flupentixol)

Indications: depressive illness (short-term use). For use in psychoses, see section 4.2.1

Cautions: cardiovascular disease (including cardiac disorders and cerebral arteriosclerosis), senile confusional states, parkinsonism, renal and hepatic disease; avoid in excitable and overactive patients; porphyria (see section 9.8.2); **interactions:** Appendix 1 (antipsychotics)

DRIVING. Drowsiness may affect performance of skilled tasks (e.g. driving); effects of alcohol enhanced

Side-effects: restlessness, insomnia; hypomania reported; rarely dizziness, tremor, visual disturbances, headache, hyperprolactinaemia, extrapyramidal symptoms

Dose: initially 1 mg (elderly 500 micrograms) in the morning, increased after 1 week to 2 mg (elderly 1 mg) if necessary. Max. 3 mg (elderly 2 mg) daily, doses above 2 mg (elderly 1 mg) being divided in 2 portions, second dose not after 4 p.m. Discontinue if no response after 1 week at maximum dosage; CHILD not recommended

COUNSELLING. Although drowsiness may occur, can also have an alerting effect so should not be taken in the evening

PoM **Depixol**® (psychoses), see section 4.2.1
PoM **Fluanxol**® (Lundbeck)

Tablets, both red, s/c, flupenthixol (as dihydrochloride) 500 micrograms, net price 60-tab pack = £2.95; 1 mg, 60-tab pack = £4.98. Label: 2, counselling, administration

NORADRENALINE RE-UPTAKE INHIBITORS

Reboxetine, a selective inhibitor of noradrenaline re-uptake, has been introduced for the treatment of depressive illness.

REBOXETINE

Indications: depressive illness

Cautions: severe renal impairment (Appendix 3), hepatic impairment (Appendix 2), manufacturer advises avoid in pregnancy and in breast-feeding, history of epilepsy, bipolar disorders, urinary retention, glaucoma; **interactions:** Appendix 1 (reboxetine)

Side-effects: insomnia, sweating, dizziness, postural hypotension, vertigo, paraesthesia, impotence, dysuria, urinary retention (mainly in men), dry mouth, constipation, tachycardia; lowering of plasma-potassium concentration on prolonged administration in the elderly

Dose: 4 mg twice daily increased if necessary after 3–4 weeks to 10 mg daily in divided doses, max. 12 mg daily; CHILD and ELDERLY not recommended

▼ PoM **Edronax**® (Pharmacia & Upjohn)
Tablets, scored, reboxetine (as mesylate) 4 mg. Net price 60-tab pack = £19.80. Counselling, driving

---

TRYPTOPHAN

Tryptophan appears to benefit some patients with resistant depression when given as adjunctive therapy but tryptophan products were withdrawn following evidence of an association with the eosinophilia-myalgia syndrome; Optimax® (Merck) has now been re-introduced for patients for whom no alternative treatment is suitable.

TRYPTOPHAN

(L-Tryptophan)

Indications: restricted to use by hospital specialists *only* for patients with severe and disabling depressive illness of more than 2 years continuous duration, *only* after an adequate trial of standard antidepressant drug treatment, and *only* as an adjunct to other antidepressant medication

Cautions: eosinophilia-myalgia syndrome has been reported with tryptophan-containing products therefore close and regular surveillance required; monitor eosinophil count, haematological changes and muscle symptomatology; pregnancy and breast-feeding; **interactions:** Appendix 1 (tryptophan)

Contra-indications: history of eosinophilia-myalgia syndrome following use of tryptophan

Side-effects: drowsiness, nausea, headache, lightheadedness; eosinophilia-myalgia syndrome, see Cautions

Dose: 1 g 3 times daily; max. 6 g daily; ELDERLY lower dose may be appropriate especially where renal or hepatic impairment; CHILD not recommended

▼ PoM **Optimax**® (Merck)
Tablets, scored, tryptophan 500 mg. Net price 84-tab pack = £16.30. Label: 3

Important. Patient and prescriber must be registered with the Optimax® Information and Clinical Support (OPTICS) Unit. A **safety questionnaire** is sent to the prescriber after **3** and **6 months** of treatment and **every 6 months** thereafter. The information is reviewed by the CSM—it is **important** that the questionnaires should be completed

4.4   Central nervous system stimulants

Central nervous system stimulants include the **amphetamines** (notably dexamphetamine) **and related drugs** (e.g. methylphenidate). They have very few indications and in particular, should **not** be used to treat depression, obesity, senility, debility, or for relief of fatigue.

Caffeine is a weak stimulant present in tea and coffee. It is included in many analgesic preparations (section 4.7.1) but does not contribute to their analgesic or anti-inflammatory effect. Over-indulgence may lead to a state of anxiety.

The **amphetamines** have a limited field of usefulness and their use should be **discouraged** as they may cause dependence and psychotic states. They have **no place** in the management of **depression** or **obesity**.

Patients with *narcolepsy* may derive benefit from treatment with dexamphetamine.

Dexamphetamine (dexamfetamine) and **methylphenidate** have been advocated (under specialist supervision) for the management of *hyperactive children*; beneficial effects have been described. However, they must be used very selectively since they retard growth and the effect of long-term therapy has not been evaluated.

Pemoline has been withdrawn recently.

DEXAMPHETAMINE SULPHATE

(Dexamfetamine Sulphate)

Indications: narcolepsy, adjunct in the management of refractory hyperkinetic states in children (under specialist supervision)

Cautions: mild hypertension (contra-indicated if moderate or severe)—monitor blood pressure; history of epilepsy (discontinue if convulsions occur); monitor growth in children (see also below); avoid abrupt withdrawal; data on safety and efficacy of long-term use not complete; porphyria (see section 9.8.2); **interactions:** Appendix 1 (sympathomimetics)

SPECIAL CAUTIONS IN CHILDREN. Monitor height and weight as growth retardation may occur during prolonged therapy (drug free periods may allow catch-up in growth but withdraw slowly to avoid inducing depression or renewed hyperactivity). In psychotic children may exacerbate behavioural disturbances and thought disorder

Contra-indications: cardiovascular disease including moderate to severe hypertension (caution if mild), hyperexcitability or agitated states, hyperthyroidism, history of drug or alcohol abuse, glaucoma, predisposition to tics or Tourette syndrome (discontinue if tics occur), pregnancy and breast-feeding

DRIVING. May affect performance of skilled tasks (e.g. driving); effects of alcohol unpredictable

Side-effects: insomnia, restlessness, irritability and excitabilitiy, nervousness, night terrors, euphoria, tremor, dizziness, headache; convulsions (see also Cautions); dependence and tolerance, sometimes psychosis; anorexia, gastrointestinal symptoms, growth retardation in chil-

---

dren (see also under Cautions); dry mouth, sweating, tachycardia (and anginal pain), palpitations, increased blood pressure; visual disturbances; cardiomyopathy reported with chronic use; central stimulants have provoked choreoathetoid movements, tics and Tourette syndrome in predisposed individuals (see also Contra-indications above); **overdosage:** see Emergency Treatment of Poisoning, p. 23

Dose: narcolepsy, 10 mg (elderly, 5 mg) daily in divided doses increased by 10 mg (elderly, 5 mg) daily at intervals of 1 week to a max. of 60 mg daily

Hyperkinesia, CHILD under 6 years not recommended, over 6 years 5–10 mg daily, increased if necessary by 5 mg at intervals of 1 week to usual max. 20 mg daily (older children have received max. 40 mg daily)

CD Dexedrine® (Evans)

Tablets, scored, dexamphetamine sulphate 5 mg. Net price 28-tab pack = 96p. Counselling, driving

---

METHYLPHENIDATE HYDROCHLORIDE

Indications: part of a comprehensive treatment programme for attention-deficit hyperactivity disorder when remedial measures alone prove insufficient (under specialist supervision)

Cautions; Contra-indications; Side-effects: see under Dexamphetamine Sulphate; other side-effects reported include rash, urticaria, fever, arthralgia, alopecia, exfoliative dermatitis, erythema multiforme, thrombocytopenic purpura, thrombocytopenia, leucopenia, (manufacturer recommends periodic complete and differential blood and platelet counts); **interactions:** Appendix 1 (sympathomimetics)

Dose: CHILD under 6 years not recommended, over 6 years, initially 5 mg 1–2 times daily, increased if necessary at weekly intervals by 5–10 mg daily to max. 60 mg daily in divided doses; discontinue if no response after 1 month, also discontinue periodically to assess child's condition (usually finally discontinued during or after puberty)

EVENING DOSE. If effect wears off in evening (with rebound hyperactivity) a dose at bedtime may be appropriate (establish need with trial bedtime dose)

CD Ritalin® (Novartis)

Tablets, scored, methylphenidate hydrochloride 10 mg, net price 30-tab pack = £5.57

COCAINE

Cocaine is a drug of addiction which causes central nervous stimulation. Its clinical use is mainly as a topical local anaesthetic (section 15.2). It has been included in analgesic elixirs for the relief of pain in palliative care but this use is obsolete. For management of cocaine poisoning, see p. 24.

4.5   Appetite suppressants

4.5.1   Bulk-forming drugs
4.5.2   Centrally acting appetite suppressants

Obesity is associated with many health problems including cardiovascular disease, diabetes mellitus, gallstones and osteoarthritis. Factors that aggravate obesity may include depression, other psychosocial problems, and drug treatment.

The main treatment of the obese patient is a suitable diet, carefully explained to the patient, with appropriate support and encouragement; the patient should also be advised to increase physical activity. Smoking cessation (while maintaining body weight) may be worthwhile before attempting supervised weight loss since cigarette smoking may be more harmful than obesity. Attendance at groups (e.g. 'weight-watchers') helps some individuals. Drugs should only be considered for those with a body mass index (BMI, patient's body-weight divided by the square of the patient's height) of 30 kg/m^2 or greater in whom at least 3 months of managed care involving supervised diet, exercise and behaviour modification fails to achieve a realistic reduction in weight; drugs should **never** be used as the sole element of treatment.

Severe obesity should be managed in an appropriate setting by staff who have been trained in the management of obesity; the patient should receive advice on diet and life-style modification and be monitored for changes in weight as well as in blood pressure, blood lipids and other associated conditions.

Thyroid hormones have **no** place in the treatment of obesity except in biochemically proven hypothyroid patients. The use of diuretics, chorionic gonadotrophin, or amphetamines is **not** appropriate for weight reduction.

4.5.1   Bulk-forming drugs

The most commonly used bulk-forming drug is **methylcellulose**. It is claimed to reduce intake by producing feelings of satiety but there is little evidence to support this claim.

METHYLCELLULOSE

Indications: adjunct in obesity (but see notes above); other indications, see section 1.6.1
Cautions: maintain adequate fluid intake
Contra-indications: gastro-intestinal obstruction
Side-effects: flatulence, abdominal distension, intestinal obstruction
Dose: see under preparations below
COUNSELLING. Preparations that swell in contact with liquid should always be carefully swallowed with water and should not be taken immediately before going to bed

Celevac® (Monmouth)

Tablets, pink, methylcellulose '450' 500 mg. Net price 112-tab pack = £2.69. Counselling, see above and dose
Dose: adjunct in obesity (but see notes above), 3 tablets, chewed or crushed, with a tumblerful of liquid half an hour before food or when hungry

---

4.5.2 Centrally acting appetite suppressants

Appetite suppressants are used as adjuncts to other methods in an appropriate setting (section 4.5). Patients prescribed these drugs should be reviewed at least at monthly intervals and a careful record kept of all treatment with appetite suppressant drugs. The patient's general practitioner should be kept informed of details of treatment and progress, if the prescription is initiated by another physician.

Dexfenfluramine and fenfluramine have been withdrawn following reports of valvular heart disease associated with their use.

Phentermine is a catecholaminergic drug with minor sympathomimetic and stimulant effects; it is licensed for use as an adjunct to the treatment of selected patients with moderate to severe obesity. Rapid weight relapse frequently occurs after short-term use of an appetite suppressant and since the use of phentermine is restricted to 12 weeks or less, this drug is not recommended for the routine management of severe obesity.

As with dexfenfluramine and fenfluramine, phentermine is associated with the rare but serious risk of pulmonary hypertension which may be insidious. Patients should be advised to report any dyspnoea or deterioration in exercise tolerance when the drug should be discontinued immediately.

CHILDREN. Centrally acting appetite suppressants should be avoided in children because of the possibility of growth suppression.

PHENTERMINE

Indications: not recommended, see notes above

Cautions: mild hypertension (avoid if moderate to severe), diabetes mellitus, history of anxiety or depression; **interactions:** Appendix 1 (sympathomimetics)

DRIVING. May impair performance of skilled tasks (e.g. driving); effects of alcohol unpredictable

Contra-indications: cardiovascular disease (including moderate to severe hypertension), glaucoma, hyperthyroidism, epilepsy, unstable personality, history of psychiatric illness; history of drug or alcohol abuse; pregnancy (congenital malformations reported with related drugs) and breast-feeding

Side-effects: see notes above; dry mouth, headache, rashes, euphoria and dependence; also insomnia, restlessness, nervousness, agitation, nausea, vomiting, dizziness, depression, psychosis, hallucinations, palpitations and tachycardia, hypertension, constipation, urinary frequency, facial oedema

Dose: 15–30 mg at breakfast time for 4–6 weeks; max. period of treatment should not exceed 3 months; ELDERLY and CHILD not recommended

CD Duromine® (3M)

Capsules, both m/r, phentermine (as resin complex) 15 mg (green/grey), net price 30-cap pack = £1.14; 30 mg (maroon/grey), 30-cap pack = £1.50. Label: 25, counselling, driving

CD Ionamin® (Torbet)

Capsules, both m/r, phentermine (as resin complex) 15 mg (grey/yellow), net price 20 = £1.11; 30 mg (yellow), 20 = £1.38. Label: 25, counselling, driving

4.6 Drugs used in nausea and vertigo

Anti-emetics should be prescribed only when the cause of vomiting is known, particularly in children, otherwise the symptomatic relief that they produce may delay diagnosis. Anti-emetics are unnecessary and sometimes harmful when the cause can be treated, e.g. as in diabetic ketoacidosis, or in excessive digoxin or antiepileptic dosage.

If antinauseant drug treatment is indicated the choice of drug depends on the aetiology of vomiting.

VESTIBULAR DISORDERS

The most effective drug for the prevention of *motion sickness* is **hyoscine**. Adverse effects (drowsiness, blurred vision, dry mouth, urinary retention) are more frequent than with the antihistamines but are not generally prominent at the doses employed. **Antihistamines** are slightly less effective, but are generally better tolerated. There is no evidence that any one antihistamine is superior to another but their duration of action and incidence of adverse effects (drowsiness and antimuscarinic effects) differ. If a sedative effect is desired **promethazine** and **dimenhydrinate** are useful, but generally a slightly less sedating antihistamine such as **cyclizine** or **cinnarizine** is preferred. **Metoclopramide** and the **phenothiazines** (except the antihistamine phenothiazine promethazine), which act selectively on the chemoreceptor trigger zone, are ineffective in motion sickness.

Vertigo and nausea associated with *Ménière's disease* and *middle-ear surgery* may be difficult to treat. **Hyoscine, antihistamines**, and **phenothiazines** (such as prochlorperazine) are effective in the prophylaxis and treatment of such conditions. **Cinnarizine** and **betahistine** have been promoted as specific treatments for Ménière's disease. In the acute attack **cyclizine** or **prochlorperazine** may be given rectally or by intramuscular injection.

Treatment of vertigo in its chronic forms is seldom fully effective but antihistamines (such as dimenhydrinate) or phenothiazines (such as prochlorperazine) may help.

For advice to avoid the inappropriate prescribing of drugs (notably phenothiazines) for dizziness in the elderly, see Prescribing for the Elderly, p. 16.

VOMITING OF PREGNANCY

Nausea in the first trimester of pregnancy does **not** require drug therapy. On rare occasions if vomiting is severe, an antihistamine or a phenothiazine (e.g. promethazine) may be required. If symptoms have not settled in 24 to 48 hours then a specialist opinion should be sought.

SYMPTOMATIC RELIEF OF NAUSEA FROM UNDERLYING DISEASE

The **phenothiazines** are dopamine antagonists and act centrally by blocking the chemoreceptor trigger zone. They are of considerable value for the prophylaxis and treatment of nausea and vomiting associated with diffuse neoplastic disease, radiation sickness, and the emesis caused by drugs such as opioid analgesics, general anaesthetics, and cytotoxic drugs. **Prochlorperazine, perphenazine,** and **trifluoperazine** are less sedating than **chlorpromazine** but severe dystonic reactions sometimes occur, especially in children. Other antipsychotic drugs including droperidol, haloperidol, and methotrimeprazine (see section 4.2.1) are also used for the relief of nausea.

Metoclopramide is an effective anti-emetic with a spectrum of activity closely resembling that of the phenothiazines but it has a peripheral action on the gut in addition to its central effect and therefore may be superior to the phenothiazines in the emesis associated with gastroduodenal, hepatic, and biliary disease. As with the phenothiazines, metoclopramide may induce acute dystonic reactions with facial and skeletal muscle spasms and oculogyric crises. These are more common in the young (especially girls and young women) and the very old, usually occur shortly after starting treatment, and subside within 24 hours of stopping the drug. Injection of an antiparkinsonian drug such as procyclidine (section 4.9.2) will abort attacks. The high-dose preparation of metoclopramide has been used for the prevention of nausea and vomiting associated with cytotoxic drug therapy.

Domperidone is used for the relief of nausea and vomiting, especially when associated with cytotoxic drug therapy. It has the advantage over metoclopramide and the phenothiazines of being less likely to cause central effects such as sedation and dystonic reactions because it does not readily cross the blood-brain barrier. It may be given for the treatment of levodopa- and bromocriptine-induced vomiting in parkinsonism (section 4.9.1). Domperidone acts at the chemoreceptor trigger zone and so is unlikely to be effective in motion sickness and other vestibular disorders.

Antihistamines are active in most of these conditions, but are not usually drugs of choice.

Nabilone is a synthetic cannabinoid with anti-emetic properties, reported to be superior to prochlorperazine. Side-effects occur frequently with standard doses.

Granisetron, ondansetron and **tropisetron** are specific (5HT$_3$) serotonin antagonists. They have a valuable role in the management of nausea and vomiting in patients receiving cytotoxics who are unable to tolerate, or whose nausea and vomiting is not controlled by, less expensive drugs.

CYTOTOXIC CHEMOTHERAPY. For *anti-emetic regimens* used in the management of nausea and vomiting induced by cytotoxic chemotherapy, see section 8.1.

ANTIHISTAMINES

CINNARIZINE
Indications: vestibular disorders, such as vertigo, tinnitus, nausea, and vomiting in Ménière's disease; motion sickness; vascular disease, see section 2.6.4

Cautions; Contra-indications; Side-effects: see under Cyclizine; also allergic skin reactions and fatigue; caution in hypotension (high doses); rarely, extrapyramidal symptoms in elderly on prolonged therapy; avoid in porphyria (see section 9.8.2)

Dose: vestibular disorders, 30 mg 3 times daily; CHILD 5–12 years half adult dose
Motion sickness, 30 mg 2 hours before travel then 15 mg every 8 hours during journey if necessary; CHILD 5–12 years half adult dose

Cinnarizine (Non-proprietary)
Tablets, cinnarizine 15 mg. Net price 20 = £1.03. Label: 2
Available from APS, Ashbourne (Cinazière®), Cox, Hillcross, Norton

Stugeron® (Janssen-Cilag)
Tablets, scored, cinnarizine 15 mg. Net price 20 = £1.07. Label: 2
Stugeron Forte®: see section 2.6.4

CYCLIZINE
Indications: nausea, vomiting, vertigo, motion sickness, labyrinthine disorders
Cautions; Contra-indications; Side-effects: drowsiness, occasional dry mouth and blurred vision; see also section 3.4.1; cyclizine may aggravate severe heart failure and counteract the haemodynamic benefits of opioids; **interactions:** Appendix 1 (antihistamines)
DRIVING. Drowsiness may affect performance of skilled tasks (e.g. driving); effects of alcohol enhanced
Dose: by mouth, cyclizine hydrochloride 50 mg up to 3 times daily; CHILD 6–12 years 25 mg
By intramuscular or intravenous injection, cyclizine lactate 50 mg 3 times daily

Valoid® (GlaxoWellcome)
Tablets, scored, cyclizine hydrochloride 50 mg. Net price 20 = 99p. Label: 2
PoM *Injection,* cyclizine lactate 50 mg/mL. Net price 1-mL amp = 57p

DIMENHYDRINATE
Indications: nausea, vomiting, vertigo, motion sickness, labyrinthine disorders
Cautions; Contra-indications; Side-effects: see under Cyclizine; porphyria (see section 9.8.2)
Dose: 50–100 mg 2–3 times daily; CHILD 1–6 years 12.5–25 mg, 7–12 years 25–50 mg
Motion sickness, first dose 30 minutes before journey

Dramamine® (Searle)
Tablets, scored, dimenhydrinate 50 mg, net price 100-tab pack = £5.13. Label: 2
Note. A 10-tab pack is on sale to the public for motion sickness

MECLOZINE HYDROCHLORIDE
Indications: see under preparations
Cautions; Contra-indications; Side-effects: see under Cyclizine

Preparations
A proprietary brand of meclozine hydrochloride tablets 12.5 mg (Sea-legs®) is on sale to the public for motion sickness

PROMETHAZINE HYDROCHLORIDE
Indications: nausea, vomiting, vertigo, labyrinthine disorders, motion sickness; other indications, see sections 3.4.1, 4.1.1, 15.1.4.1
Cautions; Contra-indications; Side-effects: see under Cyclizine but more sedating; intramuscular injection may be painful; avoid in porphyria (see section 9.8.2)
Dose: motion sickness prevention (elixir), 25 mg at bedtime on night before travelling, repeat following morning if necessary; CHILD under 2 years not recommended, 2–5 years, 5 mg at night and following morning; 5–10 years, 10 mg at night and following morning

Preparations
See section 3.4.1

PROMETHAZINE THEOCLATE
(Promethazine Teoclate)
Indications: nausea, vertigo, labyrinthine disorders, motion sickness (acts longer than the hydrochloride)
Cautions; Contra-indications; Side-effects: see under Promethazine Hydrochloride
Dose: 25–75 mg, max. 100 mg, daily; CHILD 5–10 years, 12.5–37.5 mg daily
Motion sickness prevention, 25 mg at bedtime on night before travelling *or* 25 mg 1–2 hours before travelling; CHILD 5–10 years, half adult dose
For severe vomiting in pregnancy, 25 mg at bedtime, increased if necessary to a max. of 100 mg daily (but see also Vomiting of Pregnancy in notes above)

Avomine® (Manx)
Tablets, scored, promethazine theoclate 25 mg. Net price 10-tab pack = £1.04; 28-tab pack = £3.05. Label: 2

PHENOTHIAZINES AND RELATED DRUGS

CHLORPROMAZINE HYDROCHLORIDE
Indications: nausea and vomiting of terminal illness (where other drugs have failed or are not available); other indications, see sections 4.2.1, 15.1.4.1
Cautions; Contra-indications; Side-effects: see section 4.2.1
Dose: by mouth, 10–25 mg every 4–6 hours; CHILD 500 micrograms/kg every 4–6 hours (1–5 years max. 40 mg daily, 6–12 years max. 75 mg daily)
By deep intramuscular injection 25 mg initially then 25–50 mg every 3–4 hours until vomiting stops; CHILD 500 micrograms/kg every 6–8 hours (1–5 years max. 40 mg daily, 6–12 years max. 75 mg daily)

By rectum in suppositories, chlorpromazine 100 mg every 6–8 hours [unlicensed]

Preparations
Section 4.2.1

PERPHENAZINE
Indications: severe nausea, vomiting (see notes above); other indications, section 4.2.1
Cautions; Contra-indications; Side-effects: see section 4.2.1; extrapyramidal symptoms may occur, particularly in young adults, elderly, and debilitated
Dose: 4 mg 3 times daily, adjusted according to response; max. 24 mg daily (chemotherapy-induced); ELDERLY quarter to half adult dose; CHILD under 14 years not recommended

Preparations
Section 4.2.1

PROCHLORPERAZINE
Indications: severe nausea, vomiting, vertigo, labyrinthine disorders (see notes above); other indications, section 4.2.1
Cautions; Contra-indications: see under Chlorpromazine Hydrochloride (section 4.2.1). Oral route only for children (avoid if less than 10 kg); elderly (see notes above)
Side-effects: see under Chlorpromazine Hydrochloride; extrapyramidal symptoms may occur, particularly in children, elderly, and debilitated
Dose: by mouth, nausea and vomiting, prochlorperazine maleate or mesylate, acute attack, 20 mg initially then 10 mg after 2 hours; prevention 5–10 mg 2–3 times daily; CHILD (over 10 kg only) 250 micrograms/kg 2–3 times daily
Labyrinthine disorders, 5 mg 3 times daily, gradually increased if necessary to 30 mg daily in divided doses, then reduced after several weeks to 5–10 mg daily; CHILD not recommended
By deep intramuscular injection, nausea and vomiting, 12.5 mg when required followed if necessary after 6 hours by an oral dose, as above; CHILD not recommended
By rectum in suppositories, nausea and vomiting, 25 mg followed if necessary after 6 hours by oral dose, as above; *or* due to migraine, 5 mg 3 times daily; CHILD not recommended

PoM **Prochlorperazine** (Non-proprietary)
Tablets, prochlorperazine maleate 5 mg, net price 20 = 46p. Label: 2
Available from Ashbourne (Prozière®), Cox, Hillcross, Norton
PoM **Stemetil®** (Rhône-Poulenc Rorer)
Tablets, prochlorperazine maleate 5 mg (off-white), net price 84-tab pack = £3.48; 25 mg (scored), 56-tab pack = £6.13. Label: 2
Syrup, straw-coloured, prochlorperazine mesylate 5 mg/5 mL. Net price 100-mL pack = £1.96. Label: 2

Eff sachets, granules, effervescent, sugar-free, prochlorperazine mesylate 5 mg/sachet. Net price 21-sachet pack = £3.64. Label: 2, 13

Injection, prochlorperazine mesylate 12.5 mg/mL. Net price 1-mL amp = 38p

Suppositories, prochlorperazine maleate (as prochlorperazine), 5 mg, net price 10 = £4.92; 25 mg, 10 = £6.45. Label: 2

Buccal preparation
PoM **Buccastem®** (R&C)
Tablets (buccal), pale yellow, prochlorperazine maleate 3 mg. Net price 5 × 10-tab pack = £5.75. Label: 2, counselling, administration, see under Dose below
Dose: 1–2 tablets twice daily; tablets are placed high between upper lip and gum and left to dissolve; CHILD not recommended

TRIFLUOPERAZINE
Indications: severe nausea and vomiting (see notes above); other indications, section 4.2.1

Cautions; Contra-indications; Side-effects: see section 4.2.1; extrapyramidal symptoms may occur, particularly in children, elderly, and debilitated

Dose: by mouth, 2–4 mg daily in divided doses *or* as a single dose of a modified-release preparation; max. 6 mg daily; CHILD 3–5 years up to 1 mg daily, 6–12 years up to 4 mg daily

Preparations
See section 4.2.1

DOMPERIDONE AND METOCLOPRAMIDE

DOMPERIDONE
Indications: see under Dose
CHILDREN. Use in children is restricted to nausea and vomiting following cytotoxics or radiotherapy
Cautions: renal impairment; pregnancy and breast-feeding; not recommended for routine prophylaxis of post-operative vomiting or for chronic administration; **interactions:** Appendix 1 (domperidone)

Side-effects: raised prolactin concentrations (possible galactorrhoea and gynaecomastia), reduced libido reported; rashes and other allergic reactions; acute dystonic reactions reported

Dose: by mouth, acute nausea and vomiting, (including nausea and vomiting induced by levodopa and bromocriptine), 10–20 mg every 4–8 hours, max. period of treatment 12 weeks; CHILD, nausea and vomiting following cytotoxic therapy or radiotherapy only, 200–400 micrograms/kg every 4–8 hours

Functional dyspepsia, 10–20 mg 3 times daily before food and 10–20 mg at night; max. period of treatment 12 weeks; CHILD not recommended

By rectum in suppositories, nausea and vomiting, 30–60 mg every 4–8 hours; CHILD over 2 years (following cytotoxic therapy or radiotherapy only), body-weight 10–15 kg max. 15 mg twice daily, body-weight 15.5–25 kg max. 30 mg twice daily, body-weight 25.5–35 kg max. 30 mg 3 times daily, body-weight 35.5–45 kg max. 30 mg 4 times daily; since dose needs to be divided

throughout day, suppositories may be cut in half for younger children

PoM **Motilium®** (Sanofi Winthrop)
Tablets, f/c, domperidone 10 mg (as maleate). Net price 30-tab pack = £2.46; 100-tab pack = £8.21
Suspension, sugar-free, domperidone 5 mg/5 mL. Net price 200-mL pack = £1.80
Suppositories, domperidone 30 mg. Net price 10 = £2.65

METOCLOPRAMIDE HYDROCHLORIDE
Indications: adults, nausea and vomiting, particularly in gastro-intestinal disorders (see section 1.2) and treatment with cytotoxics or radiotherapy; migraine—section 4.7.4.1
PATIENTS UNDER 20 YEARS. Use restricted to severe intractable vomiting of known cause, vomiting of radiotherapy and cytotoxics, aid to gastro-intestinal intubation, pre-medication
Cautions: hepatic and renal impairment; elderly, young adults, and children (measure dose accurately, preferably with a pipette); may mask underlying disorders such as cerebral irritation; avoid for 3–4 days following gastro-intestinal surgery, may cause acute hypertensive response in phaeochromocytoma; pregnancy and breast-feeding; porphyria (see section 9.8.2); **interactions:** Appendix 1 (metoclopramide)

Side-effects: extrapyramidal effects (especially in children/young adults), hyperprolactinaemia, occasionally tardive dyskinesia on prolonged administration; also reported, drowsiness, restlessness, diarrhoea, depression, neuroleptic malignant syndrome; cardiac conduction abnormalities reported following intravenous administration

Dose: by mouth, or by intramuscular injection or by intravenous injection over 1–2 minutes, 10 mg (5 mg in young adults 15–19 years under 60 kg) 3 times daily; CHILD up to 1 year (up to 10 kg) 1 mg twice daily, 1–3 years (10–14 kg) 1 mg 2–3 times daily, 3–5 years (15–19 kg) 2 mg 2–3 times daily, 5–9 years (20–29 kg) 2.5 mg 3 times daily, 9–14 years (30 kg and over) 5 mg 3 times daily
Note. Daily dose of metoclopramide should not normally exceed 500 micrograms/kg, particularly for children and young adults (restricted use, see above)
For diagnostic procedures, as a single dose 5–10 minutes before examination, 10–20 mg (10 mg in young adults 15–19 years); CHILD under 3 years 1 mg, 3–5 years 2 mg, 5–9 years 2.5 mg, 9–14 years 5 mg

PoM **Metoclopramide** (Non-proprietary)
Tablets, metoclopramide hydrochloride 10 mg, net price 20 = 46p
Available from Antigen, APS, Ashbourne (Gastroflux®), Berk (Primperan®), Cox, CP, Lagap (Parmid®), Norton
Oral solution, metoclopramide hydrochloride 5 mg/5 mL, net price 100-mL pack = £1.09
Available from Berk (Primperan®, sugar-free), Lagap (Parmid® sugar-free), Rosemont (sugar-free)
Injection, metoclopramide hydrochloride 5 mg/mL, net price 2-mL amp = 27p
Available from Antigen, Phoenix

PoM **Maxolon**® (Monmouth)

Tablets, scored, metoclopramide hydrochloride 5 mg, net price 84-tab pack = £4.69; 10 mg, 21-tab pack = £2.35, 84-tab pack = £9.38

Syrup, sugar-free, metoclopramide hydrochloride 5 mg/5 mL. Net price 200-mL pack = £3.83

Paediatric liquid, sugar-free, metoclopramide hydrochloride 1 mg/mL. Net price 15-mL pack with pipette = £1.51. Counselling, use of pipette

Injection, metoclopramide hydrochloride 5 mg/mL. Net price 2-mL amp = 27p

High-dose (with cytotoxic chemotherapy only)
PoM **Maxolon High Dose**® (Monmouth)

Injection, metoclopramide hydrochloride 5 mg/mL. Net price 20-mL amp = £2.67.

For dilution and use as an intravenous infusion in nausea and vomiting associated with cytotoxic chemotherapy only

Dose: by continuous intravenous infusion (preferred method), initially (before starting chemotherapy), 2–4 mg/kg over 15–20 minutes, then 3–5 mg/kg over 8–12 hours; max. in 24 hours, 10 mg/kg

By intermittent intravenous infusion, initially (before starting chemotherapy), up to 2 mg/kg over at least 15 minutes then up to 2 mg/kg over at least 15 minutes every 2 hours; max. in 24 hours, 10 mg/kg

Note. Injection of metoclopramide hydrochloride 5 mg/mL also available in 20-mL ampoules from Phoenix

Modified-release preparations
Note. All unsuitable for patients under 20 years
PoM **Gastrobid Continus**® (Napp)

Tablets, m/r, metoclopramide hydrochloride 15 mg. Net price 56-tab pack = £10.16. Label: 25

Dose: patients over 20 years, 1 tablet twice daily

PoM **Gastromax**® (Pfizer)

Capsules, m/r, orange/yellow, enclosing white to light beige pellets, metoclopramide hydrochloride 30 mg. Net price 28-cap pack = £11.55. Label: 22, 25

Dose: patients over 20 years, 1 capsule daily

PoM **Maxolon SR**® (Monmouth)

Capsules, m/r, clear, enclosing white granules, metoclopramide hydrochloride 15 mg. Net price 56-cap pack = £10.76. Label: 25

Dose: patients over 20 years, 1 capsule twice daily

Compound preparations (for migraine), section 4.7.4.1

5HT$_3$ ANTAGONISTS

GRANISETRON

Indications: see under Dose

Cautions: pregnancy and breast-feeding

Side-effects: constipation, headache, rash; transient increases in liver enzymes; hypersensitivity reactions reported

Dose: nausea and vomiting induced by cytotoxic chemotherapy or radiotherapy, *by mouth*, 1–2 mg within 1 hour before start of treatment, then 2 mg daily in 1–2 divided doses during treatment; when intravenous infusion also used, max. combined total 9 mg in 24 hours; CHILD 20 micrograms/kg (max. 1 mg) within 1 hour before start of treatment, then 20 micrograms/kg (max. 1 mg) twice daily for up to 5 days during treatment

By intravenous injection (diluted in 15 mL sodium chloride 0.9% and given over not less than 30 seconds) *or by intravenous infusion* (over 5 minutes, see Appendix 6), prevention, 3 mg before start of cytotoxic therapy (up to 2 additional 3-mg doses may be given within 24 hours); treatment, as for prevention (the two additional doses must not be given less than 10 minutes apart); max. 9 mg in 24 hours; CHILD, *by intravenous infusion*, (over 5 minutes), prevention, 40 micrograms/kg (max. 3 mg) before start of cytotoxic therapy; treatment, as for prevention—one additional dose of 40 micrograms/kg (max. 3 mg) may be given within 24 hours (not less than 10 minutes after initial dose)

Postoperative nausea and vomiting, *by intravenous injection* (diluted to 5 mL and given over 30 seconds), prevention, 1 mg before induction of anaesthesia; treatment, 1 mg, given as for prevention; max. 2 mg in one day; CHILD not recommended

PoM **Kytril**® (SmithKline Beecham)

Tablets, f/c, granisetron (as hydrochloride) 1 mg, net price 10-tab pack = £91.43; 2 mg, 5-tab pack = £91.43

Paediatric liquid, sugar-free, granisetron (as hydrochloride) 1 mg/5 mL, net price 30 mL = £54.86

Sterile solution, granisetron (as hydrochloride) 1 mg/mL, for dilution and use as injection or infusion, net price 1-mL vial = £12.00, 3-mL amp = £36.00

ONDANSETRON

Indications: see under Dose

Cautions: pregnancy and breast-feeding; moderate or severe hepatic impairment (max. 8 mg daily)

Side-effects: constipation; headache, sensation of warmth or flushing, hiccups; occasional alterations in liver enzymes; hypersensitivity reactions reported; occasional transient visual disturbances and dizziness following intravenous administration; involuntary movements, seizures, chest pain, arrhythmias, hypotension and bradycardia also reported; suppositories may cause rectal irritation

Dose: moderately emetogenic chemotherapy or radiotherapy, *by mouth*, 8 mg 1–2 hours before treatment *or by rectum*, 16 mg 1–2 hours before treatment *or by intramuscular injection or slow intravenous injection*, 8 mg immediately before treatment

then *by mouth*, 8 mg every 12 hours for up to 5 days *or by rectum*, 16 mg daily for up to 5 days

Severely emetogenic chemotherapy, *by intramuscular injection or slow intravenous injection*, 8 mg immediately before treatment, where necessary followed by 8 mg at intervals of 2–4 hours for 2 further doses (*or* followed by 1 mg/hour *by continuous intravenous infusion* for up to 24 hours)

then *by mouth*, 8 mg every 12 hours for up to 5 days *or by rectum*, 16 mg daily for up to 5 days

---

alternatively, by intravenous infusion over at least 15 minutes, 32 mg immediately before treatment *or by rectum*, 16 mg 1–2 hours before treatment *then by mouth*, 8 mg every 12 hours for up to 5 days *or by rectum*, 16 mg daily for up to 5 days

Note. Efficacy may be enhanced by addition of a single dose of dexamethasone sodium phosphate 20 mg by intravenous injection

CHILD, *by slow intravenous injection or by intravenous infusion* over 15 minutes, 5 mg/m^2 immediately before chemotherapy then, 4 mg *by mouth* every 12 hours for up to 5 days

Prevention of postoperative nausea and vomiting, *by mouth*, 16 mg 1 hour before anaesthesia *or* 8 mg 1 hour before anaesthesia followed by 8 mg at intervals of 8 hours for 2 further doses
alternatively, by intramuscular or slow intravenous injection, 4 mg at induction of anaesthesia; CHILD over 2 years, *by slow intravenous injection*, 100 micrograms/kg (max. 4 mg) before, during, or after induction of anaesthesia

Treatment of postoperative nausea and vomiting, *by intramuscular or slow intravenous injection*, 4 mg; CHILD over 2 years, *by slow intravenous injection*, 100 micrograms/kg (max. 4 mg)

PoM **Zofran**® (GlaxoWellcome)

Tablets, both yellow, f/c, ondansetron (as hydrochloride) 4 mg, net price 30-tab pack = £121.50; 8 mg, 10-tab pack = £81.00

Syrup, sugar-free, ondansetron (as hydrochloride) 4 mg/5 mL. Net price 50-mL pack = £40.50

Injection, ondansetron (as hydrochloride) 2 mg/mL, net price 2-mL amp – £6.75; 4-mL amp = £13.50

Suppositories, ondansetron 16 mg. Net price 5 = £81.00

TROPISETRON

Indications: see under Dose

Cautions: uncontrolled hypertension (has been aggravated by doses higher than recommended); pregnancy and breast-feeding

DRIVING. Dizziness or drowsiness may affect performance of skilled tasks (e.g. driving)

Side-effects: constipation, diarrhoea, abdominal pain; headache, dizziness, fatigue; hypersensitivity reactions reported (including facial flushing, urticaria, chest tightness, dyspnoea, bronchospasm and hypotension); collapse, syncope, bradycardia, cardiovascular collapse also reported (causal relationship not established)

Dose: prevention of nausea and vomiting induced by cytotoxic chemotherapy, *by slow intravenous injection or by intravenous infusion*, 5 mg shortly before chemotherapy, then 5 mg *by mouth* every morning at least 1 hour before food for 5 days; CHILD not recommended

Postoperative nausea and vomiting, *by slow intravenous injection or by intravenous infusion*, prevention, 2 mg shortly before induction of anaesthesia; treatment, 2 mg within 2 hours of the end of anaesthesia

PoM **Navoban**® (Novartis)

Capsules, white/yellow, tropisetron (as hydrochloride) 5 mg, net price 5-cap pack = £63.37; 50-cap pack = £633.65. Label: 23

Injection, tropisetron (as hydrochloride), 1 mg/mL, net price 2-mL amp = £5.72, 5-mL amp = £14.31

CANNABINOID

NABILONE

Indications: nausea and vomiting caused by cytotoxic chemotherapy, unresponsive to conventional anti-emetics (under close observation, preferably in in-patient setting)

Cautions: history of psychiatric disorder; elderly; hypertension; heart disease; adverse effects on mental state can persist for 48–72 hours after stopping; **interactions:** Appendix 1 (nabilone)

DRIVING. Drowsiness may affect performance of skilled tasks (e.g. driving); effects of alcohol enhanced

Contra-indications: severe hepatic impairment; pregnancy and breast-feeding

Side-effects: drowsiness, vertigo, euphoria, dry mouth, ataxia, visual disturbance, concentration difficulties, sleep disturbance, dysphoria, hypotension, headache and nausea; also confusion, disorientation, hallucinations, psychosis, depression, decreased coordination, tremors, tachycardia, decreased appetite, and abdominal pain

BEHAVIOURAL EFFECTS. Patients should be made aware of possible changes of mood and other adverse behavioural effects

Dose: patients over 18 years, initially 1 mg twice daily, increased if necessary to 2 mg twice daily, throughout each cycle of cytotoxic therapy and, if necessary, for 48 hours after the last dose of each cycle; max. 6 mg daily given in 3 divided doses. The first dose should be taken the night before initiation of cytotoxic treatment and the second dose 1–3 hours before the first dose of cytotoxic drug; ADOLESCENT and CHILD under 18 years not recommended

PoM **Nabilone** (Cambridge)

Capsules, blue/white, nabilone 1 mg. Net price 20-cap pack = £101.85 (hosp. only). Label: 2, counselling, behavioural effects

---

HYOSCINE

HYOSCINE HYDROBROMIDE

(Scopolamine Hydrobromide)

Indications: motion sickness; premedication, see section 15.1.3

Cautions: elderly, urinary retention, cardiovascular disease, gastro-intestinal obstruction, hepatic or renal impairment; porphyria (see section 9.8.2); pregnancy and breast-feeding; **interactions:** Appendix 1 (antimuscarinics)

DRIVING. Drowsiness may affect performance of skilled tasks (e.g. driving) and may persist for up to 24 hours or longer after removal of patch: effects of alcohol enhanced

---

Contra-indications: closed-angle glaucoma

Side-effects: drowsiness, dry mouth, dizziness, blurred vision, difficulty with micturition

Dose: motion sickness, *by mouth*, 300 micrograms 30 minutes before start of journey followed by 300 micrograms every 6 hours if required; max. 3 doses in 24 hours; CHILD 4–10 years 75–150 micrograms, over 10 years 150–300 micrograms

Note. Proprietary brands of hyoscine hydrobromide tablets (Joy-rides®, Kwells®) are on sale to the public for motion sickness

Injection, see section 15.1.3

PoM **Scopoderm TTS®** (Novartis)

Patch, self-adhesive, pink, releasing hyoscine approx. 1 mg/72 hours when in contact with skin. Net price 2 = £2.84. Label: 19, counselling, see below

Administration: motion sickness prevention, apply 1 patch to hairless area of skin behind ear 5–6 hours before journey; replace if necessary after 72 hours, siting replacement patch behind other ear; CHILD under 10 years not recommended

COUNSELLING. Explain accompanying instructions to patient and in particular emphasise advice to wash hands after handling and to wash application site after removing, and to use one at a time

---

OTHER DRUGS FOR MÉNIÈRE'S DISEASE

Betahistine has been promoted as a specific treatment for Ménière's disease.

BETAHISTINE DIHYDROCHLORIDE

Indications: vertigo, tinnitus and hearing loss associated with Ménière's disease

Cautions: asthma, history of peptic ulcer; pregnancy and breast-feeding; **interactions:** Appendix 1 (betahistine)

Contra-indications: phaeochromocytoma

Side-effects: gastro-intestinal disturbances; headache, rashes and pruritus reported

Dose: initially 16 mg 3 times daily, preferably with food; maintenance 24–48 mg daily; CHILD not recommended

PoM **Betahistine Dihydrochloride** (Non-proprietary)

Tablets, betahistine dihydrochloride 8 mg, net price 120-tab pack = £9.82; 16 mg, 84-tab pack = £18.03. Label: 21

Available from Cox, Lagap, Solvay (Serc®)

PoM **Serc®** (Solvay)

Tablets, betahistine dihydrochloride 8 mg (Serc®-8), net price 120-tab pack = £10.04; 16 mg (Serc®-16), 84-tab pack = £18.03. Label: 21

4.7   Analgesics

4.7.1   Non-opioid analgesics
4.7.2   Opioid analgesics
4.7.3   Trigeminal neuralgia
4.7.4   Antimigraine drugs

For advice on pain relief in palliative care see Prescribing in Palliative Care, p. 12.

4.7.1   Non-opioid analgesics

The non-opioid drugs, paracetamol and aspirin (and other NSAIDs), are particularly suitable for pain in musculoskeletal conditions, whereas the opioid analgesics are more suitable for severe visceral pain.

Aspirin is indicated for headache, transient musculoskeletal pain, dysmenorrhoea and pyrexia. In inflammatory conditions, most physicians prefer anti-inflammatory treatment with another NSAID which may be better tolerated and more convenient for the patient. Aspirin is used increasingly for its antiplatelet properties (section 2.9). Aspirin tablets or dispersible aspirin tablets are adequate for most purposes as they act rapidly.

Gastric irritation may be a problem; it is minimised by taking the dose after food. Enteric coated preparations are available, but have a slow onset of action and are therefore unsuitable for single-dose analgesic use (though their prolonged action may be useful for night pain).

Aspirin interacts significantly with a number of other drugs and its interaction with warfarin is a **special hazard**, see **interactions:** Appendix 1 (aspirin).

Paracetamol is similar in efficacy to aspirin, but has no demonstrable anti-inflammatory activity; it is less irritant to the stomach and for that reason is now generally preferred to aspirin, particularly in the elderly. **Overdosage** with paracetamol is particularly dangerous as it may cause hepatic damage which is sometimes not apparent for 4 to 6 days (see Emergency Treatment of Poisoning, p. 20). **Benorylate** (section 10.1.1) is an aspirin–paracetamol ester.

Nefopam may have a place in the relief of persistent pain unresponsive to other non-opioid analgesics. It causes little or no respiratory depression, but sympathomimetic and antimuscarinic side-effects may be troublesome.

Non-steroidal anti-inflammatory analgesics (NSAIDs, section 10.1.1) are particularly useful for the treatment of patients with chronic disease accompanied by pain and inflammation. Some of them are also used in the short-term treatment of mild to moderate pain including transient musculoskeletal pain but paracetamol is now often preferred, particularly in the elderly (see also p. 16). They are also suitable for the relief of pain in *dysmenorrhoea* and to treat pain caused by *secondary bone tumours,* many of which produce lysis of bone and release prostaglandins (see Prescribing in Palliative Care, p. 12). NSAIDs including ketorolac are also used for perioperative analgesia, see section 15.1.4.2.

COMPOUND ANALGESIC PREPARATIONS

Compound analgesic preparations containing paracetamol or aspirin with a *low dose* of an opioid analgesic (e.g. 8 mg of codeine phosphate per compound tablet) are commonly used, but the advantages have not been substantiated. The low dose of the opioid may be enough to cause opioid side-effects (in particular, constipation) and can complicate the treatment of **overdosage** (see p. 22) yet may not provide significant additional relief of pain.

Compound analgesic preparations containing a *full dose* of the opioid component (e.g. 30 mg of codeine phosphate per compound tablet) carry the full range of opioid side-effects (including nausea, vomiting, severe constipation, drowsiness, respiratory depression, and risk of dependence on long-term administration). For details of the **side-effects, cautions** and **contra-indications** of opioid analgesics, see p. 200 (**important**: the elderly are particularly susceptible to opioid side-effects and should receive lower doses).

In general, when assessing pain, it is necessary to weigh up carefully whether there is a need for a non-opioid and an opioid analgesic to be taken simultaneously.

Caffeine is a weak stimulant that is often included, in small doses, in analgesic preparations. It is claimed that the addition of caffeine may enhance the analgesic effect, but the alerting effect, mild habit-forming effect and possible provocation of headache may not always be desirable. Moreover, in excessive dosage or on withdrawal caffeine may itself induce headache.

DYSMENORRHOEA

Use of an oral contraceptive prevents the pain of dysmenorrhoea which is generally associated with ovulatory cycles. If treatment is necessary paracetamol or an NSAID (section 10.1.1) will generally provide adequate relief of pain. The vomiting and severe pain associated with dysmenorrhoea in women with endometriosis may call for an antiemetic (in addition to an analgesic). Antispasmodics (such as alverine citrate, section 1.2) have been advocated for dysmenorrhoea but the antispasmodic action does not generally provide significant relief. Hyoscine butylbromide (section 1.2) has also been advocated for its antispasmodic action despite the fact that its absorption following oral administration is extremely poor.

ASPIRIN

(Acetylsalicylic Acid)

Indications: mild to moderate pain, pyrexia; see also section 10.1.1; antiplatelet (section 2.9)

Cautions: asthma, allergic disease, impaired renal or hepatic function (avoid if severe), dehydration, pregnancy; elderly; G6PD-deficiency (section 9.1.5); **interactions:** Appendix 1 (aspirin)

Contra-indications: children under 12 years and in breast-feeding (Reye's syndrome, see below);

gastro-intestinal ulceration, haemophilia; not for treatment of gout

HYPERSENSITIVITY. Aspirin and other NSAIDs are **contra-indicated** in patients with a history of hypersensitivity to aspirin or any other NSAID—*which includes those* in whom attacks of *asthma, angioedema, urticaria or rhinitis* have been precipitated by aspirin or any other NSAID

REYE'S SYNDROME. Owing to an association with Reye's syndrome the CSM has recommended that aspirin-containing preparations should no longer be given to children under the age of 12 years, unless specifically indicated, e.g. for juvenile arthritis (Still's disease). It is **important** to advise families that aspirin is not a suitable medicine for children with minor illness.

Side-effects: generally mild and infrequent but high incidence of gastro-intestinal irritation with slight asymptomatic blood loss, increased bleeding time, bronchospasm and skin reactions in hypersensitive patients. Prolonged administration, see section 10.1.1. **Overdosage:** see Emergency Treatment of Poisoning, p. 20

Dose: 300–900 mg every 4–6 hours when necessary; max. 4 g daily; CHILD not recommended (see notes above)

Aspirin (Non-proprietary)
Tablets, aspirin 300 mg. Net price 20 = 9p. Label: 21, 32
Available from most generic manufacturers
Dispersible tablets, aspirin 300 mg, net price 20 = 8p; 75 mg, see section 2.9. Label: 13, 21, 32
Available from most generic manufacturers
Note. BP directs that when no strength is stated the 300-mg strength should be dispensed, and that when soluble aspirin tablets are prescribed, dispersible aspirin tablets shall be dispensed.
Suppositories, aspirin 300 mg, net price 10 = £8.40. Label: 32
Dose: 2–3 suppositories inserted every 4 hours when necessary (max. 12 suppositories in 24 hours); CHILD not recommended (see above)
Available from Aurum (who also supply a 150-mg strength)

Caprin® (Sinclair)
Tablets, e/c, f/c, pink, aspirin 300 mg, net price 100-tab pack = £4.89; 75 mg, see section 2.9. Label: 5, 25, 32

Disprin CV®: see section 2.9

Nu-Seals® Aspirin (Lilly)
Tablets, e/c, aspirin 300 mg, net price 100-tab pack = £5.80; 75 mg, see section 2.9. Label: 5, 25, 32
Note. Aspirin enteric-coated also available from Ashbourne (postMI® 75)

With codeine phosphate 8 mg

Co-codaprin (Non-proprietary)
Tablets, co-codaprin 8/400 (codeine phosphate 8 mg, aspirin 400 mg). Net price 20 = 26p. Label: 21, 32
Dose: 1–2 tablets every 4–6 hours when necessary; max. 8 tablets daily
Dispersible tablets, co-codaprin 8/400 (codeine phosphate 8 mg, aspirin 400 mg). Net price 20 = 54p. Label: 13, 21, 32
Dose: 1–2 tablets in water every 4–6 hours; max. 8 tablets daily
Available from Cox
When co-codaprin tablets or dispersible tablets are prescribed and no strength is stated tablets, or dispersible tablets, respectively, containing codeine phosphate 8 mg and aspirin 400 mg should be dispensed

---

Cautionary label wordings, see inside back cover

Prices are **net**, see p.1

Other compound preparations

PoM **Aspav**® (Hoechst Marion Roussel)

Dispersible tablets, aspirin 500 mg, mixed opium alkaloids (anhydrous morphine (as morphine hydrochloride) 5 mg, papaverine hydrochloride 600 micrograms, codeine hydrochloride 520 micrograms). Net price 20 = £2.04. Label: 2, 13, 21, 32

Dose: 1–2 tablets in water every 4–6 hours if necessary; max. 8 tablets daily

NHS PoM **Doloxene Compound**® (Lilly)

Capsules, grey/red, dextropropoxyphene napsylate 100 mg, aspirin 375 mg, caffeine 30 mg. Net price 100-cap pack = £9.22. Label: 2, 21, 32

Dose: 1 capsule 3–4 times daily; max. 4 capsules daily

NHS CD **Equagesic**® (Wyeth)

Tablets, pink/white/yellow, ethoheptazine citrate 75 mg, meprobamate 150 mg, aspirin 250 mg. Net price 100-tab pack = £4.50. Label: 2, 21, 32

Dose: muscle pain, 1–2 tablets 3–4 times daily

Preparations on sale to the public

For a list of **preparations** containing aspirin and paracetamol **on sale to the public**, see p. 197.

PARACETAMOL

Indications: mild to moderate pain, pyrexia

Cautions: hepatic and renal impairment, alcohol dependence; **interactions:** Appendix 1 (paracetamol)

Side-effects: side-effects rare, but rashes, blood disorders; acute pancreatitis reported after prolonged use; **important:** liver damage (and less frequently renal damage) following **overdosage**, see Emergency Treatment of Poisoning, p. 20

Dose: by mouth, 0.5–1 g every 4–6 hours to a max. of 4 g daily; CHILD 2 months 60 mg for post-immunisation pyrexia; otherwise under 3 months (on doctor's advice only), 10 mg/kg (5 mg/kg if jaundiced); 3 months–1 year 60–120 mg, 1–5 years 120–250 mg, 6–12 years 250–500 mg; these doses may be repeated every 4–6 hours when necessary (max. of 4 doses in 24 hours)

For full Joint Committee on Vaccination and Immunisation recommendation on post-immunisation pyrexia, see section 14.1

Rectal route, see below

Paracetamol (Non-proprietary)

Tablets, paracetamol 500 mg. Net price 20 = 9p. Label: 29, 30

Available from APS, Cox, Norton, Sterling Health (NHS Panadol®)

Soluble Tablets (= Dispersible tablets), paracetamol 500 mg. Net price 60-tab pack = £2.26. Label: 13, 29, 30

Available from Sterling Health (NHS Panadol Soluble®)

Paediatric Soluble Tablets (= Paediatric dispersible tablets), paracetamol 120 mg. Net price 24-tab pack = 82p. Label: 13, 30

Available from R&C (NHS Disprol® Soluble Paracetamol)

Paediatric Oral Solution (= Paediatric Elixir), paracetamol 120 mg/5 mL. Net price 100 mL = 37p. Label: 30

Note. Sugar-free versions are available and can be ordered by specifying 'sugar-free' on the prescription.

Available from Berk, Evans, Norton, Rosemont (NHS Paldesic®), Wallace Mfg (NHS Salzone®)

Oral Suspension 120 mg/5 mL (= Paediatric Mixture), paracetamol 120 mg/5 mL. Net price 100 mL = 43p. Label: 30

Note. BP directs that when Paediatric Paracetamol Oral Suspension or Paediatric Paracetamol Mixture is prescribed Paracetamol Oral Suspension 120 mg/5 mL should be dispensed; sugar-free versions can be ordered by specifying 'sugar-free' on the prescription

Available from Cupal (Cupanol® Paediatric, sugar-free—now called Medinol® Paediatric), Norton, R&C (Disprol® Paediatric, sugar-free), Rosemont (Paldesic®), Sterling Health (Panadol®, sugar-free), Warner Lambert (Calpol® Paediatric, Calpol® Paediatric sugar-free)

Oral Suspension 250 mg/5 mL (= Mixture), paracetamol 250 mg/5 mL. Net price 100 mL = 74p. Label: 30

Available from Cupal (Cupanol® Over 6, sugar-free—now called NHS Medinol® Over 6), Hillcross, Rosemont (Paldesic®), Warner Wellcome (NHS Calpol® 6 Plus)

Suppositories, paracetamol 125 mg, net price 10 = £11.50; 500 mg, 10 = £9.90. Label: 30

Dose: by rectum, ADULT and CHILD over 12 years 0.5–1 g up to 4 times daily, CHILD 1–5 years 125–250 mg, 6–12 years 250–500 mg

Available from Aurum (120 mg, 240 mg, 500 mg), Novex (Alvedon®, 125 mg)

Co-codamol 8/500

When co-codamol tablets, dispersible (or effervescent) tablets, or capsules are prescribed and **no strength is stated** tablets, dispersible (or effervescent) tablets, or capsules, respectively, containing codeine phosphate **8 mg** and paracetamol **500 mg** should be dispensed.

Co-codamol (Non-proprietary)

Tablets, co-codamol 8/500 (codeine phosphate 8 mg, paracetamol 500 mg) Net price 20 = 23p. Label: 29, 30

Dose: 1–2 tablets every 4–6 hours; max. 8 tablets daily; CHILD 6–12 years ½–1 tablet

Available from APS, Cox, CP, Galen, (NHS Parake®), Norton, Sterling Health (NHS Panadeine®)

Effervescent or *dispersible tablets*, co-codamol 8/500 (codeine phosphate 8 mg, paracetamol 500 mg). Net price 20 = 65p. Label: 13, 29, 30

Dose: 1–2 tablets in water every 4–6 hours; max. 8 tablets daily; CHILD 6–12 years ½–1 tablet, max 4 daily

Available from Roche Consumer Health (NHS Paracodol®), Sterwin

Note. The Drug Tariff allows tablets of co-codamol labelled 'dispersible' to be dispensed against an order for 'effervescent' and *vice versa*

Capsules, co-codamol 8/500 (codeine phosphate 8 mg, paracetamol 500 mg). Net price 30 = £2.14. Label: 29, 30

Dose: 1–2 capsules every 4 hours; max. 8 capsules daily

Available from Roche Consumer Health (NHS Paracodol®)

Co-codamol 30/500

When co-codamol tablets, dispersible (or effervescent) tablets, or capsules are prescribed and **no strength is stated** tablets, dispersible (or effervescent) tablets, or capsules, respectively, containing codeine phosphate **8 mg** and paracetamol **500 mg** should be dispensed (see preparations above).

See warnings and notes on p. 195 (**important**: special care in elderly—reduce dose)

PoM **Kapake**® (Galen)

Tablets, scored, co-codamol 30/500 (codeine phosphate 30 mg, paracetamol 500 mg). Net price 30-tab pack = £2.26 (hosp. only), 100-tab pack = £7.53. Label: 2, 29, 30

Dose: 1–2 tablets every 4 hours; max. 8 tablets daily; CHILD not recommended

PoM Solpadol® (Sanofi Winthrop)

Caplets (= tablets), co-codamol 30/500 (codeine phosphate 30 mg, paracetamol 500 mg). Net price 100-tab pack = £7.90. Label: 2, 29, 30

Dose: 2 tablets every 4 hours; max. 8 daily; CHILD not recommended

Effervescent tablets, co-codamol 30/500 (codeine phosphate 30 mg, paracetamol 500 mg). Contains 18.6 mmol Na+/tablet; avoid in *renal impairment*. Net price 100-tab pack = £9.48. Label: 2, 13, 29, 30

Dose: 2 tablets in water every 4 hours; max. 8 daily; CHILD not recommended

PoM Tylex® (Schwarz)

Capsules, co-codamol 30/500 (codeine phosphate 30 mg, paracetamol 500 mg). Net price 100-cap pack = £8.60. Label: 2, 29, 30

Dose: 1–2 capsules every 4 hours; max. 8 capsules daily; CHILD not recommended

Effervescent tablets, co-codamol 30/500 (codeine phosphate 30 mg, paracetamol 500 mg). Contains 13.6 mmol Na+/tablet; avoid in *renal impairment*. Net price 90-tab pack = £8.53. Label: 2, 13, 29, 30

Note. Contains aspartame 25 mg/tablet (see section 9.4.1)

Dose: 1–2 tablets in water every 4 hours; max. 8 tablets daily; CHILD not recommended

With methionine (co-methiamol)

A mixture of methionine and paracetamol; methionine has no analgesic activity but may prevent paracetamol-induced liver toxicity if overdose taken

Note. Pameton® (co-methiamol 250/500) now available only on direct request to SmithKline Beecham Healthcare

Paradote® (Penn)

Tablets, f/c, co-methiamol 100/500 (DL-methionine 100 mg, paracetamol 500 mg). Net price 24-tab pack = £1.05, 96-tab pack = £2.77. Label: 29, 30

Dose: 2 tablets every 4 hours; max. 8 tablets daily; CHILD 12 years and under, not recommended

With dihydrocodeine tartrate 10 mg

See notes on p. 195

PoM Co-dydramol (Non-proprietary)

Tablets, scored, co-dydramol 10/500 (dihydrocodeine tartrate 10 mg, paracetamol 500 mg). Net price 20 = 28p. Label: 21, 29, 30

Dose: 1–2 tablets every 4–6 hours; max. 8 tablets daily; CHILD not recommended

Available from APS, Cox, CP, Galen (NHS Galake®), Generics, Norton, Sterwin

When co-dydramol tablets are prescribed and no strength is stated tablets containing dihydrocodeine tartrate 10 mg and paracetamol 500 mg should be dispensed.

Note. Tablets containing paracetamol 500 mg and dihydrocodeine 7.46 mg (NHS Paramol®) are on sale to the public. The name Paramol® was formerly applied to a brand of co-dydramol tablets

With dihydrocodeine tartrate 20 or 30 mg

See warnings and notes on p. 195 (**important**: special care in elderly—reduce dose)

PoM Remedeine® (Napp)

Tablets, paracetamol 500 mg, dihydrocodeine tartrate 20 mg. Net price 112-tab pack = £12.21. Label: 2, 21, 29, 30

Dose: 1–2 tablets every 4–6 hours; max. 8 tablets daily; CHILD not recommended

Effervescent tablets, paracetamol 500 mg, dihydrocodeine tartrate 20 mg. Contains 15.2 mmol Na+/tablet; avoid in *renal impairment*. Net price 56-tab pack = £7.39. Label: 2, 13, 21, 29, 30

Dose: 1–2 tablets every 4–6 hours; max. 8 tablets daily; CHILD not recommended

Forte tablets, paracetamol 500 mg, dihydrocodeine tartrate 30 mg. Net price 56-tab pack = £7.54. Label: 2, 21, 29, 30

Dose: 1–2 tablets every 4–6 hours; max. 8 tablets daily; CHILD not recommended

Forte effervescent tablets, paracetamol 500 mg, dihydrocodeine tartrate 30 mg. Contains 15.2 mmol Na+/tablet; avoid in *renal impairment*. Net price 56-tab pack = £9.15. Label: 2, 13, 21, 29, 30

Dose: 1–2 tablets every 4–6 hours; max. 8 tablets daily; CHILD not recommended

Other compound preparations

See warnings and notes on p. 195 (**important**: special care in elderly—reduce dose)

PoM Co-proxamol (Non-proprietary)

Tablets, co-proxamol 32.5/325 (dextropropoxyphene hydrochloride 32.5 mg, paracetamol 325 mg). Net price 20 = 25p. Label: 2, 10 patient information leaflet (if available), 29, 30

Dose: 2 tablets 3–4 times daily; max. 8 tablets daily; CHILD not recommended

Available from APS, Berk, Cox (NHS Cosalgesic®), Dista (NHS Distalgesic®), Norton, Sterwin

When co-proxamol tablets are prescribed and no strength is stated tablets containing dextropropoxyphene hydrochloride 32.5 mg and paracetamol 325 mg should be dispensed.

NHS CD Fortagesic® (Sanofi Winthrop)

Tablets, pentazocine 15 mg (as hydrochloride), paracetamol 500 mg. Net price 100-tab pack = £7.00. Label: 2, 21, 29, 30

Dose: 2 tablets up to 4 times daily; CHILD 7–12 years 1 tablet every 4 hours, max. 4 tablets daily

Preparations on Sale to the Public

The following is a list of preparations on sale to the public that contain **aspirin** or **paracetamol, alone** or with **other ingredients**. Other significant ingredients (such as codeine and caffeine) are listed. For details of preparations containing ibuprofen on sale to the public, see section 10.1.1.

Important: in overdose contact **Poisons Information Services** (p. 18) for full details of the ingredients

Alka-Seltzer® (aspirin), **Alka-Seltzer® XS** (aspirin, caffeine, paracetamol), **Anadin®** (aspirin, caffeine), **Anadin Extra®**, **Anadin Extra Soluble®** (both aspirin, caffeine, paracetamol), **Anadin Maximum Strength®** (aspirin, caffeine), **Anadin Paracetamol®** (paracetamol), **Andrews Answer®** (paracetamol, caffeine), **Angettes 75®** (aspirin), **Askit®** (aspirin, aloxiprin = polymeric product of aspirin, caffeine), **Aspro®** (aspirin), **Aspro Clear®** (aspirin)

Bayer Aspirin® (aspirin), **Beechams-All-In-One®**, (paracetamol, guaphenesin, phenylephrine), **Beechams Flu-Plus Powder®**, **Beechams Hot Lemon®**, **Hot Lemon and Honey®**, **Hot Blackcurrant®** (all paracetamol, phenylephrine), **Beechams Flu-Plus Caplets®** (paracetamol, caffeine, phenylephrine), **Beechams Powders®** (aspirin, caffeine), **Beechams Powders Capsules®** With Decongestant (paracetamol, caffeine, phenylephrine), **Beecham Aspirin®**, **Beechams Powders Tablets®** (both aspirin), **Benylin 4 Flu®** (paracetamol, diphenhydramine, pseudoephedrine), **Benylin Day and Night®** (day tablets, paracetamol, phenylpropanolamine, night tablets, paracetamol, diphenhydramine), **Boots Cold & Flu Relief Tablets®** (paracetamol, caffeine, phenylephrine), **Boots Children's Cold Relief®**, **Boots Cold Relief Hot Blackcurrant®**, **Hot Lemon®** (paracetamol), **Boots Day Cold Comfort®** (paracetamol, pholcodine, pseudoephedrine), **Boots Headache and Indigestion Relief®** (paracetamol, caffeine), **Boots**

Night-Cold Comfort® (diphenhydramine, paracetamol, pholcodine, pseudoephedrine), **Boots Children's Pain Relief Syrup**® (paracetamol), **Boots Pain Relief Tablets**® (paracetamol, caffeine), **Boots Migraine Relief**® (codeine, paracetamol)
Calpol Infant®, **Calpol 6 Plus**®, **Calpol Paediatric**® (all paracetamol), **Caprin**® (aspirin), **Catarrh-Ex**® (paracetamol, caffeine, phenylephrine), **Codis 500**® (aspirin, codeine), **Coldrex Blackcurrant Powders**®, **Hot Lemon Powders**® (both paracetamol, phenylephrine), **Coldrex Tablets**® (paracetamol, caffeine, phenylephrine), **Mrs. Cullen's**® (aspirin), **Cupanol Over 6**®, **Cupanol Under 6**® (both paracetamol)
Day Nurse® (paracetamol, dextromethorphan, phenylpropanolamine), **De Witt's Analgesic Pills**® (paracetamol, caffeine), **Disprin**®, **Disprin CV**®, **Disprin Direct**® (all aspirin), **Disprin Extra**® (aspirin, paracetamol), **Disprol**® (paracetamol), **Dristan Tablets**® (aspirin, caffeine, chlorpheniramine, phenylephrine)
EP® (paracetamol, caffeine, codeine)
Fanalgic® (paracetamol), **Femigraine**® (aspirin, cyclizine), **Feminax**® (paracetamol, caffeine, codeine, hyoscine), **Fennings Children's Cooling Powders**® (paracetamol), **Flurex Bedtime**® (paracetamol, diphenhydramine, pseudoephedrine), **Fynnon**® **Calcium Aspirin** (aspirin)
Hedex® (paracetamol), **Hedex Extra**® (paracetamol, caffeine), **Hedex Headcold Caplets**® (paracetamol, caffeine, phenylephrine), **Hedex Headcold Powders**® (paracetamol, phenylephrine), **Hill's Balsam Flu Strength Hot Lemon Powders**® (paracetamol)
Infadrops® (paracetamol)
Lem-Plus Capsules® (paracetamol, caffeine, phenylephrine), **Lem-Plus Powders**® (paracetamol), **Lemsip Lemcaps**® (paracetamol, caffeine, phenylephrine), **Lemsip Cool Lemon**®, **Lemsip Flu Strength**®, **Lemsip Lemon**® or **Blackcurrant**®, **Lemsip Max Strength**®, **Lemsip Menthol Extra**® (all paracetamol, phenylephrine), **Lemsip Flu Strength Nightime**® (paracetamol, chlorpheniramine, dextromethorphan, phenylpropanolamine)
Maximum Strength Aspro Clear® (aspirin), **Medinol**® (paracetamol), **Medised**® (paracetamol, promethazine), **Midrid**® (paracetamol, isometheptene mucate), **Migraleve**® (*pink tablets*, paracetamol, codeine, buclizine, *yellow tablets*, paracetamol, codeine), **Miradol**® (paracetamol), **Mu-Cron Tablets**® (paracetamol, phenylpropanolamine)
Night Nurse® (paracetamol, dextromethorphan, promethazine), **Nurse Sykes' Powders**® (aspirin, caffeine, paracetamol)
Paldesic® (paracetamol), **Panadeine**® (paracetamol, codeine), **Panadol**®, **Panadol Baby and Infant**® (both paracetamol), **Panadol Extra**® (paracetamol, caffeine), **Panadol Junior**® (paracetamol), **Panadol Night**® (paracetamol, diphenhydramine), **Panadol Ultra**® (paracetamol, codeine), **Panaleve Junior**®, **Panaleve 6+**® (both paracetamol), **Panerel**® (paracetamol, codeine), **Paracets**® (paracetamol), **Paraclear Extra Strength**® (paracetamol, caffeine), **Paraclear**® (paracetamol), **Paracodol**® (paracetamol, codeine), **Paramin**® (paracetamol), **Paramol**® (paracetamol, dihydrocodeine), **Phensic**® (aspirin, caffeine), **Placidex**® (paracetamol), **Powerin**® (aspirin, caffeine, paracetamol), **Propain**® (paracetamol, caffeine, codeine, diphenhydramine)
Resolve® (paracetamol)
Salzone® (paracetamol), **Sinutab**® (paracetamol, phenylpropanolamine), **Sinutab Nightime**® (paracetamol, phenylpropanolamine, phenyltoloxamine), **Solpadeine**® (paracetamol, caffeine, codeine), **SP Cold Relief Capsules**® (paracetamol, caffeine, phenylephrine), **Sudafed-Co**® (paracetamol, pseudoephedrine), **Syndol**® (paracetamol, caffeine, codeine, doxylamine)
Toptabs® (aspirin, caffeine), **Tramil**® **500** (paracetamol), **Triogesic**® (paracetamol, phenylpropanolamine)
Uniflu with Gregovite C® (paracetamol, caffeine, codeine, diphenhydramine, phenylephrine)
Veganin® (aspirin, paracetamol, codeine), **Vicks**® **Coldcare** (paracetamol, dextromethorphan, phenylpropanolamine), **Vicks Medinite**® (paracetamol, dextromethorphan, doxylamine, ephedrine)

IBUPROFEN

Indications: fever and pain in children; see also section 10.1.1

Cautions; Contra-indications; Side-effects: see section 10.1.1

Dose: see section 10.1.1; CHILD, fever and pain, see below

Fever and pain in children
Junifen Sugar Free® (Crookes)
Suspension, sugar-free, ibuprofen 100 mg/5 mL, net price 150-mL pack = £2.45. Label: 21

Dose: fever and pain in children, under 1 year not recommended, 1–12 years 20 mg/kg daily in divided doses *or* 1–2 years 2.5 mL 3–4 times daily, 3–7 years 5 mL, 8–12 years 10 mL

Other preparations: see section 10.1.1

NEFOPAM HYDROCHLORIDE

Indications: moderate pain

Cautions: hepatic or renal disease, elderly, urinary retention; pregnancy and breast-feeding; **interactions:** Appendix 1 (nefopam)

Contra-indications: convulsive disorders; not indicated for myocardial infarction

Side-effects: nausea, nervousness, urinary retention, dry mouth, lightheadedness; less frequently vomiting, blurred vision, drowsiness, sweating, insomnia, tachycardia, headache; confusion and hallucinations also reported; may colour urine (pink)

Dose: *by mouth*, initially 60 mg (elderly, 30 mg) 3 times daily, adjusted according to response; usual range 30–90 mg 3 times daily; CHILD not recommended

By intramuscular injection, 20 mg every 6 hours; CHILD not recommended

Note. Nefopam hydrochloride 20 mg by injection ≡ 60 mg by mouth

PoM **Acupan**® (3M)
Tablets, f/c, nefopam hydrochloride 30 mg. Net price 90-tab pack = £11.44. Label: 2, 14
Injection, nefopam hydrochloride 20 mg/mL. Net price 1-mL amp = 73p

4.7.2   Opioid analgesics

Opioid analgesics are used to relieve moderate to severe pain particularly of visceral origin. Repeated administration may cause dependence and tolerance, but this is no deterrent in the control of pain in terminal illness, for guidelines see Prescribing in Palliative Care, p. 12.

SIDE-EFFECTS. Opioid analgesics share many side-effects though qualitative and quantitative differences exist. The most common include nausea, vomiting, constipation, and drowsiness. Larger doses produce respiratory depression and hypotension. **Overdosage**, see Emergency Treatment of Poisoning, p. 22.

INTERACTIONS. See Appendix 1 (opioid analgesics) (**important**: special hazard with *pethidine and possibly other opioids* and MAOIs).

DRIVING. Drowsiness may affect performance of skilled tasks (e.g. driving); effects of alcohol enhanced.

CHOICE. **Morphine** remains the most valuable opioid analgesic for severe pain although it frequently causes nausea and vomiting. It is the standard against which other opioid analgesics are compared. In addition to relief of pain, morphine also confers a state of euphoria and mental detachment.

Morphine is the opioid of choice for the oral treatment of *severe pain in palliative care*. It is given regularly every 4 hours (or every 12 or 24 hours as modified-release preparations). For guidelines on dosage adjustment in palliative care, see p. 12.

Buprenorphine has both opioid agonist and antagonist properties and may precipitate withdrawal symptoms, including pain, in patients dependent on other opioids. It has abuse potential and may itself cause dependence. It has a much longer duration of action than morphine and sublingually is an effective analgesic for 6 to 8 hours. Vomiting may be a problem. Unlike most opioid analgesics its effects are only partially reversed by naloxone.

Codeine is effective for the relief of mild to moderate pain but is too constipating for long-term use.

Dextromoramide is less sedating than morphine and has a short duration of action.

Diphenoxylate (in combination with atropine, as co-phenotrope) is used in acute diarrhoea (see section 1.4.2).

Dipipanone used alone is less sedating than morphine but the only preparation available contains an anti-emetic and is therefore not suitable for regular regimens in palliative care (see p. 14).

Dextropropoxyphene given alone is a very mild analgesic somewhat less potent than codeine. Combinations of dextropropoxyphene with paracetamol (co-proxamol) or aspirin have little more analgesic effect than paracetamol or aspirin alone. An important disadvantage of co-proxamol is that **overdosage** (which may be combined with alcohol) is complicated by respiratory depression and acute heart failure due to the dextropropoxyphene and by hepatotoxicity due to the paracetamol. Rapid treatment is essential (see Emergency Treatment of Poisoning, p. 22).

Diamorphine (heroin) is a powerful opioid analgesic. It may cause less nausea and hypotension than morphine. In *palliative care* the greater solubility of diamorphine allows effective doses to be injected in smaller volumes and this is important in the emaciated patient.

Dihydrocodeine has an analgesic efficacy similar to that of codeine. The dose of dihydrocodeine by mouth is usually 30 mg every 4 hours; doubling the dose to 60 mg may provide some additional pain relief but this may be at the cost of more nausea and vomiting. A 40-mg tablet is now also available.

Alfentanil, **fentanyl** and **remifentanil** are used by injection for intra-operative analgesia (section 15.1.4.3); fentanyl has been introduced recently in a transdermal drug delivery system as a self-adhesive patch which is changed every 72 hours.

Meptazinol is claimed to have a low incidence of respiratory depression. It has a reported length of action of 2 to 7 hours with onset within 15 minutes, but there is an incidence of nausea and vomiting.

Methadone is less sedating than morphine and acts for longer periods. In prolonged use, methadone should not be administered more often than twice daily to avoid the risk of accumulation and opioid overdosage. Methadone may be used instead of morphine in the occasional patient who experiences excitation (or exacerbation of pain) with morphine.

Nalbuphine has a similar efficacy to that of morphine for pain relief, but may have fewer side-effects and less abuse potential. Nausea and vomiting occur less than with other opioids but respiratory depression is similar to that with morphine.

Oxycodone is used as the pectinate in suppositories (special order from BCM Specials) for the control of *pain in palliative care*.

Papaveretum is used peri-operatively, section 15.1.4.3.

Pentazocine has both agonist and antagonist properties and precipitates withdrawal symptoms, including pain in patients dependent on other opioids. By injection it is more potent than dihydrocodeine or codeine, but hallucinations and thought disturbances may occur. It is not recommended and, in particular, should be avoided after myocardial infarction as it may increase pulmonary and aortic blood pressure as well as cardiac work.

Pethidine produces prompt but short-lasting analgesia; it is less constipating than morphine, but even in high doses is a less potent analgesic. It is not suitable for severe continuing pain. It is used for analgesia in labour, and in the neonate is associated with less respiratory depression than other opioid analgesics (probably because its action is weaker).

Phenazocine is effective in severe pain and has less tendency to increase biliary pressure than other opioid analgesics. It can be administered sublingually if nausea and vomiting are a problem.

Tramadol has been introduced recently and is claimed to produce analgesia by two mechanisms: an opioid effect and an enhancement of serotoninergic and adrenergic pathways. It is reported to have fewer of the typical opioid side-effects (notably, less respiratory depression, less constipation and less addiction potential); psychiatric reactions have been reported.

ADDICTS. Although caution is necessary addicts (and ex-addicts) may be treated with analgesics in the same way as other people when there is a real clinical need. Doctors are reminded that they do not require a special licence to prescribe opioid analgesics for addicts for relief of pain due to organic disease or injury.

MORPHINE SALTS

Indications: see notes above; acute pulmonary oedema; peri-operative analgesia (section 15.1.4.3)

Cautions: hypotension, hypothyroidism, asthma (avoid during attack) and decreased respiratory reserve, prostatic hypertrophy; pregnancy and breast-feeding; may precipitate coma in hepatic impairment (reduce dose or avoid but many such patients tolerate morphine well); reduce dose or avoid in renal impairment (see also Appendix 3), elderly and debilitated (reduce dose); convulsive disorders, dependence (severe withdrawal symptoms if withdrawn abruptly); use of cough suppressants containing opioid analgesics not generally recommended in children and should be avoided altogether in those under at least 1 year; **interactions:** Appendix 1 (opioid analgesics)

PALLIATIVE CARE. In the control of pain in terminal illness these cautions should not necessarily be a deterrent to the use of opioid analgesics

Contra-indications: avoid in acute respiratory depression, acute alcoholism and where risk of paralytic ileus; not indicated for acute abdomen; also avoid in raised intracranial pressure or head injury (in addition to interfering with respiration, affect pupillary responses vital for neurological assessment); avoid injection in phaeochromocytoma (risk of pressor response to histamine release)

Side-effects: nausea and vomiting (particularly in initial stages), constipation, and drowsiness; larger doses produce respiratory depression and hypotension; other side-effects include difficulty with micturition, ureteric or biliary spasm, dry mouth, sweating, headache, facial flushing, vertigo, bradycardia, tachycardia, palpitations, postural hypotension, hypothermia, hallucinations, dysphoria, mood changes, dependence, miosis, decreased libido or potency, rashes, urticaria and pruritus; **overdosage:** see Emergency Treatment of Poisoning, p. 22; for reversal of opioid-induced respiratory depression, see section 15.1.7.

Dose: acute pain, *by subcutaneous injection* (not suitable for oedematous patients) *or by intramuscular injection,* 10 mg every 4 hours if necessary (15 mg for heavier well-muscled patients); CHILD up to 1 month 150 micrograms/kg, 1–12 months 200 micrograms/kg, 1–5 years 2.5–5 mg, 6–12 years 5–10 mg

Postoperative pain, see section 15.1.4.3

By slow intravenous injection, quarter to half corresponding intramuscular dose

Patient controlled analgesia (PCA), consult hospital protocols

Myocardial infarction, *by slow intravenous injection* (2 mg/minute), 10 mg followed by a further 5–10 mg if necessary; elderly or frail patients, reduce dose by half

Acute pulmonary oedema, *by slow intravenous injection* (2 mg/minute) 5–10 mg

Chronic pain, *by mouth or by subcutaneous injection* (not suitable for oedematous patients) *or by intramuscular injection,* 5–20 mg regularly every 4 hours; dose may be increased according to

needs; oral dose should be approximately double corresponding intramuscular dose and triple to quadruple corresponding intramuscular *diamorphine* dose (see also Prescribing in Palliative Care, p. 12); *by rectum,* as suppositories, 15–30 mg regularly every 4 hours

Note. The doses stated above refer equally to morphine hydrochloride, sulphate, and tartrate; see below for doses of **modified-release** preparations.

Oral solutions

Note. For advice on transfer from oral solutions of morphine to modified-release preparations of morphine, see Prescribing in Palliative Care, p. 12

PoM or CD Morphine Oral Solutions

Oral solutions of morphine can be prescribed by writing the formula:

Morphine hydrochloride 5 mg
Chloroform water to 5 mL

Note. The proportion of morphine hydrochloride may be altered when specified by the prescriber; if above 13 mg per 5 mL the solution becomes **CD**. For sample prescription see Controlled Drugs and Drug Dependence, p. 7. It is usual to adjust the strength so that the dose volume is 5 or 10 mL.

Oramorph® (Boehringer Ingelheim)

PoM *Oramorph® oral solution,* morphine sulphate 10 mg/5 mL. Net price 100-mL pack = £2.31; 250-mL pack = £5.36; 500-mL pack = £9.70. Label: 2

PoM *Oramorph® Unit Dose Vials 10 mg* (oral vials), sugar-free, morphine sulphate 10 mg/5-mL vial, net price 25 vials = £3.31. Label: 2

CD *Oramorph® Unit Dose Vials 30 mg* (oral vials), sugar-free, morphine sulphate 30 mg/5-mL vial, net price 25 vials = £9.30. Label: 2

CD *Oramorph® concentrated oral solution,* sugar-free, morphine sulphate 100 mg/5 mL. Net price 30-mL pack = £6.47; 120-mL pack = £24.15 (both with calibrated dropper). Label: 2

CD *Oramorph® Unit Dose Vials 100 mg* (oral vials), sugar-free, morphine sulphate 100 mg/5-mL vial, net price 25 vials = £31.00. Label: 2

Tablets

CD Sevredol® (Napp)

Tablets, f/c, scored, morphine sulphate 10 mg (blue), net price 56-tab pack = £6.31; 20 mg (pink), 56-tab pack = £12.62; 50 mg (pale green), 56-tab pack = £31.55. Label: 2

Dose: severe pain uncontrolled by weaker opioid, 10–50 mg every 4 hours (dose adjusted according to need and tolerance); CHILD 3–5 years, 5 mg; 6–12 years, 5–10 mg

Modified release

CD Morcap® SR (Sanofi Winthrop)

Capsules, m/r, clear enclosing ivory and brown pellets, morphine sulphate 20 mg, net price 30-cap pack = £5.71, 60-cap pack = £11.42; 50 mg, 30-cap pack = £13.84, 60-cap pack = £27.68; 100 mg, 30-cap pack = £27.68, 60-cap pack = £55.37. Label: 2, counselling, see below

---

Dose: adjusted according to daily morphine requirements, for further advice on determining dose, see Palliative Care, p. 12; dosage requirements may need to be reviewed if the brand is altered

COUNSELLING. Swallow whole or open capsule and sprinkle contents on soft food

Note. Prescription must also specify 'capsules' (i.e. 'Morcap SR capsules')

CD MST Continus® (Napp)
Tablets, m/r, f/c, morphine sulphate 5 mg (white), net price 60-tab pack = £4.50; 10 mg (brown), 60-tab pack = £7.51; 15 mg (green), 60-tab pack = £13.16; 30 mg (purple), 60-tab pack = £18.03; 60 mg (orange), 60-tab pack = £35.16; 100 mg (grey), 60-tab pack = £55.67; 200 mg (green), 60-tab pack = £111.35. Label: 2, 25

Suspension (= sachet of granules to mix with water), m/r, pink, morphine sulphate 20 mg/sachet, net price 30-sachet pack = £28.60; 30 mg/sachet, 30-sachet pack = £29.72; 60 mg/sachet, 30-sachet pack = £59.44; 100 mg/sachet, 30-sachet pack = £99.07; 200 mg/sachet pack, 30-sachet pack = £198.14. Label: 2, 13

Dose: adjusted according to daily morphine requirements, for further advice on determining dose, see Palliative Care, p. 12; dosage requirements may need to be reviewed if the brand is altered

Note. Prescriptions must also specify 'tablets' or 'suspension' (i.e. 'MST Continus tablets' or 'MST Continus suspension').

CD MXL® (Napp)
Capsules, m/r, morphine sulphate 30 mg (light blue), net price 28-cap pack = £12.28; 60 mg (brown), 28-cap pack = £16.83; 90 mg (pink), 28-cap pack = £24.82; 120 mg (green), 28-cap pack = £32.82; 150 mg (blue), 28-cap pack = £41.02; 200 mg (red-brown), 28-cap pack = £51.96. Label: 2, counselling, see below

Dose: adjusted according to daily morphine requirements, for further advice on determining dose, see Palliative Care, p. 12; dosage requirements may need to be reviewed if the brand is altered

COUNSELLING. Swallow whole or open capsule and sprinkle contents on soft food

Note. Prescriptions must also specify 'capsules' (i.e. 'MXL capsules')

CD Oramorph® SR (Boehringer Ingelheim)
Tablets, m/r, f/c, morphine sulphate 10 mg (buff), net price 60-tab pack = £5.75; 30 mg (violet), 60-tab pack = £13.80; 60 mg (orange), 60-tab pack = £26.89; 100 mg (grey), 60-tab pack = £42.59. Label: 2, 25

Dose: adjusted according to daily morphine requirements, for further advice on determining dose, see Palliative Care, p. 12; dosage requirements may need to be reviewed if the brand is altered

Note. Prescriptions must also specify 'tablets' (i.e. 'Oramorph SR tablets')

CD Zomorph® (Link)
Capsules, m/r, morphine sulphate 10 mg (yellow/clear enclosing pale yellow pellets), net price 60-cap pack = £4.51; 30 mg (pink/clear enclosing pale yellow pellets), 60-cap pack = £10.82; 60 mg (orange/clear enclosing pale yellow pellets), 60-cap pack = £21.10; 100 mg (white/clear enclosing pale yellow pellets), 60-cap pack = £33.40; 200 mg (clear enclosing pale yellow pellets), 60-cap pack = £66.80. Label: 2, counselling, see below

Dose: adjusted according to daily morphine requirements, for further advice on determining doses, see Prescribing in Palliative Care, p. 12; dosage requirements may need to be reviewed if the brand is altered

COUNSELLING. Swallow whole or open capsule and sprinkle contents on soft food

Note. Prescriptions must also specify 'capsules' (i.e. 'Zomorph capsules')

Injections

CD Morphine Sulphate (Non-proprietary)
Injection, morphine sulphate 10, 15, 20, and 30 mg/mL, net price 1- and 2-mL amp (all) = 64–96p

CD Min-I-Jet® Morphine Sulphate (IMS)
Injection, morphine sulphate 10 mg/mL, net price 2-mL disposable syringe = £10.85

CD Morphine and Atropine Injection
See section 15.1.4.3

CD Morphine Sulphate Rapiject® (IMS)
Injection, morphine sulphate 1 mg/mL, net price 50-mL disposable syringe = £9.50; 2 mg/mL, 50-mL disposable syringe = £10.50

Injection with anti-emetic
CAUTION. In myocardial infarction cyclizine may aggravate severe heart failure and counteract the haemodynamic benefits of opioids, see section 4.6. **Not recommended** in palliative care, see p. 14

CD Cyclimorph® (GlaxoWellcome)
Cyclimorph-10® *Injection,* morphine tartrate 10 mg, cyclizine tartrate 50 mg/mL. Net price 1-mL amp = £1.28

Dose: by subcutaneous, intramuscular, or intravenous injection, 1 mL, repeated not more often than every 4 hours, with not more than 3 doses in any 24-hour period; CHILD 1–5 years 0.25–0.5 mL as a single dose, 6–12 years 0.5–1 mL as a single dose

Cyclimorph-15® *Injection,* morphine tartrate 15 mg, cyclizine tartrate 50 mg/mL. Net price 1-mL amp = £1.33

Dose: by subcutaneous, intramuscular, or intravenous injection, 1 mL, repeated not more often than every 4 hours, with not more than 3 doses in any 24-hour period

Suppositories

CD Morphine (Non-proprietary)
Suppositories, morphine hydrochloride or sulphate 10 mg, net price 12 = £6.12; 15 mg, 12 = £5.53; 20 mg, 12 = £7.45; 30 mg, 12 = £8.50. Label: 2

Available from Aurum, Evans, Martindale

Note. Both the strength of the suppositories and the morphine salt contained in them must be specified by the prescriber

BUPRENORPHINE

Indications: moderate to severe pain; peri-operative analgesia, see section 15.1.4.3

Cautions; Contra-indications; Side-effects: see under Morphine Salts and notes above; can give rise to mild withdrawal symptoms in patients dependent on opioids; effects only partially reversed by naloxone; **interactions:** Appendix 1 (opioid analgesics)

Dose: by sublingual administration, initially 200–400 micrograms every 8 hours, increasing if necessary to 200–400 micrograms every 6–8 hours; CHILD over 6 months, 16–25 kg, 100 micrograms; 25–37.5 kg, 100–200 micrograms; 37.5–50 kg, 200–300 micrograms

By intramuscular or slow intravenous injection, 300–600 micrograms every 6–8 hours; CHILD over 6 months 3–6 micrograms/kg every 6–8 hours (max. 9 micrograms/kg)

CD Temgesic® (R&C)

Tablets (sublingual), buprenorphine (as hydrochloride), 200 micrograms, net price 50-tab pack = £6.00; 400 micrograms, 50-tab pack = £12.00. Label: 2, 26

Injection, buprenorphine 300 micrograms (as hydrochloride)/mL. Net price 1-mL amp = 55p

---

CODEINE PHOSPHATE

Indications: mild to moderate pain

Cautions; Contra-indications; Side-effects: see under Morphine Salts and notes above; use of cough suppressants containing codeine or similar opioid analgesics not generally recommended in children and should be avoided altogether in those under 1 year; **interactions:** Appendix 1 (opioid analgesics)

Dose: by mouth, 30–60 mg every 4 hours when necessary, to a max. of 240 mg daily; CHILD 1–12 years, 3 mg/kg daily in divided doses

By intramuscular injection, 30–60 mg every 4 hours when necessary

Codeine Phosphate (Non-proprietary)

PoM *Tablets*, codeine phosphate 15 mg, net price 20 = 35p; 30 mg, 20 = 39p; 60 mg, 20 = 97p. Label: 2

Note. As for schedule 2 controlled drugs, travellers needing to take codeine phosphate preparations abroad may require a doctor's letter explaining why they are necessary

PoM *Syrup*, codeine phosphate 25 mg/5 mL. Net price 100 mL = 87p. Label: 2

CD *Injection*, codeine phosphate 60 mg/mL. Net price 1-mL amp = £1.76

Codeine Linctuses

See section 3.9.1

Note. Codeine is an ingredient of some compound analgesic preparations, section 4.7.1 and section 10.1.1 (*Codafen Continus®*)

DEXTROMORAMIDE

Indications: severe pain

Cautions; Contra-indications; Side-effects: see under Morphine Salts and notes above; only short duration of action (2–3 hours); avoid in obstetric analgesia (increased risk of neonatal depression); **interactions:** Appendix 1 (opioid analgesics)

Dose: by mouth, 5 mg increasing to 20 mg, when required

By rectum in suppositories, 10 mg when required

CD Palfium® (Boehringer Mannheim)

Tablets, both scored, dextromoramide (as tartrate) 5 mg, net price 60-tab pack = £4.66; 10 mg (peach), 60-tab pack = £9.21. Label: 2

Suppositories, dextromoramide 10 mg (as tartrate). Net price 10 = £2.29. Label: 2

DEXTROPROPOXYPHENE HYDROCHLORIDE

Indications: mild to moderate pain

Cautions; Contra-indications; Side-effects: see under Morphine Salts and notes above; occasional hepatotoxicity; porphyria (see section 9.8.2); compound preparations special hazard in overdose, see notes above; convulsions reported in overdose; contra-indicated in those who are suicidal or addiction prone; **interactions:** Appendix 1 (opioid analgesics)

Dose: 65 mg every 6–8 hours when necessary; CHILD not recommended

Note. 65 mg dextropropoxyphene hydrochloride ≡ 100 mg dextropropoxyphene napsylate

PoM **Dextropropoxyphene** (Non-proprietary)

Capsules, the equivalent of dextropropoxyphene hydrochloride 65 mg (as napsylate). Net price 20 = £1.64. Label: 2

Available from Lilly (NHS Doloxene®)

Note. Dextropropoxyphene is an ingredient of some compound analgesic preparations, section 4.7.1

DIAMORPHINE HYDROCHLORIDE

(Heroin Hydrochloride)

Indications: see notes above; acute pulmonary oedema

Cautions; Contra-indications; Side-effects: see under Morphine Salts and notes above; **interactions:** Appendix 1 (opioid analgesics)

Dose: acute pain, *by subcutaneous or intramuscular injection*, 5 mg repeated every 4 hours if necessary (up to 10 mg for heavier well-muscled patients)

By slow intravenous injection, quarter to half corresponding intramuscular dose

Myocardial infarction, *by slow intravenous injection* (1 mg/minute), 5 mg followed by a further 2.5–5 mg if necessary; elderly or frail patients, reduce dose by half

Acute pulmonary oedema, *by slow intravenous injection* (1 mg/minute) 2.5–5 mg

Chronic pain, *by mouth or by subcutaneous or intramuscular injection*, 5–10 mg regularly every 4 hours; dose may be increased according to needs; intramuscular dose should be approximately half corresponding oral dose, and quarter to third corresponding oral *morphine* dose—see also Palliative Care, p. 15; *by subcutaneous infusion* (using syringe driver), see Palliative Care, p. 14

CD Diamorphine (Non-proprietary)

Tablets, diamorphine hydrochloride 10 mg. Net price 100-tab pack = £11.20. Label: 2

Available from Aurum

Injection, powder for reconstitution, diamorphine hydrochloride. Net price 5-mg amp = £1.16, 10-mg amp = £1.34, 30-mg amp = £1.60, 100-mg amp = £4.42, 500-mg amp = £20.68

Available from Berk (Diagesil®), CP, Evans, Hillcross

CD Diamorphine Linctus

See section 3.9.1

DIHYDROCODEINE TARTRATE

Indications: moderate to severe pain

Cautions; Contra-indications; Side-effects: see under Morphine Salts and notes above

Dose: by mouth, 30 mg every 4–6 hours when necessary (see also notes above); CHILD over 4 years 0.5–1 mg/kg every 4–6 hours

By deep subcutaneous or intramuscular injection, up to 50 mg repeated every 4–6 hours if necessary; CHILD over 4 years 0.5–1 mg/kg every 4–6 hours

Dihydrocodeine (Non-proprietary)

PoM *Tablets,* dihydrocodeine tartrate 30 mg. Net price 20 = 56p. Label: 2, 21
Available from most generic manufacturers

PoM *Oral solution,* dihydrocodeine tartrate 10 mg/ 5 mL. Net price 150 mL = £2.40. Label: 2, 21
Available from Napp

CD *Injection,* dihydrocodeine tartrate 50 mg/mL. Net price 1-mL amp = £1.49
Available from Aurum, Napp (DF 118®)
Note. The brand name DF118® was formerly used for tablets of dihydrocodeine tartrate 30 mg

PoM **DF 118 Forte®** (Napp)

Tablets, dihydrocodeine tartrate 40 mg. Net price 100-tab pack = £12.05. Label: 2, 21
Dose: severe pain, 40–80 mg 3 times daily; max. 240 mg daily; CHILD not recommended

Modified release

PoM **DHC Continus®** (Napp)

Tablets, m/r, dihydrocodeine tartrate 60 mg, net price 56-tab pack = £6.58; 90 mg, 56-tab pack = £10.06, 120 mg, 56-tab pack = £13.83. Labels 2, 25
Dose: chronic severe pain, 60–120 mg every 12 hours; CHILD not recommended

Note. Dihydrocodeine is an ingredient of some compound analgesic preparations, see section 4.7.1

DIPIPANONE HYDROCHLORIDE

Indications: moderate to severe pain

Cautions; Contra-indications; Side-effects: see under Morphine Salts and notes above; **interactions:** Appendix 1 (opioid analgesics)

CD **Diconal®** (GlaxoWellcome)

Tablets, pink, scored, dipipanone hydrochloride 10 mg, cyclizine hydrochloride 30 mg. Net price 50-tab pack = £7.59. Label: 2
Dose: 1 tablet gradually increased to 3 tablets every 6 hours; CHILD not recommended
CAUTION. **Not recommended** in palliative care, see p. 14

FENTANYL

Indications: chronic intractable pain due to cancer, see below; other indications, see section 15.1.4.3

Cautions; Contra-indications; Side-effects: see under Morphine Salts and notes above; local reac-

tions such as rash, erythema and itching reported; **interactions:** Appendix 1 (opioid analgesics)
FEVER OR EXTERNAL HEAT. Monitor patients for increased side-effects if fever present (increased absorption possible); avoid exposing application site to external heat (may also increase absorption)

Administration: see under preparation, below
LONG DURATION OF ACTION. In view of the long duration of action, patients who have experienced severe side-effects should be monitored for up to 24 hours after patch removal

▼ CD **Durogesic®** (Janssen-Cilag)

Patches, self-adhesive, transparent, fentanyl, '25' patch (releasing approx. 25 micrograms/hour for 72 hours), net price 5 = £28.97; '50' patch (releasing approx. 50 micrograms/hour for 72 hours), 5 = £54.11; '75' patch (releasing approx. 75 micrograms/hour for 72 hours), 5 = £75.43; '100' patch (releasing approx. 100 micrograms/ hour for 72 hours), 5 = £92.97. Label: 2

ADMINISTRATION: apply to dry, non-irritated, non-irradiated, non-hairy skin on torso or upper arm, removing after 72 hours and siting replacement patch on a different area (avoid using the same area for several days). Patients who have not previously received a strong opioid analgesic, initial dose, one '25 micrograms/hour' patch replaced after 72 hours; patients who have received a strong opioid analgesic, initial dose based on previous 24-hour opioid requirement (oral morphine sulphate 90 mg over 24 hours ≈ one '25 micrograms/hour' patch, see data sheet for details); CHILD not recommended
Note. When starting initial evaluation of the analgesic effect should **not** be made before the system has been worn for **24 hours** (to allow for the gradual increase in plasma-fentanyl concentration)—previous analgesic therapy should be phased out gradually from time of first patch application; dose adjustment should normally be carried out in 72-hour steps of '25 micrograms/hour'. More than one patch may be used at a time for doses greater than '100 micrograms/hour' (but applied at *same time* to avoid confusion)—consider additional or alternative analgesic therapy if dose required exceeds 300 micrograms/hour (**important:** it may take 17 hours or longer for the plasma-fentanyl concentration to decrease by 50%, therefore replacement opioid therapy should be initiated at a low dose, increasing gradually).

CD **Sublimaze®**

Section 15.1.4.3

HYDROMORPHONE HYDROCHLORIDE

Indications: severe pain in cancer

Cautions: see Morphine salts and notes above; **interactions:** Appendix 1 (opioid analgesics)

Contra-indications: see Morphine salts and notes above

Side-effects: see Morphine salts and notes above

Dose: see preparations below

▼ CD **Palladone®** (Napp)

Capsules, hydromorphone hydrochloride 1.3 mg (orange/clear), net price 56-cap pack = £8.67; 2.6 mg (red/clear), 56-cap pack = £17.34. Label: 2, counselling, see below
Dose: 1.3 mg every 4 hours, increased if necessary according to severity of pain; CHILD under 12 years not recommended
COUNSELLING. Swallow whole or open capsule and sprinkle contents on soft food

▼ **CD Palladone® SR** (Napp)
Capsules, all m/r, hydromorphone hydrochloride 2 mg (yellow/clear), net price 56-cap pack = £18.42; 4 mg (pale blue/clear), 56-cap pack = £25.24; 8 mg (pink/clear), 56-cap pack = £49.22; 16 mg (brown/clear), 56-cap pack = £93.52; 24 mg (dark blue/clear), 56-cap pack = £140.30. Label: 2, counselling, see below
Dose: 4 mg every 12 hours, increased if necessary according to severity of pain; CHILD under 12 years not recommended
COUNSELLING. Swallow whole or open capsule and sprinkle contents on soft food

MEPTAZINOL
Indications: moderate to severe pain, including postoperative and obstetric pain and renal colic; peri-operative analgesia, see section 15.1.4.3
Cautions; Contra-indications; Side-effects: see under Morphine Salts and notes above; effects only partially reversed by naloxone
Dose: by mouth, 200 mg every 3–6 hours as required; CHILD not recommended
By intramuscular injection, 75–100 mg every 2–4 hours if necessary; obstetric analgesia, 100–150 mg according to patient's weight (2 mg/kg); CHILD not recommended
By slow intravenous injection, 50–100 mg every 2–4 hours if necessary; CHILD not recommended

PoM **Meptid®** (Monmouth)
Tablets, orange, f/c, meptazinol 200 mg. Net price 20 = £4.39. Label: 2
Injection, meptazinol 100 mg (as hydrochloride)/mL. Net price 1-mL amp = £1.92

METHADONE HYDROCHLORIDE
Indications: severe pain, see notes above; adjunct in treatment of opioid dependence, section 4.10
Cautions; Contra-indications; Side-effects: see under Morphine Salts and notes above; **interactions:** Appendix 1 (opioid analgesics)
Dose: by mouth or by subcutaneous or intramuscular injection, 5–10 mg every 6–8 hours, adjusted according to response; CHILD not recommended

CD Methadone (Non-proprietary)
Tablets, scored, methadone hydrochloride 5 mg. Net price 50 = £3.11. Label: 2
Available from GlaxoWellcome (Physeptone®)
Injection, methadone hydrochloride, 10 mg/mL, net price 1-mL amp = 86p, 2-mL amp = £1.55, 3.5-mL amp = £1.78, 5-mL amp = £1.92
Available from CP, Martindale, GlaxoWellcome (Physeptone®)
Linctus, section 3.9.1
Mixture 1 mg/mL, section 4.10

NALBUPHINE HYDROCHLORIDE
Indications: moderate to severe pain; peri-operative analgesia, see section 15.1.4.3
Cautions; Contra-indications; Side-effects: see under Morphine Salts and notes above; **interactions:** Appendix 1 (opioid analgesics)
Dose: by subcutaneous, intramuscular, or intravenous injection, 10–20 mg for 70 kg patient every 3–6 hours, adjusted as required; CHILD up to 300 micrograms/kg repeated once or twice as necessary
Myocardial infarction, *by slow intravenous injection,* 10–20 mg repeated after 30 minutes if necessary

Preparations
Section 15.1.4.3

PENTAZOCINE
Indications: moderate to severe pain, but see notes above
Cautions; Contra-indications; Side-effects: see under Morphine Salts and notes above; occasional hallucinations; avoid in patients dependent on opioids and in arterial or pulmonary hypertension and heart failure; porphyria (see section 9.8.2); **interactions:** Appendix 1 (opioid analgesics)
Dose: by mouth, pentazocine hydrochloride 50 mg every 3–4 hours preferably after food (range 25–100 mg); CHILD 6–12 years 25 mg
By subcutaneous, intramuscular, or intravenous injection, moderate pain, pentazocine 30 mg, severe pain 45–60 mg every 3–4 hours when necessary; CHILD over 1 year, *by subcutaneous or intramuscular injection,* up to 1 mg/kg, *by intravenous injection* up to 500 micrograms/kg
By rectum in suppositories, pentazocine 50 mg up to 4 times daily; CHILD not recommended

CD Pentazocine (Non-proprietary)
Capsules, pentazocine hydrochloride 50 mg. Net price 20 = £3.51. Label: 2, 21
Tablets, pentazocine hydrochloride 25 mg. Net price 20 = £1.58. Label: 2, 21
Injection, pentazocine 30 mg (as lactate)/mL. Net price 1-mL amp = £1.45; 2-mL amp = £2.80
Suppositories, pentazocine 50 mg (as lactate). Net price 20 = £17.33. Label: 2
Note. The brand name NHS Fortral® (Sanofi Winthrop) is used for all the above preparations of pentazocine

PETHIDINE HYDROCHLORIDE
Indications: moderate to severe pain, obstetric analgesia; peri-operative analgesia, see section 15.1.4.3
Cautions; Contra-indications; Side-effects: see under Morphine Salts and notes above; avoid in severe renal impairment; not suitable for severe continuing pain; convulsions reported in **overdosage; interactions:** Appendix 1 (opioid analgesics)
Dose: by mouth, 50–150 mg every 4 hours; CHILD 0.5–2 mg/kg
By subcutaneous or intramuscular injection, 25–100 mg, repeated after 4 hours; CHILD, *by intramuscular injection,* 0.5–2 mg/kg
By slow intravenous injection, 25–50 mg, repeated after 4 hours
Obstetric analgesia, *by subcutaneous or intramuscular injection,* 50–100 mg, repeated 1–3 hours later if necessary; max. 400 mg in 24 hours
Postoperative pain, see section 15.1.4.3

CD **Pethidine** (Non-proprietary)

Tablets, pethidine hydrochloride 50 mg, net price 20 = £1.84. Label: 2

Available from Roche

Injection, pethidine hydrochloride 50 mg/mL. Net price 1-mL amp = 39p; 2-mL amp = 39p. 10 mg/mL see section 15.1.4.3

Various strengths available from Martindale

CD **Pamergan P100®** (Martindale)

Injection, pethidine hydrochloride 50 mg, promethazine hydrochloride 25 mg/mL. Net price 2-mL amp = 69p

Dose: by intramuscular injection, for obstetric analgesia, 1–2 mL every 4 hours if necessary; severe pain, 1–2 mL every 4–6 hours if necessary; premedication, see section 15.1.4.3

Note. Although usually given intramuscularly, may be given intravenously after dilution to at least 10 mL with water for injections

---

PHENAZOCINE HYDROBROMIDE

Indications: severe pain

Cautions; Contra-indications; Side-effects: see under Morphine Salts and notes above; **interactions:** Appendix 1 (opioid analgesics)

Dose: by mouth or sublingually, 5 mg every 4–6 hours when necessary; single doses may be increased to 20 mg; CHILD not recommended

CD **Narphen®** (Napp)

Tablets, phenazocine hydrobromide 5 mg. Net price 100-tab pack = £28.51. Label: 2

TRAMADOL HYDROCHLORIDE

Indications: moderate to severe pain

Cautions; Contra-indications; Side-effects: see under Morphine Salts and notes above; in addition to hypotension, hypertension also occasionally reported; anaphylaxis, hallucinations and confusion also reported; caution if history of epilepsy (convulsions reported, usually after rapid intravenous injection); avoid in pregnancy and breast-feeding; not suitable as substitute in opioid-dependent patients; **interactions:** Appendix 1 (opioid analgesics)

GENERAL ANAESTHESIA. Not recommended for analgesia during potentially very light planes of general anaesthesia (possibly increased operative recall reported)

Dose: by mouth, 50–100 mg not more often than every 4 hours; total of more than 400 mg daily by mouth not usually required; CHILD not recommended

By intramuscular injection or by intravenous injection (over 2–3 minutes) *or by intravenous infusion*, 50–100 mg every 4–6 hours

Postoperative pain, 100 mg initially then 50 mg every 10–20 minutes if necessary during first hour to total max. 250 mg (including initial dose) in first hour, *then* 50–100 mg every 4–6 hours; max. 600 mg daily; CHILD not recommended

▼ PoM **Tramadol Hydrochloride** (Non-proprietary)

Capsules, tramadol hydrochloride 50 mg. Net price 100-cap pack = £15.20. Label: 2

Available from Ethical Generics Ltd, Galen, Norton

▼ PoM **Zamadol®** (ASTA Medica)

Capsules, tramadol hydrochloride 50 mg. Net price 100-cap pack = £15.20. Label: 2

▼ PoM **Zydol®** (Searle)

Capsules, green/yellow, tramadol hydrochloride 50 mg. Net price 100-cap pack = £17.71. Label: 2

Soluble tablets, tramadol hydrochloride 50 mg, net price 20-tab pack = £3.19, 100-tab pack = £15.95. Label: 2, 13

Injection, tramadol hydrochloride 50 mg/mL. Net price 2-mL amp = £1.30

Modified release

▼ PoM **Zamadol® SR** (ASTA Medica)

Capsules, all m/r, tramadol hydrochloride 50 mg (green), net price 60-cap pack = £8.60; 100 mg, net price 60-cap pack = £17.20; 150 mg (dark green), 60-cap pack = £25.80; 200 mg (yellow), 60-cap pack = £34.40. Label: 2

Dose: 50–100 mg twice daily increased if necessary to 150–200 mg twice daily; total of more than 400 mg daily not usually required; CHILD under 12 years not recommended

COUNSELLING. Swallow whole or open capsule and swallow contents immediately without chewing

▼ PoM **Zydol SR®** (Searle)

Tablets, all m/r, f/c, tramadol hydrochloride 100 mg, net price 60-tab pack = £19.12; 150 mg (beige), 60-tab pack = £28.68; 200 mg (orange), 60-tab pack = £38.24. Label: 2, 25

Dose: 100 mg twice daily increased if necessary to 150–200 mg twice daily; total of more than 400 mg daily by mouth not usually required; CHILD not recommended

---

4.7.3   Trigeminal neuralgia

Carbamazepine (section 4.8.1), taken during the acute stages of trigeminal neuralgia, reduces the frequency and severity of attacks. It has no effect on other forms of headache. A dose of 100 mg once or twice a day should be given initially and the dose slowly increased until the best response is obtained; most patients require 200 mg 3–4 times daily but a few may require an increased total daily dosage of up to 1.6 g. Plasma-carbamazepine concentration should be monitored when high doses are given. Occasionally extreme dizziness is encountered which is a further reason for starting treatment with a small dose and increasing it slowly.

Some cases of trigeminal neuralgia respond to **phenytoin** (section 4.8.1) given alone or in conjunction with carbamazepine. A combination of phenytoin and carbamazepine is only required in refractory cases or in those unable to tolerate high doses of carbamazepine.

Although **tricyclic antidepressants** are not indicated for true trigeminal neuralgia they are more effective than carbamazepine in *post-herpetic neuralgia* and may also be useful in *oral and facial pain*, particularly if it is associated with depression.

4.7.4   Antimigraine drugs

4.7.4.1 Treatment of the acute migraine attack
4.7.4.2 Prophylaxis of migraine

4.7.4.1 TREATMENT OF THE ACUTE MIGRAINE ATTACK

Acute attacks of migraine may be relieved by analgesics or a specific treatment such as the use of a $5HT_1$ agonist or ergotamine. An anti-emetic may also be given if nausea and vomiting are features.

ANALGESICS

Most migraine headaches respond to analgesics such as **aspirin** or **paracetamol** (section 4.7.1) but since peristalsis is often reduced during migraine attacks the medication may not be sufficiently well absorbed to be effective; dispersible or effervescent preparations should therefore preferably be used.

The NSAID **tolfenamic acid** is licensed specifically for the treatment of acute attack of migraine.

$5HT_1$ AGONISTS

Sumatriptan is a $5HT_1$ agonist; it is of considerable value in the treatment of an acute attack. It may be used during the established headache phase of an attack and should be regarded as preferred treatment in those who fail to respond to conventional analgesics. Sumatriptan is also of value in cluster headache.

Naratriptan and **zolmitriptan** have been introduced recently.

CAUTIONS. $5HT_1$ agonists should be used with caution in conditions which predispose to coronary artery disease (pre-existing cardiac disease, see Contra-indications below); hepatic impairment (see Appendix 2); pregnancy and breast-feeding. $5HT_1$ agonists are recommended as monotherapy and should not be taken concurrently with other acute migraine therapies.

CONTRA-INDICATIONS. $5HT_1$ agonists should not be used for prophylaxis and are contra-indicated in ischaemic heart disease; previous myocardial infarction; coronary vasospasm (including Prinzmetal's angina); uncontrolled hypertension.

SIDE-EFFECTS. Side-effects of the $5HT_1$ agonists include sensations of tingling, heat, heaviness, pressure, or tightness of any part of the body (including throat and chest—discontinue if intense, may be due to coronary vasoconstriction or to anaphylaxis; see also CSM advice under Sumatriptan); flushing, dizziness, feeling of weakness; fatigue; nausea and vomiting also reported.

ERGOTAMINE

The value of **ergotamine** is limited by difficulties in absorption and by its side-effects, particularly *nausea, vomiting, abdominal pain*, and *muscular cramps*; it is best avoided. The recommended doses of ergotamine preparations should **not** be exceeded and treatment should **not** be repeated at intervals of less than 4 days.

To avoid habituation the frequency of administration of ergotamine should be limited to **no more than** twice a month. It should **never** be prescribed prophylactically but in the management of cluster headache a low dose (e.g. ergotamine 1 mg at night for 6 nights in 7) is occasionally given daily for 1 to 2 weeks [unlicensed indication].

ANTI-EMETICS

Anti-emetics (section 4.6), such as **metoclopramide** by mouth or, if vomiting is likely, by intramuscular injection, or the phenothiazine and antihistamine anti-emetics, relieve the nausea associated with migraine attacks. Domperidone or prochlorperazine may be given rectally if vomiting is a problem. Metoclopramide has the added advantage of promoting gastric emptying and normal peristalsis. A single dose should be given at the onset of symptoms. Oral analgesic preparations containing metoclopramide are a convenient alternative (**important:** for warnings relating to extrapyramidal effects particularly in children and young adults, see p. 191).

OTHER DRUGS FOR MIGRAINE

Isometheptene mucate (in combination with paracetamol) is licensed for the treatment of acute attacks of migraine; other effective treatments are however available now.

ANALGESICS

Aspirin
  Section 4.7.1

Paracetamol
  Section 4.7.1

With anti-emetics
Migraleve® (Pfizer Consumer)

Tablets, all f/c, *pink tablets*, buclizine hydrochloride 6.25 mg, paracetamol 500 mg, codeine phosphate 8 mg; *yellow tablets*, paracetamol 500 mg, codeine phosphate 8 mg. Net price 48-tab Duopack (32 pink + 16 yellow) = £5.10; 48 pink = £5.56; 48 yellow = £4.70. Label: 2 (pink tablets), 17, 30

Dose: 2 pink tablets at onset of attack, or if it is imminent, then 2 yellow tablets every 4 hours if necessary; max. in 24 hours 2 pink and 6 yellow; CHILD 10–14 years, half adult dose

PoM **Migravess®** (Bayer)

Tablets, effervescent, scored, metoclopramide hydrochloride 5 mg, aspirin 325 mg. Net price 30-tab pack = £3.60. Label: 13, 17, 32

Forte tablets, effervescent, scored, metoclopramide hydrochloride 5 mg, aspirin 450 mg. Net price 30-tab pack = £4.94. Label: 13, 17, 32

Dose: tablets or Forte tablets, 2 dissolved in water at onset of attack then every 4 hours when necessary; max. 6 tablets in 24 hours; CHILD 12–15 years, half adult dose

IMPORTANT. Ingredients include metoclopramide which can cause **severe extrapyramidal effects**, particularly in children and young adults (for further details, see p. 191)

PoM **Paramax**® (Lorex)

Tablets, scored, paracetamol 500 mg, metoclopramide hydrochloride 5 mg. Net price 42-tab pack = £6.30. Label: 17, 30

Sachets, effervescent powder, sugar-free, the contents of 1 sachet = 1 tablet; to be dissolved in ¼ tumblerful of liquid before administration. Net price 42-sachet pack = £8.25. Label: 13, 17, 30

Dose: (tablets or sachets): 2 at onset of attack then every 4 hours when necessary to max. of 6 in 24 hours; YOUNG ADULT 12–19 years, 1 at onset of attack then 1 every 4 hours when necessary to max. of 3 in 24 hours (max. dose of metoclopramide 500 micrograms/kg daily)

IMPORTANT. Metoclopramide can cause **severe extrapyramidal effects**, particularly in children and young adults (for further details, see p. 191)

ERGOTAMINE TARTRATE

Indications: acute attacks of migraine and migraine variants unresponsive to analgesics

Cautions: risk of peripheral vasospasm (see advice below); elderly; should not be used for migraine prophylaxis; **interactions:** Appendix 1 (ergotamine) and under Sumatriptan (Cautions), below

PERIPHERAL VASOSPASM. Warn patient to stop treatment immediately if numbness or tingling of extremities develops and to contact doctor.

Contra-indications: peripheral vascular disease, coronary heart disease, obliterative vascular disease and Raynaud's syndrome, hepatic or renal impairment, sepsis, severe or inadequately controlled hypertension, hyperthyroidism, pregnancy and breast-feeding, porphyria (see section 9.8.2)

Side-effects: nausea, vomiting, vertigo, abdominal pain, diarrhoea, muscle cramps, and occasionally increased headache (see also notes above); precordial pain, myocardial ischaemia, rarely myocardial infarction; repeated high dosage may cause ergotism with gangrene and confusion; pleural and peritoneal fibrosis may occur with excessive use

Dose: see under preparations below

PoM **Cafergot**® (Novartis)

Tablets, ergotamine tartrate 1 mg, caffeine 100 mg. Net price 30-tab pack = £1.34. Label: 18, counselling, dosage

Dose: 1–2 tablets at onset; max. 4 tablets in 24 hours; not to be repeated at intervals of less than 4 days; max. 8 tablets in one week (but see also notes above); CHILD not recommended

Suppositories, ergotamine tartrate 2 mg, caffeine 100 mg. Net price 30 = £4.87. Label: 18, counselling, dosage

Dose: 1 suppository at onset; max. 2 in 24 hours; not to be repeated at intervals of less than 4 days; max. 4 suppositories in one week (but see also notes above); CHILD not recommended

PoM **Lingraine**® (Sanofi Winthrop)

Tablets (for sublingual use), green, ergotamine tartrate 2 mg. Net price 12 = £7.43. Label: 18, 26, counselling, dosage

Dose: 1 tablet at onset repeated after 30–60 minutes if necessary; max. 3 tablets in 24 hours and 6 tablets in one week (but see also notes above); CHILD not recommended

PoM **Medihaler-Ergotamine**® (3M)

Aerosol inhalation (oral), ergotamine tartrate 360 micrograms/metered inhalation. Net price 75-dose unit = £3.06. Label: 18, counselling, dosage

Additives: include CFC propellants

Dose: 360 micrograms (1 puff) repeated if necessary after 5 minutes; max. 6 inhalations in 24 hours and 15 inhalations in one week (but see also notes above); CHILD under 10 years not recommended

PoM **Migril**® (GlaxoWellcome)

Tablets, scored, ergotamine tartrate 2 mg, cyclizine hydrochloride 50 mg, caffeine hydrate 100 mg. Net price 20 = £11.67. Label: 2, 18, counselling, dosage

Dose: 1 tablet at onset, followed after 30 minutes by ½–1 tablet, repeated every 30 minutes if necessary; max. 4 tablets per attack and 6 tablets in one week (but see also notes above); CHILD not recommended

ISOMETHEPTENE MUCATE

Indications: migraine attack

Cautions: cardiovascular disease, hepatic and renal impairment, diabetes mellitus, hyperthyroidism; **interactions:** Appendix 1 (sympathomimetics)

Contra-indications: glaucoma, severe cardiac, hepatic and renal impairment, severe hypertension, pregnancy and breast-feeding; porphyria (see section 9.8.2)

Side-effects: dizziness, circulatory disturbances, rashes, blood disorders also reported

Midrid® (Shire)

Capsules, red, isometheptene mucate 65 mg, paracetamol 325 mg. Net price 20 = £2.38. Label: 30, counselling, dosage

Dose: migraine, 2 capsules at onset of attack, followed by 1 capsule every hour if necessary; max. 5 capsules in 12 hours; CHILD not recommended

NARATRIPTAN

Indications: acute treatment of migraine attacks

Cautions: see above; renal impairment; **interactions:** Appendix 1 (5HT₁ agonists)

DRIVING. Drowsiness may affect performance of skilled tasks (e.g. driving)

Contra-indications: see above; peripheral vascular disease

Side-effects: see above, bradycardia or tachycardia; visual disturbances

Dose: 2.5 mg as soon as possible after onset; if migraine recurs after initial response, dose may be repeated after 4 hours (patient not responding should not take second dose for same attack); max. 5 mg in 24 hours

▼ PoM **Naramig**® (GlaxoWellcome)

Tablets, f/c, green; naratriptan (as hydrochloride) 2.5 mg. Net price 6-tab pack = £24.00. Label: 3

SUMATRIPTAN

Indications: acute treatment of migraine attacks; cluster headache (subcutaneous injection only)

Cautions: see above; renal impairment; should not be taken until 24 hours after stopping an ergotamine-containing preparation (conversely, ergotamine-containing preparations should not be taken until 6 hours after sumatriptan); other **interactions:** Appendix 1 (5HT₁ agonists)

DRIVING. Drowsiness may affect performance of skilled tasks (e.g. driving)

Contra-indications: see above

Side-effects: see above; drowsiness, transient increase in blood pressure, hypotension, bradycardia or tachycardia, altered liver function tests, seizures reported

CSM advice. Following reports of chest pain and tightness (coronary vasoconstriction) CSM has emphasised that sumatriptan should **not** be used in ischaemic heart disease or Prinzmetal's angina, and that use with ergotamine should be **avoided** (see also Cautions).

Dose: by mouth, 100 mg (50 mg effective in some patients) as soon as possible after onset (patient not responding should not take second dose for same attack); dose may be repeated if migraine recurs; max. 300 mg in 24 hours

By subcutaneous injection using auto-injector, 6 mg as soon as possible after onset (patients not responding should not take second dose for same attack); dose may be repeated once after not less than 1 hour if migraine recurs; max. 12 mg in 24 hours

IMPORTANT. **Not** for intravenous injection which may cause coronary vasospasm and angina

Intranasally, 20 mg (1 spray) into one nostril as soon as possible after onset (patient not responding should not take a second dose for same attack); dose may be repeated once after not less than two hours if migraine recurs; max. 40 mg in 24 hours

PoM **Imigran**® (GlaxoWellcome)

Tablets, f/c, sumatriptan (as succinate) 50 mg, net price 6-tab pack = £29.70, 12-tab pack = £56.43; 100 mg, 3-tab pack = £24.00, 6-tab pack = £48.00. Label: 3, 10 patient information leaflet

Injection, sumatriptan (as succinate) 12 mg/mL (= 6 mg/0.5-mL syringe), net price, treatment pack (2 × 0.5-mL pre-filled syringes and auto-injector) = £41.14; refill pack (2 × 0.5-mL pre-filled syringes) = £39.14. Label: 3, 10 patient information leaflet

Nasal spray, sumatriptan 20 mg/0.1-mL unit-dose spray device. Net price 2 unit-dose vials with applicator = £16.00. Label: 3, 10 patient information leaflet

TOLFENAMIC ACID

Indications: acute attack of migraine

Cautions; Contra-indications; Side-effects: see section 10.1.1; also dysuria (most commonly in men), tremor, euphoria, and fatigue reported

Dose: see under preparations

▼ PoM **Clotam**® (Thames)

Capsules, tolfenamic acid 200 mg. Net price 10-cap pack = £10.00

Dose: 200 mg at onset repeated once after 2–3 hours if necessary

Rapid Tablets, tolfenamic acid 200 mg. Net price 10-tab pack = £15.00

Dose: 200 mg at onset repeated once after 1–2 hours if necessary

ZOLMITRIPTAN

Indications: acute treatment of migraine attacks

Cautions: see above; should not be taken within 12 hours of any other 5HT$_1$ agonist; **interactions:** Appendix 1 (5HT$_1$ agonists)

Contra-indications: see above; Wolff-Parkinson-White syndrome or arrhythmias associated with accessory cardiac conduction pathways

Side-effects: see above; drowsiness, transient increase in blood pressure; dry mouth, myalgia and muscle weakness, dysaesthesia reported

Dose: 2.5 mg as soon as possible after onset repeated after 2 hours if migraine persists or recurs (increase to 5 mg for subsequent attacks in patients not achieving satisfactory relief with 2.5-mg dose); max. 15 mg in 24 hours

▼ PoM **Zomig**® (Zeneca)

Tablets, f/c, yellow, zolmitriptan 2.5 mg, net price 3-tab pack = £12.00, 6-tab pack = £24.00

4.7.4.2 PROPHYLAXIS OF MIGRAINE

Where migraine attacks are frequent, search should be made for provocative factors such as stress or diet (chocolate, cheese, alcohol, etc.). Benzodiazepines should be avoided because of the risk of dependence. In patients with more than one attack a month, one of three main prophylactic agents may be tried: pizotifen, beta-blockers, or tricyclic antidepressants (even when the patient is not obviously depressed). Long-term treatment with any of these prophylactic drugs is undesirable; the need for continuing therapy should be reviewed at intervals of about 6 months. Oral contraceptives may precipitate or worsen migraine; patients reporting a sharp increase in frequency of migraine or focal features should be recommended alternative contraceptive measures.

Pizotifen is an antihistamine and serotonin antagonist structurally related to the tricyclic antidepressants. It affords good prophylaxis but may cause weight gain. To avoid undue drowsiness treatment may be started at 500 micrograms at night and gradually increased to 3 mg; it is rarely necessary to exceed this dose.

The **beta-blockers** propranolol, metoprolol, nadolol, and timolol (section 2.4) are all effective. Propranolol is the most commonly used in an initial dose of 40 mg 2 to 3 times daily by mouth. Beta-blockers may also be given as a single daily dose of a long-acting preparation. The value of beta-blockers is limited by their contra-indications (section 2.4) and by interaction with ergotamine (see Appendix 1, beta-blockers).

Tricyclic antidepressants (section 4.3.1) may usefully be prescribed in a dose, for example, of amitriptyline 10 mg at night, increasing to a maintenance dose of 50 to 75 mg at night.

Sodium valproate (section 4.8.1) may be effective in a dose of 300 mg twice daily; it has been associated with severe hepatic and pancreatic toxicity, although these effects are rare.

There is some evidence that the **calcium-channel blockers** (section 2.6.2), e.g. verapamil and nifedipine may be useful in migraine prophylaxis.

Cyproheptadine (section 3.4.1), an antihistamine with serotonin-antagonist and calcium channel-blocking properties, may also be tried in refractory cases.

Clonidine (*Dixarit®*) is not recommended and may aggravate depression or produce insomnia. **Methysergide** has dangerous side-effects (retroperitoneal fibrosis and fibrosis of the heart valves and pleura); **important:** it should only be administered under hospital supervision.

PIZOTIFEN
Indications: prevention of vascular headache including classical migraine, common migraine, and cluster headache
Cautions: urinary retention; closed-angle glaucoma, renal impairment; pregnancy and breast-feeding; **interactions:** Appendix 1 (pizotifen)
DRIVING. Drowsiness may affect performance of skilled tasks (e.g. driving); effects of alcohol enhanced
Side-effects: antimuscarinic effects, drowsiness, increased appetite and weight gain; occasionally nausea, dizziness; CNS stimulation may occur in children
Dose: 1.5 mg at night *or* 500 micrograms 3 times daily (but see also notes above), adjusted according to response within the usual range 0.5–3 mg daily; max. single dose 3 mg, max. daily dose 4.5 mg; CHILD up to 1.5 mg daily in divided doses; max. single dose at night 1 mg

PoM **Sanomigran®** (Novartis)
Tablets, both ivory-yellow, s/c, pizotifen (as hydrogen malate), 500 micrograms, net price 20 = £1.56; 1.5 mg, 28-tab pack = £7.78. Label. 2
Elixir, pizotifen 250 micrograms (as hydrogen malate)/5 mL. Net price 300-mL pack = £4.12. Label: 2

CLONIDINE HYDROCHLORIDE
Indications: prevention of recurrent migraine (but see notes above), vascular headache, menopausal flushing; hypertension, see section 2.5.2
Cautions: depressive illness, concurrent antihypertensive therapy; porphyria (see section 9.8.2); **interactions:** Appendix 1 (clonidine)
Side-effects: dry mouth, sedation, dizziness, nausea, nocturnal restlessness; occasionally rashes
Dose: 50 micrograms twice daily, increased after 2 weeks to 75 micrograms twice daily if necessary; CHILD not recommended

PoM **Dixarit®** (Boehringer Ingelheim)
Tablets, blue, s/c, clonidine hydrochloride 25 micrograms. Net price 112-tab pack = £7.11
PoM **Catapres®** (hypertension), see section 2.5.2

METHYSERGIDE
Indications: prevention of severe recurrent migraine and cluster headache in patients who are refractory to other treatment and whose lives are seriously disrupted (**important:** hospital supervision only, see notes above)
Cautions: history of peptic ulceration; avoid abrupt withdrawal of treatment; after 6 months withdraw (gradually over 2 to 3 weeks) for reassessment for at least 1 month (see also notes above)
Contra-indications: renal, hepatic, pulmonary, and cardiovascular disease, severe hypertension, collagen disease, cellulitis, urinary-tract disorders, cachectic or septic conditions, pregnancy, breast-feeding

Side-effects: nausea, vomiting, heartburn, abdominal discomfort, drowsiness, and dizziness occur frequently in initial treatment; mental and behavioural disturbances, insomnia, oedema, weight gain, rashes, loss of scalp hair, cramps, arterial spasm (including coronary artery spasm with angina and possible myocardial infarction), paraesthesias of extremities, postural hypotension, and tachycardia also occur; retroperitoneal and other abnormal fibrotic reactions may occur on prolonged administration, requiring immediate withdrawal of treatment
Dose: 1 mg at bedtime, gradually increased to 1–2 mg 2–3 times daily with food (see notes above); CHILD not recommended
Carcinoid syndrome, usual range, 12–20 mg daily (hospital supervision); CHILD not recommended

PoM **Deseril®** (Novartis)
Tablets, s/c, methysergide 1 mg (as maleate). Net price 60-tab pack = £5.36. Label: 2, 21

4.8   Antiepileptics
4.8.1   Control of epilepsy
4.8.2   Drugs used in status epilepticus
4.8.3   Febrile convulsions

4.8.1   Control of epilepsy
The object of treatment is to prevent the occurrence of seizures by maintaining an effective plasma concentration of the drug. Careful adjustment of doses is necessary, starting with low doses and increasing gradually until seizures are controlled or there are overdose effects.

The frequency of administration is often determined by the plasma half-life, and should be kept as low as possible to encourage better patient compliance. Most antiepileptics, when used in average dosage, may be given twice daily. Phenobarbitone and sometimes phenytoin, which have long half-lives, may often be given as a daily dose at bedtime. However, with large doses, some antiepileptics may need to be administered 3 times daily to avoid adverse effects associated with high peak plasma concentrations. Young children metabolise antiepileptics more rapidly than adults and therefore require more frequent doses and a higher amount per kilogram body-weight.

COMBINATION THERAPY. Therapy with several antiepileptic drugs concurrently should generally be avoided. Patients are best controlled with one antiepileptic. Combinations of drugs have been used on the grounds that their therapeutic effects were additive while their individual toxicity was reduced but there is no evidence for this. In fact, toxicity may be enhanced with combination therapy. A second drug should only be added to the regimen if seizures continue despite side-effects. The use of more than two antiepileptics is rarely justified. Another disadvantage of multiple therapy is that drug interactions occur between the various antiepileptics (see below). Moreover, it is illogical to combine primidone and phenobarbitone as the former is largely metabolised to phenobarbitone in the liver, which is responsible for most, if not all, of its antiepileptic action.

INTERACTIONS. Interactions between antiepileptics are complex and may enhance toxicity without a corresponding increase in antiepileptic effect. Interactions are usually caused by *hepatic enzyme induction* or *hepatic enzyme inhibition*; *displacement from protein binding sites* is not usually a problem. These interactions are highly variable and unpredictable. Plasma monitoring is therefore often advisable with combination therapy.

Interactions that occur between antiepileptics themselves are as follows:

Carbamazepine
often lowers plasma concentration of *clonazepam, lamotrigine, phenytoin* (but may also raise), *topiramate, and valproate*
sometimes lowers plasma concentration of *ethosuximide, and primidone* (but tendency for corresponding increase in phenobarbitone level)
Ethosuximide
sometimes raises plasma concentration of *phenytoin*
Lamotrigine
sometimes raises plasma concentration of *an active metabolite of carbamazepine*
Phenobarbitone *or* Primidone
often lowers plasma concentration of *carbamazepine, clonazepam, lamotrigine, phenytoin* (but may also raise), *and valproate*
sometimes lowers plasma concentration of *ethosuximide*
Phenytoin
often lowers plasma concentration of *clonazepam, carbamazepine, lamotrigine, topiramate, and valproate*
often raises plasma concentration of *phenobarbitone*
sometimes lowers plasma concentration of *ethosuximide, and primidone* (by increasing conversion to phenobarbitone)
Topiramate
sometimes raises plasma concentration of *phenytoin*
Valproate
often raises plasma concentration of *an active metabolite of carbamazepine,* and of *lamotrigine, phenobarbitone, and phenytoin* (but may also lower)
sometimes raises plasma concentration of *ethosuximide, and primidone* (and tendency for significant increase in phenobarbitone level)
Vigabatrin
often lowers plasma concentration of *phenytoin*
sometimes lowers plasma concentration of *phenobarbitone, and primidone*

For other important interactions see **Appendix 1**, and for FPA guidelines on enzyme-inducing antiepileptics and **oral contraceptives**, see section 7.3.1.

WITHDRAWAL. Abrupt withdrawal of antiepileptics, particularly the barbiturates and benzodiazepines, should be avoided, as this may precipitate severe rebound seizures. Reduction in dosage should be carried out in stages and, in the case of the barbiturates, the withdrawal process may take months. The changeover from one antiepileptic drug regimen to another should be made cautiously, withdrawing the first drug only when the new regimen has been largely established.

The decision to withdraw all antiepileptics from a seizure-free patient, and its timing, is often difficult and may depend on individual patient factors. Even in patients who have been seizure-free for several years, there is a significant risk of seizure recurrence on drug withdrawal.

DRIVING. Patients suffering from epilepsy may drive a motor vehicle (but not a heavy goods or public service vehicle) provided that they have had a seizure-free period of one year or, if subject to attacks only while asleep, have established a three-year period of asleep attacks without awake attacks. Patients affected by drowsiness should not drive or operate machinery.

PREGNANCY AND BREAST-FEEDING. During pregnancy, total plasma concentrations of antiepileptics (particularly of phenytoin) may fall, particularly in the later stages but free plasma concentrations may remain the same (or even rise). There is an increased risk of teratogenicity associated with the use of antiepileptic drugs (reduced if treatment is limited to a single drug). In view of the increased risk of neural tube and other defects associated, in particular, with **carbamazepine, phenytoin** and **valproate** women taking antiepileptic drugs who *may become pregnant* should be **informed of the possible consequences**. Those who *wish to become pregnant* should be referred to an appropriate specialist for advice. Women who become pregnant should be **counselled** and offered **antenatal screening** (alpha-fetoprotein measurement and a second trimester ultrasound scan).

To counteract the risk of neural tube defects adequate folate supplements are advised for women before and during pregnancy; to prevent recurrence of neural tube defects, women should receive folic acid 5 mg daily (see section 9.1.2)—this dose may also be appropriate for women receiving established antiepileptic drugs.

In view of the risk of neonatal bleeding associated with carbamazepine, phenobarbitone and phenytoin, prophylactic vitamin K_1 is recommended for the mother before delivery (as well as for the neonate).

Breast-feeding is acceptable with all antiepileptic drugs, taken in normal doses, with the possible exception of the barbiturates and ethosuximide, and also some of the more recently introduced ones, see also Prescribing during Breast-feeding (Appendix 5).

PARTIAL SEIZURES WITH OR WITHOUT SECONDARY GENERALISATION

Carbamazepine, sodium valproate and **phenytoin** are the drugs of choice for secondary generalised tonic-clonic seizures and for partial (focal) seizures. Phenobarbitone and primidone are also effective but are likely to be more sedating. Second-line drugs include clonazepam, clobazam, and acetazolamide. The newer drugs **gabapentin, lamotrigine,** and **vigabatrin** are now available where control is difficult to obtain and are effective in partial seizures with or without secondary generalisation. Partial epilepsy and secondarily generalised seizures are more difficult to control than tonic-clonic seizures as part of a syndrome of primary generalised epilepsy.

GENERALISED SEIZURES

TONIC-CLONIC SEIZURES (GRAND MAL). The drugs of choice for tonic-clonic seizures are **carbamazepine, phenytoin**, and **sodium valproate**. For those patients who have tonic-clonic seizures as part of the syndrome of primary generalised epilepsy, **sodium valproate** is the drug of choice. **Phenobarbitone** (phenobarbital) and **primidone** are also effective but may be more sedating. There is evidence that **lamotrigine** is also effective, where control is difficult to obtain.

ABSENCE SEIZURES (PETIT MAL). **Ethosuximide** and **sodium valproate** are the drugs of choice in simple absence seizures. Sodium valproate is also highly effective in treating the tonic-clonic seizures which may co-exist with absence seizures in primary generalised epilepsy.

MYOCLONIC SEIZURES. Myoclonic seizures (myoclonic jerks) occur in a variety of syndromes, and response to treatment varies considerably. **Sodium valproate** is the drug of choice and **clonazepam, ethosuximide**, and other antiepileptic drugs may be used. For reference to the adjunctive use of piracetam, see section 4.9.3.

ATYPICAL ABSENCE, ATONIC, AND TONIC SEIZURES. These seizure types are usually seen in childhood, in specific epileptic syndromes, or associated with cerebral damage or mental retardation. They may respond poorly to the traditional drugs. **Phenytoin, sodium valproate, lamotrigine, clonazepam, ethosuximide**, and **phenobarbitone** may be tried. Second-line antiepileptic drugs that are occasionally helpful, include **acetazolamide** and **corticosteroids**.

CARBAMAZEPINE

Carbamazepine is a drug of choice for simple and complex partial seizures and for tonic-clonic seizures secondary to a focal discharge. It has a wider therapeutic index than phenytoin and the relationship between dose and plasma concentration is linear, but monitoring of plasma concentrations may be helpful in determining optimum dosage. It has generally fewer side-effects than phenytoin or the barbiturates, but reversible blurring of vision, dizziness, and unsteadiness are dose-related, and may be dose-limiting. These side-effects may be reduced by altering the timing of medication; use of modified release tablets (*Tegretol Retard®*) also significantly lessens the incidence of dose-related side-effects. It is essential to initiate carbamazepine therapy at a low dose (100–200 mg daily) and build this up slowly with increments of 100–200 mg every two weeks.

CARBAMAZEPINE

Indications: partial and secondary generalised tonic-clonic seizures, but not primary generalised seizures; trigeminal neuralgia (section 4.7.3); prophylaxis in manic-depressive illness (4.2.3)

Cautions: hepatic or renal impairment; cardiac disease (see also Contra-indications); skin reactions (see also Side-effects), history of haematological reactions to other drugs; manufacturer recommends blood counts and hepatic and renal function tests (but evidence of practical value unsatisfactory); glaucoma; pregnancy (**important:** see p. 210 and Appendix 4 (neural tube screening)), breast-feeding (see p. 210); avoid sudden withdrawal; **Interactions:** see p. 210 and Appendix 1 (carbamazepine)

BLOOD, HEPATIC or SKIN DISORDERS. Patients or their carers should be told how to recognise signs of blood, liver, or skin disorders, and advised to seek immediate medical attention if symptoms such as fever, sore throat, rash, mouth ulcers, bruising, or bleeding develop. Leucopenia which is severe, progressive or associated with clinical symptoms requires withdrawal (if necessary under cover of suitable alternative).

Contra-indications: AV conduction abnormalities (unless paced); history of bone marrow depression, porphyria (see section 9.8.2)

Side-effects. nausea and vomiting, dizziness, drowsiness, headache, ataxia, confusion and agitation (elderly), visual disturbances (especially double vision and often associated with peak plasma concentrations), constipation or diarrhoea, anorexia; mild transient generalised erythematous rash may occur in a large number of patients (withdraw if worsens or is accompanied by other symptoms); leucopenia and other blood disorders (including thrombocytopenia, agranulocytosis and aplastic anaemia); other side-effects include cholestatic jaundice, hepatitis and acute renal failure, Stevens-Johnson syndrome, toxic epidermal necrolysis, alopecia, thromboembolism, arthralgia, fever, proteinuria, lymph node enlargement, cardiac conduction disturbances (sometimes arrhythmias), dyskinesias, paraesthesia, depression, impotence (and impaired fertility), gynaecomastia, galactorrhoea, aggression, activation of psychosis; photosensitivity; pulmonary hypersensitivity (with dyspnoea and pneumonitis), hyponatraemia and oedema also reported; suppositories may cause occasional rectal irritation

Dose: by mouth, epilepsy, initially, 100–200 mg 1–2 times daily, increased slowly (see notes above) to usual dose of 0.8–1.2 g daily in divided doses; in some cases 1.6–2 g daily may be needed; ELDERLY reduce initial dose; CHILD daily in divided doses, up to 1 year 100–200 mg, 1–5 years 200–400 mg, 5–10 years 400–600 mg, 10–15 years 0.6–1 g

By rectum, as suppositories, see below

Note. Plasma concentration for optimum response 4–12 mg/litre (20–50 micromol/litre)

PoM **Carbamazepine** (Non-proprietary)

Tablets, carbamazepine 100 mg, net price 20 = 58p; 200 mg, 20 = £1.07; 400 mg, 20 = £2.11. Label: 3, 8, counselling, blood, hepatic or skin disorder symptoms (see above), driving (see notes above)

Available from APS, Cox, Generics, Hillcross, Norton (Epimaz®)

Note. Different preparations may vary in bioavailability; to avoid reduced effect or excessive side-effects, it may be prudent to avoid changing the formulation (see also notes above on how side-effects may be reduced)

PoM **Tegretol®** (Novartis)

Tablets, all scored, carbamazepine 100 mg, net price 84-tab pack = £2.43; 200 mg, 84-tab pack = £4.50; 400 mg, 56-tab pack = £5.90. Label: 3, 8, counselling, blood, hepatic or skin disorder symptoms (see above), driving (see notes above)

Chewtabs, orange, carbamazepine 100 mg, net price 56-tab pack = £2.95; 200 mg, 56-tab pack = £5.49. Label: 3, 8, 21, 24, counselling, blood, hepatic or skin disorder symptoms (see above), driving (see notes above)

Liquid, sugar-free, carbamazepine 100 mg/5 mL. Net price 300-mL pack = £5.72. Label: 3, 8, counselling, blood, hepatic or skin disorder symptoms (see above), driving (see notes above)

Suppositories, carbamazepine 125 mg, net price 5 = £7.50; 250 mg, 5 = £10.00. Label: 3, 8, counselling, blood, hepatic or skin disorder symptoms (see above), driving (see notes above)

Dose: epilepsy, for short-term use (max. 7 days) when oral therapy temporarily not possible; suppositories of 125 mg may be considered to be approximately equivalent in therapeutic effect to tablets of 100 mg but final adjustment should always depend on clinical response (plasma concentration monitoring recommended); max. by rectum 1 g daily in 4 divided doses

PoM **Tegretol® Retard** (Novartis)

Tablets, m/r, both scored, carbamazepine 200 mg (beige-orange), net price 56-tab pack = £4.82; 400 mg (brown-orange), 56-tab pack = £9.48. Label: 3, 8, 25, counselling, blood, hepatic or skin disorder symptoms (see above), driving (see notes above)

Dose: epilepsy (ADULT and CHILD over 5 years), as above; trigeminal neuralgia, as section 4.7.3; total daily dose given in 2 divided doses

---

ETHOSUXIMIDE

Ethosuximide is the drug of choice in simple absence seizures; it may also be used in myoclonic seizures and in atypical absence, atonic, and tonic seizures.

ETHOSUXIMIDE

Indications: absence seizures

Cautions: see notes above; hepatic and renal impairment; manufacturer recommends blood counts and hepatic and renal function tests (but evidence of practical value unsatisfactory); pregnancy and breast-feeding (see notes above); avoid sudden withdrawal; porphyria (see section 9.8.2); **interactions:** Appendix 1 (ethosuximide)

BLOOD DISORDERS. Patients or their carers should be told how to recognise signs of blood disorders, and advised to seek immediate medical attention if symptoms such as fever, sore throat, mouth ulcers, bruising or bleeding develop

Side-effects: gastro-intestinal disturbances, weight loss, drowsiness, dizziness, ataxia, dyskinesia, hiccup, photophobia, headache, depression, and mild euphoria. Psychotic states, rashes, hepatic and renal changes (see Cautions), and haematological disorders such as agranulocytosis and aplastic anaemia occur rarely (blood counts required if signs or symptoms of infection); systemic lupus erythematosus and erythema multiforme (Stevens-Johnson syndrome) reported; other side-effects reported include gum hypertrophy, swelling of tongue, irritability, hyperactivity, sleep disturbances, night terrors, inability to concentrate, aggressiveness, increased libido, myopia, vaginal bleeding

Dose: ADULT and CHILD over 6 years initially, 500 mg daily, increased by 250 mg at intervals of 4–7 days to usual dose of 1–1.5 g daily; occasionally up to 2 g daily may be needed; CHILD up to 6 years initially 250 mg daily, increased gradually to usual dose of 20 mg/kg daily

Note. Plasma concentration for optimum response 40–100 mg/litre (300–700 micromol/litre)

PoM **Emeside®** (LAB)

Capsules, orange, ethosuximide 250 mg. Net price 112-cap pack = £11.15. Label: 8, counselling, blood disorders (see above), driving (see notes above)

Syrup, black currant or orange, ethosuximide 250 mg/5 mL. Net price 200-mL pack = £6.00. Label: 8, counselling, blood disorders (see above), driving (see notes above)

PoM **Zarontin®** (P-D)

Capsules, orange, ethosuximide 250 mg. Net price 50-cap pack = £4.03. Label: 8, counselling, blood disorders (see above), driving (see notes above)

Syrup, red, ethosuximide 250 mg/5 mL. Net price 300-mL pack = £5.60. Label: 8, counselling, blood disorders (see above), driving (see notes above)

LAMOTRIGINE

Lamotrigine is an antiepileptic for partial seizures and secondarily generalised tonic-clonic seizures. Lamotrigine may rarely cause serious skin rash especially in children; dose recommendations should be adhered to closely.

Lamotrigine is used either as sole treatment or as an adjunct to treatment with other antiepileptic drugs. Valproate increases plasma-lamotrigine concentration whereas the enzyme inducing antiepileptics reduce it; care is therefore required in choosing the appropriate initial dose and subsequent titration. Where the potential for interaction is not known, treatment should be initiated with lower doses such as those used with valproate.

LAMOTRIGINE

Indications: monotherapy and adjunctive treatment of partial seizures and primary and secondarily generalised tonic-clonic seizures; seizures associated with Lennox Gastaut syndrome

---

Cautions: closely monitor (including hepatic, renal and clotting parameters) and consider withdrawal if rash, fever, influenza-like symptoms, drowsiness, or worsening of seizure control develops (although causal relationship not established, lamotrigine given with other antiepileptics has been associated with rapidly progressive illness with status epilepticus, multi-organ dysfunction, disseminated intravascular coagulation and death); avoid abrupt withdrawal (taper off over 2 weeks or longer) unless serious skin reaction occurs; renal impairment; elderly; pregnancy and breast-feeding; monitor body-weight in children and review dose if necessary; **interactions**: see p. 210 and Appendix 1 (lamotrigine)

Contra-indications: hepatic impairment

Side-effects: commonly rashes (see also below)—fever, malaise, influenza-like symptoms, drowsiness and rarely hepatic dysfunction, lymphadenopathy, leucopenia, and thrombocytopenia reported in conjunction with rash; angioedema, and photosensitivity also reported; diplopia, blurred vision, conjunctivitis, dizziness, drowsiness, insomnia, headache, ataxia, tiredness, gastro-intestinal disturbances (including vomiting), irritability, aggression, tremor, agitation, confusion; headache, nausea, dizziness, diplopia and ataxia in patients also taking carbamazepine usually resolve when dose of either drug reduced

SKIN REACTIONS. Serious skin reactions including Stevens-Johnson syndrome and toxic epidermal necrolysis (rarely with fatalities) have developed in adults and especially in children; most rashes occur within 8 weeks of starting lamotrigine. The CSM has advised that factors associated with increased risk of serious skin reactions include concomitant use of valproate, initial lamotrigine dosing higher than recommended, and more rapid dose escalation than recommended.

COUNSELLING. Warn patients to see their doctor immediately if rash or influenza-like symptoms associated with hypersensitivity develop

Dose: IMPORTANT. Do not confuse the different combinations; see also notes above

Monotherapy, initially 25 mg daily for 14 days, increased to 50 mg daily for further 14 days, then increased by max. of 50–100 mg every 7–14 days; usual maintenance as monotherapy, 100–200 mg daily in 1–2 divided doses (up to 500 mg daily has been required)

Adjunctive therapy *with valproate,* initially 25 mg every other day for 14 days then 25 mg daily for further 14 days, thereafter increased by max. of 25–50 mg every 7–14 days; usual maintenance, 100–200 mg daily in 1–2 divided doses

Adjunctive therapy (with enzyme inducing drugs) *without valproate,* initially 50 mg daily for 14 days then 50 mg twice daily for further 14 days, thereafter increased by max. of 100 mg every 7–14 days; usual maintenance 200–400 mg daily in 2 divided doses (up to 700 mg daily has been required)

CHILD under 12 years, *monotherapy,* not recommended

CHILD 2–12 years, adjunctive therapy *with valproate,* initially 200 micrograms/kg daily for 14 days then 500 micrograms/kg daily for further 14 days (those weighing 12.5–25 kg may receive 5 mg on alternate days for first 14 days), thereafter increased by max. of 0.5–1 mg/kg every 7–14 days; usual maintenance 1–5 mg/kg daily in 1–2 divided doses

CHILD 2–12 years adjunctive therapy (with enzyme inducing drugs) *without valproate,* initially 2 mg/kg daily in 2 divided doses for 14 days then 5 mg/kg daily in 2 divided doses for further 14 days, thereafter increased by max. of 2–3 mg/kg every 7–14 days; usual maintenance 5–15 mg/kg daily in 2 divided doses

▼ PoM **Lamictal**® (GlaxoWellcome)

Tablets, all yellow, lamotrigine 25 mg, net price 21-tab pack (*'Valproate Add-on therapy' Starter Pack*) = £7.49, 42-tab pack (*'Monotherapy' Starter Pack*) = £14.97, 56-tab pack = £19.97; 50 mg, 42-tab pack (*'Non-valproate Add-on therapy' Starter Pack*) = £25.46, 56-tab pack = £33.95; 100 mg, 56-tab pack = £58.57; 200 mg, 56-tab pack = £99.56. Label: 8, counselling, driving (see notes above)

Dispersible tablets, lamotrigine 5 mg (scored), net price 28-tab pack = £7.96; 25 mg, 56-tab pack = £19.97; 100 mg, 56-tab pack = £58.57. Label: 8, 13, counselling, driving (see notes above)

PHENOBARBITONE AND OTHER BARBITURATES

Phenobarbitone is effective for tonic-clonic and partial seizures but may be sedative in adults and cause behavioural disturbances and hyperkinesia in children. It may be tried for atypical absence, atonic, and tonic seizures. Rebound seizures may be a problem on withdrawal. Monitoring plasma concentrations is less useful than with other drugs because tolerance occurs. **Methylphenobarbitone** is largely converted to phenobarbitone in the liver and has no advantages. **Primidone** is largely converted to phenobarbitone and this is probably responsible for its antiepileptic action. A small starting dose of primidone (125 mg) is essential, and the drug should be introduced over several weeks.

PHENOBARBITONE
(Phenobarbital)

Indications: all forms of epilepsy except absence seizures; status epilepticus, section 4.8.2

Cautions: elderly, debilitated, children, impaired renal or hepatic function, respiratory depression (avoid if severe), pregnancy and breast-feeding (see notes above); avoid sudden withdrawal; see also notes above; avoid in porphyria (see section 9.8.2); **interactions:** see p. 210 and Appendix 1 (barbiturates and primidone)

Side-effects: drowsiness, lethargy, mental depression, ataxia and allergic skin reactions; paradoxical excitement, restlessness and confusion in the elderly and hyperkinesia in children; megaloblastic anaemia (may be treated with folic acid); **overdosage:** see Emergency Treatment of Poisoning, p. 23

Dose: by mouth, 60–180 mg at night; CHILD 5–8 mg/kg daily

By intramuscular or intravenous injection, 50–200 mg, repeated after 6 hours if necessary; max. 600 mg daily; dilute injection 1 in 10 with water for injections before intravenous administration; status epilepticus, section 4.8.2

Note. For therapeutic purposes phenobarbitone and phenobarbitone sodium may be considered equivalent in effect. Plasma concentration for optimum response 15–40 mg/litre (60–180 micromol/litre)

CD [1]**Phenobarbitone Tablets,** phenobarbitone 15 mg, net price 20 = 6p; 30 mg, 20 = 8p; 60 mg, 20 = 14p. Label: 2, 8, counselling, driving (see notes above)

CD [1]**Phenobarbitone Elixir,** phenobarbitone 15 mg/5 mL in a suitable flavoured vehicle, containing alcohol 38%. Net price 100 mL = 82p. Label: 2, 8, counselling, driving (see notes above)

Note. Some hospitals supply alcohol-free formulations

CD [1]**Phenobarbitone Injection,** phenobarbitone sodium 200 mg/mL in propylene glycol 90% and water for injections 10%. Net price 1-mL amp = 99p

Note. Must be diluted before intravenous administration (see under Dose)

Available from Concord (**CD** [1]Gardenal Sodium®), Martindale; other strengths also available from Martindale.

1. See p. 7 for prescribing requirements for phenobarbitone

METHYLPHENOBARBITONE
(Methylphenobarbital)

Indications; Cautions; Side-effects: see under Phenobarbitone

Dose: 100–600 mg daily

CD Prominal® (Sanofi Winthrop)

Tablets, methylphenobarbitone 30 mg, net price 20 = 78p; 60 mg, 20 = £1.03; 200 mg, 20 = £2.20. Label: 2, 8, counselling, driving (see notes above)

PRIMIDONE

Indications: all forms of epilepsy except absence seizures; essential tremor (section 4.9.3)

Cautions; Side-effects: see under Phenobarbitone. Drowsiness, ataxia, nausea, visual disturbances, and rashes, particularly at first, usually reversible on continued administration; **interactions:** see p. 210 and Appendix 1 (barbiturates and primidone)

Dose: epilepsy, initially, 125 mg daily at bedtime, increased by 125 mg every 3 days to 500 mg daily in 2 divided doses then increased by 250 mg every 3 days to a max. of 1.5 g daily in divided doses; CHILD under 2 years, 250–500 mg daily in 2 divided doses; 2–5 years, 500–750 mg daily in 2 divided doses; 6–9 years 0.75–1 g daily in 2 divided doses

Note. Monitor plasma concentrations of derived phenobarbitone. Optimum range as for phenobarbitone.

PoM **Mysoline®** (Zeneca)

Tablets, scored, primidone 250 mg. Net price 100-tab pack = £1.77. Label: 2, 8, counselling, driving (see notes above)

Oral suspension, primidone 250 mg/5 mL. Net price 250-mL pack = £1.01. Label: 2, 8, counselling, driving (see notes above)

PHENYTOIN

Phenytoin is effective in tonic-clonic and partial seizures. It has a narrow therapeutic index and the relationship between dose and plasma concentration is non-linear; small dosage increases in some patients may produce large rises in plasma concentrations with acute toxic side-effects. Monitoring of plasma concentration greatly assists dosage adjustment. A few missed doses or a small change in drug absorption may result in a marked change in plasma concentration.

Phenytoin may cause coarse facies, acne, hirsutism, and gingival hyperplasia and so may be particularly undesirable in adolescent patients.

PHENYTOIN

Indications: all forms of epilepsy except absence seizures; trigeminal neuralgia (see also section 4.7.3)

Cautions: hepatic impairment (reduce dose), pregnancy (**important:** see notes above and Appendix 4), breast-feeding (see notes above); avoid sudden withdrawal; manufacturer recommends blood counts (but evidence of practical value unsatisfactory); avoid in porphyria (see section 9.8.2); see also notes above; **interactions:** see p. 210 and Appendix 1 (phenytoin)

BLOOD, or SKIN DISORDERS. Patients or their carers should be told how to recognise signs of blood, or skin disorders, and advised to seek immediate medical attention if symptoms such as fever, sore throat, rash, mouth ulcers, bruising, or bleeding develop. Leucopenia which is severe, progressive or associated with clinical symptoms requires withdrawal (if necessary under cover of suitable alternative)

Side-effects: nausea, vomiting, mental confusion, dizziness, headache, tremor, transient nervousness, insomnia occur commonly; rarely dyskinesias, peripheral neuropathy; ataxia, slurred speech, nystagmus and blurred vision are signs of overdosage; rashes (discontinue, if mild re-introduce cautiously but discontinue immediately if recurrence), coarse facies, acne and hirsutism, fever and hepatitis; lupus erythematosus, erythema multiforme (Stevens-Johnson syndrome), toxic epidermal necrolysis, polyarteritis nodosa; lymphadenopathy; gingival hypertrophy and tenderness; rarely haematological effects, including megaloblastic anaemia (may be treated with folic acid), leucopenia, thrombocytopenia, agranulocytosis, and aplastic anaemia; plasma calcium may be lowered (rickets and osteomalacia)

Dose: by mouth, initially 3–4 mg/kg daily *or* 150–300 mg daily (as a single dose *or* in two divided doses) increased gradually as necessary (plasma monitoring, see notes above); usual dose 200–500 mg daily; max. 600 mg daily; CHILD initially, 5 mg/kg daily in 2 divided doses, usual dose range 4–8 mg/kg daily; max. 300 mg

By intravenous injection—section 4.8.2

Note. Plasma concentration for optimum response 10–20 mg/litre (40–80 micromol/litre)

COUNSELLING. Take preferably with or after food

PoM **Phenytoin** (Non-proprietary)

Capsules, phenytoin sodium 50 mg, net price 20 = 40p; 100 mg, 20 = 56p. Label: 8, counselling, administration, blood or skin disorder symptoms (see above), driving (see notes above)

Tablets, coated, phenytoin sodium 50 mg, net price 20 = 26p; 100 mg, 20 = 31p. Label: 8, counselling, administration, blood or skin disorder symptoms (see above), driving (see notes above)

Available from APS, Berk (Pentran®), Cox

Note. On the basis of single dose tests there are no clinically relevant differences in bioavailability between available phenytoin sodium tablets and capsules but some clinics prefer patients to remain on the same brand whenever possible

PoM **Epanutin®** (P-D)

Capsules, phenytoin sodium 25 mg (white/purple), net price 20 = 39p; 50 mg (white/pink), 20 = 40p; 100 mg (white/orange), 20 = 56p; 300 mg (white/green), 20 = £1.69. Label: 8, counselling, administration, blood or skin disorder symptoms (see above), driving (see notes above)

Infatabs® (= tablets, chewable), yellow, scored, phenytoin 50 mg. Net price 20 = £1.10. Label: 8, 24, counselling, blood or skin disorder symptoms (see above), driving (see notes above)

Note. Contain phenytoin 50 mg (as against phenytoin sodium) therefore care is needed on changing to capsules or tablets containing phenytoin sodium

Suspension, red, phenytoin 30 mg/5 mL. Net price 100 mL = 71p. Label: 8, counselling, administration, blood or skin disorder symptoms (see above), driving (see notes above)

Note. Suspension of phenytoin 90 mg in 15 mL may be considered to be approximately equivalent in therapeutic effect to capsules or tablets containing phenytoin sodium 100 mg, but nevertheless care is needed in making changes

---

VALPROATE

Sodium valproate is effective in controlling tonic-clonic seizures, particularly in primary generalised epilepsy. It is a drug of choice in primary generalised epilepsy, generalised absences and myoclonic seizures, and may be tried in atypical absence, atonic, and tonic seizures. Controlled trials in partial epilepsy suggest that it has similar efficacy to that of carbamazepine and phenytoin. Plasma-valproate concentrations are not a useful index of efficacy, therefore routine monitoring is unhelpful. The drug has widespread metabolic effects, and may have dose-related side-effects. There has been concern over severe hepatic or pancreatic toxicity, although these effects are rare.

SODIUM VALPROATE

Indications: all forms of epilepsy

Cautions: monitor liver function before therapy and during first 6 months especially in patients most at risk (see also below), ensure no undue potential for bleeding before starting and before major surgery; severe renal impairment; pregnancy (**important** see notes above and Appendix 4 (neural tube screening)); breast-feeding; systemic lupus erythematosus; false-positive urine tests for ketones; avoid

sudden withdrawal; see also notes above; **interactions:** see p. 210 and Appendix 1 (valproate)

LIVER TOXICITY. Liver dysfunction (including fatal hepatic failure) has occurred in association with valproate (especially in children under 3 years of age and those with metabolic or degenerative disorders, organic brain disease or severe seizure disorders associated with mental retardation) usually in the first 6 months of therapy and usually involving multiple antiepileptic therapy (monotherapy preferred). Raised liver enzymes are not uncommon during valproate treatment and are usually transient but patients should be reassessed clinically and liver function (including prothrombin time) monitored until return to normal—an abnormally prolonged prothrombin time (particularly in association with other relevant abnormalities) requires discontinuation of treatment. Any concomitant use of salicylates should be stopped.

BLOOD OR HEPATIC DISORDERS. Patients or their carers should be told how to recognise signs of blood or liver disorders, and advised to seek immediate medical attention if symptoms develop (advice is given on patient information leaflet).

Contra-indications: active liver disease, family history of severe hepatic dysfunction, porphyria (section 9.8.2)

Side-effects: gastric irritation, nausea, ataxia and tremor; hyperammonaemia, increased appetite and weight gain; transient hair loss (regrowth may be curly), oedema, thrombocytopenia, and inhibition of platelet aggregation; impaired hepatic function leading rarely to fatal hepatic failure (see also under Cautions—withdraw treatment immediately if vomiting, anorexia, jaundice, drowsiness, or loss of seizure control occurs); rashes; sedation reported (rarely lethargy and confusion associated with too high an initial dose) and also increased alertness (occasionally aggression, hyperactivity and behavioural disturbances); rarely pancreatitis (measure plasma amylase in acute abdominal pain), leucopenia, pancytopenia, red cell hypoplasia, fibrinogen reduction; irregular periods, amenorrhoea, gynaecomastia, hearing loss, and vasculitis also reported

Dose: *by mouth*, initially, 600 mg daily given in 2 divided doses, preferably after food, increasing by 200 mg/day at 3-day intervals to a max. of 2.5 g daily in divided doses, usual maintenance 1–2 g daily (20–30 mg/kg daily); CHILD up to 20 kg, initially 20 mg/kg daily in divided doses, may be increased provided plasma concentrations monitored (above 40 mg/kg daily also monitor clinical chemistry and haematological parameters); over 20 kg, initially 400 mg daily in divided doses increased until control (usually in range of 20–30 mg/kg daily); max. 35 mg/kg daily

By intravenous injection (over 3–5 minutes) or *by intravenous infusion*, continuation of valproate treatment when oral therapy not possible, same as current dose by oral route

Initiation of valproate therapy (when oral valproate not possible), *by intravenous injection* (over 3–5 minutes), 400–800 mg (up to 10 mg/kg) followed by *intravenous infusion* up to max. 2.5 g daily; CHILD, usually 20–30 mg/kg daily, may be increased provided plasma concentrations monitored (above 40 mg/kg daily also monitor clinical chemistry and haematological parameters)

PoM **Sodium Valproate** (Non-proprietary)

Tablets, e/c, sodium valproate 200 mg, net price 20 = £1.18; 500 mg, 20 = £2.94. Label: 5, 8, 25, counselling, blood or hepatic disorder symptoms (see above), driving (see notes above)

Available from Cox, CP (Orlept®), Hillcross, Norton

Oral solution, sodium valproate 200 mg/5 mL. Net price 100 mL = £1.96. Label: 8, counselling, blood or hepatic disorder symptoms (see above), driving (see notes above)

Available from APS, CP, (Orlept®, sugar-free), Hillcross, Norton (sugar-free)

PoM **Epilim**® (Sanofi Winthrop)

Tablets (crushable), scored, sodium valproate 100 mg. Net price 20 = 78p. Label: 8, counselling, blood or hepatic disorder symptoms (see above), driving (see notes above)

Note. Sodium valproate crushable tablets also available from Hillcross

Tablets, both e/c, lilac, sodium valproate 200 mg, net price 20 = £1.28; 500 mg, 20 = £3.21. Label: 5, 8, 25, counselling, blood or hepatic disorder symptoms (see above), driving (see notes above)

Liquid, red, sugar-free, sodium valproate 200 mg/5 mL. Net price 300-mL pack = £5.89. Label: 8, counselling, blood or hepatic disorder symptoms (see above), driving (see notes above)

Syrup, red, sodium valproate 200 mg/5 mL. Net price 300-mL pack = £5.89. Label: 8, counselling, blood or hepatic disorder symptoms (see above), driving (see notes above)

PoM **Epilim Chrono**® (Sanofi Winthrop)

Tablets, m/r, all lilac, sodium valproate 200 mg (as sodium valproate and valproic acid), net price 100-tab pack = £7.70; 300 mg, 100-tab pack = £11.55; 500 mg, 100-tab pack = £19.25. Label: 8, 25, counselling, blood or hepatic disorder symptoms (see above), driving (see notes above)

Dose: ADULT and CHILD over 20 kg, as above, total daily dose given in 1–2 divided doses

PoM **Epilim**® **Intravenous** (Sanofi Winthrop)

Injection, powder for reconstitution, sodium valproate. Net price 400-mg vial (with 4-mL amp water for injections) = £8.77

Valproic acid

PoM **Convulex**® (Pharmacia & Upjohn)

Capsules, e/c, valproic acid 150 mg, net price 100-cap pack = £3.85; 300 mg, 100-cap pack = £7.70; 500 mg, 100-cap pack = £12.83. Label: 8, 25, counselling, blood or hepatic disorder symptoms (see above), driving (see notes above)

Dose: ADULT and CHILD initially 15 mg/kg daily in 2–4 divided doses, gradually increasing in steps of 5–10 mg/kg up to 30 mg/kg daily

EQUIVALENCE TO SODIUM VALPROATE. Manufacturer advises that Convulex® has a 1:1 dose relationship with products containing sodium valproate, but nevertheless care is needed in making changes.

VIGABATRIN

Vigabatrin is effective for use in chronic epilepsy not satisfactorily controlled by other antiepileptics. It is useful in tonic-clonic and partial seizures but has prominent behavioural side-effects in some patients.

VIGABATRIN

Indications: epilepsy not satisfactorily controlled by other antiepileptics, monotherapy for management of infantile spasms (West's syndrome)

Cautions: renal impairment; elderly; closely monitor neurological function; avoid sudden withdrawal (taper off over 2–4 weeks); history of psychosis or behavioural problems; **interactions:** see p. 210 and Appendix 1 (vigabatrin)

Contra-indications: pregnancy (see Appendix 4) and breast-feeding

Side-effects: drowsiness (rarely marked sedation, stupor, and confusion with non-specific slow wave EEG), fatigue, dizziness, nervousness, irritability, agitation, depression, abnormal thinking, headache, nystagmus, ataxia, tremor, paraesthesia, impaired concentration; less commonly confusion, aggression, psychosis, mania, memory disturbance, visual disturbance (e.g. diplopia); also weight gain, oedema, gastro-intestinal disturbances, alopecia, rash, urticaria; excitation and agitation in children; occasional increase in seizure frequency (especially if myoclonic), decrease in liver enzymes, slight decrease in haemoglobin; visual field defect, photophobia and retinal disorders (e.g. peripheral retinal atrophy) also reported

Dose: with current antiepileptic therapy, initially 1 g daily in single or 2 divided doses then increased according to response in steps of 500 mg; usual range 2–4 g daily—above 4 g daily (max. 6 g daily) only in exceptional circumstances with close monitoring for adverse effects; CHILD initially 40 mg/kg daily increased according to response to 80–100 mg/kg daily; *or* body-weight 10–15 kg, 0.5–1 g daily; body-weight 15–30 kg, 1–1.5 g daily; body-weight 30–50 kg, 1.5–3 g daily; body-weight over 50 kg, 2–4 g daily

Infantile spasms (West's syndrome), *monotherapy*, 60–100 mg/kg daily, adjusted according to response over 7 days; up to 150 mg/kg daily used with good tolerability

PoM **Sabril**® (Hoechst Marion Roussel)

Tablets, f/c, scored, vigabatrin 500 mg, net price 100-tab pack = £44.85. Label: 3, 8, counselling, driving (see notes above)

Powder, sugar-free, vigabatrin 500 mg/sachet. Net price 50-sachet pack = £24.33. Label: 3, 8, 13, counselling, driving (see notes above)

*Note.*The contents of a sachet should be dissolved in water or a soft drink immediately before taking

BENZODIAZEPINES

Clonazepam is occasionally used in tonic-clonic or partial seizures, but its sedative side-effects may be prominent. **Clobazam** may be used as adjunctive therapy in the treatment of epilepsy (section 4.1.2), but the effectiveness of these and other **benzodiazepines** may wane considerably after weeks or months of continuous therapy.

CLOBAZAM

Indications: adjunct in epilepsy; anxiety (short-term use)

Cautions; Contra-indications; Side-effects: see under Diazepam

Dose: epilepsy, 20–30 mg daily; max. 60 mg daily; CHILD over 3 years, not more than half adult dose

Anxiety, 20–30 mg daily in divided doses or as a single dose at bedtime, increased in severe anxiety (in hospital patients) to a max. of 60 mg daily in divided doses; ELDERLY (or debilitated) 10–20 mg daily

NHS¹ PoM **Clobazam** (Non-proprietary)

Tablets, clobazam 10 mg. Net price 30-tab pack = £9.98. Label: 2 *or* 19, 8, counselling, driving (see notes above)

1. Except for epilepsy and endorsed 'SLS'

Note. The brand name NHS *Frisium*® (Hoechst Marion Roussel) is used for clobazam tablets

CLONAZEPAM

Indications: all forms of epilepsy; myoclonus; status epilepticus, section 4.8.2

Cautions: see notes above; respiratory disease; hepatic and renal impairment; elderly and debilitated; pregnancy and breast-feeding (see notes above); avoid sudden withdrawal; porphyria (see section 9.8.2); **interactions:** see p. 210 and Appendix 1 (clonazepam)

DRIVING. Drowsiness may affect the performance of skilled tasks (e.g. driving); effects of alcohol enhanced

Contra-indications: respiratory depression; acute pulmonary insufficiency

Side-effects: drowsiness, fatigue, dizziness, muscle hypotonia, coordination disturbances; hypersalivation in infants, paradoxical aggression, irritability and mental changes; rarely, blood disorders, abnormal liver-function tests; **overdosage:** see Emergency Treatment of Poisoning, p. 23

Dose: 1 mg (elderly, 500 micrograms), initially at night for 4 nights, increased over 2–4 weeks to a usual maintenance dose of 4–8 mg daily in divided doses; CHILD up to 1 year 250 micrograms increased as above to 0.5–1 mg, 1–5 years 250 micrograms increased to 1–3 mg, 5–12 years 500 micrograms increased to 3–6 mg

PoM **Rivotril**® (Roche)

Tablets, both scored, clonazepam 500 micrograms (beige), net price 20 = 88p; 2 mg, 20 = £1.18. Label: 2, 8, counselling, driving (see notes above)

Injection, section 4.8.2

OTHER DRUGS

Acetazolamide, a carbonic anhydrase inhibitor, is a second-line drug for both tonic-clonic and partial seizures. It is occasionally helpful in atypical absence, atonic, and tonic seizures.

Piracetam (section 4.9.3) has been introduced recently as adjunctive treatment for myoclonus.

Gabapentin is a new antiepileptic which can be given as adjunctive therapy in partial epilepsy with or without secondary generalisation.

Topiramate is another new antiepileptic which can be given as adjunctive therapy in partial seizures with or without secondary generalisation.

ACETAZOLAMIDE

Indications: see notes above

Cautions; Side-effects: see section 11.6

Dose: 0.25–1 g daily in divided doses; CHILD 8–30 mg/kg daily; max. 750 mg daily

Preparations

See section 11.6

GABAPENTIN

Indications: adjunctive treatment of partial seizures with or without secondary generalisation not satisfactorily controlled with other antiepileptics

Cautions: avoid sudden withdrawal (taper off over at least 1 week); elderly (may need to reduce dose), renal impairment (reduce dose), false positive readings with some urinary protein tests; pregnancy and breast-feeding; **interactions:** Appendix 1 (gabapentin)

Side-effects: somnolence, dizziness, ataxia, fatigue, nystagmus, headache, tremor, diplopia, nausea and vomiting, rhinitis, amblyopia; also convulsions, pharyngitis, dysarthria, weight gain, dyspepsia, amnesia, nervousness, coughing; rarely pancreatitis, altered liver function tests, and Stevens-Johnson syndrome

Dose: 300 mg on first day, then 300 mg twice daily on second day, then 300 mg 3 times daily on third day, then increased according to response to 1.2 g daily (in 3 equally divided doses); if necessary may be further increased in steps of 300 mg daily (in 3 divided doses) to max. 2.4 g daily, usual range 0.9–1.2 g daily; max. period between doses should not exceed 12 hours; CHILD not recommended

▼ PoM **Neurontin**® (P-D)

Capsules, gabapentin 100 mg (white), net price 100-cap pack = £22.86; 300 mg (yellow), 100-cap pack = £53.00; 400 mg (orange), 100-cap pack = £61.33. Label: 3, 5, 8, counselling, driving (see notes above)

TOPIRAMATE

Indications: adjunctive treatment of partial seizures with or without secondary generalisation not satisfactorily controlled with other antiepileptics

Cautions: avoid abrupt withdrawal; ensure adequate hydration (especially if predisposition to nephrolithiasis); pregnancy (see notes above); renal impairment; **interactions:** see p. 210 and Appendix 1 (topiramate)

Contra-indications: breast-feeding

Side-effects: ataxia, impaired concentration, confusion, dizziness, fatigue, paraesthesia, somnolence, abnormal thinking, agitation, emotional lability (with abnormal behaviour), depression; nephrolithiasis (see Cautions); also amnesia, anorexia, aphasia, diplopia, nausea, nystagmus, speech disorder, taste alteration, abnormal vision, weight loss

Dose: initially 100 mg daily as a single dose for a week (lower dose may be used) *then* increased to 200 mg daily in 2 divided doses for a further week, *further dose increments* of 200 mg daily should be made at weekly intervals; usual dose 200–600 mg daily in 2 divided doses; max. 800 mg daily; CHILD not recommended

Note. If patient cannot tolerate titration regimen recommended above then smaller increments or longer interval between increments may be used

▼ PoM **Topamax**® (Janssen-Cilag)

Tablets, f/c, topiramate 25 mg, net price 60-tab pack = £22.02; 50 mg (light yellow), 60-tab pack = £36.17; 100 mg (yellow), 60-tab pack = £64.80; 200 mg (salmon), 60-tab pack £125.83. Label: 3, 8, counselling, driving (see notes above)

4.8.2 Drugs used in status epilepticus

Major status epilepticus should be *treated initially* with intravenous **diazepam,** used with caution because of the risk of respiratory depression; in situations where facilities for resuscitation are not immediately available, *small doses* of diazepam can be given intravenously or the drug can be administered as a rectal solution. Absorption from intramuscular injection or from suppositories is too slow for treatment of status epilepticus. When diazepam is given intravenously there may be a high risk of venous thrombophlebitis which is minimised by using an emulsion (Diazemuls®). **Clonazepam** and **lorazepam** are also used; lorazepam has the advantage of a long duration of action.

To *prevent recurrence* **phenytoin sodium** may be given by slow intravenous injection, with ECG monitoring in a dose of 15 mg/kg at a rate of not more than 50 mg/minute (in adults) followed by the maintenance dosage. Intramuscular use of phenytoin is not recommended (absorption is slow and erratic). Alternatively, **phenobarbitone sodium** (section 4.8.1) can be given by intravenous injection in a dose of 10–15 mg/kg at a rate of not more than 100 mg/minute. Other drugs which can be tried include **chlormethiazole** (clomethiazole) given by intravenous infusion. Chlormethiazole has a short half-life, and the rate of infusion can be titrated against the patient's clinical condition (see **cautions** on next page).

Paraldehyde also remains a valuable drug. Given rectally (or occasionally by deep intramuscular injection) it causes little respiratory depression and is therefore useful where facilities for resuscitation are poor.

If the above measures fail to control seizures, anaesthesia with **thiopentone** or **a non-barbiturate anaesthetic** should be instituted with full intensive care support.

DIAZEPAM

Indications: status epilepticus; convulsions due to poisoning (see Emergency Treatment of Poisoning); other indications, see sections 4.1.2, 10.2.2, 15.1.4.1

Cautions; Contra-indications; Side-effects: see section 4.1.2; hypotension and apnoea may occur; when given intravenously facilities for reversing respiratory depression with mechanical ventilation must be at hand (but see also notes above); intravenous infusion, see also below

SPECIAL CAUTIONS FOR INTRAVENOUS INFUSION. Intravenous infusion of diazepam is potentially hazardous (especially if prolonged), calling for close and constant observation and best carried out in specialist centres with intensive care facilities. Special cautions required on prolonged intravenous infusion are as for Chlormethiazole, p. 219

Dose: by intravenous injection, 10–20 mg at a rate of 0.5 mL (2.5 mg) per 30 seconds, repeated if necessary after 30–60 minutes; may be followed by *intravenous infusion* to max. 3 mg/kg over 24 hours; CHILD 200–300 micrograms/kg *or* 1 mg per year of age

By rectum as rectal solution, ADULT and CHILD over 10 kg 500 micrograms/kg; ELDERLY 250 micrograms/kg

PoM **Diazepam** (Non-proprietary)

Injection (solution), diazepam 5 mg/mL. See Appendix 6. Net price 2-mL amp = 25p

Available from CP, Roche (Valium®)

Injection (emulsion), diazepam 5 mg/mL (0.5%). See Appendix 6. Net price 2-mL amp = 76p

Available from Dumex (Diazemuls®)

Rectal tubes (= rectal solution), diazepam 2 mg/mL. Net price 1.25-mL (2.5-mg) tube = 90p, 2.5-mL (5-mg) tube = £1.27; 4 mg /mL, 2.5-mL (10-mg) tube = £1.62, 5-mL (20-mg) tube = £2.92

Available from CP (Diazepam Rectubes® 2.5 mg, 5 mg, 10 mg, 20 mg), Dumex (Stesolid® 5 mg, 10 mg), Lagap

Oral preparations, section 4.1.2

CLONAZEPAM

Indications: status epilepticus; other forms of epilepsy, and myoclonus, section 4.8.1

Cautions; Contra-indications; Side-effects: see section 4.8.1. Hypotension and apnoea may occur and resuscitation facilities must be available; intravenous infusion, see also below

SPECIAL CAUTIONS FOR INTRAVENOUS INFUSION. Intravenous infusion of clonazepam is potentially hazardous (especially if prolonged), calling for close and constant observation and best carried out in specialist centres with intensive care facilities. Special cautions required on prolonged intravenous infusion are as for Chlormethiazole, p. 219

Dose: by intravenous injection into a large vein (over 30 seconds) *or by intravenous infusion*, 1 mg, repeated if necessary; CHILD all ages, 500 micrograms

PoM **Rivotril®** (Roche)

Injection, clonazepam 1 mg/mL in solvent, for dilution with 1 mL water for injections immediately before injection or as described in Appendix 6. Net price 1-mL amp (with 1 mL water for injections) = 71p

Oral preparations, section 4.8.1

CHLORMETHIAZOLE
(Clomethiazole)

Indications: status epilepticus; other indications, see sections 4.1.1, 4.10, 15.1.4.1; eclampsia, see product literature

Cautions: see section 4.10 for general cautions; resuscitation facilities must be available; maintain clear airway (risk of mechanical obstruction in deep sedation); *rapid infusion* to be given only under direct medical supervision (risk of apnoea and hypotension—special care in those susceptible to cerebral or cardiac complications, e.g. the elderly); during *continuous infusion* sleep induced may lapse into deep unconsciousness and patient must be kept under close and constant observation; *prolonged infusion* may lead to accumulation and delay recovery, may also cause electrolyte imbalance (infusion contains only Na$^+$ 32 mmol/litre and no other electrolytes); **interactions:** Appendix 1 (anxiolytics and hypnotics)

LENNOX GASTAUT SYNDROME. Paradoxical worsening of epilepsy may occur in the Lennox Gastaut syndrome

Contra-indications: acute pulmonary insufficiency

Side-effects: nasal congestion and irritation (with sneezing), conjunctival irritation, headache; localised thrombophlebitis, tachycardia and transient fall in blood pressure (apnoea and hypotension on rapid infusion, see cautions); see also section 4.10

Dose: by intravenous infusion, as a 0.8% solution of chlormethiazole edisylate, initially 5–15 mL (40–120 mg)/minute up to a max. total dose of 40–100 mL (320–800 mg); may then be continued if necessary at a reduced rate according to response (see notes above); usual rate 0.5–1 mL (4–8 mg)/minute

CHILD   initially   0.01 mL   (80 micrograms)/kg/minute, then dose increased every 2–4 hours if necessary until seizures controlled or drowsiness occurs; if no seizure for 2 days dose gradually reduced every 4–6 hours (if seizures recur dose increased to previous level)

IMPORTANT. See cautions for intravenous infusion under Cautions (above)

PoM **Heminevrin®** (Astra)

Intravenous infusion 0.8%, chlormethiazole edisylate 8 mg/mL. Net price 500-mL bottle = £5.12

Oral preparations, section 4.10

LORAZEPAM

Indications: status epilepticus; other indications, section 4.1.2

Cautions; Contra-indications; Side-effects: see section 4.1.2; hypotension and apnoea may occur and resuscitation facilities must be available

Dose: by intravenous injection (into large vein), 4 mg; CHILD 2 mg

Preparations
Section 4.1.2

PARALDEHYDE

Indications: status epilepticus

Cautions: bronchopulmonary disease, hepatic impairment; avoid intramuscular injection near sciatic nerve (causes severe causalgia)

INTRAVENOUS INFUSION. Paraldehyde has been given by intravenous infusion (diluted in physiological saline) in specialist centres with intensive care facilities but this method of administration is no longer recommended

Side-effects: rashes; pain and sterile abscess after intramuscular injection; rectal irritation after enema

Dose: by deep intramuscular injection, as a single dose, 5–10 mL; usual max. 20 mL daily with not more than 5 mL at any one site; CHILD up to 3 months 0.5 mL, 3–6 months 1 mL, 6–12 months 1.5 mL, 1–2 years 2 mL, 3–5 years 3–4 mL, 6–12 years 5–6 mL

By intravenous infusion, formerly given in a dose of up to 4–5 mL diluted to a 4% solution with sodium chloride intravenous infusion 0.9%, but **no longer recommended**

By rectum, 5–10 mL, administered as a 10% enema in physiological saline (some centres mix paraldehyde with an equal volume of arachis (peanut) oil instead); CHILD as for intramuscular dose

Note. Do not use paraldehyde if it has a brownish colour or an odour of acetic acid. Avoid contact with rubber and plastics.

PoM **Paraldehyde** (Non-proprietary)

Injection, sterile paraldehyde 5-mL and 10-mL amp

Note. May temporarily be unavailable

PHENYTOIN SODIUM

Indications: status epilepticus; seizures in neurosurgery; arrhythmias, but now obsolete, see section 2.3.2

Cautions: hypotension and heart failure; resuscitation facilities must be available; injection solutions alkaline (irritant to tissues); see also section 4.8.1; **interactions:** see p. 210 and Appendix 1 (phenytoin)

Contra-indications: sinus bradycardia, sino-atrial block, and second- and third-degree heart block; Stokes-Adams syndrome; porphyria (section 9.8.2)

Side-effects: intravenous injection may cause cardiovascular and CNS depression (particularly if injection too rapid) with arrhythmias, hypotension, and cardiovascular collapse; alterations in respiratory function (including respiratory arrest)

Dose: *by slow intravenous injection or infusion* (with blood pressure and ECG monitoring), status epilepticus, 15 mg/kg at a rate not exceeding 50 mg per minute, as a loading dose (see also notes above). Maintenance doses of about 100 mg should be given thereafter at intervals of every 6–8 hours, monitored by measurement of plasma concentrations; rate and dose reduced according to weight; CHILD 15 mg/kg as a loading dose (neonate 15–20 mg/kg at rate of 1–3 mg/kg/minute)

Ventricular arrhythmias (but use now obsolete), *by intravenous injection* via caval catheter, 3.5–5 mg/kg at a rate not exceeding 50 mg/minute, with blood pressure and ECG monitoring; repeat once if necessary

Note. Phenytoin is now also licensed for administration by intravenous infusion (at the same rate of administration as the injection—not exceeding 50 mg/minute, for further details of the infusion, see Appendix 6). To avoid local venous irritation each injection or infusion should be both preceded and followed by an injection of sterile physiological saline through the same needle or catheter

By intramuscular injection, not recommended (see notes above)

PoM Epanutin Ready Mixed Parenteral® (P-D)
Injection, phenytoin sodium 50 mg/mL with propylene glycol 40% and alcohol 10% in water for injections. Net price 5-mL amp = £4.07
Note. Phenytoin injection also available from Antigen, Faulding DBL

Oral preparations, section 4.8.1

4.8.3   Febrile convulsions

Brief febrile convulsions need only simple treatment such as tepid sponging or bathing, or antipyretic medication, e.g. **paracetamol** (section 4.7.1). *Prolonged febrile convulsions* (those lasting 15 minutes or longer), *recurrent convulsions*, or those occurring in a child at known risk must be treated more actively, as there is the possibility of resulting brain damage. **Diazepam** is the drug of choice given either by slow intravenous injection in a dose of 250 micrograms/kg (section 4.8.2) or preferably rectally in solution (section 4.8.2) in a dose of 500 micrograms/kg (max. 10 mg), repeated if necessary. The rectal route is preferred as satisfactory absorption is achieved within minutes and administration is much easier. Suppositories are not suitable because absorption is too slow.

Intermittent prophylaxis (i.e. the anticonvulsant administered at the onset of fever) is possible in only a small proportion of children. Again **diazepam** is the treatment of choice, orally or rectally.

The exact role of continuous prophylaxis in children at risk from prolonged or complex febrile convulsions is controversial. It is probably indicated in only a small proportion of children, including those whose first seizure occurred at under 14 months or who have pre-existing neurological abnormalities or who have had previous prolonged or focal convulsions. Thus long-term anticonvulsant prophylaxis is rarely indicated.

4.9   Drugs used in parkinsonism and related disorders

4.9.1	Dopaminergic drugs used in parkinsonism
4.9.2	Antimuscarinic drugs used in parkinsonism
4.9.3	Drugs used in essential tremor, chorea, tics, and related disorders

In idiopathic Parkinson's disease, progressive degeneration of pigment-containing cells of the substantia nigra leads to deficiency of the neurotransmitter dopamine. This, in turn, results in a neurohumoral imbalance in the basal ganglia, causing the characteristic signs and symptoms of the illness to appear. The pathogenesis of this process is still obscure and current drug therapy aims simply to correct the imbalance. Although this approach fails to prevent the progression of the disease, it greatly improves the quality and expectancy of life of most patients.

The patient should be advised at the outset of the limitations of treatment and possible side-effects. About 10 to 20% of patients are unresponsive to treatment.

ELDERLY. Antiparkinsonian drugs carry a special risk of inducing confusion in the elderly. It is particularly important to initiate treatment with low doses and to use small increments.

4.9.1   Dopaminergic drugs used in parkinsonism

Levodopa, used with a **dopa-decarboxylase inhibitor**, is the treatment of choice for patients disabled by idiopathic Parkinson's disease. It is least valuable in elderly patients and in those with long-standing disease who may not tolerate a dose large enough to overcome their deficit. It is also less valuable in patients with post-encephalitic disease who are particularly susceptible to the side-effects. Parkinsonism caused by generalised degenerative brain disease does not normally respond to levodopa. It should not be used for neuroleptic-induced parkinsonism.

Levodopa, the amino-acid precursor of dopamine, acts mainly by replenishing depleted striatal dopamine. It improves bradykinesia and rigidity more than tremor. It is generally administered in conjunction with an extracerebral dopa-decarboxylase inhibitor which prevents the peripheral degradation of levodopa to dopamine but, unlike levodopa, does not cross the blood-brain barrier. Effective brain concentrations of dopamine can thereby be achieved with lower doses of levodopa. At the same time the reduced peripheral formation of dopamine decreases peripheral side-effects such as nausea and vomiting and cardiovascular effects. There is also less delay in onset of therapeutic effect and a smoother clinical response. A disadvantage is an increased incidence of abnormal involuntary movements.

The extracerebral dopa-decarboxylase inhibitors given with levodopa are benserazide (in **co-benel-dopa**) and carbidopa (in **co-careldopa**).

When co-careldopa 10/100 (10 mg of carbidopa for each 100 mg of levodopa) is used the dose of carbidopa may be insufficient to achieve full inhibition of extracerebral dopa-decarboxylase; co-careldopa 25/100 (25 mg of carbidopa for each 100 mg of levodopa) should then be used so that the daily dose of carbidopa is at least 75 mg.

Levodopa therapy should be initiated with low doses and gradually increased, by small increments, at intervals of 2 to 3 days. The final dose is usually a compromise between increased mobility and dose-limiting side-effects. Intervals between doses may be critical and should be chosen to suit the needs of the individual patient. Nausea and vomiting are rarely dose-limiting but doses should be taken after meals. Domperidone (section 4.6) may be useful in controlling vomiting. The most frequent dose-limiting side-effects of levodopa are involuntary movements and psychiatric complications. As the patient ages, the maintenance dose may need to be reduced.

During the first 6 to 18 months of levodopa therapy there may be a slow improvement in the response of the patient which is maintained for 1½ to 2 years; thereafter a slow decline may occur. Particularly troublesome is the 'on-off' effect the incidence of which increases as the treatment progresses. This is characterised by fluctuations in performance with normal performance during the 'on' period and weakness and akinesia lasting for 2 to 4 hours during the 'off' period.

'End-of-dose' deterioration may also occur where the duration of benefit after each dose becomes progressively shorter. Modified-release preparations may help with 'end-of-dose' deterioration or nocturnal immobility and rigidity.

Selegiline is a monoamine-oxidase-B inhibitor used in severe parkinsonism in conjunction with levodopa to reduce 'end-of-dose' deterioration. Early treatment with selegiline may delay the need for levodopa therapy but there is no convincing evidence that it delays disease progression. Selegiline given with levodopa may be associated with increased mortality in the longer term, but this remains to be confirmed. Selegiline need not necessarily be withdrawn from patients stabilised on treatment; sudden withdrawal of selegiline may exacerbate symptoms.

Tolcapone has recently been introduced for use as an adjunct to co-beneldopa or co-careldopa for patients who cannot be stabilised on these levodopa combinations or those who experience 'end-of-dose' deterioration; tolcapone increases the plasma-levodopa concentration.

The ergot derivatives, **bromocriptine**, **cabergoline**, **lysuride** (lisuride), and **pergolide** act by direct stimulation of surviving dopamine receptors. Although effective, they have no advantages over levodopa. They should be reserved for patients in whom levodopa alone is no longer adequate or who despite careful titration cannot tolerate levodopa. Ergot derivatives are sometimes useful in reducing 'off' periods and in ameliorating fluctuations in the later stage of Parkinson's disease. Their use is often limited by their side-effects and when used with levodopa, abnormal involuntary movements and confusional states are common; occasionally, ergot derivatives may cause neuropsychiatric effects and retroperitoneal fibrosis.

Ropinirole is a dopamine D_2 receptor agonist which improves the symptoms and signs in Parkinson's disease. Its side-effects are similar to those of bromocriptine. It is likely to be most useful as an adjunct to levodopa. The role of ropinirole and other dopamine agonists as initial therapy in Parkinson's disease remains controversial.

Amantadine has modest antiparkinsonian effects. It improves mild bradykinetic disabilities as well as tremor and rigidity. Unfortunately only a small proportion of patients derive much benefit from this drug and tolerance to its effects occurs. However it has the advantage of being relatively free from side-effects.

Apomorphine is a potent stimulator of D_1 and D_2 receptors, which is sometimes helpful in stabilising patients experiencing unpredictable 'off' periods with levodopa treatment. It is essential to establish patients on domperidone for three days before starting apomorphine. Long-term specialist supervision is advisable throughout apomorphine treatment.

LEVODOPA

Indications: parkinsonism (but not drug-induced extrapyramidal symptoms), see notes above

Cautions: pulmonary disease, peptic ulceration, cardiovascular disease, diabetes mellitus, osteomalacia, open-angle glaucoma, skin melanoma, psychiatric illness (avoid if severe). In prolonged therapy, psychiatric, hepatic, haematological, renal, and cardiovascular surveillance is advisable. Warn patients who benefit from therapy to resume normal activities gradually; avoid abrupt withdrawal; pregnancy (toxicity in *animals*) and breast-feeding; **interactions:** Appendix 1 (levodopa)

Contra-indications: closed-angle glaucoma

Side-effects: anorexia, nausea and vomiting, insomnia, agitation, postural hypotension (rarely labile hypertension), dizziness, tachycardia, arrhythmias, reddish discoloration of urine and other body fluids, rarely hypersensitivity; abnormal involuntary movements and psychiatric symptoms which include hypomania and psychosis may be dose-limiting; depression, drowsiness, headache, flushing, sweating, gastro-intestinal bleeding, peripheral neuropathy, and liver enzyme changes also reported; syndrome resembling neuroleptic malignant syndrome reported on withdrawal

Dose: initially 125–500 mg daily in divided doses after meals, increased according to response (but rarely used alone, see notes above)

PoM **Levodopa** (Cambridge)

Tablets, scored, levodopa 500 mg. Net price 20 = £4.22. Label: 14, 21

Note. The brand name Larodopa® was formerly used for levodopa tablets

CO-BENELDOPA

A mixture of benserazide hydrochloride and levodopa in mass proportions corresponding to 1 part of benserazide and 4 parts of levodopa

Indications; Cautions; Contra-indications; Side-effects: see under Levodopa and notes above

Dose: expressed as levodopa, initally 50 mg 3–4 times daily (100 mg 3 times daily in advanced disease), increased by 100 mg once or twice weekly according to response; usual maintenance dose 400–800 mg daily in divided doses after meals; ELDERLY initially 50 mg once or twice daily, increased by 50 mg every third or fourth day according to response

Note. When transferring patients from other levodopa preparations, the previous preparation should be discontinued 12 hours beforehand; 3 capsules co-beneldopa 25/100 (*Madopar 125*®) should be substituted for 2 g levodopa; if transferring from another levodopa/dopa-decarboxylase inhibitor preparation, initial dose, expressed as levodopa, should be 50 mg 3–4 times daily

PoM **Madopar**® (Roche)

Capsules 62.5, blue/grey, co-beneldopa 12.5/50 (benserazide 12.5 mg (as hydrochloride), levodopa 50 mg). Net price 100-cap pack = £7.76. Label: 14, 21

Capsules 125, blue/pink, co-beneldopa 25/100 (benserazide 25 mg (as hydrochloride), levodopa 100 mg). Net price 100-cap pack = £10.81. Label: 14, 21

Capsules 250, blue/caramel, co-beneldopa 50/200 (benserazide 50 mg (as hydrochloride), levodopa 200 mg). Net price 100-cap pack = £18.43. Label: 14, 21

Dispersible tablets 62.5, scored, co-beneldopa 12.5/50 (benserazide 12.5 mg (as hydrochloride), levodopa 50 mg). Net price 100-tab pack = £8.29. Label: 14, 21, counselling, administration, see below

Dispersible tablets 125, scored, co-beneldopa 25/100 (benserazide 25 mg (as hydrochloride) levodopa 100 mg). Net price 100-tab pack = £14.70. Label: 14, 21, counselling, administration, see below

Note. The tablets may be dispersed in water or orange squash (not orange juice) or swallowed whole

PoM **Madopar**® **CR** (Roche)

Capsules 125, m/r, dark green/light blue, co-beneldopa 25/100 (benserazide 25 mg (as hydrochloride), levodopa 100 mg). Net price 100-cap pack = £17.97. Label: 5, 14, 25

Dose: Patients not receiving levodopa therapy, initially 1 capsule 3 times daily (max. initial dose 6 capsules daily) Fluctuations in response related to plasma-levodopa concentration or to timing of dose, initially 1 capsule substituted for every 100 mg of levodopa and given at same dosage frequency, subsequently increased every 2–3 days according to response; average increase of 50%

needed over previous levodopa dose and titration may take up to 4 weeks

Supplementary dose of conventional *Madopar*® may be needed with first morning dose; if response still poor to total daily dose of *Madopar*® CR plus *Madopar*® corresponding to 1.2 g levodopa, consider alternative therapy

CO-CARELDOPA

A mixture of carbidopa and levodopa; the proportions are expressed in the form *x/y* where *x* and *y* are the strengths in milligrams of carbidopa and levodopa respectively

Indications; Cautions; Contra-indications; Side-effects: see under Levodopa and notes above

Dose: expressed as levodopa, initially 100 mg (with carbidopa 25 mg, as *Sinemet-Plus*®) 3 times daily, increased by 50–100 mg (with carbidopa 12.5–25 mg, as *Sinemet LS*® or *Sinemet-Plus*®) daily or on alternate days acccording to response, up to 800 mg (with carbidopa 200 mg) daily in divided doses

Note. Carbidopa 70–100 mg daily is necessary to achieve full inhibition of peripheral dopa-decarboxylase

Alternatively, initially 50–100 mg (with carbidopa 10–12.5 mg, as *Sinemet LS*® or *Sinemet-110*®) 3–4 times daily, increased by 50–100 mg daily or on alternate days acccording to response, up to 800 mg (with carbidopa 80–100 mg) daily in divided doses

Alternatively, initially 125 mg (with carbidopa 12.5 mg, as ½ tablet of *Sinemet-275*®) 1–2 times daily, increased by 125 mg (with carbidopa 12.5 mg) daily or on alternate days acccording to response

Note. When transferring patients from levodopa, 1 tablet co-careldopa 25/250 (*Sinemet-275*®) 3–4 times daily should be substituted for patients receiving more than 1.5 g levodopa daily; 1 tablet co-careldopa 25/100 (*Sinemet-Plus*®) 3–4 times daily should be substituted for patients receiving less than 1.5 g levodopa daily; the levodopa should be discontinued 12 hours beforehand (24 hours for modified-release preparations)

PoM **Sinemet**® (Du Pont)

Tablets (*Sinemet-110*®), blue, scored, co-careldopa 10/100 (carbidopa 10 mg (as monohydrate), levodopa 100 mg). Net price 20 = £1.71. Label: 14, 21

Tablets (*Sinemet-275*®), blue, scored, co-careldopa 25/250 (carbidopa 25 mg (as monohydrate), levodopa 250 mg). Net price 20 = £3.57. Label: 14, 21

PoM **Sinemet LS**® (Du Pont)

Tablets, yellow, scored, co-careldopa 12.5/50 (carbidopa 12.5 mg (as monohydrate), levodopa 50 mg). Net price 84-tab pack = £6.87. Label: 14, 21

Note. 2 tablets *Sinemet LS*® ≡ 1 tablet *Sinemet Plus*®

PoM **Sinemet-Plus**® (Du Pont)

Tablets, yellow, scored, co-careldopa 25/100 (carbidopa 25 mg (as monohydrate), levodopa 100 mg). Net price 20 = £2.52. Label: 14, 21

Note. The daily dose of carbidopa required to achieve full inhibition of extracerebral dopa-decarboxylase is 75 mg; co-careldopa 25/100 provides an adequate dose of carbidopa when low doses of levodopa are needed

Modified release

PoM Half Sinemet® CR (Du Pont)

Tablets, m/r, pink, co-careldopa 25/100 (carbidopa 25 mg (as monohydrate), levodopa 100 mg). Net price 56-tab pack = £18.56. Label: 14, 25

Dose: for fine adjustment of *Sinemet® CR* dose (see below)

PoM Sinemet® CR (Du Pont)

Tablets, m/r, peach, co-careldopa 50/200 (carbidopa 50 mg (as monohydrate), levodopa 200 mg). Net price 56-tab pack = £21.84. Label: 14, 25

Dose: initial treatment or fluctuations in response to conventional levodopa therapy, 1 *Sinemet® CR* tablet twice daily; both dose and interval then adjusted according to response at intervals of not less than 3 days; if transferring from existing levodopa therapy withdraw 8 hours beforehand; 1 tablet *Sinemet® CR* twice daily can be substituted for a daily dose of levodopa 300–400 mg in conventional *Sinemet®* tablets

AMANTADINE HYDROCHLORIDE

Indications: Parkinson's disease (but not drug-induced extrapyramidal symptoms); antiviral, see section 5.3

Cautions: hepatic, or renal impairment (avoid if severe), congestive heart disease (may exacerbate oedema), confused or hallucinatory states, elderly; avoid abrupt discontinuation in Parkinson's disease; **interactions:** Appendix 1 (amantadine)

DRIVING. May affect performance of skilled tasks (e.g. driving)

Contra-indications: epilepsy, history of gastric ulceration, severe renal impairment; pregnancy (toxicity in *animals*), breast-feeding

Side-effects: anorexia, nausea, nervousness, inability to concentrate, insomnia, dizziness, convulsions, hallucinations or feelings of detachment, blurred vision, gastro-intestinal disturbances, livedo reticularis and peripheral oedema; rarely leucopenia, rashes

Dose: 100 mg daily increased after one week to 100 mg twice daily (not later than 4 p.m.), usually in conjunction with other treatment

ELDERLY over 65 years, less than 100 mg daily *or* 100 mg at intervals of more than 1 day

PoM Symmetrel® (Novartis)

Capsules, red-brown, amantadine hydrochloride 100 mg. Net price 56-cap pack = £10.41. Counselling, driving

Syrup, amantadine hydrochloride 50 mg/5 mL. Net price 150-mL pack = £3.49. Counselling, driving

APOMORPHINE HYDROCHLORIDE

Indications: refractory motor fluctuations in Parkinson's disease ('off' episodes) inadequately controlled by levodopa or other dopaminergics (for capable and motivated patients under specialist supervision)

Cautions: tendency to nausea and vomiting; pulmonary, cardiovascular or endocrine disease, renal impairment; elderly and debilitated, history of postural hypotension (special care on initiation); hepatic, haemopoietic, renal, and cardiovascular monitoring; *on administration with levodopa* test initially and every 6 months for haemolytic anaemia (development calls for specialist haematological care with dose reduction and possible discontinuation); **interactions:** Appendix 1 (apomorphine)

Contra-indications: respiratory or CNS depression, hypersensitiviy to opioids; neuropsychiatric problems or dementia; not suitable if 'on' response to levodopa marred by severe dyskinesia, hypotonia or psychiatric effects; pregnancy and breast-feeding

Side-effects: dyskinesias during 'on' periods (may require discontinuation); postural instability and falls (impaired speech and balance may not improve), increasing cognitive impairment, personality change and disabling dyskinesias during 'on' phase; nausea and vomiting (see below under Dose); confusion and hallucinations (if continued, specialist observation required with possible gradual dose reduction), sedation, postural hypotension; also euphoria, light-headedness, restlessness, tremors; haemolytic anaemia with levodopa (see Cautions) and rarely eosinophilia; local reactions common (include nodule formation and possible ulceration)—rotate injection sites, dilute with sodium chloride 0.9%, consider ultrasound, ensure no infection

Dose: ADULT over 18 years, *by subcutaneous injection*, usual range (after initiation as below) 3–30 mg daily in divided doses; subcutaneous infusion may be preferable in those requiring division of injections into more than 10 doses daily; max. single dose 10 mg; ADOLESCENT (under 18 years) and CHILD not recommended

By continuous subcutaneous infusion (those requiring division into more than 10 injections daily) initially 1 mg/hour daily increased according to response (not more often than every 4 hours) in max. steps of 500 micrograms/hour to max. 4 mg/hour (15–60 micrograms/kg/hour); change infusion site every 12 hours and give during waking hours only (24-hour infusions not advised unless severe night-time symptoms)—intermittent bolus boosts also usually needed (in those with severe dyskinesias only when absolutely necessary)

Total daily dose by either route (or combined routes) max. 100 mg

REQUIREMENTS FOR INITIATION. *Hospital admission* and at least 3 days of pretreatment with domperidone, *after at least 3 days* withhold existing antiparkinsonian medication overnight to provoke 'off' episode, *determine* threshold dose, *re-establish* other antiparkinsonian drugs, *determine* effective apomorphine regimen, *teach* to administer by subcutaneous injection into lower abdomen or outer thigh at first sign of 'off' episode, *discharge* from hospital, *monitor* frequently and *adjust* dosage regimen as appropriate (domperidone may normally be withdrawn over several weeks or longer)—for full details of initiation requirements see product literature

PoM Britaject® (Britannia)

Injection, apomorphine hydrochloride 10 mg/mL, net price 2-mL amp = £7.95, 5-mL amp = £15.95; 3-mL pen injector = £25.95

BROMOCRIPTINE

Indications: parkinsonism (but not drug-induced extrapyramidal symptoms); endocrine disorders, section 6.7.1

Cautions; Side-effects: section 6.7.1

Dose: first week 1–1.25 mg at night, second week 2–2.5 mg at night, third week 2.5 mg twice daily, fourth week 2.5 mg 3 times daily then increasing by 2.5 mg every 3–14 days according to response to a usual range of 10–40 mg daily; taken with food

Preparations

See section 6.7.1

CABERGOLINE

Indications: adjunct to levodopa (with dopa-decarboxylase inhibitor) in Parkinson's disease; endocrine disorders, section 6.7.1

Cautions; Contra-indications; Side-effects: section 6.7.1

HYPOTENSIVE REACTIONS. Hypotensive reactions may be disturbing in some patients during the first few days of treatment and particular care should be exercised when driving or operating machinery; tolerance may be reduced by alcohol

Dose: initially 1 mg daily, increased by increments of 0.5–1 mg at 7 or 14 day intervals; usual range 2–6 mg daily

Note. Concurrent dose of levodopa may be decreased gradually while dose of cabergoline is increased

▼ PoM **Cabaser®** (Pharmacia & Upjohn)
Tablets, all scored, cabergoline 1 mg, net price 20-tab pack = £79.00; 2 mg, 20-tab pack = £79.00; 4 mg, 16-tab pack = £63.20. Label: 21, counselling, hypotensive reactions
Note. Dispense in original container (contains desiccant)

LYSURIDE MALEATE
(Lisuride Maleate)

Indications: Parkinson's disease

Cautions: history of pituitary tumour; history of psychotic disturbance; pregnancy; porphyria (section 9.8.2); **interactions:** Appendix 1 (lysuride)

HYPOTENSIVE REACTIONS. Hypotensive reactions may be disturbing in some patients during the first few days of treatment and particular care should be exercised when driving or operating machinery

Contra-indications: severe disturbances of peripheral circulation; coronary insufficiency

Side-effects: see notes above; nausea and vomiting; dizziness; headache, lethargy, malaise, drowsiness, psychotic reactions (including hallucinations); occasionally severe hypotension, rashes; rarely abdominal pain and constipation; Raynaud's phenomenon reported

Dose: initially 200 micrograms at bedtime with food increased as necessary at weekly intervals to 200 micrograms twice daily (midday and bedtime) then to 200 micrograms 3 times daily (morning, midday, and bedtime); further increases made by adding 200 micrograms each week first to the bedtime dose, then to the midday dose and finally to the morning dose; max. 5 mg daily in 3 divided doses after food

PoM **Revanil®** (Cambridge)
Tablets, scored, lysuride maleate 200 micrograms. Net price 100-tab pack = £24.00. Label: 21, counselling, hypotensive reactions

PERGOLIDE

Indications: adjunct to levodopa in Parkinson's disease

Cautions: arrhythmias or underlying cardiac disease, history of confusion or hallucinations, dyskinesia (may cause or exacerbate), pregnancy, breast-feeding; increase dose gradually and avoid abrupt withdrawal; porphyria (section 9.8.2); **interactions:** Appendix 1 (pergolide)

HYPOTENSIVE REACTIONS. Hypotensive reactions may be disturbing in some patients during the first few days of treatment and particular care should be exercised when driving or operating machinery

Side-effects: see notes above; hallucinations, confusion, dizziness, dyskinesia, somnolence, abdominal pain, nausea, dyspepsia, diplopia, rhinitis, dyspnoea, pleuritis, pleural effusion, pleural fibrosis, pericarditis, pericardial effusion and retroperitoneal fibrosis, insomnia, constipation or diarrhoea, hypotension, syncope, tachycardia and atrial premature contractions, rash, fever reported; neuroleptic malignant syndrome also reported

Dose: 50 micrograms daily for 2 days, increased gradually by 100–150 micrograms every third day over next 12 days, usually given in 3 divided doses; further increases of 250 micrograms every third day; usual maintenance 3 mg daily (above 5 mg daily not evaluated); during pergolide titration levodopa dose may be reduced cautiously

PoM **Celance®** (Lilly)
Tablets, all scored, pergolide (as mesylate) 50 micrograms (ivory), net price 100-tab pack = £40.34; 250 micrograms (green), 100-tab pack = £60.85; 1 mg (pink), 100-tab pack = £219.62; 14-day starter pack of 75 × 50-microgram tablets with 6 × 250-microgram tablets = £33.57. Counselling, hypotensive reactions

ROPINIROLE

Indications: Parkinson's disease, see notes above

Cautions: severe cardiovascular disease, major psychotic disorders, avoid abrupt withdrawal; **interactions:** Appendix 1 (ropinirole)

DRIVING. May affect performance of skilled tasks (e.g. driving)

Contra-indications: hepatic and severe renal impairment; pregnancy and breast-feeding

Side-effects: nausea, somnolence, leg oedema, abdominal pain, vomiting and syncope; dyskinesia, hallucinations and confusion reported in adjunctive therapy; occasionally severe hypotension and bradycardia

Dose: initially 750 micrograms daily in 3 divided doses, increased by increments of 750 micrograms at weekly intervals to 3 mg daily; further increased by increments of up to 3 mg at weekly intervals according to response; usual range 3–9 mg daily (but higher doses may be required if used with levodopa); max. 24 mg daily
Note. When administered as adjunct to levodopa, concurrent dose of levodopa may be reduced by approx. 20%

▼ PoM **Requip**® (SmithKline Beecham)
Tablets, all f/c, ropinirole (as hydrochloride) 250 micrograms, net price 210-tab pack = £39.20; 1 mg (green), 84-tab pack = £46.20; 2 mg (pink), 84-tab pack = £92.40; 5 mg (blue), 84-tab pack = £184.80. Label: 2, 21

SELEGILINE

Indications: Parkinson's disease or symptomatic parkinsonism (but not drug-induced extrapyramidal symptoms), either used alone (in early disease) or as an adjunct to levodopa therapy (but see notes above)

Cautions: peptic ulceration, uncontrolled hypertension, arrhythmias, angina, psychosis, pregnancy and breast-feeding, side-effects of levodopa may be increased, concurrent levodopa dosage may need to be reduced by 20–50%; **interactions:** Appendix 1 (selegiline)

Side-effects: hypotension, nausea and vomiting, confusion or psychosis, agitation, dry mouth, liver enzyme disturbances, sleep disturbances; difficulty in micturition and skin reactions reported

Dose: 10 mg in the morning, or 5 mg at breakfast and midday; ELDERLY see below

ELDERLY. To avoid initial confusion and agitation, it may be appropriate to start treatment with a dose of 2.5 mg daily, particularly in the elderly

PoM **Selegiline Hydrochloride** (Non-proprietary)
Tablets, selegiline hydrochloride 5 mg, net price 60-tab pack = £17.07; 10 mg, 30-tab pack = £16.41
Available from APTA Medica (Virapryl®), Berk (Stil line®), Bioglan, Cox, Hillcross, Lagap, Norton, Opus (Centrapryl®), Sanofi Winthrop

PoM **Eldepryl**® (Orion)
Tablets, both scored, selegiline hydrochloride 5 mg, net price 60-tab pack = £28.08; 10 mg, 30-tab pack = £27.20
Oral liquid, selegiline hydrochloride 10 mg/5 mL, net price 200-mL = £37.44

TOLCAPONE

Indications: adjunct to levodopa (with dopa-decarboxylase inhibitor) in Parkinson's disease

Cautions: severe renal impairment; moderate hepatic impairment (Appendix 2); monitor hepatic transaminases when starting treatment and monthly for 6 months (discontinue if hepatic transaminases significantly elevated or jaundice develops); pregnancy; **interactions:** Appendix 1 (tolcapone)

Contra-indications: breast-feeding

Side-effects: diarrhoea, nausea, dyskinesia, sleep disorders, anorexia; intensification of urine colour; increase in levodopa-associated side-effects

Dose: initially 100 mg 3 times daily, adjusted according to response up to max. of 200 mg 3 times daily

Note. The first daily dose should be taken at the same time as the levodopa-containing preparation; most patients receiving more than levodopa 600 mg daily require reduction of levodopa dose

▼ PoM **Tasmar**® (Roche)
Tablets, f/c, tolcapone 100 mg (pale yellow), net price 100-tab pack = £95.20; 200 mg (orange), 100-tab pack = £147.05. Label: 14, 25

4.9.2 Antimuscarinic drugs used in parkinsonism

Antimuscarinic drugs (less correctly termed 'anticholinergics') are the other main class of drugs used in Parkinson's disease. They are less effective than levodopa in idiopathic Parkinson's disease although they often usefully supplement its action. Patients with mild symptoms, particularly where tremor predominates, may be treated initially with antimuscarinic drugs (alone or with selegiline, section 4.9.1), levodopa being added or substituted as symptoms progress. They have value in post-encephalitic parkinsonism.

Antimuscarinic drugs exert their antiparkinsonian effect by correcting the relative central cholinergic excess thought to occur in parkinsonism as a result of dopamine deficiency. In most patients their effects are only moderate, reducing tremor and rigidity to some effect but without significant action on bradykinesia. They exert a synergistic effect when used with levodopa and are also useful in reducing sialorrhoea.

The antimuscarinic drugs also reduce the symptoms of drug-induced parkinsonism as seen, for example, with antipsychotic drugs (section 4.2.1) but there is no justification for giving them simultaneously with antipsychotics unless parkinsonian side effects occur. Tardive dyskinesia is not improved by the antimuscarinic drugs and may be made worse.

No important differences exist between the many synthetic antimuscarinic drugs available but some patients appear to tolerate one better than another. They may be taken before food if dry mouth is troublesome, or after food if gastro-intestinal symptoms predominate. Those most commonly used are **orphenadrine** and **benzhexol** (trihexyphenidyl); **benztropine** and **procyclidine** are also used. Benztropine is similar to benzhexol but is excreted more slowly; changes in dose therefore need to be carried out very gradually. Both procyclidine and benztropine may be given parenterally and are effective emergency treatment for acute drug-induced dystonic reactions which may be severe.

BENZHEXOL HYDROCHLORIDE
(Trihexyphenidyl Hydrochloride)

Indications: parkinsonism; drug-induced extrapyramidal symptoms (but not tardive dyskinesia, see notes above)

Cautions: cardiovascular disease, hepatic or renal impairment; elderly; avoid abrupt discontinuation of treatment; liable to abuse; **interactions:** Appendix 1 (antimuscarinics)

DRIVING. May affect performance of skilled tasks (e.g. driving)

Contra-indications: untreated urinary retention, closed-angle glaucoma, gastro-intestinal obstruction

Side-effects: dry mouth, gastro-intestinal disturbances, dizziness, blurred vision; less commonly urinary retention, tachycardia, hypersensitivity, nervousness, and with high doses in susceptible patients, mental confusion, excitement, and psychiatric disturbances which may necessitate discontinuation of treatment

Dose: 1 mg daily, gradually increased; usual maintenance dose 5–15 mg daily in 3–4 divided doses; ELDERLY preferably lower end of range

PoM **Benzhexol** (Non-proprietary)
Tablets, both scored, benzhexol hydrochloride 2 mg, net price 20 = 36p; 5 mg, 20 = 70p. Counselling, before or after food (see notes above), driving
Available from Genus
Note. The brand name *Artane*® was formerly used
PoM **Broflex**® (Bioglan)
Syrup, pink, benzhexol hydrochloride 5 mg/5 mL. Net price 200-mL pack = £6.36. Counselling, before or after food (see notes above), driving

BENZTROPINE MESYLATE
(Benzatropine Mesilate)
Indications; Cautions; Contra-indications; Side-effects: see under Benzhexol Hydrochloride, but causes sedation rather than stimulation; avoid in children under 3 years
Dose: by mouth, 0.5–1 mg daily usually at bedtime, gradually increased; max. 6 mg daily; usual maintenance dose 1–4 mg daily in single or divided doses; ELDERLY preferably lower end of range
By intramuscular or intravenous injection, 1–2 mg, repeated if symptoms reappear; ELDERLY preferably lower end of range

PoM **Cogentin**® (MSD)
Tablets, scored, benztropine mesylate 2 mg. Net price 20 = 29p. Label: 2
Injection, benztropine mesylate 1 mg/mL. Net price 2-mL amp = 92p

BIPERIDEN
Indications; Cautions; Contra-indications; Side-effects: see under Benzhexol Hydrochloride, but may cause drowsiness; injection may cause hypotension
Dose: by mouth, biperiden hydrochloride 1 mg twice daily, gradually increased to 2 mg 3 times daily; usual maintenance dose 3–12 mg daily in divided doses; ELDERLY preferably lower end of range
By intramuscular or slow intravenous injection, biperiden lactate 2.5–5 mg up to 4 times daily; ELDERLY preferably lower end of range

PoM **Akineton**® (Knoll)
Tablets, scored, biperiden hydrochloride 2 mg. Net price 100-tab pack = £4.60. Label: 2
Injection, biperiden lactate 5 mg/mL. Net price 1-mL amp = 69p

ORPHENADRINE HYDROCHLORIDE
Indications; Cautions; Contra-indications; Side-effects: see under Benzhexol Hydrochloride, but more euphoric; may cause insomnia; porphyria (see section 9.8.2)
Dose: 150 mg daily in divided doses, gradually increased; max. 400 mg daily; ELDERLY preferably lower end of range

PoM **Orphenadrine Hydrochloride** (Non-proprietary)
Oral solution, orphenadrine hydrochloride 50mg/5 mL. Net price 200-mL = £7.25. Counselling, driving
Available from Rosemont (sugar-free)
PoM **Biorphen**® (Bioglan)
Elixir, sugar-free, orphenadrine hydrochloride 25 mg/5 mL. Net price 200-mL pack = £7.25. Counselling, driving
PoM **Disipal**® (Yamanouchi)
Tablets, yellow, s/c, orphenadrine hydrochloride 50 mg. Net price 20 = 50p. Counselling, driving
Additives: include tartrazine

PROCYCLIDINE HYDROCHLORIDE
Indications; Cautions; Contra-indications; Side-effects: see under Benzhexol Hydrochloride
Dose: by mouth, 2.5 mg 3 times daily, gradually increased if necessary; usual max. 30 mg daily (60 mg daily in exceptional circumstances); ELDERLY preferably lower end of range
Acute dystonia, *by intramuscular injection,* 5–10 mg repeated if necessary after 20 minutes; max. 20 mg daily; *by intravenous injection,* 5 mg (usually effective within 5 minutes); an occasional patient may need 10 mg or more and may require up to half an hour to obtain relief; ELDERLY preferably lower end of dose range

PoM **Procyclidine** (Non-proprietary)
Tablets, procyclidine hydrochloride 5 mg. Net price 20 = £1.11. Counselling, driving
PoM **Arpicolin**® (Rosemont)
Syrup, sugar-free, procyclidine hydrochloride 2.5 mg/5 mL, net price 200-mL pack = £5.70; 5 mg/5 mL, 200-mL pack = £10.20. Counselling, driving
PoM **Kemadrin**® (GlaxoWellcome)
Tablets, scored, procyclidine hydrochloride 5 mg. Net price 20 = £1.17. Counselling, driving
Injection, procyclidine hydrochloride 5 mg/mL. Net price 2-mL amp = £1.49

4.9.3   Drugs used in essential tremor, chorea, tics, and related disorders

Tetrabenazine is mainly used to control movement disorders in Huntington's chorea and related disorders. It may act by depleting nerve endings of dopamine. It has useful action in only a proportion of patients and its use may be limited by the development of depression.

Haloperidol may be useful in improving motor tics and symptoms of Gilles de la Tourette syndrome and related choreas. **Pimozide** (see sec-

---

tion 4.2.1 for CSM warning) and more recently **clonidine** (section 4.7.4.2) and **sulpiride** (section 4.2.1), are also used in Gilles de la Tourette syndrome. **Benzhexol** (section 4.9.2) at high dosage may also improve some movement disorders. It is sometimes necessary to build the dose up over many weeks, to 20 to 30 mg daily or higher. **Chlorpromazine** and **haloperidol** are used to relieve intractable hiccup (section 4.2.1).

Propranolol or another beta-adrenoceptor blocking drug (section 2.4) may be useful in treating essential tremor or tremors associated with anxiety or thyrotoxicosis. Propranolol is given in a dosage of 40 mg 2 or 3 times daily, increased if necessary; 80 to 160 mg daily is usually required for maintenance.

Primidone in some cases provides relief from benign essential tremor; the dose is increased slowly to reduce side-effects.

Piracetam has been introduced recently as adjunctive treatment for myoclonus of cortical origin.

Riluzole has been introduced recently to extend life or the time to mechanical ventilation in patients with amyotrophic lateral sclerosis. Treatment should only be initiated by physicians experienced in treating motor neurone disease.

HALOPERIDOL

Indications: motor tics, adjunctive treatment in choreas and Gilles de la Tourette syndrome; other indications, section 4.2.1

Cautions; Contra-indications; Side-effects: section 4.2.1

Dose: by mouth, 0.5–1.5 mg 3 times daily adjusted according to the response; 10 mg daily or more may occasionally be necessary in Gilles de la Tourette syndrome; CHILD, Gilles de la Tourette syndrome up to 10 mg daily

Preparations
Section 4.2.1

PIRACETAM

Indications: adjunctive treatment of cortical myoclonus

Cautions: avoid abrupt withdrawal; elderly; renal impairment (avoid if severe)

Contra-indications: hepatic and severe renal impairment; pregnancy and breast-feeding

Side-effects: diarrhoea, weight gain; somnolence, insomnia, nervousness, depression; hyperkinesia; rash

Dose: initially 7.2 g daily in 2–3 divided doses, increased according to response by 4.8 g daily every 3–4 days to max. 20 g daily (subsequently, attempts should be made to reduce dose of concurrent therapy); CHILD under 16 years not recommended

ORAL SOLUTION. Follow the oral solution with a glass of water (or soft drink) to reduce bitter taste.

▼ PoM **Nootropil**® (UCB Pharma)
Tablets, f/c, scored, piracetam 800 mg, net price 90-tab pack = £15.80; 1.2 g, 56-tab pack = £14.74. Label: 3
Oral solution, piracetam, 333.3 mg/mL, net price 300-mL pack = £21.93. Label: 3

PRIMIDONE

Indications: essential tremor; epilepsy, see section 4.8.1

Cautions; Contra-indications; Side-effects: section 4.8.1

Dose: essential tremor, initially 50 mg daily increased gradually over 2–3 weeks according to response; max. 750 mg daily

Preparations
Section 4.8.1

RILUZOLE

Indications: to extend life or the time to mechanical ventilation for patients with amyotrophic lateral sclerosis, initiated by specialist physicians experienced in the management of motor neurone disease

Cautions: history of abnormal hepatic function (see product literature for details); **interactions:** Appendix 1 (riluzole)

BLOOD DISORDERS. Patients or their carers should be told how to recognise signs of neutropenia and advised to seek immediate medical attention if symptoms such as fever occur; white blood cell counts should be determined in febrile illness: neutropenia requires discontinuation of riluzole

DRIVING. Dizziness or vertigo may affect performance of skilled tasks (e.g. driving)

Contra-indications: hepatic and renal impairment; pregnancy and breast-feeding

Side-effects: nausea, vomiting, asthenia, tachycardia, somnolence, headache, dizziness, vertigo, pain, paraesthesia, alterations in liver function tests

Dose: 50 mg twice daily; CHILD not recommended

▼ PoM **Rilutek**® (Rhône-Poulenc Rorer)
Tablets, f/c, riluzole 50 mg. Net price 56-tab pack = £286.00. Counselling, blood disorders, driving

TETRABENAZINE

Indications: movement disorders due to Huntington's chorea, senile chorea, and related neurological conditions

Cautions: pregnancy; avoid in breast-feeding; **interactions:** Appendix 1 (tetrabenazine)

DRIVING. May affect performance of skilled tasks (e.g. driving)

Side-effects: drowsiness, gastro-intestinal disturbances, depression, extrapyramidal dysfunction, hypotension

Dose: initially 12.5 mg twice daily (elderly 12.5 mg daily) gradually increased to 12.5–25 mg 3 times daily; max. 200 mg daily

PoM **Tetrabenazine** (Cambridge)

Tablets, pale yellow-buff, scored, tetrabenazine 25 mg. Net price 120-tab pack = £17.71. Label: 2

Note. The brand name Nitoman® was formerly used for tetrabenazine preparations

---

TORSION DYSTONIAS AND OTHER INVOLUNTARY MOVEMENTS

BOTULINUM A TOXIN-HAEMAGGLUTININ COMPLEX

Indications: see under preparations below

Cautions: as a biological product bear in mind potential for anaphylaxis; do not give with (or before) aminoglycoside antibiotics or spectinomycin; other specific cautions, see below; other **interactions:** Appendix 1 (botulinum toxin)

SPECIFIC CAUTIONS WHEN TREATING BLEPHAROSPASM OR HEMIFACIAL SPASM. Avoid deep or misplaced injections—relevant anatomy (and any alterations due to previous surgery) must be understood before injecting; reduced blinking can lead to corneal exposure, persistent epithelial defect and corneal ulceration (especially in those with VIIth nerve disorders)—careful testing of corneal sensation in previously operated eyes, avoidance of injection in lower lid area and vigorous treatment of epithelial defect needed

SPECIFIC CAUTIONS WHEN TREATING TORTICOLLIS. Only for specialists experienced in diagnosis and management of torticollis and who have received training (provided by Speywood) in administering Dysport®; patients with defective neuromuscular transmission (risk of excessive muscle weakness)

COUNSELLING. All patients should be alerted to possible side-effects

Contra-indications: generalised disorders of muscle activity (e.g. myasthenia gravis); pregnancy and breast-feeding

Side-effects: increased electrophysiologic jitter in some distant muscles; misplaced injections may paralyse nearby muscle groups and excessive doses may paralyse distant muscles; rash; antibody formation (substantial deterioration in response); transient burning sensation after injection

SPECIFIC SIDE-EFFECTS WHEN TREATING BLEPHAROSPASM OR HEMIFACIAL SPASM. Ptosis, lacrimation and irritation (including dry eye, lagophthalmos and photophobia); also ectropion, keratitis, diplopia and entropion; angle-closure glaucoma reported; bruising, ecchymosis and swelling of soft eyelid tissues minimised by applying gentle pressure at injection site immediately after injection

SPECIFIC SIDE-EFFECTS WHEN TREATING TORTICOLLIS. Dysphagia and pooling of saliva (occurs most frequently after injection into sternomastoid muscle); dry mouth, voice changes, weakness of neck muscles; generalised muscle weakness, diplopia and blurred vision; rarely respiratory difficulties (associated with high doses); CSM has warned of persistent dysphagia and sequelae (including death)—**important**, see also under Cautions

Dose: see under preparations below (**important:** specific to **each individual preparation** and **not interchangeable**)

▼ PoM **Botox®** (Allergan)

Injection, powder for reconstitution, botulinum A toxin-haemagglutinin complex, net price 100-unit vial = £135.00

Dose: Blepharospasm, into medial and lateral orbicularis oculi of upper lid and lateral orbicularis oculi of lower lid (additional sites in brow area, lateral orbicularis and upper facial area may also be injected if spasms interfere with vision), initially 1.25–2.5 units at each site (total of up to 25 units per eye) increased to max. 5 units per site, if response inadequate (e.g. not longer than 2 months); total dose should not exceed 100 units every 12 weeks; CHILD not recommended

Hemifacial spasm or VIIth nerve disorders, as for unilateral blepharospasm (other affected facial muscles being injected with initial doses of 1.25–2.5 units); electromyographic control may be needed to identify affected small circumoral muscles; CHILD not recommended

IMPORTANT. Botox® is licensed **only** for blepharospasm and hemifacial spasm; it is **not** licensed for torticollis

DURATION OF ACTION. Initial effect usually within 3 days with peak after 1–2 weeks. Injections need to be repeated approximately every 12 weeks.

PoM **Dysport®** (Speywood)

Injection, powder for reconstitution, botulinum A toxin-haemagglutinin complex, net price 500-unit vial = £172.50

Dose: Blepharospasm, initially 20 units medially and 40 units laterally into junction between preseptal and orbital parts of both upper and lower orbicularis oculi of each eye (total of 120 units per eye)—see package insert for diagram to aid placement of injections; subsequently, dose may need to be reduced to 20 units medially and 20 units laterally as above (total of 80 units per eye); dose may be further reduced to total of 60 units per eye by omitting medial lower lid injection; CHILD not recommended

Hemifacial spasm, as for unilateral blepharospasm, above; CHILD not recommended

DURATION OF ACTION (BLEPHAROSPASM AND HEMIFACIAL SPASM). Initial effect usually within 2–4 days with peak within 2 weeks. Injections need to be repeated approximately every 8 weeks.

Torticollis, administration by specialist experienced in diagnosis and management (see also Cautions above),

Spasmodic torticollis, initially 500 units divided between 2–3 most active neck muscles

Rotational torticollis, initially 350 units into splenius capitis muscle (ipsilateral to direction of chin/head rotation) and 150 units into sternomastoid muscle (contralateral to rotation)

Laterocollis, initially 350 units into ipsilateral splenius capitis muscle and 150 units into ipsilateral sternomastoid muscle; if associated *with shoulder elevation*, ipsilateral trapezoid or levator scapulae muscles may also require treatment (according to visible hypertrophy of muscle or electromyographic findings); if 3 muscles require treatment, inject 300 units into splenius capitis muscle, 100 units into sternomastoid muscle and 100 units into third muscle

Retrocollis, initially, 250 units into each splenius capitis muscle *then* after 6 weeks may be followed by bilateral trapezius injections (up to 250 units per muscle)—bilateral splenii injections may increase risk of neck muscle weakness

Subsequent injections adjusted according to response and side-effects; max. 1000 units

CHILD not recommended

DURATION OF ACTION (TORTICOLLIS). Initial effect usually within 1 week. Injections need to be repeated every 8–12 weeks or as required

---

4.10   Drugs used in substance dependence

This section includes drugs used in alcohol dependence, cigarette smoking, and opioid dependence.

The health departments of the UK have produced a report, *Drug Misuse and Dependence* which contains guidelines on clinical management.

Drug Misuse and Dependence, London, HMSO, 1991 can be obtained from:

> The Publications Centre
> PO Box 276, London SW8 5DT
> Telephone orders, 0171-873 9090

or from HMSO bookshops and through all good booksellers.

It is **important** to be aware that *people who misuse drugs* may be at risk not only from the intrinsic toxicity of the drug itself but also from the practice of injecting preparations intended for administration by mouth. Excipients used in the production of oral dose forms are usually insoluble and may lead to *abscess formation at the site of injection*, or even to *necrosis and gangrene*; moreover, deposits in the heart or lungs may lead to *severe cardiac or pulmonary toxicity*. Additional hazards include *infection* following the use of a dirty needle or an unsterilised diluent.

ALCOHOL DEPENDENCE

Disulfiram (Antabuse®) is used as an adjunct to the treatment of alcohol dependence. It gives rise to extremely unpleasant systemic reactions after the ingestion of even small amounts of alcohol because it leads to accumulation of acetaldehyde in the body. Reactions include flushing of the face, throbbing headache, palpitations, tachycardia, nausea, vomiting, and, with large doses of alcohol, arrhythmias, hypotension, and collapse. Even the small amounts of alcohol included in many oral medicines may be sufficient to precipitate a reaction (even toiletries containing alcohol should be avoided). It may be advisable for patients to carry a card warning of the danger of administration of alcohol.

Benzodiazepines (section 4.1) are used to attenuate withdrawal symptoms but they also have a dependence potential. To minimise the risk of dependence, administration should be for a limited period only (e.g. **chlordiazepoxide** 10–50 mg 4 times daily, gradually reducing over 7–14 days).

Chlormethiazole (clomethiazole) can be used in the management of withdrawal but again has a dependence potential. It should not be prescribed if the patient is likely to continue drinking alcohol.

Acamprosate is a new drug which, in combination with counselling, may be helpful in maintaining abstinence in alcohol-dependent patients. It should be initiated as soon as possible *after* abstinence has been achieved and should be maintained if the patient relapses. Continued alcohol abuse, however, negates the therapeutic benefit of acamprosate.

ACAMPROSATE CALCIUM

Indications: maintenance of abstinence in alcohol dependence

Cautions: continued alcohol abuse (risk of treatment failure)

Contra-indications: renal and severe hepatic impairment; pregnancy and breast-feeding

Side-effects: diarrhoea, nausea, vomiting, abdominal pain, pruritus, occasionally maculopapular rash, rarely bullous skin reactions; fluctuation in libido

Dose: ADULT 18–65 years, 60 kg and over, 666 mg 3 times daily; less than 60 kg, 666 mg at breakfast, 333 mg at midday and 333 mg at night

TREATMENT COURSE. Treatment should be initiated as soon as possible after alcohol withdrawal period and maintained if patient relapses; recommended treatment period 1 year

▼ PoM **Campral EC®** (Lipha)
Tablet, e/c, acamprosate calcium 333 mg. Net price 84-tab pack = £24.95. Label: 21, 25
Electrolytes: Ca²⁺ 0.8 mmol/tablet

CHLORMETHIAZOLE
(Clomethiazole)

Indications: see under Dose; insomnia, restlessness and agitation in the elderly (section 4.1.1); status epilepticus (section 4.8.2); sedation during regional anaesthesia (section 15.1.4.1); eclampsia, see product literature

Cautions: cardiac and respiratory disease (confusional state may indicate hypoxia); history of drug abuse, marked personality disorder, pregnancy and breast-feeding; elderly (excessive sedation with higher doses); hepatic impairment (especially if severe since sedation can mask hepatic coma); renal impairment; avoid prolonged use (and abrupt withdrawal thereafter); **interactions:** Appendix 1 (anxiolytics and hypnotics)

SPECIAL CAUTIONS FOR INTRAVENOUS INFUSION. Resuscitation facilities must be available; maintain clear airway (risk of mechanical obstruction in deep sedation); *rapid infusion* to be given only under direct medical supervision (risk of apnoea and hypotension—special care in those susceptible to cerebral or cardiac complications, e.g. the elderly); during *continuous infusion* sleep induced may lapse into deep unconsciousness and patient must be kept under close and constant observation; *prolonged infusion* may lead to accumulation and delay recovery, may also cause electrolyte imbalance (infusion contains only Na⁺ 32 mmol/litre and no other electrolytes)

DRIVING. Drowsiness may persist the next day and affect performance of skilled tasks (e.g. driving); effects of alcohol enhanced

Contra-indications: acute pulmonary insufficiency; alcohol-dependent patients who continue to drink

Side-effects: nasal congestion and irritation (with sneezing), conjunctival irritation, headache; rarely, paradoxical excitement, confusion, dependence; gastro-intestinal disturbances, rash, urticaria, bullous eruption, anaphylaxis, alterations in liver enzymes also reported; on *intravenous infusion*, localised thrombophlebitis, tachycardia and

---

transient fall in blood pressure (apnoea and hypotension on rapid infusion, see Cautions)

Dose: *by mouth,* alcohol withdrawal, initially 2–4 capsules, if necessary repeated after some hours; day 1 (first 24 hours), 9–12 capsules in 3–4 divided doses;
day 2, 6–8 capsules in 3–4 divided doses;
day 3, 4–6 capsules in 3–4 divided doses; then gradually reduced over days 4–6; total treatment for not more than 9 days

Note. In terms of therapeutic effect 1 capsule ≡ 5 mL syrup

By intravenous infusion, acute alcohol withdrawal, when oral administration not practicable, as a 0.8% solution of chlormethiazole edisylate, initially 3–7.5 mL (24–60 mg)/minute until shallow sleep induced (from which patient can be easily awakened) then reduced to 0.5–1 mL (4–8 mg)/minute to achieve lowest possible rate to maintain shallow sleep and adequate spontaneous respiration; urgent deep sedation (direct medical supervision only) 40–100 mL (320–800 mg) over 3–5 minutes then reduced to maintenance as indicated above

IMPORTANT. See special cautions for intravenous infusion under Cautions (above)

PoM **Heminevrin®** (Astra)
Capsules, grey-brown, chlormethiazole base 192 mg in an oily basis. Net price 60-cap pack = £4.34. Label: 19
Syrup, sugar-free, chlormethiazole edisylate 250 mg/5 mL. Net price 300-mL pack = £3.63. Label: 19
Intravenous infusion 0.8%, chlormethiazole edisylate 8 mg/mL. Net price 500-mL bottle = £5.12

DISULFIRAM

Indications: adjunct in the treatment of chronic alcohol dependence (under specialist supervision)
Cautions: ensure that alcohol not consumed for at least 24 hours before initiating treatment; see also notes above; alcohol challenge **not** recommended on routine basis (if considered essential—specialist units only with resuscitation facilities); hepatic or renal impairment, respiratory disease, diabetes mellitus, epilepsy; **interactions:** Appendix 1 (disulfiram)

ALCOHOL REACTION. Patients should be warned of unpredictable and occasionally severe nature of disulfiram-alcohol interactions. Reactions can occur within 10 minutes and last several hours (may require intensive supportive therapy—oxygen should be available). Patients should not ingest alcohol at all and should be warned of possible presence of alcohol in liquid medicines, remedies, tonics, foods and even in toiletries (alcohol should also be avoided for at least 1 week after stopping)

Contra-indications: cardiac failure, coronary artery disease, history of cerebrovascular accident, hypertension, psychosis, severe personality disorder, suicide risk, pregnancy, breast-feeding
Side-effects: initially drowsiness and fatigue; nausea, vomiting, halitosis, reduced libido; rarely psychotic reactions (depression, paranoia, schizophrenia, mania), allergic dermatitis, peripheral neuritis, hepatic cell damage

Dose: 800 mg as a single dose on first day, reducing over 5 days to 100–200 mg daily; should not be continued for longer than 6 months without review; CHILD not recommended

PoM **Antabuse®** (Dumex)
Tablets, scored, disulfiram 200 mg. Net price 50-tab pack = £19.25. Label: 2, counselling, alcohol reaction

---

CIGARETTE SMOKING

Nicotine chewing gum, patches or nasal spray may be used as an adjunct to counselling but are not generally available on the NHS.

NICOTINE PRODUCTS

Indications: adjunct to smoking cessation
Cautions: cardiovascular disease (avoid if severe); hyperthyroidism; diabetes mellitus; phaeochromocytoma; renal and hepatic impairment; history of gastritis and peptic ulcers; *patches,* exercise may increase absorption and side-effects, skin disorders (patches should not be placed on broken skin); should not smoke or use nicotine replacement products in combination; **interactions:** Appendix 1 (nicotine and tobacco)

DRIVING. The nasal spray should not be used when driving or operating machinery (sneezing or watering eyes could contribute to accident)

Contra-indications: severe cardiovascular disease (including severe arrhythmias or immediate post-myocardial infarction period); recent cerebrovascular accident (including transient ischaemic attacks); pregnancy and breast-feeding; *patches,* chronic generalised skin disease (patches should not be placed on broken skin); patches not for occasional smokers
Side-effects: nausea, dizziness, headache and cold and influenza-like symptoms, palpitations, dyspepsia, insomnia, vivid dreams, myalgia; other side-effects reported include chest pain, blood pressure changes, anxiety and irritability, somnolence and impaired concentration, dysmenorrhoea; *with patches,* skin reactions (discontinue if severe)—vasculitis also reported; *with spray,* nasal irritation, nose bleeds, watering eyes, ear sensations; *with gum,* increased salivation, aphthous ulceration (sometimes with swelling of tongue); *spray* or *gum,* throat irritation
Dose: see under preparations, below

Note. Proprietary brands of nicotine products on sale to the public include *Boots Nicotine Gum* 2 mg, 4 mg and *Boots NRT Patch* 5 mg/16 hours, 10 mg/16 hours, 15 mg/16 hours

NHS **Niconil®** (Elan)
Patches, self-adhesive, nicotine, *'11 mg' patch* (releasing approx. 11 mg/24 hours), net price 7 = £8.54; *'22 mg' patch* (releasing approx. 22 mg/24 hours), starter pack = £8.54, 7 = £8.54

ADMINISTRATION. apply to dry, non-hairy skin on trunk or upper arm, removing after 24 hours and siting replacement patch on different area (avoid using the same area for several days); initially '22 mg' patch daily usually for 4 weeks; then '11 mg' patch for 2 weeks; review treatment if abstinence not achieved in 3 months; CHILD not recommended

NHS **Nicorette®** (Pharmacia & Upjohn)
Nicorette chewing gum, sugar-free, nicotine (as resin) 2 mg, net price pack of 15 = £1.49; pack of 30 = £2.98; pack of 105 = £8.05

Prices are **net**, see p. 1

Nicorette plus chewing gum, sugar-free, nicotine (as resin) 4 mg, net price pack of 15 = £1.70; pack of 30 = £3.98; pack of 105 = £10.80

Note. Also available in mint flavour

Dose: initially one 2-mg piece (**Nicorette®**) chewed slowly for approx. 30 minutes, when urge to smoke occurs; patients needing more than 15 pieces of 2 mg daily may need the 4-mg strength (**Nicorette Plus®**); max. 15 pieces of 4-mg strength daily; withdraw gradually after 3 months; CHILD not recommended

Nicorette patches, self-adhesive, all beige, nicotine, '*5 mg*' patch (releasing approx. 5 mg/16 hours), net price 7 = £7.20; '*10 mg*' patch (releasing approx. 10 mg/16 hours), 7 = £8.36; '*15 mg*' patch (releasing approx. 15 mg/16 hours), 7 = £9.07,

ADMINISTRATION: apply on waking to dry, non-hairy skin on hip, chest or upper arm, removing after approx. 16 hours, usually when retiring; site next patch on different area (avoid using same area for several days); initially '15-mg' patch for 16 hours daily for 8 weeks then '10-mg' patch for 16 hours daily for 2 weeks then '5-mg' patch for 16 hours daily for 2 weeks; review treatment if abstinence not achieved in 3 months; CHILD not recommended

PoM *Nicorette nasal spray*, nicotine 500 micrograms/metered spray. Net price 200-spray unit = £10.99

ADMINISTRATION: Apply 1 spray into each nostril as required to max. twice an hour for 16 hours daily (max. 64 sprays daily) for 8 weeks, then reduce gradually over next 4 weeks (reduce by half at end of first 2 weeks, stop altogether at end of next 2 weeks); max. treatment length 3 months; CHILD under 16 years not recommended

Nicorette inhalator (nicotine-impregnated plug for use in inhalator mouthpiece), nicotine 10 mg/cartridge. Net price 6-cartridge (starter) pack = £3.39, 42-cartridge (refill) pack = £11.37

ADMINISTRATION: Inhale when urge to smoke occurs; initially use between 6 and 12 cartridges daily for up to 8 weeks, then reduce number of cartridges used by half over next 2 weeks and then stop altogether at end of further 2 weeks; review treatment if abstinence not achieved in 3 months; CHILD under 18 years not recommended

NHS **Nicotinell®** (Novartis Consumer Health)

NHS*Chewing gum*, sugar-free, nicotine 2 mg, net price pack of 24 = £2.57; pack of 96 = £7.70

Note. Also available in mint flavour

Dose: initially one 2-mg piece chewed slowly for approx. 30 minutes, when urge to smoke occurs; max. 15 pieces daily; withdraw gradually after 3 months; CHILD not recommended

TTS Patches, self-adhesive, all yellowish-ochre, nicotine, '*10*' patch (releasing approx. 7 mg/24 hours), net price 7 = £8.25; '*20*' patch (releasing approx. 14 mg/24 hours), 7 = £8.68; '*30*' patch (releasing approx. 21 mg/24 hours), 7 = £9.12

ADMINISTRATION: apply to dry, non-hairy skin on trunk or upper arm, removing after 24 hours and siting replacement patch on a different area (avoid using the same area for several days); individuals smoking 20 cigarettes daily or fewer, initially '20' patch daily; individuals smoking more than 20 cigarettes daily, initially '30' patch daily; withdraw gradually, reducing dose every 3–4 weeks; review treatment if abstinence not achieved in 3 months; CHILD under 18 years not recommended

OPIOID DEPENDENCE

Methadone is an opioid *agonist*. It can be substituted for opioids such as diamorphine, preventing the onset of withdrawal symptoms; it is itself addictive and should only be prescribed for those who are physically dependent on opioids. It is administered in a single daily dose usually as methadone mixture 1 mg/mL. The dose is adjusted according to the degree of dependence with the aim of gradual reduction.

Naltrexone is an opioid *antagonist*. It blocks the action of opioids such as diamorphine and precipitates withdrawal symptoms in opioid-dependent subjects. Since the euphoric action of opioid agonists is blocked by naltrexone it is given to former addicts as an aid to relapse prevention.

Lofexidine has been recently introduced for the alleviation of symptoms in patients undergoing opioid withdrawal. Like clonidine it appears to act centrally to produce a reduction in sympathetic tone but reduction in blood pressure is less marked.

LOFEXIDINE HYDROCHLORIDE

Indications: management of symptoms of opioid withdrawal

Cautions: severe coronary insufficiency, recent myocardial infarction, cerebrovascular disease, marked bradycardia (monitor pulse rate frequently); renal impairment; history of depression (on longer treatment); pregnancy and breast-feeding; withdraw gradually over 2–4 days (or longer) to minimise risk of rebound hypertension and associated symptoms; **interactions:** Appendix 1 (lofexidine)

Side-effects: drowsiness, dry mucous membranes (particularly dry mouth, throat and nose), hypotension, bradycardia, rebound hypertension on withdrawal (see Cautions); sedation and coma in overdosage

Dose: initially, 200 micrograms twice daily, increased as necessary in steps of 200–400 micrograms daily to max. 2.4 mg daily; recommended duration of treatment 7–10 days if no opioid use (but longer may be required); withdraw gradually over 2–4 days or longer; CHILD not recommended

PoM **BritLofex®** (Britannia)

Tablets, peach, f/c, lofexidine hydrochloride 200 micrograms. Net price 60-tab pack = £77.95. Label: 2

METHADONE HYDROCHLORIDE

Indications: adjunct in treatment of opioid dependence, see notes above; analgesia, section 4.7.2

Cautions; Contra-indications; Side-effects: section 4.7.2; **overdosage:** see Emergency Treatment of Poisoning, p. 22

IMPORTANT: Methadone, even in low doses is a **special hazard** for children; non-dependent adults are also at risk; dependent adults are at risk if tolerance is incorrectly assessed during induction

INCOMPATIBILITY: Syrup preserved with hydroxybenzoate esters may be incompatible with methadone hydrochloride.

Dose: initially 10–20 mg daily, increased by 10–20 mg daily until no signs of withdrawal or intoxication; usual dose 40–60 mg daily; CHILD not recommended (see also important note above)

CD Methadone (Non-proprietary)

Mixture 1 mg/mL, methadone hydrochloride 1 mg/mL, net price 30 mL = 46p, 50 mL = 76p, 100 mL = £1.52, 500 mL = £7.59. Label: 2

Available from Hillcross, Link (*Methex®*), Martindale, Rosemont (*Metharose®*, sugar-free), Thornton & Ross—taste and colour of different formulations may vary slightly

IMPORTANT. This preparation is 2½ times the strength of Methadone Linctus and is intended only for drug dependent persons for whom treatment may be ordered on form FP10(HP)(ad) or FP10(MDA), or in Scotland on forms HBP(A) or GP10. The title includes the strength and prescriptions should be written accordingly

Injection and *Tablets*, section 4.7.2

Linctus, see section 3.9.1

CD Methadose® (Rosemont)

Oral concentrate, methadone hydrochloride 10 mg/mL (blue), net price 200 mL = £17.84; 20 mg/mL (brown), 200 mL = £35.68. Label: 2

Note. The final strength of the methadone mixture to be dispensed to the patient must be specified on the prescription

IMPORTANT. Care is required in prescribing and dispensing the **correct strength** since any confusion could lead to an overdose; this preparation should be dispensed only **after dilution** as appropriate with *Methadose® Diluent* (life of diluted solution 3 months) and is for drug dependent persons for whom treatment may be ordered on form FP10(HP)(ad) or FP10(MDA), or in Scotland on forms HBP(A)

NALTREXONE HYDROCHLORIDE

Indications: adjunct to prevent relapse in detoxified formerly opioid-dependent patients (who have remained opioid-free for at least 7–10 days)

Cautions: hepatic and renal impairment; liver function tests needed before and during treatment; test for opioid dependence with naloxone; avoid concomitant use of opioids but increased dose of opioid analgesic may be required for pain (monitor for opioid intoxication); pregnancy, breast-feeding

WARNING FOR PATIENTS. Patients need to be warned that an attempt to overcome the block could result in acute opioid intoxication

Contra-indications: patients currently dependent on opioids; acute hepatitis or liver failure

Side-effects: nausea, vomiting, abdominal pain; anxiety, nervousness, sleeping difficulty, headache, reduced energy; joint and muscle pain; less frequently, loss of appetite, diarrhoea, constipation, increased thirst; chest pain; increased sweating and lachrymation; increased energy, 'feeling down', irritability, dizziness, chills; delayed ejaculation, decreased potency; rash; occasionally, liver function abnormalities; reversible idiopathic thrombocytopenia reported

Dose: (initiate in specialist clinics only) 25 mg initially then 50 mg daily; the total weekly dose may be divided and given on 3 days of the week for improved compliance (e.g. 100 mg on Monday and Wednesday, and 150 mg on Friday); CHILD not recommended

PoM **Nalorex®** (Du Pont)

Tablets, yellow, f/c, scored, naltrexone hydrochloride 50 mg. Net price 50-tab pack = £79.49

4.11   Drugs for dementia

Donepezil is a reversible inhibitor of acetylcholinesterase for the symptomatic treatment of mild to moderate dementia in Alzheimer's disease only. It may slow the rate of cognitive and non-cognitive deterioration in about 40% of patients. It has no effect in patients with other causes of confusion or dementia.

DONEPEZIL HYDROCHLORIDE

Indications: mild to moderate dementia in Alzheimer's disease

Cautions: sick sinus syndrome or other supraventricular conduction abnormalities; patients at risk of developing peptic ulcers; asthma, obstructive airways disease; pregnancy and breast-feeding; **interactions:** Appendix 1 (parasympathomimetics)

Side-effects: nausea, vomiting, diarrhoea, fatigue, insomnia, muscle cramps, less frequently headache, dizziness; rarely syncope, bradycardia, sinoatrial block and atrioventricular block; minor increase in plasma-creatine kinase concentration; potential for bladder outflow obstruction, convulsions

Dose: 5 mg once daily at bedtime, increased if necessary after one month to 10 mg daily; max. 10 mg daily

▼ PoM **Aricept®** (Eisai, Pfizer)

Tablets, f/c, donepezil hydrochloride 5 mg, net price 28-tab pack = £68.32; 10 mg (yellow), 28-tab pack = £95.76.

5: Drugs used in the treatment of
INFECTIONS

In this chapter, drug treatment is discussed under the following headings:

5.1 Antibacterial drugs
5.2 Antifungal drugs
5.3 Antiviral drugs
5.4 Antiprotozoal drugs
5.5 Anthelmintics

Notifiable diseases

Doctors must notify the Proper Officer of the local authority (usually the consultant in communicable disease control) when attending a patient suspected of suffering from any of the diseases listed below; a form is available from the Proper Officer.

Anthrax	Mumps
Cholera	Ophthalmia neonatorum
Diphtheria	Paratyphoid fever
Dysentery (amoebic or bacillary)	Plague
	Poliomyelitis, acute
Encephalitis, acute	Rabies
Food poisoning	Relapsing fever
Haemorrhagic fever (viral)	Rubella
Hepatitis, viral	Scarlet fever
Leprosy	Smallpox
Leptospirosis	Tetanus
Malaria	Tuberculosis
Measles	Typhoid fever
Meningitis	Typhus
Meningococcal septicaemia (without meningitis)	Whooping cough
	Yellow fever

5.1 Antibacterial drugs

5.1.1 Penicillins
5.1.2 Cephalosporins, cephamycins and other beta-lactam antibiotics
5.1.3 Tetracyclines
5.1.4 Aminoglycosides
5.1.5 Macrolides
5.1.6 Clindamycin
5.1.7 Some other antibiotics
5.1.8 Sulphonamides and trimethoprim
5.1.9 Antituberculous drugs
5.1.10 Antileprotic drugs
5.1.11 Metronidazole and tinidazole
5.1.12 4-Quinolones
5.1.13 Urinary-tract infections

CHOICE OF A SUITABLE DRUG. Before selecting an antibiotic the clinician must first consider two factors—the patient and the known or likely causative organism. Factors related to the patient which must be considered include history of allergy, renal and hepatic function, resistance to infection (i.e. whether immunocompromised), ability to tolerate drugs by mouth, severity of illness, ethnic origin, age and, if female, whether pregnant, breast-feeding or taking an oral contraceptive.

The known or likely organism and its antibiotic sensitivity, in association with the above factors, will suggest one or more antibiotics, the final choice depending on the microbiological, pharmacological, and toxicological properties.

An example of a rational approach to the selection of an antibiotic is treatment of a urinary-tract infection in a patient complaining of nausea in early pregnancy. The organism is reported as being resistant to ampicillin but sensitive to nitrofurantoin (can cause nausea), gentamicin (can only be given by injection and best avoided in pregnancy), tetracycline (causes dental discoloration) and co-trimoxazole (folate antagonist therefore theoretical teratogenic risk), and cephalexin. The safest antibiotics in pregnancy are the penicillins and cephalosporins; therefore, cephalexin would be indicated for this patient.

The principles involved in selection of an antibiotic must allow for a number of variables including changing renal and hepatic function, increasing bacterial resistance, and new information on side-effects. Duration of therapy, dosage, and route of administration depend on site, type and severity of infection.

ANTIBIOTIC POLICIES. Many hospitals limit the antibiotics that may be used to achieve reasonable economy consistent with adequate cover, and to reduce the development of resistant organisms. An authority may indicate a range of drugs for general use, and permit other drugs only on the advice of the microbiologist or physician responsible for the control of infectious diseases.

BEFORE STARTING THERAPY. The following precepts should be considered before starting:

Viral infections should not be treated with antibiotics.

Samples should be taken for culture and sensitivity testing; **'blind'** prescribing of an antibiotic for a patient ill with unexplained pyrexia usually leads to further difficulty in establishing the diagnosis.

An up-to-date knowledge of **prevalent organisms** and their current sensitivity is of great help in choosing an antibiotic before bacteriological confirmation is available.

The **dose** of an antibiotic will vary according to a number of factors including age, weight, renal function, and severity of infection. The prescribing of the so-called 'standard' dose in serious infections may result in failure of treatment or even death of the patient therefore it is important to prescribe a dose appropriate to the condition. On the other hand, for an antibiotic with a narrow margin between the toxic and therapeutic dose (e.g. an aminoglycoside) it is also important to avoid an excessive dose and plasma concentration monitoring may be required.

The **route** of administration of an antibiotic will often depend on the severity of the infection. Life-threatening infections require intravenous therapy. Whenever possible painful intramuscular injections should be avoided in children.

Duration of therapy depends on the nature of the infection and the response to treatment. Courses should not be unduly prolonged as they are wasteful and may lead to side-effects; in many cases a 5-day course is sufficient. However, in certain infections such as tuberculosis or chronic osteomyelitis it is necessary to continue treatment for relatively long periods. Conversely a single dose of an antibiotic may cure uncomplicated urinary-tract infections.

SUPERINFECTION. In general, broad-spectrum antibacterial drugs such as the cephalosporins are more likely to be associated with adverse reactions related to the selection of resistant organisms e.g. *fungal infections* or *antibiotic-associated colitis* (pseudomembranous colitis); other problems associated with superinfection include vaginitis and pruritus ani.

THERAPY. Suggested treatment is shown in table 1. When the pathogen has been isolated treatment may be changed to a more appropriate antibiotic if necessary. If no bacterium is cultured the antibiotic can be continued or stopped on clinical grounds. Infections for which prophylaxis is useful are listed in table 2.

Table 1. Summary of antibacterial therapy

Gastro-intestinal system
Gastro-enteritis
Antibiotic not usually indicated
Frequently self-limiting and may not have bacterial aetiology
Campylobacter enteritis
Ciprofloxacin *or* erythromycin
Invasive salmonellosis
Ciprofloxacin *or* trimethoprim
Includes severe infections which may be invasive
Shigellosis
Ciprofloxacin *or* trimethoprim
Antibiotic not indicated for mild cases. Ciprofloxacin should be used for trimethoprim-resistant strains
Typhoid fever
Ciprofloxacin *or* chloramphenicol
Infections from Indian subcontinent, Middle-East, and South-East Asia may be chloramphenicol-resistant and ciprofloxacin may be more appropriate
Antibiotic-associated colitis (pseudomembranous colitis)
Oral metronidazole *or* oral vancomycin
Biliary-tract infection
Gentamicin *or* a cephalosporin
Peritonitis
Gentamicin (*or* a cephalosporin) + metronidazole (*or* clindamycin)
Peritoneal dialysis-associated peritonitis
Vancomycin[2] + gentamicin added to dialysis fluid (*or* vancomycin added to dialysis fluid + oral ciprofloxacin)
Discontinue any antibiotic not required when sensitivity known; treat usually for 14 days or longer

Cardiovascular system
Endocarditis caused by Penicillin-sensitive streptococci (e.g. viridans streptococci)
Benzylpenicillin (*or* vancomycin[2] if penicillin-allergic) + low-dose gentamicin (i.e. 60–80 mg twice daily)
Treat for up to 4 weeks; stop gentamicin after 2 weeks if organism fully sensitive to penicillin. Oral amoxycillin[1] may be substituted for benzylpenicillin after 2 weeks
Endocarditis caused by Streptococci with reduced sensitivity to penicillin e.g. *Enterococcus (Streptococcus) faecalis*
Benzylpenicillin (*or* vancomycin[2] if penicillin-allergic) + low-dose gentamicin (i.e. 60–80 mg twice daily)
Treat for 4 weeks
Endocarditis caused by Staphylococcus aureus (and *Staphylococcus epidermidis*)
Flucloxacillin + *either* gentamicin *or* fusidic acid (*or* vancomycin[2] alone if penicillin-allergic)
Treat for at least 4 weeks; stop gentamicin after 2 weeks

Respiratory system
Haemophilus influenzae epiglottitis
Cefotaxime *or* chloramphenicol
Give intravenously
Exacerbations of chronic bronchitis
Amoxycillin[1] *or* trimethoprim *or* tetracycline
Note that 20% of pneumococci and 15% of *Haemophilus influenzae* strains tetracycline-resistant; 15% *H. influenzae* strains amoxycillin-resistant
Uncomplicated pneumonia
Amoxycillin[1] (*or* benzylpenicillin if previously healthy chest *or* erythromycin[3] if penicillin-allergic)
Add flucloxacillin if staphylococcus suspected, e.g. in influenza or measles; add erythromycin[3] if atypical pneumonia suspected; pneumococci with decreased penicillin sensitivity being isolated but not yet common in UK
Severe pneumonia of unknown aetiology
Erythromycin[3] + cefuroxime *or* cefotaxime
Add flucloxacillin if staphylococcus suspected
Suspected atypical pneumonia
Erythromycin[3]
Severe Legionella infections may require addition of rifampicin or a 4-quinolone; tetracycline is an alternative for chlamydial and mycoplasma infections; treat for at least 10–14 days
Hospital-acquired pneumonia
A broad-spectrum cephalosporin (e.g. cefotaxime or ceftazidime) *or* an antipseudomonal penicillin + an aminoglycoside

Central nervous system
Meningitis: Initial 'blind' therapy
If meningococcal disease suspected, general practitioners advised to give a single dose of benzylpenicillin before urgent transportation to hospital (see under Benzylpenicillin, section 5.1.1.1)
Meningitis caused by Meningococci
Benzylpenicillin *or* cefotaxime
Give rifampicin for 2 days before hospital discharge
Meningitis caused by Pneumococci
Cefotaxime
Substitute benzylpenicillin if organism penicillin-sensitive; if organism highly penicillin- and cephalosporin-resistant, add vancomycin
Meningitis caused by Haemophilus influenzae
Cefotaxime *or* chloramphenicol
For *H. influenzae* type b give rifampicin for 4 days before hospital discharge
Meningitis caused by Listeria
Amoxycillin[1] + gentamicin

---

1. Where amoxycillin is suggested ampicillin or an ester of ampicillin (see section 5.1.1.3) may be used.
2. Where vancomycin is suggested teicoplanin may be used.
3. Where erythromycin is suggested another macrolide (e.g. azithromycin or clarithromycin) may be used.

Table 1. Summary of antibacterial therapy *(continued)*

Urinary tract

Acute pyelonephritis or prostatitis

Trimethoprim *or* gentamicin *or* cephalosporin *or* a 4-quinolone

Treat prostatitis with trimethoprim or a 4-quinolone for 4 weeks

'Lower' urinary-tract infection

Trimethoprim *or* amoxycillin[1] *or* nitrofurantoin *or* oral cephalosporin

Genital system

Syphilis

Procaine penicillin (*or* tetracycline *or* doxycycline *or* erythromycin if penicillin-allergic)

Treat with procaine penicillin for 10–21 days, treat with tetracycline, doxycycline or erythromycin for 14–21 days

Gonorrhoea

Amoxycillin[1] with probenecid (*or* spectinomycin *or* a 4-quinolone if penicillin-allergic)

Single-dose treatment in uncomplicated infection; choice depends on locality where infection acquired; contact-tracing recommended; remember chlamydia

Uncomplicated genital chlamydial infection, non-gonococcal urethritis and non-specific genital infection

Doxycycline *or* erythromycin

Treat with doxycycline for 7–21 days or erythromycin for 7–14 days; alternatively treat with azithromycin 1 g as a single dose; contact tracing recommended

Pelvic inflammatory disease

Metronidazole + doxycycline (*or* erythromycin)

Treat with metronidazole for 7–14 days and with doxycycline (or erythromycin) for 14–21 days; severely ill patients may require a cephalosporin such as cefotaxime + doxycyline; remember gonorrhoea

Blood

Septicaemia: Initial 'blind' therapy

Aminoglycoside + a broad-spectrum penicillin *or* a 'third-generation' cephalosporin (e.g. cefotaxime or ceftazidime) alone *or* meropenem alone *or* imipenem (with cilastatin as *Primaxin*®) alone

In immunocompromised, aminoglycoside + a broad-spectrum penicillin *or* a 'third-generation' cephalosporin (e.g. cefotaxime or ceftazidime) alone

Choice depends on local resistance patterns and clinical presentation; use aminoglycoside + broad-spectrum penicillin if pseudomonas suspected; add metronidazole if anaerobic infection suspected; add flucloxacillin or vancomycin[2] if Gram-positive infection suspected

Meningococcal septicaemia

Benzylpenicillin *or* cefotaxime

If meningococcal disease suspected, general practitioners advised to give a single dose of benzylpenicillin before urgent transportation to hospital (see under Benzylpenicillin, section 5.1.1.1); give rifampicin for 2 days before hospital discharge

Musculoskeletal system

Osteomyelitis and septic arthritis

Clindamycin alone *or* flucloxacillin + fusidic acid. If *Haemophilus influenzae* give amoxycillin[1] *or* cefuroxime

Under 5 years of age may be *H. influenzae*. Treat acute disease for at least 6 weeks and chronic infection for at least 12 weeks

Eye

Purulent conjunctivitis

Chloramphenicol *or* gentamicin eye-drops

Ear, nose, and oropharynx

Dental infections

Phenoxymethylpenicillin (*or* amoxycillin[1]) *or* erythromycin *or* metronidazole

Tetracycline for chronic destructive forms of periodontal disease

Sinusitis

Amoxycillin[1] *or* doxycycline *or* erythromycin[3]

Treat for 2 weeks

Otitis externa

Flucloxacillin

Otitis media

Amoxycillin[1] (*or* erythromycin[3] if penicillin-allergic)

Initial parenteral therapy (in severe infections) with benzylpenicillin, then oral therapy with phenoxymethylpenicillin; under 5 years of age may be *Haemophilus influenzae*; many infections are caused by viruses

Throat infections

Phenoxymethylpenicillin (*or* erythromycin[3] if penicillin-allergic) *or* oral cephalosporin

Avoid amoxycillin if possibility of glandular fever, see section 5.1.1.3; initial parenteral therapy (in severe infection) with benzylpenicillin, then oral therapy with phenoxymethylpenicillin *or* amoxycillin[1]; treat beta-haemolytic streptococcal infections for at least 10 days. Most infections are caused by viruses

Skin

Impetigo

Topical fusidic acid or mupirocin; oral flucloxacillin *or* erythromycin if widespread

Topical treatment for 7 days usually adequate; max. duration of topical treatment 10 days

Erysipelas

Phenoxymethylpenicillin

Cellulitis

Phenoxymethylpenicillin + flucloxacillin (*or* erythromycin alone if penicillin-allergic) *or* co-amoxiclav alone

Severe cellulitis may require parenteral benzylpenicillin + flucloxacillin or co-amoxiclav alone

Animal bites

Co-amoxiclav

Cleanse wound thoroughly; for tetanus prone wound, give human tetanus immunoglobulin (with adsorbed tetanus vaccine if necessary, according to immunisation history), see under Tetanus Vaccines, section 14.4

Acne—see section 13.6

---

1. Where amoxycillin is suggested ampicillin or an ester of ampicillin (see section 5.1.1.3) may be used.
2. Where vancomycin is suggested teicoplanin may be used.
3. Where erythromycin is suggested another macrolide (e.g. azithromycin or clarithromycin) may be used.

Table 2. Summary of antibacterial prophylaxis

Prevention of recurrence of rheumatic fever
Phenoxymethylpenicillin 250 mg twice daily *or* sulphadiazine 1 g daily (500 mg daily for patients under 30 kg)

Prevention of secondary case of meningococcal meningitis[1]
Rifampicin 600 mg every 12 hours for 2 days; CHILD 10 mg/kg (under 1 year, 5 mg/kg) every 12 hours for 2 days
or ciprofloxacin 500 mg as a single dose [not licensed for this indication]; CHILD obtain further advice[1]
or i/m ceftriaxone 250 mg as a single dose [not licensed for this indication]; CHILD under 12 years 125 mg

Prevention of secondary case of *Haemophilus influenzae* type b disease[1]
Rifampicin 600 mg once daily for 4 days (optimum regimen for adults); CHILD over 3 months 20 mg/kg once daily for 4 days (max. 600 mg daily)

Prevention of secondary case of diphtheria in non-immune patient
Erythromycin 500 mg every 6 hours for 7–10 days; CHILD up to 2 years 125 mg every 6 hours, 2–8 years 250 mg every 6 hours

Prevention of whooping cough
ADULT and CHILD erythromycin 50 mg/kg (max. 2 g) daily in 4 divided doses for 7–10 days

Prevention of pneumococcal infection in asplenia or in patients with sickle cell disease
Phenoxymethylpenicillin 500 mg every 12 hours; CHILD under 5 years 125 mg every 12 hours, 6–12 years 250 mg every 12 hours—if cover also needed for *H. influenzae* in CHILD give amoxycillin instead (under 5 years 125 mg every 12 hours, over 5 years 250 mg every 12 hours)

Prevention of endocarditis[2] in patients with heart-valve lesion, septal defect, patent ductus, or prosthetic valve

Dental procedures[3] *under local or no anaesthesia*, patients who have not received more than a single dose of a penicillin[4] in the previous month, including those with a prosthetic valve (but not those who have had endocarditis), oral amoxycillin 3 g 1 hour before procedure; CHILD under 5 years quarter adult dose; 5–10 years half adult dose

patients who are penicillin-allergic or have received more than a single dose of a penicillin[4] in the previous month, oral clindamycin[5] 600 mg 1 hour before procedure; CHILD under 5 years quarter adult dose; 5–10 years half-adult dose

patients who have had endocarditis, amoxycillin + gentamicin, as under general anaesthesia

Dental procedures[3] *under general anaesthesia*, *no special risk* (including patients who have not received more than a single dose of a penicillin in the previous month),
either i/v amoxycillin 1 g at induction, then oral amoxycillin 500 mg 6 hours later; CHILD under 5 years quarter adult dose; 5–10 years half adult dose
or oral amoxycillin 3 g 4 hours before induction then oral amoxycillin 3 g as soon as possible after procedure; CHILD under 5 years quarter adult dose; 5–10 years half adult dose
or oral amoxycillin 3 g + oral probenecid 1 g 4 hours before procedure

special risk (patients with a prosthetic valve or who have had endocarditis), i/v amoxycillin 1 g + i/v gentamicin 120 mg at induction, then oral amoxycillin 500 mg 6 hours later; CHILD under 5 years amoxycillin quarter adult dose, gentamicin 2 mg/kg; 5–10 years amoxycillin half adult dose, gentamicin 2 mg/kg

patients who are penicillin-allergic or who have received more than a single dose of a penicillin in the previous month,
either i/v vancomycin 1 g over at least 100 minutes then i/v gentamicin 120 mg at induction or 15 minutes before procedure; CHILD under 10 years vancomycin 20 mg/kg, gentamicin 2 mg/kg
or i/v teicoplanin 400 mg + gentamicin 120 mg at induction or 15 minutes before procedure; CHILD under 14 years teicoplanin 6 mg/kg, gentamicin 2 mg/kg
or i/v clindamycin[5] 300 mg over at least 10 minutes at induction or 15 minutes before procedure then oral or i/v clindamycin 150 mg 6 hours later; CHILD under 5 years quarter adult dose; 5–10 years half adult dose

1. For details of those who should receive chemoprophylaxis contact a consultant in communicable disease control (or a consultant in infectious diseases or the local public health laboratory). Unless there has been mouth to mouth contact, hospital workers do not generally require chemoprophylaxis.
2. Advice on the prevention of endocarditis reflects the recommendations of a Working Party of the British Society for Antimicrobial Chemotherapy, *Lancet*, 1982, **2**, 1323–26; *idem*, 1986, **1**, 1267; *idem*, 1990, **335**, 88–9; *idem*, 1992, **339**, 1292–93; also *J Antimicrob Chemother*, 1993; **31**, 437–8
3. Dental procedures that require antibiotic prophylaxis are, *extractions, scaling*, and *surgery involving gingival tissues*. Antibiotic prophylaxis for dental procedures may be supplemented with *chlorhexidine gluconate gel 1%* or *chlorhexidine gluconate mouthwash 0.2%*, used 5 minutes before procedure
4. For multistage procedures a max. of 2 single doses of a penicillin may be given in a month; alternative drugs should be used for further treatment and the penicillin should not be used again for 3–4 months
5. If **clindamycin** is used, periodontal or other multistage procedures should not be repeated at intervals of less than 2 weeks

Table 2. Summary of antibacterial prophylaxis
(continued)

Prevention of **endocarditis**[1] in patients with
heart-valve lesion, septal defect, patent ductus,
or prosthetic valve

Upper respiratory-tract procedures, as for dental
procedures; post-operative dose may be given
parenterally if swallowing is painful

Genito-urinary procedures, as for *special risk*
patients undergoing dental procedures under general
anaesthesia except that clindamycin is not given, see
above; if urine infected, prophylaxis should also
cover infective organism

**Obstetric, gynaecological and gastro-intestinal
procedures** (prophylaxis required for patients with
prosthetic valves or those who have had endocarditis
only), as for genito-urinary procedures

Joint prostheses and dental treatment

Advice of a Working Party of the British Society for
Antimicrobial Chemotherapy is that patients with
prosthetic joint implants (including total hip replacements) do not require antibiotic prophylaxis for dental treatment. The Working Party considers that it is
unacceptable to expose patients to the adverse effects
of antibiotics when there is no evidence that such
prophylaxis is of any benefit, but that those who
develop any intercurrent infection require prompt
treatment with antibiotics to which the infecting
organisms are sensitive.

The Working Party has commented that joint infections have rarely been shown to follow dental procedures and are even more rarely caused by oral
streptococci.

Dermatological procedures

Advice of a Working Party of the British Society for
Antimicrobial Chemotherapy is that patients who
undergo dermatological procedures do not require
antibacterial prophylaxis against endocarditis.

**Immunosuppression and indwelling intraperito-
neal catheters**

Advice of a Working Party of the British Society for
Antimicrobial Chemotherapy is that patients who are
immunosuppressed (including transplant patients)
and patients with indwelling intraperitoneal catheters
do not require antibiotic prophylaxis for dental treatment provided there is no other indication for
prophylaxis.

The Working Party has commented that there is little
evidence that dental treatment is followed by infection in immunosuppressed and immunodeficient
patients nor is there evidence that dental treatment is
followed by infection in patients with indwelling
intraperitoneal catheters.

---

1. Advice on the prevention of endocarditis reflects the
recommendations of a Working Party of the British
Society for Antimicrobial Chemotherapy, *Lancet*, 1982,
2, 1323–26; *idem*, 1986, **1**, 1267; *idem*, 1990, **335**, 88–9;
idem, 1992, **339**, 1292–93; also *J Antimicrob Chemother*, 1993; **31**, 437–8

Prevention of **gas-gangrene** in high lower-limb
amputations or following major trauma
   Benzylpenicillin 300–600 mg every 6 hours for 5
   days *or* if penicillin-allergic metronidazole
   500 mg every 8 hours

Prevention of **tuberculosis** in susceptible close
contacts
   Isoniazid 300 mg daily for 6 months; CHILD isoniazid 5–10 mg/kg daily (max. 300 mg daily)
   or isoniazid 300 mg daily + rifampicin 600 mg
   daily (450 mg if less than 50 kg) for 3 months;
   CHILD isoniazid 5–10 mg/kg daily (max. 300 mg
   daily) + rifampicin 10 mg/kg daily (max. 600 mg
   daily)

Prevention of infection in **abdominal surgery**
   Operations on stomach or oesophagus for carcinoma, or cholecystectomy in patients with possibly infected bile
   Single dose of gentamicin *or* a cephalosporin
   given in 2 hours before operation
   Resections of colon and rectum for carcinoma, and
   resections in inflammatory bowel disease
   Single dose of *either* gentamicin + metronidazole
   or cefuroxime + metronidazole given in 2 hours
   before operation
   Hysterectomy
   Metronidazole as suppository *or* single i/v dose

5.1.1   Penicillins

   5.1.1.1 Benzylpenicillin and
          phenoxymethylpenicillin
   5.1.1.2 Penicillinase-resistant penicillins
   5.1.1.3 Broad-spectrum penicillins
   5.1.1.4 Antipseudomonal penicillins

The penicillins are bactericidal and act by interfering with bacterial cell wall synthesis. They diffuse
well into body tissues and fluids, but penetration
into the cerebrospinal fluid is poor except when the
meninges are inflamed. They are excreted in the
urine in therapeutic concentrations. Probenecid (see
section 10.1.4) blocks the renal tubular excretion of
the penicillins, producing higher and more prolonged plasma concentrations; it is not recommended in children under 2 years of age.

   The most important side-effect of the penicillins
is hypersensitivity, which causes rashes and, occasionally, anaphylaxis, which can be fatal. Patients
who are allergic to one penicillin will be allergic to
all as the hypersensitivity is related to the basic
penicillin structure. A rare but serious toxic effect
of the penicillins is encephalopathy due to cerebral
irritation. This may result from excessively high
doses or in patients with severe renal failure. The
penicillins should **not** be given by intrathecal injection as they can cause encephalopathy which may
be fatal.

   Prices are **net**, see p.1

A second problem relating to high doses of penicillin, or normal doses given to patients with renal failure, is the accumulation of electrolyte since most injectable penicillins contain either sodium or potassium.

Diarrhoea frequently occurs during oral penicillin therapy. It is most common with ampicillin and its derivatives, which can also cause antibiotic-associated colitis.

5.1.1.1 BENZYLPENICILLIN AND PHENOXYMETHYLPENICILLIN

Benzylpenicillin (Penicillin G), the first of the penicillins, remains an important and useful antibiotic but is inactivated by bacterial penicillinases (beta-lactamases). It is effective for streptococcal, pneumococcal, gonococcal, and meningococcal infections and also for anthrax, diphtheria, gas-gangrene, leptospirosis, tetanus, and treatment of Lyme disease in children. Pneumococci, meningococci, and gonococci which have decreased sensitivity to penicillin have been isolated; benzylpenicillin is no longer drug of first choice for pneumococcal meningitis. Benzylpenicillin is inactivated by gastric acid and absorption from the gut is low; therefore it is best given by injection. Benzylpenicillin may cause convulsions after high doses by intravenous injection or in renal failure.

Procaine penicillin (procaine benzylpenicillin) is a sparingly soluble salt of benzylpenicillin. It is used in intramuscular depot preparations which provide therapeutic tissue concentrations for up to 24 hours. It is the preferred choice for the treatment of yaws and syphilis; neurosyphilis requires special consideration.

Phenoxymethylpenicillin (Penicillin V) has a similar antibacterial spectrum to benzylpenicillin, but is less active. It is gastric acid-stable, so is suitable for oral administration. It should not be used for serious infections because absorption can be unpredictable and plasma concentrations variable. It is indicated principally for respiratory-tract infections in children, for streptococcal tonsillitis, and for continuing treatment after one or more injections of benzylpenicillin when clinical response has begun. It should not be used for meningococcal or gonococcal infections. Phenoxymethylpenicillin is used for prophylaxis against streptococcal infections following rheumatic fever and against pneumococcal infections following splenectomy or in sickle cell disease.

BENZYLPENICILLIN
(Penicillin G)

Indications: throat infections, otitis media, streptococcal endocarditis, meningococcal meningitis, pneumonia (see table 1); prophylaxis in limb amputation

Cautions: history of allergy; renal impairment; **interactions:** Appendix 1 (penicillins)

Contra-indications: penicillin hypersensitivity

Side-effects: hypersensitivity reactions including urticaria, fever, joint pains, rashes, angioedema, anaphylaxis, serum sickness-like reactions, haemolytic anaemia and interstitial nephritis; neutropenia, thrombocytopenia, coagulation disorders and central nervous system toxicity reported (especially with high doses or in severe renal impairment); paraesthesia with prolonged use; diarrhoea and antibiotic-associated colitis

Dose: by intramuscular or by slow intravenous injection or by infusion, 1.2 g daily in 4 divided doses, increased if necessary to 2.4 g daily or more (see also below); PREMATURE INFANT and NEONATE, 50 mg/kg daily in 2 divided doses; INFANT 1–4 weeks, 75 mg/kg daily in 3 divided doses; CHILD 1 month–12 years, 100 mg/kg daily in 4 divided doses (higher doses may be required, see also below)

Bacterial endocarditis, *by slow intravenous injection or by infusion,* 7.2 g daily in 4–6 divided doses

Meningococcal meningitis, *by slow intravenous injection or by infusion,* 2.4 g every 4–6 hours; PREMATURE INFANT and NEONATE, 100 mg/kg daily in 2 divided doses; INFANT 1–4 weeks, 150 mg/kg daily in 3 divided doses; CHILD 1 month–12 years, 180–300 mg/kg daily in 4–6 divided doses

Important. If meningococcal disease is suspected general practitioners are advised to give a single injection of benzylpenicillin by intramuscular or by intravenous injection before transporting the patient urgently to hospital. Suitable doses are: ADULT 1.2 g; INFANT 300 mg; CHILD 1–9 years 600 mg, 10 years and over as for adult. In confirmed **penicillin allergy**, cefotaxime (section 5.1.2) may be an alternative

Prophylaxis in limb amputation, section 5.1, table 2

By intrathecal injection, **not** recommended

Note. Benzylpenicillin doses in BNF may differ from those in data sheet

PoM **Crystapen®** (Britannia)
Injection, powder for reconstitution, benzylpenicillin sodium (unbuffered). Net price 600-mg vial = 44p, 2-vial 'GP pack' = £1.99
Electrolytes: Na+ 1.68 mmol/600-mg vial

PHENOXYMETHYLPENICILLIN
(Penicillin V)

Indications: tonsillitis, otitis media, erysipelas; rheumatic fever and pneumococcal infection prophylaxis (see table 2)

Cautions; Contra-indications; Side-effects: see under Benzylpenicillin; **interactions:** Appendix 1 (penicillins)

Dose: 500 mg every 6 hours increased to 750 mg every 6 hours in severe infections; CHILD, every 6 hours, up to 1 year 62.5 mg, 1–5 years 125 mg, 6–12 years 250 mg

Rheumatic fever and pneumococcal infection prophylaxis, section 5.1, table 2

PoM **Phenoxymethylpenicillin** (Non-proprietary)
Tablets, phenoxymethylpenicillin (as potassium salt) 250 mg, net price 20 = 33p. Label: 9, 23
Available from APS (Apsin®), Berk, Cox, Generics, Kent (Tenkicin®), Lagap

Oral solution, phenoxymethylpenicillin (as potassium salt) for reconstitution with water, net price 125 mg/5 mL, 100 mL = 89p; 250 mg/5 mL, 100 mL = £1.09. Label: 9, 23

Available from APS (Apsin®), Cox, Generics, Kent (Tenkicin®)

PROCAINE PENICILLIN
(Procaine benzylpenicillin)
Indications: penicillin-sensitive infections
Cautions; Contra-indications; Side-effects: see under Benzylpenicillin; **not** for intravenous administration
Dose: see below

PoM **Bicillin®** (Yamanouchi)
Injection, powder for reconstitution, procaine penicillin 1.8 g, benzylpenicillin sodium 360 mg. Net price 6-mL multidose vial = £2.70

Electrolytes: Na+ 1 mmol/vial
Dose: when reconstituted with 4.6 mL water for injections, 1 mL (procaine penicillin 300 mg, benzylpenicillin sodium 60 mg) every 12–24 hours by intramuscular injection
Primary syphilis, by intramuscular injection, 3 mL (4 mL in patients over 80 kg) daily for 10 days (14 days for secondary or latent syphilis)
Note. Reconstitution with 4.6 mL water for injections produces 6 mL

5.1.1.2 PENICILLINASE-RESISTANT PENICILLINS

Most staphylococci are now resistant to benzylpenicillin because they produce penicillinases. **Cloxacillin** and **flucloxacillin**, however, are not inactivated by these enzymes and are thus effective in infections caused by penicillin-resistant staphylococci, which is the sole indication for their use. They are acid-stable and can, therefore, be given by mouth as well as by injection.

Flucloxacillin is better absorbed from the gut than cloxacillin; cloxacillin is available only in combination with ampicillin (section 5.1.1.3). For CSM warning on cholestatic jaundice see under Flucloxacillin.

Staphylococcus aureus strains resistant to methicillin [now discontinued] (methicillin-resistant *Staph. aureus*, MRSA) and to cloxacillin have emerged in many hospitals; some of these organisms are only sensitive to vancomycin (section 5.1.7). Other alternatives include rifampicin and teicoplanin.

Temocillin is a new penicillin with activity against penicillinase-producing Gram-negative bacteria (except *Pseudomonas aeruginosa*); it is not active against Gram-positive bacteria.

FLUCLOXACILLIN
Indications: infections due to penicillinase-producing staphylococci including otitis externa; adjunct in pneumonia, impetigo, cellulitis and in staphylococcal endocarditis (section 5.1 table 1)

Cautions; Contra-indications; Side-effects: see under Benzylpenicillin (section 5.1.1.1); hepatitis and cholestatic jaundice reported (see also CSM advice below); caution in porphyria (see section 9.8.2)
CHOLESTATIC JAUNDICE. CSM has advised that cholestatic jaudice may occur up to several weeks after treatment with flucloxacillin has been stopped. Administration for more than 2 weeks and increasing age are risk factors
Dose: by mouth, 250 mg every 6 hours, at least 30 minutes before food
By intramuscular injection, 250 mg every 6 hours
By slow intravenous injection or by infusion, 0.25–1 g every 6 hours
Doses may be doubled in severe infections
CHILD, any route, under 2 years quarter adult dose; 2–10 years half adult dose

PoM **Flucloxacillin** (Non-proprietary)
Capsules, flucloxacillin (as sodium salt) 250 mg, net price 20 = £1.56; 500 mg, 20 = £2.94. Label: 9, 23

Available from APS, Ashbourne (*Fluclomix*®), Berk (*Ladropen*®), Cox, Galen (*Galfloxin*®), Kent, Lagap, Norton, Opus (*Zoxin*®), Yamanouchi (*Stafoxil*®)
Oral solution (= elixir or syrup), flucloxacillin (as sodium salt) for reconstitution with water, 125 mg/5 mL. Net price 100 mL = £3.11. Label: 9, 23

Available from APS, Berk (*Ladropen*®), Cox, Kent, Norton
Injection, powder for reconstitution, flucloxacillin (as sodium salt). Net price 250-mg vial = 75p; 500-mg vial = £1.71

Available from Berk (*Ladropen*®)
PoM **Floxapen®** (Beecham)
Capsules, both black/caramel, flucloxacillin (as sodium salt) 250 mg, net price 20-cap pack = £5.08, 28-cap pack = £7.11; 500 mg, 28-cap pack = £14.25. Label: 9, 23

Syrup, flucloxacillin (as magnesium salt) for reconstitution with water, 125 mg/5 mL, net price 100 mL = £3.65; 250 mg/5 mL, 100 mL = £7.30. Label: 9, 23

Injection, powder for reconstitution, flucloxacillin (as sodium salt). Net price 250-mg vial = £1.02; 500-mg vial = £2.04; 1-g vial = £4.08

Electrolytes: Na+ 0.57 mmol/250-mg vial, 1.13 mmol/500-mg vial, 2.26 mmol/1-g vial

TEMOCILLIN
Indications: infections due to penicillinase-producing Gram-negative bacteria except pseudomonas
Cautions; Contra-indications; Side-effects: see under Benzylpenicillin (section 5.1.1.1)
Dose: by intramuscular injection or by intravenous injection (over 3–4 minutes) *or by intravenous infusion,* 1–2 g every 12 hours
Acute uncomplicated urinary-tract infections, 1 g daily as a single dose

PoM **Temopen®** (Bencard)

Injection, powder for reconstitution, temocillin (as sodium salt). Net price 1-g vial = £15.00

Electrolytes: Na⁺ 5 mmol/g

5.1.1.3 BROAD-SPECTRUM PENICILLINS

Ampicillin is active against certain Gram-positive and Gram-negative organisms but is inactivated by penicillinases including those produced by *Staphylococcus aureus* and by common Gram-negative bacilli such as *Escherichia coli*. Almost all staphylococci, 50% of *E. coli* strains and 15% of *Haemophilus influenzae* strains are now resistant. The likelihood of resistance should therefore be considered before using ampicillin for the 'blind' treatment of infections; in particular, it should not be used for hospital patients without checking sensitivity.

Ampicillin is well excreted in the bile and urine. It is principally indicated for the treatment of exacerbations of chronic bronchitis and middle ear infections, both of which are usually due to *Streptococcus pneumoniae* and *H. influenzae*, and for urinary-tract infections (section 5.1.13) and gonorrhoea.

Ampicillin can be given by mouth but less than half the dose is absorbed, and absorption is further decreased by the presence of food in the gut. Higher plasma concentrations are obtained with the ampicillin ester **pivampicillin**; its absorption is little affected by the presence of food, and the incidence of diarrhoea is less than with ampicillin.

Maculopapular rashes commonly occur with ampicillin (and amoxycillin) but are not usually related to true penicillin allergy. They almost always occur in patients with glandular fever; broad-spectrum penicillins should not therefore be used for 'blind' treatment of a sore throat. Rashes are also common in patients with chronic lymphatic leukaemia; rashes may also be more common in patients infected with the human immunodeficiency virus (HIV) although initial reports have not been confirmed.

Amoxycillin (amoxicillin) is a derivative of ampicillin which differs by only one hydroxyl group and has a similar antibacterial spectrum. It is better absorbed than ampicillin when given by mouth, producing higher plasma and tissue concentrations; unlike ampicillin, absorption is not affected by the presence of food in the stomach. Amoxycillin is used for endocarditis prophylaxis (section 5.1, table 2); it may also be used for the treatment of Lyme disease in children.

Co-amoxiclav consists of amoxycillin with the beta-lactamase inhibitor clavulanic acid. Clavulanic acid itself has no significant antibacterial activity but, by inactivating penicillinases, it makes the combination active against penicillinase-producing bacteria that are resistant to amoxycillin. These include most *Staph. aureus*, 50% of *E. coli* strains, and up to 15% of *H. influenzae* strains, as well as many *Bacteroides* and *Klebsiella* spp. Co-amoxiclav should be reserved for infections likely, or known, to be caused by amoxycillin resistant penicillinase-producing strains; for CSM warning on cholestatic jaundice see under Co-amoxiclav.

Combinations of ampicillin with flucloxacillin (as co-fluampicil) and ampicillin with cloxacillin (*Ampiclox®*) are available.

AMOXYCILLIN

(Amoxicillin)

Indications: see under Ampicillin; also endocarditis prophylaxis; adjunct in listerial meningitis (section 5.1, table1)

Cautions; Contra-indications; Side-effects: see under Ampicillin

Dose: by mouth, 250 mg every 8 hours, doubled in severe infections; CHILD up to 10 years, 125 mg every 8 hours, doubled in severe infections
Severe or recurrent purulent respiratory infection, 3 g every 12 hours
Endocarditis prophylaxis, section 5.1, table 2

Short-course oral therapy
Dental abscess, 3 g repeated after 8 hours
Urinary-tract infections, 3 g repeated after 10–12 hours
Gonorrhoea, single dose of 2–3 g with probenecid 1 g
Otitis media, CHILD 3–10 years, 750 mg twice daily for 2 days
By intramuscular injection, 500 mg every 8 hours; CHILD, 50–100 mg/kg daily in divided doses
By intravenous injection or infusion, 500 mg every 8 hours increased to 1 g every 6 hours; CHILD, 50–100 mg/kg daily in divided doses

PoM **Amoxycillin** (Non-proprietary)

Capsules, amoxycillin (as trihydrate) 250 mg, net price 20 = 74p; 500 mg, 20 = £1.05. Label: 9
Available from APS, Ashbourne (*Amix®*), Berk (*Almodan®*), Cox, Eastern (*Amoram®*), Galen (*Galenamox®*), Hillcross, Kent, Lagap, Norton, Rima (*Rimoxallin®*)

Oral suspension, amoxycillin (as trihydrate) for reconstitution with water, 125 mg/5 mL, net price 100 mL = 89p; 250 mg/5 mL, 100 mL = £1.48. Label: 9

Note. Sugar-free versions are available and can be ordered by specifying 'sugar-free' on the prescription
Available from APS, Ashbourne (*Amix®*), Berk (*Almodan®*), Cox, Eastern (*Amoram®*), Galen (*Galenamox®*), Hillcross, Kent, Lagap, Norton, Rima (*Rimoxallin®*)

Sachets, sugar-free, amoxycillin 3 g (as trihydrate)/sachet, net price 2-sachet pack = £4.55, 14-sachet pack = £31.39. Label: 9, 13
Available from Hillcross, Kent, Norton

PoM **Amoxil®** (Bencard)

Capsules, both maroon/gold, amoxycillin (as trihydrate), 250 mg, net price 21-cap pack = £4.04; 500 mg, 21-cap pack = £8.09. Label: 9

Dispersible tablets, sugar-free, amoxycillin 500 mg (as trihydrate). Net price 21-tab pack = £9.33. Label: 9, 13

Fiztab (= chewable tablets), sugar-free, amoxycillin (as trihydrate) 125 mg, net price 20-tab pack = £2.42; 250 mg, 20-tab pack = £4.84. Label: 9, 10 patient information leaflet

Note. Dose form not suitable for children under 3 years

Syrup SF, both sugar-free, amoxycillin (as trihydrate) for reconstitution with water, 125 mg/5 mL, net price 100 mL = £2.42; 250 mg/5 mL, 100 mL = £4.84. Label: 9

Paediatric suspension, amoxycillin 125 mg (as trihydrate)/1.25 mL when reconstituted with water. Net price 20 mL = £3.63. Label: 9, counselling, use of pipette

Sachets SF, powder, sugar-free, amoxycillin 750 mg (as trihydrate)/sachet, net price 4-sachet pack = £3.15; 3 g/sachet, 2-sachet pack = £5.20. Label: 9, 13

Injection, powder for reconstitution, amoxycillin (as sodium salt). Net price 250-mg vial = 36p; 500-mg vial = 66p; 1-g vial = £1.31
Electrolytes: Na⁺ 3.3 mmol/g

AMPICILLIN

Indications: urinary-tract infections, otitis media, sinusitis, chronic bronchitis, invasive salmonellosis, gonorrhoea

Cautions: history of allergy; renal impairment; erythematous rashes common in glandular fever, chronic lymphatic leukaemia, and possibly HIV infection (see notes above); **interactions:** Appendix 1 (penicillins)

Contra-indications: penicillin hypersensitivity

Side-effects: nausea, diarrhoea; rashes (discontinue treatment); rarely, antibiotic-associated colitis; see also under Benzylpenicillin (section 5.1.1.1)

Dose: by mouth, 0.25–1 g every 6 hours, at least 30 minutes before food

Gonorrhoea, 2–3.5 g as a single dose with probenecid 1 g

Urinary-tract infections, 500 mg every 8 hours

By intramuscular injection or intravenous injection or infusion, 500 mg every 4–6 hours; higher doses in meningitis

CHILD under 10 years, any route, half adult dose

PoM **Ampicillin** (Non-proprietary)
Capsules, ampicillin 250 mg, net price 20 = 69p; 500 mg, 20 = £1.29. Label: 9, 23
Available from APS, Berk (*Vidopen*®), Cox, Kent, Lagap, Norton, Rima (*Rimacillin*®)
Oral suspension, ampicillin 125 mg/5 mL when reconstituted with water, net price 100 mL = 84p; 250 mg/5 mL, 100 mL = £1.05. Label: 9, 23
Available from APS, Berk, Cox, Kent, Lagap, Norton, Rima (*Rimacillin*®)

PoM **Penbritin**® (Beecham)
Capsules, both black/red, ampicillin (as trihydrate) 250 mg, net price 28-cap pack = £2.26; 500 mg, 20 = £3.13. Label: 9, 23
Syrup, ampicillin (as trihydrate) for reconstitution with water, 125 mg/5 mL, net price 100 mL = £1.20; 250 mg/5 mL, 100 mL = £2.39. Label: 9, 23
Paediatric suspension, ampicillin 125 mg (as trihydrate)/1.25 mL. Net price 25 mL = £2.23. Label: 9, 23, counselling, use of pipette
Injection, powder for reconstitution, ampicillin (as sodium salt). Net price 500-mg vial = 74p
Electrolytes: Na⁺ 1.47 mmol/500-mg vial

With cloxacillin
PoM **Ampiclox**® (Beecham)
Capsules, black/purple, ampicillin 250 mg (as trihydrate), cloxacillin 250 mg (as sodium salt). Net price 20-cap pack = £7.00. Label: 9, 23
Dose: 1–2 capsules every 4–6 hours
Syrup, ampicillin 125 mg (as trihydrate), cloxacillin 125 mg (as sodium salt)/5 mL when reconstituted with water. Net price 100 mL = £5.00. Label: 9, 23
Dose: 10–20 mL every 4–6 hours; CHILD 1 month–2 years, quarter adult dose; 2–12 years, half adult dose
Injection, ampicillin 250 mg (as sodium salt), cloxacillin 250 mg (as sodium salt). Net price per vial = £1.49
Electrolytes: Na⁺ 1.32 mmol/vial
Dose: by intramuscular injection or intravenous injection or infusion, 1–2 vials every 4–6 hours; CHILD up to 2 years quarter adult dose, 2–10 years half adult dose

PoM **Ampiclox Neonatal**® (Beecham)
Suspension, sugar-free, ampicillin 60 mg (as trihydrate), cloxacillin 30 mg (as sodium salt)/0.6 mL when reconstituted with water. Net price 10 mL = £2.27. Label: 9, counselling, use of pipette
Dose: 0.6 mL every 4 hours
Injection, ampicillin 50 mg (as sodium salt), cloxacillin 25 mg (as sodium salt). Net price per vial = 42p.
Electrolytes: Na⁺ <0.5 mmol/vial
Dose: NEONATE and PREMATURE INFANT, by intramuscular injection or by intravenous injection or infusion, 1 vial every 8 hours

With flucloxacillin
See Co-fluampicil

CO-AMOXICLAV

A mixture of amoxycillin (as the trihydrate or as the sodium salt) and clavulanic acid (as potassium clavulanate); the proportions are expressed in the form *x*/*y* where *x* and *y* are the strengths in milligrams of amoxycillin and clavulanic acid respectively

Indications: infections due to penicillinase-producing strains (where amoxycillin alone not appropriate) including respiratory-tract infections, genito-urinary and abdominal infections, cellulitis, animal bites, severe dental infection with spreading cellulitis

Cautions: see under Ampicillin and notes above; also caution in hepatic impairment (monitor hepatic function), pregnancy
CHOLESTATIC JAUNDICE. CSM has advised that cholestatic jaundice has been identified as an adverse reaction occuring either during, or shortly after, the use of co-amoxiclav. An epidemiological study has shown that the risk of acute liver toxicity was about 6 times greater with co-amoxiclav than with amoxycillin. Cholestatic jaundice is more common in patients above the age of 65 years and in males; these reactions have only rarely been reported in children. Jaundice is usually self-limiting and very rarely fatal. The duration of treatment should be appropriate to the indication and should not usually exceed 14 days

Contra-indications: penicillin hypersensitivity, history of co-amoxiclav-associated or penicillin-associated jaundice or hepatic dysfunction

Side-effects: see under Ampicillin; hepatitis, cholestatic jaundice (see above); erythema multiforme (including Stevens-Johnson syndrome), toxic epidermal necrolysis, exfoliative dermatitis, vasculitis reported; rarely prolongation of bleeding time, dizziness, headache, convulsions (particularly with high doses or in renal impairment); superficial staining of teeth with suspension, phlebitis at injection site

Dose: by mouth, expressed as amoxycillin, 250 mg every 8 hours, dose doubled in severe infections; CHILD see under preparations below (under 6 years Augmentin® '125/31 SF' suspension; 6–12 years Augmentin® '250/62 SF' suspension *or* for short-term treatment with twice daily dosage in CHILD 2 months–12 years Augmentin-Duo® 400/57 suspension)

Severe dental infections (but not generally first-line, see notes above), expressed as amoxycillin, 250 mg every 8 hours for 5 days

By intravenous injection over 3–4 minutes *or by intravenous infusion*, expressed as amoxycillin, 1 g every 8 hours increased to 1 g every 6 hours in more serious infections; INFANTS up to 3 months 25 mg/kg every 8 hours (every 12 hours in the perinatal period and in premature infants); CHILD 3 months–12 years, 25 mg/kg every 8 hours increased to 25 mg/kg every 6 hours in more serious infections

Surgical prophylaxis, expressed as amoxycillin, 1 g at induction; for high risk procedures (e.g. colorectal surgery) a further 2–3 doses may be given every 8 hours in first 24 hours (longer if significantly increased risk of infection)

PoM **Augmentin®** (Beecham)
Tablets 375 mg, f/c, co-amoxiclav 250/125 (amoxycillin 250 mg as trihydrate, clavulanic acid 125 mg as potassium salt). Net price 21-tab pack = £9.79. Label: 9
Tablets 625 mg, f/c, co-amoxiclav 500/125 (amoxycillin 500 mg as trihydrate, clavulanic acid 125 mg as potassium salt). Net price 21-tab pack = £14.30. Label: 9
Dispersible tablets, sugar-free, co-amoxiclav 250/125 (amoxycillin 250 mg as trihydrate, clavulanic acid 125 mg as potassium salt). Net price 21-tab pack = £10.99. Label: 9, 13
Suspension '125/31 SF', sugar-free, co-amoxiclav 125/31 (amoxycillin 125 mg as trihydrate, clavulanic acid 31 mg as potassium salt)/5 mL when reconstituted with water. Net price 100 mL = £4.57. Label: 9
Note. Suspension contains aspartame 12.5 mg/5 mL (see section 9.4.1)
Dose: CHILD 1–6 years (10–18 kg) 5 mL every 8 hours *or* INFANT and CHILD up to 6 years 0.8 mL/kg daily in 3 divided doses; in severe infections dose increased to 1.6 mL/kg daily in 3 divided doses
Suspension '250/62 SF', sugar-free, co-amoxiclav 250/62 (amoxycillin 250 mg as trihydrate, clavulanic acid 62 mg as potassium salt)/5 mL when reconstituted with water. Net price 100 mL = £6.42. Label: 9
Note. Suspension contains aspartame 12.5 mg/5 mL (see section 9.4.1)
Dose: CHILD 6–12 years (18–40 kg) 5 mL every 8 hours *or* 0.4 mL/kg daily in 3 divided doses; in severe infections dose increased to 0.8 mL/kg daily in 3 divided doses

Injection 600 mg, powder for reconstitution, co-amoxiclav 500/100 (amoxycillin 500 mg as sodium salt, clavulanic acid 100 mg as potassium salt). Net price per vial = £1.49
Electrolytes: Na⁺ 1.6 mmol, K⁺ 0.5 mmol/600-mg vial
Injection 1.2 g, powder for reconstitution, co-amoxiclav 1000/200 (amoxycillin 1 g as sodium salt, clavulanic acid 200 mg as potassium salt). Net price per vial = £2.97
Electrolytes: Na⁺ 3.1 mmol, K⁺ 1 mmol/1.2-g vial

PoM **Augmentin-Duo®** (SmithKline Beecham)
Suspension '400/57', sugar-free, co-amoxiclav 400/57 (amoxycillin 400 mg as trihydrate, clavulanic acid 57 mg as potassium salt)/5 mL when reconstituted with water. Net price 35 mL = £4.57, 70 mL = £6.42. Label: 9
Note. Suspension contains aspartame 12.5 mg/5 mL (see section 9.4.1)
Dose: CHILD 2 months–2 years 0.15 mL/kg twice daily, 2–6 years (13–21 kg) 2.5 mL twice daily, 7–12 years (22–40 kg) 5 mL twice daily, doubled in severe infections

CO-FLUAMPICIL

A mixture of equal parts by mass of flucloxacillin and ampicillin

Indications: mixed infections involving penicillinase-producing staphylococci
Cautions; Contra-indications; Side-effects: see under Ampicillin and Flucloxacillin
Dose: by mouth, co-fluampicil, 250/250 every 6 hours, dose doubled in severe infections; CHILD under 10 years half adult dose, dose doubled in severe infections
By intramuscular or slow intravenous injection or by intravenous infusion, co-fluampicil 250/250 every 6 hours, dose doubled in severe infections; CHILD under 2 years quarter adult dose, 2–10 years half adult dose, dose doubled in severe infections

PoM **Co-fluampicil** (Non-proprietary)
Capsules, co-fluampicil 250/250 (flucloxacillin 250 mg as sodium salt, ampicillin 250 mg as trihydrate). Net price 20 = £4.55. Label: 9, 22
Available from Cox, Generics (Flu-Amp®), Kent, Norton
PoM **Magnapen®** (Beecham)
Capsules, black/turquoise, co-fluampicil 250/250 (flucloxacillin 250 mg as sodium salt, ampicillin 250 mg as trihydrate). Net price 20-cap pack = £6.15. Label: 9, 22
Syrup, co-fluampicil 125/125 (flucloxacillin 125 mg as magnesium salt, ampicillin 125 mg as trihydrate)/5 mL when reconstituted with water. Net price 100 mL = £4.99. Label: 9, 22
Injection 500 mg, powder for reconstitution, co-fluampicil 250/250 (flucloxacillin 250 mg as sodium salt, ampicillin 250 mg as sodium salt). Net price per vial = £1.33
Electrolytes: Na⁺ 1.3 mmol/vial

PIVAMPICILLIN

Indications: see under Ampicillin
Cautions; Contra-indications; Side-effects: see under Ampicillin; hepatic and renal function tests required in long-term use; avoid in porphyria (see section 9.8.2) and in carnitine deficiency

Dose: 500 mg every 12 hours, doubled in severe infections; CHILD 3 months–1 year 40–60 mg/kg daily in 2–3 divided doses; 1–5 years 350–525 mg daily; 6–10 years 525–700 mg daily; doses can be doubled in severe infections

PoM **Pondocillin®** (Leo)
Tablets, f/c, pivampicillin 500 mg. Net price 20 = £4.22. Label: 5, 9, 21
Suspension, sugar-free, pivampicillin 175 mg/5 mL when reconstituted with water. Net price 100 mL = £2.77. Label: 5, 9, 21

5.1.1.4 ANTIPSEUDOMONAL PENICILLINS

The carboxypenicillin, **ticarcillin**, is principally indicated for serious infections caused by *Pseudomonas aeruginosa* although it also has activity against certain other Gram-negative bacilli including *Proteus* spp. and *Bacteroides fragilis*.

Ticarcillin is now available only in combination with clavulanic acid (section 5.1.1.3); the combination (*Timentin®*) is active against beta-lactamase-producing bacteria resistant to ticarcillin.

The ureidopenicillins, **azlocillin** and **piperacillin**, have a broad spectrum and are both more active than ticarcillin against *Ps. aeruginosa*.

Tazocin® (piperacillin with the beta-lactamase inhibitor tazobactam) is active against beta-lactamase-producing bacteria resistant to the ureidopenicillins.

For pseudomonas septicaemias (especially in neutropenia or endocarditis) these antipseudomonal penicillins should be given with an aminoglycoside (e.g. gentamicin or netilmicin, section 5.1.4) since they have a synergistic effect. Penicillins and aminoglycosides must not, however, be mixed in the same syringe or infusion.

Owing to the sodium content of many of these antibiotics, high doses may lead to hypernatraemia.

AZLOCILLIN
Indications: infections due to *Pseudomonas aeruginosa*, see notes above
Cautions; Contra-indications; Side-effects: see under Benzylpenicillin (section 5.1.1.1); **interactions:** Appendix 1 (penicillins)
Dose: by intravenous injection, 2 g every 8 hours
Serious infections, *by intravenous infusion*, 5 g every 8 hours; PREMATURE INFANT 50 mg/kg every 12 hours; NEONATE 100 mg/kg every 12 hours; INFANT 7 days–1 year 100 mg/kg every 8 hours; CHILD 1–14 years 75 mg/kg every 8 hours

PoM **Securopen®** (Bayer)
Injection, powder for reconstitution, azlocillin (as sodium salt). Net price 1-g vial = £2.36; 2-g vial = £2.94
Electrolytes: Na⁺ 1.08 mmol/500-mg vial, 2.17 mmol/1-g vial, 4.33 mmol/2-g vial
Infusion, powder for reconstitution, azlocillin (as sodium salt). Net price 5 g vial = £8.10 (also available with 50 mL water for injections, transfer needle, and infusion bag)
Electrolytes: Na⁺ 10.84 mmol/5-g vial

PIPERACILLIN
Indications: infections due to *Pseudomonas aeruginosa*, see notes above; surgical prophylaxis
Cautions; Contra-indications; Side-effects: see under Benzylpenicillin (section 5.1.1.1); renal impairment (reduce dose; see Appendix 3); erythema multiforme and Stevens-Johnson syndrome reported rarely; leucopenia with prolonged use
Dose: by deep intramuscular injection or by intravenous injection over 3–5 minutes *or by intravenous infusion*, 100–150 mg/kg daily (in divided doses), increased to 200–300 mg/kg daily in severe infections, and to at least 16 g daily in life-threatening infections; single doses over 2 g intravenous route only; NEONATE *by intravenous injection* over 3–5 minutes *or by intravenous infusion*, aged up to 7 days *or* over 7 days but under 2 kg, 150 mg/kg daily in 3 divided doses; aged over 7 days and over 2 kg, 300 mg/kg daily in 3–4 divided doses; CHILD 1 month–12 years, 100–200 mg/kg daily in 3–4 divided doses, increased in severe infections to 200–300 mg/kg daily in 3–4 divided doses
Surgical prophylaxis, *by deep intramuscular injection or by intravenous injection* over 3–5 minutes *or by intravenous infusion*, 2 g just before surgery (or, in caesarean section, when umbilical cord clamped) followed by at least 2 doses of 2 g at 4 or 6 hour intervals within 24 hours of surgery
Acute gonorrhoea, *by deep intramuscular injection*, 2 g as a single dose

PoM **Pipril®** (Lederle)
Injection, powder for reconstitution, piperacillin (as sodium salt). Net price 1-g vial = £2.79; 2-g vial = £5.53
Infusion, powder for reconstitution, piperacillin 4 g (as sodium salt), with 50-mL bottle water for injections and transfer needle. Net price complete unit = £11.65
Electrolytes: Na⁺ 1.85 mmol/g

With tazobactam
PoM **Tazocin®** (Lederle)
Injection 2.25 g, powder for reconstitution, piperacillin 2 g (as sodium salt), tazobactam 250 mg (as sodium salt). Net price per vial = £7.24
Electrolytes: Na⁺ 4.69 mmol/2.25-g vial
Injection 4.5 g, powder for reconstitution, piperacillin 4 g (as sodium salt), tazobactam 500 mg (as sodium salt). Net price per vial = £13.16; infusion pack (4.5-g infusion bottle, 50-mL bottle water for injections and transfer needle) = £14.48
Electrolytes: Na⁺ 9.37 mmol/4.5-g vial
Dose: lower respiratory-tract, urinary-tract, intra-abdominal and skin infections, and septicaemia, ADULT and CHILD over 12 years, *by intravenous injection* over 3–5 minutes *or by intravenous infusion*, 2.25–4.5 g every 6–8 hours, usually 4.5 g every 8 hours; CHILD under 12 years, not yet recommended

TICARCILLIN
Indications: infections due to *Pseudomonas* and *Proteus* spp, see notes above

Cautions; Contra-indications; Side-effects: see under Benzylpenicillin (section 5.1.1.1)

Dose: see under preparation

With clavulanic acid

Note. For a CSM warning on cholestatic jaundice possibly associated with clavulanic acid, see under Co-amoxiclav p. 241.

PoM **Timentin®** (Beecham)

Injection 1.6 g, powder for reconstitution, ticarcillin 1.5 g (as sodium salt), clavulanic acid 100 mg (as potassium salt). Net price per vial = £3.04

Injection 3.2 g, powder for reconstitution, ticarcillin 3 g (as sodium salt), clavulanic acid 200 mg (as potassium salt). Net price per vial = £6.08

Electrolytes: Na+ 16 mmol, K+ 1 mmol/3.2-g vial

Dose: by intravenous infusion, 3.2 g every 6–8 hours increased to every 4 hours in more severe infections; CHILD 80 mg/kg every 6–8 hours (every 12 hours in neonates)

5.1.2 Cephalosporins, cephamycins, and other beta-lactam antibiotics

Antibiotics discussed in this section include the **cephalosporins**, such as cefotaxime, ceftazidime, cefuroxime, cephalexin and cephradine, the **cephamycin**, cefoxitin, the **monobactam**, aztreonam, and the **carbapenems** imipenem (a thienamycin derivative) and meropenem.

CEPHALOSPORINS AND CEPHAMYCINS

The cephalosporins are broad-spectrum antibiotics which are used for the treatment of septicaemia, pneumonia, meningitis, biliary-tract infections, peritonitis, and urinary-tract infections. All have a similar antibacterial spectrum although individual agents have differing activity against certain organisms. The pharmacology of the cephalosporins is similar to that of the penicillins, excretion being principally renal and blocked by probenecid.

The principal side-effect of the cephalosporins is hypersensitivity and about 10% of penicillin-sensitive patients will also be allergic to the cephalosporins. Haemorrhage due to interference with blood clotting factors has been associated with several cephalosporins.

Cephradine (cefradine) and **cephazolin** (cefazolin) have generally been replaced by the newer cephalosporins mentioned below.

Cefuroxime and **cephamandole** (cefamandole) are 'second generation' cephalosporins and are less susceptible than the earlier cephalosporins to inactivation by beta-lactamases. They are, therefore, active against certain bacteria which are resistant to the other drugs and have greater activity against *Haemophilus influenzae* and *Neisseria gonorrhoeae.*

Cefotaxime, **ceftazidime**, **cefodizime** and **ceftriaxone** are 'third generation' cephalosporins with greater activity than the 'second generation' cephalosporins against certain Gram-negative bacteria. However, they are less active than cefuroxime and cephamandole against Gram-positive bacteria, most

notably *Staphylococcus aureus*. Their broad antibacterial spectrum may encourage superinfection with resistant bacteria or fungi.

Ceftazidime has good activity against pseudomonas. It is also active against other Gram-negative bacteria.

Ceftriaxone has a longer half-life than other cephalosporins and therefore only needs once daily administration. Indications include serious infections such as septicaemia, pneumonia, and meningitis. The calcium salt of ceftriaxone forms a precipitate in the gall bladder which may rarely cause symptoms but these usually resolve when the antibiotic is stopped.

Cefpirome is indicated for urinary-tract, lower respiratory-tract and skin infections, bacteraemia, and infections associated with neutropenia.

Cefoxitin, a cephamycin antibiotic, is active against bowel flora including *Bacteroides fragilis* and because of this it has been recommended for abdominal sepsis such as peritonitis.

ORALLY ACTIVE CEPHALOSPORINS. The orally active 'first generation' cephalosporins, **cephalexin** (cefalexin), **cephradine**, and **cefadroxil** and the 'second generation' cephalosporin, **cefaclor** have a similar antimicrobial spectrum. They are useful for urinary-tract infections which do not respond to other drugs or which occur in pregnancy, respiratory-tract infections, sinusitis, and skin and soft-tissue infections. Cefaclor has good activity against *H. influenzae*, but is associated with protracted skin reactions especially in children. Cefadroxil has a longer duration of action than the other cephalosporins but poor activity against *H. influenzae*. **Cefuroxime axetil**, an ester of the 'second generation' cephalosporin cefuroxime, has the same antibacterial spectrum as the parent compound.

Cefixime has a longer duration of action than the other cephalosporins that are active by mouth. It is presently only licensed for acute infections. **Ceftibuten** is similar to cefixime but is less active against pneumococci.

Cefpodoxime proxetil, is more active than the other oral cephalosporins against respiratory bacterial pathogens and it is licensed for upper and lower respiratory-tract infections.

CEFACLOR

Indications: infections due to sensitive Gram-positive and Gram-negative bacteria, but see notes above

Cautions: penicillin sensitivity; renal impairment (see Appendix 3); pregnancy and breast-feeding (but appropriate to use); false positive urinary glucose (if tested for reducing substances) and false positive Coombs' test; **interactions:** Appendix 1 (cephalosporins)

Contra-indications: cephalosporin hypersensitivity; porphyria (see section 9.8.2)

Side-effects: diarrhoea and rarely antibiotic-associated colitis (CSM has warned both more likely with higher doses), nausea and vomiting, abdominal discomfort, headache; allergic reactions including rashes, pruritus, urticaria, serum sickness-like reactions with rashes, fever and arthralgia, and anaphylaxis; erythema multiforme, toxic epidermal necrolysis reported; disturbances in liver enzymes, transient hepatitis and cholestatic jaundice; other side-effects reported include eosinophilia and blood disorders (including thrombocytopenia, leucopenia, agranulocytosis, aplastic anaemia and haemolytic anaemia); reversible interstitial nephritis, hyperactivity, nervousness, sleep disturbances, confusion, hypertonia, and dizziness

Dose: 250 mg every 8 hours, doubled for severe infections; max. 4 g daily; CHILD over 1 month, 20 mg/kg daily in 3 divided doses, doubled for severe infections, max. 1 g daily; *or* 1 month–1 year, 62.5 mg every 8 hours; 1–5 years, 125 mg; over 5 years, 250 mg; doses doubled for severe infections

PoM **Cefaclor** (Non-proprietary)
Capsules, cefaclor (as monohydrate) 250 mg, net price 21-cap pack = £6.80; 500 mg 21-cap pack = £22.74. Label: 9
Available from Cox, Ethical Generics Ltd, Galen (*Keftid*®), Hillcross, Kent
Suspension, cefaclor (as monohydrate) for reconstitution with water, 125 mg/5 mL, net price 100 mL = £5.16; 250 mg/5 mL, 100 mL = £10.32. Label: 9
Note. Sugar-free versions are available and can be ordered by specifying 'sugar-free' on the prescription
Available from Ethical Generics Ltd, Galen (*Keftid*®), Hillcross

PoM **Distaclor**® (Dista)
Capsules, cefaclor (as monohydrate) 500 mg (violet/grey), net price 20 = £21.66. Label: 9
Suspension, both pink, cefaclor (as monohydrate) for reconstitution with water, 125 mg/5 mL, net price 100 mL = £5.16; 250 mg/5 mL, 100 mL = £10.32. Label: 9

PoM **Distaclor MR**® (Dista)
Tablets, m/r, both blue, cefaclor (as monohydrate) 375 mg. Net price 14-tab pack = £6.93. Label: 9, 21, 25
Dose: 375 mg every 12 hours with food, dose doubled for pneumonia
Lower urinary-tract infections, 375 mg every 12 hours with food

CEFADROXIL
Indications: see under Cefaclor; see also notes above
Cautions; Contra-indications; Side-effects: see under Cefaclor
Dose: patients over 40 kg, 0.5–1 g twice daily; skin, soft tissue, and simple urinary-tract infections, 1 g daily; CHILD under 1 year, 25 mg/kg daily in divided doses; 1–6 years, 250 mg twice daily; over 6 years, 500 mg twice daily

PoM **Baxan**® (Bristol-Myers)
Capsules, cefadroxil 500 mg (as monohydrate). Net price 20 = £5.64. Label: 9
Suspension, cefadroxil (as monohydrate) for reconstitution with water, 125 mg/5 mL, net price 60 mL = £1.75; 250 mg/5 mL, 60 mL = £3.48; 500 mg/5 mL, 60 mL = £5.21. Label: 9

CEFIXIME
Indications: see under Cefaclor and notes above
Cautions; Contra-indications; Side-effects: see under Cefaclor
Dose: ADULT and CHILD over 10 years, 200–400 mg daily as a single dose or in 2 divided doses; CHILD over 6 months 8 mg/kg daily as a single dose or in 2 divided doses *or* 6 months–1 year 75 mg daily; 1–4 years 100 mg daily; 5–10 years 200 mg daily

PoM **Suprax**® (Rhône-Poulenc Rorer)
Tablets, f/c, scored, cefixime 200 mg. Net price 7-tab pack = £10.94. Label: 9
Paediatric oral suspension, cefixime 100 mg/5 mL when reconstituted with water. Net price 37.5 mL (with double-ended spoon for measuring 3.75 mL or 5 mL since dilution not recommended) = £7.18; 75 mL = £12.89. Label: 9

CEFODIZIME
Indications: see under Dose
Cautions; Contra-indications; Side-effects: see under Cefaclor
Dose: by intramuscular or intravenous injection or by intravenous infusion, lower respiratory-tract infection (including pneumonia and broncho-pneumonia), 1 g every 12 hours
Upper and lower urinary-tract infections (including acute and chronic pyelonephritis and cystitis), 1 g every 12 hours *or* 2 g daily (as a single dose); single doses over 1 g intravenous route only

PoM **Timecef**® (Hoechst Marion Roussel)
Injection, powder for reconstitution, cefodizime (as sodium salt), net price 1-g vial = £11.04
Electrolytes: Na+ 3.18 mmol/g

CEFOTAXIME
Indications: see under Cefaclor; surgical prophylaxis; Haemophilus epiglottitis and meningitis (see section 5.1 table 1); see also notes above
Cautions; Contra-indications; Side-effects: see under Cefaclor
Dose: by intramuscular or intravenous injection or by intravenous infusion, 1 g every 12 hours increased up to 12 g daily in 3–4 divided doses in severe infections (doses greater than 6 g daily for sensitive pseudomonal infections); NEONATE, 50 mg/kg daily in 2–4 divided doses increased to 150–200 mg/kg daily in severe infections; CHILD, 100–150 mg/kg daily in 2–4 divided doses increased up to 200 mg/kg daily in very severe infections
Gonorrhoea, 1 g as a single dose

PoM **Claforan**® (Hoechst Marion Roussel)
Injection, powder for reconstitution, cefotaxime (as sodium salt). Net price 500-mg vial = £2.41; 1-g vial = £4.85; 2-g vial = £9.65
Electrolytes: Na+ 2.09 mmol/g

CEFOXITIN

Indications: see under Cefaclor; surgical prophylaxis; more active against Gram-negative bacteria
Cautions; Contra-indications; Side-effects: see under Cefaclor
Dose: by deep intramuscular or by slow intravenous injection or by infusion, 1–2 g every 6–8 hours, increased up to 12 g daily in divided doses for infections requiring higher doses; CHILD up to 1 week 20–40 mg/kg every 12 hours, 1–4 weeks 20–40 mg/kg every 8 hours, over 1 month 20–40 mg/kg every 6–8 hours, increased up to 200 mg/kg daily in divided doses (max. 12 g daily) in severe infections; intravenous route recommended for children
Uncomplicated urinary-tract infection, *by deep intramuscular injection,* 1 g every 12 hours for 10 days
Uncomplicated gonorrhoea, *by deep intramuscular injection,* 2 g as a single dose with probenecid 1 g by mouth
Surgical prophylaxis, *by deep intramuscular injection or by intravenous injection or infusion,* 2 g 30–60 minutes before surgery, dose repeated every 6 hours for usual max. 24 hours; CHILD 30–40 mg/kg 30–60 minutes before surgery, dose repeated every 6 hours for usual max. 24 hours (second and third doses every 8–12 hours in NEONATES); intravenous route recommended for children

PoM **Mefoxin**® (MSD)
Injection, powder for reconstitution, cefoxitin (as sodium salt). Net price 1-g vial = £4.92; 2-g vial = £9.84
Electrolytes: Na+ 2.3 mmol/g

CEFPIROME

Indications: see under Cefaclor and notes above
Cautions; Contra-indications; Side-effects: see under Cefaclor; interference with creatinine assays using picrate method; taste disturbance shortly after injection reported
Dose: by intravenous injection or infusion, complicated upper and lower urinary-tract, skin and soft-tissue infections, 1 g every 12 hours increased to 2 g every 12 hours in very severe infections
Lower respiratory-tract infections, 1–2 g every 12 hours
Severe infections including bacteraemia and septicaemia and infections in neutropenic patients, 2 g every 12 hours
CHILD under 12 years not recommended

PoM **Cefrom**® (Hoechst Marion Roussel)
Injection, powder for reconstitution, cefpirome (as sulphate), net price 1-g vial = £10.75; 2-g vial = £21.50

CEFPODOXIME

Indications: respiratory-tract infections but in pharyngitis and tonsillitis reserved for infections which are recurrent, chronic, or resistant to other antibiotics

Cautions; Contra-indications; Side-effects: see under Cefaclor
Dose: upper respiratory-tract infections, 100 mg twice daily with food (200 mg twice daily in sinusitis)
Lower respiratory-tract infections (including bronchitis and pneumonia), 100–200 mg twice daily with food
CHILD under 15 days not recommended, 15 days–6 months 8 mg/kg daily in 2 divided doses, 6 months–2 years 40 mg twice daily, 3–8 years 80 mg twice daily, over 9 years 100 mg twice daily

PoM **Orelox**® (Hoechst Marion Roussel)
Tablets, f/c, cefpodoxime 100 mg (as cefpodoxime proxetil). Net price 10-tab pack = £9.26. Label: 5, 9, 21
Oral suspension, cefpodoxime (as proxetil) for reconstitution with water, 40 mg/5 mL, net price 50 mL = £6.50, 100 mL = £10.89. Label: 5, 9, 21
Note. Suspension contains aspartame (see section 9.4.1)

CEFTAZIDIME

Indications: see under Cefaclor; see also notes above
Cautions; Contra-indications; Side-effects: see under Cefaclor
Dose: by deep intramuscular injection or intravenous injection or infusion, 1 g every 8 hours *or* 2 g every 12 hours; 2 g every 8–12 hours in severe infections; single doses over 1 g intravenous route only; elderly usual max. 3 g daily; CHILD, up to 2 months 25–60 mg/kg daily in 2 divided doses, over 2 months 30–100 mg/kg daily in 2–3 divided doses; up to 150 mg/kg daily (max. 6 g daily) in 3 divided doses if immunocompromised or meningitis; intravenous route recommended for children
Urinary-tract and less serious infections, 0.5–1 g every 12 hours
Pseudomonal lung infection in cystic fibrosis, ADULT with normal renal function 100–150 mg/kg daily in 3 divided doses; CHILD up to 150 mg/kg daily (max. 6 g daily) in 3 divided doses; intravenous route recommended for children
Surgical prophylaxis, prostatic surgery, 1 g at induction of anaesthesia repeated if necessary when catheter removed

PoM **Fortum**® (GlaxoWellcome)
Injection, powder for reconstitution, ceftazidime (as pentahydrate), with sodium carbonate, net price 250-mg vial = £2.48, 500-mg vial = £4.95, 1-g vial = £9.90, 2-g vial (for injection and for infusion, both) = £19.80, 3-g vial (for injection or infusion) = £29.00; *infusion kit,* 2-g vial, 50-mL bag sodium chloride intravenous infusion, transfer needle, swab, sealing cap, and label, complete kit = £20.82; *Monovial,* 2 g vial (with transfer needle) = £19.80
Electrolytes: Na+ 2.3 mmol/g
PoM **Kefadim**® (Lilly)
Injection, powder for reconstitution, ceftazidime (as pentahydrate), with sodium carbonate, net price 500-mg vial = £4.95, 1-g vial = £9.90, 2-g vial (for injection and for infusion, both) = £19.80
Electrolytes: Na+ 2.3 mmol/g

CEFTIBUTEN

Indications: see under Cefaclor and notes above

Cautions; Contra-indications; Side-effects: see under Cefaclor

Dose: ADULT and CHILD over 10 years (over 45 kg) 400 mg daily as a single dose; CHILD over 6 months, as oral suspension, 9 mg/kg daily as a single dose *or* see under oral suspension below

PoM **Cedax®** (Schering-Plough)

Capsules, ceftibuten (as dihydrate) 400 mg, net price 5-cap pack = £13.03, 7-cap pack = £17.50. Label: 9

Oral suspension, ceftibuten (as dihydrate) for reconstitution with water, 90 mg/5 mL, net price 60 mL = £7.63; 180 mg/5 mL, 60 mL = £15.26. Label: 9

Dose: as oral suspension containing 90 mg/5 mL, CHILD 6 months–1 year 5 mL daily as a single dose, 1–3 years 8 mL daily, 3–6 years 10 mL daily

As oral suspension containing 180 mg/5 mL, CHILD 3–6 years 5 mL daily as a single dose, 6–10 years 8 mL daily, over 10 years 10 mL daily

CEFTRIAXONE

Indications: see under Cefaclor and notes above; surgical prophylaxis

Cautions: see under Cefaclor; severe renal impairment (Appendix 3); hepatic impairment if accompanied by renal impairment (Appendix 2); premature neonates; may displace bilirubin from serum albumin, administer over 60 minutes in neonates (see also Contra-indications)

Contra-indications: see under Cefaclor; neonates with jaundice, hypoalbuminaemia, acidosis or impaired bilirubin binding

Side-effects: see under Cefaclor; calcium ceftriaxone precipitates in urine (particularly in very young, dehydrated or those who are immobilised) or in gall bladder—consider discontinuation if symptomatic; rarely prolongation of prothrombin time

Dose: by deep intramuscular injection, or by intravenous injection over at least 2–4 minutes, *or by intravenous infusion,* 1 g daily as a single dose; 2–4 g daily as a single dose in severe infections; intramuscular doses over 1 g divided between more than one site

INFANT and CHILD 20–50 mg/kg daily as a single dose; up to 80 mg/kg daily as a single dose in severe infections; doses of 50 mg/kg and over by intravenous infusion only; NEONATES *by intravenous infusion* over 60 minutes, 20–50 mg/kg daily as a single dose

Uncomplicated gonorrhoea, *by deep intramuscular injection,* 250 mg as a single dose

Surgical prophylaxis, *by deep intramuscular injection or by intravenous injection* over at least 2–4 minutes, 1 g as a single dose; colorectal surgery, *by intramuscular or by intravenous injection* over at least 2–4 minutes *or by intravenous infusion,* 2 g; intramuscular doses over 1 g divided between more than one site

Prophylaxis of meningococcal meningitis, section 5.1 (table 2)

PoM **Rocephin®** (Roche)

Injection, powder for reconstitution, ceftriaxone (as sodium salt), net price 250-mg vial = £2.87; 1-g vial = £11.46; 2-g vial = £22.92

Electrolytes: Na⁺ 3.6 mmol/g

CEFUROXIME

Indications: see under Cefaclor; surgical prophylaxis; more active against *Haemophilus influenzae* and *Neisseria gonorrhoeae*

Cautions; Contra-indications; Side-effects: see under Cefaclor

Dose: by mouth (as cefuroxime axetil), 250 mg twice daily in most infections including mild to moderate lower respiratory-tract infections (e.g. bronchitis); doubled for more severe lower respiratory-tract infections or if pneumonia suspected

Urinary-tract infection, 125 mg twice daily, doubled in pyelonephritis

Gonorrhoea, 1 g as a single dose

CHILD over 3 months, 125 mg twice daily, if necessary doubled in child over 2 years with otitis media

By intramuscular injection or intravenous injection or infusion, 750 mg every 6–8 hours; 1.5 g every 6–8 hours in severe infections; single doses over 750 mg intravenous route only

CHILD usual dose 60 mg/kg daily (range 30–100 mg/kg daily) in 3–4 divided doses (2–3 divided doses in neonates)

Gonorrhoea, 1.5 g as a single dose by intramuscular injection (divided between 2 sites)

Surgical prophylaxis, 1.5 g by intravenous injection at induction; may be supplemented with 750 mg intramuscularly 8 and 16 hours later (abdominal, pelvic, and orthopaedic operations) *or* followed by 750 mg intramuscularly every 8 hours for further 24–48 hours (cardiac, pulmonary, oesophageal, and vascular operations)

Meningitis, 3 g intravenously every 8 hours; CHILD, 200–240 mg/kg daily (in 3–4 divided doses) reduced to 100 mg/kg daily after 3 days or on clinical improvement; NEONATE, 100 mg/kg daily reduced to 50 mg/kg daily

PoM **Zinacef®** (GlaxoWellcome)

Injection, powder for reconstitution, cefuroxime (as sodium salt). Net price 250-mg vial = 88p; 750-mg vial = £2.64; 1.5-g vial (for injection and for infusion) = £5.29; *infusion kit,* 750-mg vial, 50-mL bag sodium chloride intravenous infusion, transfer needle, swab, sealing cap, and label, complete kit = £3.67; *Zinacef/Metronidazole infusion kit,* 750-mg vial, 100-mL bag metronidazole 5 mg/mL, transfer needle, swab, sealing cap and label, complete kit = £3.77

Electrolytes: Na⁺ 1.8 mmol/750-mg vial

PoM **Zinnat®** (GlaxoWellcome)

Tablets, both f/c, cefuroxime 125 mg (as cefuroxime axetil), net price 14-tab pack = £4.73; 250 mg, 14-tab pack = £9.45. Label: 9, 21, 25

Suspension, cefuroxime (as cefuroxime axetil) 125 mg/5 mL when reconstituted with water. Net price 70 mL = £5.40. Label: 9, 21

Sachets, cefuroxime (as cefuroxime axetil) 125 mg/sachet, net price 14-sachet pack = £5.40. Label: 9, 13, 21

CEPHALEXIN
(Cefalexin)

Indications: see under Cefaclor

Cautions; Contra-indications; Side-effects: see under Cefaclor

Dose: 250 mg every 6 hours *or* 500 mg every 8–12 hours increased to 1–1.5 g every 6–8 hours for severe infections; CHILD, 25 mg/kg daily in divided doses, doubled for severe infections, max. 100 mg/kg daily; *or* under 1 year, 125 mg every 12 hours; 1–5 years, 125 mg every 8 hours; 6–12 years, 250 mg every 8 hours

Prophylaxis of recurrent urinary-tract infection, ADULT 125 mg at night

PoM **Cephalexin** (Non-proprietary)

Capsules, cephalexin 250 mg, net price 20 = £2.21; 500 mg, 20 = £4.23. Label: 9

Available from APS, Berk (Kiflone®), Cox, Hillcross, Kent (Tenkorex®)

Tablets, cephalexin 250 mg, net price 20 = £2.24; 500 mg, 20 = £4.19. Label: 9

Available from APS, Berk (Kiflone®), Cox, Hillcross, Kent (Tenkorex®), Norton

Oral suspension, cephalexin for reconstitution with water, 125 mg/5 mL, net price 100 mL = £1.27; 250 mg/5 mL, 100 mL = £2.48. Label: 9

Available from APS, Berk (Kiflone®), Cox, Hillcross, Kent (Tenkorex®)

PoM **Ceporex®** (GlaxoWellcome)

Capsules, both caramel/grey, cephalexin 250 mg, net price 28-cap pack = £4.47; 500 mg, 28-cap pack = £8.72. Label: 9

Tablets, all pink, f/c, cephalexin 250 mg, net price 28-tab pack = £4.47; 500 mg, 28-tab pack = £8.72; 1 g (scored), 14-tab pack = £8.72. Label: 9

Syrup, all orange, cephalexin for reconstitution with water, 125 mg/5 mL, net price 100 mL = £1.59; 250 mg/5 mL, 100 mL = £3.19; 500 mg/5 mL, 100 mL = £6.19. Label: 9

PoM **Keflex®** (Lilly)

Capsules, cephalexin 250 mg (green/white), net price 28-cap pack = £3.57; 500 mg (pale green/dark green), 21-cap pack = £5.23. Label: 9

Tablets, both peach, cephalexin 250 mg, net price 28-tab pack = £3.57; 500 mg (scored), 21-tab pack = £5.23. Label: 9

Suspension, cephalexin for reconstitution with water, 125 mg/5 mL (pink), net price 100 mL = £1.27; 250 mg/5 mL (orange), 100 mL = £2.55. Label: 9

CEPHAMANDOLE
(Cefamandole)

Indications: see under Cefaclor; surgical prophylaxis

Cautions; Contra-indications; Side-effects: see under Cefaclor

Dose: by deep intramuscular injection or by intravenous injection over 3–5 minutes *or by intravenous infusion,* 0.5–2 g every 4–8 hours; CHILD over 1 month, 50–100 mg/kg daily in 3–6 divided doses increased to 150 mg/kg daily for severe infections

Surgical prophylaxis, by intramuscular or intravenous injection, 1–2 g 30–60 minutes before surgery followed by 1–2 g every 6 hours for 24–48 hours (up to 72 hours for implantation of prostheses)

PoM **Kefadol®** (Dista)

Injection, powder for reconstitution, cephamandole (as nafate) with sodium carbonate. Net price 1-g vial = £3.91

Electrolytes: Na+ 3.35 mmol/1-g vial

CEPHAZOLIN
(Cefazolin)

Indications: see under Cefaclor; surgical prophylaxis

Cautions; Contra-indications; Side-effects: see under Cefaclor

Dose: by intramuscular injection or intravenous injection or infusion, 0.5–1 g every 6–12 hours; CHILD, 25–50 mg/kg daily (in divided doses), increased to 100 mg/kg daily in severe infections

PoM **Kefzol®** (Lilly)

Injection, powder for reconstitution, cephazolin (as sodium salt). Net price 500-mg vial = £2.45; 1-g vial = £3.91

Electrolytes: Na+ 2.1 mmol/g

CEPHRADINE
(Cefradine)

Indications: see under Cefaclor; surgical prophylaxis

Cautions; Contra-indications; Side-effects: see under Cefaclor

Dose: by mouth, 250–500 mg every 6 hours *or* 0.5–1 g every 12 hours; CHILD, 25–50 mg/kg daily in divided doses

By deep intramuscular injection or by intravenous injection over 3–5 minutes *or by intravenous infusion,* 0.5–1 g every 6 hours, increased to 8 g daily in severe infections; CHILD 50–100 mg/kg daily in 4 divided doses

Surgical prophylaxis, by deep intramuscular injection or by intravenous injection over 3–5 minutes, 1–2 g immediately prior to surgery

PoM **Velosef®** (Squibb)

Capsules, cephradine 250 mg (orange/blue), net price 20-cap pack = £3.55; 500 mg (blue), 20-cap pack = £7.00. Label: 9

Syrup, cephradine 250 mg/5 mL when reconstituted with water. Net price 100 mL = £4.22. Label: 9

Injection, powder for reconstitution, cephradine. Net price 500-mg vial = 99p; 1-g vial = £1.95

OTHER BETA-LACTAM ANTIBIOTICS

Aztreonam is a monocyclic beta-lactam ('monobactam') antibiotic with an antibacterial spectrum limited to Gram-negative aerobic bacteria including *Pseudomonas aeruginosa, Neisseria meningitidis,* and *Haemophilus influenzae;* it should not be used alone for 'blind' treatment since it is not active against Gram-positive organisms. Aztreonam is also effective against *Neisseria gonorrhoeae* (but not against concurrent chlamydial infection). Side-effects are similar to those of the other beta-lactams although aztreonam may be less likely to cause hypersensitivity in penicillin-sensitive patients.

Imipenem, a carbapenem, has a broad spectrum of activity which includes many aerobic and anaerobic Gram-positive and Gram-negative bacteria. Imipenem is partially inactivated in the kidney by enzymatic activity and is therefore administered in combination with **cilastatin**, a specific enzyme inhibitor, which blocks its renal metabolism. Side-effects are similar to those of other beta-lactam antibiotics; neurotoxicity has been observed at very high dosage or in renal failure. **Meropenem** is similar to imipenem but is stable to the renal enzyme which inactivates imipenem and therefore can be given without cilastatin. Meropenem has less seizure-inducing potential and can be used to treat central nervous system infection.

AZTREONAM

Indications: Gram-negative infections including *Pseudomonas aeruginosa*, *Haemophilus influenzae*, and *Neisseria meningitidis*

Cautions: hypersensitivity to beta-lactam antibiotics; hepatic impairment; reduce dose in renal impairment; **interactions:** Appendix 1 (aztreonam)

Contra-indications: aztreonam hypersensitivity; pregnancy and breast-feeding

Side-effects: nausea, vomiting, diarrhoea, abdominal cramps; mouth ulcers, altered taste; jaundice and hepatitis; blood disorders (including thrombocytopenia and neutropenia); urticaria and rashes

Dose: *by deep intramuscular injection or by intravenous injection* over 3–5 minutes *or by intravenous infusion,* 1 g every 8 hours *or* 2 g every 12 hours; 2 g every 6–8 hours for severe infections (including systemic *Pseudomonas aeruginosa* and lung infections in cystic fibrosis); single doses over 1 g intravenous route only

CHILD over 1 week, *by intravenous injection or infusion,* 30 mg/kg every 6–8 hours increased in severe infections for child of 2 years or older to 50 mg/kg every 6–8 hours; max. 8 g daily

Urinary-tract infections, 0.5–1 g every 8–12 hours

Gonorrhoea/cystitis, *by intramuscular injection,* 1 g as a single dose

PoM **Azactam**® (Squibb)

Injection, powder for reconstitution, aztreonam. Net price 500-mg vial = £4.48; 1-g vial = £8.95; 2-g vial = £17.90

IMIPENEM WITH CILASTATIN

Indications: aerobic and anaerobic Gram-positive and Gram-negative infections; surgical prophylaxis; not indicated for CNS infections

Cautions: hypersensitivity to other beta-lactam antibiotics; renal impairment; CNS disorders (e.g. epilepsy); pregnancy; **interactions:** Appendix 1 (*Primaxin*®)

Contra-indications: hypersensitivity to imipenem or cilastatin; breast-feeding

Side-effects: nausea, vomiting, diarrhoea (antibiotic-associated colitis reported), taste disturbances; blood disorders, positive Coombs test; allergic reactions (with rash, pruritus, urticaria, fever, anaphylactic reactions, rarely toxic epidermal necrolysis); myoclonic activity, convulsions, confusion and mental disturbances reported; slight increases in liver enzymes and bilirubin reported; increases in serum creatinine and blood urea; red coloration of urine in children reported; local reactions: erythema, pain and induration, and thrombophlebitis

Dose: *by deep intramuscular injection,* mild to moderate infections, in terms of imipenem, 500–750 mg every 12 hours; gonococcal urethritis or cervicitis, 500 mg as a single dose

By intravenous infusion, in terms of imipenem, 1–2 g daily (in 3–4 divided doses); less sensitive organisms, up to 50 mg/kg daily (to max. 4 g daily); CHILD 3 months and older, 60 mg/kg (up to max. of 2 g) daily in 4 divided doses

Surgical prophylaxis, *by intravenous infusion,* 1 g at induction of anaesthesia repeated after 3 hours, supplemented in high risk (e.g. colorectal) surgery by doses of 500 mg 8 and 16 hours after induction

PoM **Primaxin**® (MSD)

Intramuscular injection, powder for reconstitution, imipenem (as monohydrate) 500 mg with cilastatin (as sodium salt) 500 mg. Net price 15-mL vial = £15.00

Electrolytes: Na⁺ 1.47 mmol/vial

Intravenous infusion, powder for reconstitution, imipenem (as monohydrate) 250 mg with cilastatin (as sodium salt) 250 mg. Net price 60-mL vial = £9.00

Electrolytes: Na⁺ 0.86 mmol/vial

Intravenous infusion, powder for reconstitution, imipenem (as monohydrate) 500 mg with cilastatin (as sodium salt) 500 mg. Net price 120-mL vial = £15.00; *Monovial,* 20-mL vial (with transfer needle) = £15.00

Electrolytes: Na⁺ 1.72 mmol/vial

MEROPENEM

Indications: aerobic and anaerobic Gram-positive and Gram-negative infections

Cautions: hypersensitivity to penicillins, cephalosporins and other beta-lactam antibiotics; hepatic impairment (monitor liver function); renal impairment; pregnancy and breast-feeding

Contra-indications: hypersensitivity to meropenem

Side-effects: nausea, vomiting, diarrhoea (antibiotic-associated colitis reported), abdominal pain; disturbances in liver function tests; thrombocytopenia (reduction in partial thromboplastin time reported), positive Coombs' test, eosinophilia, neutropenia; headache, paraesthesia; rash, pruritus, urticaria; convulsions reported, local reactions including pain and thrombophlebitis at injection site

Dose: by intravenous injection over 5 minutes *or by intravenous infusion*, 500 mg every 8 hours, dose doubled in hospital-acquired pneumonia, peritonitis, septicaemia and infections in neutropenic patients; CHILD 3 months–12 years 10–20 mg/kg every 8 hours, over 50 kg body weight adult dose

Meningitis, 2 g every 8 hours; CHILD 3 months–12 years 40 mg/kg every 8 hours, over 50 kg body weight adult dose

Exacerbations of chronic lower respiratory-tract infection in cystic fibrosis, up to 2 g every 8 hours; CHILD 4–18 years 25–40 mg/kg every 8 hours

PoM **Meronem**® (Zeneca)
Injection, powder for reconstitution, meropenem (as trihydrate), net price 250-mg vial = £10.00; 500-mg vial = £15.00; 1-g vial = £30.00
Intravenous infusion, powder for reconstitution, meropenem (as trihydrate), with 100-mL mini-bag sodium chloride 0.9%, net price 500-mg vial = £16.00; 1-g vial = £31.00
Electrolytes: Na⁺ 3.9 mmol/g

5.1.3   Tetracyclines
The tetracyclines are broad-spectrum antibiotics whose value has decreased owing to increasing bacterial resistance. They remain, however, the treatment of choice for infections caused by chlamydia (trachoma, psittacosis, salpingitis, urethritis, and lymphogranuloma venereum), rickettsia (including Q-fever), brucella (doxycycline with either streptomycin or rifampicin), and the spirochaete, *Borrelia burgdorferi* (Lyme disease). They are also used in respiratory and genital mycoplasma infections, in acne, in destructive (refractory) periodontal disease, in exacerbations of chronic bronchitis (because of their activity against *Haemophilus influenzae*), and for leptospirosis in penicillin hypersensitivity (as an alternative to erythromycin).

Microbiologically, there is little to choose between the various tetracyclines, the only exception being **minocycline** which has a broader spectrum; it is active against *Neisseria meningitidis* and has been used for meningococcal prophylaxis but is no longer recommended because of side-effects including dizziness and vertigo (see section 5.1, table 2 for current recommendations).

The tetracyclines are deposited in growing bone and teeth (being bound to calcium) causing staining and occasionally dental hypoplasia, and should **not** be given to children under 12 years or to pregnant or breast-feeding women. With the exception of **doxycycline** and **minocycline** the tetracyclines may exacerbate renal failure and should **not** be given to patients with kidney disease. Absorption of tetracyclines is decreased by milk (except doxycycline and minocycline), antacids, and calcium, iron and magnesium salts.

TETRACYCLINE
Indications: exacerbations of chronic bronchitis; brucellosis (see also notes above), chlamydia, mycoplasma, and rickettsia; pleural effusions due to malignancy or cirrhosis; acne vulgaris, rosacea (section 13.6)

Cautions: hepatic impairment (avoid intravenous administration); renal impairment (see Appendix 3); rarely causes photosensitivity; **interactions:** Appendix 1 (tetracyclines)
Contra-indications: renal impairment (see Appendix 3), pregnancy and breast-feeding (see also Appendixes 4 and 5), children under 12 years of age, systemic lupus erythematosus
Side-effects: nausea, vomiting, diarrhoea; erythema (discontinue treatment); headache and visual disturbances may indicate benign intracranial hypertension; hepatotoxicity, pancreatitis and antibiotic-associated colitis reported; see also notes above
Dose: by mouth, 250 mg every 6 hours, increased in severe infections to 500 mg every 6–8 hours
Acne, see section 13.6
Primary, secondary, or latent syphilis, 500 mg every 6 hours for 14–21 days
Non-gonococcal urethritis, 500 mg every 6 hours for 7–14 days (21 days if failure or relapse following the first course)
COUNSELLING. Tablets or capsules should be swallowed whole with plenty of fluid while sitting or standing
By intravenous infusion, 500 mg every 12 hours; max. 2 g daily
Pleural effusions, see under *Achromycin*® intravenous infusion

PoM **Tetracycline** (Non-proprietary)
Tablets, coated, tetracycline hydrochloride 250 mg. Net price 20 = 32p. Label: 7, 9, 23, counselling, posture, see above
Available from Cox, Hillcross, Kent, Norton
PoM **Achromycin**® (Lederle)
Capsules, orange, tetracycline hydrochloride 250 mg. Net price 20 = 96p. Label: 7, 9, 23, counselling, posture, see above
Intravenous infusion, powder for reconstitution, tetracycline hydrochloride. Net price 500-mg vial = £1.98
Dose: infections, see above
Recurrent pleural effusions, by intrapleural instillation, 500 mg in 30–50 mL sodium chloride intravenous infusion 0.9%
PoM **Sustamycin**® (Syner-Med)
Capsules, m/r, light blue/dark blue, tetracycline hydrochloride 250 mg. Net price 50-cap pack = £6.00. Label: 7, 9, 23, 25
Dose: 2 capsules initially, then 1 every 12 hours
PoM **Tetrachel**® (Berk)
Capsules, orange, tetracycline hydrochloride 250 mg. Net price 20 = 49p. Label: 7, 9, 23, counselling, posture, see above

Compound preparations
PoM **Deteclo**® (Lederle)
Tablets, blue, f/c, tetracycline hydrochloride 115.4 mg, chlortetracycline hydrochloride 115.4 mg, demeclocycline hydrochloride 69.2 mg. Net price 20 = £2.48. Label: 7, 9, 11, 23, counselling, posture, see above
Dose: 1 tablet every 12 hours; 3–4 tablets daily in more severe infections

---

DEMECLOCYCLINE HYDROCHLORIDE

Indications: see under Tetracycline; also inappropriate secretion of antidiuretic hormone, section 6.5.2

Cautions; Contra-indications; Side-effects: see under Tetracycline, but photosensitivity is more common; reversible nephrogenic diabetes insipidus reported

Dose: 150 mg every 6 hours *or* 300 mg every 12 hours

PoM **Ledermycin**® (Lederle)
Capsules, red, demeclocycline hydrochloride 150 mg. Net price 20 = £4.13. Label: 7, 9, 11, 23

DOXYCYCLINE

Indications: see under Tetracycline; brucellosis (with rifampicin); also chronic prostatitis and sinusitis; pelvic inflammatory disease (with metronidazole, section 5.1, table 1); malaria (section 5.4.1); acne, rosacea (section 13.6)

Cautions; Contra-indications; Side-effects: see under Tetracycline, but may be used in renal impairment; photosensitivity reported (avoid exposure to sunlight or sun lamps); avoid in porphyria (see section 9.8.2)

Dose: 200 mg on first day, then 100 mg daily; severe infections (including refractory urinary-tract infections), 200 mg daily
Acne, 50 mg daily for 6–12 weeks or longer
Uncomplicated genital chlamydia, non-gonococcal urethritis, 100 mg twice daily for 7–21 days (14–21 days in pelvic inflammatory disease)
COUNSELLING. Capsules should be swallowed whole with plenty of fluid during meals while sitting or standing

PoM **Doxycycline** (Non-proprietary)
Capsules, doxycycline (as hydrochloride) 50 mg, net price 28-cap pack = £7.27; 100 mg, 20 = £5.92. Label: 6, 9, 11, 27, counselling, posture, see above
Available from APS, Ashbourne (*Demix*®), Berk (*Cyclodox*®), Cox, Hillcross, ISIS (*Ramysis*®), Kent, Lagap (*Doxylar*®), Norton

PoM **Vibramycin**® (Invicta)
Capsules, doxycycline (as hydrochloride) 50 mg (green/ivory), net price 28-cap pack = £7.74, 56-cap pack (*Acne Pack*) = £17.80; 100 mg (green), 8-cap pack = £4.18. Label: 6, 9, 11, 27, counselling, posture, see above

PoM **Vibramycin-D**® (Invicta)
Dispersible tablets, off-white, doxycycline 100 mg. Net price 8-tab pack = £4.91. Label: 6, 9, 11, 13

LYMECYCLINE

Indications; Cautions; Contra-indications; Side-effects: see under Tetracycline
Dose: 408 mg every 12 hours

PoM **Tetralysal 300**® (Galderma)
Capsules, lymecycline 408 mg (≡tetracycline 300 mg). Net price 28-cap pack = £4.97. Label: 6, 9

MINOCYCLINE

Indications: see under Tetracycline; also meningococcal carrier state

Cautions; Contra-indications: see under Tetracycline, but may be used in renal impairment; if treatment continued for longer than 6 months, monitor for hepatotoxicity and for systemic lupus erythematosus—discontinue if these develop or if pre-existing systemic lupus erythematosus worsens

Side-effects: see under Tetracycline; also dizziness and vertigo (more common in women); severe exfoliative rashes, pigmentation (sometimes irreversible) discolouration of conjunctiva, tears and sweat, systemic lupus erythematosus and liver damage reported

Dose: 100 mg twice daily
Acne, 50 mg twice daily *or* 100 mg once daily for minimum course of 6 weeks (discontinue if no satisfactory response after 6 months)
Gonorrhoea, initially 200 mg then 100 mg every 12 hours for at least 4 days in men; women may require longer treatment
Prophylaxis of asymptomatic meningococcal carrier state (but no longer recommended, see notes above), 100 mg twice daily for 5 days usually followed by rifampicin

PoM **Minocycline** (Non-proprietary)
Capsules, minocycline (as hydrochloride) 50 mg, net price 56-cap pack = £17.20; 100 mg, 28-cap pack = £14.74. Label: 6, 9
Available from Merck (*Aknemin*®)
Tablets, minocycline (as hydrochloride) 50 mg, net price 84 tab pack = £16.46; 100 mg, 20 = £8.15, Label: 6, 9
Available from APS, Ashbourne (*Blemix*®), Berk (*Cyclomin*®), Cox, CP, Hillcross, Kent, Lederle (*Minocin*®), Norton

PoM **Minocin MR**® (Lederle)
Capsules, m/r, orange/brown (enclosing yellow and orange pellets), minocycline (as hydrochloride) 100 mg. Net price 56-cap pack = £32.03. Label: 6, 25
Dose: acne, 1 capsule daily

OXYTETRACYCLINE

Indications; Cautions; Contra-indications; Side-effects: see under Tetracycline; avoid in porphyria (see section 9.8.2)
Dose: 250–500 mg every 6 hours

PoM **Oxytetracycline** (Non-proprietary)
Tablets, coated, oxytetracycline dihydrate 250 mg, net price 20 = 26p. Label: 7, 9, 23
Available from APS, Ashbourne (*Oxytetramix*®), Berk (*Berkmycen*®, contain tartrazine), Cox, DDSA (*Oxymycin*®), Kent, Norton

PoM **Terramycin**® (Pfizer)
Capsules, yellow, oxytetracycline 250 mg (as hydrochloride). Net price 28-cap pack = 96p. Label: 7, 9, 23
Tablets, yellow, s/c, oxytetracycline 250 mg (as dihydrate). Net price 28-tab pack = 96p. Label: 7, 9, 23

5.1.4   Aminoglycosides

These include amikacin, gentamicin, kanamycin, neomycin, netilmicin, streptomycin, and tobramycin. All are bactericidal and active against some Gram-positive and many Gram-negative organisms. Amikacin, gentamicin, and tobramycin are also active against *Pseudomonas aeruginosa*; streptomycin is active against *Mycobacterium tuberculosis* and is now almost entirely reserved for tuberculosis (section 5.1.9).

The aminoglycosides are not absorbed from the gut (although there is a risk of absorption in inflammatory bowel disease and liver failure) and must therefore be given by injection for systemic infections.

Excretion is principally via the kidney and accumulation occurs in renal impairment.

Most side-effects of this group of antibiotics are dose-related therefore care must be taken with dosage and whenever possible treatment should not exceed 7 days. The important side-effects are ototoxicity, and nephrotoxicity; they occur most commonly in the elderly and in patients with renal failure.

If there is impairment of renal function (or high pre-dose plasma concentrations) the interval between doses must be increased; if the renal impairment is severe the dose itself should be reduced as well.

Aminoglycosides may impair neuromuscular transmission and should not be given to patients with myasthenia gravis; large doses given during surgery have been responsible for a transient myasthenic syndrome in patients with normal neuromuscular function.

Aminoglycosides should not be given with potentially ototoxic diuretics (e.g. frusemide and ethacrynic acid); if concurrent use is unavoidable administration of the aminoglycoside and of the diuretic should be separated by as long a period as practicable.

Plasma concentrations. Plasma concentration monitoring avoids both excessive and subtherapeutic concentrations thus preventing toxicity and ensuring efficacy. Concentrations should be measured approximately 1 hour after intramuscular or intravenous administration and also just before the next dose.

If possible plasma aminoglycoside concentrations should be measured in all patients and **must** be determined in *infants*, in *elderly*, in *obesity*, and in *cystic fibrosis, or* if *high doses* are being given, *or* if there is *renal impairment, or* if treatment lasts *longer than 7 days*.

Once daily dosage. Although aminoglycosides are generally given in 2–3 divided doses during the 24 hours, *once daily administration* has been shown to reduce the risk of toxicity (while ensuring adequate plasma concentrations) but **expert advice** about dosage and plasma concentrations should be obtained.

Gentamicin is the most important of the aminoglycosides and is widely used for the treatment of serious infections. It is the aminoglycoside of choice in the UK. It has a broad spectrum but is inactive against anaerobes and has poor activity against haemolytic streptococci and pneumococci. When used for the 'blind' therapy of undiagnosed serious infections it is usually given in conjunction with a penicillin and/or metronidazole.

The daily dose is up to 5 mg/kg given in divided doses every 8 hours (if renal function is normal); whenever possible treatment should not exceed 7 days. Higher doses are occasionally indicated for serious infections, especially in the neonate or the compromised host. A lower dose of 80 mg twice daily (60 mg for lighter or elderly patients) in association with benzylpenicillin is sufficient for endocarditis due to oral streptococci (often termed *Streptococcus viridans*) and gut streptococci.

Amikacin is a derivative of kanamycin and has one important advantage over gentamicin in that it is stable to 8 of the 9 classified aminoglycoside-inactivating enzymes whereas gentamicin is inactivated by 5. It is principally indicated for the treatment of serious infections caused by Gram-negative bacilli resistant to gentamicin.

Kanamycin has been superseded by other aminoglycosides.

Netilmicin has similar activity to gentamicin, but may cause less ototoxicity in those needing treatment for longer than 10 days. Netilmicin is active against a number of gentamicin-resistant Gram-negative bacilli but is less active against *Ps. aeruginosa* than gentamicin or tobramycin.

Tobramycin is similar to gentamicin. It is slightly more active against *Ps. aeruginosa* but shows less activity against certain other Gram-negative bacteria.

Neomycin is too toxic for parenteral administration and can only be used for infections of the skin or mucous membranes or to reduce the bacterial population of the colon prior to bowel surgery or in hepatic failure. Oral administration may lead to malabsorption. Small amounts of neomycin may be absorbed from the gut in patients with hepatic failure and, as these patients may also be uraemic, cumulation may occur with resultant ototoxicity.

Pregnancy. Where possible, the aminoglycosides should be avoided in pregnancy as they cross the placenta and can cause fetal eighth nerve damage.

GENTAMICIN

Indications: septicaemia and neonatal sepsis; meningitis and other CNS infections; biliary-tract infection, acute pyelonephritis or prostatitis, endocarditis caused by *Strep. viridans* or *Strep. faecalis* (with a penicillin); pneumonia in hospital patients, adjunct in listerial meningitis (section 5.1, table 1)

Cautions: renal impairment, infants and elderly (adjust dose and monitor renal, auditory and vestibular function together with plasma gentamicin concentrations); avoid prolonged use; see also notes above; **interactions:** Appendix 1 (aminoglycosides)

Contra-indications: pregnancy, myasthenia gravis

Side-effects: vestibular and auditory damage, nephrotoxicity; rarely, hypomagnesaemia on prolonged therapy, antibiotic-associated colitis; also reported, nausea, vomiting, rash; see also notes above

Dose: by intramuscular or by slow intravenous injection over at least 3 minutes *or by intravenous infusion,* 2–5 mg/kg daily (in divided doses every 8 hours), see also notes above; reduce dose and measure plasma concentrations in renal impairment

CHILD up to 2 weeks, 3 mg/kg every 12 hours; 2 weeks–12 years, 2 mg/kg every 8 hours

By intrathecal injection, 1 mg daily (increased if necessary to 5 mg daily), with 2–4 mg/kg daily *by intramuscular injection* (in divided doses every 8 hours)

Endocarditis prophylaxis, section 5.1, table 2

Note. One-hour ('peak') concentration should not exceed 10 mg/litre; pre-dose ('trough') concentration should be less than 2 mg/litre

PoM **Gentamicin** (Non-proprietary)
Injection, gentamicin (as sulphate), net price 40 mg/mL, 1-mL amp = £1.40, 2-mL amp = £1.54, 2-mL vial = £1.54
Available from Faulding DBL

PoM **Cidomycin**® (Hoechst Marion Roussel)
Injection, gentamicin 40 mg (as sulphate)/mL. Net price 2-mL amp or vial = £1.55
Paediatric injection, gentamicin 10 mg (as sulphate)/mL. Net price 2-mL vial = 65p
Intrathecal injection, gentamicin 5 mg (as sulphate)/mL. Net price 1-mL amp = 77p

PoM **Genticin**® (Roche)
Injection, gentamicin 40 mg (as sulphate)/mL. Net price 2-mL amp = £1.58

PoM **Isotonic Gentamicin Injection** (Baxter)
Intravenous infusion, gentamicin 800 micrograms (as sulphate)/mL in sodium chloride intravenous infusion 0.9%. Net price 100 mL (80-mg) Viaflex® bag = £1.61
Electrolytes: Na$^+$ 15.4 mmol/100-mL bag

AMIKACIN

Indications: serious Gram-negative infections resistant to gentamicin

Cautions; Contra-indications; Side-effects: see under Gentamicin

Dose: by intramuscular or by slow intravenous injection or by infusion, 15 mg/kg daily in 2 divided doses, see also notes above

Note. One-hour ('peak') concentration should not exceed 30 mg/litre; pre-dose ('trough') concentration should be less than 10 mg/litre

PoM **Amikacin** (Non-proprietary)
Injection, amikacin (as sulphate) 250 mg/mL. Net price 2-mL vial = £9.64
Electrolytes: Na$^+$ 0.56 mmol/500-mg vial
Available from Faulding DBL

PoM **Amikin**® (Bristol-Myers)
Injection, amikacin (as sulphate) 250 mg/mL. Net price 2-mL vial = £10.14
Electrolytes: Na$^+$ < 0.5 mmol/vial

Paediatric injection, amikacin (as sulphate) 50 mg/mL. Net price 2-mL vial = £2.36
Electrolytes: Na$^+$ < 0.5 mmol/vial

KANAMYCIN

Indications: superseded by other aminoglycosides (see notes above)

Cautions; Contra-indications; Side-effects: see under Gentamicin

Dose: by intramuscular injection, 250 mg every 6 hours *or* 500 mg every 12 hours, see also notes above

By intravenous infusion, 15–30 mg/kg daily in divided doses every 8–12 hours, see also notes above

Note. One-hour ('peak') concentration should not exceed 30 mg/litre; pre-dose ('trough') concentration should be less than 10 mg/litre

PoM **Kannasyn**® (Sanofi Winthrop)
Powder (for preparing injections), kanamycin (as acid sulphate). Net price 1-g vial = £23.77

NEOMYCIN SULPHATE

Indications: bowel sterilisation prior to surgery, see also notes above

Cautions; Contra-indications; Side-effects: see under Gentamicin but too toxic for systemic use, see notes above; avoid in intestinal obstruction and in renal impairment

Dose: by mouth, bowel sterilisation, 1 g every 4 hours

Hepatic coma, up to 4 g daily in divided doses usually for a max. 14 days

PoM **Mycifradin**® (Pharmacia & Upjohn)
Tablets, neomycin sulphate 500 mg. Net price 20 = £3.60

PoM **Nivemycin**® (Knoll)
Tablets, neomycin sulphate 500 mg. Net price 20 = £2.17

NETILMICIN

Indications: serious Gram-negative infections resistant to gentamicin

Cautions; Contra-indications; Side-effects: see under Gentamicin

Dose: by intramuscular injection or by intravenous injection over 3–5 minutes *or by intravenous infusion,* 4–6 mg/kg daily, as a single daily dose or in divided doses every 8 or 12 hours; in severe infections, up to 7.5 mg/kg daily in divided doses every 8 hours (reduced as soon as clinically indicated, usually within 48 hours) NEONATE up to 1 week, 3 mg/kg every 12 hours; INFANT over 1 week, 2.5–3 mg/kg every 8 hours; CHILD 2–2.5 mg/kg every 8 hours

Urinary-tract infection, 150 mg as a single daily dose for 5 days

Gonorrhoea, 300 mg as a single dose

Note. For divided daily dose regimens, one-hour ('peak') concentration should not exceed 12 mg/litre; pre-dose ('trough') concentration should be less than 2 mg/litre

PoM **Netillin**® (Schering-Plough)

Injection, netilmicin (as sulphate) 10 mg/mL, net price 1.5-mL (15-mg) amp = £1.49; 50 mg/mL, 1-mL (50-mg) amp = £2.21; 100 mg/mL, 1-mL (100-mg) amp = £2.88; 1.5-mL (150-mg) amp = £4.11, 2-mL (200-mg) amp = £5.33

TOBRAMYCIN

Indications: see under Gentamicin and notes above

Cautions; Contra-indications; Side-effects: see under Gentamicin

Dose: by intramuscular injection or by slow intravenous injection or by intravenous infusion, 3 mg/kg daily in divided doses every 8 hours, see also notes above; in severe infections up to 5 mg/kg daily in divided doses every 6–8 hours (reduced to 3 mg/kg as soon as clinically indicated); NEONATE 2 mg/kg every 12 hours; CHILD over 1 week 2–2.5 mg/kg every 8 hours

Urinary-tract infection, *by intramuscular injection*, 2–3 mg/kg daily as a single dose

Note. One-hour ('peak') concentration should not exceed 10 mg/litre; pre-dose ('trough') concentration should be less than 2 mg/litre

PoM **Tobramycin** (Non-proprietary)

Injection, tobramycin (as sulphate) 40 mg/mL, net price 1-mL (40-mg) vial = £3.22, 2-mL (80-mg) vial = £5.78

Available from Faulding DBL

PoM **Nebcin**® (Lilly)

Injection, tobramycin (as sulphate) 10 mg/mL, net price 2-mL (20-mg) vial = £2.38; 40 mg/mL, 1-mL (40-mg) vial = £3.22, 2-mL (80-mg) vial = £5.78

5.1.5   Macrolides

Erythromycin has an antibacterial spectrum that is similar but not identical to that of penicillin; it is thus an alternative in penicillin-allergic patients.

Indications for erythromycin include respiratory infections, whooping cough, legionnaires' disease, and campylobacter enteritis. It has activity against gut anaerobes and has been used with neomycin for prophylaxis before bowel surgery. It is active against many penicillin-resistant staphylococci but some are now also resistant to erythromycin; it has poor activity against *Haemophilus influenzae*. Erythromycin is also active against chlamydia and mycoplasmas.

Erythromycin causes nausea, vomiting, and diarrhoea in some patients; in mild to moderate infections this can be avoided by giving a lower dose (250 mg 4 times daily) but if a more serious infection, such as Legionella pneumonia, is suspected higher doses are needed.

Azithromycin is a macrolide with slightly less activity than erythromycin against Gram-positive bacteria but enhanced activity against some Gram-negative organisms including *H. influenzae*. Plasma concentrations are very low but tissue concentrations are much higher. It has a long tissue half-life and once daily dosage is recommended.

Clarithromycin is an erythromycin derivative with slightly greater activity than the parent compound. Tissue concentrations are higher than with erythromycin. It is given twice daily.

Azithromycin and clarithromycin cause fewer gastro-intestinal side-effects than erythromycin.

Spiramycin is also a macrolide (see section 5.4.7).

ERYTHROMYCIN

Indications: alternative to penicillin in hypersensitive patients; campylobacter enteritis, pneumonia, legionnaires' disease, syphilis, non-gonococcal urethritis, chronic prostatitis, acne vulgaris and rosacea (see section 13.6); diphtheria and whooping cough prophylaxis

Cautions: hepatic and renal impairment; prolongation of QT interval (ventricular tachycardia reported); porphyria (see section 9.8.2); pregnancy (not known to be harmful) and breast-feeding (only small amounts in milk); **interactions:** Appendix 1 (erythromycin and other macrolides)

ARRHYTHMIAS. Avoid concomitant administration with astemizole or terfenadine, see also pp. 142 and 143; also avoid with cisapride (see p. 34).[other interactions, Appendix 1]

Contra-indications: estolate contra-indicated in liver disease

Side-effects: nausea, vomiting, abdominal discomfort, diarrhoea (antibiotic-associated colitis reported); urticaria, rashes and other allergic reactions; reversible hearing loss reported after large doses; cholestatic jaundice and cardiac effects (including chest pain and arrhythmias) also reported

Dose: by mouth, ADULT and CHILD over 8 years, 250–500 mg every 6 hours *or* 0.5–1 g every 12 hours (see notes above); up to 4 g daily in severe infections; CHILD up to 2 years 125 mg every 6 hours, 2–8 years 250 mg every 6 hours, doses doubled for severe infections

Acne, see section 13.6

Early syphilis, 500 mg 4 times daily for 14–21 days

Non-gonococcal urethritis, 500 mg 2–4 times daily for 7–14 days

By intravenous infusion, ADULT and CHILD severe infections, 50 mg/kg daily by continuous infusion *or* in divided doses every 6 hours; mild infections (oral treatment not possible), 25 mg/kg daily

PoM **Erythromycin** (Non-proprietary)

Tablets, e/c, erythromycin 250 mg, net price 20 = 82p; 500 mg, 20 = £1.80. Label: 5, 9, 25

Available from Abbott, APS, Ashbourne (Rommix®), Berk (Erycen®), Cox, Kent, Norton

PoM **Erythromycin Ethyl Succinate** (Non-proprietary)

Oral suspension, erythromycin (as ethyl succinate) for reconstitution with water 125 mg/5 mL, net price 100 mL = £1.07; 250 mg/5 mL, 100 mL = £1.78; 500 mg/5 mL, 100 mL = £3.02. Label: 9

Note. Sugar-free versions are available and can be ordered by specifying 'sugar-free' on the prescription

Available from APS, Ashbourne (Rommix®), Berk, Cox, Hillcross, Kent, Lagap, Norton, Rosemont (Arpimycin®)

PoM **Erythromycin Lactobionate** (Non-proprietary)

Intravenous infusion, powder for reconstitution, erythromycin (as lactobionate), net price 1-g vial = £9.90

Available from Abbott, Faulding DBL

PoM **Erymax®** (Elan)

Capsules, opaque orange/clear orange, enclosing orange and white e/c pellets, erythromycin 250 mg. Net price 30-cap pack = £6.08. Label: 5, 9, 25

Dose: 1 every 6 hours *or* 2 every 12 hours; acne, 1 twice daily then 1 daily after 1 month

PoM **Erymin®** (Elan)

Oral Suspension, m/r (polymer-coated suspension in soya oil), erythromycin (as ethyl succinate), 250 mg/5 mL. Net price 70 mL = £5.32. Label: 9, 23

Dose: ADULT and CHILD over 8 years, 625 mg every 12 hours, doubled in severe infections; CHILD up to 2 years 125 mg every 12 hours, 2–8 years 250 mg every 12 hours, doses doubled in severe infections

Note. Contains aspartame (see section 9.4.1)

PoM **Erythrocin®** (Abbott)

Tablets, both f/c, erythromycin (as stearate), 250 mg, net price 20 = £2.65; 500 mg, 20 = £5.46. Label: 9

PoM **Erythroped®** (Abbott)

Suspension, erythromycin (as ethyl succinate) for reconstitution with water, 125 mg/5 mL (*Suspension PI*), net price 140 mL = £2.81; 250 mg/5 mL, 140 mL = £5.32; 500 mg/5 mL (*Suspension forte*), 140 mL = £9.43. Label: 9

Suspension SF, sugar-free, erythromycin (as ethyl succinate) for reconstitution with water, 125 mg/5 mL (*Suspension PI SF*), net price 140 mL = £2.89; 250 mg/5 mL, 140 mL = £5.63. Label: 9

Granules, erythromycin (as ethyl succinate), 250 mg/sachet, net price 28-sachet pack = £6.64; 500 mg/sachet (*Granules forte*), 28-sachet pack = £10.75. Label: 9, 13

PoM **Erythroped A®** (Abbott)

Tablets, yellow, f/c, erythromycin 500 mg (as ethyl succinate). Net price 28-tab pack = £9.26. Label: 9

PoM **Ilosone®** (Dista)

Capsules, ivory/red, erythromycin 250 mg (as estolate). Net price 20 = £6.26. Label: 9

Tablets, pink, erythromycin 500 mg (as estolate). Net price 12-tab pack = £7.48. Label: 9

PoM **Tiloryth®** (Tillomed)

Capsules, enclosing e/c microgranules, erythromycin 250 mg. Net price 30-cap pack = £6.08. Label 5, 9, 25

AZITHROMYCIN

Indications: respiratory-tract infections; otitis media; skin and soft-tissue infections; uncomplicated genital chlamydial infections

Cautions; Side-effects: see under Erythromycin; caution in pregnancy and breast-feeding; photosensitivity and mild neutropenia reported; **interactions:** Appendix 1 (erythromycin and other macrolides)

Contra-indications: hepatic impairment

Dose: 500 mg once daily for 3 days; CHILD over 6 months 10 mg/kg once daily for 3 days; *or* body-weight 15–25 kg, 200 mg once daily for 3 days; body-weight 26–35 kg, 300 mg once daily for 3 days; body-weight 36–45 kg, 400 mg once daily for 3 days

Genital chlamydial infections, 1 g as a single dose

PoM **Zithromax®** (Richborough)

Capsules, azithromycin (as dihydrate) 250 mg. Net price 4-cap pack = £8.95, 6-cap pack = £13.43. Label: 5, 9, 23

Oral suspension, azithromycin (as dihydrate) 200 mg/5 mL when reconstituted with water. Net price 15-mL pack = £5.08, 22.5-mL pack = £7.62, 30-mL pack = £13.80. Label: 5, 9, 23

CLARITHROMYCIN

Indications: respiratory-tract infections, mild to moderate skin and soft tissue infections; adjunct in the treatment of duodenal ulcers by eradication of *Helicobacter pylori*—see section 1.3

Cautions; Side-effects: see under Erythromycin; reduce dose in renal impairment; caution in pregnancy and breast-feeding; also reported, headache, taste disturbances, stomatitis, glossitis, cholestasis, jaundice, hepatitis, and Stevens-Johnson syndrome; on intravenous infusion, local tenderness, phlebitis; **interactions:** Appendix 1 (erythromycin and other macrolides)

ARRHYTHMIAS. Avoid concomitant administration with astemizole or terfenadine, see also pp. 142 and 143, also avoid with cisapride (see p. 34) [other interactions, Appendix 1]

Dose: by mouth, 250 mg every 12 hours for 7 days, increased in severe infections to 500 mg every 12 hours for up to 14 days; CHILD body-weight under 8 kg, 7.5 mg/kg twice daily; 8–11 kg (1–2 years), 62.5 mg twice daily, 12–19 kg (3–6 years), 125 mg twice daily; 20–29 kg (7–9 years), 187.5 mg twice daily; 30–40 kg (10–12 years), 250 mg twice daily

Eradication of *H. pylori*, see section 1.3

By intravenous infusion into larger proximal vein, 500 mg twice daily; CHILD not recommended

PoM **Klaricid®** (Abbott)

Tablets, both yellow, f/c, clarithromycin 250 mg, net price 14-tab pack = £11.24; 500 mg, 14-tab pack = £22.49, 20-tab pack = £32.13. Label: 9

Paediatric suspension, clarithromycin 125 mg/5 mL when reconstituted with water. Net price 70 mL = £6.00, 100 mL = £10.32. Label: 9

Intravenous infusion, powder for reconstitution, clarithromycin. Net price 500-mg vial = £12.14

Electrolytes: Na⁺ < 0.5 mmol/500-mg vial

PoM **Klaricid XL®** (Abbott)

Tablets, m/r, yellow, clarithromycin 500 mg, net price 7-tab pack = £11.24, 14-tab pack = £22.48. Label: 9, 21, 25

Dose: 500 mg once daily (doubled in severe infections) for 7–14 days

5.1.6   Clindamycin

Clindamycin has only a limited use because of serious side-effects. Its most serious toxic effect is antibiotic-associated colitis (section 1.5) which may be fatal and is most common in middle-aged and elderly women, especially following operation. Although it can occur with most antibiotics it is more frequently seen with clindamycin. Patients should therefore discontinue treatment immediately if diarrhoea develops.

Clindamycin is active against Gram-positive cocci, including penicillin-resistant staphylococci and also against many anaerobes, especially *Bacteroides fragilis*. It is well concentrated in bone and excreted in bile and urine.

Clindamycin is recommended for staphylococcal joint and bone infections such as osteomyelitis, and intra-abdominal sepsis. Clindamycin is also used for endocarditis prophylaxis (section 5.1, table 2).

CLINDAMYCIN
Indications: staphylococcal bone and joint infections, peritonitis; endocarditis prophylaxis, section 5.1, table 2
Cautions: discontinue immediately if diarrhoea or colitis develops; hepatic or renal impairment; monitor liver and renal function on prolonged therapy and in neonates and infants; pregnancy; breast-feeding (Appendix 5); avoid rapid intravenous administration; **interactions:** Appendix 1 (clindamycin)
Contra-indications: diarrhoeal states
Side-effects: diarrhoea (discontinue treatment), abdominal discomfort, nausea, vomiting, antibiotic-associated colitis; jaundice and altered liver function tests; neutropenia, eosinophilia, agranulocytosis and thrombocytopenia reported; rash, urticaria, erythema multiforme, exfoliative and vesiculobullous dermatitis reported; pain, induration, and abscess after intramuscular injection; thrombophlebitis after intravenous injection
Dose: by mouth, 150–300 mg every 6 hours; up to 450 mg every 6 hours in severe infections; CHILD, 3–6 mg/kg every 6 hours
COUNSELLING. Patients should discontinue immediately and contact doctor if diarrhoea develops; capsules should be swallowed with a glass of water.
By deep intramuscular injection or by intravenous infusion, 0.6–2.7 g daily (in 2–4 divided doses); life-threatening infection, up to 4.8 g daily; single doses above 600 mg by intravenous infusion only; single doses by intravenous infusion not to exceed 1.2 g
CHILD over 1 month, 15–40 mg/kg daily in 3–4 divided doses; severe infections, at least 300 mg daily regardless of weight
Endocarditis prophylaxis, section 5.1, Table 2

PoM **Dalacin C**® (Pharmacia & Upjohn)
Capsules, clindamycin (as hydrochloride) 75 mg (lavender), net price 24-cap pack = £6.21; 150 mg, (lavender/maroon), 24-cap pack = £11.43. Label: 9, 27, counselling, see above (diarrhoea)

Paediatric suspension, off-white, clindamycin (as palmitate hydrochloride) 75 mg/5 mL when reconstituted with purified water (freshly boiled and cooled). Net price 100 mL = £6.62. Label: 9, 27, counselling, see above (diarrhoea)
Injection, clindamycin (as phosphate) 150 mg/mL. Net price 2-mL amp = £5.17; 4-mL amp = £10.29

5.1.7   Some other antibiotics

Antibacterials discussed in this section include chloramphenicol, fusidic acid, spectinomycin, glycopeptide antibiotics (vancomycin and teicoplanin), and the polymyxin, colistin.

CHLORAMPHENICOL

Chloramphenicol is a potent broad-spectrum antibiotic; however, it is associated with serious haematological side-effects when given systemically and should therefore be reserved for the treatment of life-threatening infections, particularly those caused by *Haemophilus influenzae,* and also for typhoid fever.

Eye-drops of chloramphenicol (section 11.3.1) are useful for bacterial conjunctivitis.

CHLORAMPHENICOL
Indications: see notes above
Cautions: avoid repeated courses and prolonged treatment; reduce doses in hepatic or renal impairment; blood counts required before and periodically during treatment; monitor plasma-chloramphenicol concentration in neonates (see below); **interactions:** Appendix 1 (chloramphenicol)
Contra-indications: pregnancy (see also Appendix 4), breast-feeding, porphyria (section 9.8.2)
Side-effects: blood disorders including reversible and irreversible aplastic anaemia (with reports of resulting leukaemia), peripheral neuritis, optic neuritis, erythema multiforme, nausea, vomiting, diarrhoea, stomatitis, glossitis; nocturnal haemoglobinuria reported; grey syndrome (abdominal distension, pallid cyanosis, circulatory collapse) may follow excessive doses in neonates with immature hepatic metabolism
Dose: by mouth or by intravenous injection or infusion, 50 mg/kg daily in 4 divided doses (exceptionally, can be doubled for severe infections such as septicaemia and meningitis, providing high doses reduced as soon as clinically indicated); CHILD, haemophilus epiglottitis and pyogenic meningitis, 50–100 mg/kg daily in divided doses (high dosages decreased as soon as clinically indicated); INFANTS under 2 weeks 25 mg/kg daily (in 4 divided doses), 2 weeks–1 year 50 mg/kg daily (in 4 divided doses)
Note. Plasma concentration monitoring required in neonates and preferred in those under 4 years of age; recommended peak plasma concentration (measured approx. 1 hour after intravenous injection or infusion) 15–25 mg/litre; pre-dose ('trough') concentration should not exceed 15 mg/litre

---

PoM **Chloramphenicol** (Non-proprietary)
Capsules, chloramphenicol 250 mg. Net price 60 = £12.88
Available from Sussex

PoM **Kemicetine®** (Pharmacia & Upjohn)
Injection, powder for reconstitution, chloramphenicol (as sodium succinate). Net price 1-g vial = £1.21
Electrolytes: Na⁺ 3.14 mmol/g

FUSIDIC ACID

Fusidic acid and its salts are narrow-spectrum antibiotics. The only indication for their use is in infections caused by penicillin-resistant staphylococci, especially osteomyelitis, as they are well concentrated in bone; they are also used for staphylococcal endocarditis (section 5.1, table 1). A second antistaphylococcal antibiotic is usually required to prevent emergence of resistance.

SODIUM FUSIDATE
Indications: see notes above
Cautions: liver-function tests required
Side-effects: nausea, vomiting, rashes, reversible jaundice, especially after high dosage or rapid infusion (withdraw therapy if persistent)
Dose: see under Preparations, below

PoM **Fucidin®** (Leo)
Tablets, f/c, sodium fusidate 250 mg. Net price 20 = £13.54. Label: 9
Dose: as sodium fusidate, 500 mg every 8 hours, doubled for severe infections
Suspension, off-white, fusidic acid 250 mg/5 mL. Net price 50 mL = £7.58. Label: 9, 21
Dose: as fusidic acid, ADULT 750 mg every 8 hours; CHILD up to 1 year 50 mg/kg daily (in 3 divided doses), 1–5 years 250 mg every 8 hours, 5–12 years 500 mg every 8 hours
Note. Fusidic acid is incompletely absorbed and doses recommended for suspension are proportionately higher than those for sodium fusidate tablets
Intravenous infusion, powder for reconstitution, sodium fusidate 500 mg (≡ fusidic acid 480 mg), with buffer. Net price per vial (with diluent) = £8.15
Electrolytes: Na⁺ 3.1 mmol/vial when reconstituted with buffer
Dose: as sodium fusidate, by intravenous infusion, ADULT over 50 kg, 500 mg 3 times daily; ADULT under 50 kg and CHILD, 6–7 mg/kg 3 times daily

SPECTINOMYCIN

Spectinomycin is active against Gram-negative organisms, including *N. gonorrhoeae*. Its only indication is the treatment of gonorrhoea caused by penicillin-resistant organisms or in a penicillin-allergic patient.

SPECTINOMYCIN
Indications: see notes above
Cautions: pregnancy and breast-feeding; **interactions:** Appendix 1 (spectinomycin)
Side-effects: nausea, dizziness, urticaria, fever
Dose: by deep intramuscular injection, 2 g; up to 4 g in difficult-to-treat cases and in geographical areas of resistance; CHILD over 2 years, if no alternative treatment, 40 mg/kg

PoM **Trobicin®** (Pharmacia & Upjohn)
Injection, powder for reconstitution, spectinomycin (as hydrochloride). Net price 2-g vial (with diluent) = £8.16

VANCOMYCIN AND TEICOPLANIN

The glycopeptide antibiotics vancomycin and teicoplanin have bactericidal activity against aerobic and anaerobic Gram-positive bacteria.

Vancomycin is used by the intravenous route in the prophylaxis and treatment of endocarditis and other serious infections caused by Gram-positive cocci including multi-resistant staphylococci; however there are increasing reports of vancomycin-resistant enterococci. It has a relatively long duration of action and can therefore be given every 12 hours; plasma concentrations should be monitored (especially in patients with renal impairment in whom the dose may need marked reduction). It is ototoxic and nephrotoxic. Vancomycin (added to dialysis fluid) is also used in the treatment of peritoneal dialysis-associated peritonitis [unlicensed route] (table 1 section 5.1). Vancomycin is **not effective** by mouth for systemic infections.

Vancomycin is effective in the treatment of antibiotic-associated colitis (pseudomembranous colitis, see also section 1.5) for which it is given by mouth; a dose of 125 mg every 6 hours for 7 to 10 days is considered to be adequate. Vancomycin should **not** be given by mouth for systemic infections since it is not significantly absorbed.

Teicoplanin is very similar to vancomycin but has a significantly longer duration of action allowing once daily administration. Unlike vancomycin, teicoplanin can be given by intramuscular as well as by intravenous injection.

VANCOMYCIN
Indications: see notes above
Cautions: avoid rapid infusion (risk of anaphylactoid reactions, see Side-effects); rotate infusion sites; renal impairment; elderly; avoid if history of deafness; blood counts, urinalysis and renal function tests required in all patients; monitor auditory function and plasma-vancomycin concentration in elderly or if renal impairment; pregnancy and breast-feeding; systemic absorption may follow oral administration especially in inflammatory bowel disorders or following multiple doses; **interactions:** Appendix 1 (vancomycin)
Side-effects: after parenteral administration: nephrotoxicity including renal failure and interstitial nephritis; ototoxicity (discontinue if tinnitus occurs); blood disorders including neutropenia (usually after 1 week or cumulative dose of 25 g), rarely agranulocytosis and thrombocytopenia; nausea; chills; fever; eosinophilia, anaphylaxis, rashes (including exfoliative dermatitis, Stevens-Johnson syndrome and vasculitis); phlebitis (irritant to tissue); on rapid infusion, severe hypotension (including shock and cardiac arrest), wheezing, dyspnoea, urticaria, pruritus, flushing

of the upper body ('red man' syndrome), pain and muscle spasm of back and chest

Dose: *by mouth,* antibiotic-associated colitis, 125 mg every 6 hours for 7–10 days, see notes above; CHILD 5 mg/kg every 6 hours, over 5 years, half adult dose

Note. Oral paediatric dose is lower than that on product literature but is adequate

By intravenous infusion, 500 mg over at least 60 minutes every 6 hours *or* 1 g over at least 100 minutes every 12 hours; NEONATE up to 1 week, 15 mg/kg initially then 10 mg/kg every 12 hours; INFANT 1–4 weeks, 15 mg/kg initially then 10 mg/kg every 8 hours; CHILD over 1 month, 10 mg/kg every 6 hours

Endocarditis prophylaxis, section 5.1, table 2

Note. Plasma concentration monitoring required; peak plasma concentration (measured 2 hours after intravenous infusion) should not exceed 30 mg/litre; pre-dose ('trough') concentration should not exceed 10 mg/litre

PoM **Vancomycin** (Non-proprietary)

Capsules, vancomycin (as hydrochloride) 125 mg, net price 28-cap pack = £88.31; 250 mg, 28-cap pack = £176.62. Label: 9

Available from Dumex

Injection, powder for reconstitution, vancomycin (as hydrochloride), for use as an infusion, net price 500-mg vial = £6.50; 1-g vial = £12.99

Note. Can be used to prepare solution for oral administration

Available from Antigen, Dumex, Faulding DBL

PoM **Vancocin®** (Lilly)

Matrigel capsules, vancomycin (as hydrochloride) 125 mg (blue/peach), net price 20-cap pack = £63.08; 250 mg (blue/grey), 20-cap pack = £126.16. Label: 9

Injection, powder for reconstitution, vancomycin (as hydrochloride), for use as an infusion. Net price 250-mg vial = £4.76; 500-mg vial = £8.66; 1-g vial = £17.32

Note. Can be used to prepare solution for oral administration

TEICOPLANIN

Indications: potentially serious Gram-positive infections including endocarditis, dialysis-associated peritonitis, and serious infections due to *Staphylococcus aureus*; prophylaxis in endocarditis and in orthopaedic surgery at risk of infection with Gram-positive organisms

Cautions: vancomycin sensitivity; blood counts and liver and kidney function tests required; reduce dose in renal impairment (and monitor renal and auditory function on prolonged administration or if other nephrotoxic or neurotoxic drugs given); pregnancy and breast-feeding

Side-effects: nausea, vomiting, diarrhoea; rash, fever, bronchospasm, anaphylactic reactions; dizziness, headache; blood disorders including eosinophilia, leucopenia, and thrombocytopenia; disturbances in liver enzymes, transient increase of serum creatinine; tinnitus, mild hearing loss, and vestibular disorders also reported; local reactions include erythema, pain, and thrombophlebitis

Dose: *by intravenous injection or infusion,* 400 mg initially, subsequently 200 mg daily; severe infections, 400 mg every 12 hours for 3 doses initially, subsequently 400 mg daily; subsequent doses can be given *by intramuscular injection;* higher doses may be required in patients of over 85 kg and in severe burns or endocarditis (see product literature)

CHILD over 2 months *by intravenous injection or infusion,* initially 10 mg/kg every 12 hours for 3 doses, subsequently 6 mg/kg daily (severe infections or in neutropenia, 10 mg/kg daily); subsequent doses can be given *by intramuscular injection* (but intravenous administration preferred in children); NEONATE *by intravenous infusion,* initially a single dose of 16 mg/kg, subsequently 8 mg/kg daily

Endocarditis prophylaxis, section 5.1, table 2

Orthopaedic surgery prophylaxis, *by intravenous injection,* 400 mg at induction of anaesthesia

PoM **Targocid®** (Hoechst Marion Roussel)

Injection, powder for reconstitution, teicoplanin, net price 200-mg vial (with diluent) = £26.05; 400-mg vial (with diluent) = £52.10

Electrolytes: Na⁺ < 0.5 mmol/200- and 400-mg vial

POLYMYXINS

The polymyxin antibiotic, **colistin**, is active against Gram-negative organisms, including *Pseudomonas aeruginosa.* It is **not** absorbed by mouth and thus needs to be given by injection to obtain a systemic effect; however, it is toxic and has few, if any, indications for systemic use.

Colistin is used by mouth in bowel sterilisation regimens in neutropenic patients (usually with nystatin); it is **not** recommended for gastro-intestinal infections. It is also given by inhalation of a nebulised solution as an adjunct to standard antibiotic therapy.

Both colistin and polymyxin B are included in some preparations for topical application.

COLISTIN

Indications: see notes above

Cautions: renal impairment; porphyria (see section 9.8.2); **interactions:** Appendix 1 (colistin)

Contra-indications: myasthenia gravis; pregnancy; breast-feeding

Side-effects: perioral and peripheral paraesthesia, vertigo, muscle weakness, apnoea, nephrotoxicity; rarely vasomotor instability, slurred speech, visual disturbance, confusion and psychosis; neurotoxicity reported with excessive doses; bronchospasm on inhalation

Dose: *by mouth,* bowel sterilisation, 1.5–3 million units every 8 hours

By intramuscular injection or intravenous injection or infusion, 2 million units every 8 hours (but see notes above)

By inhalation of nebulised solution, patients over 40 kg, 1 million units every 12 hours; patients under 40 kg, 500 000 units every 12 hours

Note. Colistin doses in BNF may differ from those in product literature

PoM **Colomycin®** (Pharmax)

Tablets, scored, colistin sulphate 1.5 million units. Net price 50 = £65.11

Syrup, colistin sulphate 250 000 units/5 mL when reconstituted with water. Net price 80 mL = £3.88

Injection, powder for reconstitution, colistin sulphomethate sodium. Net price 500 000-unit vial = £1.27; 1 million-unit vial = £1.88

Electrolytes: (before reconstitution) Na⁺ <0.5 mmol/500 000- and 1 million-unit vial

5.1.8 Sulphonamides and trimethoprim

The importance of the sulphonamides has decreased as a result of increasing bacterial resistance and their replacement by antibiotics which are generally more active and less toxic.

Sulphamethoxazole (sulfamethoxazole) and trimethoprim are used in combination (as **co-trimoxazole**) because of their synergistic activity, but see below for important CSM recommendations limiting the use of this combination.

> **CSM recommendations.** Co-trimoxazole should be limited to the role of drug of choice in *Pneumocystis carinii* pneumonia; it is also indicated for *toxoplasmosis* and *nocardiasis*. It should now only be considered for use in *acute exacerbations of chronic bronchitis* and *infections of the urinary tract* when there is good bacteriological evidence of sensitivity to co-trimoxazole and good reason to prefer this combination to a single antibiotic; similarly it should only be used in *acute otitis media in children* when there is good reason to prefer it. Review of the safety of co-trimoxazole using spontaneous adverse drug reaction data has indicated that the profile of reported adverse reactions with trimethoprim is similar to that with co-trimoxazole; *blood and generalised skin disorders* are the most serious reactions with both drugs and predominantly have been reported to occur in **elderly patients**. A recent large post-marketing study has demonstrated that such reactions are very rare with co-trimoxazole; the study did not distinguish between co-trimoxazole and trimethoprim with respect to serious hepatic, renal, blood or skin disorders.

Trimethoprim can be used alone for urinary- and respiratory-tract infections and for prostatitis, shigellosis, and invasive salmonella infections.

Side-effects of the sulphonamides include rashes, Stevens-Johnson syndrome (erythema multiforme), renal failure (especially with the less soluble preparations), and blood dyscrasias, notably marrow depression and agranulocytosis.

The **longer-acting sulphonamide**, sulfametopyrazine (sulfalene) which is highly bound to plasma proteins, has the advantage of requiring less frequent administration, but toxic effects due to accumulation are more likely to occur.

For *topical preparations* of sulphonamides used in the treatment of burns see section 13.10.1.1.

CO-TRIMOXAZOLE

A mixture of trimethoprim and sulphamethoxazole in the proportions of 1 part to 5 parts

Indications: see CSM recommendations above

Cautions: hepatic and renal impairment; maintain adequate fluid intake; avoid in blood disorders (unless under specialist supervision); monitor blood counts on prolonged treatment; discontinue immediately if blood disorders or rash develop; elderly (see CSM recommendations above); asthma; G6PD deficiency (see section 9.1.5); pregnancy (see Appendix 4) and breast-feeding; avoid in infants under 6 weeks (except for treatment or prophylaxis of pneumocystis pneumonia); **interactions:** Appendix 1 (co-trimoxazole)

Contra-indications: hepatic or renal failure; porphyria (see section 9.8.2)

Side-effects: nausea, vomiting; rash (including Stevens-Johnson syndrome, toxic epidermal necrolysis, photosensitivity)—discontinue immediately; blood disorders (including neutropenia, thrombocytopenia, rarely agranulocytosis and purpura)—discontinue immediately; rarely, allergic reactions, diarrhoea, glossitis, stomatitis, anorexia, arthralgia, myalgia; also reported, liver damage including jaundice and hepatic necrosis, pancreatitis, antibiotic-associated colitis, eosinophilia, cough and shortness of breath, pulmonary infiltrates, aseptic meningitis, headache, depression, convulsions, ataxia, tinnitus, megaloblastic anaemia due to trimethoprim, electrolyte disturbances, crystalluria, renal disorders including interstitial nephritis

Dose: by mouth, 960 mg every 12 hours, increased to 1.44 g in severe infections; 480 mg every 12 hours if treated for more than 14 days; CHILD, every 12 hours, 6 weeks–5 months, 120 mg; 6 months–5 years, 240 mg; 6–12 years, 480 mg

By intravenous infusion, 960 mg every 12 hours increased to 1.44 g every 12 hours in severe infections; CHILD 36 mg/kg daily in 2 divided doses increased to 54 mg/kg daily in severe infections

Treatment of *pneumocystis carinii* infections (undertaken where facilities for appropriate monitoring available consult microbiologist and product literature), *by mouth or by intravenous infusion*, 120 mg/kg daily in 2–4 divided doses for 14 days

Note. 480 mg of co-trimoxazole consists of sulphamethoxazole 400 mg and trimethoprim 80 mg

PoM **Co-trimoxazole** (Non-proprietary)

Tablets, co-trimoxazole 480 mg, net price 20 =61p; 960 mg, 20 = £5.05. Label: 9

Available from APS, Ashbourne (Comixco®), Cox, DDSA (Fectrim®, Fectrim® Forte), Hillcross, Kent, Norton

Dispersible tablets, co-trimoxazole 480 mg. Net price 20 = £1.77. Label: 9, 13

Available from APS

Paediatric oral suspension, co-trimoxazole 240 mg/5 mL. Net price 100 mL = £1.12. Label: 9

Available from APS, Ashbourne (Comixco®), Lagap (Laratrim®), Norton, Rosemont (Chemotrim®)

Oral suspension, co-trimoxazole 480 mg/5 mL. Net price 100 mL = £3.50. Label: 9

Available from Kent, Lagap (Laratrim®)

Cautionary label wordings, see inside back cover

Prices are **net**, see p.1

Strong sterile solution, co-trimoxazole 96 mg/mL. For dilution and use as an intravenous infusion. Net price 5-mL amp = £1.58, 10-mL amp = £3.06
Available from Faulding DBL

PoM **Septrin®** (GlaxoWellcome)
Tablets, co-trimoxazole 480 mg. Net price 20 = £3.34. Label: 9
Dispersible tablets, orange, sugar-free, co-trimoxazole 480 mg. Net price 20 = £3.55. Label: 9, 13
Forte tablets, scored, co-trimoxazole 960 mg. Net price 20 = £5.05. Label: 9
Adult suspension, co-trimoxazole 480 mg/5 mL. Net price 100 mL = £4.74. Label: 9
Paediatric suspension, sugar-free, co-trimoxazole 240 mg/5 mL. Net price 100 mL = £2.63. Label: 9
Intravenous infusion, co-trimoxazole 96 mg/mL. To be diluted before use. Net price 5-mL amp = £1.59

SULFAMETOPYRAZINE
(Sulfalene)
Indications: urinary-tract infections, chronic bronchitis
Cautions; Contra-indications; Side-effects: see under Co-trimoxazole
Dose: 2 g once weekly

PoM **Kelfizine W®** (Pharmacia & Upjohn)
Tablets, sulfametopyrazine 2 g. Tablets to be taken in water. Net price 5-tab pack = £6.68. Label: 9, 13

SULPHADIAZINE
(Sulfadiazine)
Indications: prevention of rheumatic fever recurrence, toxoplasmosis [unlicensed]—see section 5.4.7
Cautions; Contra-indications; Side-effects: see under Co-trimoxazole; avoid in severe renal impairment
Dose: prevention of rheumatic fever, *by mouth*, 1 g daily (500 mg daily for patients less than 30kg)

PoM **Sulphadiazine** (Non-proprietary)
Tablets, sulphadiazine 500 mg. Net price 56-tab pack = £14.99. Label: 9, 27
Available from CP
Injection, sulphadiazine (as sodium salt) 250 mg/mL. Net price 4-mL amp = £2.00
Available from Rhône-Poulenc Rorer

SULPHADIMIDINE
(Sulfadimidine)
Indications: urinary-tract infections
Cautions; Contra-indications; Side-effects: see under Co-trimoxazole
Dose: by mouth, 2 g initially, then 0.5–1 g every 6–8 hours

PoM **Sulphadimidine** (Non-proprietary)
Tablets, sulphadimidine 500 mg. Net price 20 = 60p. Label: 9, 27
Available from Sussex

TRIMETHOPRIM
Indications: urinary-tract infections, acute and chronic bronchitis
Cautions: renal impairment, breast-feeding, predisposition to folate deficiency, manufacturer recommends blood counts on long-term therapy (but evidence of practical value unsatisfactory); neonates (specialist supervision required); porphyria (see section 9.8.2); **interactions:** Appendix 1 (trimethoprim)
BLOOD DISORDERS. On long-term treatment, patients and their carers should be told how to recognise signs of blood disorders and advised to seek immediate medical attention if symptoms such as fever, sore throat, rash, mouth ulcers, purpura, bruising or bleeding develop
Contra-indications: severe renal impairment, pregnancy, blood dyscrasias
Side-effects: gastro-intestinal disturbances including nausea and vomiting, pruritus, rashes, depression of haematopoiesis; rarely erythema multiforme, toxic epidermal necrolysis; aseptic meningitis reported
Dose: by mouth, acute infections, 200 mg every 12 hours; CHILD, twice daily, 2–5 months 25 mg, 6 months–5 years 50 mg, 6–12 years 100 mg
Chronic infections and prophylaxis, 100 mg at night; CHILD 1–2 mg/kg at night
By slow intravenous injection or infusion, 150–250 mg every 12 hours; CHILD under 12 years, 6–9 mg/kg daily in 2–3 divided doses

PoM **Trimethoprim** (Non-proprietary)
Tablets, trimethoprim 100 mg, net price 20 =40p; 200 mg, 20 = 69p. Label: 9
Available from APS, Ashbourne (Triprimix®), Berk (Trimopan®), Cox, Kent, Lagap (Trimogal®), Norton
PoM **Ipral®** (Squibb)
Tablets, trimethoprim 100 mg, net price 20 = 80p; 200 mg, 20 = £1.71. Label: 9
PoM **Monotrim®** (Solvay)
Tablets, both scored, trimethoprim 100 mg, net price 20 = 82p; 200 mg, 20 = £1.44. Label: 9
Suspension, sugar-free, trimethoprim 50 mg/5 mL. Net price 100 mL = £1.77. Label: 9
Injection, trimethoprim (as lactate) 20 mg/mL. Net price 5-mL amp = £1.11
PoM **Trimopan®** (Berk)
Suspension, sugar-free, trimethoprim 50 mg/5 mL. Net price 100 mL = £2.34. Label: 9

5.1.9   Antituberculous drugs

Tuberculosis is treated in two phases—an *initial phase* using at least three drugs and a *continuation phase* using two drugs. Treatment requires specialised knowledge, particularly where the disease involves resistant organisms or non-respiratory organs.

The regimens given below are recommended by experts in the treatment of tuberculosis and the Joint Tuberculosis Committee of the British Thoracic Society for the treatment of tuberculosis in the UK; variations occur in other countries.

INITIAL PHASE. The concurrent use of at least three drugs during the initial phase is designed to reduce the population of viable bacteria as rapidly as possible and to prevent the emergence of drug-resistant bacteria. Treatment of choice for the initial phase is the daily use of isoniazid, rifampicin, pyrazinamide and ethambutol; ethambutol can be omitted from the regimen if the risk of resistance to isoniazid is low (e.g. those who have not been treated previously for tuberculosis, those who are not immunosuppressed, and those who have not been in contact with organisms known to be drug resistant). Streptomycin is now rarely used in the UK but it may be added if the organism is resistant to isoniazid. The initial phase drugs should be continued for 2 months. Where a positive culture for *M. tuberculosis* has been obtained, but susceptibility results are not available after 2 months, treatment with pyrazinamide (and ethambutol if appropriate) should be continued until full susceptibility is confirmed, even if this is for longer than 2 months.

CONTINUATION PHASE. After the initial phase, treatment is continued for a further 4 months with isoniazid and rifampicin; longer treatment may be necessary for meningitis, or for resistant organisms.

Recommended dosage for standard unsupervised 6-month regimen

Isoniazid (for 6 months)	ADULT 300 mg daily; CHILD 5–10 mg/kg (max. 300 mg) daily
Rifampicin (for 6 months)	ADULT under 50 kg 450 mg daily, 50 kg and over 600 mg daily: CHILD 10 mg/kg daily
Pyrazinamide (for first 2 months only)	ADULT under 50 kg 1.5 g, 50 kg and over 2 g daily; CHILD 35 mg/kg daily
¹Ethambutol (for first 2 months only)	ADULT and CHILD 15 mg/kg daily

1. Ethambutol may be omitted from the regimen if the risk of resistance is low

PREGNANCY AND BREAST-FEEDING. The standard regimen (above) may be used during pregnancy and breast-feeding; pyridoxine supplements are advisable. Streptomycin should not be given in pregnancy.

CHILDREN. Children are given isoniazid, rifampicin, and pyrazinamide for the first 2 months followed by isoniazid and rifampicin during the next 4 months. Ethambutol should be included in the first 2 months in children with a high risk of resistant infection (see Initial Phase, above). However, care is needed in young children because of the difficulty in testing eyesight and in obtaining reports of visual symptoms (see below).

SUPERVISED TREATMENT. Treatment needs to be fully supervised in patients who cannot be relied upon to comply with the treatment regimen. These patients are given isoniazid, rifampicin, pyrazinamide and ethambutol (or streptomycin) 3 times a week under supervision for the first 2 months followed by isoniazid and rifampicin three times a week for a further 4 months.

Recommended dosage for intermittent supervised treatment

Isoniazid (for 6 months)	ADULT and CHILD 15 mg/kg 3 times a week
Rifampicin (for 6 months)	ADULT 600–900 mg 3 times a week; CHILD 15 mg/kg 3 times a week
Pyrazinamide (for first 2 months only)	ADULT under 50 kg 2 g 3 times a week, 50 kg and over 2.5 g; CHILD 50 mg/kg 3 times a week *or* ADULT under 50 kg 3 g twice a week, 50 kg and over 3.5 g; CHILD 75 mg/kg twice a week
¹Ethambutol (for first 2 months only)	ADULT and CHILD 30 mg/kg 3 times a week *or* ADULT and CHILD 45 mg/kg twice a week

1. Ethambutol may be omitted from the regimen if the risk of resistance is low

IMMUNOCOMPROMISED PATIENTS. Immunocompromised patients may develop tuberculosis owing to reactivation of previously latent disease or to new infection. Multi-resistant *Mycobacterium tuberculosis* may be present or the infection may be caused by other mycobacteria e.g. *M. avium* complex in which case specialist advice is needed. Culture should always be carried out and the type of organism and its sensitivity confirmed. Confirmed *M. tuberculosis* infection sensitive to first-line drugs should be treated with a standard 6-month regimen; after completion of treatment, patients should be closely monitored.

MONITORING. Since isoniazid, rifampicin and pyrazinamide are associated with liver toxicity (see Appendix 2), *hepatic function* should be checked before treatment with these drugs. Those with pre-existing liver disease should have frequent checks particularly in the first 2 months. If there is no evidence of liver disease (and pre-treatment liver function is normal), further checks are only necessary if the patient develops fever, malaise, vomiting, jaundice or unexplained deterioration during treatment. In view of the need to comply fully with antituberculous treatment on the one hand and to guard against serious liver damage on the other, patients and their carers should be informed carefully how to recognise signs of liver disorders and advised to discontinue treatment and seek **immediate** medical attention should symptoms of liver disease occur.

Renal function should be checked before treatment with antituberculous drugs and appropriate dosage adjustments made. Streptomycin or ethambutol should preferably be avoided in patients with renal impairment, but if used require dose reduction and possibly drug concentration monitoring (see Appendix 3).

Visual acuity should be tested before ethambutol is used (see below).

> Major causes of treatment failure are incorrect prescribing by the physician and inadequate compliance by the patient. Avoid both excessive and inadequate dosage. Treatment should be supervised by a specialist physician.

Isoniazid is cheap and highly effective. Like rifampicin it should always be included in any antituberculous regimen unless there is a specific contra-indication. Its only common side-effect is peripheral neuropathy which is more likely to occur where there are pre-existing risk factors such as diabetes, alcoholism, chronic renal failure, malnutrition and HIV infection. In these circumstances pyridoxine 10 mg daily should be given prophylactically from the start of treatment. Other side-effects such as hepatitis (important: see Monitoring above) and psychosis are rare.

Rifampicin is a key component of any antituberculous regimen. Like isoniazid it should always be included unless there is a specific contra-indication.

During the first two months of rifampicin administration transient disturbance of liver function with elevated serum transaminases is common but generally does not require interruption of treatment. Occasionally more serious liver toxicity requires a change of treatment particularly in those with pre-existing liver disease (important: see Monitoring above).

On intermittent treatment six toxicity syndromes have been recognised—influenza-like, abdominal, and respiratory symptoms, shock, renal failure, and thrombocytopenic purpura—and can occur in 20 to 30% of patients.

Rifampicin induces hepatic enzymes which accelerate the metabolism of several drugs including oestrogens, corticosteroids, phenytoin, sulphonylureas, and anticoagulants; **interactions:** Appendix 1 (rifamycins). **Important:** the effectiveness of oral contraceptives is reduced and alternative family planning advice should be offered (see section 7.3.1).

Rifabutin, a newly introduced rifamycin, is indicated for *prophylaxis* against *M. avium* complex infections in patients with a low CD4 count; it is also licensed for the *treatment* of non-tuberculous mycobacterial disease and pulmonary tuberculosis. As with rifampicin it induces hepatic enzymes and the effectiveness of oral contraceptives is reduced requiring alternative family planning methods.

Pyrazinamide is a bactericidal drug only active against intracellular dividing forms of *Mycobacterium tuberculosis*; it exerts its main effect only in the first two or three months. It is particularly useful in tuberculous meningitis because of good meningeal penetration. It is not active against *M. bovis*. Serious liver toxicity may occasionally occur (important: see Monitoring above).

Ethambutol is included in a treatment regimen if resistance is suspected; it can be omitted if the risk of resistance is low.

Side-effects of ethambutol are largely confined to visual disturbances in the form of loss of acuity, colour blindness, and restriction of visual fields. These toxic effects are more common where excessive dosage is used or if the patient's renal function is impaired. The earliest features of ocular toxicity are subjective and patients should be advised to discontinue therapy immediately if they develop deterioration in vision and promptly seek further advice. Early discontinuation of the drug is almost always followed by recovery of eyesight. Patients who cannot understand warnings about visual side-effects should, if possible, be given an alternative drug. In particular, ethambutol should be used with caution in children until they are at least 5 years old and capable of reporting symptomatic visual changes accurately.

Visual acuity should be tested by Snellen chart before treatment with ethambutol.

Streptomycin is now rarely used in the UK except for resistant organisms. It is given intramuscularly in a dose of 15 mg/kg (max. 1 g) daily. Plasma drug concentrations should be measured, particularly in patients with impaired renal function in whom streptomycin must be used with great care. Side-effects increase after a cumulative dose of 100 g, which should only be exceeded in exceptional circumstances.

Drug-resistant tuberculosis should be treated by a specialist physician with experience in such cases, and where appropriate facilities for infection-control exist. Second-line drugs available for infections caused by resistant organisms, or when first-line drugs cause unacceptable side-effects, include capreomycin, cycloserine, newer macrolides (e.g. azithromycin and clarithromycin), 4-quinolones (e.g. ciprofloxacin and ofloxacin) and prothionamide (protionamide) (no longer on UK market). Advice on the availability of second-line antituberculous drugs can be obtained from Regional Drug Information Services.

CAPREOMYCIN

Indications: in combination with other drugs, tuberculosis resistant to first-line drugs

Cautions: renal, hepatic, or auditory impairment; monitor renal, hepatic, auditory, and vestibular function and electrolytes; pregnancy (teratogenic in *animals*) and breast-feeding; **interactions:** Appendix 1 (capreomycin)

Side-effects: hypersensitivity reactions including urticaria and rashes; leucocytosis or leucopenia, rarely thrombocytopenia; changes in liver function tests; nephrotoxicity, electrolyte disturbances; hearing loss with tinnitus and vertigo; neuromuscular block after large doses, pain and induration at injection site

Dose: by deep intramuscular injection, 1 g daily (not more than 20 mg/kg) for 2–4 months, then 1 g 2–3 times each week

PoM **Capastat®** (Dista)
Injection, powder for reconstitution, capreomycin sulphate 1 million units (≡ capreomycin approx. 1 g). Net price per vial = £17.25

CYCLOSERINE

Indications: in combination with other drugs, tuberculosis resistant to first-line drugs

Cautions: discontinue (or reduce dose) if allergic dermatitis or symptoms of CNS toxicity; reduce dose in renal impairment (avoid if severe); monitor haematological, renal, and hepatic function; pregnancy and breast-feeding; **interactions:** Appendix 1 (cycloserine)

Contra-indications: severe renal impairment, epilepsy, depression, severe anxiety, psychotic states, alcohol dependence, porphyria (see section 9.8.2)

Side-effects: mainly neurological, including headache, dizziness, vertigo, drowsiness, tremor, convulsions; psychosis, depression; rashes; megaloblastic anaemia; changes in liver function tests

Dose: initially 250 mg every 12 hours for 2 weeks increased according to blood concentration and response to max. 500 mg every 12 hours; CHILD initially 10 mg/kg daily adjusted according to blood concentration and response

Note. Blood concentration monitoring required especially in renal impairment or if dose exceeds 500 mg daily or if signs of toxicity; blood concentration should not exceed 30 mg/litre

PoM **Cycloserine** (Lilly)
Capsules, red/grey cycloserine 250 mg, net price 100-cap pack = £220.69. Label: 2, 8

ETHAMBUTOL HYDROCHLORIDE

Indications: tuberculosis, in combination with other drugs

Cautions: reduce dose in renal impairment; elderly; pregnancy; warn patients to report visual changes—see notes above

Contra-indications: young children (see notes), optic neuritis, poor vision

Side-effects: optic neuritis, red/green colour blindness, peripheral neuritis, rarely rash, pruritus, urticaria, thrombocytopenia

Dose: see notes above

PoM **Ethambutol** (Non-proprietary)
Tablets, ethambutol hydrochloride 100 mg (yellow), net price 100-tab pack = £9.03; 400 mg (grey), 100-tab pack = £32.30. Label: 8
Available from Genus
Note. The brand name Myambutol® was formerly used

ISONIAZID

Indications: tuberculosis, in combination with other drugs; prophylaxis—section 5.1, table 2

Cautions: hepatic impairment (monitor hepatic function, see also below); renal impairment; slow acetylator status (increased risk of side-effects); epilepsy; history of psychosis; alcoholism; pregnancy and breast-feeding; porphyria (see section 9.8.2); **interactions:** Appendix 1 (isoniazid)
HEPATIC DISORDERS. Patients or their carers should be told how to recognise signs of liver disorder, and advised to discontinue treatment and seek immediate medical attention if symptoms such as persistent nausea, vomiting, malaise or jaundice develop

Contra-indications: drug-induced liver disease

Side-effects: nausea, vomiting; peripheral neuritis with high doses (pyridoxine prophylaxis, see notes above), optic neuritis, convulsions, psychotic episodes; hypersensitivity reactions including fever, erythema multiforme, purpura; agranulocytosis; hepatitis (especially over age of 35); systemic lupus erythematosus-like syndrome, pellagra, hyperglycaemia, and gynaecomastia reported

Dose: by mouth or by intramuscular or intravenous injection, see notes above

PoM **Isoniazid** (Non-proprietary)
Tablets, isoniazid 50 mg, net price 20 = £1.51; 100 mg, 20 = 40p. Label: 8, 22
Available from APS, Norton

Elixir (BPC), isoniazid 50 mg, citric acid monohydrate 12.5 mg, sodium citrate 60 mg, concentrated anise water 0.05 mL, compound tartrazine solution 0.05 mL, glycerol 1 mL, double-strength chloroform water 2 mL, water to 5 mL. Label: 8, 22
'Special order' [unlicensed] product; contact Martindale, Rosemont, or regional hospital manufacturing unit

Injection, isoniazid 25 mg/mL. Net price 2-mL amp = £2.91
Available from Cambridge

PYRAZINAMIDE

Indications: tuberculosis in combination with other drugs

Cautions: hepatic impairment (monitor hepatic function, see also below); renal impairment; diabetes; gout; **interactions:** Appendix 1 (pyrazinamide)
HEPATIC DISORDERS. Patients or their carers should be told how to recognise signs of liver disorder, and advised to discontinue treatment and seek immediate medical attention if symptoms such as persistent nausea, vomiting, malaise or jaundice develop

Contra-indications: liver damage, porphyria (see section 9.8.2)

Side-effects: hepatotoxicity including fever, anorexia, hepatomegaly, jaundice, liver failure; nausea, vomiting, arthralgia, sideroblastic anaemia, urticaria

Dose: see notes above

PoM **Zinamide®** (MSD)
Tablets, scored, pyrazinamide 500 mg. Net price 20 = £1.44. Label: 8

RIFABUTIN

Indications: see under Dose

Cautions: see under Rifampicin; renal impairment (Appendix 3)

Side-effects: nausea, vomiting; leucopenia, thrombocytopenia, anaemia, rarely haemolysis; raised liver enzymes, jaundice, rarely hepatitis; uveitis following high doses or administration with drugs which raise plasma concentration—see also **interactions:** Appendix 1 (rifamycins); arthralgia, myalgia, influenza-like syndrome, dyspnoea; also hypersensitivity reactions including fever, rash, eosinophilia, bronchospasm, shock; urine, saliva and other body secretions coloured orange-red; asymptomatic corneal opacities reported with long-term use

Dose: prophylaxis of *Mycobacterium avium* complex infections in immunosuppressed patients with low CD4 count (see product literature), 300 mg daily as a single dose

Treatment of non-tuberculous mycobacterial disease, in combination with other drugs, 450–600 mg daily as a single dose for up to 6 months after cultures negative

Treatment of pulmonary tuberculosis, in combination with other drugs, 150–450 mg daily as a single dose for at least 6 months

CHILD not recommended

PoM **Mycobutin®** (Pharmacia & Upjohn)

Capsules, red-brown, rifabutin 150 mg. Net price 30-cap pack = £82.29. Label: 8, 14, counselling, lenses, see under Rifampicin

RIFAMPICIN

Indications: see under Dose

Cautions: reduce dose in hepatic impairment (see Appendix 2; liver function tests and blood counts in hepatic disorders and on prolonged therapy, see also below); renal impairment (if above 600 mg daily); pregnancy and breast-feeding (see notes above and Appendixes 4 and 5); **important:** advise patients on oral contraceptives to use additional means (see also section 7.3.1); discolours soft contact lenses; see also notes above; **interactions:** Appendix 1 (rifamycins)

Note. If treatment interrupted re-introduce with low dosage and increase gradually; discontinue permanently if serious side-effects develop

HEPATIC DISORDERS. Patients or their carers should be told how to recognise signs of liver disorder, and advised to discontinue treatment and seek immediate medical attention if symptoms such as persistent nausea, vomiting, malaise or jaundice develop

Contra-indications: jaundice, porphyria (see section 9.8.2)

Side-effects: gastro-intestinal symptoms including anorexia, nausea, vomiting, diarrhoea (antibiotic-associated colitis reported); those occurring mainly on intermittent therapy include influenza-like symptoms (with chills, fever, dizziness, bone pain), respiratory symptoms (including shortness of breath), collapse and shock, haemolytic anaemia, acute renal failure, and thrombocytopenic purpura; alterations of liver function, jaundice; flushing, urticaria, and rashes; other side-effects reported include oedema, muscular weakness and myopathy, leucopenia, eosinophilia, menstrual disturbances; urine, saliva, and other body secretions coloured orange-red; thrombophlebitis reported if infusion used for prolonged period

Dose: brucellosis, legionnaires' disease and serious staphylococcal infections, in combination with other drugs, *by mouth or by intravenous infusion,* 0.6–1.2 g daily (in 2–4 divided doses)

Tuberculosis, in combination with other drugs, notes above

Leprosy, section 5.1.10

Prophylaxis of meningococcal meningitis and *Haemophilus influenzae* (type b) infection, section 5.1, table 2

PoM **Rifampicin** (Non-proprietary)

Capsules, rifampicin 150 mg, net price 20 = £3.46; 300 mg, 20 = £7.05. Label: 8, 14, 22, counselling, see lenses above

Available from APS, Generics

PoM **Rifadin®** (Hoechst Marion Roussel)

Capsules, rifampicin 150 mg (blue/red), net price 20 = £3.73; 300 mg (red), 20 = £7.45. Label: 8, 14, 22, counselling, see lenses above

Syrup, red, rifampicin 100 mg/5 mL. Net price 120 mL = £3.62. Label: 8, 14, 22, counselling, see lenses above

Intravenous infusion, powder for reconstitution, rifampicin. Net price 600-mg vial (with solvent) = £7.80

Electrolytes: Na⁺ < 0.5 mmol/vial

PoM **Rimactane®** (Novartis)

Capsules, rifampicin 150 mg (red), net price 56-tab pack = £11.39; 300 mg (red/brown), 56-tab pack = £22.77. Label: 8, 14, 22, counselling, see lenses above

Syrup, red, rifampicin 100 mg/5 mL. Net price 100 mL = £3.06. Label: 8, 14, 22, counselling, see lenses above

Intravenous infusion, powder for reconstitution, rifampicin (as sodium salt). Net price 300-mg vial (with diluent) = £8.01

Electrolytes: Na⁺ < 0.5 mmol/vial

Note. Owing to risk of contact sensitisation care must be taken to avoid contact during preparation and infusion

Combined preparations

PoM **Rifater®** (Hoechst Marion Roussel)

Tablets, pink-beige, s/c, rifampicin 120 mg, isoniazid 50 mg, pyrazinamide 300 mg. Net price 20 = £4.29. Label: 8, 14, 22, counselling, see lenses above

Dose: initial treatment of pulmonary tuberculosis, patients up to 40 kg 3 tablets daily preferably before breakfast, 40–49 kg 4 tablets daily, 50–64 kg 5 tablets daily, 65 kg or more, 6 tablets daily; not suitable for use in children

PoM **Rifinah 150®** (Hoechst Marion Roussel)

Tablets, pink, rifampicin 150 mg, isoniazid 100 mg. Net price 84-tab pack = £16.18. Label: 8, 14, 22, counselling, see lenses above

Dose: ADULT under 50 kg, 3 tablets daily, preferably before breakfast

PoM **Rifinah 300®** (Hoechst Marion Roussel)

Tablets, orange, rifampicin 300 mg, isoniazid 150 mg. Net price 56-tab pack = £21.38. Label: 8, 14, 22, counselling, see lenses above

Dose: ADULT 50 kg and over, 2 tablets daily, preferably before breakfast

PoM **Rimactazid 150®** (Novartis)

Tablets, pink, s/c, rifampicin 150 mg, isoniazid 100 mg. Net price 84-tab pack = £16.42. Label: 8, 14, 22, counselling, see lenses above

Additives: include gluten

Dose: ADULT under 50 kg, 3 tablets daily, preferably before breakfast

PoM **Rimactazid 300®** (Novartis)

Tablets, orange, s/c, rifampicin 300 mg, isoniazid 150 mg. Net price 56-tab pack = £21.71. Label: 8, 14, 22, counselling, see lenses above

Additives: include gluten

Dose: ADULT 50 kg and over, 2 tablets daily, preferably before breakfast

STREPTOMYCIN

Indications: tuberculosis, in combination with other drugs; adjunct to doxycycline in brucellosis
Cautions; Contra-indications; Side-effects: see under Aminoglycosides, section 5.1.4; also hypersensitivity reactions, paraesthesia of mouth
Dose: by deep intramuscular injection, tuberculosis, see notes above; brucellosis, expert advice essential

PoM **Streptomycin Sulphate** (Evans)
Injection, powder for reconstitution, streptomycin (as sulphate). Net price 1-g vial = £5.62

5.1.10 Antileprotic drugs

Advice from a member of the Panel of Leprosy Opinion is essential for the treatment of leprosy (Hansen's disease). Details of the Panel can be obtained from the Department of Health telephone 0171-972 4480.

The World Health Organization has made recommendations to overcome the problem of dapsone resistance and to prevent the emergence of resistance to other antileprotic drugs. Drugs recommended are **dapsone**, **rifampicin** (section 5.1.9), and **clofazimine**. Other drugs with significant activity against *Mycobacterium leprae* include ofloxacin, minocycline and clarithromycin, but none of these are as active as rifampicin; at present they should be reserved as second-line drugs for leprosy.

A three-drug regimen is recommended for *multibacillary leprosy* (lepromatous, borderline-lepromatous, and borderline leprosy) and a two-drug regimen for *paucibacillary leprosy* (borderline-tuberculoid, tuberculoid, and indeterminate). The following regimens are widely used throughout the world (with minor local variations):

Multibacillary leprosy (3 drug regimen)

Rifampicin	600 mg once-monthly, supervised (450 mg for adults weighing less than 35 kg)
Dapsone	100 mg daily, self-administered (50 mg daily or 1–2 mg/kg daily for adults weighing less than 35 kg)
Clofazimine	300 mg once-monthly, supervised, *and* 50 mg daily (or 100 mg on alternate days), self-administered

Multibacillary leprosy should be treated for at least 2 years and, wherever possible, continued up to smear negativity. It should be continued unchanged during both type I (reversal) or type II (erythema nodosum leprosum) reactions. During reversal reactions neuritic pain or weakness can herald the rapid onset of permanent nerve damage. Treatment with prednisolone (initially 40–60 mg daily) should be instituted at once. Mild type II reactions may respond to aspirin or chloroquine. Severe type II reactions may require corticosteroids; increased doses of clofazimine 100 mg 3 times daily for the first month with subsequent reductions, are also useful but may take 4–6 weeks to attain full effect.

Paucibacillary leprosy (2-drug regimen)

Rifampicin	600 mg once-monthly, supervised (450 mg for those weighing less than 35 kg)
Dapsone	100 mg daily, self-administered (50 mg daily or 1–2 mg/kg daily for adults weighing less than 35 kg)

Paucibacillary leprosy should be treated for 6 months. If treatment is interrupted the regimen should be recommenced where it was left off to complete the full course.

Neither the multibacillary nor the paucibacillary antileprosy regimen is sufficient to treat tuberculosis.

DAPSONE

Indications: leprosy, dermatitis herpetiformis
Cautions: cardiac or pulmonary disease; anaemia (treat severe anaemia before starting); G6PD-deficiency (including breast-feeding of affected children, section 9.1.5); pregnancy; avoid in porphyria (section 9.8.2); **interactions:** Appendix 1 (dapsone)
Side-effects: (dose-related and uncommon at doses used for leprosy), haemolysis, methaemoglobinaemia, neuropathy, allergic dermatitis (rarely including toxic epidermal necrolysis and Stevens-Johnson syndrome), anorexia, nausea, vomiting, headache, insomnia, psychosis, hepatitis, agranulocytosis; dapsone syndrome (rash with fever and eosinophilia)—discontinue immediately (may progress to exfoliative dermatitis, hepatitis, hypoalbuminaemia, psychosis and death)
Dose: leprosy, 1–2 mg/kg daily, see notes above
Dermatitis herpetiformis, see specialist literature

PoM **Dapsone** (Non-proprietary)
Tablets, dapsone 50 mg, net price 20 = 54p; 100 mg, 20 = 73p. Label: 8
Available from Cox

CLOFAZIMINE

Indications: leprosy
Cautions: hepatic and renal impairment; pregnancy and breast-feeding; may discolour soft contact lenses; avoid if persistent abdominal pain and diarrhoea
Side-effects: nausea, vomiting (hospitalise if persistent), abdominal pain; headache, tiredness; brownish-black discoloration of lesions and skin including areas exposed to light; reversible hair discoloration; dry skin; red discoloration of faeces, urine and other body fluids; also rash, pruritus, photosensitivity, acne-like eruptions, anorexia, eosinophilic enteropathy, bowel obstruction, dry eyes, dimmed vision, macular and subepithelial corneal pigmentation; elevation of blood sugar, weight loss, splenic infarction lymphadenopathy
Dose: leprosy, see notes above
Lepromatous lepra reactions, dosage increased to 300 mg daily for max. of 3 months

---

Cautionary label wordings, see inside back cover

Prices are **net**, see p.1

PoM **Lamprene®** (Novartis)

Capsules, brown, clofazimine 100 mg. Net price 100-cap pack = £6.66. Label: 8, 14, 21

5.1.11   Metronidazole and tinidazole

Metronidazole is an antimicrobial drug with high activity against anaerobic bacteria and protozoa; indications include trichomonal vaginitis (section 5.4.3), bacterial vaginosis (notably *Gardnerella vaginalis* infections), and *Entamoeba histolytica* and *Giardia lamblia* infections (section 5.4.2). It is also used for surgical and gynaecological sepsis in which its activity against colonic anaerobes, especially *Bacteroides fragilis*, is important. Metronidazole is also effective in the treatment of antibiotic-associated colitis (pseudomembranous colitis, see also section 1.5) in a dose of 400 mg by mouth three times daily. Topical metronidazole (section 13.10.1.2) reduces the odour produced by anaerobic bacteria in fungating tumours; it is also used in the management of rosacea (section 13.6).

Tinidazole is similar to metronidazole but has a longer duration of action.

METRONIDAZOLE

Indications: anaerobic infections (including dental), see under Dose below; protozoal infections, section 5.4.2

Cautions: disulfiram-like reaction with alcohol, hepatic impairment and hepatic encephalopathy; pregnancy and breast-feeding (manufacturer advises avoidance of high-dose regimens); clinical and laboratory monitoring advised if treatment exceeds 10 days; **interactions:** Appendix 1 (metronidazole)

Side-effects: nausea, vomiting, unpleasant taste, furred tongue, and gastro-intestinal disturbances; rashes, urticaria and angioedema; rarely drowsiness, headache, dizziness, ataxia, darkening of urine, and anaphylaxis; on prolonged or intensive therapy peripheral neuropathy, transient epileptiform seizures, and leucopenia

Dose: anaerobic infections (usually treated for 7 days), *by mouth, either* 800 mg initially then 400 mg every 8 hours *or* 500 mg every 8 hours; *by rectum*, 1 g every 8 hours for 3 days, then 1 g every 12 hours; *by intravenous infusion*, 500 mg every 8 hours; CHILD, any route, 7.5 mg/kg every 8 hours

Leg ulcers and pressure sores, *by mouth*, 400 mg every 8 hours for 7 days

Bacterial vaginosis, *by mouth*, 400–500 mg twice daily for 7 days *or* 2 g as a single dose

Acute ulcerative gingivitis, *by mouth*, 200–250 mg every 8 hours for 3 days; CHILD 1–3 years 50 mg every 8 hours for 3 days; 3–7 years 100 mg every 12 hours; 7–10 years 100 mg every 8 hours

Acute dental infections, *by mouth*, 200 mg every 8 hours for 3–7 days

Surgical prophylaxis, *by mouth*, 400 mg every 8 hours started 24 hours before surgery, then continued postoperatively *by intravenous infusion* or *by rectum* (see below) until oral administration can be resumed; CHILD 7.5 mg/kg every 8 hours

By rectum, 1 g every 8 hours; CHILD 125–250 mg every 8 hours

By intravenous infusion, 500 mg shortly before surgery then every 8 hours until oral administration can be started; CHILD, 7.5 mg/kg every 8 hours

PoM **Metronidazole** (Non-proprietary)

Tablets, metronidazole 200 mg, net price 20 =43p; 400 mg, 20 = 97p. Label: 4, 9, 21, 25, 27

Available from APS, Cox, DDSA (Vaginyl®), Hillcross, Kent, Lagap (Metrolyl®), Norton, Rosemont

Tablets, metronidazole 500 mg, net price 21-tab pack = £3.50. Label: 4, 9, 21, 25, 27

Available from Dumex

Suspension, metronidazole (as benzoate) 200 mg/ 5 mL. Net price 100 mL = £4.14. Label: 4, 9, 23

Available from Hillcross, Rosemont

Intravenous infusion, metronidazole 5 mg/mL. Net price 20-mL amp = £1.70, 100-mL container = £3.57

Available from Braun, Faulding DBL, Phoenix

PoM **Anabact®:** see section 13.10.1.2

PoM **Flagyl®** (Rhône-Poulenc Rorer)

Tablets, both f/c, ivory, metronidazole 200 mg, net price 21-tab pack = £2.14; 400 mg, 14-tab pack = £3.03. Label: 4, 9, 21, 25, 27

Intravenous infusion, metronidazole 5 mg/mL. Net price 100-mL Viaflex® bag = £3.41

Electrolytes: Na⁺ 13.6 mmol/100-mL bag

Suppositories, metronidazole 500 mg, net price 10 = £7.26; 1 g, 10 = £11.02. Label: 4, 9

PoM **Flagyl S®** (Rhône-Poulenc Rorer)

Suspension, metronidazole (as benzoate) 200 mg/ 5 mL. Net price 100 mL = £5.34. Label: 4, 9, 23

PoM **Metrogel®:** see section 13.10.1.2

PoM **Metrolyl®** (Lagap)

Intravenous infusion, metronidazole 5 mg/mL. Net price 100-mL Steriflex® bag = £4.50

Electrolytes: Na⁺ 14.53 mmol/100-mL bag

Suppositories, metronidazole 500 mg, net price 10 = £4.25; 1 g, 10 = £6.80. Label: 4, 9

PoM **Metrotop®:** see section 13.10.1.2

PoM **Rozex®:** see section 13.10.1.2

With antifungal

PoM **Flagyl Compak®** (Rhône-Poulenc Rorer)

Treatment pack, tablets, off-white, f/c, metronidazole 400 mg, with pessaries, yellow, nystatin 100 000 units. Net price 14 tablets and 14 pessaries (with applicator) = £5.23

Dose: for mixed trichomonal and candidal infections, 1 tablet twice daily for 7 days and 1 pessary inserted twice daily for 7 days *or* 1 pessary at night for 14 nights

---

TINIDAZOLE

Indications: anaerobic infections, see under Dose below; protozoal infections, section 5.4.2

Cautions; Side-effects: see under Metronidazole; pregnancy (manufacturer advises avoidance in first trimester)

Dose: anaerobic infections *by mouth*, 2 g initially, followed by 1 g daily *or* 500 mg twice daily, usually for 5–6 days

Bacterial vaginosis and acute ulcerative gingivitis, a single 2-g dose

Abdominal surgery prophylaxis, a single 2-g dose approximately 12 hours before surgery

---

PoM **Fasigyn®** (Pfizer)
Tablets, f/c, tinidazole 500 mg. Net price 20-tab pack = £11.50. Label: 4, 9, 21, 25

5.1.12 4-Quinolones

Antibacterials discussed in this section include ciprofloxacin, ofloxacin, and the urinary antiseptics cinoxacin, nalidixic acid, and norfloxacin.

Nalidixic acid, **cinoxacin**, and **norfloxacin** are effective in uncomplicated urinary-tract infections.

Ciprofloxacin is active against both Gram-positive and Gram-negative bacteria. It is particularly active against Gram-negative bacteria, including salmonella, shigella, campylobacter, neisseria, and pseudomonas. Ciprofloxacin only has moderate activity against Gram-positive bacteria such as *Streptococcus pneumoniae* and *Strep. faecalis*; it is not the drug of first choice for pneumococcal pneumonia. It is active against chlamydia and some mycobacteria. Most anaerobic organisms are not susceptible. Uses for ciprofloxacin include infections of the respiratory (but not for pneumococcal pneumonia, see above) and urinary tracts, and of the gastro-intestinal system (including typhoid fever), and gonorrhoea and septicaemia caused by sensitive organisms. Although licensed for skin and soft tissue infections there is a high incidence of staphylococcal resistance and it should be avoided in methicillin-resistant *Staphylococcus aureus* (MRSA) infections.

Ofloxacin is used for urinary-tract infections, lower respiratory-tract infections, gonorrhoea, and non-gonococcal urethritis and cervicitis.

CAUTIONS. 4-Quinolones should be used with caution in patients with epilepsy, a history of epilepsy, or conditions that predispose to seizures, in hepatic or renal impairment (see Appendixes 2 and 3), in pregnancy, during breast-feeding, and in children or adolescents (arthropathy has developed in weight-bearing joints in young *animals*). The CSM has warned that 4-quinolones may induce **convulsions** in patients with or without a history of convulsions; taking NSAIDs at the same time may also induce them. Other **interactions**: Appendix 1 (4-quinolones).

> **CSM advice (tendon damage)**
> At the first sign of pain or inflammation, patients taking 4-quinolones should discontinue the treatment and rest the affected limb until tendon symptoms have resolved.

SIDE-EFFECTS. Side-effects of the 4-quinolones include nausea, vomiting, abdominal pain, diarrhoea (rarely antibiotic-associated colitis), headache, dizziness, sleep disorders, rash, pruritus, fever, anaphylaxis, photosensitivity, increase in blood urea and creatinine, transient disturbances in liver enzymes and bilirubin, arthralgia and myalgia, blood disorders (including eosinophilia, leucopenia, thrombocytopenia, and altered prothrombin concentration). Less frequent side-effects include anorexia, restlessness, depression, hallucinations, confusion, and disturbances in vision, taste, hearing

and smell; also isolated reports of intracranial hypertension and tendon damage (especially in the elderly and those taking corticosteroids, see also CSM advice above). Side-effects that have been reported to the CSM also include haemolytic anaemia, renal impairment, hepatic dysfunction, anaphylaxis, and hypoglycaemia. The drug should be **discontinued** if mental, neurological or hypersensitivity reactions occur with the first dose.

CIPROFLOXACIN

Indications: Gram-negative and Gram-positive infections, see notes above; surgical prophylaxis in upper gastro-intestinal procedures

Cautions; Side-effects: see notes above; avoid excessive alkalinity of urine and ensure adequate fluid intake (risk of crystalluria); not recommended in children or growing adolescents; caution in G6PD deficiency (see section 9.1.5); anaphylaxis reported, also reported dyspepsia, flatulence, dysphagia, tremor, convulsions, jaundice and hepatitis with necrosis, renal failure, nephritis, vasculitis, urticaria, erythema nodosum, Stevens-Johnson syndrome, Lyell syndrome, petechiae, haemorrhagic bullae, tenosynovitis and tachycardia; pain and phlebitis at injection site; **interactions**: Appendix 1 (4-quinolones)

DRIVING. May impair performance of skilled tasks (e.g. driving); effects of alcohol enhanced

Dose: by mouth, respiratory-tract infections, 250–750 mg twice daily

Urinary-tract infections, 250–500 mg twice daily (100 mg twice daily for 3 days in acute uncomplicated cystitis in women)

Gonorrhoea, 250 mg as a single dose; 500 mg may be required in resistant cases

Pseudomonal lower respiratory-tract infection in cystic fibrosis, 750 mg twice daily

Most other infections, 500–750 mg twice daily

Surgical prophylaxis, 750 mg 60–90 minutes before procedure

Prophylaxis of meningococcal meningitis [not licensed], section 5.1, table 2

By intravenous infusion (over 30–60 minutes; 400 mg over 60 minutes), 200–400 mg twice daily

Pseudomonal lower respiratory-tract infection in cystic fibrosis, 400 mg twice daily

Urinary-tract infections, 100 mg twice daily

Gonorrhoea, 100 mg as a single dose

CHILD not recommended (see above) but where benefit outweighs risk, *by mouth*, 7.5–15 mg/kg daily in 2 divided doses *or by intravenous infusion*, 5–10 mg/kg daily in 2 divided doses

PoM **Ciproxin®** (Baypharm)
Tablets, all f/c, ciprofloxacin (as hydrochloride) 100 mg, net price 6-tab pack = £2.80; 250 mg (scored), 10-tab pack = £7.50, 20-tab pack = £15.00; 500 mg (scored), 10-tab pack = £14.20, 20-tab pack = £28.40; 750 mg, 10-tab pack = £20.00. Label: 6, 9, 25, counselling, driving

Intravenous infusion, ciprofloxacin (as lactate) 2 mg/mL, in sodium chloride 0.9%, net price 50-mL bottle = £10.18, 100-mL bottle = £19.85, 200-mL bottle = £29.00

Electrolytes: Na+ 15.4 mmol/100-mL bottle

Intravenous infusion (*Flexibag*), ciprofloxacin (as lactate) 2 mg/mL, in glucose 5%, net price 100-mL infusion bag = £20.85, 200-mL infusion bag = £30.45

CINOXACIN

Indications: urinary-tract infections

Cautions; Side-effects: see notes above; avoid in severe renal impairment; also reported, perineal burning, Stevens-Johnson syndrome; **interactions:** Appendix 1 (4-quinolones)

DRIVING. May impair performance of skilled tasks (e.g. driving)

Dose: 500 mg every 12 hours; prophylaxis, 500 mg at night

PoM **Cinobac**® (Lilly)

Capsules, green/orange, cinoxacin 500 mg. Net price 14-cap pack = £10.41. Label: 9, counselling, driving

NALIDIXIC ACID

Indications: urinary-tract infections

Cautions; Side-effects: see notes above; avoid in porphyria (see section 9.8.2) and if history of convulsive disorders, avoid strong sunlight, false positive urinary glucose (if tested for reducing substances); monitor blood counts, renal and liver function if treatment exceeds 2 weeks; caution in G6PD deficiency (see section 9.1.5); also reported toxic psychosis and convulsions, weakness, increased intracranial pressure, paraesthesia, cranial nerve palsy, cholestasis, metabolic acidosis; **interactions:** Appendix 1 (4-quinolones)

Dose: 1 g every 6 hours for 7 days, reduced in chronic infections to 500 mg every 6 hours; CHILD over 3 months max. 50 mg/kg daily in divided doses; reduced in prolonged therapy to 30 mg/kg daily

PoM **Nalidixic Acid** (Non-proprietary)

Tablets, nalidixic acid 500 mg. Net price 56-tab pack = £12.83. Label: 9, 11
Available from Norton

PoM **Mictral**® (Sanofi Winthrop)

Granules, effervescent, nalidixic acid 660 mg, sodium citrate (as sodium citrate and citric acid) 4.1 g/sachet (Na^+ 41 mmol/sachet). Net price 9-sachet pack = £5.48. Label: 9, 11, 13

Dose: 1 sachet in water 3 times daily for 3 days

PoM **Negram**® (Sanofi Winthrop)

Tablets, beige, nalidixic acid 500 mg. Net price 56-tab pack = £12.83. Label: 9, 11

Suspension, pink, sugar-free, nalidixic acid 300 mg/5 mL. Net price 150 mL = £12.85. Label: 9, 11

PoM **Uriben**® (Rosemont)

Suspension, pink, nalidixic acid 300 mg/5 mL. Net price 200 mL = £16.95; 500 mL = £40.10. Label: 9, 11

NORFLOXACIN

Indications: see under Dose

Cautions; Side-effects: see notes above; caution in G6PD deficiency (section 9.1.5); avoid in prepubertal children and growing adolescents; also reported, anorexia, depression, anxiety, tinnitus, toxic epidermal necrolysis, exfoliative dermatitis, erythema multiforme (Stevens-Johnson syndrome); **interactions:** Appendix 1 (4-quinolones)

DRIVING. May impair performance of skilled tasks (e.g. driving)

Dose: urinary-tract infections, 400 mg twice daily for 7–10 days (for 3 days in uncomplicated lower urinary-tract infections)

Chronic relapsing urinary-tract infections, 400 mg twice daily for up to 12 weeks; may be reduced to 400 mg once daily if adequate suppression within first 4 weeks

PoM **Utinor**® (MSD)

Tablets, scored, norfloxacin 400 mg. Net price 6-tab pack = £2.88, 14-tab pack = £6.72. Label: 6, 9, counselling, driving

OFLOXACIN

Indications: see under Dose

Cautions; Side-effects: see notes above; caution in history of psychiatric illness, in diabetes, and in G6PD deficiency (section 9.1.5); avoid strong sunlight; avoid in epilepsy or history of epilepsy and in children and adolescents; also reported, tachycardia, transient hypotension, inflammation and rupture of tendons, erythema multiforme, Lyell syndrome, vasculitic reactions, angioedema, anxiety, unsteady gait and tremor, paraesthesia, hypaesthesia, neuropathy, extrapyramidal symptoms, psychotic reactions (discontinue treatment—see notes above); agranulocytosis and pancytopenia; very rarely changes in blood sugar; isolated cases of pneumonitis, interstitial nephritis; on intravenous infusion, hypotension and local reactions (including thrombophlebitis); **interactions:** Appendix 1 (4-quinolones)

DRIVING. May affect performance of skilled tasks (e.g. driving); effects enhanced by alcohol

Dose: by mouth, urinary-tract infections, 200–400 mg daily preferably in the morning, increased if necessary in upper urinary-tract infections to 400 mg twice daily

Lower respiratory-tract infections, 400 mg daily preferably in the morning, increased if necessary to 400 mg twice daily

Skin and soft-tissue infections, 400 mg twice daily

Uncomplicated gonorrhoea, 400 mg as a single dose

Non-gonococcal urethritis and cervicitis, 400 mg daily in single or divided doses

By intravenous infusion (over at least 30 minutes for each 200 mg), complicated urinary-tract infection, 200 mg daily

Lower respiratory-tract infection, 200 mg twice daily

Septicaemia, 200 mg twice daily

Skin and soft-tissue infections, 400 mg twice daily

Severe or complicated infections, dose may be increased to 400 mg twice daily

PoM **Tarivid**® (Hoechst Marion Roussel)

Tablets, f/c, scored, ofloxacin 200 mg, net price 10-tab pack = £10.26, 20-tab pack = £20.50; 400 mg (yellow), 5-tab pack = £10.24, 10-tab pack = £20.43. Label: 6, 9, 11, counselling, driving

Intravenous infusion, ofloxacin (as hydrochloride) 2 mg/mL, net price 50-mL bottle = £15.41; 100-mL bottle = £22.01 (both hosp. only)

5.1.13 Urinary-tract infections

Urinary-tract infection is more common in women than in men; when it occurs in men there is frequently an underlying abnormality of the renal tract. Recurrent episodes of infection are an indication for radiological investigation especially in children in whom untreated pyelonephritis may lead to permanent kidney damage.

Escherichia coli is the most common cause of urinary-tract infection. Less common causes include Proteus and Klebsiella spp. *Pseudomonas aeruginosa* infections are almost invariably associated with functional or anatomical abnormalities of the renal tract. *Staphylococcus epidermidis* and *Enterococcus faecalis* infection may complicate catheterisation or instrumentation. Whenever possible a specimen of urine should be collected for culture and sensitivity testing before starting antibiotic therapy.

Uncomplicated lower urinary-tract infections often respond to ampicillin, nalidixic acid, nitrofurantoin, or trimethoprim given for 5–7 days; those caused by fully sensitive bacteria respond to two 3-g doses of amoxycillin (section 5.1.1.3). Bacterial resistance, however, especially to ampicillin (to which approximately 50% of *E. coli* are now resistant), has increased the importance of urine culture prior to therapy. Alternatives for resistant organisms include co-amoxiclav (amoxycillin with clavulanic acid), an oral cephalosporin, and ciprofloxacin. Hexamine should **not** be used as it is only bacteriostatic, requires acid urine, and frequently causes side-effects.

Long-term low dose therapy may be required in selected patients to prevent *recurrence of infection*; indications include frequent relapses and significant kidney damage. Trimethoprim, nitrofurantoin and cephalexin have been recommended for long-term therapy.

Acute pyelonephritis can be associated with septicaemia and is best treated initially by injection of a broad-spectrum antibiotic such as aztreonam, cefuroxime, ciprofloxacin, or gentamicin especially if the patient is vomiting or severely ill.

Prostatitis can be difficult to cure and requires treatment for several weeks with an antibiotic which penetrates prostatic tissue such as trimethoprim, erythromycin, or ciprofloxacin.

Where infection is localised and associated with an indwelling *catheter* a bladder instillation is often effective (see section 7.4.4).

Patients with *heart-valve lesions* undergoing instrumentation of the urinary tract should be given a parenteral antibiotic to prevent bacteraemia and endocarditis (section 5.1, table 2).

Urinary-tract infection in *pregnancy* may be asymptomatic and requires prompt treatment to prevent progression to acute pyelonephritis. Penicillins and cephalosporins can be given in pregnancy but trimethoprim, sulphonamides, 4-quinolones, and tetracyclines should be avoided.

In *renal failure* antibiotics normally excreted by the kidney accumulate with resultant toxicity unless the dose is reduced. This applies especially to the aminoglycosides which should be used with great caution; tetracyclines, hexamine, and nitrofurantoin should be avoided altogether.

NITROFURANTOIN

Indications: urinary-tract infections

Cautions: anaemia; diabetes mellitus; electrolyte imbalance; vitamin B and folate deficiency; pulmonary disease; hepatic impairment; monitor lung and liver function on long-term therapy, especially in the elderly; susceptibility to peripheral neuropathy; false positive urinary glucose (if tested for reducing substances); urine may be coloured yellow or brown; **interactions:** Appendix 1 (nitrofurantoin)

Contra-indications: impaired renal function, infants less than 3 months old, G6PD deficiency (including pregnancy at term, and breast-feeding of affected infants, see section 9.1.5 and Appendixes 4 and 5), porphyria (see section 9.8.2)

Side-effects: anorexia, nausea, vomiting, and diarrhoea; acute and chronic pulmonary reactions (may be associated with lupus erythematosus-like syndrome); peripheral neuropathy; also reported, angioedema, urticaria, rash and pruritus; rarely, cholestatic jaundice, hepatitis, exfoliative dermatitis, erythema multiforme, pancreatitis, arthralgia, blood disorders (including agranulocytosis, thrombocytopenia, and aplastic anaemia), benign intracranial hypertension, and transient alopecia

Dose: acute uncomplicated infection, 50 mg every 6 hours with food for 7 days; CHILD over 3 months, 3 mg/kg daily in 4 divided doses

Severe chronic recurrent infection, 100 mg every 6 hours with food for 7 days (dose reduced or discontinued if severe nausea)

Prophylaxis (but see Cautions), 50–100 mg at night; CHILD over 3 months, 1 mg/kg at night

PoM **Nitrofurantoin** (Non-proprietary)

Tablets, nitrofurantoin 50 mg and 100 mg. Label: 9, 14, 21

Available from Biorex, Cox, Kent

PoM **Furadantin**® (Procter & Gamble Pharm.)

Tablets, all yellow, scored, nitrofurantoin 50 mg, net price 20 = £1.96; 100 mg, 20 = £3.62. Label: 9, 14, 21

PoM **Macrobid**® (Procter & Gamble Pharm.)

Capsules, m/r, blue/yellow, nitrofurantoin 100 mg (as nitrofurantoin macrocrystals and nitrofurantoin monohydrate). Net price 14-cap pack = £4.89. Label: 9, 14, 21, 25

Dose: uncomplicated urinary-tract infection, 1 capsule twice daily with food

Genito-urinary surgical prophylaxis, 1 capsule twice daily on day of procedure and for 3 days after

PoM **Macrodantin**® (Procter & Gamble Pharm.)

Capsules, nitrofurantoin 50 mg (yellow/white), net price 30-cap pack = £3.05; 100 mg (yellow), 20 = £3.84. Label: 9, 14, 21

HEXAMINE HIPPURATE

(Methenamine hippurate)

Indications: prophylaxis and long-term treatment of recurrent urinary-tract infections

Cautions: pregnancy; avoid concurrent administration with sulphonamides (risk of crystalluria) or urinary alkalinising agents; **interactions:** Appendix 1 (hexamine)

Contra-indications: severe renal impairment, dehydration, metabolic acidosis

Side-effects: gastro-intestinal disturbances, bladder irritation, rash

Dose: 1 g every 12 hours (may be increased in patients with catheters to 1 g every 8 hours); CHILD 6–12 years 500 mg every 12 hours

Hiprex® (3M)

Tablets, scored, hexamine hippurate 1 g. Net price 60-tab pack = £7.40. Label: 9

5.2   Antifungal drugs

Fungal infections are frequently associated with a defect in host resistance which should, if possible, be corrected otherwise drug therapy may fail. Similarly, treatment of dermatophyte infection may be unsuccessful until the animal source has been removed or controlled.

For local treatment of fungal infections see also sections 7.2.2 (genital), 7.4.4 (bladder), 11.3.2 (eye), 12.1.1 (ear), 12.3.2 (oropharynx), and 13.10.2 (skin).

POLYENE ANTIFUNGALS. The polyene antifungals include amphotericin and nystatin.

Amphotericin is not absorbed from the gut and is the only polyene antibiotic which can be given parenterally. It is used for the treatment of systemic fungal infections and is active against most fungi and yeasts. It is highly protein bound and penetrates poorly into body fluids and tissues. When given parenterally amphotericin is toxic and side-effects are common.

A formulation of amphotericin encapsulated in liposomes (*AmBisome*®) is available and is apparently significantly less toxic than the parent compound. Amphotericin is also available as a complex with sodium cholesteryl sulphate (*Amphocil*®). Another lipid formulation (*Abelcet*®) has also recently been introduced. All are recommended for systemic mycoses when amphotericin alone is contra-indicated because of toxicity, especially nephrotoxicity.

Nystatin is not absorbed when given by mouth and is too toxic for parenteral use. It is active against a number of yeasts and fungi but is principally used for *Candida albicans* infections of skin and mucous membranes. It is also used in the treatment of intestinal candidiasis.

IMIDAZOLE ANTIFUNGALS. The imidazole antifungals include clotrimazole, econazole, fenticonazole, isoconazole, ketoconazole, miconazole, sulconazole, and tioconazole; they are active against a wide range of fungi and yeasts. Their main indications are vaginal candidiasis and dermatophyte infections. Clotrimazole, econazole, fenticonazole, isoconazole, sulconazole, and tioconazole are used for local treatment.

Miconazole is used for local treatment and can be given by mouth for oral and intestinal infection.

Ketoconazole is significantly better absorbed after oral administration than the other imidazoles, but has been associated with fatal hepatotoxicity. The CSM has advised that prescribers should weigh the potential benefits of ketoconazole treatment against the liver damage risk and should carefully monitor patients both clinically and biochemically. It should **not** be given for superficial fungal infections.

TRIAZOLE ANTIFUNGALS. The triazole antifungals include fluconazole and itraconazole which are absorbed by mouth.

Fluconazole is an oral triazole antifungal indicated for local and systemic candidiasis and cryptococcal infections.

Itraconazole is indicated for oropharyngeal and vulvovaginal candidiasis, pityriasis versicolor, and tinea corporis and pedis; it is metabolised in the liver and should not be given to patients with a history of liver disease. It is also indicated for systemic fungal infections (including aspergillosis, candidiasis, and cryptococcosis) where other antifungal drugs are inappropriate or ineffective.

OTHER ANTIFUNGALS. **Flucytosine** is a synthetic antifungal drug which is only active against yeasts and has been used for the treatment of systemic candidiasis, cryptococcosis, and torulopsosis. Side-effects are uncommon but bone-marrow depression can occur and weekly blood counts are necessary during prolonged therapy. Synergy has been demonstrated with amphotericin. Resistance to flucytosine is not uncommon and can develop during therapy; sensitivity testing is, therefore, essential before and during treatment.

Griseofulvin is selectively concentrated in keratin and is the drug of choice for widespread or intractable dermatophyte infections. It is well absorbed from the gut but is inactive when applied topically. It is more effective in skin than in nail infections and treatment must be continued for several weeks or even months. Side-effects are uncommon.

Terbinafine, an allylamine antifungal, has recently been introduced for ringworm and nail fungal infections where oral treatment is considered appropriate.

AMPHOTERICIN
(Amphotericin B)

Indications: See under Dose

Cautions: when given parenterally, toxicity common (close supervision necessary and test dose required); hepatic and renal-function tests, blood counts, and plasma electrolyte monitoring required; corticosteroids (avoid except to control reactions); pregnancy and breast-feeding; frequent change of injection site (irritant); avoid rapid infusion (risk of arrhythmias); **interactions:** Appendix 1 (amphotericin)

ANAPHYLAXIS. The CSM has advised that anaphylaxis occurs rarely with any intravenous amphotericin product and a test dose is advisable before the first infusion; the patient should be carefully observed for about 30 minutes after the test dose. Prophylactic antipyretics or hydrocortisone should only be used in patients who have previously experienced acute adverse reactions (in whom continued treatment with amphotericin is essential)

Side-effects: when given parenterally, anorexia, nausea and vomiting, diarrhoea, epigastric pain; febrile reactions, headache, muscle and joint pain; anaemia; disturbances in renal function (including hypokalaemia and hypomagnesaemia) and renal toxicity; also cardiovascular toxicity (including arrhythmias), blood disorders, neurological disorders (including hearing loss, diplopia, convulsions, peripheral neuropathy), abnormal liver function (discontinue treatment), rash, anaphylactoid reactions (see anaphylaxis, above)

Dose: by mouth, intestinal candidiasis, 100–200 mg every 6 hours

Oral and perioral infections, see section 12.3.2

By intravenous infusion, see under preparations, below

PoM **Fungilin®** (Squibb)
Tablets, yellow, scored, amphotericin 100 mg. Net price 56-tab pack = £8.32. Label: 9

Lozenges see section 12.3.2

Suspension, yellow, sugar-free, amphotericin 100 mg/mL. Net price 12 mL = £2.31. Label: 9, counselling, use of pipette

PoM **Fungizone®** (Squibb)
Intravenous infusion, powder for reconstitution, amphotericin (as sodium deoxycholate complex). Net price 50-mg vial = £3.70.
Electrolytes: Na⁺ < 0.5 mmol/vial
Dose: by intravenous infusion, systemic fungal infections, initial test dose of 1 mg over 20–30 minutes then 250 micrograms/kg daily, gradually increased if tolerated to 1 mg/kg daily; max. (severe infection) 1.5 mg/kg daily or on alternate days
Note. Prolonged treatment usually necessary; if interrupted for longer than 7 days recommence at 250 micrograms/kg daily and increase gradually

Lipid formulations
▼ PoM **Abelcet®** (Liposome Company)
Intravenous infusion, amphotericin 5 mg/mL as lipid complex with L-α-dimyristoylphosphatidylcholine and L-α-dimyristoylphosphatidylglycerol. Net price 20-mL vial = £86.00 (hosp. only)
Dose: severe invasive candidiasis; severe systemic fungal infections in patients not responding to conven-

tional amphotericin or to other antifungal drugs or where toxicity or renal impairment precludes conventional amphotericin, including invasive aspergillosis, cryptococcal meningitis and disseminated cryptococcosis in HIV patients, by intravenous infusion, ADULT and CHILD, initial test dose 1 mg over 15 minutes then 5 mg/kg daily for at least 14 days

PoM **AmBisome®** (NeXstar)
Intravenous infusion, powder for reconstitution, amphotericin 50 mg encapsulated in liposomes. Net price 50-mg vial = £145.00
Electrolytes: Na⁺ < 0.5 mmol/vial
Dose: severe systemic or deep mycoses where toxicity (particularly nephrotoxicity) precludes use of conventional amphotericin, by intravenous infusion, ADULT and CHILD initial test dose 1 mg over 10 minutes then 1 mg/kg daily as a single dose increased gradually if necessary to 3 mg/kg daily as a single dose
Visceral leishmaniasis, see product literature

PoM **Amphocil®** (Zeneca)
Intravenous infusion, powder for reconstitution, amphotericin as a complex with sodium cholesteryl sulphate. Net price 50-mg vial = £109.00, 100-mg vial = £199.00
Electrolytes: Na⁺ < 0.5 mmol/vial
Dose: severe systemic or deep mycoses where toxicity or renal failure preclude use of conventional amphotericin, by intravenous infusion, ADULT and CHILD initial test dose 2 mg over 10 minutes then 1 mg/kg daily as a single dose increased gradually if necessary to 3–4 mg/kg daily as a single dose

FLUCONAZOLE

Indications: see under Dose

Cautions: renal impairment; pregnancy (toxicity at high doses in *animal* studies) and breast-feeding; raised liver enzymes (review need for treatment if raised significantly, possible risk of hepatic necrosis); **interactions:** Appendix 1 (antifungals, imidazole and triazole)

ARRHYTHMIAS. Avoid concomitant administration with astemizole or terfenadine, see also pp. 142 and 143; also avoid with cisapride (see p. 34) [other interactions, Appendix 1]

Side-effects: nausea, abdominal discomfort, diarrhoea, and flatulence; occasionally abnormalities of liver enzymes; rarely rash (discontinue treatment or monitor closely if infection invasive or systemic); angioedema, anaphylaxis, bullous lesions, toxic epidermal necrolysis, and Stevens-Johnson syndrome reported; severe cutaneous reactions in AIDS patients also reported

Dose: vaginal candidiasis and candidal balanitis, *by mouth,* a single dose of 150 mg

Mucosal candidiasis (except genital), *by mouth,* 50 mg daily (100 mg daily in unusually difficult infections) given for 7–14 days in oropharyngeal candidiasis (max. 14 days except in severely immunocompromised patients); for 14 days in atrophic oral candidiasis associated with dentures; for 14–30 days in other mucosal infections (e.g. oesophagitis, candiduria, non-invasive bronchopulmonary infections); CHILD *by mouth or by intravenous infusion,* 3–6 mg/kg on first day then 3 mg/kg daily (every 72 hours in NEONATE up to 2 weeks old, every 48 hours in neonate 2–4 weeks old)

Tinea pedis, corporis, cruris, pityriasis versicolor, and dermal candidiasis, *by mouth,* 50 mg daily for

2–4 weeks (for up to 6 weeks in tinea pedis); max. duration of treatment 6 weeks

Invasive candidal infections (including candidaemia and disseminated candidiasis) and cryptococcal infections (including meningitis), *by mouth or intravenous infusion*, 400 mg initially then 200 mg daily, increased if necessary to 400 mg daily; treatment continued according to response (at least 6–8 weeks for cryptococcal meningitis); CHILD 6–12 mg/kg daily (every 72 hours in NEONATE up to 2 weeks old, every 48 hours in neonate 2–4 weeks old)

Prevention of relapse of cryptococcal meningitis in AIDS patients after completion of primary therapy, *by mouth or by intravenous infusion*, 100–200 mg daily

Prevention of fungal infections in immunocompromised patients following cytotoxic chemotherapy or radiotherapy, *by mouth or by intravenous infusion*, 50–400 mg daily adjusted according to risk; 400 mg daily if high risk of systemic infections e.g. following bone-marrow transplantation; commence treatment before anticipated onset of neutropenia and continue for 7 days after neutrophil count in desirable range; CHILD according to extent and duration of neutropenia, 3–12 mg/kg daily (every 72 hours in NEONATE up to 2 weeks old, every 48 hours in neonate 2–4 weeks old)

Diflucan® (Pfizer)

PoM[1] *Capsules*, fluconazole 50 mg (blue/white), net price 7-cap pack = £16.61; 150 mg (blue), single-capsule pack = £7.12; 200 mg (purple/white), 7-cap pack = £66.42. Label: 50 and 200 mg, 9

1. Can be sold to the public for vaginal candidiasis in women aged 16–60 years, in a container or packaging containing not more than 150 mg and labelled to show a max. dose of 150 mg; a proprietary brand (Diflucan® One) containing a single 150-mg capsule is on sale to the public

PoM *Oral suspension*, fluconazole for reconstitution with water, 50 mg/5 mL, net price 35 mL = £16.61; 200 mg/5 mL, 35 mL = £66.42. Label: 9

PoM *Intravenous infusion*, fluconazole 2 mg/mL in sodium chloride intravenous infusion 0.9%, net price 25-mL bottle = £7.32; 100-mL bottle = £29.28
Electrolytes: Na$^+$ 15 mmol/100-mL bottle

FLUCYTOSINE

Indications: systemic yeast and fungal infections; adjunct to amphotericin (or fluconazole) in cryptococcal meningitis, adjunct to amphotericin in severe systemic candidiasis and in other severe or long-standing infections

Cautions: renal impairment (reduce dose and monitor plasma concentrations), elderly, blood disorders, liver- and kidney-function tests and blood counts required (weekly in renal impairment or blood disorders); pregnancy, breast-feeding

Side-effects: nausea, vomiting, diarrhoea, rashes; less frequently confusion, hallucinations, convulsions, headache, sedation, vertigo, alterations in liver function tests (hepatitis and hepatic necrosis reported); blood disorders including thrombocytopenia, leucopenia, and aplastic anaemia reported

Dose: *by intravenous infusion* over 20–40 minutes, ADULT and CHILD, 200 mg/kg daily in 4 divided doses usually for not more than 7 days; extremely sensitive organisms, 100–150 mg/kg daily may be sufficient; treat for at least 4 months in cryptococcal meningitis

Note. For plasma concentration monitoring blood should be taken shortly before starting the next infusion; plasma concentration for optimum response 25–50 mg/litre (200–400 micromol/litre)—should not be allowed to exceed 80 mg/litre (620 micromol/litre)

PoM **Alcobon®** (Roche)

Intravenous infusion, flucytosine 10 mg/mL. Net price 250-mL infusion bottle = £18.21 (hosp. only)

Electrolytes: Na$^+$ 34.5 mmol/250-mL bottle
Note. Flucytosine tablets may be available on a named-patient basis from Bell and Croyden

GRISEOFULVIN

Indications: dermatophyte infections of the skin, scalp, hair and nails, where topical therapy has failed or is inappropriate

Cautions: rarely aggravation or precipitation of systemic lupus erythematosus; breast-feeding; **interactions:** Appendix 1 (griseofulvin)

DRIVING. May impair performance of skilled tasks (e.g. driving); effects of alcohol enhanced

Contra-indications: liver failure, lupus erythematosus and related conditions, porphyria (see section 9.8.2); pregnancy (**avoid** pregnancy **during** and for **1 month after** treatment; manufacturer now also states that a man should not father a child within 6 months of treatment)

Side-effects: headache, nausea, vomiting, rashes, photosensitivity; dizziness, fatigue, agranulocytosis and leucopenia reported; lupus erythematosus, erythema multiforme, toxic epidermal necrolysis, peripheral neuropathy, confusion and impaired co-ordination also reported

Dose: 500 mg daily, in divided doses or as a single dose, in severe infection dose may be doubled, reducing when response occurs; CHILD, 10 mg/kg daily in divided doses or as a single dose

PoM **Fulcin®** (Zeneca)

Tablets, griseofulvin 125 mg (scored), net price 20 = 61p; 500 mg (f/c), 20 = £2.29. Label: 9, 21, counselling, driving

Oral suspension, brown, griseofulvin 125 mg/5 mL. Net price 100 mL = £1.10. Label: 9, 21, counselling, driving

PoM **Grisovin®** (GlaxoWellcome)

Tablets, both f/c, griseofulvin 125 mg, net price 20 = 47p; 500 mg, 20 = £1.75. Label: 9, 21, counselling, driving

ITRACONAZOLE

Indications: oropharyngeal and vulvovaginal candidiasis; pityriasis versicolor and other dermatophyte infections; onychomycosis; histoplasmosis; alternative where other antifungal drugs inappropriate or ineffective in systemic infections (aspergillosis, candidiasis and cryptococcosis including cryptococcal meningitis), and in maintenance treatment of AIDS patients to prevent relapse of underlying fungal infection; prevention of fungal infection in neutropenia when standard therapy inappropriate

Cautions: liver disease (Appendix 2); liver function tests required if history of liver disease or if treatment exceeds 1 month or if anorexia, nausea, vomiting, fatigue, abdominal pain or dark urine develop (discontinue if test abnormal); renal impairment (bioavailability may be reduced); absorption reduced in AIDS and neutropenia (monitor plasma-itraconazole concentration and increase dose if necessary); discontinue treatment if peripheral neuropathy; pregnancy (Appendix 4) and breast-feeding; **interactions:** Appendix 1 (antifungals, imidazole and triazole)

ARRHYTHMIAS. Avoid concomitant administration with astemizole or terfenadine, see also pp. 142 and 143; also avoid with cisapride (see p. 34) [other interactions, Appendix 1]

Side-effects: nausea, abdominal pain, dyspepsia, constipation (diarrhoea with oral liquid), headache, dizziness, raised liver enzymes, menstrual disorders; allergic reactions (including pruritus, rash, urticaria and angioedema), hepatitis and cholestatic jaundice (especially if treatment exceeds 1 month), peripheral neuropathy (discontinue treatment), and Stevens-Johnson syndrome reported; on prolonged use hypokalaemia, oedema and hair loss reported

Dose: oropharyngeal candidiasis, 100 mg daily (200 mg daily in AIDS or neutropenia) for 15 days; see also under *Sporanox*® oral liquid below
Vulvovaginal candidiasis, 200 mg twice daily for 1 day
Pityriasis versicolor, 200 mg daily for 7 days
Tinea corporis and tinea cruris, *either* 100 mg daily for 15 days *or* 200 mg daily for 7 days
Tinea pedis and tinea manuum, 100 mg daily for 30 days
Onychomycosis, *either* 200 mg daily for 3 months or course ('pulse') of 200 mg twice daily for 7 days, subsequent courses repeated after 21-day interval; fingernails two courses, toenails three courses
Histoplasmosis, 200 mg 1–2 times daily
Alternative in systemic infections, 200 mg once daily (candidiasis 100–200 mg once daily) increased in invasive or disseminated disease and in cryptococcal meningitis to 200 mg twice daily
Maintenance in AIDS patients and prophylaxis in neutropenia, 200 mg once daily, increased to 200 mg twice daily if low plasma-itraconazole concentration (see Cautions)
CHILD and ELDERLY not recommended

Oral liquid, itraconazole 10 mg/mL. Net price 150 mL (with 10-mL measuring cup) = £52.28. Label: 9, counselling, administration

Dose: oral or oesophageal candidiasis in HIV-positive or other immunocompromised patients, 20 mL (2 measuring cups) daily in 1–2 divided doses for 1 week (continue for another week if no response)
Fluconazole-resistant oral or oesophageal candidiasis, 20–40 mL (2–4 measuring cups) daily in 1–2 divided doses for 2 weeks (continue for another 2 weeks if no response)
COUNSELLING. Do not take with food; swish around mouth and swallow, do not rinse afterwards

KETOCONAZOLE

Indications: systemic mycoses, serious chronic resistant mucocutaneous candidiasis, serious resistant gastro-intestinal mycoses, chronic resistant vaginal candidiasis, resistant dermatophyte infections of skin or finger nails (not toe nails); prophylaxis of mycoses in immunosuppressed patients

Cautions: **important:** monitor liver function clinically and biochemically—for treatment lasting longer than 14 days perform liver function tests before starting, 14 days after starting, then at monthly intervals (for details see product literature)—for CSM advice see p. 270; avoid in porphyria (see section 9.8.2); **interactions:** Appendix 1 (antifungals, imidazole and triazole)

ARRHYTHMIAS. Avoid concomitant administration with astemizole or terfenadine, see also pp. 142 and 143; also avoid with cisapride (see p. 34) [other interactions, Appendix 1]

Contra-indications: hepatic impairment; pregnancy (teratogenicity in *animal* studies, packs carry a warning to avoid in pregnancy) and breast-feeding

Side-effects: nausea, vomiting, abdominal pain; headache, rashes, urticaria, pruritus; rarely angio-edema, thrombocytopenia, paraesthesia, photophobia, dizziness, alopecia, gynaecomastia and oligospermia; fatal liver damage—see also under Cautions, risk of developing hepatitis greater if given for longer than 14 days

Dose: 200 mg once daily with food, usually for 14 days; if response inadequate after 14 days continue until at least 1 week after symptoms have cleared and cultures become negative; max. 400 mg daily.
CHILD, 3 mg/kg daily
Chronic resistant vaginal candidiasis, 400 mg daily with food for 5 days

---

PoM **Sporanox**® (Janssen-Cilag)
Capsules, blue/pink, enclosing coated beads, itraconazole 100 mg. Net price 4-cap pack = £5.99; 15-cap pack = £22.46; 28-cap pack (Sporanox-Pulse®) = £41.93; 60-cap pack = £89.84. Label: 5, 9, 21, 25

PoM **Nizoral**® (Janssen-Cilag)
Tablets, scored, ketoconazole 200 mg. Net price 30-tab pack = £15.69. Label: 5, 9, 21
Suspension, pink, ketoconazole 100 mg/5 mL. Net price 100 mL with pipette = £7.16. Label: 5, 9, 21, counselling, use of pipette

---

MICONAZOLE
Indications: see under Dose
Cautions: pregnancy and breast-feeding; avoid in porphyria (see section 9.8.2); **interactions:** Appendix 1 (antifungals, imidazole and triazole) ARRHYTHMIAS. Avoid concomitant administration with astemizole or terfenadine, see also pp. 142 and 143; also avoid with cisapride (see p. 34) [other interactions, Appendix1]
Contra-indications: hepatic impairment
Side-effects: nausea and vomiting, diarrhoea (usually on long-term treatment); rarely allergic reactions; isolated reports of hepatitis
Dose: prevention and treatment of oral and intestinal fungal infections, 5–10 mL in the mouth after food 4 times daily; retain near lesions before swallowing; CHILD under 2 years, 2.5 mL twice daily, 2–6 years, 5 mL twice daily, over 6 years, 5 mL 4 times daily
Localised lesions, smear on affected area with clean finger

PoM **¹ Daktarin®** (Janssen-Cilag)
Oral gel, sugar-free, orange-flavoured, miconazole 24 mg/mL. Net price 15-g tube = £2.27, 80-g tube = £5.00. Label: 9, counselling advised, hold in mouth, after food
1. 15-g tube can be sold to public

NYSTATIN
Indications: candidiasis
Side-effects: nausea, vomiting, diarrhoea at high doses; oral irritation and sensitisation; rash (including urticaria) and rarely Stevens-Johnson syndrome reported
Dose: by mouth, intestinal candidiasis 500 000 units every 6 hours, doubled in severe infections; CHILD 100 000 units 4 times daily
Prophylaxis, 1 million units daily; NEONATE 100 000 units daily as a single dose
For use as a mouthwash in oral candidiasis, see section 12.3.2

PoM **Nystatin** (Non-proprietary)
Oral suspension, nystatin 100 000 units/mL. Net price 30 mL = £1.98. Label: 9, counselling use of pipette
Available from Hillcross, Kent, Lagap, Opus (Infestat®), Rosemont (sugar-free, Nystamont®)
PoM **Nystan®** (Squibb)
Tablets, brown, s/c, nystatin 500 000 units. Net price 56-tab pack = £4.70. Label: 9
Pastilles—see section 12.3.2
Pessaries—see section 7.2.2
Suspension, yellow, nystatin 100 000 units/mL. Net price 30 mL with pipette = £2.05. Label: 9, counselling, use of pipette
Suspension, gluten-, lactose-, and sugar-free, nystatin 100 000 units/mL when reconstituted with water. Net price 24 mL with pipette = £1.67. Label: 9, counselling, use of pipette

TERBINAFINE
Indications: dermatophyte infections of the nails, ringworm infections (including tinea pedis, cruris, and corporis) where oral therapy appropriate (due to site, severity or extent)
Cautions: hepatic and renal impairment; pregnancy, breast-feeding; **interactions:** Appendix 1 (terbinafine)
Side-effects: abdominal discomfort, loss of appetite, nausea, diarrhoea; headache; rash and urticaria occasionally with arthralgia or myalgia; serious skin reactions including Stevens-Johnson syndrome and toxic epidermal necrolysis reported (discontinue treatment if progressive skin rash); also reported, taste disturbance, photosensitivity, and rarely liver toxicity including jaundice, cholestasis and hepatitis
Dose: 250 mg daily usually for 2–6 weeks in tinea pedis, 2–4 weeks in tinea cruris, 4 weeks in tinea corporis, 6 weeks–3 months or longer in nail infections; CHILD not recommended

PoM **Lamisil®** (Novartis)
Tablets, off-white, scored, terbinafine 250 mg (as hydrochloride), net price 14-tab pack = £23.16, 28-tab pack = £44.66. Label: 9

5.3   Antiviral drugs
The specific therapy of virus infections is generally unsatisfactory and treatment is, therefore, primarily symptomatic. Fortunately, the majority of infections resolve spontaneously in the immunocompetent. For **interferon** preparations used in hepatitis B and C infections, see section 8.2.4.

HERPES SIMPLEX AND VARICELLA–ZOSTER

Aciclovir is active against herpes viruses but does not eradicate them. It is effective only if started at the onset of infection. Uses of aciclovir include the systemic treatment of varicella–zoster (chickenpox–shingles) and the systemic and topical treatment of herpes simplex infections of the skin and mucous membranes (including initial and recurrent genital herpes); it is also used topically in the eye. It can be life-saving in herpes simplex and varicella–zoster infections in the immunocompromised, and is also used in the immunocompromised for prevention of recurrence and prophylaxis. Aciclovir may also be given by mouth to immunocompetent adults and older adolescents with chickenpox; it is not generally indicated for immunocompetent children in whom the disease is milder. See also section 11.3.3 (eye) and section 13.10.3 (skin, including herpes labialis).

Famciclovir, a prodrug of penciclovir, is similar to aciclovir and it is recommended for herpes zoster and initial and recurrent genital herpes. Penciclovir itself is used as a cream for herpes simplex labialis (section 13.10.3). **Valaciclovir** is an ester of aciclovir which is licensed for herpes zoster and for herpes simplex infections of the skin and mucous membranes (including initial and recurrent genital herpes).

Idoxuridine (section 13.10.3) is also only effective if started at the onset of infection; it is too toxic for systemic use. It has been used topically in the treatment of herpes simplex lesions of the skin and external genitalia with variable results; it has also been used topically in the treatment of zoster, but evidence of its value is dubious.

Inosine pranobex has been used by mouth for herpes simplex infections; its effectiveness has not been established.

Amantadine has been used by mouth for herpes zoster but, again, its effectiveness has not been established. Amantadine may be used for prophylaxis during an outbreak of influenza A **only** in:

unimmunised patients in 'at risk' groups (see under Influenza vaccine, section 14.4), for 2 weeks while the vaccine takes effect

patients in 'at risk' groups for whom immunisation is contra-indicated, for the duration of the outbreak

health care workers and other key personnel (to prevent disruption of service), during an epidemic

The Joint Committee on Vaccination and Immunisation has advised that amantadine should not be used for both prophylaxis and treatment of influenza in the same household (risk of resistance).

ACICLOVIR
(Acyclovir)

Indications: herpes simplex and varicella–zoster (see also under Dose)

Cautions: maintain adequate hydration; renal impairment (see Appendix 3); pregnancy and breast-feeding; **interactions:** Appendix 1 (aciclovir and famciclovir)

Side-effects: rashes; gastro-intestinal disturbances; rises in bilirubin and liver enzymes, increases in blood urea and creatinine, decreases in haematological indices, headache, neurological reactions (including dizziness), fatigue; on intravenous infusion, severe local inflammation (sometimes leading to ulceration), also confusion, hallucinations, agitation, tremors, somnolence, psychosis, convulsions and coma

Dose: by mouth,

Herpes simplex, treatment, 200 mg (400 mg in the immunocompromised or if absorption impaired) 5 times daily, usually for 5 days; CHILD under 2 years, half adult dose, over 2 years, adult dose

Herpes simplex, prevention of recurrence, 200 mg 4 times daily *or* 400 mg twice daily possibly reduced to 200 mg 2 or 3 times daily and interrupted every 6–12 months

Herpes simplex, prophylaxis in the immunocompromised, 200–400 mg 4 times daily; CHILD under 2 years, half adult dose, over 2 years, adult dose

Varicella and herpes zoster, treatment, 800 mg 5 times daily for 7 days; CHILD, varicella, 20 mg/kg (max. 800 mg) 4 times daily for 5 days *or* under 2 years 200 mg 4 times daily, 2–5 years 400 mg 4 times daily, over 6 years 800 mg 4 times daily

By intravenous infusion, treatment of herpes simplex in the immunocompromised, severe initial genital herpes, and varicella–zoster, 5 mg/kg every 8 hours usually for 5 days, doubled to 10 mg/kg every 8 hours in varicella–zoster in the immunocompromised and in simplex encephalitis (usually given for 10 days in encephalitis); prophylaxis of herpes simplex in the immunocompromised, 5 mg/kg every 8 hours

NEONATE up to 3 months, herpes simplex, 10 mg/kg every 8 hours usually for 10 days; CHILD 3 months–12 years, herpes simplex or varicella–zoster, 250 mg/m^2 every 8 hours usually for 5 days, doubled to 500 mg/m^2 every 8 hours for varicella–zoster in the immunocompromised and in simplex encephalitis (usually given for 10 days in encephalitis)

By topical application, see sections 13.10.3 (skin) and 11.3.3 (eye)

PoM **Aciclovir** (Non-proprietary)

Tablets, aciclovir 200 mg, net price 25-tab pack = £18.95; 400 mg, 56-tab pack = £70.85; 800 mg, 35-tab pack £96.57. Label:9

Available from CP, Dominion, Ethical Generics Ltd, Lennon, Opus (Virovir®)

Dispersible tablets, aciclovir 200 mg, net price 25-tab pack = £20.80; 400 mg, 56-tab pack = £74.09; 800 mg, 35-tab pack = £83.60. Label: 9

Available from Cox, Hillcross, Norton

Intravenous infusion, powder for reconstitution, aciclovir (as sodium salt). Net price 250-mg vial = £9.27; 500-mg vial = £17.19

Electrolytes: Na⁺ 1.1 mmol/250-mg vial

Available from Lennon

Intravenous infusion, aciclovir (as sodium salt), net price 250 mg/10 mL vial = £10.37; 500 mg/20 mL vial = £19.21; 1 g/40 mL vial = £40.44

Electrolytes: Na⁺ 1.16 mmol/250-mg vial

Available from Faulding DBL

PoM **Zovirax®** (GlaxoWellcome)

Tablets, all dispersible, aciclovir 200 mg (blue), net price 25-tab pack = £28.89; 400 mg (pink), 56-tab pack = £105.95; 800 mg (scored, *Shingles Treatment Pack*), 35-tab pack = £107.30. Label: 9

Suspension, both off-white, sugar-free, aciclovir 200 mg/5 mL, net price 125 mL = £28.89; 400 mg/5 mL (*Chickenpox Treatment*) 50 mL = £16.14. Label: 9

Intravenous infusion, powder for reconstitution, aciclovir (as sodium salt). Net price 250-mg vial = £10.91; 500-mg vial = £20.22

Electrolytes: Na⁺ 1.1 mmol/250-mg vial

AMANTADINE HYDROCHLORIDE

Indications: see under Dose; parkinsonism, see section 4.9.1

Cautions; Contra-indications; Side-effects: see section 4.9.1

Dose: herpes zoster (but see notes above), 100 mg twice daily for 14 days, if necessary extended for a further 14 days for post-herpetic pain

Influenza A (see also notes above), ADULT and CHILD over 10 years, treatment, 100 mg daily for 4–5 days; prophylaxis, 100 mg daily usually for 6 weeks *or* with influenza vaccination for 2–3 weeks after vaccination

ELDERLY over 65 years, less than 100 mg daily *or* 100 mg at intervals of more than 1 day

Preparations

See section 4.9.1

FAMCICLOVIR

Note. Famciclovir is a pro-drug of penciclovir

Indications: treatment of herpes zoster, acute genital herpes simplex and suppression of recurrent genital herpes

Cautions: renal impairment; pregnancy and breast-feeding; **interactions:** Appendix 1 (aciclovir and famciclovir)

Side-effects: nausea, vomiting; headache; rarely dizziness, confusion; rash

Dose: herpes zoster, 250 mg 3 times daily for 7 days *or* 750 mg once daily for 7 days
Genital herpes, first episode, 250 mg 3 times daily for 5 days; recurrent infection, 125 mg twice daily for 5 days; suppression, 250 mg twice daily (interrupted every 6–12 months)
CHILD not recommended

PoM **Famvir**® (SmithKline Beecham)
Tablets, all f/c, famciclovir 125 mg, net price 10-tab pack = £28.12; 250 mg, 15-tab pack = £84.35, 21-tab pack = £118.18; 56-tab pack = £314.90; 750 mg, 7-tab pack = £107.35. Label: 9

INOSINE PRANOBEX

Indications: see under Dose

Cautions: avoid in renal impairment; history of gout or hyperuricaemia

Side-effects: reversible increases in serum and urinary uric acid

Dose: mucocutaneous herpes simplex, 1 g 4 times daily for 7–14 days
Adjunctive treatment of genital warts, 1 g 3 times daily for 14–28 days

PoM **Imunovir**® (Ardern)
Tablets, inosine pranobex 500 mg. Net price 100 = £39.50. Label: 9

VALACICLOVIR

Note. Valaciclovir is a pro-drug of aciclovir

Indications: treatment of herpes zoster and of herpes simplex infections of skin and mucous membranes including initial and recurrent genital herpes

Cautions: maintain adequate hydration; renal impairment (see Appendix 3); pregnancy and breast-feeding; **interactions:** Appendix 1 (aciclovir and famciclovir)

Side-effects: as a pro-drug of aciclovir it is anticipated that side-effects will be comparable; nausea and headache reported

Dose: herpes zoster, 1 g 3 times daily for 7 days
Herpes simplex, first episode, 500 mg twice daily for 5 days (up to 10 days if severe); recurrent infection, 500 mg twice daily for 5 days
CHILD not recommended

PoM **Valtrex**® (GlaxoWellcome)
Tablets, valaciclovir (as hydrochloride) 500 mg. Net price 10-tab (*HS Treatment*) pack = £23.50, 42-tab (*Shingles Treatment*) pack = £98.50. Label: 9

HUMAN IMMUNODEFICIENCY VIRUS

There is no cure for infection caused by the human immunodeficiency virus (HIV) but there are a number of drugs which slow the progression of HIV infection.

PRINCIPLES OF TREATMENT. Drugs for HIV infection are potentially toxic and expensive; treatment should be undertaken only by those experienced in their use. Treatment is aimed at reducing the plasma viral load as much as possible and for as long as possible; it should be started before the immune system is irreversibly damaged. The need for early drug treatment should, however, be balanced against the development of toxicity. The development of drug resistance is prevented by using a combination of drugs; such combinations should be chosen to have synergistic or additive activity while ensuring that their toxicity is not additive. It should be borne in mind that advice on the management of HIV infection is subject to rapid change.

INITIATION OF TREATMENT. The optimum time for initiation of antiviral treatment will depend on the CD4 cell count, the plasma viral load, and clinical symptoms. Initiation treatment with a **combination** of zidovudine with *either* didanosine *or* zalcitabine *or* lamivudine has been used; combinations involving the use of three drugs (including a protease inhibitor *or* a non-nucleoside reverse transcriptase inhibitor) have been recommended and may be appropriate in high plasma viral load.

SWITCHING THERAPY. Deterioration of the condition (including clinical and virological changes) may require either switching therapy or adding another antiviral drug. The choice of an alternative regimen depends on factors such as the response to previous treatment, tolerance and the possibility of cross-resistance.

POST-EXPOSURE PROPHYLAXIS. Treatment with antiviral drugs may be appropriate following occupational exposure to HIV-contaminated material. Immediate expert advice should be sought in such cases; national guidelines on post-exposure prophylaxis for healthcare workers have been developed (by the Chief Medical Officer's Expert Advisory Group on AIDS) and local ones may also be available.

DRUGS USED FOR HIV INFECTION. **Zidovudine**, a nucleoside reverse transcriptase inhibitor (or 'nucleoside analogue'), was the first of the anti-HIV drugs; it penetrates the blood-brain barrier and may be useful in preventing the AIDS dementia complex. Other nucleoside reverse transcriptase inhibitors include **didanosine**, **lamivudine**, **stavudine**, and **zalcitabine**.

The protease inhibitors, **indinavir**, **ritonavir** and **saquinavir** have been introduced recently. Ritonavir, indinavir and possibly saquinavir inhibit the cytochrome P450 enzyme system and therefore have a potential for significant drug interactions.

Non-nucleoside reverse transcriptase inhibitors are not on the UK market (but may be available on a named-patient basis).

NUCLEOSIDE REVERSE TRANSCRIPTASE INHIBITORS

DIDANOSINE
(ddI, DDI)

Indications: progressive or advanced HIV infection preferably in combination with other antiretroviral drugs

Cautions: history of pancreatitis (extreme caution, see also below); peripheral neuropathy or hyperuricaemia (see under Side-effects); monitor liver enzymes (suspend if significant elevation); hepatic and renal impairment (see Appendixes 2 and 3); pregnancy; dilated retinal examinations recommended (especially in children) every 6 months, or if visual changes occur; **interactions;** Appendix 1 (didanosine)

PANCREATITIS. If symptoms of pancreatitis develop or if serum amylase is raised (even if asymptomatic) suspend treatment until diagnosis of pancreatitis excluded; on return to normal values re-initiate treatment only if essential (using low dose increased gradually if appropriate). Whenever possible avoid concomitant treatment with other drugs known to cause pancreatic toxicity (e.g. intravenous pentamidine isethionate); monitor closely if concomitant therapy unavoidable. Since significant elevations of triglycerides cause pancreatitis monitor closely if elevated

Contra-indications: breast-feeding

Side-effects: pancreatitis (see also under Cautions); peripheral neuropathy especially in advanced HIV infection—suspend (reduced dose may be tolerated when symptoms resolve); asymptomatic hyperuricaemia (suspend treatment if measures to reduce uric acid concentration fail); diarrhoea (occasionally serious); also reported, nausea, vomiting, dry mouth, hypersensitivity reactions, retinal and optic nerve changes (especially in children), diabetes mellitus, liver failure

Dose: ADULT under 60 kg 125 mg every 12 hours, 60 kg and over 200 mg every 12 hours; CHILD over 3 months, 120 mg/m^2 every 12 hours (90 mg/m^2 every 12 hours in combination with zidovudine)

PoM **Videx**® (Bristol-Myers)

Tablets, both with calcium and magnesium antacids, didanosine 25 mg, net price 60-tab pack = £28.60; 100 mg, 60-tab pack = £88.00; 150 mg, 60-tab pack = £132.00. Label: 23, counselling, administration, see below

Additives: contains aspartame equivalent to phenylalanine 36.5 mg per tablet (see section 9.4.1)

Note. Antacids in formulation may affect absorption of other drugs—see **interactions:** Appendix 1 (antacids and adsorbents)

COUNSELLING. To ensure sufficient antacid, each dose to be taken as 2 tablets (CHILD under 1 year 1 tablet) chewed thoroughly, crushed or dispersed in water; clear apple juice may be added for flavouring

LAMIVUDINE
(3TC)

Indications: progressive HIV infection, in combination with other antiretroviral drugs

Cautions: renal impairment (see Appendix 3), hepatic disease due to chronic hepatitis B infection (risk of rebound hepatitis on discontinuation); pregnancy (manufacturer recommends avoid in first trimester); **interactions:** Appendix 1 (lamivudine)

Contra-indications: breast-feeding

Side-effects: nausea, vomiting, diarrhoea, abdominal pain; cough; headache, insomnia; malaise, musculoskeletal pain; nasal symptoms; peripheral neuropathy reported; rarely pancreatitis (discontinue); neutropenia and anaemia (in combination with zidovudine); thrombocytopenia; raised liver enzymes and serum amylase reported

Dose: 150 mg every 12 hours (preferably not taken with food); CHILD under 12 years, safety and efficacy not established

▼ PoM **Epivir**® (GlaxoWellcome)

Tablets, f/c, lamivudine 150 mg. Net price 60-tab pack = £171.30.

Oral solution, lamivudine 10 mg/mL. Net price 240-mL pack = £46.63.

STAVUDINE
(d4T)

Indications: progressive or advanced HIV infection, see notes above

Cautions: history of peripheral neuropathy (see below); history of pancreatitis or concomitant use with other drugs associated with pancreatitis; renal impairment (see Appendix 3); pregnancy; monitor liver enzymes (reduce dose if significant elevation); **interactions:** Appendix 1 (stavudine)

PERIPHERAL NEUROPATHY. Suspend if peripheral neuropathy develops—characterised by persistent numbness, tingling or pain in feet or hands; if symptoms resolve satisfactorily on withdrawl, resume treatment at half previous dose

LIVER ENZYMES. If liver enzymes raised significantly, manage as for peripheral neuropathy, above

Contra-indications: breast-feeding

Side-effects: peripharal neuropathy (dose-related, see above); pancreatitis; nausea, vomiting, diarrhoea, constipation, anorexia, abdominal discomfort; chest pain; dyspnoea; headache, dizziness, insomnia, mood changes; asthenia, musculoskeletal pain; influenza-like symptoms, rash and other allergic reactions; lymphadenopathy; neoplasms; elevated liver enzymes (see above) and serum amylase; neutropenia, thrombocytopenia

Dose: ADULT under 60 kg, 30 mg every 12 hours preferably at least 1 hour before food; 60 kg and over, 40 mg every 12 hours; CHILD over 3 months, under 30 kg, 1 mg/kg every 12 hours; 30 kg and over, adult dose

---

▼ PoM **Zerit®** (Bristol-Myers)

Capsules, stavudine 15 mg (yellow/red), net price 56-cap pack = £153.87; 20 mg (brown), 56-cap pack = £159.19; 30 mg (light orange/dark orange), 56-cap pack = £166.94; 40 mg (dark orange), 56-cap pack = £171.98 (all hosp. only)

Oral solution, cherry-flavoured, stavudine for reconstitution with water, 1 mg/mL, net price 200 mL = £24.35

ZALCITABINE
(ddC, DDC)

Indications: advanced HIV infection in adults intolerant of zidovudine (low haemoglobin concentration, symptomatic anaemia or low neutrophil count) or in whom zidovudine has failed (clinical deterioration, rapidly worsening immunological status), see also notes above

Cautions: patients at risk of developing peripheral neuropathy (see below); pancreatitis (see also below)—monitor serum amylase in those with history of elevated serum amylase, pancreatitis, alcohol abuse, or receiving parenteral nutrition; cardiomyopathy, history of congestive cardiac failure; hepatotoxicity (see below); pregnancy (women of childbearing age should use effective contraception during treatment); renal impairment; **interactions:** Appendix 1 (zalcitabine)

PERIPHERAL NEUROPATHY. Discontinue immediately if peripheral neuropathy develops—characterised by numbness and burning dysaesthesia possibly followed by sharp shooting pains or severe continuous burning and potentially irreversible pain; extreme caution and close monitoring required in those at risk of peripheral neuropathy (especially those with low CD4 cell count for whom risk is greater)

PANCREATITIS. Discontinue permanently if clinical pancreatitis develops; suspend if raised serum amylase associated with dysglycaemia, rising triglyceride, decreasing serum calcium or other signs of impending pancreatitis until pancreatitis excluded; suspend if treatment required with another drug known to cause pancreatic toxicity (e.g. intravenous pentamidine isethionate); caution and close monitoring if history of pancreatitis (or of elevated serum amylase) or if risk of pancreatitis

HEPATOTOXICITY. Potentially life-threatening lactic acidosis and severe hepatomegaly with steatosis reported therefore caution in liver disease, liver enzyme abnormalities, or history of alcohol abuse or hepatitis; suspend or discontinue if deterioration in liver function tests, hepatic steatosis, progressive hepatomegaly or unexplained lactic acidosis

Contra-indications: peripheral neuropathy (see also above); breast-feeding

Side-effects: peripheral neuropathy (discontinue immediately, see also above); oral ulcers, nausea, vomiting, dysphagia, anorexia, diarrhoea, abdominal pain, constipation; pharyngitis; headache, dizziness; myalgia, arthralgia; rash, pruritus, sweating, weight loss, fatigue, fever, rigors, chest pain, anaemia, leucopenia, neutropenia, thrombocytopenia, disorders of liver function; less frequently pancreatitis (see also above), oesophageal ulcers (suspend treatment if no response to treatment for specific organisms); jaundice and hepatocellular damage (see also under Cautions); other less frequent side-effects include taste disturbances, tachycardia, cardiomyopathy, dyspnoea, asthenia, tremor, movement disorders, mood changes, hearing and visual disturbances, alopecia, hyperuricaemia and renal disorders

Dose: 750 micrograms every 8 hours; CHILD under 13 years safety and efficacy not established

▼ PoM **Hivid®** (Roche)

Tablets, both f/c, zalcitabine 375 micrograms (beige), net price 100-tab pack = £104.20; 750 micrograms (grey), 100-tab pack = £158.71

ZIDOVUDINE
(Azidothymidine, AZT)

Note. The abbreviation AZT which has sometimes been used for zidovudine has also been used for another drug

Indications: management of advanced human immunodeficiency virus (HIV) disease such as acquired immunodeficiency syndrome (AIDS) or AIDS-related complex; early symptomatic or asymptomatic HIV infection with markers indicating risk of disease progression (see also notes above); symptomatic or asymptomatic HIV-infected children with markers indicating significant immune suppression; consider for prevention of maternal-fetal HIV transmission (by treating pregnant women and their newborn infants)

Cautions: haematological toxicity (blood tests at least every 2 weeks for first 3 months then at least once a month, early disease with good bone marrow reserves may require less frequent tests e.g. every 1–3 months); vitamin B_{12} deficiency (increased risk of neutropenia); reduce dose or interrupt treatment according to data sheet if anaemia or myelosuppression; renal impairment; hepatic impairment, monitor closely patients at risk of liver disease (especially obese women) including those with hepatomegaly and hepatitis; risk of lactic acidosis, see Side-effects; elderly; pregnancy; breast-feeding not recommended during treatment; **interactions:** Appendix 1 (zidovudine)

Contra-indications: abnormally low neutrophil counts or haemoglobin values (see data sheet); neonates with hyperbilirubinaemia requiring treatment other than phototherapy, or with raised transaminase (see data sheet)

Side-effects: anaemia (may require transfusion), neutropenia, and leucopenia (all more frequent with high dose and advanced disease); also include, nausea and vomiting, anorexia, abdominal pain, dyspepsia, headache, rash, fever, myalgia, paraesthesia, neuropathy, insomnia, malaise, and asthenia; also reported, convulsions (and other cerebral effects), myopathy, pigmentation of nail, skin and oral mucosa, pancytopenia (with bone marrow hypoplasia and rarely thrombocytopenia), liver disorders including fatty change and raised bilirubin and liver enzymes (suspend treatment if progressive hepatomegaly or rapidly elevating plasma aminotransferase), lactic acidosis (with tachypnoea, dyspnoea, and reduced plasma bicarbonate—suspend treatment)

Dose: by mouth, various dosages *including* 500–600 mg daily in 2–5 divided doses *or* 1 g daily in 2 divided doses; CHILD over 3 months 120–180 mg/m² every 6 hours (max. 200 mg every 6 hours)

Prevention of maternal-fetal HIV transmission, women over 14 weeks gestation, *by mouth,* 100 mg 5 times daily until beginning of labour *then* during labour and delivery, *by intravenous infusion* initially 2 mg/kg over 1 hour *then* 1 mg/kg/hour until umbilical cord clamped (for planned caesarean section, start intravenous infusion 4 hours before operation); newborn INFANT starting within 12 hours of birth, *by mouth,* 2 mg/kg every 6 hours continued until 6 weeks old (or if unable to take by mouth, *by intravenous infusion* over 30 minutes, 1.5 mg/kg every 6 hours)

Patients temporarily unable to take zidovudine by mouth, *by intravenous infusion* over 1 hour, 1–2 mg/kg every 4 hours (approximating to 1.5–3 mg/kg every 4 hours by mouth) usually for not more than 2 weeks

PoM **Retrovir**® (GlaxoWellcome)
Capsules, zidovudine 100 mg (white/blue band), net price 100 = £124.95; 250 mg (blue/white/dark blue band), 40-cap pack = £124.95
Tablets, zidovudine 300 mg, net price 60 = £224.90
Syrup, zidovudine 50 mg/5 mL. Net price 200-mL pack with 10-mL oral syringe = £24.99
Injection, zidovudine 10 mg/mL. For dilution and use as an intravenous infusion. Net price 20-mL vial = £12.54

PROTEASE INHIBITORS

INDINAVIR

Indications: progressive or advanced HIV infection, in combination with nucleoside analogues
Cautions: hepatic impairment (see Appendix 2); ensure adequate hydration to reduce risk of nephrolithiasis; haemophilia (possible increased bleeding); pregnancy; metabolism of many drugs inhibited if administered concomitantly, **interactions:** Appendix 1 (indinavir)
Contra-indications: breast-feeding
Side-effects: nausea, vomiting, diarrhoea, abdominal discomfort, dry mouth, taste disturbances; headache, dizziness, insomnia; myalgia, asthenia, paraesthesia; rash, pruritus, dry skin, hyperpigmentation; nephrolithiasis (may require interruption or discontinuation), dysuria, haematuria, crystalluria, proteinuria; elevated liver enzymes and bilirubin, hepatitis; blood disorders including neutropenia, haemolytic anaemia; increased blood glucose
Dose: 800 mg every 8 hours (600 mg every 8 hours if receiving concurrent ketoconazole *or* in hepatic impairment), CHILD safety and efficacy not established

▼ PoM **Crixivan**® (MSD)
Capsules, indinavir (as sulphate), 200 mg net price 360-cap pack = £242.40; 400 mg 180-cap pack = £242.40. Counselling, administration
COUNSELLING. Administer 1 hour before or 2 hours after a meal; may be administered with a low-fat, light meal; in combination with didanosine, allow 1 hour between each drug (antacids in didanosine tablets reduce absorption of indinavir)
Note. Containers include desiccant canisters

RITONAVIR

Indications: progressive or advanced HIV infection, in combination with nucleoside analogues
Cautions: hepatic impairment; haemophilia (possible increased bleeding); pregnancy; metabolism of many drugs inhibited and toxicity increased if administered concomitantly, **interactions:** Appendix 1 (ritonavir)
Contra-indications: severe hepatic impairment; breast-feeding
Side-effects: nausea, vomiting, diarrhoea (may impair absorption—close monitoring required), abdominal pain, taste disturbances, dyspepsia, anorexia, throat irritation; vasodilatation; headache, circumoral and peripheral paraesthesia, hyperaesthesia, dizziness, sleep disturbances, asthenia, rash, leucopenia; raised liver enzymes, bilirubin, triglycerides, cholesterol, lipids and uric acid; occasionally flatulence, eructation, dry mouth and ulceration, cough, anxiety, fever, pain, myalgia, weight loss, decreased thyroxine, sweating, pruritus, electrolyte disturbances, increased blood glucose, anaemia, neutropenia, increased prothrombin time
Dose: 600 mg every 12 hours, CHILD under 12 years, safety and efficacy not established

▼ PoM **Norvir**® (Abbott)
Capsules, ritonavir 100 mg. Net price 336-cap pack = £337.39. Label: 21
Oral solution, sugar-free, ritonavir 400 mg/5 mL. Net price 5 x 90-mL packs (with measuring cup) = £403.20. Label: 21, counselling, administration
COUNSELLING. Oral solution contains 43% alcohol; bitter taste can be masked by mixing with chocolate milk; do not mix with water, measuring cup must be dry

SAQUINAVIR

Indications: progressive or advanced HIV infection, in combination with nucleoside analogues
Cautions: severe hepatic or renal impairment; haemophilia (possible increased bleeding); pregnancy; **interactions:** Appendix 1 (saquinavir)
Contra-indications: breast-feeding
Side-effects: diarrhoea, buccal and mucosal ulceration, abdominal discomfort, nausea; headache, peripheral neuropathy, asthenia; rash and other skin eruptions, rarely Stevens-Johnson syndrome; other rare side-effects include thrombocytopenia and other blood disorders, seizures, liver damage, pancreatitis and nephrolithiasis; reports of elevated creatine phosphokinase, increased or decreased blood glucose, raised liver enzymes and neutropenia when used in combination therapy

---

Dose: 600 mg every 8 hours (within 2 hours after a meal); CHILD under 16 years, safety and efficacy not established

▼ PoM **Invirase**® (Roche)
Capsules, brown/green, saquinavir (as mesylate) 200 mg. Net price 270-cap pack = £302.86. Label: 21

CYTOMEGALOVIRUS (CMV)

Ganciclovir is related to aciclovir but is more active against cytomegalovirus; it is also much more toxic than aciclovir. It should therefore only be prescribed when the potential benefit outweighs the risks. It is administered by intravenous infusion. Capsules are available for *maintenance treatment* of CMV retinitis in AIDS patients following intravenous therapy if the condition is stable. Ganciclovir causes profound myelosuppression when given with zidovudine; the two should not normally be given together particularly during initial ganciclovir therapy.

Foscarnet is also active against cytomegalovirus; it is toxic and can cause renal impairment in up to 50% of patients.

Cidofovir is a DNA polymerase chain inhibitor which is given for CMV retinitis in AIDS patients when ganciclovir and foscarnet are contra-indicated; it is given in combination with probenecid. It is nephrotoxic.

CIDOFOVIR

Indications: cytomegalovirus retinitis in AIDS patients for whom other drugs are inappropriate

Cautions: monitor renal function (serum creatinine and urinary protein) and neutrophil count within 24 hours before each dose; pretreatment with probenecid and prior hydration with intravenous fluids necessary to minimise potential nephrotoxicity (see below); diabetes mellitus (increased risk of ocular hypotony); hepatic impairment

NEPHROTOXICITY. Do not initiate treatment in renal impairment (assess creatinine clearance and proteinuria—consult product literature); discontinue treatment and hydrate with intravenous fluids if deterioration of renal function occurs—consult product literature

Contra-indications: renal impairment (creatinine clearance 55 mL/minute or less); concomitant administration of potentially nephrotoxic drugs; pregnancy (avoid pregnancy during and after treatment, men should not father a child during or within 3 months of treatment), breast-feeding

Side-effects: dose-dependent nephrotoxicity (see Cautions above); neutropenia, fever, asthenia, alopecia, nausea, decreased intraocular pressure; for side-effects related to probenecid see section 10.1.4

Dose: by *intravenous infusion* over 1 hour, initial (induction) treatment, 5 mg/kg once weekly for 2 weeks (give probenecid and intravenous fluids with each dose, see below); CHILD not recommended

Maintenance treatment, beginning 2 weeks after completion of induction, *by intravenous infusion* over 1 hour, 5 mg/kg once every 2 weeks (give probenecid and intravenous fluids with each dose, see below)

PROBENECID CO-TREATMENT, *by mouth* (preferably after food), probenecid 2 g 3 hours before cidofovir infusion followed by probenecid 1 g at 2 hours and 1 g at 8 hours after the end of cidofovir infusion (total probenecid 4 g); for cautions, contra-indications and side-effects of probenecid see section 10.1.4

PRIOR HYDRATION, sodium chloride 0.9%, *by intravenous infusion,* at least 1 litre over 1 hour immediately before cidofovir infusion (an additional 1 litre may be given over 1–3 hours, starting at the same time as the cidofovir infusion, if tolerated)

▼ PoM **Vistide**® (Pharmacia & Upjohn)
Intravenous infusion, cidofovir 75 mg/mL, net price 5-mL vial = £570.00
CAUTION IN HANDLING. Wear gloves and safety glasses and prepare infusion in a laminar flow biological safety cabinet; if solution comes into contact with skin or mucosa immediately wash with water

GANCICLOVIR

Indications: life-threatening or sight-threatening cytomegalovirus infections in immunocompromised patients only; prevention of cytomegalovirus disease during immunosuppressive therapy following organ transplantation

Cautions: close monitoring of blood counts (see product literature); history of cytopenia; low platelet count; concomitant use of myelosuppressants or drugs which inhibit rapid cell replication; potential carcinogen and teratogen; renal impairment; ensure adequate hydration during administration; vesicant—infuse into vein with adequate flow preferably via a plastic cannula; limited experience in children (possible risk of long-term carcinogenic or reproductive toxicity—not for neonatal or congenital cytomegalovirus disease); **interactions:** see notes above and Appendix 1 (ganciclovir)

Contra-indications: pregnancy (includes effective contraception during treatment and barrier contraception for men during and for 90 days after treatment); breast-feeding (until 72 hours after last dose); hypersensitivity to ganciclovir or aciclovir; abnormally low neutrophil or platelet counts (see product literature)

Side-effects: most frequent, leucopenia and thrombocytopenia; less frequent, anaemia, pancytopenia, fever, rash, abnormal liver function tests; also chills, oedema, infections, malaise; nausea, vomiting, mouth ulcers, dyspepsia, dysphagia, diarrhoea, anorexia, gastro-intestinal haemorrhage, abdominal pain; chest pain, arrhythmias, hypertension, hypotension, deep thrombophlebitis, migraine, vasodilation; dyspnoea; psychosis, confusion, mood disturbances, nervousness, dry mouth, drowsiness, dizziness, abnormal gait, ataxia, paraesthesia, tremor, headache, coma; eosinphilia; decrease in blood glucose; haematuria, raised serum creatinine and blood urea nitrogen; breast pain, urinary frequency, urinary-tract infection, aspermatogenesis; myasthenia, myalgia; disturbances in taste and vision, eye pain, deafness; retinal detachment in AIDS patients with retinitis; alopecia, acne, sweating, rash, pruritus, urticaria; local inflammation, pain and phlebitis at injection site

Dose: *by intravenous infusion* over 1 hour, initial (induction) treatment, 5 mg/kg every 12 hours for 14–21 days for treatment or for 7–14 days for prevention; maintenance (for patients at risk of relapse of retinitis) 6 mg/kg daily on 5 days per week *or* 5 mg/kg daily every day; if retinitis progresses initial induction treatment may be repeated

Maintenance treatment in AIDS patients where retinitis stable (following at least 3 weeks of intravenous ganciclovir), *by mouth*, 1 g 3 times daily with food *or* 500 mg 6 times daily with food

In renal impairment, consult product literature

PoM **Cymevene**® (Roche)

Capsules, green, ganciclovir 250 mg, net price 84-cap pack = £265.65. Label: 21

Intravenous infusion, powder for reconstitution, ganciclovir (as sodium salt). Net price 500-mg vial = £35.58

Electrolytes: Na⁺ 2 mmol/500-mg vial

CAUTION IN HANDLING. Wear gloves and safety glasses when reconstituting; if solution contacts skin or mucosa immediately wash with soap and water

FOSCARNET SODIUM

Indications: cytomegalovirus retinitis in AIDS patients; mucocutaneous herpes simplex virus infections unresponsive to aciclovir in immunocompromised patients

Cautions: renal impairment (reduce dose or avoid if severe); monitor electrolytes, particularly calcium and magnesium; monitor serum creatinine every second day during induction and every week during maintenance; ensure adequate hydration; avoid rapid infusion

Contra-indications: pregnancy, breast-feeding

Side-effects: nausea, vomiting, diarrhoea (occasionally constipation and dyspepsia), abdominal pain, anorexia; changes in blood pressure and ECG; headache, fatigue, mood disturbances (including psychosis), asthenia, paraesthesia, convulsions, tremor, dizziness, and other neurological disorders; rash; impairment of renal function including acute renal failure; hypocalcaemia (sometimes symptomatic) and other electrolyte disturbances; abnormal liver function tests; decreased haemoglobin concentration, leucopenia, granulocytopenia, thrombocytopenia; thrombophlebitis if given undiluted by peripheral vein; genital irritation and ulceration (due to high concentrations excreted in urine); isolated reports of pancreatitis

Dose: CMV retinitis induction, *by intravenous infusion*, 60 mg/kg every 8 hours for 2–3 weeks then maintenance, 60 mg/kg daily, increased to 90–120 mg/kg if tolerated; if retinitis progresses on maintenance dose, repeat induction regimen

Mucocutaneous herpes simplex infection, *by intravenous infusion*, 40 mg/kg every 8 hours for 2–3 weeks or until lesions heal

PoM **Foscavir**® (Astra)

Intravenous infusion, foscarnet sodium hexahydrate 24 mg/mL, net price 250-mL bottle = £31.35, 500-mL bottle = £52.24

RESPIRATORY SYNCYTIAL VIRUS

Tribavirin inhibits a wide range of DNA and RNA viruses. It is given by inhalation for the treatment of severe bronchiolitis caused by the respiratory syncytial virus in infants, especially when they have other serious diseases. It is also effective in Lassa fever.

TRIBAVIRIN
(Ribavirin)

Indications: severe respiratory syncytial virus bronchiolitis in infants and children

Cautions: maintain standard supportive respiratory and fluid management therapy; monitor electrolytes closely; monitor equipment for precipitation; pregnant women (and those planning pregnancy) should avoid exposure to aerosol

Contra-indications: pregnancy

Side-effects: reticulocytosis, anaemia; also worsening respiration, bacterial pneumonia, and pneumothorax reported

Dose: *by aerosol inhalation or nebulisation* (via small particle aerosol generator) of solution containing 20 mg/mL, for 12–18 hours for at least 3 days; max. 7 days

PoM **Virazid**® (ICN)

Inhalation, tribavirin 6 g for reconstitution with 300 mL water for injections. Net price 3 × 6-g vials = £739.60

5.4   Antiprotozoal drugs

5.4.1	Antimalarials
5.4.2	Amoebicides
5.4.3	Trichomonacides
5.4.4	Antigiardial drugs
5.4.5	Leishmaniacides
5.4.6	Trypanocides
5.4.7	Drugs for toxoplasmosis
5.4.8	Drugs for pneumocystis pneumonia

Advice on specific problems available from:

Malaria Reference	
Laboratory	0171-927 2437 (prophylaxis only)
Birmingham	0121-766 6611
Glasgow	0141-946 7120
Liverpool	0151-708 9393
London	0171-530 3500 (treatment)
	0171-388 9600 (travel prophylaxis)
	0181-200 6868 extn 3421 (travel prophylaxis)
Oxford	(01865) 225217
Recorded advice	
for Travellers	0891 600350
(49p/minute standard rate, 39p/minute cheap rate)	

5.4.1   Antimalarials

Recommendations on the prophylaxis and treatment of malaria reflect guidelines agreed by UK malaria specialists.

The centres listed above should be consulted for advice on special problems.

TREATMENT OF MALARIA

If the infective species is **not known**, or if the infection is **mixed**, initial treatment should be with quinine or mefloquine (or rarely with halofantrine) as for *falciparum malaria*.

FALCIPARUM MALARIA (TREATMENT)

Falciparum malaria (malignant malaria) is caused by *Plasmodium falciparum*. In most parts of the world *P. falciparum* is now resistant to chloroquine which should not therefore be given for treatment[1].

Quinine, **mefloquine**, *Malarone*® or **halofantrine** can be given *by mouth* if the patient can swallow tablets and there are no serious manifestations (e.g. impaired consciousness); quinine should be given *by intravenous infusion* (see below) if the patient is seriously ill or unable to take tablets.

Oral. The adult dosage regimen for **quinine** *by mouth* is:

600 mg (of quinine salt[2]) every 8 hours for 7 days *and* (if quinine resistance known or suspected) *followed by*

either Fansidar® 3 tablets as a single dose

or (if *Fansidar*®-resistant) **doxycycline** 200 mg daily for at least 7 days.

Alternatively **mefloquine**, *Malarone*® or **halofantrine** (**important:** see warnings on p. 287) may be given instead of quinine but resistance has been reported in several countries. It is not necessary to give *Fansidar*® or doxycycline after mefloquine or halofantrine treatment.

---

1. For chloroquine-sensitive strains of falciparum malaria chloroquine *by mouth* is effective in the dosage schedule outlined under benign malarias but it should **not** be used unless there is an **unambiguous exposure history** in one of the few remaining areas of chloroquine sensitivity.

If the patient with a *chloroquine-sensitive infection* is seriously ill, chloroquine is given *by continuous intravenous infusion*. The dosage (for adults and children) is chloroquine 10 mg/kg (of base) infused over 8 hours, followed by three 8-hour infusions of 5 mg/kg (of base) each. *Oral therapy* is started as soon as possible to complete the course; the total cumulative dose for the course should be 25 mg/kg of base.

2. Valid for quinine hydrochloride, dihydrochloride, and sulphate; not valid for quinine bisulphate which contains a correspondingly smaller amount of quinine.

3. In intensive care units the loading dose can alternatively be given as quinine salt[2] 7 mg/kg infused over 30 minutes followed immediately by 10 mg/kg over 4 hours then (after 8 hours) maintenance dose as described.

4. **Important:** the loading dose of 20 mg/kg should **not** be used if the patient has received quinine (or quinidine) or mefloquine during the previous 24 hours—**for additional warnings** relating to halofantrine, see p. 287

5. Maintenance dose should be reduced to 5–7 mg/kg of salt if parenteral treatment is required for more than 48 hours.

The adult dosage regimen for **mefloquine** *by mouth* is:

20–25 mg/kg (of mefloquine base) as a single dose (up to maximum 1.5 g) *or preferably* as 2–3 divided doses 6–8 hours apart.

Malarone® (atovaquone and proguanil hydrochloride) has been introduced recently; the adult dose *by mouth* is:

4 tablets once daily for 3 days.

Halofantrine is now rarely used (see warnings on p. 287) the adult dosage regimen *by mouth* is:

1.5 g of halofantrine hydrochloride divided into three doses of 500 mg given at intervals of 6 hours (on an empty stomach); this course should be repeated after an interval of 1 week.

Parenteral. If the patient is seriously ill, **quinine** should be given *by intravenous infusion*. The adult dosage regimen for quinine *by infusion* is:

loading dose[3] of 20 mg/kg[4] (up to maximum 1.4 g) of quinine salt[2] infused over 4 hours *then after 8–12 hours* maintenance dose of 10 mg/kg[5] (up to maximum 700 mg) of quinine salt[2] infused over 4 hours every 8–12 hours (until patient can swallow tablets to complete the 7-day course) *either followed by Fansidar*® *or* doxycycline as above. Alternatively, after at least 2–3 days' treatment with a parenteral quinine salt, treatment may be completed with mefloquine by mouth started at least 12 hours after parenteral quinine salt has been administered.

CHILDREN.

Oral. **Quinine** is well tolerated by children although the salts are bitter. The dosage regimen for quinine *by mouth* for children is:

10 mg/kg (of quinine salt[2]) every 8 hours for 7 days *then* (if quinine resistance known or suspected)

Fansidar® as a single dose: up to 4 years ½ tablet, 5–6 years 1 tablet, 7–9 years 1½ tablets, 10–14 years 2 tablets.

Alternatively **mefloquine** or *Malarone*® (or **halofantrine** but now rarely used—see warnings on p. 287) may be given instead of quinine; it is not necessary to give *Fansidar*® after mefloquine or halofantrine treatment. The dosage regimen for mefloquine *by mouth* for children is calculated on a mg/kg basis as for adults (see above). The dosage regimen for *Malarone*® *by mouth* for children over 40 kg is the same as for adults (see above); the dosage regimen for *Malarone*® for smaller children is reduced as follows:

weight under 11 kg, no suitable dose form

weight 11–20 kg, 1 tablet daily for 3 days

weight 21–30 kg, 2 tablets daily for 3 days

weight 31–40kg, 3 tablets daily for 3 days.

The dosage regimen for halofantrine *by mouth* (**important:** see warnings on p. 287) for children over 37 kg is the same as for adults (see above); the dosage regimen for halofantrine for smaller children is reduced as follows:

weight under 23 kg, no suitable dose form;

weight 23–31 kg, 3 doses of 250 mg at intervals of 6 hours;

weight 32–37 kg, 3 doses of 375 mg at intervals of 6 hours.

This course of halofantrine should be repeated after an interval of 1 week.

Parenteral. The dosage regimen for quinine *by intravenous infusion* for children is calculated on a mg/kg basis as for adults (see above).

PREGNANCY. Falciparum malaria is particularly dangerous in pregnancy, especially in the last trimester. The adult treatment doses of oral and intravenous quinine given above (including the loading dose) can safely be given to pregnant women. Halofantrine is contra-indicated in pregnancy and doxycycline should be avoided (causes dental discoloration); *Fansidar*® and mefloquine are also best avoided until more information is available.

BENIGN MALARIAS (TREATMENT)

Benign malaria is usually caused by *Plasmodium vivax* and less commonly by *P. ovale* and *P. malariae*. **Chloroquine**[6] is the drug of choice for the treatment of benign malarias (but chloroquine-resistant *P. vivax* infection has been reported from New Guinea and some adjacent islands).

The adult dosage regimen for **chloroquine** *by mouth* is:

initial dose of 600 mg (of base) *then*

a single dose of 300 mg after 6 to 8 hours *then*

a single dose of 300 mg daily for 2 days

(approximate total cumulative dose of 25 mg/kg of base)

Chloroquine alone is adequate for *P. malariae* infections but in the case of *P. vivax* and *P. ovale*, a *radical cure* (to destroy parasites in the liver and thus prevent relapses) is required. This is achieved with **primaquine**[7] in an adult dosage of 15 mg daily for 14 to 21 days given after the chloroquine; a 21-day (or even longer) course may be needed for Chesson-type strains of *P. vivax* from south-east Asia and western Pacific.

---

6. Mefloquine is also active in benign malarias (but is not required since chloroquine is usually effective); Halofantrine is active against *P. vivax* but is not generally used; as with chloroquine a radical cure is required for *P. vivax* and *P. ovale* infections.

7. Before starting primaquine blood should be tested for glucose-6-phosphate dehydrogenase (G6PD) activity since the drug can cause haemolysis in G6PD-deficient patients. In G6PD deficiency primaquine, in a dose for adults of 30 mg once a week (children 500–750 micrograms/kg once a week) for 8 weeks, has been found useful and without undue harmful effects.

CHILDREN. The dosage regimen of chloroquine for benign malaria in children is:

initial dose of 10 mg/kg (of base) *then*

a single dose of 5 mg/kg after 6–8 hours *then*

a single dose of 5 mg/kg daily for 2 days

For a *radical cure* children are then given primaquine[7] in a dose of 250 micrograms/kg daily.

PREGNANCY. The adult treatment doses of chloroquine can be given for benign malaria. In the case of *P. vivax* or *P. ovale*, however, the radical cure with primaquine should be **postponed** until the pregnancy is over; instead chloroquine should be continued at a dose of 600 mg each week during the pregnancy.

PROPHYLAXIS AGAINST MALARIA

The recommendations on prophylaxis reflect guidelines agreed by UK malaria specialists; the advice is aimed at residents of the UK who travel to endemic areas for short stays. The choice of drug (see next page) takes account of:

risk of exposure to malaria;

extent of drug resistance;

efficacy of the recommended drugs;

side-effects of the drugs;

patient-related criteria (e.g. age, pregnancy, renal or hepatic impairment).

PROTECTION AGAINST BITES **Prophylaxis is relative and not absolute**, and breakthrough can occur with any of the drugs recommended. Personal protection against being bitten is very important. Mosquito nets impregnated with permethrin provide the most effective barrier protection against insects; coils, mats and vaporised insecticides are also useful. Diethyltoluamide (DEET) in lotions, sprays or roll-on formulations is safe and effective when applied to the skin but the protective effect only lasts for a few hours. Long sleeves and trousers worn after dusk also provide protection.

LENGTH OF PROPHYLAXIS. In order to determine tolerance and to establish habit, prophylaxis should be started one week (preferably 2–3 weeks in the case of mefloquine) before travel into an endemic area (or if not possible at earliest opportunity up to 1 or 2 days before travel); it should be continued for **at least 4 weeks after leaving**.

In those requiring long-term prophylaxis, chloroquine and proguanil may be used for periods of over 5 years. Mefloquine is licenced for up to 1 year (although it has been used for up to 2 years without undue problems). Specialist advice should be sought for long-term prophylaxis and especially for travel to areas where chloroquine, proguanil or mefloquine are inappropriate.

RETURN FROM MALARIAL REGION. It is important to be aware that **any illness** that occurs within 1 year and **especially within 3 months of return might be malaria** even if all recommended precautions against malaria were taken. Travellers should be **warned** of this and told that if they develop any ill-

---

ness **particularly within 3 months** of their return they should go **immediately** to a doctor and specifically mention their exposure to malaria.

CHILDREN. The following prophylactic doses are based on guidelines agreed by UK malaria experts and may differ from advice in data sheets. If in doubt telephone centres listed on p. 281.

		Fraction of adult dose	
Age	Weight (kg)	Chloroquine Proguanil	Maloprim®
0–5 weeks		⅛	—
6 weeks–11 months		¼	—
1–5 years	10–19	½	¼
6–11 years	20–39	¾	½
12 years	40	adult dose	adult dose

Note. Weight is a better guide than age for children over 6 months old. Specialist advice should be obtained for use of *Maloprim*® in children under 1 year of age.

For children's doses of mefloquine see p. 288.

Prophylaxis is required in **breast-fed infants**; although antimalarials are excreted in milk, the amounts are too variable to give reliable protection.

EPILEPSY. Both chloroquine and mefloquine are unsuitable for malaria prophylaxis in subjects with a history of epilepsy. In areas *without chloroquine resistance* proguanil 200 mg daily alone is recommended; in areas *with chloroquine resistance* doxycycline may be considered [unlicensed indication, specialist advice needed] but its metabolism may be influenced by antiepileptics (see **interactions:** Appendix 1 (tetracyclines). *Maloprim*® may be another alternative; it should be supplemented with folic acid (5 mg daily) in those taking phenytoin or phenobarbitone.

RENAL IMPAIRMENT. Avoidance (or dosage reduction) of proguanil is recommended since it is excreted by the kidneys. Chloroquine is only partially excreted by the kidneys and reduction of the dose for prophylaxis is not required except in severe impairment. Mefloquine is considered to be appropriate to use in renal impairment and does not require dosage reduction. Doxycycline is also considered to be appropriate [unlicensed indication, specialist advice needed].

PREGNANCY. Chloroquine and proguanil may be given in usual doses in areas where *P. falciparum* strains are sensitive; in the case of proguanil, folic acid 5 mg daily should be given. Mefloquine should be avoided in the first trimester (see p. 288). *Maloprim*® is also contra-indicated in the first trimester; folate supplements should be given if *Maloprim*® is prescribed in the second and third trimester. The centres listed on p. 281 should be consulted for advice on prophylaxis in resistant areas.

SPECIFIC RECOMMENDATIONS

Where a journey requires two regimens, the regimen for the higher risk area should be used for the whole journey. Those travelling to remote or little-visited areas may require expert advice.

> **Risk may vary in different parts of a country— check under all risk levels**

> WARNING. Settled immigrants (or long-term visitors) to the UK may be unaware that they will have **lost their immunity** and also that the areas where they previously lived **may now be malarious**

North Africa and the Middle East

VERY LOW RISK. Risk *very low* in Abu Dhabi, Algeria, tourist areas of Egypt, Libya, Morocco, Tunisia, most tourist areas of Turkey:

> no prophylaxis recommended but consider malaria if fever presents

LOW RISK. Risk *low* in southern border areas of Azerbaijan, Egypt (El Fayoum only, June–October), rural north Iraq (May–November), north border of Syria (May–October), Turkey (plain around Adana, Side, south-east Anatolia, March–November), south border areas of Tajikistan:

preferably

> chloroquine 300 mg (as base) once weekly

or
(if chloroquine not appropriate)

> proguanil hydrochloride 200 mg once daily

RISK. Risk *present* and *chloroquine resistance present* in Afghanistan (below 2000 m, May–November), Iran (March–November), Oman, Saudi Arabia (except Northern, Eastern and Central Provinces, Asir plateau, and western border cities where very little risk), northern rural United Arab Emirates, Yemen:

both

> chloroquine 300 mg (as base) once weekly

and

> proguanil hydrochloride 200 mg once daily

Sub-Saharan Africa

VERY HIGH RISK. Risk *very high* (or *locally very high*) and *chloroquine resistance very widespread* in Angola, Benin, Burkina Faso, Burundi, Cameroon, Central African Republic, Chad, Comoros,

Congo, Djibouti, Equatorial Guinea, Eritrea, Ethiopia, Gabon, Gambia[1], Ghana, Guinea, Guinea-Bissau, Ivory Coast, Kenya[1], Liberia, Madagascar, Malawi, Mali, Mozambique, Niger, Nigeria, Principe, Rwanda, São Tomé, Senegal, Sierra Leone, Somalia, Sudan, Swaziland, Tanzania[1], Togo, Uganda, Zaïre, Zambia, Zimbabwe (Zambezi valley, see also below):

preferably

mefloquine 250 mg once weekly

or
(if mefloquine not appropriate)

both
chloroquine 300 mg (as base) once weekly
and
proguanil hydrochloride 200 mg once daily

1. Visitors for periods of 2 weeks or less to tourist resorts of Gambia (between January and May), of coastal Kenya and coastal Tanzania can take chloroquine plus proguanil; however, mefloquine provides better protection and is recommended for longer visits, higher exposure risk (e.g. backpacking, staying in rural areas, safaris) and for Gambia between June and December

RISK. Risk *present* (in *parts of country*) and *some chloroquine resistance* in northern half of Botswana (November–June), Mauritania (all year in southern half; July–October in northern half), northern third of Namibia (November–June), north-east part of South Africa (low altitude areas of north and eastern Transvaal and eastern Natal to 100 kilometres north of Durban), areas below 1200 m in Zimbabwe (November–June; all year in Zambezi valley *where mefloquine preferable*).

preferably

both
chloroquine 300 mg (as base) once weekly
and
proguanil hydrochloride 200 mg once daily

or
(if chloroquine plus proguanil not appropriate)

mefloquine 250 mg once weekly

Note. In Zimbabwe and neighbouring countries, Maloprim® (also known as Deltaprim®) prophylaxis is used by local residents (sometimes with chloroquine).

No prophylaxis recommended for Cape Verde and non-rural areas of Mauritius (but consider malaria if fever presents); *chloroquine prophylaxis* appropriate for rural areas of **Mauritius**

South Asia

HIGH RISK. Risk *high* and *chloroquine resistance high* in Bangladesh (only in Chittagong Hill Tracts):

preferably

mefloquine 250 mg once weekly

or
(if mefloquine not appropriate)

both
chloroquine 300 mg (as base) once weekly
and
proguanil hydrochloride 200 mg once daily

VARIABLE RISK. Risk *variable* and *chloroquine resistance usually moderate* in Bangladesh (except in Chittagong Hill Tracts, see above; no risk in Dhaka city), southern districts of Bhutan, India (no risk in mountain states of north), Nepal (below 1300 m; no risk in Kathmandu), Pakistan (below 2000 m), Sri Lanka (no risk in and just south of Colombo):

both
chloroquine 300 mg (as base) once weekly
and
proguanil hydrochloride 200 mg once daily

South-East Asia

VERY LOW RISK. Risk *very low* in Bali, Brunei, main tourist areas of China (but *substantial risk* in Yunnan and Hainan, see below; *chloroquine prophylaxis* appropriate for other remote areas), Hong Kong, Malaysia (but *variable risk* in Sabah, and in deep forests, see below), Sarawak (but *variable risk* in deep forests, see below), Singapore (no risk), Thailand (Bangkok, main tourist centres and rural areas not near borders—**important:** regional risk exists, see under Low but significant risk, below):

no prophylaxis recommended but consider malaria if fever presents

VARIABLE RISK. Risk *variable* and *some chloroquine resistance* in Indonesia (very low risk in Bali and cities but *substantial risk* in Irian Jaya, see below), rural Philippines below 600 m (no risk in Cebu, Leyte, Bohol, Catanduanes), deep forests of peninsular Malaysia and Sarawak, Sabah:

both
chloroquine 300 mg (as base) once weekly
and
proguanil hydrochloride 200 mg once daily

SUBSTANTIAL RISK. Risk *substantial* and *drug resistance common* in Cambodia (**important:** specialist advice needed for western provinces, see below), China (Yunnan and Hainan; *chloroquine prophylaxis* appropriate for other remote areas), Irian Jaya, Laos, Myanmar (formerly Burma), Vietnam (no risk in cities, Red River delta area, coastal plain north of Nha Trang):

> mefloquine 250 mg once weekly

LOW BUT SIGNIFICANT RISK. Risk *low but significant* because *mefloquine resistance prevalent* in western provinces of Cambodia, borders of Thailand with Cambodia and Myanmar, and Ko Chang:

> doxycycline 100 mg once daily
> [unlicensed indication—specialist advice
> needed and not for longer than 3 months]

Oceania
RISK. Risk *high* and *chloroquine resistance high* in Papua New Guinea (below 1800 m), Solomon Islands, Vanuatu:

preferably

> doxycycline 100 mg once daily [unlicensed]

or

> mefloquine 250 mg once weekly

Latin America and Caribbean
VARIABLE TO LOW RISK. Risk *variable to low* in Argentina (small area in north-west only), rural Belize (except Belize district), rural Costa Rica (below 500 m), Dominican Republic, El Salvador, Guatemala (below 1500 m), Haiti, Honduras, some rural areas of Mexico (not regularly visited by tourists), Nicaragua, Panama (west of Panama Canal but *variable to high risk* east of Panama Canal, see below), rural Paraguay (October–May):

preferably

> chloroquine 300 mg (as base) once weekly

or
(if chloroquine not appropriate)

> proguanil hydrochloride 200 mg once daily

VARIABLE TO HIGH RISK. Risk *variable to high* and *chloroquine resistance present* in rural areas of Bolivia (below 2500 m), Ecuador (below 1500 m), Panama (east of Panama Canal), rural areas of Peru

(below 1500 m), rural areas of Venezuela (except on coast, Caracas free of malaria):

preferably

> **both**
> chloroquine 300 mg (as base) once weekly
> **and**
> proguanil hydrochloride 200 mg once daily

or
(if chloroquine plus proguanil not appropriate)

> mefloquine 250 mg once weekly

Note. Maloprim® plus chloroquine prophylaxis is also an alternative

---

HIGH RISK. Risk *high* and *marked chloroquine resistance* in Bolivia (Amazon basin area), Brazil (throughout 'Legal Amazon' area which includes the Amazon basin region, Mato Grosso and Maranhao only; elsewhere *very low risk*—no prophylaxis), Colombia (most areas below 800 m), French Guiana, all interior regions of Guyana, Surinam (except Paramaribo and coast), Venezuela (Amazon basin area):

preferably

> mefloquine 250 mg once weekly

or
(if mefloquine not appropriate)

> **both**
> chloroquine 300 mg (as base) once weekly
> **and**
> proguanil hydrochloride 200 mg once daily

STANDBY TREATMENT. Adults travelling for prolonged periods to areas of chloroquine-resistance who are unlikely to have easy access to medical care should carry a standby treatment course. Self-medication should be **avoided** if medical help is accessible; prophylaxis should be continued during and after the attack.

In order to avoid excessive self-medication, the traveller should be provided with **written instructions** that urgent medical attention should be sought if fever (38°C or more) develops 7 days (or more) after arriving in a malarious area and that self treatment is indicated if medical help is not immediately available or the condition is worsening.

In view of the continuing emergence of resistant strains and of the different regimens required for different areas expert advice should be sought on the best treatment course for an individual traveller.

CHLOROQUINE

Chloroquine is used for the *prophylaxis of malaria* in areas of the world where the *risk of chloroquine resistant falciparum malaria is still low*. It is also used with proguanil when chloroquine resistant falciparum malaria is present although this regimen may not be that of first choice (see specific recommendations by country, pp. 284–6). Chloroquine is also combined with *Maloprim*® in some areas.

Chloroquine is **no longer recommended** for the *treatment of falciparum malaria* owing to widespread resistance, nor is it recommended if the infective species is *not known* or if the infection is *mixed*; in these cases treatment should be with quinine, mefloquine or rarely halofantrine (for details, see pp. 282–3). It is still recommended for the *treatment of benign malarias* (for details, see p. 283).

CHLOROQUINE

Indications: chemoprophylaxis and treatment of malaria, see notes above; rheumatoid arthritis and lupus erythematosus—see section 10.1.3

Cautions: hepatic impairment, renal impairment (see notes above), pregnancy (but for malaria benefit outweighs risk, see Appendix 4, Antimalarials), may exacerbate psoriasis, neurological disorders (avoid for prophylaxis if history of epilepsy, see notes above), may aggravate myasthenia gravis, severe gastro-intestinal disorders, G6PD deficiency (see section 9.1.5); ophthalmic examination and long-term therapy, see under Chloroquine, section 10.1.3; avoid concurrent therapy with hepatotoxic drugs and with halofantrine (see CSM advice under Halofantrine)—other **interactions**: Appendix 1 (chloroquine)

Side-effects: gastro-intestinal disturbances, headache; also convulsions, visual disturbances, depigmentation or loss of hair, skin reactions (rashes, pruritus); rarely, bone-marrow suppression; other side-effects (not usually associated with malaria prophylaxis or treatment), see under Chloroquine, section 10.1.3; very toxic in **overdosage**—immediate advice from poisons centres essential (see also p. 22)

Dose: see notes above

COUNSELLING. Warn travellers about **importance** of avoiding mosquito bites, **importance** of taking prophylaxis regularly, and **importance** of immediate visit to doctor if ill within 1 year and **especially** within 3 months of return. For details, see notes above

PoM *Avloclor® (Zeneca)
Tablets, scored, chloroquine phosphate 250 mg (≡ chloroquine base 155 mg). Net price 20-tab pack = £1.11. Label: 5, counselling, prophylaxis, see above

* Can be sold to the public provided it is licensed and labelled for the prophylaxis of malaria

Nivaquine® (Rhône-Poulenc Rorer)
PoM* *Tablets,* f/c, yellow, chloroquine sulphate 200 mg (≡ chloroquine base 150 mg). Net price 28-tab pack = £1.22. Label: 5, counselling, prophylaxis, see above

PoM* *Syrup,* golden, chloroquine sulphate 68 mg/5 mL (≡ chloroquine base 50 mg/5 mL). Net price 100 mL = £2.56. Label: 5, counselling, prophylaxis, see above

* Can be sold to the public provided it is licensed and labelled for the prophylaxis of malaria

PoM *Injection,* chloroquine sulphate 54.5 mg/mL (≡ chloroquine base 40 mg/mL). Net price 5-mL amp = 69p

Halofantrine is not suitable for the *prophylaxis of malaria.*

Halofantrine is licensed for the *treatment of falciparum malaria* but is now rarely used—see warnings below (for details on the treatment of falciparum malaria, see pp. 282–3). It should not be used for the *treatment of benign malarias,* as chloroquine is usually effective. It should not be used where mefloquine has been used for prophylaxis.

HALOFANTRINE HYDROCHLORIDE

Indications: treatment of uncomplicated chloroquine-resistant falciparum malaria or of chloroquine-resistant vivax malaria, but see notes above

Cautions: no experience of use in cerebral or complicated malaria; cardiac disease (see below); **interactions:** see below and Appendix 1 (halofantrine)

ARRHYTHMIAS. Halofantrine prolongs QT interval and has a potential for inducing hazardous arrhythmias in susceptible individuals, especially if dose excessive or if taken with food (which enhances absorption). It should **not** be used for standby treatment. Recommendations of the **CSM** are that halofantrine:

should **not** be taken with meals;
should **not** be taken with other drugs which may induce arrhythmias (e.g. *chloroquine, mefloquine, quinine, tricyclic antidepressants, antipsychotics, certain antiarrhythmics* and *antihistamines such as astemizole and terfenadine*);
should **not** be taken with drugs causing electrolyte disturbances;
should **not** be administered to those with known prolongation of the QT interval;
should **not** be administered to those with any form of cardiac disease associated with QT interval prolongation or ventricular arrhythmias (e.g. coronary heart disease, cardiomyopathy, and congenital heart disease)

Contra-indications: cardiac disorders including family history of congenital QT interval prolongation (**important:** see also above); other conditions associated with prolonged QT interval (e.g. hypokalaemia, hypomagnesaemia or other electrolyte disorders, thiamine deficiency); unexpected syncopal attacks; pregnancy and breast-feeding (avoid during treatment)

Side-effects: diarrhoea, abdominal pain, nausea, vomiting; transient elevation of serum transaminases; pruritus, rash, intravascular haemolysis, and hypersensitivity reactions also reported; **important:** ventricular arrhythmias (see also above)

Dose: see notes above

PoM **Halfan**® (SK&F)
Tablets, scored, halofantrine hydrochloride 250 mg. Net price 12-tab pack = £13.96. Label: 23

Mefloquine is used for the *prophylaxis of malaria* in areas of the world where there is a *high risk of chloroquine-resistant falciparum malaria* (for details, see specific recommendations by country, pp. 284–6).

Mefloquine is used for the *treatment of falciparum malaria* (or if the infective species is *not known* or if the infection is *mixed*) (for details, see pp. 282–3). It is also effective for the *treatment of benign malarias*, but is not required as chloroquine is usually effective. Mefloquine should not be used for treatment if it has been used for prophylaxis.

MEFLOQUINE

Indications: chemoprophylaxis of malaria, treatment of uncomplicated falciparum malaria and chloroquine-resistant vivax malaria, see notes above

Cautions: exclude pregnancy before starting chemoprophylaxis (see also under Contra-indications); avoid for chemoprophylaxis in severe hepatic impairment; cardiac conduction disorders; epilepsy (avoid for prophylaxis); not recommended in infants under 3 months (5 kg); halofantrine must not be given with or after mefloquine (danger of fatal arrhythmias—see also under Halofantrine); other **interactions:** Appendix 1 (mefloquine)

DRIVING. Dizziness or a disturbed sense of balance may affect performance of skilled tasks (e.g. driving); effects may persist for up to 3 weeks

Contra-indications: chemoprophylaxis in first trimester of pregnancy (teratogenic in *animals*, **avoid** pregnancy **during** and for **3 months after**), breast-feeding, and history of neuropsychiatric disorders, including depression, or convulsions, or family history of epilepsy; hypersensitivity to quinine

Side-effects: nausea, vomiting, diarrhoea, abdominal pain; dizziness, loss of balance, headache, sleep disorders (insomnia, drowsiness, abnormal dreams); also neuropsychiatric reactions (including sensory and motor neuropathies, tremor, ataxia, anxiety, depression, panic attacks, agitation, hallucinations, overt psychosis, convulsions), tinnitus and vestibular disorders, visual disturbances, circulatory disorders (hypotension and hypertension), tachycardia, bradycardia, cardiac conduction disorders, muscle weakness, myalgia, arthralgia, rash, urticaria, pruritus, alopecia, disturbances in liver function tests, asthenia, malaise, fatigue, fever, loss of appetite, leucopenia or leucocytosis, thrombocytopenia; rarely Stevens-Johnson syndrome, AV block and encephalopathy

CSM recommendation. Patients should be informed about adverse reactions associated with mefloquine and advised that, if these occur, they should seek medical advice on alternative antimalarials before the next dose is due

Dose: chemoprophylaxis, starting 1–3 weeks before departure (see p. 283) and continued for 4 weeks after leaving malarious area, ADULT and CHILD over 45 kg 250 mg each week; CHILD 5–19 kg (3 months–5 years) quarter adult dose, 20–30 kg (6–8 years) half adult dose, 31–45 kg (9–14 years) three-quarters adult dose

LONG-TERM CHEMOPROPHYLAXIS. Mefloquine prophylaxis can be taken for up to 1 year

Treatment, see notes above

COUNSELLING. See CSM recommendation above. Also warn travellers about **importance** of avoiding mosquito bites, **importance** of taking prophylaxis regularly, and **importance** of immediate visit to doctor if ill within 1 year and **especially** within 3 months of return. For details, see notes above

PoM [1] **Lariam**® (Roche)

Tablets, scored, mefloquine (as hydrochloride) 250 mg. Net price 8-tab pack = £14.53. Label: 21, 25, 27, counselling, driving, prophylaxis, see above

1. Prescriptions may be referred to Health Authorities to investigate circumstances under which written since prescriptions for chemoprophylaxis of malaria may not be reimbursable

---

PRIMAQUINE

Primaquine is used to eliminate the liver stages of *P. vivax or P. ovale following chloroquine treatment* (for details, see p. 283).

PRIMAQUINE

Indications: adjunct in the treatment of *Plasmodium vivax* and *P. ovale* malaria (eradication of liver stages)

Cautions: G6PD deficiency (see notes above); systemic diseases associated with granulocytopenia (e.g. rheumatoid arthritis, lupus erythematosus); pregnancy and breast-feeding; **interactions:** Appendix 1 (primaquine)

Side-effects: nausea, vomiting, abdominal pain; less commonly methaemoglobinaemia, haemolytic anaemia especially in G6PD deficiency

Dose: see notes above

Primaquine (Non-proprietary)

Tablets, primaquine (as phosphate) 7.5 mg

Available from Durbin [unlicensed—special order]

PROGUANIL

Proguanil is used (usually *with chloroquine*, but occasionally *alone*) for the *prophylaxis of malaria*, (for details, see specific recommendations by country, see pp. 284–6).

Proguanil used alone is not suitable for the *treatment of malaria*; a combination of atovaquone and proguanil is, however, licensed for the treatment of acute uncomplicated falciparum malaria.

PROGUANIL HYDROCHLORIDE

Indications: chemoprophylaxis of malaria

Cautions: renal impairment (see notes under Prophylaxis against malaria and Appendix 3); pregnancy (folate supplements needed); **interactions:** Appendix 1 (proguanil)

Side-effects: mild gastric intolerance and diarrhoea; occasionally mouth ulcers and stomatitis; skin reaction and hair loss reported

Dose: see notes above

COUNSELLING. Warn travellers about **importance** of avoiding mosquito bites, **importance** of taking prophylaxis regularly, and **importance** of immediate visit to doctor if ill within 1 year and **especially** within 3 months of return. For details, see notes above

---

Paludrine® (Zeneca)
Tablets, scored, proguanil hydrochloride 100 mg.
Net price 98-tab pack = £7.43. Label: 21, counselling, prophylaxis, see above

PROGUANIL HYDROCHLORIDE WITH ATOVAQUONE
Indications: treatment of acute, uncomplicated falciparum malaria, particularly where resistance to other antimalarial drugs is suspected
Cautions: acute renal failure, diarrhoea or vomiting (reduced absorption of atovaquone), pregnancy; avoid breast-feeding; efficacy not evaluated in cerebral or complicated malaria (including hyperparasitaemia, pulmonary oedema or renal failure); **interactions:** see Appendix 1 (proguanil, atovaquone)
Side-effects: nausea, vomiting, diarrhoea, abdominal pain, anorexia; headache, cough, occasionally elevated liver enzymes
Dose: see under preparation

▼ PoM **Malarone®** (GlaxoWellcome)
Tablets, pink, f/c, proguanil hydrochloride 100 mg, atovaquone 250 mg. Net price 12-tab pack = £24.00. Label: 21
Dose: ADULT and CHILD over 40 kg, 4 tablets once daily for 3 days; CHILD 11–20 kg 1 tablet daily for 3 days; 21–30 kg 2 tablets once daily for 3 days; 31–40 kg 3 tablets once daily for 3 days

PYRIMETHAMINE

Pyrimethamine should not be used alone, but is used with sulfadoxine (in *Fansidar®*) and with dapsone (in *Maloprim®*).
Fansidar® is not recommended for the *prophylaxis of malaria*, but it is used in the treatment of *falciparum malaria* and can be used *with (or following) quinine.*
Maloprim® is used with *chloroquine* for the *prophylaxis of malaria* in certain areas where there is a *high risk of chloroquine-resistant falciparum malaria* (for details see specific recommendations by country, see pp. 284–6). *Maloprim®* is not suitable for the *treatment of malaria.*

PYRIMETHAMINE
Indications: malaria (but used only in combined preparations incorporating dapsone or sulfadoxine); toxoplasmosis [not licensed]—section 5.4.7
Cautions: hepatic or renal impairment, folate supplements in pregnancy, breast-feeding, blood counts required with prolonged treatment; **interactions:** Appendix 1 (pyrimethamine)
Side-effects: depression of haematopoiesis with high doses, rashes, insomnia
Dose: malaria, no dose stated because not recommended
Toxoplasmosis, section 5.4.7

PoM **Daraprim®** (GlaxoWellcome)
Tablets, scored, pyrimethamine 25 mg. Net price 30-tab pack = £2.22

PYRIMETHAMINE WITH SULFADOXINE
Indications: adjunct to quinine in treatment of *Plasmodium falciparum* malaria (see notes above); **not** recommended for prophylaxis
Cautions; Contra-indications; Side-effects: see under Pyrimethamine and under Co-trimoxazole (section 5.1.8); contra-indicated in sulphonamide allergy; pregnancy and breast-feeding (see Appendixes 4 and 5); severe side-effects on long-term use therefore not recommended for prophylaxis; pulmonary infiltrates (e.g. eosinophilic or allergic alveolitis) reported—discontinue if cough or shortness of breath
Dose: treatment, see notes above
Prophylaxis, not recommended by UK malaria experts

PoM **Fansidar®** (Roche)
Tablets, scored, pyrimethamine 25 mg, sulfadoxine 500 mg. Net price 10-tab pack = £2.77

PYRIMETHAMINE WITH DAPSONE
Indications: prophylaxis of *Plasmodium falciparum* malaria (limited use, see notes above)
Cautions; Contra-indications; Side-effects: see under Pyrimethamine and under Dapsone (section 5.1.10); contra-indicated in sulphonamide allergy; caution in G6PD deficiency (see section 9.1.5); pregnancy (see notes under Prophylaxis against Malaria and Appendix 4) and breast-feeding (see Appendix 5); side-effects including methaemoglobinaemia, thrombocytopenia, mononucleosis-like syndrome, psychosis, jaundice, pneumonia with eosinophilic pulmonary infiltration, and on prolonged treatment hypoalbuminaemia reported
Dose: malaria prophylaxis, see notes above
COUNSELLING. Warn travellers about **importance** of avoiding mosquito bites, **importance** of taking prophylaxis regularly, and **importance** of immediate visit to doctor if ill within 1 year and **especially** within 3 months of return. For details, see notes above

PoM **Maloprim®** (GlaxoWellcome)
Tablets, scored, pyrimethamine 12.5 mg, dapsone 100 mg. Net price 30-tab pack = £2.76. Counselling, prophylaxis, see above

QUININE

Quinine is not suitable for the *prophylaxis of malaria.*
Quinine is used for the *treatment of falciparum malaria* (or if the infective species is *not known* or if the infection is *mixed*) (for details see pp. 282–3).

QUININE
Indications: falciparum malaria; nocturnal leg cramps, see section 10.2.2
Cautions: atrial fibrillation, conduction defects, heart block, pregnancy (but appropriate for treatment of malaria); monitor blood glucose concentration during parenteral treatment; G6PD deficiency (see section 9.1.5); avoid concurrent administration with halofantrine (see CSM advice under Halofantrine), other **interactions:** Appendix 1 (quinine)

Contra-indications: haemoglobinuria, optic neuritis

Side-effects: cinchonism, including tinnitus, headache, hot and flushed skin, nausea, abdominal pain, rashes, visual disturbances (including temporary blindness), confusion; hypersensitivity reactions including angioedema, blood disorders (including thrombocytopenia and intravascular coagulation), and acute renal failure; hypoglycaemia (especially after parenteral administration); cardiovascular effects (see Cautions); very toxic in **overdosage**—immediate advice from poisons centres essential (see also p. 22)

Dose: see notes above

Note. Quinine (anhydrous base) 100 mg ≡ quinine bisulphate 169 mg ≡ quinine dihydrochloride 122 mg ≡ quinine hydrochloride 122 mg ≡ quinine sulphate 121 mg. Quinine bisulphate 300-mg tablets are available but provide smaller amounts of quinine than the dihydrochloride, hydrochloride, or sulphate

PoM **Quinine Sulphate** (Non-proprietary)
Tablets, coated, quinine sulphate 200 mg, net price 20 = 76p; 300 mg, 20 = 82p
Available from APS, Cox, CP, Hillcross, Kent

PoM **Quinine Dihydrochloride** (Non-proprietary)
Injection, quinine dihydrochloride 300 mg/mL. For dilution and use as an infusion. 1- and 2-mL amps
Available from Martindale (special order) or from specialist centres (see p. 281)
Note. Intravenous injection of quinine is so hazardous that it has been superseded by infusion

TETRACYCLINES

Doxycycline (section 5.1.3) is used for the *prophylaxis of malaria* [unlicensed indication—specialist advice needed] in areas of *widespread mefloquine and chloroquine resistance* and also as a second-line drug for those who are unable to take chloroquine or mefloquine (for details, see specific recommendations by country, pp. 284–6).

Doxycycline is also used as an *adjunct to quinine in the treatment of falciparum malaria* (for details see pp. 282–3).

5.4.2 Amoebicides

Metronidazole is the drug of choice for *acute invasive amoebic dysentery* since it is very effective against vegetative forms of *Entamoeba histolytica* in ulcers; it is given in an adult dose of 800 mg three times daily for 5 days. **Tinidazole** is also effective. Metronidazole and tinidazole are also active against amoebae which have migrated to the liver. Treatment with metronidazole (or tinidazole) is followed by a 10-day course of diloxanide furoate.

Diloxanide furoate is the drug of choice for asymptomatic patients with *E. histolytica* cysts in the faeces; metronidazole and tinidazole are relatively ineffective. Diloxanide furoate is relatively free from toxic effects and the usual course is of 10 days, given alone for chronic infections or following metronidazole or tinidazole treatment.

For *amoebic abscesses* of the liver **metronidazole** is effective in doses of 400 mg 3 times daily for 5–10 days; tinidazole is an alternative. The course may be repeated after 2 weeks if necessary. Aspiration of the abscess is indicated where it is suspected that it may rupture or where there is no improvement after 72 hours of metronidazole; the aspiration may need to be repeated. Aspiration aids penetration of metronidazole and, for abscesses with more than 100 mL of pus, if carried out in conjunction with drug therapy, may reduce the period of disability.

Rarely, where metronidazole and tinidazole appear to be ineffective, dehydroemetine may be used (but the risk of side-effects is much greater). Diloxanide furoate is not effective against hepatic amoebiasis, but a 10-day course should be given at the completion of metronidazole or tinidazole treatment to destroy any amoebae in the gut.

DILOXANIDE FUROATE
Indications: chronic amoebiasis—see notes
Side-effects: flatulence, vomiting, urticaria, pruritus
Dose: 500 mg every 8 hours for 10 days; CHILD 20 mg/kg daily in 3 divided doses.
See also notes above

PoM **Furamide®** (Knoll)
Tablets, scored, diloxanide furoate 500 mg, net price 15-tab pack = £1.92. Label: 9

METRONIDAZOLE
Indications: see under Dose below; anaerobic infections, section 5.1.11
Cautions; Side-effects: section 5.1.11
Dose: by mouth, invasive intestinal amoebiasis, 800 mg every 8 hours for 5 days; CHILD 1–3 years 200 mg every 8 hours; 3–7 years 200 mg every 6 hours; 7–10 years 400 mg every 8 hours
Extra-intestinal amoebiasis (including liver abscess) and symptomless amoebic cyst passers, 400–800 mg every 8 hours for 5–10 days; CHILD 1–3 years 100–200 mg every 8 hours; 3–7 years 100–200 mg every 6 hours; 7–10 years 200–400 mg every 8 hours
Urogenital trichomoniasis, 200 mg every 8 hours for 7 days *or* 400–500 mg every 12 hours for 7 days, *or* 800 mg in the morning and 1.2 g at night for 2 days, *or* 2 g as a single dose; CHILD 1–3 years 50 mg every 8 hours for 7 days; 3–7 years 100 mg every 12 hours; 7–10 years 100 mg every 8 hours
Giardiasis, 2 g daily for 3 days *or* 500 mg twice daily for 7–10 days; CHILD 1–3 years 500 mg daily for 3 days; 3–7 years 600–800 mg daily; 7–10 years 1 g daily

Preparations
Section 5.1.11

TINIDAZOLE
Indications: see under Dose below; anaerobic infections, section 5.1.11
Cautions; Side-effects: section 5.1.11

Dose: intestinal amoebiasis, 2 g daily for 2–3 days; CHILD 50–60 mg/kg daily for 3 days
Amoebic involvement of liver, 1.5–2 g daily for 3–5 days; CHILD 50–60 mg/kg daily for 5 days
Urogenital trichomoniasis and giardiasis, single 2-g dose (repeated once if necessary); CHILD single dose of 50–75 mg/kg

Preparations
Section 5.1.11

5.4.3 Trichomonacides

Metronidazole (section 5.4.2) is the treatment of choice for *Trichomonas vaginalis* infection.

If metronidazole is ineffective, **tinidazole** may be tried; it is usually given as a single 2-g dose, with food. A further 2-g dose may be given if there is no clinical improvement.

Alcohol should be avoided during treatment with both metronidazole and tinidazole.

5.4.4 Antigiardial drugs

Metronidazole (section 5.4.2) is the treatment of choice for *Giardia lamblia* infections, given by mouth in a dosage of 2 g daily for 3 days or 400 mg every 8 hours for 5 days.

Alternative treatments are **tinidazole** (section 5.4.2) 2 g as a single dose or **mepacrine hydrochloride** 100 mg every 8 hours for 5–7 days.

MEPACRINE HYDROCHLORIDE
Indications: giardiasis; discoid lupus erythematosus—section 10.1.3
Cautions: hepatic impairment, elderly, history of psychosis; avoid in psoriasis; **interactions:** Appendix 1 (mepacrine)
Side-effects: gastro-intestinal disturbances; dizziness, headache; with large doses nausea, vomiting and occasionally transient acute toxic psychosis and CNS stimulation; on prolonged treatment yellow discoloration of skin and urine, chronic dermatoses (including severe exfoliative dermatitis), hepatitis, aplastic anaemia; also reported blue/black discoloration of palate and nails and corneal deposits with visual disturbances
Dose: giardiasis, 100 mg every 8 hours for 5–7 days; CHILD 2 mg/kg every 8 hours

Mepacrine Hydrochloride
Tablets, mepacrine hydrochloride 100 mg. Label: 4, 9, 14, 21
Available from BCM Specials [unlicensed—special order]

5.4.5 Leishmaniacides

Cutaneous leishmaniasis frequently heals spontaneously but if skin lesions are extensive or unsightly, treatment is indicated, as it is in visceral leishmaniasis (kala-azar).

Sodium stibogluconate, an organic pentavalent antimony compound, is the treatment of choice for visceral leishmaniasis. The dose is 20 mg/kg daily (max. 850 mg) for at least 20 days by intramuscular or intravenous injection; the dosage varies with different geographical regions and expert advice should be obtained. Skin lesions are treated for 10 days.

Pentamidine isethionate (pentamidine isetionate) (section 5.4.8) has been used in antimony-resistant visceral leishmaniasis, but although the initial response is often good, the relapse rate is high; it is associated with serious side-effects. Other treatments include paromomycin (not on UK Market, available from IDIS) or the liposomal amphotericin *AmBisome®* (section 5.2).

SODIUM STIBOGLUCONATE
Indications: leishmaniasis
Cautions: hepatic impairment; pregnancy; intravenous injections must be given slowly over 5 minutes (to reduce risk of local thrombosis) and stopped if coughing or substernal pain; mucocutaneous disease (see below); heart disease (withdraw if conduction disturbances occur); treat intercurrent infection (e.g. pneumonia)
MUCOCUTANEOUS DISEASE. Successful treatment of mucocutaneous leishmaniasis may induce severe inflammation around the lesions (may be life-threatening if pharyngeal or tracheal involvement)—may require corticosteroid
Contra-indications: significant renal impairment; breast-feeding
Side-effects: anorexia, nausea, vomiting, abdominal pain; ECG changes; headache, lethargy, myalgia; raised liver enzymes; coughing and substernal pain (see Cautions); rarely anaphylaxis; also reported, fever, sweating, flushing, vertigo, bleeding from nose or gum, jaundice, rash; pain and thrombosis on intravenous administration, intramuscular injection also painful
Dose: see notes above

PoM **Pentostam®** (GlaxoWellcome)
Injection, sodium stibogluconate equivalent to pentavalent antimony 100 mg/mL. Net price 100-mL bottle = £68.01

5.4.6 Trypanocides
The prophylaxis and treatment of trypanosomiasis is difficult and differs according to the strain of organism. Expert advice should therefore be obtained.

5.4.7 Drugs for toxoplasmosis
Most infections caused by *Toxoplasma gondii* are self-limiting, and treatment is not necessary. Exceptions are patients with eye involvement (toxoplasma choroidoretinitis), and those who are immunosuppressed. Toxoplasmic encephalitis is a common complication of AIDS. The treatment of choice is a combination of pyrimethamine and sulphadiazine (sulfadiazine), given for several weeks (expert advice **essential**). Pyrimethamine is a folate antagonist, and adverse reactions to this combination are relatively common (folinic acid supplements and weekly blood counts needed). Alternative regimens use combinations of pyrimethamine with clindamycin or clarithromycin or azithromycin. Long-term secondary prophylaxis is required after treatment of toxoplasmosis in AIDS.

If toxoplasmosis is acquired in pregnancy, transplacental infection may lead to severe disease in the fetus. Spiramycin (not on UK market, available from IDIS) may reduce the risk of transmission of maternal infection to the fetus.

5.4.8   Drugs for Pneumocystis pneumonia

Pneumonia caused by *Pneumocystis carinii* occurs in immunosuppressed or severely debilitated patients. It is the commonest cause of pneumonia in AIDS. **Co-trimoxazole** (section 5.1.8) in high dosage is the drug of choice for the treatment of pneumocystis pneumonia. **Pentamidine isethionate** (pentamidine isetionate) is an alternative to co-trimoxazole and is particularly indicated for patients with a history of adverse reactions to, or who have not responded to, co-trimoxazole. Pentamidine isethionate is a potentially toxic drug that can cause severe hypotension during or immediately after administration; it should only be administered by those experienced in its use. Pentamidine isethionate is given by intravenous infusion but can also be administered by inhalation which reduces side-effects (although systemic absorption may still occur).

Intermittent *prophylactic inhalation* of pentamidine isethionate may prevent relapse but co-trimoxazole is easier to administer and just as effective (in a dose of 960 mg twice daily) for prophylaxis.

Atovaquone has recently become available for the treatment of mild to moderate Pneumocystis pneumonia in patients who are intolerant of co-trimoxazole.

Trimetrexate is an alternative in AIDS patients who are intolerant of co-trimoxazole and pentamidine isethionate or who do not respond to these drugs. Trimetrexate is a potent dihydrofolate reductase inhibitor and must be given with calcium folinate (see below).

ATOVAQUONE

Indications: treatment of mild to moderate *Pneumocystis carinii* pneumonia in patients intolerant of co-trimoxazole

Cautions: initial diarrhoea and difficulty in taking with food may reduce absorption (and require alternative therapy); other causes of pulmonary disease should be sought and treated; elderly; hepatic and renal impairment; pregnancy; avoid breast-feeding; **interactions:** Appendix 1 (atovaquone)

Side-effects: diarrhoea, nausea, vomiting; headache, insomnia; rash, fever; elevated liver enzymes and amylase; anaemia, neutropenia; hyponatraemia

Dose: see under preparations

PoM **Wellvone®** (GlaxoWellcome)
Tablets, yellow, f/c, atovaquone 250 mg. Net price 189-tab pack = £377.14. Label: 21
  Dose: 750 mg 3 times daily with food (particularly high fat) for 21 days; CHILD not recommended
Suspension, sugar-free, fruit-flavoured, atovaquone 750 mg/5 mL. Net price 210 mL = £377.14. Label: 21
  Dose: 750 mg twice daily with food (particularly high fat) for 21 days; CHILD not recommended

With proguanil hydrochloride
See section 5.4.1

PENTAMIDINE ISETHIONATE
(Pentamidine isetionate)

Indications: see under Dose (should only be given by specialists)

Cautions: risk of severe hypotension following administration (establish baseline blood pressure and administer with patient lying down; monitor blood pressure closely during administration, and at regular intervals, until treatment concluded); hepatic and renal impairment; hypertension or hypotension; hyperglycaemia or hypoglycaemia; leucopenia, thrombocytopenia, or anaemia; pregnancy and breast-feeding; carry out laboratory monitoring according to product literature; care required to protect personnel during handling and administration

Side-effects: severe reactions, sometimes fatal, due to hypotension, hypoglycaemia, pancreatitis, and arrhythmias; also leucopenia, thrombocytopenia, acute renal failure, hypocalcaemia; also reported: azotaemia, abnormal liver-function tests, anaemia, hyperkalaemia, nausea and vomiting, dizziness, syncope, flushing, hyperglycaemia, rash, and taste disturbances; Stevens-Johnson syndrome reported; on inhalation, bronchoconstriction (may be prevented by prior use of bronchodilators), cough, shortness of breath, and wheezing; discomfort, pain, induration, abscess formation, and muscle necrosis at injection site

Dose: Pneumocystis carinii pneumonia, *by intravenous infusion,* 4 mg/kg daily for at least 14 days (reduced according to product literature in renal impairment)
By inhalation of nebulised solution (using suitable equipment—consult product literature) 600 mg pentamidine isethionate daily for 3 weeks; secondary prevention, 300 mg every 4 weeks *or* 150 mg every 2 weeks
Visceral leishmaniasis (kala-azar, section 5.4.5), *by deep intramuscular injection,* 3–4 mg/kg on alternate days to max. total of 10 injections; course may be repeated if necessary
Cutaneous leishmaniasis, *by deep intramuscular injection,* 3–4 mg/kg once or twice weekly until condition resolves (but see also section 5.4.5)
Trypanosomiasis, *by deep intramuscular injection or intravenous infusion,* 4 mg/kg daily or on alternate days to total of 7–10 injections
  Note. Direct bolus intravenous injection should be avoided whenever possible and **never** given rapidly; intramuscular injections should be deep and preferably given into the buttock

PoM **Pentacarinat®** (JHC)

Injection, powder for reconstitution, pentamidine isethionate. Net price 300-mg vial = £34.28

Nebuliser solution, pentamidine isethionate. Net price 300-mg bottle = £36.20

CAUTION IN HANDLING. Pentamidine isethionate is toxic and personnel should be adequately protected during handling and administration—consult product literature

TRIMETREXATE

Indications: treatment of moderate to severe *Pneumocystis carinii* pneumonia in AIDS patients intolerant of, or refractory to, standard therapy or for whom standard therapy is contra-indicated (specialist use only)

Cautions: administer calcium folinate during treatment and for 72 hours after last dose (to avoid potentially serious or life-threatening bone-marrow suppression, oral and gastro-intestinal ulceration, and renal and hepatic dysfunction); suspend myelosupressive drugs (e.g. zidovudine) to administer therapeutic doses of trimetrexate; hepatic and renal impairment; **interactions:** Appendix 1 (trimetrexate)

MONITORING. Monitor at least twice weekly full blood count, renal and hepatic function; interrupt treatment if significant change in renal or hepatic function (see product literature); adjust dose of trimetrexate and calcium folinate if significant haematological toxicity (see product literature)

Contra-indications: pregnancy (following administration to woman or man, avoid conception for **at least 6 months** after treatment), breast-feeding

Side-effects: blood disorders including thrombocytopenia, granulocytopenia and anaemia (dose modification may be necessary, see also monitoring, above); vomiting, diarrhoea, oral and gastro-intestinal mucosal ulceration (discontinue if interfering with eating and drinking); fever (discontinue if uncontrolled by antipyretics); confusion, rarely seizures; disturbances in liver enzymes; disturbances in plasma calcium, potassium and magnesium reported; rash, anaphylaxis very rarely reported; rarely local irritation at injection site

Dose: by intravenous infusion, 45 mg/m^2 daily for 21 days together with calcium folinate *by mouth* or *by intravenous injection* (over 5–10 minutes), 20 mg/m^2 every 6 hours for 24 days

Note. Calcium folinate must not be given with trimetrexate in the same intravenous line (administer either before or after trimetrexate infusion)

▼ PoM **Neutrexin®** (Speywood)

Injection, powder for reconstitution, trimetrexate (as glucuronate). Net price 25-mg vial = £33.86

5.5 Anthelmintics

5.5.1 Drugs for threadworms
5.5.2 Ascaricides
5.5.3 Drugs for tapeworm infections
5.5.4 Drugs for hookworms
5.5.5 Schistosomicides
5.5.6 Filaricides
5.5.7 Drugs for cutaneous larva migrans
5.5.8 Drugs for strongyloidiasis

Advice on prophylaxis and treatment of helminth infections is available from:

Birmingham	0121-766 6611
Glasgow	0141-946 7120
Liverpool	0151-708 9393
London	0171-387 4411 (treatment)

5.5.1 Drugs for threadworms
(pinworms, *Enterobius vermicularis*)

Anthelmintics are effective in threadworm infections, but their use needs to be combined with hygienic measures to break the cycle of auto-infection. All members of the family require treatment.

Adult threadworms do not live for longer than 6 weeks and for development of fresh worms, ova must be swallowed and exposed to the action of digestive juices in the upper intestinal tract. Direct multiplication of worms does not take place in the large bowel. Adult female worms lay ova on the peri-anal skin which causes pruritus; scratching the area then leads to ova being transmitted on fingers to the mouth, often via food eaten with unwashed hands. Washing hands and scrubbing nails before each meal and after each visit to the toilet is essential. A bath taken immediately after rising will remove ova laid during the night.

Mebendazole is the drug of choice for patients of all ages over 2 years. It is given as a single dose; as reinfection is very common, a second dose may be given after 2–3 weeks.

Piperazine salts are preferably given daily for 7 days (followed by a second course if necessary 7 days later); single-dose preparations are also available.

MEBENDAZOLE

Indications: threadworm, roundworm, whipworm, and hookworm infections

Cautions: pregnancy (toxicity in *rats*), breast-feeding; **interactions:** Appendix 1 (mebendazole)

Note. The package insert in the Vermox® pack includes the statement that it is not suitable for women known to be pregnant or children under 2 years

Side-effects: rarely abdominal pain, diarrhoea; hypersensitivity reactions (including exanthema, rash, urticaria, and angioedema) reported

Dose: threadworms, ADULT and CHILD over 2 years, 100 mg as a single dose; if reinfection occurs second dose may be needed after 2–3 weeks; CHILD under 2 years, not yet recommended

Whipworms, ADULT and CHILD over 2 years, 100 mg twice daily for 3 days; CHILD under 2 years, not yet recommended

Roundworms—section 5.5.2

Hookworms—section 5.5.4

PoM [1]**Vermox**® (Janssen-Cilag)
Tablets, orange, scored, chewable, mebendazole 100 mg. Net price 6-tab pack = £1.53
Suspension, mebendazole 100 mg/5 mL. Net price 30 mL = £1.77
1. Can be sold to the public if supplied for oral use in the treatment of enterobiasis in adults and children over 2 years provided its container or package is labelled to show a max. single dose of 100 mg and it is supplied in a container or package containing not more than 800 mg; proprietary brands on sale to the public include *Ovex*® and *Pripsen*® *Mebendazole.*

PIPERAZINE

Indications: threadworm and roundworm infections

Cautions: renal impairment (avoid if severe), liver disease, neurological disease; epilepsy, pregnancy (see also Appendix 4—packs on sale to the general public carry a warning to avoid in epilepsy and pregnancy)

Side-effects: nausea, vomiting, colic, diarrhoea, allergic reactions including urticaria, bronchospasm, and rare reports of Stevens-Johnson syndrome and angioedema; rarely dizziness, muscular incoordination ('worm wobble'); drowsiness, confusion and clonic contractions in patients with neurological or renal abnormalities

Dose: see under Preparations, below

Piperazine Citrate (Non-proprietary)
Elixir, piperazine hydrate 750 mg/5 mL (as citrate) Available from Cupal (Expelix®), De Witt (De Witt's Worm Syrup), Seton (Pripsen® Worm Elixir)
Dose: threadworms, 15 mL once daily for 7 days; CHILD under 2 years (on doctor's advice only) 0.3–0.5 mL/kg once daily for 7 days, 2–3 years 5 mL once daily for 7 days, 4–6 years 7.5 mL once daily for 7 days, 7–12 years 10 mL once daily for 7 days; repeat course after 1 week if necessary
Roundworms, 30 mL as a single dose; CHILD under 1 year (on doctor's advice only) 0.8 mL/kg as a single dose, 1–3 years 10 mL as a single dose, 4–5 years 15 mL as a single dose, 6–8 years 20 mL as a single dose, 9–12 years 25 mL as a single dose; repeat dose after 2 weeks

Pripsen® (Seton)
Oral powder, cream, piperazine phosphate 4 g and sennosides 15.3 mg/sachet. Net price two-dose sachet pack = £1.31. Label: 13
Dose: threadworms, stirred into a small glass of milk or water and drunk immediately, ADULT and CHILD over 6 years, 1 sachet, repeat after 14 days; INFANT 3 months–1 year, one-third sachet (2.5 mL powder), repeat after 14 days; CHILD 1–6 years, two-thirds sachet (5 mL powder), repeat after 14 days
Roundworms, first dose as for threadworms; repeat at monthly intervals for up to 3 months if reinfection risk

5.5.2   Ascaricides
(common roundworm infections)

Levamisole (not on UK market, available from IDIS) is very effective against *Ascaris lumbricoides* and is generally considered to be the drug of choice. It is very well tolerated; mild nausea or vomiting has been reported in about 1% of treated patients; it is given as a single dose of 120–150 mg in adults.

Mebendazole (section 5.5.1) is also active against ascaris; the usual dose is 100 mg twice daily for 3 days. **Piperazine** may be given in a single adult dose equivalent to 4–4.5 g of piperazine hydrate see Piperazine, above.

5.5.3   Drugs for tapeworm infections

TAENICIDES

Niclosamide is the most widely used drug for tapeworm infections and side-effects are limited to occasional gastro-intestinal upset, lightheadedness, and pruritus; it is not effective against larval worms. Fears of developing cysticercosis in *Taenia solium* infections have proved unfounded. All the same, it is wise to anticipate this possibility by using an anti-emetic on wakening.

Praziquantel (*Biltricide*®, not on UK market, available from Bayer) is as effective as niclosamide and is given as a single dose of 10–20 mg/kg after a light breakfast (a single dose of 25 mg/kg for *Hymenolepis nana*).

NICLOSAMIDE
Indications: tapeworm infections—see notes above and under Dose
Side-effects: nausea, retching, abdominal pain; lightheadedness; pruritus
Dose: *Taenia solium,* ADULT and CHILD over 6 years 2 g as a single dose after a light breakfast followed by a purgative after 2 hours; CHILD under 2 years 500 mg, 2–6 years 1 g
T. saginata and *Diphyllobothrium latum,* as for *T. solium* but half the dose may be taken after breakfast and the remainder 1 hour later followed by a purgative 2 hours after last dose
Hymenolepis nana, ADULT and CHILD over 6 years 2 g as a single dose on first day then 1 g daily for 6 days; CHILD under 2 years 500 mg on first day then 250 mg daily for 6 days, 2–6 years 1 g on first day then 500 mg daily for 6 days
COUNSELLING. Tablets should be chewed thoroughly (or crushed) before washing down with water

Yomesan® (Bayer)
Tablets, yellow, chewable, niclosamide 500 mg. Net price 4-tab pack = £1.41. Label: 4, 24, counselling, administration

HYDATID DISEASE

Cysts caused by *Echinococcus granulosus* grow slowly and asymptomatic patients do not always require treatment. Surgical treatment remains the

---

method of choice in many situations. **Albendazole** is used in conjunction with surgery to reduce the risk of recurrence or as primary treatment in inoperable cases. Alveolar echinococcosis due to *E. multilocularis* is usually fatal if untreated. Surgical removal with albendazole cover is the treatment of choice, but where effective surgery is impossible, repeated cycles of albendazole (for a year or more) may help. Careful monitoring of liver function is particularly important during drug treatment.

ALBENDAZOLE

Indications: adjunct to surgery in hydatid cysts caused by *Echinococcus granulosus* or *E. multilocularis*, or primary treatment if surgery not possible; strongyloidiasis (section 5.5.8)

Cautions: blood counts and liver function tests before treatment and twice during each cycle; breast-feeding; exclude pregnancy before starting treatment (non-hormonal contraception during and for 1 month after treatment)

Contra-indications: pregnancy (see also Cautions)

Side-effects: gastro-intestinal disturbances, headache, dizziness, changes in liver enzymes; rarely reversible alopecia; rash, fever, blood disorders including leucopenia and pancytopenia reported; allergic shock if cyst leakage; convulsions and meningism in cerebral disease

Dose: E. granulosus, ADULT over 60 kg, medical treatment, 800 mg daily in divided doses for 28 days followed by 14 tablet-free days; up to 3 cycles of treatment may be given

Adjunct in surgical treatment, *pre-surgery*, 800 mg daily in divided doses for 28 days followed by 14 tablet-free days, repeat cycle once before surgery; *post-surgery* (if viable cysts after pre-surgery treatment, or if no pre-surgery treatment, or if only short pre-surgery course), 800 mg daily in divided doses for 28 days followed by 14 tablet-free days, repeat cycle once

E. multilocularis, ADULT over 60 kg, 800 mg daily in divided doses for 28 days followed by 14 tablet-free days; prolonged treatment may be required, see notes above

PoM **Eskazole®** (SmithKline Beecham)

Tablets, orange, scored, chewable, albendazole 400 mg. Net price 60-tab pack = £72.00. Label: 9

5.5.4 Drugs for hookworms
(ancylostomiasis, necatoriasis)

Hookworms live in the upper small intestine and draw blood from the point of their attachment to their host. An iron-deficiency anaemia may thereby be produced and, if present, effective treatment of the infection requires not only expulsion of the worms but treatment of the anaemia.

Mebendazole (section 5.5.1) has a useful broad-spectrum activity, and is effective against hookworms; the usual dose is 100 mg twice daily for 3 days.

5.5.5 Schistosomicides
(bilharziasis)

Adult *Schistosoma haematobium* worms live in the genito-urinary veins and adult *S. mansoni* in those of the colon and mesentery. *S. japonicum* is more widely distributed in veins of the alimentary tract and portal system.

Praziquantel (*Biltricide®*, Bayer, not on UK market) is effective against all human schistosomes. The dose is 40 mg/kg in 2 divided doses 4–6 hours apart on one day (60 mg/kg in 3 divided doses on one day for *S. japonicum* infections). No serious toxic effects have been reported. Of all the available schistosomicides, it has the most attractive combination of effectiveness, broad-spectrum activity, and low toxicity.

Metriphonate (metrifonate) (*Bilarcil®*, Bayer, not on UK market) is effective against *S. haematobium* infections only; it may be used if praziquantel is not available.

Hycanthone, lucanthone, niridazole, oxamniquine, and stibocaptate have now been superseded.

5.5.6 Filaricides

Diethylcarbamazine (Hetrazan®, *Lederle*) is effective against microfilariae and adults of *Loa loa*, *Wuchereria bancrofti*, and *Brugia malayi*. To minimise reactions treatment is commenced with a dose of diethylcarbamazine citrate 1 mg/kg on the first day and increased gradually over 3 days to 6 mg/kg daily in divided doses; this dosage is maintained for 21 days and usually gives a radical cure for these infections. Close medical supervision is necessary particularly in the early phase of treatment.

In heavy infections there may be a febrile reaction, and in heavy *Loa loa* infection there is a small risk of encephalopathy. In such cases treatment must be given under careful in-patient supervision and stopped at the first sign of cerebral involvement (and specialist advice sought).

Ivermectin (Mectizan®, *MSD*, not on UK market) is very effective in *onchocerciasis* and it is now the drug of choice. A single dose of 150 micrograms/kg by mouth produces a prolonged reduction in microfilarial levels. Retreatment at intervals of 6 to 12 months depending on symptoms must be given until the adult worms die out. Reactions are usually slight and most commonly take the form of temporary aggravation of itching and rash. Diethylcarbamazine or suramin should no longer be used for onchocerciasis because of their toxicity.

5.5.7 Drugs for cutaneous larva migrans
(creeping eruption)

Dog and cat hookworm larvae may enter human skin where they produce slowly extending itching tracks usually on the foot. Single tracks can be treated with topical thiabendazole (no commercial preparation available). Multiple infections respond to **ivermectin** (*Mectizan®*, MSD, not on UK market), **albendazole** [unlicensed indication] or **thiabendazole** (tiabendazole) (section 5.5.8) by mouth.

5.5.8   Drugs for strongyloidiasis

Adult *Strongyloides stercoralis* live in the gut and produce larvae which penetrate the gut wall and invade the tissues, setting up a cycle of auto-infection. **Thiabendazole** (tiabendazole) is the drug of choice for adults (but side-effects are much more marked in the elderly); it is given at a dosage of 25 mg/kg (max. 1.5 g) every 12 hours for 3 days. **Albendazole** (section 5.5.3) is an alternative with fewer side-effects; it is given in a dose of 400 mg twice daily for 3 days, repeated after 3 weeks if necessary. **Ivermectin** (Mectizan®, *MSD*, not on UK market) in a dose of 200 micrograms/kg daily for 2 days may be the most effective drug for chronic *Strongyloides* infection.

THIABENDAZOLE
(Tiabendazole)

Indications: strongyloidiasis, cutaneous and visceral larva migrans, dracontiasis, symptoms of trichinosis; secondary treatment for threadworm when mixed with above infestations; adjunct in hookworm, whipworm, or roundworm (but not suitable for mixed infections involving roundworms—risk of migration); not for prophylactic use

Cautions: hepatic or renal impairment, elderly; discontinue if hypersensitivity reactions occur; correct anaemia, dehydration or malnutrition preferably before treatment; **interactions**: Appendix 1 (thiabendazole)

DRIVING. May impair performance of skilled tasks (e.g. driving)

Contra-indications: pregnancy (teratogenesis in *animal* studies) and breast-feeding

Side-effects: include anorexia, nausea, vomiting, dizziness, diarrhoea, headache, pruritus, drowsiness; hypersensitivity reactions including fever, chills, angioedema, rashes, erythema multiforme and Stevens-Johnson syndrome; rarely tinnitus, collapse, parenchymal liver damage (may be severe and irreversible), visual disorders

Dose: see notes above

PoM **Mintezol**® (MSD)
Tablets, orange, chewable, thiabendazole 500 mg. Net price 6-tab pack = 62p. Label: 3, 21, 24

6: Drugs used in the treatment of disorders of the
ENDOCRINE SYSTEM

In this chapter, drug treatment is discussed under the following headings:

6.1   Drugs used in diabetes

CHOICE OF TREATMENT. About 25% of diabetics require insulin treatment; apart from those presenting in ketoacidosis, insulin is needed by most of those with a rapid onset of symptoms, weight loss, weakness, and sometimes vomiting, often associated with ketonuria. The majority of those who are obese can be managed by restriction of carbohydrate or energy intake alone or with the subsequent administration of oral hypoglycaemic drugs. Most children require insulin from the outset.

6.1.1   Insulins

6.1.1.1 Short-acting insulins
6.1.1.2 Intermediate- and long-acting insulins
6.1.1.3 Hypodermic equipment

Insulin plays a key role in the body's regulation of carbohydrate, fat, and protein metabolism. Diabetes mellitus is due to a deficiency in insulin synthesis and secretion. Patients are generally described as insulin-dependent diabetics (type 1) or non-insulin-dependent diabetics (type 2), although many of the latter need insulin to maintain satisfactory control.

Insulin is a polypeptide hormone of complex structure. It is extracted mainly from pork pancreas and purified by crystallisation; it is also made biosynthetically by recombinant DNA technology using *Escherichia coli* or semisynthetically by enzymatic modification of porcine material (see under Human Insulins, below). All insulin preparations are to a greater or lesser extent immunogenic in man but immunological resistance to insulin action is uncommon.

Insulin is inactivated by gastro-intestinal enzymes, and must therefore be given by injection; the subcutaneous route is ideal for most circumstances. It is usually injected into the upper arms, thighs, buttocks, or abdomen; there may be increased absorption from a limb site if the limb is used in strenuous exercise following the injection. Insulin is most readily administered by injection devices ('pens') (section 6.1.1.3) which hold the insulin in a cartridge and meter the required dose. The more conventional syringe and needle is still preferred by many and is also required for insulins not available in cartridge form. Subcutaneous insulin injections generally cause no problems although fat hypertrophy is not rare; to some extent it can be avoided by rotating the injection sites. Local allergic reactions are now scarcely seen.

Insulin can also be given by continuous subcutaneous infusion using soluble insulin in an infusion pump. This technique has a limited place in the treatment of diabetes, and provides for continuous basal insulin infusion with prandial boosts. There are many disadvantages to the technique. Patients using it must be well-motivated, reliable, and able to monitor their own blood glucose, and must have access to expert advice both day and night.

MANAGEMENT OF DIABETIC PATIENTS. The aim of treatment is to achieve the best possible control of plasma-glucose concentration without making the patient obsessional, whilst avoiding disabling hypoglycaemia; close co-operation is needed between the patient and the medical team since good control reduces the incidence of complications. Mixtures of insulin preparations may be required and appropriate combinations have to be worked out for the individual patient.

For ill patients with acute-onset diabetes, treatment should be started with short-acting soluble insulin given 2 to 4 times a day. For those less severely ill, treatment should be started with a medium-acting insulin or a mixture of premixed short- and medium-acting insulins given twice daily; 8 units twice daily is a suitable initial dose for most ambulant patients. Insulin requirements may be affected by variations in lifestyle, concurrent infection, and use of corticosteroids. In pregnancy insulin requirements should be assessed frequently by an experienced diabetes physician.

Many patients now monitor their own blood glucose concentrations using blood glucose strips preferably with an electronic meter. Since blood glucose concentrations oscillate substantially throughout the day, 'normoglycaemia' cannot always be achieved throughout a 24-hour period without causing damaging hypoglycaemia. It is therefore best to recommend that patients should maintain blood glucose concentrations of between 4 and 10 mmol/litre for most of the time, while accepting that on occasions, for brief periods, they will be above these values; strenuous efforts should be made to prevent blood glucose concentration from falling below 4 mmol/litre. Patients should be advised to look for 'peaks' and 'troughs' of blood glucose, and to adjust their insulin dosage only once or twice weekly. A measure of the total glycated (or glycosylated) haemoglobin (HbA_1) or a specific fraction (HbA_{1c}) provides a good indication of long-term glycaemic control. Overall it is ideal to aim for an HbA_{1c} concentration of less than 7% (normal range 4–6%) or an HbA_1 of less than 8.8% (normal range 5.0–7.5%) although this is not always possible without causing disabling hypoglycaemia. Fructosamine can also be used to assess control: this is a simpler and cheaper but less reliable measurement of glycated serum proteins.

The energy and carbohydrate intake must be adequate to allow normal growth and development but obesity must be avoided. The carbohydrate intake must be regulated and should be distributed throughout the day. Fine control of plasma glucose can be achieved by moving portions of carbohydrate from one meal to another without altering the total intake.

Insulin doses are determined on an individual basis, by gradually increasing the dose but avoiding troublesome hypoglycaemic reactions.

There are 3 main types of insulin preparations:

1. those of **short** duration which have a relatively rapid onset of action, namely soluble forms of insulin and insulin lispro;
2. those with an **intermediate** action, e.g. Isophane Insulin Injection and Insulin Zinc Suspension; and
3. those whose action is slower in onset and lasts for **long** periods, e.g. Human Ultratard®.

The *duration of action* of different insulin preparations varies considerably from one patient to another, and needs to be assessed for every individual. The type of insulin used and its dose and frequency of administration depend on the particular needs of the patient. Most patients are best started on insulins of intermediate action twice daily and a short-acting insulin can be added later to cover any hyperglycaemia which may follow breakfast or evening meal.

EXAMPLES OF RECOMMENDED INSULIN REGIMENS

---

1. Short-acting insulin *mixed* with Intermediate-acting insulin: twice daily (before meals)

2. Short-acting insulin *mixed* with Intermediate-acting insulin: before breakfast
   Short-acting insulin: before evening meal
   Intermediate-acting insulin: at bedtime

3. Short-acting insulin: three times daily (before breakfast, midday and evening meal)
   Intermediate-acting insulin: at bedtime

4. Intermediate-acting insulin *with or without* Short-acting insulin: once daily either before breakfast or at bedtime suffices for some non-insulin dependent (type 2) diabetic patients needing insulin

---

HUMAN INSULINS. There are differences in the amino-acid sequence in animal insulins, human insulins and the human insulin analogue, insulin lis-

pro. Most available insulins are either porcine in origin or of human sequence prepared either by modification of porcine material (emp) or biosynthetically (crb, prb, or pyr). Preparations of human sequence insulin should theoretically be less immunogenic, but in trials no real advantage has been shown.

HYPOGLYCAEMIA. Hypoglycaemia is a potential hazard for all patients receiving insulin, therefore much of their instruction must be directed towards avoiding it. For advice on the treatment of hypoglycaemia, see section 6.1.4

The conversion from beef to human sequence insulin should always be undertaken with specialist advice; it is usual to reduce the total dose by about 10%, with careful monitoring for the first few days. When changing from porcine to human sequence insulin, a dose change is not usually needed, but careful monitoring is advised.

Loss of warning of hypoglycaemia is a common problem among insulin-treated patients and can be a serious hazard, especially for drivers. The cause is not known, but very tight control of diabetes appears to lower the blood glucose concentration needed to trigger hypoglycaemic symptoms. Betablockers can also blunt hypoglycaemic awareness (and can delay recovery).

Some patients have reported loss of warning of hypoglycaemia after transfer to human insulin. Patients should be warned of this possibility and if they believe that human insulin is responsible for their loss of warning it is reasonable to transfer them back to porcine insulin and at the same time to re-educate them about avoiding hypoglycaemia. When prescribing insulin great care should be taken to specify whether a human or an animal preparation is required. Indications for changing from animal to human preparations must be very carefully considered in the light of these reported problems. Beef insulin preparations are still available for patients who specifically request them.

A very small number of insulin-dependent diabetic patients have been reported to have died in bed without known cause. There is no evidence that human insulin was responsible and the cause is still under investigation.

DRIVING. Car drivers need to be particularly careful to avoid hypoglycaemia (see also above) and should be warned of the problems. They should normally check their blood glucose concentration before driving and, on long journeys, at intervals of approximately two hours and they should ensure that a supply of sugar is always available in the car. If hypoglycaemia occurs a car driver should switch off the ignition until recovery is complete, which may take up to 15 minutes or longer. Driving is not permitted when hypoglycaemic awareness has been lost.

DIABETES AND SURGERY. When an insulin-dependent diabetic patient requires surgery that is likely to require an intravenous infusion for longer than 12 hours the following regimen provides for intravenous administration of insulin (for an indefinite period).

Give an injection of the patient's **usual insulin** *on the night before the operation.*

Early on the day of the operation, start an intravenous infusion of glucose 5% containing potassium chloride 10 mmol per litre (provided that the patient is not hyperkalaemic) and run at a constant rate appropriate to the patient's fluid requirements (usually 125 mL per hour); make up a solution of **soluble insulin** 1 unit/mL in sodium chloride 0.9% and infuse intravenously using a syringe pump piggy-backed to the intravenous infusion.

The rate of the insulin infusion should normally be:
Blood glucose < 4 mmol/litre, *give* 0.5 units/hour
Blood glucose 4–15 mmol/litre, *give* 2 units/hour
Blood glucose 15–20 mmol/litre, *give* 4 units/hour
Blood glucose > 20 mmol/litre, *review*

In resistant cases (such as patients who are shocked or severely ill or those receiving corticosteroids or sympathomimetics) 2–4 times these rates or even more may be needed.

If a syringe pump is not available **soluble insulin** 16 units/litre should be added to the intravenous infusion of glucose 5% containing potassium chloride 10 mmol per litre (provided the patient is not hyperkalaemic) and the infusion run at the rate appropriate to the patient's fluid requirements (usually 125 mL per hour) with the insulin dose adjusted as follows:

Blood glucose < 4 mmol/litre, *give* 8 units/litre
Blood glucose 4–15 mmol/litre, *give* 16 units/litre
Blood glucose 15–20 mmol/litre, *give* 32 units/litre
Blood glucose > 20 mmol/litre, *review*

The rate of intravenous infusion depends on the volume depletion, cardiac function, age, and other factors. Blood glucose concentration should be measured pre-operatively then every 2 hours until stable then every 6 hours. Intravenous insulin lasts for only a few minutes therefore infusion must not be stopped unless the patient becomes frankly hypoglycaemic (blood glucose < 3 mmol/litre) in which case it should be stopped for up to 30 minutes. The amount of potassium chloride required in the infusion needs to be assessed by regular measurement of serum electrolytes. Sodium chloride 0.9% infusion should be substituted for glucose 5% if the blood glucose is persistently above 15 mmol/litre.

After recovery, once the patient starts to eat and drink, give subcutaneous insulin *before breakfast* and stop intravenous insulin 30 minutes later; the dose may need to be 10–20% more than usual if the patient is still in bed or unwell. If the patient was not previously receiving insulin, initially give 30–40 units daily in four divided doses using soluble before meals and intermediate-acting at bedtime and adjust amount from day to day. Patients with hyperglycaemia often relapse after conversion back to subcutaneous insulin calling for one of the following approaches:

additional doses of soluble insulin at any of the four injection times (before meals or bedtime) *or*
temporary addition of intravenous insulin infusion (while continuing the subcutaneous regimen) until blood glucose concentration is satisfactory *or*
complete reversion to the intravenous regimen (especially if the patient is unwell).

UNITS. The word 'unit' should **not** be abbreviated.

6.1.1.1 SHORT-ACTING INSULINS

Soluble Insulin is a short-acting form of insulin. For maintenance regimens it is usual to inject it 15 to 30 minutes before meals.

Soluble insulin is the only appropriate form of insulin for use in diabetic emergencies and at the time of surgery. It has the great advantage that it can be given intravenously and intramuscularly, as well as subcutaneously.

When injected subcutaneously, soluble insulin has a rapid onset of action (after 30 to 60 minutes), a peak action between 2 and 4 hours, and a duration of action of up to 8 hours. Human sequence preparations tend to have a more rapid onset and a shorter overall duration.

When injected intravenously, soluble insulin has a very short half-life of only about 5 minutes and its effect disappears within 30 minutes.

The recently introduced human insulin analogue, **insulin lispro**, has a shorter duration of action than soluble insulin; as a result, compared to soluble insulin fasting and preprandial blood-glucose concentration is a little higher, postprandial blood-glucose concentration is a little lower, and mild (though not severe) hypoglycaemia occurs slightly less frequently. Subcutaneous injection of insulin lispro may prove convenient to those who wish to inject close to a meal and it may be an advantage to those prone to pre-lunch hypoglycaemia.

SOLUBLE INSULIN

(Insulin Injection; Neutral Insulin)
A sterile solution of insulin (i.e. bovine or porcine) or of human insulin; pH 6.6–8.0
Indications: diabetes mellitus; diabetic ketoacidosis (section 6.1.3)
Cautions: see notes above; reduce dose in renal impairment; **interactions:** Appendix 1 (antidiabetics)
Side-effects: see notes above; local reactions and fat hypertrophy at injection site; overdose causes hypoglycaemia
Dose: by subcutaneous, intramuscular, or intravenous injection or intravenous infusion, according to patient's requirements
COUNSELLING. Show bottle to patient and confirm that patient is expecting the version dispensed

Highly purified animal
Hypurin® Bovine Neutral (CP)
Injection, soluble insulin (bovine, highly purified) 100 units/mL. Net price 10-mL vial = £16.80; 5 × 1.5-mL cartridge = £12.60

Hypurin® Porcine Neutral (CP)
Injection, soluble insulin (porcine, highly purified) 100 units/mL. Net price 10-mL vial = £16.80; 5 × 1.5-mL cartridge = £12.60

Pork Velosulin® (Novo Nordisk, GlaxoWellcome)
Injection, soluble insulin (porcine, highly purified) 100 units/mL. Net price 10-mL vial = £6.58

Human sequence
Human Actrapid® (Novo Nordisk)
Injection, soluble insulin (human, pyr) 100 units/mL. Net price 10-mL vial = £9.98; *Penfil®* cartridge (for NHS *NovoPen®* devices) 5 × 1.5-mL = £9.87, 5 × 3-mL = £22.87; 5 × 3-mL *Actrapid®* prefilled disposable injection devices (range 2–78 units, allowing 2-unit dosage adjustments) = £26.33

Human Velosulin® (Novo Nordisk, GlaxoWellcome)
Injection, soluble insulin (human, emp) 100 units/mL. Net price 10-mL vial = £9.98

Humulin S® (Lilly)
Injection, soluble insulin (human, prb) 100 units/mL. Net price 10-mL vial = £10.98; 5 × 1.5-mL cartridge (for NHS *B-D Pen®*) = £9.13; 5 × 3-mL cartridge (for NHS *B-D Pen® 3 mL*) = £18.26; 5 × 3-mL *Humaject S®* prefilled disposable injection devices (range 2–96 units, allowing 2-unit dosage adjustment) = £23.70

Mixed preparations, see Biphasic Insulin and Biphasic Isophane Insulin (section 6.1.1.2)

INSULIN LISPRO
(Recombinant human insulin analogue)
Indications: diabetes mellitus
Cautions; Side-effects: see under Soluble Insulin
Dose: by subcutaneous injection, according to patient's response
COUNSELLING. Show bottle to patient and confirm that patient is expecting the version dispensed

▼ **Humalog®** (Lilly)
Injection, insulin lispro (recombinant human insulin analogue) 100 units/mL. Net price 10-mL vial = £15.71; 5 × 1.5-mL cartridge (for NHS *B-D Pen®* or NHS *Diapen®*) = £13.39

6.1.1.2 INTERMEDIATE- AND LONG-ACTING INSULINS

When given by subcutaneous injection intermediate- and long-acting insulins have an onset of action of approximately 1–2 hours, a maximal effect at 4–12 hours, and a duration of 16–35 hours. Some are given twice daily in conjunction with short-acting (soluble) insulin, and others are given once daily, particularly in elderly patients. They can be mixed with soluble insulin in the syringe, essentially retaining the properties of the two components, although there may be some blunting of the initial effect of the soluble insulin component (especially on mixing with protamine zinc insulin, see below).

Isophane Insulin is a suspension of insulin with protamine which is of particular value for initiation of twice-daily insulin regimens. Patients usually mix isophane with soluble insulin but ready-mixed preparations may be appropriate (**Biphasic Isophane Insulin**).

Insulin Zinc Suspension (Crystalline) has a more prolonged duration of action; it may be used independently or in **Insulin Zinc Suspension** (30% amorphous, 70% crystalline).

Protamine Zinc Insulin is usually given once daily in conjunction with short-acting (soluble) insulin. It has the drawback of binding with the soluble insulin when mixed in the same syringe, and is now rarely used.

INSULIN ZINC SUSPENSION
(Insulin Zinc Suspension (Mixed); I. Z. S.)
A sterile neutral suspension of bovine and/or porcine insulin or of human insulin in the form of a complex obtained by the addition of a suitable zinc salt; consists of rhombohedral crystals (10–40 microns) and of particles of no uniform shape (not exceeding 2 microns)
Indications: diabetes mellitus (long acting)
Cautions; Side-effects: see under Soluble Insulin (section 6.1.1.1)
Dose: by subcutaneous injection, according to patient's requirements
COUNSELLING. Show bottle to patient and confirm that patient is expecting the version dispensed

Highly purified animal
Hypurin® Bovine Lente (CP)
Injection, insulin zinc suspension (bovine, highly purified) 100 units/mL. Net price 10-mL vial = £16.80

Lentard MC® (Novo Nordisk)
Injection, insulin zinc suspension (bovine and porcine, highly purified) 100 units/mL. Net price 10-mL vial = £5.78

Human sequence
Human Monotard® (Novo Nordisk)
Injection, insulin zinc suspension (human, pyr) 100 units/mL. Net price 10-mL vial = £9.98

Humulin Lente® (Lilly)
Injection, insulin zinc suspension (human, prb) 100 units/mL. Net price 10-mL vial = £12.08

INSULIN ZINC SUSPENSION (CRYSTALLINE)
(Cryst. I. Z. S.)
A sterile neutral suspension of bovine insulin or of human insulin in the form of a complex obtained by the addition of a suitable zinc salt; consists of rhombohedral crystals (10–40 microns)
Indications: diabetes mellitus (long acting)
Cautions; Side-effects: see under Soluble Insulin (section 6.1.1.1)
Dose: by subcutaneous injection, according to patient's requirements
COUNSELLING. Show bottle to patient and confirm that patient is expecting the version dispensed

Human sequence
Human Ultratard® (Novo Nordisk)
Injection, insulin zinc suspension, crystalline (human, pyr) 100 units/mL. Net price 10-mL vial = £9.98
Humulin Zn® (Lilly)
Injection, insulin zinc suspension, crystalline (human, prb) 100 units/mL. Net price 10-mL vial = £12.08

ISOPHANE INSULIN
(Isophane Insulin Injection; Isophane Protamine Insulin Injection; Isophane Insulin (NPH))
A sterile suspension of bovine or porcine insulin or of human insulin in the form of a complex obtained by the addition of protamine sulphate or another suitable protamine
Indications: diabetes mellitus (intermediate acting)
Cautions; Side-effects: see under Soluble Insulin (section 6.1.1.1); protamine may cause allergic reactions
Dose: by subcutaneous injection, according to patient's requirements
COUNSELLING. Show bottle to patient and confirm that patient is expecting the version dispensed

Highly purified animal
Hypurin® Bovine Isophane (CP)
Injection, isophane insulin (bovine, highly purified) 100 units/mL. Net price 10-mL vial = £16.80; 5 × 1.5-mL cartridge = £12.60
Hypurin® Porcine Isophane (CP)
Injection, isophane insulin (porcine, highly purified) 100 units/mL. Net price 10-mL vial = £16.80; 5 × 1.5-mL cartridge = £12.60
Pork Insulatard® (Novo Nordisk, GlaxoWellcome)
Injection, isophane insulin (porcine, highly purified) 100 units/mL. Net price 10-mL vial = £6.58

Human sequence
Human Insulatard® ge (Novo Nordisk)
Injection, isophane insulin (human, pyr) 100 units/ mL. Net price 10-mL vial = £9.98; Penfill® cartridge (for NHS Novopen® devices) 5 × 1.5-mL = £9.87, 5 × 3-mL = £22.87; 5 × 3-mL prefilled disposable injection devices (range 2–78 units allowing 2-unit dosage adjustment) = £26.33
Humulin I® (Lilly)
Injection, isophane insulin (human, prb) 100 units/ mL. Net price 10-mL vial = £9.98; 5 × 1.5-mL cartridge (for NHS *B-D Pen®*) = £9.13; 5 × 3-mL cartridge (for NHS *B-D Pen®* 3 mL) = £18.26; 5 × 3-mL *Humaject I®* prefilled disposable injection devices (range 2–96 units, allowing 2-unit dosage adjustment) = £23.70

Mixed preparations, see Biphasic Isophane Insulin (below)

PROTAMINE ZINC INSULIN
(Protamine Zinc Insulin Injection)
A sterile suspension of insulin in the form of a complex obtained by the addition of a suitable protamine and zinc chloride; this preparation was included in BP 1980 but is not included in BP 1988
Indications: diabetes mellitus (long acting)
Cautions; Side-effects: see under Soluble Insulin (section 6.1.1.1); protamine may cause allergic reactions; see also notes above
Dose: by subcutaneous injection, according to patient's requirements
COUNSELLING. Show bottle to patient and confirm that patient is expecting the version dispensed

Hypurin® Bovine Protamine Zinc (CP)
Injection, protamine zinc insulin (bovine, highly purified) 100 units/mL. Net price 10-mL vial = £16.80

BIPHASIC INSULINS

BIPHASIC ISOPHANE INSULIN
(Biphasic Isophane Insulin Injection)
A sterile buffered suspension of porcine insulin complexed with protamine sulphate (or another suitable protamine) in a solution of porcine insulin *or* a sterile buffered suspension of human insulin complexed with protamine sulphate (or another suitable protamine) in a solution of human insulin
Indications: diabetes mellitus (intermediate acting)
Cautions; Side-effects: see under Soluble Insulin (section 6.1.1.1); protamine may cause allergic reactions
Dose: by subcutaneous injection, according to the patient's requirements
COUNSELLING. Show bottle to patient and confirm that patient is expecting the version dispensed

Highly purified animal
Hypurin® Porcine Biphasic Isophane 30/70 Mix (CP)
Injection, biphasic isophane insulin (porcine, highly purified), 30% soluble, 70% isophane, 100 units/mL. Net price 10-mL vial = £16.80; 5 × 1.5-ml cartridge = £12.60
Pork Mixtard 30® (Novo Nordisk, GlaxoWellcome)
Injection, biphasic isophane insulin (porcine, highly purified), 30% soluble, 70% isophane, 100 units/mL. Net price 10-mL vial = £6.58

Human sequence
Human Mixtard® 30 ge (Novo Nordisk)
Injection, biphasic isophane insulin (human, pyr), 30% soluble, 70% isophane, 100 units/mL. Net price 10-mL vial = £9.98
Human Mixtard® 10 (Novo Nordisk)
Injection, biphasic isophane insulin (human, pyr), 10% soluble, 90% isophane, 100 units/mL. Net price *Penfill®* cartridge (for NHS *Novopen®* devices) 5 × 1.5-mL = £9.87, 5 × 3-mL = £22.87; 5 × 3-mL prefilled disposable injection devices (range 2–78 units, allowing 2-unit dosage adjustment) = £26.33

Human Mixtard® 20 (Novo Nordisk)

Injection, biphasic isophane insulin (human, pyr), 20% soluble, 80% isophane, 100 units/mL. Net price *Penfill®* cartridge (for NHS *Novopen®* devices) 5 × 1.5-ml = £9.87, 5 × 3-mL = £22.87; 5 × 3-mL prefilled disposable injection devices (range 2–78 units, allowing 2-unit dosage adjustment) = £26.33

Human Mixtard® 30 (Novo Nordisk)

Injection, biphasic isophane insulin (human, pyr), 30% soluble, 70% isophane, 100 units/mL. Net price *Penfill®* cartridge (for NHS *Novopen®* devices) 5 × 1.5-mL = £9.87, 5 × 3-mL = £22.87; 5 × 3-mL prefilled disposable injection devices (range 2–78 units, allowing 2-unit dosage adjustment) = £26.33

Human Mixtard® 40 (Novo Nordisk)

Injection, biphasic isophane insulin (human, pyr), 40% soluble, 60% isophane, 100 units/mL. Net price *Penfill®* cartridge (for NHS *Novopen®* devices) 5 × 1.5-mL = £9.87, 5 × 3-mL = £22.87; 5 × 3-mL prefilled disposable injection devices (range 2–78 units, allowing 2-unit dosage adjustments) = £26.33

Human Mixtard® 50 (Novo Nordisk)

Injection, biphasic isophane insulin (human, pyr), 50% soluble, 50% isophane, 100 units/mL. Net price 10-mL vial = £9.98; *Penfill®* cartridge (for NHS *Novopen®* devices) 5 × 1.5-mL = £9.87, 5 × 3-mL = £22.87; 5 × 3-mL prefilled disposable injection devices (range 2–78 units, allowing 2-unit dosage adjustment) = £26.33

Humulin M1® (Lilly)

Injection, biphasic isophane insulin (human, prb), 10% soluble, 90% isophane, 100 units/mL. Net price 10-mL vial = £12.08; 5 × 1.5-mL cartridge (for NHS *B-D Pen®* or NHS *Diapen®*) = £10.04; 5 × 3-mL cartridge (for NHS *B-D Pen® 3 mL*) = £18.26; 5 × 3-mL *Humaject M1®* prefilled disposable injection devices (range 2–96 units, allowing 2-unit dosage adjustment) = £23.70

Humulin M2® (Lilly)

Injection, biphasic isophane insulin (human, prb), 20% soluble, 80% isophane, 100 units/mL. Net price 10-mL vial = £10.98; 5 × 1.5-mL cartridge (for NHS *B-D Pen®* or NHS *Diapen®*) = £9.13; 5 × 3-mL cartridge (for NHS *B-D Pen® 3 mL*) = £18.26; 5 × 3-mL *Humaject M2®* prefilled disposable injection devices (range 2–96 units, allowing 2-unit dosage adjustment) = £23.70

Humulin M3® (Lilly)

Injection, biphasic isophane insulin (human, prb), 30% soluble, 70% isophane, 100 units/mL. Net price 10-mL vial = £9.98; 5 × 1.5-mL cartridge (for NHS *B-D Pen®* or NHS *Diapen®*) = £9.13; 5 × 3-mL cartridge (for NHS *B-D Pen® 3 mL*) = £18.26; 5 × 3-mL *Humaject M3®* prefilled disposable injection devices (range 2–96 units, allowing 2-unit dosage adjustment) = £23.70

Humulin M4® (Lilly)

Injection, biphasic isophane insulin (human, prb), 40% soluble, 60% isophane, 100 units/mL. Net price 10-mL vial = £12.08; 5 × 1.5-mL cartridge (for NHS *B-D Pen®* or NHS *Diapen®*) = £10.04; 5 × 3-mL cartridge (for NHS *B-D Pen® 3 mL*) =

£18.26; 5 × 3-mL *Humaject M4®* prefilled disposable injection devices (range 2–96 units, allowing 2-unit dosage adjustment) = £23.70

Humulin M5® (Lilly)

Injection, biphasic isophane insulin (human, prb), 50% soluble, 50% isophane, 100 units/mL. Net price 10-mL vial = £12.08; 5 × 1.5-mL cartridge (for NHS *B-D Pen®* or NHS *Diapen®*) = £10.04

6.1.1.3 HYPODERMIC EQUIPMENT

Patients should be advised on the safe disposal of lancets, single-use syringes, and needles. Suitable arrangements for the safe disposal of contaminated waste must be made before these products are prescribed for patients who are carriers of infectious diseases.

Injection devices

NHS Autopen® (Owen Mumford)

Injection device, for use with Lilly and Novo Nordisk 1.5-mL insulin cartridges; allows adjustment of dosage in multiples of one unit, max. 16 units (single unit version); two units, max. 32 units (two unit version). Net price (both) = £13.96

NHS B-D Pen® (Becton Dickinson)

Injection devices, for use with Lilly insulin cartridges; *B-D Pen®* (for 1.5-mL cartridges) allows adjustment of dosage in multiples of one unit, max. 30 units, net price = £23.86 (also available from clinics); *B-D Pen® 3 mL* (for 3-mL cartridges) allows adjustment of dosage in multiples of one unit, max. 69 units (available only from clinics)

NHS Diapen® (Lilly)

Injection devices for use with *Humulin®* 1.5-mL insulin cartridges; allows adjustment of dosage in multiples of one unit, max.18 units (*Diapen® 1*); two units, max. 36 units (*Diapen® 2*). Net price (both) = £49.00

NHS NovoPen® (Novo Nordisk)

Injection devices, for use with *Penfill®* insulin cartridges; allows adjustment of dosage in multiples of 2 units, max. 36 units (*NovoPen® II*) *or* 1 unit, max. 40 units (*NovoPen® Classic, NovoPen® Fun, NovoPen® 3*). Available only from clinics

NHS Penject® (Hypoguard)

Injection device, for use with B-D U100 1mL syringe; allows adjustment of dosage in multiples of two units. Net price = £21.25

Lancets— sterile, single use

Type A (Drug Tariff). Cylindrical mount fluted longitudinally; compatible with NHS Autoclix® (BM Diagnostics), NHS B-D Lancer® (Becton Dickinson), NHS Glucolet® (Bayer Diagnostics), NHS Monojector® (Sherwood), NHS Penlet® II (Lifescan) and NHS Soft Touch® (BM Diagnostics) finger-pricking devices

Available from Bayer (Baylet®, net price 100-lancet pack = £3.19; 200-lancet pack = £6.08), Becton Dickinson (B-D Microfine® +, net price 200-lancet pack = £6.13), Gainor Medical (Cleanlet® 25, net price 100-lancet pack = £3.19; 200-lancet pack = £6.08), Owen Mumford (Unilet G® Superlite net price 100-lancet pack = £3.17; 200-lancet pack = £6.01; Unilet® Universal Comfort-Touch, net price 100-lancet pack = £3.17; 200-lancet pack = £6.01), Sherwood (Monolet®, net price 100-lancet pack = £3.28; 200-lancet pack = £6.24; Monolet Extra®, net price 100-lancet pack = £3.28)

Type B (Drug Tariff). Cylindrical mount with concentric ribs; compatible with NHS Autolet® (Owen Mumford)

and NHS Glucolet® (Bayer Diagnostics) finger-pricking devices

Available from Bayer Diagnostics (Ames®, net price 100-lancet pack = £3.19; 200-lancet pack = £6.08), Gainor Medical (Cleanlet® 25XL, net price 100-lancet pack = £3.19; 200-lancet pack = £6.08), Owen Mumford (Unilet® Superlite, net price 100-lancet pack = £3.17; 200-lancet pack = £6.01; Unilet® Universal Comfer-Touch, net price 100-lancet pack = £3.17; 200-lancet pack = £6.01)

Needles

Hypodermic Needle , Sterile single use (Drug Tariff). For use with re-usable glass syringe, sizes 0.5 mm (25G), 0.45 mm (26G), 0.4 mm (27G). Net price 100-needle pack = £2.20

Available from Becton Dickinson (Microlance®), Sherwood (Monoject®)

Needle Clipping (Chopping) Device (Drug Tariff). Consisting of a clipper to remove needle from its hub and container from which cut-off needles cannot be retrieved; designed to hold 1200 needles, not suitable for use with lancets. Net price = £1.08

Available from Becton Dickinson (B-D Safe-clip®)

Syringes

Clickcount® (Hypoguard). Calibrated glass with Luer taper conical fitting, supplied with dosage chart and strong box for blind patients for whom the Pre-Set syringe is unsuitable. Net price 1 mL = £17.42

Hypodermic Syringe (Drug Tariff). Calibrated glass with Luer taper conical fitting, for use with U100 insulin. Net price 0.5 mL and 1 mL = £13.21

Available from Rand Rocket (Abcare®)

Pre-Set U100 Insulin Syringe (Drug Tariff). Calibrated glass with Luer taper conical fitting, supplied with dosage chart and strong box, for blind patients. Net price 1 mL = £20.11

Available from Rand Rocket

U100 Insulin Syringe with Needle (Drug Tariff). Disposable with fixed or separate needle for single use or single patient-use, colour coded orange, 0.45 mm (26G), 0.4 mm (27G), 0.36 mm (28G), 0.33 mm (29G). Net price 10 (with needle) , 0.3 mL = £1.19; 0.5 mL = £1.15; 1 mL = £1.16

Available from Becton Dickinson (B-D Micro-Fine®+, Plastipak®), Braun (Omnikan®), Rand Rocket (Clinipak®), Sherwood (Monoject® Ultra), Steriseal (Insupak®), Terumo (Myjector®)

Syringe carrying case (Drug Tariff). For use with Clickcount® and Hypodermic insulin syringe. Net price 1 = £1.93; screw cap (to convert for use with Pre-Set U 100 insulin syringe) = 71p

6.1.2   Oral antidiabetic drugs

6.1.2.1 Sulphonylureas
6.1.2.2 Biguanides
6.1.2.3 Other antidiabetics

Oral antidiabetic drugs are used for non-insulin-dependent (type 2) diabetes; they should not be prescribed until patients have been shown not to respond adequately to at least three months' restriction of energy and carbohydrate intake and an increase in physical activity. They should be used to augment the effect of diet and exercise, and not to replace them.

6.1.2.1 SULPHONYLUREAS

The sulphonylureas act mainly by augmenting insulin secretion and consequently are effective only when some residual pancreatic beta-cell activity is present; during long-term administration they also have an extrapancreatic action. All may lead to hypoglycaemia 4 hours or more after food but this is usually an indication of overdose, and is relatively uncommon.

There are several sulphonylureas but there is no evidence for any difference in their effectiveness. Only **chlorpropamide** has appreciably more side-effects, mainly because of its very prolonged duration of action and the consequent hazard of hypoglycaemia (but also as a result of the common and unpleasant chlorpropamide-alcohol flush phenomenon). Selection of an individual sulphonylurea depends otherwise on the age of the patient and renal function (see below), or more generally just on personal preference.

Elderly patients are particularly prone to the dangers of hypoglycaemia when long-acting sulphonylureas are used; **chlorpropamide**, and also **glibenclamide**, should be avoided in these patients and replaced by others, such as **gliclazide** or **tolbutamide**.

CAUTIONS AND CONTRA-INDICATIONS. These drugs tend to encourage weight gain and should be prescribed only if poor control and symptoms persist despite adequate attempts at dieting; metformin should be considered in obese patients. They should not be used during breast-feeding, and caution is needed in the elderly and those with hepatic and renal insufficiency because of the hazard of hypoglycaemia. The short-acting tolbutamide may be used in renal impairment, as may gliquidone and gliclazide which are principally metabolised and inactivated in the liver but careful monitoring of blood-sugar concentration is essential; care is required to choose the smallest possible dose that produces adequate control of blood glucose. Sulphonylureas should be avoided in porphyria (section 9.8.2).

Insulin therapy should be instituted temporarily during intercurrent illness (such as myocardial infarction, coma, infection, and trauma) and during surgery since control of diabetes with the sulphonylureas is often inadequate in such circumstances. Insulin therapy is also usually substituted during pregnancy (see also Appendix 4). Sulphonylureas are contra-indicated in the presence of ketoacidosis.

SIDE-EFFECTS. These are generally mild and infrequent and include gastro-intestinal disturbances and headache.

Chlorpropamide may cause facial flushing after drinking alcohol; this effect is not normally witnessed with other sulphonylureas. Chlorpropamide may also enhance antidiuretic hormone and very rarely cause hyponatraemia.

Sensitivity reactions (usually in first 6–8 weeks of therapy) include transient rashes, which rarely progress to erythema multiforme and exfoliative dermatitis, fever, and jaundice; photosensitivity has also rarely been reported with chlorpropamide. Blood disorders are rare too but include thrombocytopenia, agranulocytosis, and aplastic anaemia. All these phenomena are very rare.

CHLORPROPAMIDE

Indications: diabetes mellitus (for use in diabetes insipidus, see section 6.5.2)

Cautions; Contra-indications; Side-effects: see notes above; **interactions:** Appendix 1 (antidiabetics)

Dose: initially 250 mg daily (elderly patients 100–125 mg but avoid—see notes above), adjusted according to response; max. 500 mg daily; taken with breakfast

PoM **Chlorpropamide** (Non-proprietary)
Tablets, chlorpropamide 100 mg, net price 20 = 18p; 250 mg, 20 = 28p. Label: 4
Available from APS, Cox, CP, Kent

GLIBENCLAMIDE

Indications: diabetes mellitus

Cautions; Contra-indications; Side-effects: see notes above; **interactions:** Appendix 1 (antidiabetics)

Dose: initially 5 mg daily (elderly patients 2.5 mg (but see also notes above)), adjusted according to response; max. 15 mg daily; taken with breakfast

PoM **Glibenclamide** (Non-proprietary)
Tablets, glibenclamide 2.5 mg, net price 20 = 34p; 5 mg, 20 = 46p
Available from APS (Libanil®), Ashbourne (Diabetamide®), Berk (Calabren®), Cox, CP, Generics, Hillcross, Kent (Gliken®), Lagap (Malix®), Norton
PoM **Daonil®** (Hoechst Marion Roussel)
Tablets, scored, glibenclamide 5 mg. Net price 28-tab pack = £2.63
PoM **Semi-Daonil®** (Hoechst Marion Roussel)
Tablets, scored, glibenclamide 2.5 mg. Net price 28-tab pack = £1.58
PoM **Euglucon®** (Hoechst Marion Roussel)
Tablets, glibenclamide 2.5 mg, net price 28-tab pack = £1.58; 5 mg (scored), 28-tab pack = £2.63

GLICLAZIDE

Indications: diabetes mellitus

Cautions; Contra-indications; Side-effects: see notes above; **interactions:** Appendix 1 (antidiabetics)

Dose: initially, 40–80 mg daily, adjusted according to response; up to 160 mg as a single dose, with breakfast; higher doses divided; max. 320 mg daily

PoM **Gliclazide** (Non-proprietary)
Tablets, scored, gliclazide 80 mg, net price 28-tab pack = £3.27, 60-tab pack = £7.00
Available from Cox, Generics, Hillcross, Norton

PoM **Diamicron®** (Servier)
Tablets, scored, gliclazide 80 mg, net price 60-tab pack = £7.00

GLIMEPIRIDE

Indications: diabetes mellitus

Cautions: see notes above; regular hepatic and haematological monitoring; **interactions**: Appendix 1 (antidiabetics)

Contra-indications: see notes above; severe liver impairment (Appendix 2); severe renal impairment (Appendix 3); pregnancy (toxicity in *animal* studies; see also Appendix 4) and breast-feeding

Side-effects: see notes above; increase in liver enzymes and deterioration of liver function with cholestasis, icterus and hepatitis; severe hypersensitivity reactions and allergic vasculitis reported; decrease in plasma-sodium concentration

Dose: initially 1 mg daily, adjusted according to response in 1-mg steps at 1–2 week intervals up to max. 6 mg daily; taken shortly before or with first main meal

Note. If changing from other oral hypoglycaemic drugs, the strength and half-life of the previous drug must be taken into account and, if necessary, a washout period of a few days between drugs should be considered to minimise hypoglycaemia

▼ PoM **Amaryl®** (Hoechst Marion Roussel)
Tablets, all scored, glimepiride 1 mg (pink), net price 30-tab pack = £9.30; 2 mg (green) 30-tab pack = £15.30; 3 mg (yellow) 30-tab pack = £23.10; 4 mg (blue) 30-tab pack = £30.60

GLIPIZIDE

Indications: diabetes mellitus

Cautions; Contra-indications; Side-effects: see notes above; **interactions:** Appendix 1 (antidiabetics)

Dose: initially 2.5–5 mg daily, adjusted according to response; max. 40 mg daily; up to 15 mg may be given as a single dose before breakfast; higher doses divided

PoM **Glipizide** (Non-proprietary)
Tablets, glipizide 5 mg. Net price 56-tab pack = £3.49
Available from Hillcross
PoM **Glibenese®** (Pfizer)
Tablets, scored, glipizide 5 mg. Net price 56-tab pack = £3.63
PoM **Minodiab®** (Pharmacia & Upjohn)
Tablets, glipizide 2.5 mg, net price 60-tab pack = £3.31; 5 mg (scored), 60-tab pack = £3.54

GLIQUIDONE

Indications: diabetes mellitus

Cautions; Contra-indications; Side-effects: see notes above; **interactions:** Appendix 1 (antidiabetics)

Dose: initially 15 mg daily before breakfast, adjusted to 45–60 mg daily in 2 or 3 divided doses; max. single dose 60 mg, max. daily dose 180 mg

PoM **Glurenorm®** (Sanofi Winthrop)
Tablets, scored, gliquidone 30 mg. Net price 100-tab pack = £17.54

TOLAZAMIDE

Indications: diabetes mellitus
Cautions; Contra-indications; Side-effects: see notes above; **interactions:** Appendix 1 (antidiabetics)
Dose: initially 100–250 mg daily with breakfast adjusted according to response; max. 1 g daily; higher doses divided

PoM **Tolanase®** (Pharmacia & Upjohn)
Tablets, both scored, tolazamide 100 mg, net price 100-tab pack = £5.65; 250 mg, 100-tab pack = £12.29

TOLBUTAMIDE

Indications: diabetes mellitus
Cautions; Contra-indications; Side-effects: see notes above; **interactions:** Appendix 1 (antidiabetics)
Dose: 0.5–1.5 g (max. 2 g) daily in divided doses (see notes above)

PoM **Tolbutamide** (Non-proprietary)
Tablets, tolbutamide 500 mg. Net price 20 = 36p
Available from APS, Cox, CP, Hillcross, Norton
PoM **Rastinon®** (Hoechst Marion Roussel)
Tablets, scored, tolbutamide 500 mg. Net price 100-tab pack = £3.33

6.1.2.2 BIGUANIDES

Metformin, the only available biguanide, has a different mode of action from the sulphonylureas, and is not interchangeable with them. It exerts its effect mainly by decreasing gluconeogenesis and by increasing peripheral utilisation of glucose; since it only acts in the presence of endogenous insulin it is only effective in diabetics with some residual functioning pancreatic islet cells. Metformin is used in the treatment of non-insulin-dependent diabetics when strict dieting and sulphonylurea treatment have failed to control diabetes, especially in overweight patients, in whom it may be used first. It can be used alone or with a sulphonylurea. An important advantage of metformin is that hypoglycaemia is not usually a problem; other advantages are the lower incidence of weight gain and lower plasma insulin levels. It does not exert a hypoglycaemic action in non-diabetic subjects unless given in overdose. Gastro-intestinal side-effects are initially common, and may persist in some patients, particularly when very high doses such as 3 g daily are given.

Metformin may provoke lactic acidosis which is most likely to occur in patients with renal impairment; it should not be used in patients with even mild renal impairment. Metformin should also be avoided (or discontinued) in other situations which might predispose to lactic acidosis, e.g. severe

dehydration, infection, shock, severe heart failure, myocardial infarction, hepatic impairment, alcohol dependency, use of x-ray contrast media, pregnancy and breast-feeding. Insulin treatment is almost always required in medical and surgical emergencies; insulin should also be substituted before elective surgery.

METFORMIN HYDROCHLORIDE

Indications: diabetes mellitus (see notes above)
Cautions: see notes above; **interactions:** Appendix 1 (antidiabetics)
Contra-indications: hepatic or renal impairment (withdraw if renal impairment suspected), predisposition to lactic acidosis, heart failure, severe infection or trauma, dehydration, alcohol dependence; pregnancy, breast-feeding
Side-effects: anorexia, nausea, vomiting, diarrhoea (usually transient), lactic acidosis (withdraw treatment), decreased vitamin-B_{12} absorption
Dose: 500 mg every 8 hours *or* 850 mg every 12 hours with or after food; max. 3 g daily in divided doses though most physicians limit this to 2 g daily (see notes above)

PoM **Metformin** (Non-proprietary)
Tablets, coated, metformin hydrochloride 500 mg, net price 20 = 40p; 850 mg, 20 = 66p. Label: 21
Available from APS, Berk, Cox, CP, Hillcross, Lagap (Orabet®), Lennon, Norton, Opus (Glucamet®)
PoM **Glucophage®** (Lipha)
Tablets, f/c, metformin hydrochloride 500 mg, net price 84-tab pack = £2.00; 850 mg, 56-tab pack = £2.22. Label: 21

6.1.2.3 OTHER ANTIDIABETICS

Acarbose, an inhibitor of intestinal alpha glucosidases, delays the digestion and absorption of starch and sucrose. It has a small but significant effect in lowering blood glucose and is used either on its own or as an adjunct to metformin or to sulphonylureas when they prove inadequate. Postprandial hyperglycaemia in insulin-dependent diabetes can be reduced by acarbose, but it has been little used for this purpose. Flatulence deters some from using acarbose although this side-effect tends to decrease with time.

Guar gum, if taken in adequate quantities, results in some reduction of postprandial plasma-glucose concentrations in diabetes mellitus, probably by retarding carbohydrate absorption. It is also used to relieve symptoms of the dumping syndrome.

ACARBOSE

Indications: diabetes mellitus inadequately controlled by diet or by diet with oral hypoglycaemic agents
Cautions: monitor hepatic transaminase levels (higher doses); may enhance hypoglycaemic effects of insulin and sulphonylureas (hypoglycaemic episodes may be treated with oral glucose but not with sucrose); **interactions:** Appendix 1 (antidiabetics)

Contra-indications: pregnancy and breast-feeding; inflammatory bowel disease (e.g. ulcerative colitis, Crohn's disease), partial intestinal obstruction (or predisposition); hepatic impairment, severe renal impairment; hernia, history of abdominal surgery

Side-effects: flatulence, soft stools, diarrhoea (may need to reduce dose or withdraw), abdominal distention and pain; rarely abnormal liver function tests and skin reactions; jaundice and hepatitis reported

Note. Antacids not recommended for treating side-effects (unlikely to be beneficial)

Dose: 50 mg daily initially (to minimise side-effects) increased to 50 mg 3 times daily, then increased if necessary after 6–8 weeks to 100 mg 3 times daily; max. 200 mg 3 times daily; CHILD under 12 years not recommended

COUNSELLING. The tablets should either be chewed with first mouthful of food or swallowed whole with a little liquid immediately before food. In order to counteract possible hypoglycaemia, patients receiving insulin or a sulphonylurea as well as acarbose need to carry glucose (not sucrose—acarbose interferes with sucrose absorption)

PoM **Glucobay®** (Bayer)

Tablets, acarbose 50 mg, net price 90-tab pack = £14.10; 100 mg (scored). 90-tab pack = £17.70. Counselling, administration

GUAR GUM

Indications: see notes above

Cautions: maintain adequate fluid intake; **interactions:** Appendix 1 (guar gum)

COUNSELLING. Preparations that swell in contact with liquid should always be carefully swallowed with water and should not be taken immediately before going to bed.

Contra-indications: gastro-intestinal obstruction

Side-effects: flatulence, abdominal distension, intestinal obstruction

Guarem® (Rybar)

Granules, ivory, sugar-free, guar gum 5 g/sachet, net price 50 sachets = £8.70; 100 sachets = £15.67. Label: 13, counselling, administration

Dose: 5 g stirred into 200 mL fluid 3 times daily immediately before main meals (or sprinkled on food and eaten accompanied by 200 mL fluid)

6.1.3   Diabetic ketoacidosis

Soluble insulin, the only form of insulin that may be given intravenously, is used in the management of diabetic ketoacidotic and hyperosmolar non-ketotic coma. It is preferable to use the type of soluble insulin that the patient has been using previously. It is necessary to achieve and to maintain an adequate plasma-insulin concentration until the metabolic disturbance is brought under control.

Insulin is best given by *intravenous infusion*, using an infusion pump, and diluted to 1 unit/mL (care in mixing, see Appendix 6). Adequate plasma concentrations can usually be maintained with infusion rates of 6 units/hour for adults and 0.1 units/kg/ hour for children. Blood glucose is expected to

decrease by about 5 mmol/hour; if the response is inadequate the infusion rate can be doubled or quadrupled. When the plasma glucose has fallen to 10 mmol/litre the infusion rate can be reduced to 3 units/hour for adults (about 0.02 units/kg/hour for children) and continued until the patient is ready to take food by mouth. The insulin infusion should not be stopped before subcutaneous insulin has been started.

No matter how large, a bolus intravenous injection of insulin can only provide an adequate plasma concentration for a short time, therefore if facilities for intravenous infusion are not available the insulin is given by *intramuscular injection*. An initial loading dose of 20 units intramuscularly is followed by 6 units intramuscularly every hour until the plasma glucose concentration has fallen to 10 mmol/litre; intramuscular injections are then given every 2 hours. Although absorption of insulin is usually rapid after intramuscular injection, it may be impaired in the presence of hypotension and poor tissue perfusion; moreover depots of insulin may build up during treatment therefore late hypoglycaemia should be watched for and treated appropriately.

Intravenous replacement of fluid and electrolytes with **sodium chloride** intravenous infusion is an essential part of the management of ketoacidosis; **potassium chloride** is included in the infusion as appropriate to prevent the hypokalaemia induced by the insulin. **Sodium bicarbonate** infusion (1.26% or 2.74%) is only used in cases of extreme acidosis and shock since the acid-base disturbance is normally corrected by the insulin. **Glucose** solution (5%) is infused once the blood glucose has decreased below 10 mmol/litre but insulin infusion must continue. For glucose, see section 9.2.2.

6.1.4   Treatment of hypoglycaemia

Initially glucose 10–20 g is given by mouth either in liquid form or as granulated sugar or sugar lumps. Glucose 10 g is available from 2 teaspoons sugar, 3 sugar lumps, milk 200 mL, and non-diet versions of *Lucozade®Sparkling Glucose Drink* 50 mL, *Coca-Cola®* 90 mL, *Ribena®* 15 mL (to be diluted). If necessary this may be repeated in 10–15 minutes.

If hypoglycaemia causes unconsciousness, 25– 50 mL of **glucose intravenous infusion 50%** (section 9.2.2) should be given intravenously into a large vein through a large-gauge needle; care is required since this concentration is highly irritant especially if extravasation occurs. Glucose intravenous infusion 10% or 20% may be used but larger volumes are required.

Glucagon can be given as an alternative to parenteral glucose in hypoglycaemia. It is a polypeptide hormone produced by the alpha cells of the islets of Langerhans. Its action is to increase plasma glucose concentration by mobilising glycogen stored in the liver. It has the advantage that it can be injected by any route (intramuscular, subcutaneous, or intravenous) in a dose of 1 mg (1 unit) in circumstances when an intravenous injection of glucose would be difficult or impossible to administer. It may be issued to close relatives of insulin-treated patients for emergency use in hypoglycaemic attacks. It is often advisable to prescribe on an 'if necessary' basis to hospitalised insulin-treated patients, so that it may be given rapidly by the nurses during an hypoglycaemic emergency. If not effective in 10 minutes intravenous glucose should be given.

GLUCAGON

Indications: see notes above and under Dose
Cautions: see notes above, insulinoma, glucagonoma; ineffective in chronic hypoglycaemia, starvation, and adrenal insufficiency
Contra-indications: phaeochromocytoma
Side-effects: nausea, vomiting, diarrhoea, hypokalaemia, rarely hypersensitivity reactions
Dose: by subcutaneous, intramuscular, or intra venous injection, adults and children 0.5–1 unit; if no response within 10 minutes intravenous glucose must be given
Diagnostic aid, consult product literature
Beta-blocker poisoning, see p. 22
Note. 1 unit of glucagon = 1 mg of glucagon or glucagon hydrochloride

PoM **Glucagon Injection** (Non-proprietary)
Injection powder for reconstitution, glucagon (as hydrochloride, with lactose). Net price 1-unit (1-mg) vial (Lilly) = £7.81
Note. If given in doses higher than 2 units (as in beta-blocker poisoning p. 22) reconstitute with water for injection instead of diluent

▼ PoM **GlucaGen®** (Novo Nordisk)
Injection, powder for reconstitution, glucagon (rys) as hydrochloride with lactose. Net price 1-mg vial with water for injection = £17.95 (hosp. only), with prefilled syringe containing water for injection (GlucaGen® Kit) = £19.95

CHRONIC HYPOGLYCAEMIA

Diazoxide, administered by mouth, is useful in the management of patients with chronic hypoglycaemia from excess endogenous insulin secretion, either from an islet cell tumour or islet cell hyperplasia. It has no place in the management of acute hypoglycaemia.

DIAZOXIDE

Indications: chronic intractable hypoglycaemia (for use in hypertensive crisis see section 2.5.1)
Cautions: ischaemic heart disease, pregnancy, labour, impaired renal function; haematological examinations and blood pressure monitoring required during prolonged treatment; growth, bone, and developmental checks in children; **interactions:** Appendix 1 (diazoxide)
Side-effects: anorexia, nausea, vomiting, hyperuricaemia, hypotension, oedema, tachycardia, arrhythmias, extrapyramidal effects; hypertrichosis on prolonged treatment
Dose: by mouth, ADULT and CHILD, initially 5 mg/kg daily in 2–3 divided doses

PoM **Eudemine®** (Evans)
Tablets, diazoxide 50 mg. Net price 20 = £7.68

6.1.5 Treatment of diabetic nephropathy and neuropathy

DIABETIC NEPHROPATHY

Regular review of diabetic patients should include an annual test for urinary protein (using *Albustix®*). If this test is negative, the urine should be tested for microalbuminuria (the earliest sign of nephropathy). If reagent strip tests (NHS *Micral-Test®*) are used and prove positive, the result should be confirmed on an overnight or 24-hour urine sample by radio-immunoassay. It is recommended that all diabetic patients with nephropathy causing albuminuria and all insulin-dependent patients with establised microalbuminuria (at least 3 positive tests) should be treated with an ACE inhibitor (section 2.5.5.1) even if the blood pressure is normal; in any case, to minimise the risk of renal deterioration, the blood pressure must always be maintained below 140 mmHg systolic and 90 mmHg diastolic.

ACE inhibitors may potentiate the hypoglycaemic effect of insulin and oral antidiabetic drugs; this effect is more likely during the first weeks of combined treatment and in patients with renal impairment.

Thiazides (section 2.2.1) have an adverse effect on blood glucose and lipids (although this problem is less marked with the lower doses now given) and should be avoided in diabetes unless the blood pressure cannot be controlled by alternative antihypertensives. Beta-blockers (section 2.4) can lead to a small deterioration of glucose tolerance and they also interfere with metabolic and autonomic responses to hypoglycaemia; cardioselective beta-blockers (see p. 74) may be preferable (but even cardioselective beta-blockers should be avoided in those with frequent episodes of hypoglycaemia).

DIABETIC NEUROPATHY

Note. Several recommendations in this section involve non-licensed indications
Optimal diabetic control is beneficial for the management of *painful neuropathy.* Most patients should be treated with insulin, and relief can probably be accelerated by continuous insulin infusion. **Non-opioid analgesics** such as aspirin and paracetamol (section 4.7.1) are indicated for pain. Relief may also be obtained with the **tricyclic antidepressants,** amitriptyline, imipramine, and nortriptyline (section 4.3.1) with or without a low dose of a **phenothiazine** (section 4.2). **Carbamazepine** (section 4.8.1) or mexiletine may be useful. **Capsaicin** applied topically as a cream (section 10.3.2) is now licensed for painful diabetic neuropathy and may have some effect.

In *autonomic neuropathy* diabetic diarrhoea can often be aborted by 2 or 3 doses of **tetracycline** 250 mg (section 5.1.3). Otherwise **codeine phosphate** (section 1.4.2) is the best drug, but other antidiarrhoeal preparations can be tried. **Anti-emetics** or **cisapride** may control vomiting in gastroparesis. In the rare cases where they do not, erythromycin (especially when given intravenously) has been shown to be of benefit but further studies are needed. (**Important**: erythromycin and cisapride must not be given together—risk of dangerous arrhythmias).

In *neuropathic postural hypotension* an increased salt intake and the use of the **mineralocorticoid** fludrocortisone 100 to 400 micrograms daily (section 6.3.1) help by increasing plasma volume but uncomfortable oedema is a common side-effect. Fludrocortisone can also be combined with **flurbiprofen** (section 10.1.1) and **ephedrine hydrochloride** (section 3.1.1.2).

Gustatory sweating can be treated with **antimuscarinics** such as propantheline bromide (section 1.2); side-effects are common. In some patients with *neuropathic oedema*, **ephedrine hydrochloride** 30 to 60 mg three times daily offers impressive relief.

6.1.6 Diagnostic and monitoring agents for diabetes mellitus

BLOOD GLUCOSE MONITORING

Blood glucose monitoring gives a direct measure of the glucose concentration at the time of the test and can detect hypoglycaemia as well as hyperglycaemia. Patients should be properly trained in the use of blood glucose monitoring systems and to take appropriate action on the results obtained. Inadequate understanding of the normal fluctuations in blood glucose may lead to confusion and inappropriate action. It is ideal for patients to observe the 'peaks' and 'troughs' of blood glucose over 24 hours and make adjustments of their insulin no more than once or twice weekly. Daily alterations to the insulin dose are highly undesirable (except during illness).

Blood glucose monitoring is best carried out by means of a meter. Visual colour comparison is often used but is much less satisfactory. Meters give a more precise reading and are useful for patients with poor eyesight or who are colour blind.

Note. In the UK blood-glucose concentration is expressed in mmol/litre and the British Diabetic Association advises that these units should be used for self-monitoring of blood glucose. In other European countries units of mg/100 mL (or mg/dL) are commonly used.

It is advisable to check that the meter is pre-set in the correct units.

Test strips
Biocare Glucose VT® (Biocare)

Reagent strips, for blood glucose monitoring, visual range (1.1–44.4 mmol/litre). Net price 50-strip pack = £8.50

BM-Accutest® (BM Diagnostics)

Reagent strips, for blood glucose monitoring, range (1.1–33.3 mmol/litre), for use with NHS Accutrend® meter only. Net price 50-strip pack = £13.57

BM-Test 1–44® (BM Diagnostics)

Reagent strips, for blood glucose monitoring, visual range (1–44 mmol/litre) meter range (0.5–27.7 mmol/litre), suitable for use with NHS Reflolux® S. Net price 50-strip pack = £14.29

Easistix® BG (Eastern)

Reagent strips, for blood glucose monitoring, visual range (0.5–28 mmol/litre). Net price 50-strip pack = £12.00

Esprit® Biosensor (Bayer Diagnostics)

Sensor discs, for blood glucose monitoring, range (0.6–33.3 mmol/L), for use with NHS Esprit® meter only. Net price 5 × 10 disc-pack = £13.75

ExacTech® (MediSense)

Biosensor strips, for blood glucose monitoring, range (2.2–25 mmol/litre), for use with NHS ExacTech® meter only. Net price 50-strip pack = £13.45

Glucostix® (Bayer Diagnostics)

Reagent strips, for blood glucose monitoring, visual range (1–44 mmol/litre) meter range (2–22 mmol/litre), suitable for use with NHS Glucometer® GX. Net price 50-strip pack = £14.27

Glucotide® (Bayer Diagnostics)

Reagent strips, for blood glucose monitoring, range (0.6–33.3 mmol/litre), for use with NHS Glucometer® 4 meter only. Net price 50-strip pack = £13.57

Hypoguard® GA (Hypoguard)

Reagent strips, for blood glucose monitoring, visual range (1–22 mmol/litre), meter range (0–22 mmol/litre), suitable for use with NHS Hypocount® GA. Net price 50-strip pack = £12.21

Hypoguard® Supreme (Hypoguard)

Reagent strips, for blood glucose monitoring, visual range 1–22 mmol/litre, meter range (2–22 mmol/litre), suitable for use with NHS Hypocount® Supreme meter. Net price 50-strip pack = £12.73

MediSense G2® (MediSense)

Sensor strips, for blood glucose monitoring, range (1.1–33.3 mmol/litre) for use with NHS MediSense Card® or NHS MediSense Pen® meters only. Net price 50-strip pack = £12.93

Medi-Test® Glycaemie C (BHR)

Reagent strips, for blood glucose monitoring, visual range (1.1–44.4 mmol/litre), meter range (1.1–33.3 mmol/litre), suitable for use with NHS Glycotronic® C meter. Net price 50-strip pack = £12.95

One Touch® (LifeScan)

Reagent strips, for blood glucose monitoring, range (0–33.3 mmol/litre), for use with NHS *One Touch®* II, *Profile* and *Basic* meters only. Net price 50-strip pack = £13.62

Meters
NHS **Accutrend®** (BM Diagnostics)

Meters for blood glucose monitoring for use with BM-Accutest® test strips. Accutrend = £34.00, Accutrend Alpha = £29.00, Accutrend Mini = £25.00, Accutrend DM = £149.00

NHS **Esprit®** (Bayer Diagnostics)

Meter for blood glucose monitoring (for use with Esprit® Biosensor test sensor discs) = £45.00

NHS **ExacTech®** (MediSense)

Meters (Sensor) for blood glucose monitoring for use with ExacTech® test strips. ExacTech Card = £24.00, ExacTech Card starter pack = £34.00, ExacTech Pen = £24.00, ExacTech Pen starter pack = £34.00

NHS **Glucometer®** (Bayer Diagnostics)

Meters for blood glucose monitoring, Glucometer 4 (for use with Glucotide® test strips) = £35.00; Glucometer GX (for use with Glucostix® test strips) = £29.00

NHS **Glycotronic® C** (BHR)

Meter for blood glucose monitoring (for use with Medi-Test® Glycaemic C test strips) = £31.00

NHS **Hypocount**® (Hypoguard)
  Meters for blood glucose monitoring, Hypocount GA (for use with Hypoguard GA® test strips) = £24.95, Hypocount® Supreme (for use with Hypoguard® Supreme test strips) = £34.95

NHS **MediSense**® (MediSense)
  Meters (Sensor) for blood glucose monitoring for use with MediSense G2® test strips. MediSense Card = £35.00, MediSense Pen = £35.00

NHS **One Touch**® (LifeScan)
  Meters for blood glucose monitoring for use with One Touch® test strips. *One Touch*® *II* system pack = £49.00, *One Touch*® *Basic* system pack = £34.00, *One Touch*® *Profile* system pack = £49.00, *One Touch*® *Basic* meter only = £29.00

NHS **Reflolux**® **S** (BM Diagnostics)
  Meter for blood glucose monitoring (for use with BM-Test 1–44® test strips) = £29.00

URINALYSIS

Urine testing for glucose is useful in patients who find blood glucose monitoring difficult. Tests for glucose range from reagent strips specific to glucose to reagent tablets which detect all reducing sugars. Few patients still use *Clinitest*; *Clinistix* is suitable for screening purposes only. Tests for ketones by patients are rarely required unless they become unwell.

Microalbuminuria can be detected with NHS *Micral-Test*® but this should be followed by confirmation in the laboratory, since false positive results are common.

Glucose
Clinistix® (Bayer Diagnostics)
  Reagent strips, for detection of glucose in urine. Net price 50-strip pack = £2.82
Clinitest® (Bayer Diagnostics)
  Reagent tablets, for detection of glucose and other reducing substances in urine. Pocket set (test tube, dropper and 36 tablets), net price = £3.62, 36-tab pack = £1.80, 6-test tube pack = £2.04, 6-dropper pack = £2.04, NHS test tube rack set (6 tubes and 2 droppers) = £5.46
Diabur Test 5000® (BM Diagnostics)
  Reagent strips, for detection of glucose in urine. Net price 50-strip pack = £2.33
Diastix® (Bayer Diagnostics)
  Reagent strips, for detection of glucose in urine. Net price 50-strip pack = £2.40
Easistix® **UG** (Eastern)
  Reagent strips, for detection of glucose in urine. Net price 50-strip pack = £1.99
Medi-Test® **Glucose** (BHR)
  Reagent strips, for detection of glucose in urine. Net price 50-strip pack = £1.99

Ketones
Acetest® (Bayer Diagnostics)
  Reagent tablets, for detection of ketones in urine. Net price 100-tab pack = £3.24
Ketostix® (Bayer Diagnostics)
  Reagent strips, for detection of ketones in urine. Net price 50-strip pack = £2.54
Ketur Test® (BM Diagnostics)
  Reagent strips, for detection of ketones in urine. Net price 50-strip pack = £2.24

Protein
Albustix® (Bayer Diagnostics)
  Reagent strips, for detection of protein in urine. Net price 50-strip pack = £3.49

Albym Test® (BM Diagnostics)
  Reagent strips, for detection of protein in urine. Net price 50-strip pack = £3.00

Other reagent strips available for urinalysis include NHS BM-Test-GP® (glucose and protein—BM Diagnostics), NHS Ketodiastix® (glucose and ketones—Bayer Diagnostics), NHS Medi-Test Combi 2® (glucose and protein—BHR), NHS Micral-Test II® (albumin—BM Diagnostics), NHS Microbumintest® (albumin—Bayer Diagnostics), NHS Uristix® (glucose and protein—Bayer Diagnostics)

GLUCOSE TOLERANCE TEST

The **glucose** tolerance test is used in the diagnosis of diabetes mellitus. This generally involves giving anhydrous glucose 75 g (equivalent to Glucose BP 82.5g) by mouth to the fasting patient, and measuring plasma concentrations at intervals.

The appropriate amount of glucose should be given with at least 300 mL fluid. Anhydrous glucose 75 g may alternatively be given as 389 mL of *Lucozade*® *Sparkling Glucose Drink* (SmithKline Beecham Healthcare) or as 116 mL *Hycal*® (Smith-Kline Beecham Healthcare) with extra fluid to administer a total volume of at least 300 mL.

6.2   Thyroid and antithyroid drugs

6.2.1   Thyroid hormones
6.2.2   Antithyroid drugs

6.2.1   Thyroid hormones

Thyroid hormones are used in hypothyroidism (myxoedema), and also in diffuse non-toxic goitre, Hashimoto's thyroiditis (lymphadenoid goitre), and thyroid carcinoma. Neonatal hypothyroidism requires prompt treatment for normal development.

Thyroxine sodium (levothyroxine sodium) is the treatment of choice for *maintenance* therapy. The initial dose should not exceed 100 micrograms daily, preferably before breakfast, or 25 to 50 micrograms in elderly patients or those with cardiac disease, increased by 25 to 50 micrograms at intervals of at least 4 weeks. The usual maintenance dose to relieve hypothyroidism is 100 to 200 micrograms daily which can be administered as a single dose.

In infants a daily dose of 10 micrograms/kg up to a maximum of 50 micrograms daily should be given; subsequent therapy should reach 100 micrograms daily by 5 years and 100–200 micrograms by 12 years, guided by clinical response, growth assessment, and measurements of plasma thyroxine and thyroid-stimulating hormone.

Liothyronine sodium has a similar action to thyroxine but is more rapidly metabolised; 20 micrograms is equivalent to 100 micrograms of thyroxine. Its effects develop after a few hours and disappear within 24 to 48 hours of discontinuing treatment. It may be used in *severe hypothyroid states* when a rapid response is desired.

Liothyronine by intravenous injection is the treatment of choice in *hypothyroid coma*. Adjunctive therapy includes intravenous fluids, hydrocortisone, and antibiotics; assisted ventilation is often required.

THYROXINE SODIUM
(Levothyroxine sodium)
Indications: hypothyroidism
Cautions: panhypopituitarism or predisposition to adrenal insufficiency from other causes (initiate corticosteroid therapy before starting thyroxine), elderly, cardiovascular disorders (myocardial insufficiency or ECG evidence of myocardial infarction, see Initial Dosage below), diabetes insipidus, diabetes mellitus (dosage increase may be needed for antidiabetic drugs including insulin); pregnancy (monitor serum thyrotrophin levels—dosage adjustment may be necessary) and breast-feeding (see Appendix 5); **interactions:** Appendix 1 (thyroxine)
INITIAL DOSAGE. A pre-therapy ECG is valuable as changes induced by hypothyroidism may be confused with evidence of ischaemia. If too rapid an increase of metabolism is produced (causing diarrhoea, nervousness, rapid pulse, insomnia, tremors and sometimes anginal pain where there is latent myocardial ischaemia), reduce dose or withhold for 1–2 days and start again at a lower dose
Contra-indications: thyrotoxicosis
Side-effects: usually at excessive dosage (see Initial Dosage above) include anginal pain, arrhythmias, palpitation, skeletal muscle cramps, tachycardia, diarrhoea, vomiting, tremors, restlessness, excitability, insomnia, headache, flushing, sweating, excessive loss of weight and muscular weakness
Dose: ADULT, initially 50–100 micrograms (50 micrograms for those over 50 years) daily, preferably before breakfast, adjusted in steps of 50 micrograms every 3–4 weeks until normal metabolism maintained (usually 100–200 micrograms daily); where there is cardiac disease, initially 25 micrograms daily *or* 50 micrograms on alternate days, adjusted in steps of 25 micrograms every 4 weeks; CHILD (see also notes above), congenital hypothyroidism, 25 micrograms daily adjusted in steps of 25 micrograms every 2–4 weeks until mild toxic symptoms appear then reduce dose slightly; juvenile myxoedema (child over 1 year), initially 2.5–5 micrograms/kg daily

PoM **Thyroxine** (Non-proprietary)
Tablets, thyroxine sodium 25 micrograms, net price 20 = 32p; 50 micrograms, 20 = 6p; 100 micrograms, 20 = 6p
Various strengths available from APS, Cox, CP, Goldshield (including Eltroxin®), Kent, Norton

LIOTHYRONINE SODIUM
(L-Tri-iodothyronine sodium)
Indications: see notes above
Cautions; Contra-indications; Side-effects: see under Thyroxine Sodium; has a more rapid effect

Dose: by mouth, initially 20 micrograms daily gradually increased to 60 micrograms daily in 2–3 divided doses; elderly patients should receive smaller initial doses, gradually increased; CHILD, adult dose reduced in proportion to body-weight
By slow intravenous injection, hypothyroid coma, 5–20 micrograms repeated every 12 hours or more frequently (every 4 hours if necessary); alternatively 50 micrograms initially then 25 micrograms every 8 hours reducing to 25 micrograms twice daily

PoM **Tertroxin®** (Link)
Tablets, scored, liothyronine sodium 20 micrograms. Net price 100-tab pack = £14.92
PoM **Triiodothyronine** (Link)
Injection, powder for reconstitution, liothyronine sodium (with dextran). Net price 20-microgram amp = £31.63

6.2.2   Antithyroid drugs

Antithyroid drugs are used for hyperthyroidism either to prepare patients for thyroidectomy or for long-term management. In the UK carbimazole is the most commonly used drug. Propylthiouracil may be used in patients who suffer sensitivity reactions to carbimazole as sensitivity is not necessarily displayed to both drugs. Both drugs act primarily by interfering with the synthesis of thyroid hormones.

> **CSM warning (neutropenia and agranulocytosis)**
>
> Doctors are reminded of the importance of recognising bone marrow suppression induced by carbimazole and the need to stop treatment promptly.
>
> 1. Patient should be asked to report symptoms and signs suggestive of infection, especially sore throat.
>
> 2. A white blood cell count should be performed if there is any clinical evidence of infection.
>
> 3. Carbimazole should be stopped promptly if there is clinical or laboratory evidence of neutropenia.

Carbimazole is given in a daily dose of 20 to 60 mg and maintained at this dose until the patient becomes euthyroid, usually after 4 to 8 weeks; the dose may then be progressively reduced to a maintenance of between 5 and 15 mg daily; therapy is usually given for 18 months. Children may be given an initial dose of 15 mg daily, adjusted according to response. Rashes are common, and propylthiouracil may then be substituted. Pruritus and rashes can also be treated with antihistamines without discontinuing therapy, however patients should be advised to report any sore throat immediately because of the rare complication of agranulocytosis (see CSM warning, above).

Propylthiouracil is given in a daily dose of 300 to 600 mg and maintained on this dose until the patient becomes euthyroid; the dose may then be progressively reduced to a maintenance of between 50 and 150 mg daily.

Although antithyroid drugs have a short half-life they need only be given once daily because of their prolonged effect on the thyroid. Over-treatment

---

with the rapid development of hypothyroidism is not uncommon and should be avoided particularly during pregnancy since it can cause fetal goitre.

A combination of carbimazole, 20 to 60 mg daily with thyroxine, 50 to 150 micrograms daily, may be used in a *blocking-replacement regimen*; therapy is again usually given for 18 months. The blocking-replacement regimen is **not** suitable during pregnancy.

Before partial thyroidectomy **iodine** may be given for 10 to 14 days in addition to carbimazole or propylthiouracil to assist control and reduce vascularity of the thyroid. Iodine should not be used for long-term treatment since its antithyroid action tends to diminish.

Radioactive sodium iodide (^{131}I) solution is used increasingly for the treatment of thyrotoxicosis at all ages, particularly where medical therapy or compliance is a problem, in patients with cardiac disease, and in patients who relapse after thyroidectomy.

Propranolol is useful for rapid relief of thyrotoxic symptoms and may be used in conjunction with antithyroid drugs or as an adjunct to radioactive iodine. Beta-blockers are also useful in neonatal thyrotoxicosis and in supraventricular arrhythmias due to hyperthyroidism. Propranolol may be used in conjunction with iodine to prepare mildly thyrotoxic patients for surgery but it is still preferable to make the patient euthyroid with carbimazole before surgery. Laboratory tests of thyroid function are not altered by beta-blockers. Most experience in treating thyrotoxicosis has been gained with propranolol but **nadolol** is also used. For doses and preparations of beta-blockers see section 2.4.

Thyrotoxic crisis ('thyroid storm') requires emergency treatment with intravenous administration of fluids, propranolol (5 mg) and hydrocortisone (100 mg every 6 hours, as sodium succinate), as well as oral iodine solution and carbimazole or propylthiouracil which may need to be administered by nasogastric tube.

PREGNANCY AND BREAST-FEEDING. Radioactive iodine therapy is contra-indicated during pregnancy. Propylthiouracil and carbimazole can be given but the blocking-replacement regimen (see above) is **not** suitable. Both propylthiouracil and carbimazole cross the placenta and in high doses may cause fetal goitre and hypothyroidism—the lowest dose that will control the hyperthyroid state should be used (requirements in Graves' disease tend to fall during pregnancy). Rarely, carbimazole has been associated with aplasia cutis of the neonate.

Carbimazole and propylthiouracil appear in breast milk but this does not preclude breast-feeding as long as neonatal development is closely monitored and the lowest effective dose is used.

CARBIMAZOLE

Indications: hyperthyroidism
Cautions: large goitre; liver disorders, pregnancy, breast-feeding (see notes)

Side-effects: nausea, mild gastrointestinal disturbances, headache, rashes and pruritus, arthralgia; rarely alopecia, agranulocytosis **(see CSM warning above)**, jaundice
Dose: see notes above

COUNSELLING. Warn patient to tell doctor immediately if sore throat, mouth ulcers, bruising, fever, malaise, or non-specific illness develops

PoM **Neo-Mercazole®** (Roche)
Tablets, both pink, carbimazole 5 mg, net price 100-tab pack = £3.01; 20 mg, 100-tab pack = £11.15. Counselling, blood disorder symptoms

IODINE AND IODIDE

Indications: thyrotoxicosis (pre-operative)
Cautions: pregnancy, children; not for long-term treatment
Contra-indications: breast feeding
Side-effects: hypersensitivity reactions including coryza-like symptoms, headache, lachrymation, conjunctivitis, pain in salivary glands, laryngitis, bronchitis, rashes; on prolonged treatment depression, insomnia, impotence; goitre in infants of mothers taking iodides

Aqueous Iodine Oral Solution (Lugol's Solution), iodine 5%, potassium iodide 10% in purified water, freshly boiled and cooled, total iodine 130 mg/mL. Net price 100 mL = £1.55. Label: 27
Dose: 0.1–0.3 mL 3 times daily well diluted with milk or water

PROPYLTHIOURACIL

Indications: hyperthyroidism
Cautions: see under Carbimazole; reduce dose in renal impairment (Appendix 3)
Side-effects: see under Carbimazole; urticaria, leucopenia; rarely cutaneous vasculitis, thrombocytopenia, aplastic anaemia, hepatitis, lupus erythematous-like syndromes
Dose: see notes above

PoM **Propylthiouracil** (Non-proprietary)
Tablets, propylthiouracil 50 mg. Net price 20 = £8.80
Available from CP, Hillcross, Norton

6.3 Corticosteroids
6.3.1 Replacement therapy
6.3.2 Glucocorticoid therapy

6.3.1 Replacement therapy

The adrenal cortex normally secretes hydrocortisone (cortisol) which has glucocorticoid activity and weak mineralocorticoid activity. It also secretes the mineralocorticoid aldosterone.

In deficiency states, physiological replacement is best achieved with a combination of **hydrocortisone** (section 6.3.2) and the mineralocorticoid **fludrocortisone**; hydrocortisone alone does not usually provide sufficient mineralocorticoid activity for complete replacement.

In *Addison's disease* or following adrenalectomy, **hydrocortisone** 20 to 30 mg daily by mouth is usually required. This is given in 2 doses, the larger in the morning and the smaller in the evening, mimicking the normal diurnal rhythm of cortisol secretion. The optimum daily dose is determined on the basis of clinical response. Glucocorticoid therapy is supplemented by fludrocortisone 50 to 300 micrograms daily.

In *acute adrenocortical insufficiency*, **hydrocortisone** is given intravenously (preferably as sodium succinate) in doses of 100 mg every 6 to 8 hours in sodium chloride intravenous infusion 0.9%.

In *hypopituitarism* glucocorticoids should be given as in adrenocortical insufficiency, but since the production of aldosterone is also regulated by the renin-angiotensin system a mineralocorticoid is not usually required. Additional replacement therapy with thyroxine (section 6.2.1) and sex hormones (section 6.4) should be given as indicated by the pattern of hormone deficiency.

Corticosteroid cover for *adrenalectomy*, for *hypophysectomy* or for operations on patients on long-term treatment with corticosteroids is determined logically from the knowledge that in a normal person major stress will not lead to the secretion of more than 300 mg of cortisol in 24 hours; once the stress is over, cortisol production rapidly returns to its usual level of approximately 20 mg per 24 hours. A simple way of mimicking this is to administer hydrocortisone. On the day of operation hydrocortisone 100 mg (usually as the sodium succinate) is given by intramuscular or intravenous injection with the premedication, and repeated every 8 hours. In the absence of complications, the dose can be halved every 24 hours until a normal maintenance dose of 20 to 30 mg per 24 hours is reached on the fifth postoperative day.

FLUDROCORTISONE ACETATE

Indications: mineralocorticoid replacement in adrenocortical insufficiency

Cautions; Contra-indications; Side-effects: section 6.3.2

Dose: adrenocortical insufficiency, 50–300 micrograms daily; CHILD 5 micrograms/kg daily

PoM **Florinef**® (Squibb)
Tablets, pink, scored, fludrocortisone acetate 100 micrograms. Net price 56-tab pack = £2.69. Label: 10 steroid card

6.3.2   Glucocorticoid therapy

In comparing the relative potencies of corticosteroids in terms of their anti-inflammatory (glucocorticoid) effects it should be borne in mind that high glucocorticoid activity in itself is of no advantage unless it occurs in conjunction with relatively low mineralocorticoid activity so that the effect on water and electrolytes is not also increased. The mineralocorticoid activity of **fludrocortisone** (section 6.3.1) is so high that its anti-inflammatory

activity is of no clinical relevance. The table below shows equivalent anti-inflammatory doses.

Equivalent Anti-inflammatory Doses of Corticosteroids

This table takes no account of mineralocorticoid effects, nor does it take account of variations in duration of action

Prednisolone 5 mg
≡ Betamethasone 750 micrograms
≡ Cortisone acetate 25 mg
≡ Deflazacort 6 mg
≡ Dexamethasone 750 micrograms
≡ Hydrocortisone 20 mg
≡ Methylprednisolone 4 mg
≡ Prednisone 5 mg
≡ Triamcinolone 4 mg

The mineralocorticoid effects of **cortisone** and **hydrocortisone** are too high for them to be used on a long-term basis for disease suppression since fluid retention would be too great, but they are suitable for adrenal replacement therapy (section 6.3.1); hydrocortisone is preferred because cortisone is only active after conversion in the liver to hydrocortisone. Hydrocortisone is used on a short-term basis by intravenous injection for the emergency management of some conditions. The relatively moderate anti-inflammatory potency of hydrocortisone also makes it a first-choice topical corticosteroid for the management of inflammatory skin conditions because side-effects (both topical and those associated with absorption) are less marked (see section 13.4); cortisone is not active topically.

Prednisolone has predominantly glucocorticoid activity and is the corticosteroid most commonly used by mouth for long-term disease suppression. **Prednisone** has a similar level of glucocorticoid activity but is only active after conversion in the liver to prednisolone; it is therefore not recommended.

Betamethasone and **dexamethasone** have very high glucocorticoid activity in conjunction with insignificant mineralocorticoid activity. This makes them particularly suitable for high-dose therapy in conditions where water retention would be a disadvantage (e.g. *cerebral oedema*).

They also have a long duration of action and this, coupled with their lack of mineralocorticoid action makes them particularly suitable for conditions which require suppression of corticotrophin secretion (e.g. *congenital adrenal hyperplasia*). Some esters of betamethasone and of **beclomethasone** exert a considerably more marked topical effect (e.g. on the skin or the lungs) than when given by mouth; use is made of this to obtain topical effects without corresponding systemic activity (e.g. for skin applications and asthma inhalations).

Deflazacort is a newly introduced corticosteroid with high glucocorticoid activity; it is derived from prednisolone.

DISADVANTAGES OF CORTICOSTEROIDS

Overdosage or prolonged use may exaggerate some of the normal physiological actions of corticoster-

---

oids leading to mineralocorticoid and glucocorticoid side-effects.

Mineralocorticoid side-effects include *hypertension, sodium and water retention and potassium loss*. They are most marked with fludrocortisone, but are significant with cortisone, hydrocortisone, corticotrophin, and tetracosactrin. Mineralocorticoid actions are negligible with the high potency glucocorticoids, betamethasone and dexamethasone, and occur only slightly with methylprednisolone, prednisolone, prednisone, and triamcinolone.

Glucocorticoid side-effects include *diabetes* and *osteoporosis*, which is a danger, particularly in the elderly, as it may result in osteoporotic fractures for example of the hip or vertebrae; in addition administration of high doses is associated with *avascular necrosis* of the femoral head. *Mental disturbances* may occur; a serious paranoid state or depression with risk of suicide may be induced, particularly in patients with a history of mental disorder. *Euphoria* is frequently observed. *Muscle wasting* (proximal myopathy) may also occur. Corticosteroid therapy is also weakly linked with *peptic ulceration* (the potential advantage of soluble or enteric-coated preparations to reduce the risk is speculative only).

High doses of corticosteroids may cause *Cushing's syndrome*, with moon face, striae, and acne; it is usually reversible on withdrawal of treatment, but this must always be gradually tapered to avoid symptoms of acute adrenal insufficiency (**important:** see also Adrenal Suppression p. 314).

In children, administration of corticosteroids may result in *suppression of growth*. Corticosteroids given in high dosage during *pregnancy* may affect adrenal development in the child (but see also Appendix 4).

Modification of tissue reactions may result in spread of *infection*; suppression of clinical signs may allow diseases such as septicaemia or tuberculosis to reach an advanced stage before being recognised—**important:** see also Infections p. 314.

Adrenal atrophy can persist for years after stopping prolonged corticosteroid therapy, therefore any illness or surgical emergency may require temporary reintroduction of corticosteroid therapy to compensate for lack of sufficient adrenocortical response. Anaesthetists **must** therefore know whether a patient is taking or has been taking corticosteroids to avoid a precipitous fall in blood pressure during anaesthesia or in the immediate postoperative period. Patients should therefore carry cards giving details of their dosage and possible complications.

> Following concern about severe chickenpox associated with systemic corticosteroids, the CSM has issued a notice that **every** patient prescribed a *systemic* corticosteroid should receive the patient information leaflet supplied by the relevant manufacturer. Steroid cards may not be available currently; new cards may become available with revised wording.

For other references to the adverse effects of corticosteroids see section 11.4 (eye) and section 13.4 (skin).

CLINICAL MANAGEMENT

Dosage of corticosteroids varies widely in different diseases and in different patients. If the use of a corticosteroid can save or prolong life, as in *exfoliative dermatitis, pemphigus, acute leukaemia* or *acute transplant rejection*, high doses may need to be given, because the complications of therapy are likely to be less serious than the effects of the disease itself.

When long-term corticosteroid therapy is used in relatively benign chronic diseases such as *rheumatoid arthritis* the danger of treatment may become greater than the disabilities produced by the disease. To minimise side-effects the maintenance dose should be kept as low as possible (see also section 10.1.2.1).

When potentially less harmful measures are ineffective corticosteroids are used topically for the treatment of *inflammatory conditions of the skin* (section 13.4). Corticosteroids should be avoided or used only under specialist supervision in *psoriasis* (section 13.5).

Corticosteroids are used both topically (by rectum) and systemically (by mouth or intravenously) in the management of *ulcerative colitis* and *Crohn's disease* (section 1.5 and section 1.7.2).

Use can be made of the mineralocorticoid activity of fludrocortisone to treat *postural hypotension* in autonomic neuropathy (section 6.1.5).

Very high doses of corticosteroids have been given by intravenous injection in *septic shock*. However a recent study (using methylprednisolone sodium succinate) did not demonstrate efficacy and, moreover, suggested a higher mortality in some subsets of patients given the high-dose corticosteroid therapy.

Dexamethasone and betamethasone have little if any mineralocorticoid action and their long duration of action makes them particularly suitable for suppressing corticotrophin secretion in *congenital adrenal hyperplasia* where the dose should be tailored to clinical response and by measurement of adrenal androgens and 17-hydroxyprogesterone. In common with all glucocorticoids their suppressive action on the hypothalamic-pituitary-adrenal axis is greatest and most prolonged when they are given at night. In most normal subjects a single dose of 1 mg of dexamethasone at night, depending on weight, is sufficient to inhibit corticotrophin secretion for 24 hours. This is the basis of the 'overnight dexamethasone suppression test' for diagnosing Cushing's syndrome.

Betamethasone and dexamethasone are also appropriate for conditions where water retention would be a disadvantage, as for example in treating traumatic *cerebral oedema* with doses of 12 to 20 mg daily.

In acute hypersensitivity reactions such as *angioedema* of the upper respiratory tract and *anaphylactic shock*, corticosteroids are indicated as an adjunct to emergency treatment with adrenaline (section 3.4.3). In such cases hydrocortisone (as sodium succinate) by intravenous injection in a dose of 100 to 300 mg may be required.

Corticosteroids are preferably used by inhalation in the management of *asthma* (section 3.2) but systemic therapy in association with bronchodilators is required for the emergency treatment of severe acute asthma (section 3.1.1).

Corticosteroids may also be useful in conditions such as *rheumatic fever*, *chronic active hepatitis*, and *sarcoidosis*; they may also lead to remissions of acquired *haemolytic anaemia*, and some cases of the *nephrotic syndrome* (particularly in children) and *thrombocytopenic purpura*.

Corticosteroids can improve the prognosis of serious conditions such as *systemic lupus erythematosus*, *temporal arteritis*, and *polyarteritis nodosa*; the effects of the disease process may be suppressed and symptoms relieved, but the underlying condition is not cured, although it may ultimately burn itself out. It is usual to begin therapy in these conditions at fairly high dose, such as 40 to 60 mg prednisolone daily, and then to reduce the dose to the lowest commensurate with disease control.

For other references to the use of corticosteroids see section 11.4 (eye), section 12.1.1 (otitis externa), section 12.2.1 (allergic rhinitis), and section 12.3.1 (aphthous ulcers).

ADMINISTRATION

Whenever possible *local treatment* with creams, intra-articular injections, inhalations, eye-drops, or enemas should be used in preference to *systemic treatment*. The suppressive action of a corticosteroid on cortisol secretion is least when it is given in the morning, therefore in an attempt to reduce pituitary-adrenal suppression a corticosteroid (usually prednisolone) should normally be taken as a single dose in the morning. In an attempt to reduce pituitary-adrenal suppression further, the total dose for two days can sometimes be taken as a single dose on alternate days; alternate-day administration has not been very successful in the management of asthma (section 3.2). Pituitary-adrenal suppression can also be reduced by means of intermittent therapy with short courses. In some conditions it may be possible to reduce the dose of corticosteroid by adding a small dose of an immunosuppressive drug (section 8.2.1).

PREDNISOLONE

Indications: suppression of inflammatory and allergic disorders; see also notes above; inflammatory bowel disease, section 1.5; asthma, section 3.2; immunosuppression, section 8.2.2; rheumatic disease, section 10.1.2

Cautions: adrenal suppression (see below), infection (see below), children and adolescents (growth retardation which may be irreversible—prolonged or continuous treatment rarely justified), elderly (side-effects more serious—close supervision required particularly on long-term

treatment); frequent monitoring required in those with history of tuberculosis (or X-ray changes), hypertension, recent myocardial infarction (rupture reported), congestive heart failure, liver failure, renal impairment, diabetes mellitus including family history, osteoporosis (post-menopausal women at special risk), glaucoma (including family history), severe affective disorders (particularly those with previous history of steroid-induced psychosis), epilepsy, peptic ulceration, hypothyroidism, history of steroid myopathy; pregnancy and breast-feeding (see Appendixes 4 and 5); **interactions:** Appendix 1 (corticosteroids)

ADRENAL SUPPRESSION. During prolonged therapy *adrenal atrophy* may develop and persist for years after stopping. Abrupt withdrawal after a prolonged period may lead to adrenal insufficiency, hypotension or death; however in most asthma patients (who continue to receive other appropriate treatment, section 3.1), abrupt withdrawal after courses of up to 3 weeks has not resulted in adverse effects. Where withdrawal needs to be gradual the dose must be tapered off over weeks or months depending on dosage and duration of therapy. Withdrawal may also be associated with fever, myalgia, arthralgia, rhinitis, conjunctivitis, painful itchy skin nodules and loss of weight.

Any significant intercurrent illness, trauma, or surgical procedure requires a temporary increase in dosage, or if already stopped, a temporary re-introduction of corticosteroid.

Patients should carry a steroid treatment card giving clear guidance on precautions to be taken to minimise risk and providing details of prescriber, drug, dosage and duration of treatment.

INFECTIONS. Susceptibility and severity of infections may be increased and clinical presentation may be atypical. Serious infections such as *septicaemia* and *tuberculosis* may reach an advanced stage before being recognised. *Amoebiasis* or *strongyloidiasis* may be activated or exacerbated (exclude before initiating corticosteroid in those at risk or with suggestive symptoms). *Ocular infections* (fungal or viral) may also be exacerbated (see also section 11.4.1).

Chickenpox: unless they have had chickenpox, patients receiving oral or parenteral corticosteroids for purposes other than replacement should be regarded as being *at risk of severe chickenpox*. Manifestations of fulminant illness include pneumonia, hepatitis and disseminated intravascular coagulation; rash is not necessarily a prominent feature. Patients (or parents of children) at risk should be advised *to avoid close personal contact* with chickenpox or herpes zoster and *to seek urgent medical attention* if exposed to chickenpox. Passive immunisation with varicella-zoster immunoglobulin (see section 14.5) is needed by exposed non-immune patients receiving systemic corticosteroids or who have used them within the previous 3 months (preferably given within 3 days of exposure and not later than 10 days). If chickenpox is confirmed, the illness warrants specialist care and urgent treatment. Corticosteroids should not be stopped (dosage may need to be increased). Currently there is no good evidence that topical, inhaled or rectal corticosteroids are associated with an increased risk of severe chickenpox.

Measles: Patients should be advised to take particular care to avoid exposure to measles and to seek medical advice without delay if exposure occurs; prophylaxis with intramuscular normal immunoglobulin (see section 14.5) may be needed.

Contra-indications: systemic infection (unless specific antimicrobial therapy given); avoid live virus vaccines in those receiving immunosuppressive doses (serum antibody response diminshed)

Side-effects: minimised by using lowest effective dose for minimum period possible; *gastro-intestinal effects* include dyspepsia, peptic ulceration (with perforation), abdominal distension, acute pancreatitis, oesophageal ulceration and candidiasis; *musculoskeletal effects* include proximal myopathy, osteoporosis, vertebral and long bone fractures, avascular osteonecrosis, tendon rupture; *endocrine effects* include adrenal suppression, menstrual irregularities and amenorrhoea, Cushing's syndrome (with high doses, usually reversible on withdrawal), hirsutism, weight gain, negative nitrogen and calcium balance, increased appetite; increased susceptibility to and severity of infection; *neuropsychiatric effects* include euphoria, psychological dependence, depression, insomnia, increased intracranial pressure with papilloedema in children (usually after withdrawal), psychosis and aggravation of schizophrenia, aggravation of epilepsy; *ophthalmic effects* include glaucoma, papilloedema, posterior subcapsular cataracts, corneal or scleral thinning and exacerbation of ophthalmic viral or fungal disease; *other side-effects* include impaired healing, skin atrophy, bruising, striae, telangiectasia, acne, myocardial rupture following recent myocardial infarction, fluid and electrolyte disturbance, leucocytosis, hypersensitivity reactions (including anaphylaxis), thromboembolism, nausea, malaise, hiccups

Dose: by mouth, initially, up to 10–20 mg daily (severe disease, up to 60 mg daily), preferably taken in the morning after breakfast; can often be reduced within a few days but may need to be continued for several weeks or months

Maintenance, usual range, 2.5–15 mg daily, but higher doses may be needed; cushingoid side-effects increasingly likely with doses above 7.5 mg daily

By intramuscular injection, prednisolone acetate, 25–100 mg once or twice weekly (for preparation see section 10.1.2.2)

PoM **Prednisolone** (Non-proprietary)
Tablets, prednisolone 1 mg, net price 20 = 19p; 5 mg, 20 = 31p. Label: 10 steroid card, 21
Available from APS, Cox, CP, Hillcross, Norton, Hoechst Marion Roussel (Precortisyl®)
Tablets, both e/c, prednisolone 2.5 mg (brown), net price 30-tab pack = 26p; 5 mg (red), 30-tab pack = 43p. Label: 5, 10 steroid card, 25
Available from APS, Biorex, Cox, Lagap, Norton (2.5 mg), Pfizer (Deltacortril Enteric®)
Injection, see section 10.1.2.2
PoM **Precortisyl Forte®** (Hoechst Marion Roussel)
Tablets, scored, prednisolone 25 mg. Net price 56-tab pack = £4.26. Label: 10 steroid card, 21
PoM **Prednesol®** (GlaxoWellcome)
Tablets, pink, scored, soluble, prednisolone 5 mg (as sodium phosphate). Net price 100-tab pack = £5.76. Label: 10 steroid card,13, 21

BETAMETHASONE

Indications: suppression of inflammatory and allergic disorders; congenital adrenal hyperplasia; cerebral oedema; see also notes above; ear, section 12.1.1; eye, section 11.4.1; nose, section 12.2.1

Cautions; Contra-indications; Side-effects: see notes above and under Prednisolone

Dose: by mouth, usual range 0.5–5 mg daily. See also Administration (above)

By intramuscular injection or slow intravenous injection or infusion, 4–20 mg, repeated up to 4 times in 24 hours; CHILD, *by slow intravenous injection,* up to 1 year 1 mg, 1–5 years 2 mg, 6–12 years 4 mg

PoM **Betnelan®** (Evans)
Tablets, scored, betamethasone 500 micrograms. Net price 100-tab pack – £3.63. Label: 10 steroid card, 21
PoM **Betnesol®** (Evans)
Tablets, pink, scored, soluble, betamethasone 500 micrograms (as sodium phosphate). Net price 100-tab pack = £3.20. Label: 10 steroid card, 13, 21
Injection, betamethasone 4 mg (as sodium phosphate)/mL. Net price 1-mL amp = 65p. Label: 10 steroid card

CORTISONE ACETATE

Indications: see under Dose but now superseded, see also notes above
Cautions; Contra-indications; Side-effects: see notes above and under Prednisolone
Dose: by mouth, for replacement therapy, 25 37.5 mg daily in divided doses

PoM **Cortisyl®** (Hoechst Marion Roussel)
Tablets, scored, cortisone acetate 25 mg. Net price 56-tab pack = £3.24. Label: 10 steroid card, 21

DEFLAZACORT

Indications: suppression of inflammatory and allergic disorders
Cautions; Contra-indications; Side-effects: see notes above and under Prednisolone
Dose: usual maintenance 3–18 mg daily (acute disorders, initially up to 120 mg daily). See also Administration (above)
CHILD 0.25–1.5 mg/kg daily (or on alternate days). See also Administration (above).

▼ PoM **Calcort®** (Shire)
Tablets, deflazacort 6 mg, net price 60-tab pack = £20.57; 30 mg, 30-tab pack = £28.50. Label: 5, 10 steroid card

DEXAMETHASONE

Indications: suppression of inflammatory and allergic disorders; shock; diagnosis of Cushing's disease, congenital adrenal hyperplasia; cerebral oedema; see also notes above; rheumatic disease, section 10.1.2; eye, section 11.4.1

Cautions; Contra-indications; Side-effects: see notes above and under Prednisolone; perineal irritation may follow intravenous administration of the phosphate ester

Dose: by mouth, usual range 0.5–10 mg daily. See also Administration (above)

Chemotherapy emesis, see section 8.1

By intramuscular injection or slow intravenous injection or infusion (as dexamethasone phosphate), initially 0.5–20 mg; CHILD 200–500 micrograms/kg daily

Cerebral oedema (as dexamethasone phosphate), *by intravenous injection,* 10 mg initially, then 4 mg *by intramuscular injection* every 6 hours as required for 2–10 days

PoM **Dexamethasone** (Organon)

Tablets, dexamethasone 500 micrograms, net price 20 = 64p; 2 mg, 20 = £1.73. Label: 10 steroid card, 21

Injection, dexamethasone sodium phosphate 5 mg/mL (≡ dexamethasone 4 mg/mL ≡ dexamethasone phosphate 4.8 mg/mL). Net price 1-mL amp = 83p; 2-mL vial = £1.27. Label: 10 steroid card

PoM **Decadron®** (MSD)

Tablets, scored, dexamethasone 500 micrograms. Net price 30-tab pack = 96p. Label: 10 steroid card, 21

Injection, dexamethasone phosphate 4 mg/mL (≡ dexamethasone 3.33 mg/mL ≡ dexamethasone sodium phosphate 4.17 mg/mL). Net price 2-mL vial = £1.76. Label: 10 steroid card

Note. Injection containing dexamethasone phosphate 4 mg/mL (as sodium phosphate) is also available from Faulding DBL

PoM **Decadron Shock-Pak®** (MSD)

Injection, dexamethasone 20 mg/mL (≡ dexamethasone sodium phosphate 25 mg/mL). Net price 5-mL vial = £15.13. Label: 10 steroid card

Note. Injection containing dexamethasone 20 mg/mL is also available from Faulding DBL

Dose: shock, by intravenous injection or infusion, 2–6 mg/kg, repeated if necessary after 2–6 hours (but see section 6.3.2)

HYDROCORTISONE

Indications: adrenocortical insufficiency (section 6.3.1); shock; see also notes above; hypersensitivity reactions (such as anaphylactic shock and angioedema), section 3.4.5; inflammatory bowel disease, section 1.5; haemorrhoids, section 1.7.2; rheumatic disease, section 10.1.2; eye, 11.4.1; skin, section 13.4

Cautions; Contra-indications; Side-effects: see notes above and under Prednisolone; perineal irritation may follow intravenous administration of the phosphate ester

Dose: by mouth, replacement therapy, 20–30 mg daily in divided doses—see section 6.3.1; CHILD 10–30 mg

By intramuscular injection or slow intravenous injection or infusion, 100–500 mg, 3–4 times in 24 hours or as required; CHILD *by slow intravenous injection* up to 1 year 25 mg, 1–5 years 50 mg, 6–12 years 100 mg

PoM **Hydrocortone®** (MSD)

Tablets, scored, hydrocortisone 10 mg, net price 30-tab pack = 70p; 20 mg, 30-tab pack = £1.07. Label: 10 steroid card, 21

PoM **Efcortesol®** (GlaxoWellcome)

Injection, hydrocortisone 100 mg (as sodium phosphate)/mL. Net price 1-mL amp = 75p; 5-mL amp = £3.40. Label: 10 steroid card

Note. Perineal irritation may follow intravenous injection of the phosphate ester

PoM **Solu-Cortef®** (Pharmacia & Upjohn)

Injection, powder for reconstitution, hydrocortisone (as sodium succinate). Net price 100-mg vial (with 2-mL amp water for injections) = £1.02; without water for injections = 96p. Label: 10 steroid card

METHYLPREDNISOLONE

Indications: suppression of inflammatory and allergic disorders; cerebral oedema; see also notes above; rheumatic disease, section 10.1.2; skin, section 13.4

Cautions; Contra-indications; Side-effects: see notes above and under Prednisolone; rapid intravenous administration of large doses has been associated with cardiovascular collapse

Dose: by mouth, usual range 2–40 mg daily. See also Administration (above)

By intramuscular injection or slow intravenous injection or infusion, initially 10–500 mg; graft rejection, up to 1 g daily *by intravenous infusion* for up to 3 days

PoM **Methylprednisolone** (Non-proprietary)

Injection, powder for reconstitution, methylprednisolone (as sodium succinate). Net price 500-mg vial = £14.85; 1-g vial = £28.28

Available from Faulding DBL

PoM **Medrone®** (Pharmacia & Upjohn)

Tablets, scored, methylprednisolone 2 mg (pink), net price 30-tab pack = £2.69; 4 mg, 30-tab pack = £5.16; 16 mg, 30-tab pack = £14.31; 100 mg (blue), 20-tab pack = £40.27. Label: 10 steroid card, 21

PoM **Solu-Medrone®** (Pharmacia & Upjohn)

Injection, powder for reconstitution, methylprednisolone (as sodium succinate) (all with solvent). Net price 40-mg vial = £1.32; 125-mg vial = £3.96; 500-mg vial = £8.00; 1-g vial = £14.42; 2-g vial = £27.38. Label: 10 steroid card

Intramuscular depot

PoM **Depo-Medrone®** (Pharmacia & Upjohn)

Injection (aqueous suspension), methylprednisolone acetate 40 mg/mL. Net price 1-mL vial = £2.73; 2-mL vial = £4.90; 3-mL vial = £7.11. Label: 10 steroid card

Dose: by deep intramuscular injection into gluteal muscle, 40–120 mg, a second injection may be given after 2–3 weeks if required

PREDNISONE

Indications: suppression of inflammatory and allergic disorders; see also notes above

Cautions; Contra-indications; Side-effects: see notes above and under Prednisolone; avoid in liver disease

Dose: see Prednisolone

PoM **Prednisone** (Non-proprietary)

Tablets, prednisone 5 mg, net price 20 = 47p. Label: 10 steroid card, 21

TRIAMCINOLONE

Indications: suppression of inflammatory and allergic disorders; see also notes above; rheumatic disease, section 10.1.2; mouth, section 12.3.1; skin, section 13.4

Cautions; Contra-indications; Side-effects: see notes above and under Prednisolone; triamcinolone in high dosage has a greater tendency to cause proximal myopathy and should be avoided in chronic therapy

Dose: by deep intramuscular injection, into gluteal muscle, 40 mg of acetonide for depot effect, repeated at intervals according to the patient's response; max. single dose 100 mg

PoM **Kenalog**® (Squibb)

Injection (aqueous suspension), triamcinolone acetonide 40 mg/mL. Net price 1-mL vial (intramuscular/intra-articular) = £1.70; 1-mL syringe (intramuscular only) – £2.11; 2-mL syringe (intramuscular only) = £3.66. Label: 10 steroid card

6.4 Sex hormones

Sex hormones are described under the following section headings:

6.4.1 Female sex hormones
6.4.2 Male sex hormones and antagonists
6.4.3 Anabolic steroids

6.4.1 Female sex hormones

6.4.1.1 Oestrogens and HRT
6.4.1.2 Progestogens

6.4.1.1 OESTROGENS AND HRT

Oestrogens are necessary for the development of female secondary sexual characteristics; they also stimulate myometrial hypertrophy with endometrial hyperplasia.

In terms of oestrogenic activity *natural oestrogens* (oestradiol (estradiol), oestrone (estrone), and oestriol (estriol)) have a more appropriate profile for hormone replacement therapy (HRT) than *synthetic oestrogens* (ethinyloestradiol (ethinylestradiol), mestranol, and stilboestrol (diethylstilbestrol)); the profile of *conjugated oestrogens* resembles that of natural oestrogens.

Oestrogen therapy is given cyclically or continuously for a number of gynaecological conditions. If long-term therapy is required a progestogen should

be added to prevent cystic hyperplasia of the endometrium and possible transformation to cancer. This addition of a progestogen is not necessary if the patient has had a hysterectomy or in the case of tibolone.

Oestrogens are no longer used to *suppress lactation* because of their association with thromboembolism.

HORMONE REPLACEMENT THERAPY

Menopausal *vasomotor symptoms* and menopausal *vaginitis* are alleviated by administration of small doses of oestrogen. There is also good evidence that small doses of oestrogen given for several years starting in the perimenopausal period will diminish postmenopausal *osteoporosis* and reduce the incidence of *stroke and myocardial infarction.* There is an increased risk of *endometrial cancer* (countered by a progestogen) and, after some years of use, possibly an increased risk of *breast cancer* (see below).

Hormone replacement therapy (HRT) is indicated for menopausal women whose lives are inconvenienced by *vaginal atrophy* or *vasomotor instability.* Vaginal atrophy may respond to a short course of vaginal oestrogen preparation given for a few weeks and repeated if necessary. Systemic therapy is needed for vasomotor symptoms and should be given for at least a year; in a woman with a uterus a progestogen should be added to reduce the risk of endometrial cancer. HRT is also indicated for women with *early natural or surgical menopause (before age 45),* since they are at high risk of osteoporosis; HRT should be given to the age of at least 50 and possibly for a further 10 years (but risk of breast cancer, see below).

Long-term HRT is almost certainly favourable in risk-benefit terms for menopausal women *without a uterus* because they do not require progestogen therapy; it should probably be continued for about 10 years (but risk of breast cancer, see below). The picture is less clear for menopausal women *with a uterus* because the need for administration of progestogen may blunt the protective effect of low-dose oestrogen against myocardial infarction and stroke; any effect of the progestogen (favourable or otherwise) on breast cancer is not yet known. Nevertheless, risk factors for osteoporosis should be borne in mind and, if there are several, consideration given to HRT. Risk factors include recent corticosteroid therapy or any disease predisposing to osteoporosis, family history, thinness, lack of exercise, alcoholism or smoking, and fracture of a hip or forearm before the age of 65; women of Afro-Caribbean origin appear to be less susceptible than those who are white or of Asian origin.

RISK OF BREAST CANCER. Following publication of an analysis of pooled original data, the CSM has advised that the increased risk of breast cancer is related to the duration of HRT use and that this excess risk disappears within about 5 years of stopping. Women who use HRT for a short time around the menopause have a very low excess risk. Breast cancers in HRT users were less likely to have spread beyond the breast than those in non-users.

About 45 in every 1000 women aged 50 years not using HRT will have breast cancer diagnosed over the next 20 years; in those using HRT for 5 years, this figure rises by 2 extra cases in 1000, in those using HRT for 10 years 6 extra cases in 1000 and in those using HRT for 15 years 12 extra cases in 1000.

The CSM's view is that these results do not provide a reason for women to stop their treatment but the results do emphasise the importance of breast awareness and regular mammograms.

RISK OF VENOUS THROMBOEMBOLISM. Recent studies show an increased risk of deep vein thrombosis and of pulmonary embolism in women currently taking HRT. The view of the CSM is that the new data do not change the overall positive balance between benefits and risks of treatment for most women. The CSM has advised that there is no need for *women without predisposing factors* for venous thromboembolism to stop taking HRT. In *women who have predisposing factors* (such as a personal or family history of deep vein thrombosis or pulmonary embolism, severe varicose veins, obesity, surgery, trauma or prolonged bed-rest) it may be prudent to review the need for HRT as in some cases the risks of HRT may be expected to exceed the benefits.

CHOICE. The choice of oestrogen for HRT is not straightforward and depends on an overall balance of indication, risk, and convenience. Oestrogen deficient vaginitis in a woman with a uterus can be treated for only a few weeks with an oestrogen, without addition of cyclical progestogen; this constraint includes vaginal preparations (section 7.2.1) since a significant amount is absorbed through the vaginal mucosa. Oestrogen therapy alone is suitable for long-term continuous therapy in a woman without a uterus. A woman with a uterus requires oestrogen with cyclical progestogen for the last 10 to 13 days of the cycle (or administration of a preparation which combines both oestrogenic and progestogenic activity). Oral preparations of oestrogen are subject to first-pass metabolism, therefore subcutaneous or transdermal administration reflects more closely endogenous hormone activity. In the case of subcutaneous implants, recurrence of vasomotor symptoms at supraphysiological plasma concentrations may occur; moreover, there is evidence of prolonged endometrial stimulation after discontinuation (calling for continued cyclical progestogen).

Provided that calcium intake is adequate calcium supplements (section 9.5.1) do not confer additional benefit on HRT.

CONTRACEPTION. HRT does **not** provide contraception and a woman is considered potentially fertile for *2 years after her last menstrual period* if she is *under 50 years*, and for *1 year* if she is *over 50 years*. A woman who is under 50 years and free of

all risk factors for venous and arterial disease can use a low-oestrogen combined oral contraceptive pill (section 7.3.1) to provide both *relief of menopausal symptoms* and *contraception*; it is recommended that the oral contraceptive be stopped at 50 years of age since there are more suitable alternatives. If any potentially fertile woman needs to use HRT, *non-hormonal contraceptive measures* (such as condoms, or by this age, contraceptive foam, section 7.3.3) are necessary.

Although follicle-stimulating hormone (FSH) measurements can be used as a guide to determine fertility, high measurements on their own (particularly under the age of 50 years) do not necessarily correlate with ovarian failure. Thus, a woman *aged 50 years using HRT* who has a raised FSH measurement (possibly only to about 25 units/litre) during the oestrogen-only phase should continue to use non-hormonal contraceptive measures. After stopping the HRT she should have two further measurements in the next month. If these FSH measurements are above 40 units/litre and the woman has menopausal symptoms the chances of ovulation appear to be low enough to discontinue all contraception. Similarly, a woman *aged 50 years using the combined oral contraceptive pill*, with a raised FSH measurement at the end of the 7-day pill-free interval, should stop the pill and use a non-hormonal contraceptive pending further measurements; two further high measurements in the month after stopping, together with menopausal symptoms, are an indication of an extremely low probability of conception.

SURGERY. Surgery is a predisposing factor for venous thromboembolism and it may be prudent to review the need for HRT (see above). Oestrogenic activity may persist after discontinuation of oestradiol implants (see above).

OESTROGENS FOR HRT

Note. Relates only to small amounts of oestrogens given for hormone replacement therapy

Indications: see notes above and under preparations

Cautions: prolonged exposure to unopposed oestrogens may increase risk of development of endometrial cancer (see notes above); migraine (or migraine-like headaches); history of breast nodules or fibrocystic disease—closely monitor breast status (risk of breast cancer, see notes above); pre-existing uterine fibroids may increase in size, symptoms of endometriosis may be exacerbated; predisposing factors to thromboembolism (see notes above); increased risk of gall bladder disease reported; porphyria (see section 9.8.2); **interactions:** Appendix 1 (oestrogens)

OTHER CONDITIONS. The product literature advises caution in other conditions including hypertension, cardiac or renal disease, diabetes, asthma, epilepsy, melanoma, otosclerosis, multiple sclerosis and systemic lupus erythematosus. Evidence for caution in these conditions is unsatisfactory and many women with these conditions may stand to benefit from HRT.

Contra-indications: pregnancy; oestrogen-dependent cancer, active thrombophlebitis or thromboembolic disorders, liver disease (where liver function tests have failed to return to normal), Dubin-Johnson and Rotor syndromes (or monitor closely), undiagnosed vaginal bleeding, breast-feeding

Side-effects: nausea and vomiting, weight changes, breast enlargement and tenderness, pre-menstrual-like syndrome, fluid retention, changes in liver function, cholestatic jaundice, rashes and chloasma, depression, headache, contact lenses may irritate; transdermal delivery systems may cause contact sensitisation (possible severe hypersensitivity reaction on continued exposure), and headache has been reported on vigorous exercise

WITHDRAWAL BLEEDING. Cyclical HRT (where a progestogen is taken for 10–14 days of each 28-day oestrogen treatment cycle) usually results in a *regular withdrawal bleed* towards the end of the progestogen. The aim of continuous combined HRT (where a combination of oestrogen and progestogen is taken, usually in a single tablet, throughout each 28-day treatment cycle) is to avoid bleeding, but *irregular bleeding* may occur during the early treatment stages (if it continues endometrial abnormality should be excluded and consideration given to cyclical HRT instead)

Dose: see under preparations

COUNSELLING ON PATCHES. Patch should be removed after 3–4 days (or once a week in case of 7-day patch) and replaced with fresh patch on slightly different site; recommended sites: clean, dry, unbroken areas of skin on trunk below waistline; not to be applied on or near breasts or under waistband. If patch falls off in bath allow skin to cool before applying new patch

---

Women with Uterus

The following preparations contain a **progestogen** as well as an **oestrogen** and are therefore suitable for a woman with an **intact uterus**; they are **not** suitable for use as (or with) hormonal contraceptives

Conjugated oestrogens with progestogen

PoM **Premique®** (Wyeth)

Premique® tablets, s/c, blue, conjugated oestrogen 625 micrograms, medroxyprogesterone acetate 5 mg. Net price 3 × 28-tab pack = £22.62

Dose: menopausal symptoms and osteoporosis prophylaxis, if uterus intact, 1 tablet daily on a continuous basis, starting on 1st day of menstruation (or any time if cycles have ceased or are infrequent)

Note. Unsuitable for use in perimenopausal women or within 12 months of last menstrual period; may cause irregular bleeding in early stages of treatment—if bleeding continues exclude endometrial abnormality and consider changing to cycle therapy, see below

Premique® Cycle Calendar pack, 28 maroon (s/c) tablets, conjugated oestrogens 625 micrograms; 14 white tablets, medroxyprogesterone acetate 10 mg. Net price 3 × 42-tab pack = £22.62

Dose: menopausal symptoms and osteoporosis prophylaxis, if uterus intact, 1 maroon tablet daily on a continuous basis starting on 1st day of menstruation (or at any time if cycles have ceased or are infrequent) and 1 white tablet daily on days 15–28 of each 28-day treatment cycle; subsequent courses are repeated without interval

PoM **Prempak-C®** (Wyeth)

Prempak C® 0.625 Calendar pack, all s/c, 28 maroon tablets, conjugated oestrogens 625 micrograms; 12 light brown tablets, norgestrel 150 micrograms (≡ levonorgestrel 75 micrograms). Net price 3 × 40-tab pack = £13.38

Dose: menopausal symptoms and osteoporosis prophylaxis, if uterus intact, 1 maroon tablet daily on continuous basis, starting on 1st day of menstruation (or at any time if cycles have ceased or are infrequent), and 1 brown tablet daily on days 17–28 of each 28-day treatment cycle; subsequent courses are repeated without interval

Prempak C® 1.25 Calendar pack, all s/c, 28 yellow tablets, conjugated oestrogens 1.25 mg; 12 light brown tablets, norgestrel 150 micrograms (≡ levonorgestrel 75 micrograms). Net price 3 × 40-tab pack = £13.38

Dose: see under 0.625 Calendar pack, but taking 1 yellow tablet daily on continuous basis (instead of 1 maroon tablet) if symptoms not fully controlled with lower strength

Mestranol with progestogen

PoM **Menophase®** (Searle)

Tablets, 5 pink, mestranol 12.5 micrograms; 8 orange, mestranol 25 micrograms; 2 yellow, mestranol 50 micrograms; 3 green, mestranol 25 micrograms and norethisterone 1 mg; 6 blue, mestranol 30 micrograms and norethisterone 1.5 mg; 4 lavender, mestranol 20 micrograms and norethisterone 750 micrograms. Net price per pack = £3.25

Dose: menopausal symptoms and osteoporosis prophylaxis, if uterus intact 1 tablet daily, starting with a pink tablet on Sunday, then in sequence (without interruption)

Oestradiol with progestogen

PoM **Climagest®** (Novartis)

Climagest® 1-mg tablets, 16 grey-blue, oestradiol valerate 1 mg; 12 white, oestradiol valerate 1 mg and norethisterone 1 mg. Net price 28-tab pack = £4.38; 3 × 28-tab pack = £12.75

Dose: menopausal symptoms, 1 grey-blue tablet daily for 16 days, starting on 1st day of menstruation (or at any time if cycles have ceased or are infrequent) then 1 white tablet for 12 days; subsequent courses are repeated without interval

Climagest® 2-mg tablets, 16 blue, oestradiol valerate 2 mg; 12 yellow, oestradiol valerate 2 mg and norethisterone 1 mg. Net price 28-tab pack = £4.38; 3 × 28-tab pack = £12.75

Dose: see Climagest® 1-mg, but starting with 1 blue tablet daily (instead of 1 grey-blue tablet) if symptoms not controlled with lower strength

PoM **Climesse®** (Novartis)

Tablets, pink, oestradiol valerate 2 mg, norethisterone 700 micrograms. Net price 1 × 28-tab pack = £7.90; 3 × 28-tab pack = £23.70

Dose: menopausal symptoms and osteoporosis prophylaxis, if uterus intact, 1 tablet daily on a continuous basis

Note. Unsuitable for use in the perimenopause or within 12 months of the last menstrual period; may cause irregular bleeding in early stages of treatment—if bleeding continues exclude endometrial abnormality and consider changing to cyclical HRT

PoM **Cyclo-Progynova®** (ASTA Medica)

Cyclo-Progynova® 1-mg Tablets, all s/c, 11 beige, oestradiol valerate 1 mg; 10 brown, oestradiol valerate 1 mg and levonorgestrel 250 micrograms. Net price per pack = £3.50

Dose: menopausal symptoms, if uterus intact, 1 beige tablet daily for 11 days, starting on 5th day of menstruation (or at any time if cycles have ceased or are infre-

---

quent), then 1 brown tablet daily for 10 days, followed by a 7-day interval

Cyclo-Progynova® 2-mg Tablets, all s/c, 11 white, oestradiol valerate 2 mg; 10 brown, oestradiol valerate 2 mg and norgestrel 500 micrograms (≡ levonorgestrel 250 micrograms). Net price per pack = £3.50

Dose: menopausal symptoms and osteoporosis prophylaxis as *Cyclo-Progynova® 1-mg*, but starting with 1 white tablet daily for 11 days, then 1 brown tablet daily for 10 days, followed by a 7-day interval

PoM **Elleste-Duet®** (Searle)

Elleste-Duet® 1-mg tablets, 16 white, oestradiol 1 mg; 12 green, oestradiol 1 mg and norethisterone acetate 1 mg. Net price 3 × 28-tab pack = £9.72

Dose: menopausal symptoms, 1 white tablet daily for 16 days starting on day 2 of menstruation (or at any time if cycles have ceased or are infrequent), then 1 green tablet daily for 12 days; subsequent courses are repeated without interval

Elleste-Duet® 2-mg tablets, 16 orange, oestradiol 2 mg; 12 grey, oestradiol 2 mg, norethisterone acetate 1 mg. Net price 3 × 28-tab pack = £9.72

Dose: menopausal symptoms and osteoporosis prophylaxis, 1 orange tablet daily for 16 days, starting on day 2 of menstruation (or at any time if cycles have ceased or are infrequent) then 1 grey tablet daily for 12 days; subsequent courses are repeated without interval

Elleste-Duet Conti® tablets, grey, oestradiol 2 mg, norethisterone acetate 1 mg. Net price 3 × 28–tab pack = £18.09.

Dose: menopausal symptoms, if uterus intact, 1 tablet daily on a continuous basis (if changing from cyclical HRT begin treatment at the end of scheduled bleed)

Note. Unsuitable for use in the perimenopause or within 12 months of the last menstrual period; may cause irregular bleeding in early stages of treatment—if bleeding continues exclude endometrial abnormality and consider changing to cyclical HRT

PoM **Estracombi®** (Novartis)

Combination pack, self-adhesive patches of *Estraderm TTS® 50* (releasing oestradiol approx. 50 micrograms/24 hours) and of *Estragest TTS®* (releasing oestradiol approx. 50 micrograms/24 hours and norethisterone acetate 250 micrograms/24 hours); net price 1-month pack (4 of each) = £11.14, 3-month pack (12 of each) = £33.42. Counselling, administration

Dose: menopausal symptoms and osteoporosis prophylaxis, if uterus intact, starting within 5 days of onset of menstruation (or any time if cycles have ceased or are infrequent), 1 *Estraderm TTS® 50* patch to be applied twice weekly for 2 weeks followed by 1 *Estragest TTS®* patch twice weekly for 2 weeks; subsequent courses are repeated without interval

PoM **Estrapak 50®** (Novartis)

Calendar pack, self-adhesive patches, releasing oestradiol approx. 50 micrograms/24 hours, and tablets, red, norethisterone acetate 1 mg; net price 1-month pack (8 patches plus 12 tablets) = £9.48, 3-month pack (24 patches plus 36 tablets) = £28.44. Counselling, administration

Dose: menopausal symptoms and osteoporosis prophylaxis, if uterus intact, starting within 5 days of onset of menstruation (or at any time if cycles have ceased or are infrequent), apply 1 patch twice weekly on continuous basis, and take 1 tablet daily on days 15–26 of each 28-day treatment cycle

PoM **Evorel® Conti** (Janssen-Cilag)

Patches, self-adhesive, (releasing oestradiol approx. 50 micrograms/24 hours and norethisterone acetate approx. 170 micrograms/24 hours). Net price 8-patch pack = £12.90. Counselling, administration

Dose: menopausal symptoms, if uterus intact, 1 patch to be applied twice weekly on a continuous basis

PoM **Evorel® Pak** (Janssen-Cilag)

Calendar pack, 8 self-adhesive patches (releasing oestradiol approx. 50 micrograms/24 hours) and 12 tablets, norethisterone 1 mg. Net price per pack = £8.45. Counselling, administration

Dose: menopausal symptoms, if uterus intact, apply 1 patch twice weekly on a continuous basis (increased if necessary to 2 patches twice weekly after first month) and take 1 tablet daily on days 15–26 of each 28-day treatment cycle

PoM **Evorel® Sequi** (Janssen-Cilag)

Combination pack, 4 self-adhesive patches of *Evorel® 50* (releasing oestradiol approx. 50 micrograms/24 hours) and 4 self-adhesive patches of *Evorel® Conti* (releasing oestradiol approx. 50 micrograms/24 hours and norethisterone acetate approx. 170 micrograms/24 hours). Net price 8-patch pack = £11.00. Counselling, administration

Dose: menopausal symptoms, if uterus intact, 1 *Evorel® 50* patch to be applied twice weekly for 2 weeks followed by 1 *Evorel® Conti* patch twice weekly for 2 weeks; subsequent courses are repeated without interval

PoM **Femapak®** (Solvay)

Femapak® 40 combination pack of 8 self-adhesive patches of *Fematrix® 40* (releasing oestradiol approx. 40 micrograms/24 hours) and 14 tablets of *Duphaston®* (dydrogesterone 10 mg). Net price per pack = £8.45. Counselling, administration

Dose: menopausal symptoms, if uterus intact, starting within 5 days of onset of menstruation (or any time if cycles have ceased or are infrequent), apply 1 patch twice weekly on a continuous basis and take 1 tablet daily on days 15–28 of each 28-day treatment cycle

Femapak® 80 combination pack of 8 self-adhesive patches of *Fematrix® 80* (releasing oestradiol approx. 80 micrograms/24 hours) and 14 tablets of *Duphaston®* (dydrogesterone 10 mg). Net price per pack = £8.95. Counselling, administration

Dose: menopausal symptoms and osteoporosis prophylaxis, if uterus intact, starting within 5 days of onset of menstruation (or any time if cycles have ceased or are infrequent), apply 1 patch twice weekly on a continuous basis and take 1 tablet daily on days 15–28 of each 28-day treatment cycle

PoM **Femoston®** (Solvay)

Femoston® 1/10 tablets, both f/c, 14 white, oestradiol 1 mg; 14 grey, oestradiol 1 mg, dydrogesterone 10 mg. Net price 28-tab pack = £4.99; 3 × 28-tab pack = £14.97

Dose: menopausal symptoms, if uterus intact, 1 white tablet daily for 14 days, starting within 5 days of onset of menstruation (or any time if cycles have ceased or are infrequent) then 1 grey tablet for 14 days; subsequent courses are repeated without interval

Femoston® 2/10 tablets, both f/c, 14 orange, oestradiol 2 mg; 14 yellow, oestradiol 2 mg, dydrogesterone 10 mg. Net price 28-tab pack = £4.99; 3 × 28-tab pack = £14.97

Dose: menopausal symptoms and osteoporosis prophylaxis, if uterus intact, 1 orange tablet daily for 14 days, starting within 5 days of onset of menstruation (or any time if cycles have ceased or are infrequent) then 1 yellow tablet daily for 14 days; subsequent courses are repeated without interval; where therapy is required for control of menopausal symptoms alone, *Femoston® 1/10* is given initially and *Femoston® 2/10* substituted if symptom control is not achieved

Femoston® 2/20 tablets, both f/c, 14 orange, oestradiol 2 mg; 14 blue, oestradiol 2 mg, dydrogesterone 20 mg. Net price 28-tab pack = £7.48; 3 × 28-tab pack = £22.44

Dose: see *Femoston® 2/10*, but taking 1 blue tablet (instead of 1 yellow tablet) if withdrawal bleed is early or endometrial biopsy shows inadequate progestational response

PoM **Kliofem**® (Novo Nordisk)

Tablets, yellow, oestradiol 2 mg, norethisterone acetate 1 mg. Net price 3 × 28-tab pack = £25.95

Dose: menopausal symptoms and osteoporosis prophylaxis, if uterus intact, 1 tablet daily on a continuous basis; start at end of scheduled bleed if changing from sequential HRT

Note. Unsuitable for use in the perimenopause or within 12 months of the last menstrual period; may cause irregular bleeding in first 6 cycles—if bleeding continues, discontinue or change to sequential HRT

PoM **Nuvelle**® (Schering Health)

Tablets, all s/c, 16 white, oestradiol valerate 2 mg; 12 pink, oestradiol valerate 2 mg and levonorgestrel 75 micrograms. Net price 3 × 28-tab pack = £13.77

Dose: menopausal symptoms and osteoporosis prophylaxis, 1 white tablet daily for 16 days, starting on 5th day of menstruation (or any time if cycles have ceased or are infrequent) then 1 pink tablet daily for 12 days; subsequent courses are repeated without interval

PoM **Nuvelle**® **TS** (Schering Health)

Combination pack of self-adhesive patches of *Nuvelle*® *TS Phase I* (releasing oestradiol approx. 80 micrograms/24 hours) and of *Nuvelle*® *TS Phase II* (releasing oestradiol approx. 50 micrograms/24 hours and levonorgestrel approx. 20 micrograms/24 hours); net price 1-month pack (4 of each) = £11.00. Counselling, administration

Dose: menopausal symptoms, if uterus intact, starting within 5 days of onset of menstruation (or any time if cycles have ceased or are infrequent) 1 *Phase I* patch to be applied twice weekly for 2 weeks followed by 1 *Phase II* patch twice weekly for 2 weeks; subsequent courses are repeated without interval

PoM **Tridestra**® (Sanofi Winthrop)

Tablets, 70 white, oestradiol valerate 2 mg; 14 blue, oestradiol valerate 2 mg and medroxyprogesterone acetate 20 mg; 7 yellow, inactive. Net price 91-tab pack = £24.90

Dose: menopausal symptoms and osteoporosis prophylaxis, if uterus intact 1 white tablet daily for 70 days, then 1 blue tablet daily for 14 days, then 1 yellow tablet daily for 7 days; subsequent courses are repeated without interval

Oestradiol and oestriol with progestogen

PoM **Trisequens**® (Novo Nordisk)

Trisequens® tablets, 12 blue, oestradiol 2 mg, oestriol 1 mg; 10 white, oestradiol 2 mg, oestriol 1 mg, norethisterone acetate 1 mg; 6 red, oestradiol 1 mg, oestriol 500 micrograms. Net price 3 × 28-tab pack = £20.55

Dose: menopausal symptoms and osteoporosis prophylaxis, if uterus intact, 1 blue tablet daily, starting on 5th day of menstruation (or at any time if cycles have ceased or are infrequent), then 1 tablet daily in sequence (without interruption)

Trisequens Forte® tablets, 12 yellow, oestradiol 4 mg, oestriol 2 mg; 10 white, oestradiol 4 mg, oestriol 2 mg, norethisterone acetate 1 mg; 6 red, oestradiol 1 mg, oestriol 500 micrograms. Net price 3 × 28-tab pack = £20.55

Dose: menopausal symptoms, see under Trisequens®, starting with 1 yellow tablet daily (instead of 1 blue tablet) if symptoms not fully controlled with lower strength

Estropipate with progestogen

PoM **Improvera**® (Pharmacia & Upjohn)

Tablets, both scored, 28 peach, estropipate 1.5 mg; 12 white, medroxyprogesterone acetate 10 mg. Net price per pack = £11.85

Dose: menopausal symptoms and osteoporosis prophylaxis, if uterus intact, 1 peach tablet daily on a continu-

ous basis starting on 5th day of menstruation (or at any time if cycles have ceased or are infrequent) and 1 white tablet on days 17–28 of each 28-day treatment cycle; subsequent courses are repeated without interval

Women without Uterus

The following preparations do **not** contain a **progestogen**; if the uterus is intact they need to be given with a progestogen in which case packs incorporating a suitable progestogen tablet are preferred (see above).

Conjugated oestrogens only

PoM **Premarin**® (Wyeth)

Tablets, all s/c, conjugated oestrogens 625 micrograms (maroon), net price 3 × 28-tab pack = £7.36; 1.25 mg (yellow), 3 × 28-tab pack = £9.99

Dose: menopausal symptoms and osteoporosis prophylaxis, (with progestogen for 12–14 days per cycle if uterus intact), 0.625–1.25 mg daily

Note. Premarin® tablets 2.5 mg (purple, net price 3 × 28-tab pack = £10.64) are still available, but no longer have a product licence for palliative care in breast cancer (and provide a higher dose than that having a product licence for osteoporosis prophylaxis)

Oestradiol only

PoM **Oestradiol Implants** (Organon)

Implant, oestradiol 25 mg, net price each = £9.59; 50 mg, each = £19.16; 100 mg, each = £33.40

Dose: by implantation, oestrogen replacement, and osteoporosis prophylaxis (with cyclical progestogen on 10–13 days of each cycle if uterus intact, see notes above), 25–100 mg as required (usually every 4–8 months) according to oestrogen levels—check before each implant

PoM **Climaval**® (Novartis)

Tablets, oestradiol valerate 1 mg (grey-blue), net price 1 × 28-tab pack = £2.34, 3 × 28-tab pack = £7.02; 2 mg (blue), 1 × 28-tab pack = £2.34, 3 × 28-tab pack = £7.02

Dose: menopausal symptoms (if patient has had a hysterectomy), 1–2 mg daily

PoM **Dermestril**® (Sanofi Winthrop)

Patches, self-adhesive, oestradiol, '25' patch (releasing approx. 25 micrograms/24 hours), net price 8-patch pack = £5.75; '50' patch (releasing approx. 50 micrograms/24 hours), 8-patch pack = £6.35; '100' patch (releasing approx. 100 micrograms/24 hours), 8-patch pack = £6.99. Counselling, administration

Dose: menopausal symptoms, 1 patch to be applied every 3–4 days on a continuous basis; give progestogen for 10–12 days a month (unless patient has had hysterectomy); therapy should be initiated with '50' patch for first month, subsequently adjusted to lowest effective dose

PoM **Elleste-Solo**® (Searle)

Elleste-Solo® *1-mg tablets*, oestradiol 1 mg. Net price 3 × 28-tab pack = £5.34

Dose: menopausal symptoms, with progestogen for 12–14 days per cycle if uterus intact, 1 mg daily

Note. Elleste-Solo® tablets can be given continuously or cyclically (21 days out of 28)

Elleste-Solo® *2-mg tablets*, oestradiol 2 mg. Net price 3 × 28-tab pack = £5.34

Dose: menopausal symptoms not controlled with lower strength and osteoporosis prophylaxis, with progestogen for 12–14 days per cycle if uterus intact, 2 mg daily

Note. Elleste-Solo® tablets can be given continuously or cyclically (21 days out of 28)

PoM **Estraderm MX**® (Novartis)

Patches, self-adhesive, oestradiol, *MX 25 patch* (releasing approx. 25 micrograms/24 hours), net price 8-patch pack = £6.75, 24-patch pack = £20.25; *MX 50 patch* (releasing approx. 50 micrograms/24 hours), 8-patch pack = £7.45, 24-patch pack = £22.35, 20-patch pack (hosp. only) = £16.76; *MX 100 patch* (releasing approx. 100 micrograms/24 hours), 8-patch pack = £8.20, 24-patch pack = £24.60. Counselling, administration

Dose: menopausal symptoms (and osteoporosis prophylaxis in case of Estraderm MX® 50 **only**), 1 patch to be applied twice weekly on a continuous basis; give progestogen for 12 days a month (unless patient has had hysterectomy); therapy should be initiated with MX 50 for first month, subsequently adjusted to lowest effective dose

PoM **Estraderm TTS**® (Novartis)

Patches, self-adhesive, oestradiol, *TTS 25 patch* (releasing approx. 25 micrograms/24 hours), net price, 8-patch pack = £6.75, 24-patch pack = £20.25; *TTS 50 patch* (releasing approx. 50 micrograms/24 hours), 8-patch pack = £7.45, 24-patch pack = £22.35; *TTS 100 patch* (releasing approx. 100 micrograms/24 hours), 8-patch pack = £8.20, 24-patch pack = £24.60, 20-patch pack (hosp. only) = £16.76 . Counselling, administration

Dose: menopausal symptoms (and osteoporosis prophylaxis in case of Estraderm TTS® 50 **only**), 1 patch to be applied twice weekly on continuous basis; give progestogen for 12 days a month (unless patient has had hysterectomy); therapy should be initiated with TTS 50 for first month, subsequently adjusted to lowest effective dose

PoM **Evorel**® (Janssen-Cilag)

Patches, self-adhesive, oestradiol, '*25' patch* (releasing approx. 25 micrograms/24 hours), net price 8-patch pack = £6.75; '*50' patch* (releasing approx. 50 micrograms/24 hours), 8-patch pack = £7.45; '*75' patch* (releasing approx. 75 micrograms/24 hours), 8-patch pack = £7.90; '*100' patch* (releasing approx. 100 micrograms/24 hours), 8-patch pack = £8.20. Counselling, administration

Dose: menopausal symptoms, 1 patch to be applied twice weekly on a continuous basis; give progestogen for 12 days a month (unless patient has had hysterectomy); therapy should be initiated with '*50' patch* for first month, subsequently adjusted to lowest effective dose

PoM **Fematrix**® (Solvay)

Fematrix® *40 patch*, self-adhesive, oestradiol, '*40' patch* (releasing approx. 40 micrograms/24 hours). Net price 8-patch pack = £6.45. Counselling, administration

Dose: menopausal symptoms, 1 patch to be applied twice weekly on a continuous basis starting within 5 days of onset of menstruation (or at any time if cycles have ceased or are infrequent); give progestogen for 12–14 days of each cycle (unless patient has had hysterectomy); '*80' patch* may be used if required (subsequently adjusted to lowest effective dose)

Fematrix® *80 patch*, self-adhesive, oestradiol (releasing approx. 80 micrograms/24 hours). Net price 8-patch pack = £6.95. Counselling, administration

Dose: menopausal symptoms and osteoporosis prophylaxis, as for *Fematrix*® *40*; therapy should be initiated with *Fematrix*® *40* in those with menopausal symptoms, prolonged oestrogen deficiency or anticipated intolerance to higher strength

PoM **FemSeven**® (Merck)

Patches, self-adhesive, releasing oestradiol approx. 50 micrograms/24 hours. Net price 4-patch pack =

£6.44, 12-patch pack = £18.72. Counselling, administration

Dose: menopausal symptoms and osteoporosis prophylaxis, 1 patch to be applied once a week on a continuous basis, increased if necessary after first month to max. 2 patches/week; give progestogen for 12 days a month (unless patient has had hysterectomy)

PoM **Menorest**® (Rhône-Poulenc Rorer)

Patches, self-adhesive, oestradiol, '*37.5' patch* (releasing approx. 37.5 micrograms/24 hours), net price 8-patch pack = £6.34; '*50' patch* (releasing approx. 50 micrograms/24 hours), 8-patch pack = £6.44; '*75' patch* (releasing approx. 75 micrograms/24 hours), 8-patch pack = £7.50. Counselling administration

Dose: menopausal symptoms, 1 patch to be applied every 3–4 days on a continuous basis; give progestogen on 12 days a month (unless patient has had hysterectomy); therapy should be initiated with '*50' patch* for first month, subsequently adjusted to lowest effective dose

PoM **Oestrogel**® (Hoechst Marion Roussel)

Gel, oestradiol 0.06%. Net price 64-dose aerosol pack (includes CFC propellants) = £7.95, 64-dose Pump-Pack (CFC-free) = £7.95. Counselling, administration

Dose: menopausal symptoms, 2 measures once daily to be applied over an area twice that of the template provided; may be increased after one month to max. 4 measures; give progestogen for 12 days a month (unless patient has had hysterectomy)

COUNSELLING. Apply gel to clean, dry, intact areas of skin such as arms, shoulders or inner thighs and allow to dry for 5 minutes before covering skin with clothing. Not to be applied on or near breasts or on vulval region. Avoid skin contact with another person (particularly male) and avoid other skin products or washing the area for at least 1 hour after application

PoM **Progynova**® (Schering Health)

Tablets, both s/c, oestradiol valerate 1 mg (beige), net price 28-tab pack = £2.34, 3 × 28-tab pack = £7.02; 2 mg (blue), 28-tab pack = £2.34, 3 × 28-tab pack = £7.02

Dose: menopausal symptoms (if patient has had a hysterectomy), 1–2 mg daily; osteoporosis prophylaxis, 2 mg daily

PoM **Progynova**® **TS** (Schering Health)

Patches, self-adhesive, *Progynova*® TS (releasing oestradiol approx. 50 micrograms/24 hours), net price 12-patch pack = £19.32; *Progynova*® *TS forte* (releasing oestradiol approx. 100 micrograms/24 hours), 12-patch pack = £25.00. Counselling, administration

Dose: menopausal symptoms, 1 patch to be applied once a week on a continuous or cyclical basis (1 patch per week for three weeks followed by a 7-day patch-free interval); give progestogen for 12 days a month (unless patient has had hysterectomy)

PoM **Sandrena**® (Organon)

Gel, oestradiol (0.1%), 500 microgram/500 mg sachet, net price 28-sachet pack = £5.95, 1 mg/1 g sachet, 28-sachet pack = £6.85. Counselling, administration

Dose: menopausal symptoms, 1mg to be applied once daily over area 1–2 times size of palm; dose may be adjusted after 2–3 cycles to a usual dose of 0.5–1.5 mg daily; give progestogen for 10–12 days a month (unless patient has had hysterectomy)

COUNSELLING. Apply gel to intact areas of skin such as lower trunk or thighs, using right and left sides on alternate days. Wash hands after application. Not to be applied on the breasts or face and avoid contact with eyes. Allow area of application to dry for 5 minutes and do not wash area for at least 1 hour

---

PoM **Zumenon®** (Solvay)
Tablets, f/c, oestradiol 1 mg, net price 84-tab pack = £7.65; 2 mg (orange), 84-tab pack = £7.65
Dose: menopausal symptoms, with progestogen for 10–14 days per cycle if uterus intact, starting on day 5 of menstruation (or any time if cycles have ceased or are infrequent) 1–4 mg daily; osteoporosis prophylaxis, 2 mg daily

Oestradiol, oestriol and oestrone only
PoM **Hormonin®** (Shire)
Tablets, pink, oestradiol 600 micrograms, oestriol 270 micrograms, oestrone 1.4 mg. Net price 90-tab pack = £6.44
Dose: menopausal symptoms and osteoporosis prophylaxis, with progestogen for 12–13 days per cycle if uterus intact, 1–2 tablets daily
Note. Hormonin® tablets can be given continuously or cyclically (21 days out of 28)

Oestriol only
PoM **Ovestin®** (Organon)
Tablets, scored, oestriol 1 mg. Net price 30-tab pack = £4.40. Label: 25
Dose: genito-urinary symptoms associated with oestrogen-deficiency states, 0.5–3 mg daily, as single dose, for up to 1 month, then 0.5–1 mg daily until restoration of epithelial integrity (short-term use)

Estropipate only
PoM **Harmogen®** (Pharmacia & Upjohn)
Tablets, peach, scored, estropipate 1.5 mg. Net price 28-tab pack = £3.14
Dose: menopausal symptoms and osteoporosis prophylaxis, 1.5 mg daily on continuous basis (with progestogen for 10–13 days per 28-day cycle if uterus intact); up to 3 mg daily (in single or divided doses) for vasomotor symptoms and menopausal vaginitis

TIBOLONE

Tibolone combines oestrogenic and progestogenic activity with weak androgenic activity. It is indicated for the treatment of vasomotor symptoms of the menopause and osteoporosis prophylaxis. It is given continuously, without cyclical progestogen.

TIBOLONE

Indications: vasomotor symptoms in oestrogen deficiency, osteoporosis prophylaxis; see also under Dose
Cautions: renal impairment, epilepsy, migraine, diabetes mellitus, hypercholesterolaemia; withdraw if signs of thromboembolic disease, abnormal liver function tests or cholestatic jaundice; see also Note below; **interactions:** Appendix 1 (tibolone)
Contra-indications: hormone-dependent tumours, history of cardiovascular or cerebrovascular disease (e.g. thrombophlebitis, thrombo-embolism), uninvestigated vaginal bleeding, severe liver disease, pregnancy, breast-feeding
Side-effects: weight changes, ankle oedema, dizziness, seborrhoeic dermatitis, vaginal bleeding, headache, abdominal pain, gastro-intestinal disturbances, increased facial hair; depression, arthralgia, myalgia, migraine, visual disturbances, liver-function changes, rash and pruritus also reported

Dose: vasomotor symptoms in oestrogen deficiency and osteoporosis prophylaxis, 2.5 mg daily
Note. Unsuitable for use in the premenopause and as (or with) an oral contraceptive; also unsuitable for use within 12 months of the last menstrual period (may cause irregular bleeding); induce withdrawal bleeding with a progestogen if transferring from another form of HRT

PoM **Livial®** (Organon)
Tablets, tibolone 2.5 mg. Net price 28-tab pack = £13.66; 3 × 28-tab pack = £40.98

ETHINYLOESTRADIOL

Ethinyloestradiol (ethinylestradiol) has been used as hormone replacement for menopausal symptoms in a dose of 10–20 micrograms daily. This has now been largely replaced by more appropriate forms of oestrogen.

Ethinyloestradiol is occasionally used, under **specialist supervision**, for the management of *hereditary haemorrhagic telangiectasia* (but evidence of any beneficial effect is uncertain). Side-effects include nausea, fluid retention, and thrombosis. Impotence and gynaecomastia occur in men.

For use in breast cancer, see section 8.3.1.

ETHINYLOESTRADIOL
(Ethinylestradiol)
Indications: see notes above
Cautions; Contra-indications; Side-effects: cardiovascular disease (sodium retention with oedema, thromboembolism), hepatic impairment (jaundice), feminising effects in men; see also under Combined Oral Contraceptives (section 7.3.1), and under Oestrogen for HRT (above)
Dose: see notes above

PoM **Ethinyloestradiol** (Non-proprietary)
Tablets, ethinyloestradiol 10 micrograms, net price 20 = £2.16; 50 micrograms, 20 = £3.19; 1 mg, 20 = £6.21
Available from Norton

6.4.1.2 PROGESTOGENS

There are two main groups of progestogen, *progesterone and its analogues* (dydrogesterone, hydroxyprogesterone, and medroxyprogesterone) and *testosterone analogues* (norethisterone and norgestrel). The newer progestogens (desogestrel, norgestimate, and gestodene) are all derivatives of norgestrel; levonorgestrel is the active isomer of norgestrel and has twice its potency. Progesterone and its analogues are less androgenic than the testosterone derivatives and neither progesterone nor dydrogesterone causes virilisation. Other synthetic derivatives are variably metabolised into testosterone and oestrogen; thus side-effects vary with the preparation and the dose.

Where *endometriosis* requires drug treatment, it may respond to a progestogen, e.g. norethisterone, administered on a continuous basis. Danazol, gestrinone, and gonadorelin analogues are also available (section 6.7.2).

Although oral progestogens have been used widely for *menorrhagia* they are relatively ineffective compared with tranexamic acid (section 2.11) or, particularly where dysmenorrhoea is also a factor, mefenamic acid (section 10.1.1); the levonorgestrel-releasing intra-uterine device (section 7.3.2.3) may be particularly useful for women also requiring contraception [currently licensed only as a contraceptive]. Oral progestogens have also been used for *severe dysmenorrhoea*, but where contraception is also required in younger women the best choice is a combined oral contraceptive (section 7.3.1).

Progestogens have also been advocated for the alleviation of *premenstrual symptoms*, but no convincing physiological basis for such treatment has been shown.

Progestogens have been used in *habitual abortion* but there is no evidence of benefit. If they are used for this purpose they should be of the true progesterone-derivative type, e.g. **hydroxyprogesterone hexanoate** (hydroxyprogesterone caproate) to avoid any masculinisation of a female fetus.

HORMONE REPLACEMENT THERAPY. In post-menopausal women receiving *long-term oestrogen therapy for hormone replacement*, a progestogen needs to be added to prevent cystic hyperplasia of the endometrium and possible transformation to cancer; it can be added on a cyclical or a continuous basis. Combined packs incorporating suitable progestogen tablets are available, see p. 319.

ORAL CONTRACEPTION. Desogestrel, ethynodiol (etynodiol), gestodene, levonorgestrel, norethisterone, and norgestimate are used in *combined oral contraceptives* and in *progestogen-only contraceptives* (see sections 7.3.1 and 7.3.2).

CANCER. Progestogens also have a role in *neoplastic disease* (see section 8.3.2).

DYDROGESTERONE

Indications: see under Dose and notes above

Cautions; Contra-indications; Side-effects: see under Medroxyprogesterone Acetate and notes above; breakthrough bleeding may occur (increase dose)

Dose: endometriosis, 10 mg 2–3 times daily from 5th to 25th day of cycle or continuously

Infertility, irregular cycles, 10 mg twice daily from 11th to 25th day for at least 6 cycles (but not recommended)

Habitual abortion, 10 mg twice daily from day 11 to day 25 of cycle until conception, then continuously until 20th week of pregnancy and gradually reduced (but see notes above)

Dysfunctional uterine bleeding, 10 mg twice daily (together with an oestrogen) for 5–7 days to arrest bleeding; 10 mg twice daily (together with an oes-

trogen) from 11th to 25th day of cycle to prevent bleeding

Dysmenorrhoea (but see notes above), 10 mg twice daily from 5th to 25th day of cycle

Amenorrhoea, 10 mg twice daily from 11th to 25th day of cycle with oestrogen therapy from 1st to 25th day of cycle

Premenstrual syndrome, 10 mg twice daily from 12th to 26th day of cycle increased if necessary (but not recommended, see notes above)

Hormone replacement therapy, with continuous oestrogen therapy, see under *Duphaston*® HRT below

PoM Duphaston® (Solvay)
Tablets, scored, dydrogesterone 10 mg. Net price 60-tab pack = £11.87

PoM Duphaston® HRT (Solvay)
Tablets, scored, dydrogesterone 10 mg. Net price 42-tab pack = £8.31
Dose: 10 mg daily on days 15–28 of each 28-day oestrogen HRT cycle, increased to 10 mg twice daily if withdrawal bleed is early or endometrial biopsy shows inadequate progestational response

---

HYDROXYPROGESTERONE HEXANOATE
(Hydroxyprogesterone Caproate)

Indications: habitual abortion but see notes above

Cautions; Contra-indications; Side-effects: see under Medroxyprogesterone acetate and notes above

Dose: by slow intramuscular injection, 250–500 mg weekly during first half of pregnancy

PoM Proluton Depot® (Schering Health)
Injection (oily), hydroxyprogesterone hexanoate 250 mg/mL. Net price 1-mL amp = £2.35; 2-mL amp = £3.69

MEDROXYPROGESTERONE ACETATE

Indications: see under Dose; contraception (section 7.3.2.2); malignant disease (section 8.3.2)

Cautions: diabetes, hypertension, cardiac or renal disease; **interactions:** Appendix 1 (progestogens)

Contra-indications: pregnancy, undiagnosed vaginal bleeding, hepatic impairment or active liver disease, severe arterial disease, breast or genital tract carcinoma; porphyria (section 9.8.2)

Side-effects: acne, urticaria, fluid retention, weight changes, gastro-intestinal disturbances, changes in libido, breast discomfort, premenstrual symptoms, irregular menstrual cycles; also depression, insomnia, somnolence, alopecia, hirsutism, anaphylactoid-like reaction; rarely jaundice

Dose: by mouth, 2.5–10 mg daily for 5–10 days beginning on 16th–21st day of cycle, repeated for 2 cycles in dysfunctional uterine bleeding and 3 cycles in secondary amenorrhoea

Mild to moderate endometriosis, 10 mg 3 times daily for 90 consecutive days, beginning on 1st day of cycle

---

PoM **Provera®** (Pharmacia & Upjohn)

Tablets, all scored, medroxyprogesterone acetate 2.5 mg (orange), net price 30-tab pack = £1.93; 5 mg (blue), 10-tab pack = £1.29; 10 mg (white), 10-tab pack = £2.59, 90-tab pack = £23.20

Combined preparations
Section 6.4.1.1

NORETHISTERONE

Indications: see under Dose; HRT (section 6.4.1.1); contraception (section 7.3.1 and section 7.3.2); malignant disease (section 8.3.2)

Cautions; Contra-indications; Side-effects: see under Medroxyprogesterone Acetate but more virilising and greater incidence of liver disturbances and jaundice; avoid in pregnancy; exacerbation of epilepsy and migraine

Dose: endometriosis 10 mg daily starting on 5th day of cycle (increased if spotting occurs to 20–25 mg daily, reduced once bleeding has stopped)
Menorrhagia (but see notes above), 5 mg 3 times daily for 10 days to arrest bleeding; to prevent bleeding 5 mg twice daily from 19th to 26th day
Dysmenorrhoea (but see notes above), 5 mg 3 times daily from 5th to 24th day for 3–4 cycles
Premenstrual syndrome, 5 mg 2–3 times daily from 19th to 26th day for several cycles (but not recommended, see notes above)
Postponement of menstruation, 5 mg 3 times daily starting 3 days before anticipated onset (menstruation occurs 2–3 days after stopping)
Progestogenic opposition of menopausal oestrogen HRT, see under *Micronor® HRT,* below

Tablets of 5 mg
Note. **Not** licensed for HRT purposes
PoM **Menzol®** (Schwarz)

Tablets, scored, norethisterone 5 mg. Net price 3 × 24-tab (8-day) 'Planapak' = £7.70; 3 × 60-tab (20-day) 'Planapak' – £19.35
PoM **Primolut N®** (Schering Health)

Tablets, norethisterone 5 mg. Net price 30-tab pack = £2.16
PoM **Utovlan®** (Searle)

Tablets, scored, norethisterone 5 mg. Net price 90-tab pack = £6.48
Note. Norethisterone 5 mg tablets are also available from Cox

Tablets of 1 mg for HRT purposes
PoM **Micronor® HRT** (Janssen-Cilag)

Tablets, norethisterone 1 mg. Net price 3 × 12-tab pack = £3.75
Dose: 1 tablet daily on days 15–26 of each 28-day oestrogen HRT cycle

Combined preparations
Section 6.4.1.1

PROGESTERONE

Indications: see under preparations
Cautions: diabetes, breast-feeding, hypertension; hepatic, cardiac, or renal disease; **interactions:** Appendix 1 (progestogens)

Contra-indications: undiagnosed vaginal bleeding, missed or incomplete abortion, severe arterial disease, mammary carcinoma; porphyria (see section 9.8.2)
Side-effects: acne, urticaria, fluid retention, weight changes, gastro-intestinal disturbances, changes in libido, breast discomfort, premenstrual symptoms, irregular menstrual cycles; also chloasma, depression, pyrexia, insomnia, somnolence, alopecia, hirsutism; rarely jaundice. Injection may be painful

PoM **Crinone®** (Wyeth)

Vaginal gel, progesterone 45 mg/application (4%), net price 6 = £11.60; 90 mg/application (8%), 15 = £40.32
Dose: by vagina, progesterone deficiency, insert 1 applicatorful of 4% gel on alternate mornings from day 15 to day 25 of cycle
Menopausal symptoms, insert 1 applicatorful of 4% gel on alternate days for the last 12 days of oestrogen therapy in each cycle (section 6.4.1.1)
Infertility due to inadequate luteal phase, insert 1 applicatorful of 8% gel daily starting either after documented ovulation or on day 18–21 of cycle
In vitro fertilisation, daily application of 8% gel, continued for 30 days after laboratory evidence of pregnancy
PoM **Cyclogest®** (Shire)

Pessaries, progesterone 200 mg, net price 15 = £5.27; 400 mg, 15 = £7.63
Dose: by vagina or rectum, premenstrual syndrome, 200 mg daily to 400 mg twice daily starting at day 12–14 and continued until onset of menstruation (but not recommended, see notes above); rectally if barrier methods of contraception are used, or if vaginal infection
PoM **Gestone®** (Ferring)

Injection, progesterone 25 mg/mL, net price 1-mL amp = 34p; 50 mg/mL, 1-mL amp = 44p, 2-mL amp = 58p
Dose: by deep intramuscular injection into buttock, embryo transfer, consult product literature

6.4.2 Male sex hormones and antagonists

Androgens cause masculinisation; they may be used as replacement therapy in castrated adults and in those who are hypogonadal due to either pituitary or testicular disease. In the normal male they inhibit pituitary gonadotrophin secretion and depress spermatogenesis. Androgens also have an anabolic action which led to the development of anabolic steroids (section 6.4.3).

Androgens are useless as a treatment of impotence and impaired spermatogenesis unless there is associated hypogonadism; they should not be given until the hypogonadism has been properly investigated. Treatment should be under expert supervision.

When given to patients with hypopituitarism they can lead to normal sexual development and potency but not to fertility. If fertility is desired, the usual treatment is with gonadotrophins or pulsatile gonadotrophin-releasing hormone (section 6.5.1) which will stimulate spermatogenesis as well as androgen production.

Caution should be used when androgens or chorionic gonadotrophin are used in treating boys

---

with delayed puberty since the fusion of epiphyses is hastened and may result in short stature.

Intramuscular depot preparations of **testosterone esters** are preferred for replacement therapy. Testosterone enanthate or propionate or alternatively Sustanon®, which consists of a mixture of testosterone esters and has a longer duration of action, may be used. Satisfactory replacement therapy can sometimes be obtained with 1 mL of Sustanon 250®, given by intramuscular injection once a month, although more frequent dose intervals are often necessary. Implants of testosterone have been superseded for hypogonadism but are still occasionally used. Menopausal women are also sometimes given implants of testosterone (in a dose of 50–100 mg every 4–8 months) as an adjunct to hormone replacement therapy.

Of the orally active preparations, **testosterone undecanoate** and **mesterolone** are available. Testosterone patches are now also available.

TESTOSTERONE AND ESTERS

Indications: see under preparations

Cautions: cardiac, renal, or hepatic impairment (see Appendix 2), elderly, ischaemic heart disease, hypertension, epilepsy, migraine, skeletal metastases (risk of hypercalcaemia), pre-pubital boys (see notes above); **interactions:** Appendix 1 (testosterone)

Contra-indications: breast cancer in men, prostate cancer, hypercalcaemia, pregnancy, breast-feeding, nephrosis

Side-effects: prostate abnormalities and prostate cancer, headache, depression, gastro-intestinal bleeding, nausea, cholestatic jaundice, changes in libido, anxiety, generalised paraesthesia, electrolyte disturbances including sodium retention with oedema and hypercalcaemia; increased bone growth; androgenic effects such as hirsuitism, male pattern baldness, seborrhoea, acne, excessive frequency and duration of penile erections, precocious sexual development and premature closure of epiphyses in pre-pubertal males, virilism in women, and suppression of spermatogenesis in men; *with patches,* local irritation and allergic reactions

Oral
PoM **Restandol®** (Organon)
Capsules, red-brown, testosterone undecanoate 40 mg in oily solution. Net price 28-cap pack = £8.69; 56-cap pack = £17.38. Label: 21, 25
Dose: androgen deficiency, 120–160 mg daily for 2–3 weeks; maintenance 40–120 mg daily

Intramuscular
PoM **Primoteston Depot®** (Cambridge)
Injection (oily), testosterone enanthate 250 mg/ mL. Net price 1-mL amp = £6.67
Dose: by slow intramuscular injection, hypogonadism, initially 250 mg every 2–3 weeks; maintenance 250 mg every 3–6 weeks
Breast cancer, 250 mg every 2–3 weeks

PoM **Sustanon 100®** (Organon)
Injection (oily), testosterone propionate 20 mg, testosterone phenylpropionate 40 mg, and testosterone isocaproate 40 mg/mL. Net price 1-mL amp = £1.22
Note. Contains arachis (peanut) oil
Dose: by deep intramuscular injection, androgen deficiency, 1 mL every 2 weeks
PoM **Sustanon 250®** (Organon)
Injection (oily), testosterone propionate 30 mg, testosterone phenylpropionate 60 mg, testosterone isocaproate 60 mg, and testosterone decanoate 100 mg/mL. Net price 1-mL amp = £2.87
Note. Contains arachis (peanut) oil
Dose: by deep intramuscular injection, androgen deficiency, 1 mL usually every 3 weeks
PoM **Virormone®** (Ferring)
Injection, testosterone propionate 50 mg/mL. Net price 2-mL amp = 46p
Dose: by intramuscular injection, androgen deficiency, 50 mg 2–3 times weekly
Delayed puberty, 50 mg weekly
Breast cancer, 100 mg 2–3 times weekly

Implant
PoM **Testosterone** (Organon)
Implant, testosterone 100 mg, net price = £7.40; 200 mg = £13.79
Dose: by implantation, male hypogonadism, 100–600 mg; 600 mg usually maintains plasma testosterone levels within the normal range for 4–5 months
Menopausal women, see notes above

Patch
▼ PoM **Andropatch®** (SmithKline Beecham)
Patches, self-adhesive, releasing testosterone approx. 2.5 mg/24 hours, net price 60-patch pack = £48.00; releasing testosterone approx. 5 mg/ 24 hours, net price 30-patch pack = £48.00. Counselling, administration
Dose: androgen deficiency in men associated with primary or secondary hypogonadism, apply to clean, dry, unbroken skin on back, abdomen, upper arms or thighs, removing after 24 hours and siting replacement patch on a different area (with an interval of 7 days before using the same site); initially apply patches equivalent to testosterone 5 mg/24 hours (2.5 mg/24 hours in non-virilised patients) at night (approx. 10 p.m.), then adjust to 2.5 mg to 7.5 mg every 24 hours according to plasma-testosterone concentration (those with a body-weight over 130 kg may require 7.5 mg every 24 hours)

MESTEROLONE

Indications: see under Dose
Cautions; Contra-indications; Side-effects: see under Testosterone Esters; spermatogenesis unimpaired
Dose: androgen deficiency, 25 mg 3–4 times daily for several months, reduced to 50–75 mg daily in divided doses for maintenance

PoM **Pro-Viron®** (Schering Health)
Tablets, scored, mesterolone 25 mg. Net price 30-tab pack = £4.75

ANTI-ANDROGENS

Cyproterone acetate is an anti-androgen used in the treatment of severe hypersexuality and sexual deviation in the male. It inhibits spermatogenesis and produces reversible infertility (but is not a male contraceptive); abnormal sperm forms are produced. Fully informed consent is recommended and an initial spermatogram. As hepatic tumours have been produced in *animal* studies, careful consideration should be given to the risk/benefit ratio before treatment. Cyproterone acetate is also used as an adjunct in prostatic cancer (section 8.3.4) and in the treatment of acne and hirsutism in women (section 13.6.2).

Finasteride is a specific inhibitor of the enzyme 5α-reductase which metabolises testosterone into the more potent androgen, dihydrotestosterone. This inhibition of testosterone metabolism leads to reduction in prostate size, with improvement in urinary flow rate and in obstructive symptoms. It is an alternative to alpha-blockers (section 7.4.1) particularly in men with a significantly enlarged prostate.

CYPROTERONE ACETATE

Indications: see notes above; prostate cancer, section 8.3.4.2

Cautions: ineffective for male hypersexuality in chronic alcoholism (relevance to prostate cancer not known); blood counts initially and throughout treatment; monitor hepatic function regularly (liver function tests should be performed before treatment, see also under Side-effects below); monitor adrenocortical function regularly; diabetes mellitus (see also Contra-indications)

DRIVING. May impair performance of skilled tasks (e.g. driving)

Contra-indications: (do not apply in prostate cancer) hepatic disease, severe diabetes (with vascular changes); sickle-cell anaemia, malignant or wasting disease, severe depression, history of thrombo-embolic disorders; youths under 18 years (may arrest bone maturation and testicular development)

Side-effects: fatigue and lassitude, breathlessness, weight changes, reduced sebum production (may clear acne), changes in hair pattern, gynaecomastia (rarely leading to galactorrhoea and benign breast nodules); rarely osteoporosis; inhibition of spermatogenesis (see notes above); hepatotoxicity reported (including jaundice, hepatitis and hepatic failure usually in men given 200–300 mg daily for prostatic cancer, see section 8.3.4.2 for details and warnings)

Dose: male hypersexuality, 50 mg twice daily after food

PoM **Androcur®** (Schering Health)
Tablets, scored, cyproterone acetate 50 mg. Net price 56-tab pack = £32.23. Label: 3, 21
Note. Tablets containing cyproterone acetate 50 mg are also available from Cox, Generics, Hillcross, Lagap

FINASTERIDE

Indications: benign prostatic hyperplasia

Cautions: obstructive uropathy, prostate cancer (may decrease markers such as prostate specific antigen); use of condoms recommended if sexual partner is pregnant or is likely to become pregnant (finasteride excreted in semen); women of child-bearing potential should avoid handling crushed or broken tablets

Side-effects: impotence, decreased libido and ejaculate volume, breast tenderness and enlargement, hypersensitivity reactions (including lip swelling and rash)

Dose: 5 mg daily, review treatment after 6 months (may require several months treatment before benefit is obtained)

PoM **Proscar®** (MSD)
Tablets, blue, f/c, finasteride 5 mg. Net price 28-tab pack = £24.90

6.4.3   Anabolic steroids

All the anabolic steroids have some androgenic activity but they cause less virilisation than androgens in women. Their protein-building property led to the hope that they might be widely useful in medicine but this hope has not been realised. Their use as body builders or tonics is quite unjustified; they are abused by some athletes.

Anabolic steroids have also been given for osteoporosis in women but are no longer advocated for this purpose.

Anabolic steroids are used in the treatment of some aplastic anaemias (section 9.1.3) and to reduce the itching of *chronic biliary obstruction* (see Prescribing in Palliative Care p. 13).

NANDROLONE

Indications: osteoporosis in postmenopausal women (but not recommended, see notes above); aplastic anaemia, section 9.1.3

Cautions: cardiac and renal impairment, hepatic impairment (see Appendix 2), hypertension, diabetes mellitus, epilepsy, migraine; monitor skeletal maturation in young patients; skeletal metastases (risk of hypercalcaemia); **interactions:** Appendix 1 (anabolic steroids)

Contra-indications: severe hepatic impairment, prostate cancer, male breast cancer, pregnancy and breast-feeding, porphyria (section 9.8.2)

Side-effects: acne, sodium retention with oedema, virilisation with high doses including voice changes (sometimes irreversible), amenorrhoea, inhibition of spermatogenesis, premature epiphyseal closure; abnormal liver-function tests reported with high doses; liver tumours reported occasionally on prolonged treatment with anabolic steroids

Dose: see below

PoM **Deca-Durabolin®** (Organon)
Injection (oily), nandrolone decanoate 25 mg/mL, net price 1-mL amp = £1.92; 50 mg/mL, 1-mL amp = £3.71
Note. Contains arachis (peanut) oil
Dose: by deep intramuscular injection, 50 mg every 3 weeks
PoM **Deca-Durabolin 100®** see section 9.1.3

STANOZOLOL

Indications: see under Dose

Cautions: cardiac or renal impairment; premature closure of epiphyses in children; peliosis hepatis and hepatic tumours reported on long-term treatment; breast cancer (possibility of hypercalcaemia); monitor liver function, haematocrit and haemoglobin; diabetes mellitus (possible dosage adjustments for oral hypoglycaemic drugs and avoid in insulin-dependent diabetes); **interactions:** Appendix 1 (anabolic steroids)

Contra-indications: pregnancy, breast-feeding, established liver disease (if history of jaundice—liver function tests before starting treatment); prostate cancer, insulin-dependent diabetes mellitus; not indicated for treatment of loss of appetite, unexplained weight loss, or failure to thrive in children; porphyria (section 9.8.2)

Side-effects: androgenic effects (generally mild and reversible on stopping treatment) include acne, hirsutism, amenorrhoea, sodium retention with oedema; voice change—usually at higher dosage (discontinue); menstrual irregularity, headache, muscle cramp, dyspepsia, rash, hair loss, euphoria, depression, increased haematocrit and haemoglobin; cholestatic jaundice and rarely peliosis hepatis and hepatic tumours also reported; changes in liver enzymes, in lipoproteins, and in thyroid hormones; also premature epiphyseal closure (on prolonged treatment)

Dose: by mouth, vascular manifestations of Behcet's disease, 10 mg daily

Hereditary angioedema, 2.5–10 mg daily to control attacks, reduced for maintenance (2.5 mg 3 times weekly may be sufficient); CHILD 1–6 years initially 2.5 mg daily, 6–12 years initially 2.5–5 mg daily, reduced for maintenance

Note. In hereditary angioedema restricted to well-established cases who have experienced serious attacks (and not for premenopausal women except in life-threatening situations)

PoM **Stromba**® (Sanofi Winthrop)

Tablets, scored, stanozolol 5 mg. Net price 56-tab pack = £26.26

6.5   Hypothalamic and pituitary hormones and anti-oestrogens

Hypothalamic and pituitary hormones are described under the following section headings:

6.5.1   Hypothalamic and anterior pituitary hormones and anti-oestrogens

6.5.2   Posterior pituitary hormones and antagonists

> Use of preparations in these sections requires detailed prior investigation of the patient and *should be reserved for specialist centres.*

6.5.1   Hypothalamic and anterior pituitary hormones and anti-oestrogens

ANTI-OESTROGENS

The anti-oestrogens **clomiphene** (clomifene) and **tamoxifen** (section 8.3.4.1) are used in the treatment of female infertility due to oligomenorrhoea or secondary amenorrhoea (e.g. associated with polycystic ovarian disease). They induce gonadotrophin release by occupying oestrogen receptors in the hypothalamus, thereby interfering with feedback mechanisms; chorionic gonadotrophin is sometimes used as an adjunct. Patients should be warned that there is a risk of multiple pregnancy (*rarely* more than twins).

CLOMIPHENE CITRATE

(Clomifene Citrate)

Indications: anovulatory infertility—see notes above

Cautions: see notes above; polycystic ovary syndrome (cysts may enlarge during treatment), ovarian hyperstimulation syndrome, uterine fibroids, ectopic pregnancy, incidence of multiple births increased (consider ultrasound monitoring), visual symptoms (discontinue and initiate ophthalmological examination)

CSM Advice. The CSM has recommended that clomiphene should not normally be used for longer than 6 cycles (possible increased risk of ovarian cancer in patients treated for longer than recommended).

Contra-indications: hepatic disease, ovarian cysts, hormone dependent tumours or abnormal uterine bleeding of undetermined cause, pregnancy

Side-effects: visual disturbances (withdraw), ovarian hyperstimulation (withdraw), hot flushes, abdominal discomfort, occasionally nausea, vomiting, depression, insomnia, breast tenderness, headache, intermenstrual spotting, menorrhagia, endometriosis, convulsions, weight gain, rashes, dizziness, hair loss

Dose: 50 mg daily for 5 days, starting within about 5 days of onset of menstruation (preferably on 2nd day) or at any time (normally preceded by a progestogen-induced withdrawal bleed) if cycles have ceased; second course of 100 mg daily for 5 days may be given in absence of ovulation; most patients who are going to respond will do so to first course; 3 courses should constitute adequate therapeutic trial; long-term cyclical therapy not recommended—see CSM advice, above

PoM **Clomid**® (Hoechst Marion Roussel)

Tablets, yellow, scored, clomiphene citrate 50 mg. Net price 30-tab pack = £11.27; 100-tab pack = £32.80

PoM **Serophene**® (Serono)

Tablets, scored, clomiphene citrate 50 mg. Net price 10-tab pack = £4.12; 30-tab pack = £11.56; 100-tab pack = £33.64

ANTERIOR PITUITARY HORMONES

CORTICOTROPHINS

Tetracosactrin (tetracosactide) an analogue of corticotrophin (ACTH) is used to test adrenocortical function; corticotrophin itself is no longer commercially available in the UK. Failure of the plasma cortisol concentration to rise after intramuscular administration indicates adrenocortical insufficiency.

Both corticotrophin and tetracosactrin were formerly used as alternatives to corticosteroids in conditions such as Crohn's disease or rheumatoid arthritis; their value was limited by the variable and unpredictable therapeutic response and by the waning of their effect with time.

TETRACOSACTRIN
(Tetracosactide)

Indications: see notes above

Cautions; Contra-indications; Side-effects: as for corticosteroids, see section 6.3.2; important risk of anaphylaxis (medical supervision; see product literature)

PoM **Synacthen®** (Novartis)
Injection, tetracosactrin   250 micrograms   (as acetate)/mL. Net price 1-mL amp – £1.03p
Dose: diagnostic (30-minute test), *by intramuscular or intravenous injection,* 250 micrograms as a single dose

PoM **Synacthen Depot®** (Novartis)
Injection (aqueous suspension), tetracosactrin 1 mg (as acetate)/mL, with zinc phosphate complex; also contains benzyl alcohol. Net price 1-mL amp = £2.09
Dose: diagnostic (5-hour test), *by intramuscular injection,* 1 mg as a single dose
Note. Formerly used therapeutically by intramuscular injection, in an initial dose of 1 mg daily (or every 12 hours in acute cases); reduced to 1 mg every 2–3 days, then 1 mg weekly (or 500 micrograms every 2–3 days) but value was limited (see notes above)

GONADOTROPHINS

Follicle-stimulating hormone (FSH) and luteinising hormone (LH) together (as in **human menopausal gonadotrophin**) or follicle-stimulating hormone alone (as in **urofollitrophin** (urofollitropin) or **follitropin**), are used in the treatment of infertile women with proven hypopituitarism or who have not responded to clomiphene, or in superovulation treatment for assisted conception (such as *in vitro* fertilisation).

The gonadotrophins are also occasionally used in the treatment of oligospermia associated with hypopituitarism. There is no justification for their use in primary gonadal failure.

Chorionic gonadotrophin has also been used in delayed puberty in the male to stimulate endogenous testosterone production, but has little advantage over testosterone (section 6.4.2).

CHORIONIC GONADOTROPHIN
(Human Chorionic Gonadotrophin; HCG)

A preparation of a glycoprotein fraction secreted by the placenta and obtained from the urine of pregnant women having the action of the pituitary luteinising hormone

Indications: see notes above

Cautions: see notes above; cardiac or renal impairment, asthma, epilepsy, migraine

Side-effects: oedema (particularly in males—reduce dose), headache, tiredness, mood changes, gynaecomastia, local reactions; sexual precocity with high doses; may aggravate ovarian hyperstimulation

Dose: by subcutaneous or intramuscular injection, according to patient's response

PoM **Choragon®** (Ferring)
Injection, powder for reconstitution, chorionic gonadotrophin. Net price 5000-unit amp (with solvent) = £3.50. For intramuscular injection

PoM **Pregnyl®** (Organon)
Injection, powder for reconstitution, chorionic gonadotrophin. Net price 1500-unit amp = £2.48; 5000-unit amp = £3.69 (both with solvent). For intramuscular injection

PoM **Profasi®** (Serono)
Injection, powder for reconstitution, chorionic gonadotrophin. Net price 2000-unit amp = £2.10; 5000-unit amp = 3.70; 10 000-unit amp = £7.39 (all with solvent). For subcutaneous or intramuscular injection

FOLLITROPIN ALFA and BETA
(Recombinant human follicle stimulating hormone)

Indications: see notes above

Cautions; Side-effects: see under Human Menopausal Gonadotrophins

Dose: by subcutaneous injection, according to patient's response

Follitropin alfa
▼ PoM **Gonal-F®** (Serono)
Injection, powder for reconstitution, follitropin alfa. Net price 75-unit amp = £29.17; 150-unit amp = £58.34 (both with diluent)

Follitropin beta
▼ PoM **Puregon®** (Organon)
Injection, powder for reconstitution, follitropin beta. Net price 50-unit amp = £21.10; 100-unit amp = £42.20; 150-unit amp = £56.99 (all with solvent); kit containing auto-injector device available from manufacturer
Note. For subcutaneous or intramuscular injection

HUMAN MENOPAUSAL GONADOTROPHINS

Purified extract of human post-menopausal urine containing follicle-stimulating hormone (FSH) and luteinising hormone (LH); the relative *in vivo* activity is designated as a ratio; the 1:1 ratio is also known as menotrophin

Indications: see notes above

Cautions: ovarian cysts, adrenal or thyroid disorders, hyperprolactinoma or pituitary tumour

Side-effects: ovarian hyperstimulation, multiple pregnancy; local reactions
Dose: by deep intramuscular injection, according to patient's response

PoM **Humegon®** (Organon)
Injection, powder for reconstitution, menotrophin as follicle-stimulating hormone 75 units, luteinising hormone 75 units, net price per amp = £8.80; follicle-stimulating hormone 150 units, luteinising hormone 150 units, 1 amp = £16.00 (both with solvent)

PoM **Menogon®** (Ferring)
Injection, powder for reconstitution, menotrophin as follicle-stimulating hormone 75 units, luteinising hormone 75 units, net price per amp (with solvent) = £9.90

PoM **Normegon®** (Organon)
Injection, powder for reconstitution. human menopausal gonadotrophins as follicle-stimulating hormone 75 units, luteinising hormone 25 units, net price per amp = £10.21; follicle-stimulating hormone 150 units, luteinising hormone 50 units, 1 amp = £20.41 (both with solvent)

PoM **Pergonal®** (Serono)
Injection, powder for reconstitution, menotrophin as follicle-stimulating hormone 75 units, luteinising hormone 75 units. Net price per amp (with solvent) = £10.18

UROFOLLITROPHIN
(Urofollitropin)
Extract of the urine of postmenopausal women containing follicle-stimulating hormone
Indications: see notes above
Cautions; Side-effects: see under Human Menopausal Gonadotrophins
Dose: by subcutaneous or intramuscular injection, according to patient's response

PoM **Metrodin High Purity®** (Serono)
Injection, powder for reconstitution, urofollitrophin as follicle-stimulating hormone, net price 75-unit amp = £18.62; 150-unit amp = £37.24 (both with solvent). For subcutaneous or intramuscular injection

PoM **Orgafol®** (Organon)
Injection, powder for reconstitution, urofollitrophin as follicle-stimulating hormone, net price 75-unit amp (with solvent) = £9.50. For intramuscular injection

GROWTH HORMONE
Growth hormone is used in the treatment of growth hormone deficiency (including short stature in Turner syndrome); only the human type is effective since growth hormone is species specific. Growth hormone of human origin (HGH; somatotrophin) has been replaced by a growth hormone of human sequence, **somatropin**, produced using recombinant DNA technology.

SOMATROPIN
(Synthetic Human Growth Hormone)
Indications: see under Dose
Cautions: diabetes mellitus (adjustment of antidiabetic therapy may be necessary), papilloedema (see under Side-effects), relative deficiencies of other pituitary hormones (notably hypothyroidism—periodic thyroid function tests recommended), history of malignant disease, slipped epiphysis of the hip (monitor for limping), resolved intracranial hypertension (monitor closely), avoid in pregnancy (interrupt treatment if pregnancy occurs)
Contra-indications: evidence of tumour activity (complete antitumour therapy and ensure intracranial lesions inactive before starting); not to be used after renal transplantation or for growth promotion in children with closed epiphyses
Side-effects: funduscopy for papilloedema recommended if severe or recurrent headache, visual problems, nausea and vomiting occur—if papilloedema confirmed consider benign intracranial hypertension (rare cases reported); fluid retention (peripheral oedema, arthralgia, myalgia), antibody formation, hypothyroidism, transient reactions at injection site; leukaemia in children with growth hormone deficiency also reported
Dose: by subcutaneous injection, weekly dosage tailored for each individual and given in 3, 6 or 7 divided doses (rotate injection sites to prevent lipoatrophy); alternatively *by intramuscular injection,* weekly dosage given in 3 divided doses (but more painful)
Gonadal dysgenesis (Turner syndrome), 0.6–1 unit/kg weekly (18–28 units/m² body-surface area weekly) in divided doses given by subcutaneous injection
Insufficient secretion of growth hormone in children, 0.5–0.7 units/kg weekly (14–20 units/m² body-surface area weekly) in divided doses given by subcutaneous or intramuscular injection
Chronic renal insufficiency in children (renal function decreased to less than 50%), approx. 1 unit/kg weekly (30 units/m² body-surface area weekly) divided into daily subcutaneous injections, higher doses may be needed; adjustment may be required after 6 months
Adult growth hormone deficiency, initially 0.125 units/kg weekly (divided into daily subcutaneous injections) gradually increased if required to max. 0.25 units/kg weekly; use minimum effective dose (requirements may decrease with age)

PoM **Genotropin®** (Pharmacia & Upjohn)
Injection, powder for reconstitution, somatropin (rbe), net price 4-unit vial (with diluent) = £30.50. For subcutaneous injection
Injection, two-compartment cartridge containing powder for reconstitution, somatropin (rbe) and diluent. Net price 16-unit cartridge = £122.00, 36-unit cartridge = £274.50. For use with NHS *Genotropin® Pen* device (available free of charge from clinics). For subcutaneous injection

---

KabiQuick injection, two-compartment single-dose syringe containing powder for reconstitution, somatropin (rbe) and diluent. Net price 2-unit syringe = £16.00, 3-unit syringe = £24.00, 4-unit syringe = £32.00. For subcutaneous injection

KabiVial injection, two-compartment cartridge containing powder for reconstitution, somatropin (rbe) and diluent. Net price 4-unit vial = £30.50, 16-unit vial = £122.00. For subcutaneous injection

PoM **Humatrope**® (Lilly)

Injection, powder for reconstitution, somatropin (rbe), net price 4-unit vial (with diluent) = £30.50; 16-unit vial (with diluent) = £122.00; 18-unit cartridge = £137.25; 36-unit cartridge = £274.50; 72-unit cartridge = £549.00. Cartridges supplied with diluent and for use with NHS *Humatro-Pen*® *II* (available free of charge from clinics). For subcutaneous or intramuscular injection

PoM **Norditropin**® (Novo Nordisk)

Injection, powder for reconstitution, somatropin (epr), net price 12-unit vial (with diluent) = £89.21. For subcutaneous injection (intramuscular route rarely used)

PenSet 12 injection, powder for reconstitution, somatropin (epr), net price 12-unit vial (with diluent in cartridge and needle) = £93.68. For use with NHS *Nordiject*® *12* device (available free of charge from clinics). For subcutaneous injection

PenSet 24 injection, powder for reconstitution, somatropin (epr), net price 24-unit vial (with diluent in cartridge and needle) = £187.35. For use with NHS *Nordiject*® *24* device (available free of charge from clinics). For subcutaneous injection

PoM **Saizen**® (Serono)

Injection, powder for reconstitution, somatropin (rmc), net price 4-unit vial (with diluent) = £30.50; 10-unit vial (with diluent) = £76.25. For subcutaneous or intramuscular injection

PoM **Zomacton**® (Ferring)

Injection, powder for reconstitution, somatropin (rbe), net price 12-unit vial (with diluent) = £83.28. For subcutaneous injection

---

HYPOTHALAMIC HORMONES

Gonadorelin when injected intravenously in normal subjects leads to a rapid rise in plasma concentrations of both luteinising hormone (LH) and follicle-stimulating hormone (FSH). It has not proved to be very helpful, however, in distinguishing hypothalamic from pituitary lesions. Gonadorelin is also used for treatment of infertility, particularly in the female. **Gonadorelin analogues** are indicated in endometriosis and infertility (section 6.7.2) and in breast and prostate cancer (section 8.3.4).

Protirelin may be of value in difficult cases of hyperthyroidism but has been superseded largely by immunoassays. Failure of plasma thyrotrophin (TSH) concentration to rise after intravenous injection indicates excess circulating thyroid hormones. Impaired or absent responses also occur in some euthyroid patients with single adenoma, multinodu-

lar goitre, or endocrine exophthalmos; patients with hypopituitarism show a reduced or delayed rise.

Sermorelin, an analogue of growth hormone releasing hormone (somatorelin, GHRH), has recently been introduced as a diagnostic test for secretion of growth hormone.

GONADORELIN

(Gonadotrophin-releasing hormone; GnRH; LH–RH)

Indications: see preparations below

Side-effects: rarely, nausea, headache, abdominal pain, increased menstrual bleeding; rarely, hypersensitivity reaction on repeated administration of large doses; irritation at injection site

Dose: see under preparations

PoM **Fertiral**® (Hoechst Marion Roussel)

Injection, gonadorelin 500 micrograms/mL. Net price 2-mL amp = £33.44

For amenorrhoea and infertility due to abnormal release of LH–RH (endogenous gonadorelin), *by pulsatile subcutaneous infusion*, initially 10–20 micrograms over 1 minute, repeated every 90 minutes until conception occurs or for max. of 6 months; *pulsatile intravenous infusion* (in association with heparin) may be required

PoM **HRF**® (Monmouth)

Injection, powder for reconstitution, gonadorelin. Net price 100-microgram vial (with diluent) = £13.45 (hosp. only)

For assessment of pituitary function (adults), *by subcutaneous or intravenous injection*, 100 micrograms

PoM **Relefact LH-RH**® (Hoechst Marion Roussel)

Injection, gonadorelin 100 micrograms/mL. Net price 1-mL amp = £9.44

For assessment of pituitary function, *by intravenous injection*, 100 micrograms

---

PROTIRELIN

(Thyrotrophin-releasing hormone; TRH)

Indications: assessment of thyroid function and thyroid stimulating hormone reserve

Cautions: severe hypopituitarism, myocardial ischaemia, bronchial asthma and obstructive airways disease, pregnancy

Side-effects: after rapid intravenous administration desire to micturate, flushing, dizziness, nausea, strange taste; transient increase in pulse rate and blood pressure; rarely bronchospasm

Dose: by intravenous injection, 200 micrograms; CHILD 1 microgram/kg

PoM **TRH-Cambridge**® (Cambridge)

Injection, protirelin 100 micrograms/mL. Net price 2-mL amp = £7.09 (hosp. only)

SERMORELIN

Indications: see notes above

Cautions: epilepsy; discontinue growth hormone therapy 1–2 weeks before test; untreated hypothyroidism, antithyroid drugs; obesity, hyperglycaemia, elevated plasma fatty acids; avoid preparations which affect release of growth horm-

---

one (includes those affecting release of somato-statin, insulin or glucocorticoids and cyclo-oxygenase inhibitors such as aspirin and indo-methacin)

Contra-indications: pregnancy and breast-feeding

Side-effects: occasional facial flushing and pain at injection site

Dose: by intravenous injection, 1 microgram/kg in the morning after an overnight fast

▼ PoM **Geref 50**® (Serono)

Injection, powder for reconstitution, sermorelin 50 micrograms (as acetate). Net price per amp (with solvent) = £55.00

6.5.2   Posterior pituitary hormones and antagonists

POSTERIOR PITUITARY HORMONES

DIABETES INSIPIDUS. **Vasopressin** (antidiuretic hormone, ADH) is used in the treatment of *pituitary* ('cranial') *diabetes insipidus* as its analogues **lypressin** or **desmopressin**. Dosage is tailored to produce a slight diuresis every 24 hours to avoid water intoxication. Treatment may be required for a limited period only in diabetes insipidus following trauma or pituitary surgery.

Desmopressin has a longer duration of action than vasopressin or lypressin; unlike vasopressin and lypressin it has no vasoconstrictor effect. It is given by mouth or intranasally for maintenance therapy, and by injection in the postoperative period or in unconscious patients. Desmopressin is also used in the differential diagnosis of diabetes insipidus. Following a dose of 2 micrograms intramuscularly or 20 micrograms intranasally, restoration of the ability to concentrate urine after water deprivation confirms a diagnosis of cranial diabetes insipidus. Failure to respond occurs in nephrogenic diabetes insipidus.

In *nephrogenic* and *partial pituitary diabetes insipidus* benefit may be gained from the paradoxical antidiuretic effect of thiazides (see section 2.2.1) e.g. chlorthalidone 100 mg twice daily reduced to maintenance dose of 50 mg daily.

Chlorpropamide (section 6.1.2.1) is also useful in partial pituitary diabetes insipidus, and probably acts by sensitising the renal tubules to the action of remaining endogenous vasopressin; it is given in doses of up to 350 mg daily in adults and 200 mg daily in children, care being taken to avoid hypo-glycaemia. Carbamazepine (see section 4.8.1) is also sometimes useful (in a dose of 200 mg once or twice daily) [unlicensed]; its mode of action may be similar to that of chlorpropamide.

OTHER USES. Desmopressin injection is also used to boost factor VIII concentrations in mild to moderate haemophilia. For a comment on use of desmopressin in nocturnal enuresis see section 7.4.2.

Vasopressin infusion is used to control variceal bleeding in portal hypertension, prior to more definitive treatment and with variable results. Terli-pressin, a derivative of vasopressin, is used similarly.

Oxytocin, another posterior pituitary hormone, is indicated in obstetrics (see section 7.1.1).

VASOPRESSIN

Indications: pituitary diabetes insipidus; bleeding from oesophageal varices

Cautions: heart failure, asthma, epilepsy, migraine or other conditions which might be aggravated by water retention; renal impairment (see also contra-indications); pregnancy; avoid fluid overload

Contra-indications: vascular disease (especially disease of coronary arteries) unless extreme caution, chronic nephritis (until reasonable blood nitrogen concentrations attained)

Side-effects: pallor, nausea, belching, abdominal cramps, desire to defaecate, hypersensitivity reactions, constriction of coronary arteries (may cause anginal attacks and myocardial ischaemia)

Dose: by subcutaneous or intramuscular injection, diabetes insipidus, 5–20 units every four hours

By intravenous infusion, initial control of variceal bleeding, 20 units over 15 minutes

Synthetic vasopressin

PoM **Pitressin**® (Goldshield)

Injection, argipressin (synthetic vasopressin) 20 units/mL. Net price 1-mL amp = £12.50 (hosp. only)

DESMOPRESSIN

Indications: see under Dose

Cautions: see under Vasopressin; less pressor activity, but still considerable caution in renal impairment, in cardiovascular disease and in hypertension (not indicated for nocturnal enuresis or nocturia in these circumstances); elderly (avoid for nocturnal enuresis and nocturia in those over 65 years); also considerable caution in cystic fibrosis; in nocturia and nocturnal enuresis limit fluid intake to minimum and only to satisfy thirst for 8 hours after dose; in nocturia periodic blood pressure and weight checks needed to monitor for fluid overload; **interactions:** Appendix 1 (desmopressin)

HYPONATRAEMIC CONVULSIONS. The CSM has advised that patients being treated for primary nocturnal enuresis should be warned to avoid fluid overload (including during swimming) and to stop taking desmopressin during an episode of vomiting or diarrhoea (until fluid balance normal). The risk of hyponatraemic convulsions can also be minimised by keeping to the recommended starting doses and by avoiding concomitant use of drugs which increase secretion of vasopressin (e.g. tricyclic anti-depressants)

Contra-indications: cardiac insufficiency and other conditions treated with diuretics

Side-effects: fluid retention, and hyponatraemia (in more serious cases with convulsions) on administration without restricting fluid intake; stomach pain, headache, nausea, vomiting, and epistaxis also reported

---

Dose: by mouth

Diabetes insipidus, treatment, ADULT and CHILD, initially 300 micrograms daily (in three divided doses); maintenance, 300–600 micrograms daily; range 0.2–1.2 mg daily

Primary nocturnal enuresis (with normal urine concentrating ability), ADULT and CHILD over 5 years (preferably over 7 years), 200 micrograms at bedtime, only increased to 400 micrograms if lower dose not effective (**important:** see also Cautions); withdraw for at least one week for reassessment after 3 months

Postoperative polyuria/polydipsia, adjust dose according to urine osmolality

Intranasally

Diabetes insipidus, diagnosis, ADULT and CHILD, 20 micrograms

Diabetes insipidus, treatment, ADULT, 10–40 micrograms daily (in one or two divided doses); CHILD, 5–20 micrograms; infants may require lower doses

Primary nocturnal enuresis (with normal urine concentrating ability), ADULT and CHILD over 5 years (preferably over 7 years), initially 20 micrograms at bedtime, only increased to 40 micrograms if lower dose not effective (**important:** see also Cautions); withdraw for at least one week for reassessment after 3 months

Nocturia associated with multiple sclerosis (when other treatments have failed), ADULT (under 65 years), 10–20 micrograms at bedtime (**important:** see also cautions), dose not to be repeated within 24 hours

Renal function testing (empty bladder at time of testing), ADULT, 40 micrograms; CHILD 1–15 years, 20 micrograms; under 1 year, 10 micrograms (restrict fluid intake to 50% at next two feeds to avoid fluid overload)

By injection

Diabetes insipidus, diagnosis (*subcutaneous or intramuscular*), ADULT and CHILD, 2 micrograms

Diabetes insipidus, treatment (*subcutaneous, intramuscular or intravenous*), ADULT, 1–4 micrograms daily; CHILD 400 nanograms

Renal function testing (*subcutaneous or intramuscular*), ADULT and CHILD, 2 micrograms

Mild to moderate haemophilia and von Willebrands disease, post lumbar puncture headache, fibrinolytic response testing, consult product literature

PoM **DDAVP®** (Ferring)

Tablets, both scored, desmopressin acetate 100 micrograms, net price 90-tab pack = £45.95; 200 micrograms, 90-tab pack = £91.90. Counselling, fluid intake, see above

Intranasal solution, desmopressin acetate 100 micrograms/mL. Net price 2.5-mL dropper bottle and catheter = £9.50. Counselling, fluid intake, see above

Injection, desmopressin acetate 4 micrograms/mL. Net price 1-mL amp = £1.07

PoM **Desmotabs®** (Ferring)

Tablets, scored, desmopressin acetate 200 micrograms, net price 28-tab pack = £29.00. Counselling, fluid intake, see above

PoM **Desmospray®** (Ferring)

Nasal spray, desmopressin acetate 10 micrograms/metered spray. Net price 6-mL unit = £28.00. Counselling, fluid intake, see above

Note. Children requiring dose of less than 10 micrograms should be given *DDAVP®* intranasal solution

LYPRESSIN

Indications: pituitary diabetes insipidus
Cautions; Contra-indications; Side-effects: see under Vasopressin; less hypersensitivity; also nasal congestion with ulceration of mucosa
Dose: intranasally, 5–10 units 3–4 times daily

PoM **Syntopressin®** (Novartis)

Nasal spray, lypressin 50 units/mL, 5 units/squeeze. Net price 5-mL bottle = £3.40

TERLIPRESSIN

Indications: bleeding from oesophageal varices
Cautions; Contra-indications; Side-effects: see under Vasopressin, but effects are milder
Dose: by intravenous injection, 2 mg followed by 1 or 2 mg every 4 to 6 hours until bleeding is controlled, for up to 72 hours

PoM **Glypressin®** (Ferring)

Injection, terlipressin, powder for reconstitution. Net price 1-mg vial with 5 mL diluent = £19.00 (hosp. only)

ANTIDIURETIC HORMONE ANTAGONISTS

Demeclocycline (section 5.1.3) may be used in the treatment of hyponatraemia resulting from inappropriate secretion of antidiuretic hormone. It is thought to act by directly blocking the renal tubular effect of antidiuretic hormone. Initially 0.9 to 1.2 g is given daily in divided doses, reduced to 600–900 mg daily for maintenance.

6.6 Drugs affecting bone metabolism

6.6.1 Calcitonin
6.6.2 Bisphosphonates

See also calcium (section 9.5.1.1), phosphorus (section 9.5.2), vitamin D (section 9.6.4), and oestrogens in postmenopausal osteoporosis (section 6.4.1.1).

6.6.1 Calcitonin

Calcitonin is involved with parathyroid hormone in the regulation of bone turnover and hence in the maintenance of calcium balance and homoeostasis.

It is used to lower the plasma-calcium concentration in some patients with hypercalcaemia (notably when associated with malignant disease). In the treatment of severe Paget's disease of bone it is used mainly for relief of pain but it is also effective in relieving some of the neurological complications, for example deafness. The prolonged use of **porcine calcitonin** can lead to the production of neutralising antibodies. **Salcatonin** (synthetic salmon calcitonin) is less immunogenic and thus more suitable for long-term therapy. When changing treatment in Paget's disease, calcitonin (pork) 80 units is equivalent to salcatonin 50 units.

CALCITONIN (PORK)

Indications: Paget's disease of bone; hypercalcaemia

Cautions: see notes above; may contain trace of thyroid; skin test if history of allergy; pregnancy and breast-feeding (avoid—inhibits lactation in *animals*)

Side-effects: nausea, vomiting, flushing, tingling of hands, unpleasant taste, inflammatory reactions at injection site

Dose: hypercalcaemia, *by subcutaneous or intramuscular injection*, initially 4 units/kg daily adjusted according to clinical and biochemical response (higher doses more conveniently given as salcatonin, see below)

Paget's disease of bone, *by subcutaneous or intramuscular injection*, dose range 80 units 3 times weekly to 160 units daily in single or divided doses; in patients with bone pain or nerve compression syndromes, 80–160 units daily for 3–6 months

PoM **Calcitare®** (Rhône-Poulenc Rorer)
Injection, powder for reconstitution, porcine calcitonin. Net price 160-unit vial (with gelatin diluent) = £13.40

SALCATONIN
(Calcitonin (salmon))

Indications: see under Dose (all short term)

Cautions; Side-effects: see under Calcitonin (pork) and notes above

Dose: hypercalcaemia, *by subcutaneous or intramuscular injection*, range from 5–10 units/kg daily *to* 400 units every 6–8 hours adjusted according to clinical and biochemical response (no additional benefit with over 8 units/kg every 6 hours); *by slow intravenous infusion* (Miacalcic® only), 5–10 units/kg over at least 6 hours

Paget's disease of bone, *by subcutaneous or intramuscular injection*, dose range 50 units 3 times weekly to 100 units daily, in single or divided doses; in patients with bone pain or nerve compression syndromes, 50–100 units daily for 3–6 months

Bone pain in neoplastic disease, *by subcutaneous or intramuscular injection*, 200 units every 6 hours *or* 400 units every 12 hours for 48 hours; may be repeated at discretion of physician

Postmenopausal osteoporosis, *by subcutaneous or intramuscular injection*, 100 units daily with dietary calcium and vitamin D supplements (see sections 9.5.1.1 and 9.6.4)

PoM **Calsynar®** (Rhône-Poulenc Rorer)
Injection, salcatonin 100 units/mL in saline/acetate, net price 1-mL amp = £7.92; 200 units/mL in saline/acetate, 2-mL vial = £28.47
For subcutaneous or intramuscular injection only

PoM **Miacalcic®** (Novartis)
Injection, salcatonin 50 units/mL, net price 1-mL amp = £3.56; 100 units/mL, 1-mL amp = £7.13; 200 units/mL, 2-mL vial = £25.62
For subcutaneous or intramuscular injection and for dilution and use as an intravenous infusion

6.6.2   Bisphosphonates

Bisphosphonates are used mainly in the treatment of *Paget's disease* of bone. They are adsorbed onto hydroxyapatite crystals, so slowing both their rate of growth and dissolution, and reduce the increased rate of bone turnover associated with the disease. They are also used in the treatment of *hypercalcaemia of malignancy* (section 9.5.1.2). Bisphosphonates may also have an important role in treating *osteoporosis in postmenopausal women.* Disodium etidronate (as *Didronel PMO®*) is also licensed for the prevention and treatment of corticosteroid-induced osteoporosis.

ALENDRONIC ACID

Indications: postmenopausal osteoporosis

Cautions: upper gastro-intestinal disorders (dysphagia, symptomatic oesophageal disease, gastritis, duodenitis, or ulcers—see also under Contraindications and Side-effects); correct disturbances of calcium and mineral metabolism (e.g. vitamin-D deficiency, hypocalcaemia) before starting; exclude other causes of osteoporosis; **interactions:** Appendix 1 (bisphosphonates)

Contra-indications: abnormalities of oesophagus and other factors which delay emptying (e.g. stricture or achalasia), hypocalcaemia, renal impairment, pregnancy and breast-feeding; inability to stand or sit upright for 30 minutes (see Counselling below)

Side-effects: oesophageal reactions (see below), abdominal pain and distension, diarrhoea or constipation, flatulence, musculoskeletal pain, headache; rarely rash, erythema, transient decrease in serum calcium and phosphate; nausea, vomiting, peptic ulceration and hypersensitivity reactions (including urticaria and angioedema) also reported

OESOPHAGEAL REACTIONS. Severe oesophageal reactions (oesophagitis, oesophageal ulcers and oesophageal erosions) have been reported; patients should be advised to stop taking the tablets and to seek medical attention if they develop symptoms of oesophageal irritation such as dysphagia, new or worsening heartburn, pain on swallowing or retrosternal pain

Dose: 10 mg daily at least 30 minutes before breakfast

COUNSELLING. Swallow the tablets whole with a full glass of water on an empty stomach at least 30 minutes before breakfast (and any other oral medication); stand or sit upright for at least 30 minutes and do not lie down until after eating breakfast. Do not take the tablets at bedtime or before rising.

▼ PoM **Fosamax**® (MSD)

Tablets, alendronic acid 10 mg (as alendronate sodium). Net price 28-tab pack = £25.69. Counselling, administration

DISODIUM ETIDRONATE

Indications: see under Dose

Cautions: reduce dose in mild renal impairment (avoid if moderate to severe); **interactions:** Appendix 1 (bisphosphonates)

Contra-indications: moderate to severe renal impairment; pregnancy and breast-feeding; not indicated for osteoporosis in presence of hypercalcaemia or hypercalciuria or for osteomalacia

Side-effects: nausea, diarrhoea or constipation, abdominal pain; asymptomatic hypocalcaemia; increased bone pain in Paget's disease, also increased risk of fractures with high doses in Paget's disease (discontinue if fractures occur); rarely skin reactions (including angioedema urticaria and pruritus), transient hyperphosphataemia, headache, paraesthesia, peripheral neuropathy reported; blood disorders (including leucopenia, agranulocytosis and pancytopenia) also reported

Dose: Paget's disease of bone, *by mouth,* 5 mg/kg as a single daily dose for up to 6 months; doses above 10 mg/kg daily for up to 3 months may be used with caution but doses above 20 mg/kg daily are not recommended; after interval of not less than 3 months may be repeated where evidence of reactivation—including biochemical indices (avoid premature retreatment)

MONITORING. Serum phosphate, serum alkaline phosphatase and (if possible) urinary hydroxyproline should be measured before starting and at intervals of 3 months—consult product literature for further details

Osteoporosis, see under *Didronel PMO*®

COUNSELLING. Avoid food for at least 2 hours before and after oral treatment, particularly calcium-containing products e.g. milk; also avoid iron and mineral supplements and antacids

PoM **Didronel**® (Procter & Gamble Pharm.)

Tablets, disodium etidronate 200 mg. Net price 60-tab pack = £43.88. Counselling, food and calcium (see above)

With calcium carbonate

For cautions and side-effects of calcium carbonate see section 9.5.1.1

PoM **Didronel PMO**® (Procter & Gamble Pharm.)

Tablets, 14 white, disodium etidronate 400 mg; 76 pink, effervescent, calcium carbonate 1.25 g (*Cacit*®). Net price per pack = £40.20. Label: 10 patient information leaflet, counselling, food and calcium (see above)

Dose: treatment of osteoporosis, prevention of bone loss in postmenopausal women (particularly if hormone replacement therapy inappropriate), and prevention and treatment of corticosteroid-induced osteoporosis, given in 90-day cycles, 1 *Didronel*® tablet daily for 14 days, then 1 *Cacit*® tablet daily for 76 days

DISODIUM PAMIDRONATE

Disodium pamidronate was formerly called aminohydroxypropylidenediphosphonate disodium (APD)

Indications: see under Dose

Cautions: renal impairment—monitor renal function in those with pre-existing renal disease or predisposition to renal impairment (e.g. in multiple myeloma or tumour-induced hypercalcaemia); cardiac disease (especially in elderly); previous thyroid surgery (risk of hypocalcaemia); monitor serum electrolytes, calcium and phosphate—possibility of convulsions due to electrolyte changes; avoid concurrent use with other bisphosphonates; **interactions:** Appendix 1 (bisphosphonates)

DRIVING. Patients should be warned against driving or operating machinery immediately after treatment (somnolence or dizziness may occur)

Contra-indications: pregnancy and breast-feeding

Side-effects: hypocalcaemia (rarely symptomatic), hypophosphataemia, transient rise in body temperature, fever and influenza-like symptoms (sometimes accompanied by malaise, rigors, fatigue and flushes); occasionally transient bone pain, arthralgia, myalgia, nausea, vomiting, headache, lymphocytopenia, hypomagnesaemia; rarely muscle cramps, anorexia, abdominal pain, diarrhoea, constipation, dyspepsia, agitation, confusion, dizziness, insomnia, somnolence, lethargy, anaemia, leucopenia, hypotension or hypertension, rash, pruritus, hyperkalaemia or hypokalaemia, hypernatraemia; isolated cases of seizures, hallucinations, thrombocytopenia, haematuria, acute renal failure, deterioration of pre-existing renal disease, conjunctivitis and other ocular symptoms, abnormal liver function tests, reactivation of herpes simplex and zoster reported; also local reactions at injection site

Dose: by slow intravenous infusion (via cannula in a relatively large vein), see also Appendix 6

Hypercalcaemia of malignancy, according to serum calcium concentration 15–60 mg in single infusion or in divided doses over 2–4 days; max. 90 mg per treatment course

Osteolytic lesions and bone pain in bone metastases associated with breast cancer or multiple myeloma, 90 mg every 4 weeks (or every 3 weeks to coincide with chemotherapy in breast cancer)

Paget's disease of bone, 30 mg once a week for 6 weeks (total dose 180 mg) *or* 30 mg in first week then 60 mg every other week (total dose 210 mg); max. total 360 mg (in divided doses of 60 mg) per treatment course; may be repeated every 6 months

CALCIUM AND VITAMIN D SUPPLEMENTS. Oral supplements are advised for those with Paget's disease at risk of calcium or vitamin D deficiency (e.g. through malabsorption or lack of exposure to sunlight) to minimise potential risk of hypocalcaemia

---

Cautionary label wordings, see inside back cover   Prices are **net,** see p.1

PoM **Aredia Dry Powder**® (Novartis)
Injection, powder for reconstitution, disodium pamidronate, for use as an infusion. Net price 15-mg vial = £27.27; 30-mg vial = £54.53; 90-mg vial = £155.80 (all with diluent). Counselling, driving, see above

SODIUM CLODRONATE

Indications: see under Dose
Cautions: monitor renal and hepatic function and white cell count; also monitor serum calcium and phosphate periodically; renal dysfunction reported in patients receiving concomitant NSAIDs; maintain adequate fluid intake during treatment; **interactions:** Appendix 1 (bisphosphonates)
Contra-indications: moderate to severe renal impairment; pregnancy and breast-feeding
Side-effects: nausea, diarrhoea; asymptomatic hypocalcaemia; skin reactions
Dose: osteolytic lesions, hypercalcaemia and bone pain associated with skeletal metastases in patients with breast cancer or multiple myeloma, *by mouth*, 1.6 g daily in single or 2 divided doses increased if necessary to a max. of 3.2 g daily
COUNSELLING. Avoid food for 1 hour before and after treatment, particularly calcium-containing products e.g. milk; also avoid iron and mineral supplements and antacids; maintain adequate fluid intake
Hypercalcaemia of malignancy, *by slow intravenous infusion*, 300 mg daily for max. 7–10 days *or* by single-dose infusion of 1.5 g

PoM **Bonefos**® (Boehringer Ingelheim)
Capsules, yellow, sodium clodronate 400 mg. Net price 30-cap pack = £45.59, 112-cap pack = £170.23, 120-cap pack = £182.39. Counselling, food and calcium
Tablets, f/c, scored, sodium clodronate 800 mg. Net price 10-tab pack = £30.40; 60-tab pack = £182.39. Counselling, food and calcium
Concentrate (= intravenous solution), sodium clodronate 60 mg/mL, for dilution and use as infusion. Net price 5-mL amp = £14.43

PoM **Loron**® (Boehringer Mannheim)
Loron® capsules, sodium clodronate 400 mg. Net price 30-cap pack = £45.59, 112-cap pack = £170.23, 120-cap pack = £182.39. Label: 10 patient information leaflet, counselling, food and calcium
Loron 520® tablets, f/c, scored, sodium clodronate 520 mg. Net price 10-tab pack = £30.40; 60-tab pack = £182.39. Label: 10 patient information leaflet, counselling, food and calcium
Dose: 2 tablets daily in single or two divided doses; may be increased to max. 4 tablets daily
Note. Due to greater bioavailability one *Loron 520*® tablet (520 mg) is equivalent to two *Loron*® capsules (2 × 400 mg)

PoM **Loron**® for infusion (Boehringer Mannheim)
Intravenous solution, sodium clodronate 30 mg/mL, for dilution and use as infusion. Net price 10-mL amp = £14.43

TILUDRONIC ACID

Indications: Paget's disease of bone
Cautions: renal impairment (monitor renal function regularly, see under Contra-indications); correct disturbances of calcium metabolism (e.g. vitamin D deficiency, hypocalcaemia) before starting; avoid concomitant use of indomethacin; **interactions:** Appendix 1 (bisphosphonates)
Contra-indications: severe renal impairment, juvenile Paget's disease, pregnancy and breast-feeding
Side-effects: stomach pain, nausea, diarrhoea; rarely asthenia, dizziness, headache and skin reactions
Dose: 400 mg daily as a single dose for 12 weeks; may be repeated if necessary after 6 months
COUNSELLING. Avoid food for 2 hours before and after treatment, particularly calcium-containing products e.g. milk; also avoid antacids

▼ PoM **Skelid**® (Sanofi Winthrop)
Tablets, tiludronic acid (as tiludronate disodium) 200 mg. Net price 28-tab pack = £99.00. Counselling, food and calcium

6.7   Other endocrine drugs

This section includes:
    6.7.1   Bromocriptine and other dopamine-receptor stimulants
    6.7.2   Danazol, gestrinone, and gonadorelin analogues
    6.7.3   Metyrapone and trilostane

6.7.1   Bromocriptine and other dopamine-receptor stimulants

Bromocriptine is a stimulant of dopamine receptors in the brain; it also inhibits release of prolactin by the pituitary. Bromocriptine is used for the treatment of galactorrhoea and cyclical benign breast disease, and for the treatment of prolactinomas (when it reduces both plasma prolactin concentration and tumour size). Bromocriptine also inhibits the release of growth hormone and is sometimes used in the treatment of acromegaly, the success rate is much lower than with prolactinomas.

Cabergoline has actions and uses similar to those of bromocriptine, but its duration of action is longer. Its profile of side-effects appears to differ from that of bromocriptine, which means that patients intolerant of bromocriptine may be able to tolerate cabergoline (and *vice versa*).

Quinagolide has been introduced recently; its actions and uses are similar to those of bromocriptine, but its profile of side-effects differs slightly.

SUPPRESSION OF LACTATION. Although bromocriptine and cabergoline are licensed to suppress lactation, they are **not** recommended for routine suppression (or for the relief of symptoms of post-partum pain and engorgement) that can be adequately treated with simple analgesics and breast support. Quinagolide is not licensed for the suppression of lactation.

BROMOCRIPTINE

Indications: see notes above and under Dose; parkinsonism, section 4.9.1

Cautions: specialist evaluation—monitor for pituitary enlargement, particularly during pregnancy, annual gynaecological assessment (postmenopausal, every 6 months), monitor for peptic ulceration in acromegalic patients; contraceptive advice if appropriate (oral contraceptives may increase prolactin concentration); caution in patients with history of serious mental disorders (especially psychotic disorders) or with cardiovascular disease or Raynaud's syndrome and monitor for retroperitoneal fibrosis; porphyria (section 9.8.2); **interactions:** Appendix 1 (bromocriptine and cabergoline)

HYPOTENSIVE REACTIONS. Hypotensive reactions may be disturbing in some patients during the first few days of treatment and particular care should be exercised when driving or operating machinery; tolerance may be reduced by alcohol

Contra-indications: hypersensitivity to bromocriptine or other ergot alkaloids; toxaemia of pregnancy and hypertension in postpartum women or in puerperium (see also below); advise women not to breast-feed if lactation prevention fails

POSTPARTUM OR PUERPERIUM. Should not be used postpartum or in puerperium in women with high blood pressure, coronary artery disease or symptoms (or history) of serious mental disorder; monitor blood pressure carefully (especially during first few days) in postpartum women. Very rarely hypertension, myocardial infarction, seizures or stroke (both sometimes preceded by severe headache) and mental disorders have been reported in postpartum women given bromocriptine for lactation suppression—caution with antihypertensive therapy and avoid other ergot alkaloids. Discontinue immediately if hypertension, unremitting headache or signs of CNS toxicity develop

Side-effects: nausea, vomiting, constipation, headache, dizziness, postural hypotension, drowsiness, vasospasm of fingers and toes particularly in patients with Raynaud's syndrome; *high doses,* confusion, psychomotor excitation, hallucinations, dyskinesia, dry mouth, leg cramps, pleural effusions (may necessitate withdrawal of treatment), retroperitoneal fibrosis reported (monitoring required)

Dose: prevention/suppression of lactation (but see notes above and under Contra-indications), 2.5 mg on 1st day (prevention) or daily for 2–3 days (suppression); then 2.5 mg twice daily for 14 days

Hypogonadism/galactorrhoea, infertility, initially 1–1.25 mg at bedtime, increased gradually; usual dose 7.5 mg daily in divided doses, increased if necessary to a max. of 30 mg daily. Usual dose in infertility without hyperprolactinaemia, 2.5 mg twice daily

Cyclical benign breast disease and cyclical menstrual disorders (particularly breast pain), 1–1.25 mg at bedtime, increased gradually; usual dose 2.5 mg twice daily

Acromegaly, initially 1–1.25 mg at bedtime, increase gradually to 5 mg every 6 hours

Prolactinoma, initially 1–1.25 mg at bedtime; increased gradually to 5 mg every 6 hours (occasional patients may require up to 30 mg daily) CHILD under 15, not recommended

PoM **Bromocriptine** (Non-proprietary)

Tablets, bromocriptine (as mesylate), 2.5 mg, net price 30-tab pack = £5.28. Label: 21, counselling, hypotensive reactions
Available from APS, Berk, Cox, Kent, Norton

PoM **Parlodel®** (Novartis)

Tablets, both scored, bromocriptine (as mesylate) 1 mg, net price 100-tab pack = £9.05; 2.5 mg, 30-tab pack = £5.28. Label: 21, counselling, hypotensive reactions

Capsules, bromocriptine (as mesylate) 5 mg (blue/white), net price 100-cap pack = £34.34; 10 mg (white), 100-cap pack = £63.53. Label: 21, counselling, hypotensive reactions

CABERGOLINE

Indications: see notes above and under Dose

Cautions: see under Bromocriptine; peptic ulcer, gastro-intestinal bleeding; severe hepatic impairment; fibrotic lung disease; monthly pregnancy tests during the amenorrhoeic period; advise non-hormonal contraception if pregnancy not desired (see also Contra-indications); **interactions:** Appendix 1 (bromocriptine and cabergoline)

HYPOTENSIVE REACTIONS. Hypotensive reactions may be disturbing in some patients during the first few days of treatment and particular care should be exercised when driving or operating machinery; tolerance may be reduced by alcohol

Contra-indications: see under Bromocriptine; exclude pregnancy before starting and avoid until at least 1 month after successful treatment (ovulatory cycles persist for 6 months)—discontinue if pregnancy occurs during treatment (specialist advice needed)

Side-effects: see under Bromocriptine (but profile of side-effects may differ, see notes above); dyspepsia, epigastric and abdominal pain, breast pain, palpitations, angina, epistaxis, peripheral oedema, hemianopia, asthenia, erythromelalgia, hot flushes, depression

Dose: prevention of lactation (but see notes above), during first day postpartum, 1 mg as a single dose; suppression of established lactation (but see notes above) 250 micrograms every 12 hours for 2 days

Hyperprolactinaemic disorders, 500 micrograms weekly (as a single dose *or* as 2 divided doses on separate days) increased at monthly intervals in steps of 500 micrograms until optimal therapeutic response (usually 1 mg weekly, range 0.25–2 mg weekly) with monthly monitoring of serum prolactin levels; reduce initial dose and increase more gradually if patient intolerant; over 1 mg weekly give as divided doses; up to 4.5 mg weekly has been used in hyperprolactinaemic patients
Parkinsonism, section 4.9.1
CHILD under 16 years, not recommended

▼ PoM **Dostinex**® (Pharmacia & Upjohn)
Tablets, scored, cabergoline 500 micrograms. Net price 8-tab pack = £31.46. Label: 21, counselling, hypotensive reactions

QUINAGOLIDE
Indications: see notes above and under Dose
Cautions; Contra-indications; Side-effects: see under Bromocriptine (but profile of side-effects may differ, see notes above); hypersensitivity to quinagolide (but not ergot alkaloids); syncope, anorexia, abdominal pain, diarrhoea, insomnia, oedema, flushing and nasal congestion also reported; advise non-hormonal contraception if pregnancy not desired; discontinue if pregnancy occurs during treatment (specialist advice needed); **interactions:** Appendix 1 (quinagolide)
HYPOTENSIVE REACTIONS. Hypotensive reactions may be disturbing in some patients during the first few days of treatment—monitor blood pressure for a few days after starting treatment and following dosage increases; particular care should be exercised when driving or operating machinery; tolerance may be reduced by alcohol
Dose: hyperprolactinaemia, 25 micrograms at bedtime for 3 days; increased at intervals of 3 days in steps of 25 micrograms to usual maintenance dose of 75–150 micrograms daily; for doses higher than 300 micrograms daily increase in steps of 75–150 micrograms at intervals of not less than 4 weeks
CHILD not recommended

PoM **Norprolac**® (Novartis)
Tablets, quinagolide (as hydrochloride) 75 micrograms (white), net price 30-tab pack = £57.00; 150 micrograms (white), 30-tab pack = £100.00; starter pack of 3 × 25-microgram tabs (pink) with 3 × 50-microgram tabs (blue) = £5.00. Label: 21, counselling, hypotensive reactions

6.7.2   Danazol, gestrinone and gonadorelin analogues

Danazol inhibits pituitary gonadotrophins; it combines androgenic activity with antioestrogenic and antiprogestogenic activity. It is used in the treatment of *endometriosis* and has also been used for *mammary dysplasia*, and *gynaecomastia* where other measures have proved unsatisfactory; it has been used for *menorrhagia* and other *menstrual disorders* but in view of its side-effects, treatment with other drugs may be preferable (see section 6.4.1.2). It may also be effective in the long-term management of *hereditary angioedema* [unlicensed indication].

Gestrinone has general actions similar to those of danazol and is indicated for the treatment of endometriosis.

DANAZOL
Indications: see notes above and under Dose
Cautions: cardiac, hepatic, or renal impairment (avoid if severe), elderly, polycythaemia, epilepsy, diabetes mellitus, hypertension, migraine, lipoprotein disorder, history of thrombosis or thromboembolic disease; withdraw if virilisation

(may be irreversible on continued use); non-hormonal contraceptive methods should be used, if appropriate; **interactions:** Appendix 1 (danazol)
Contra-indications: pregnancy, ensure that patients with amenorrhoea are not pregnant; breast-feeding; severe hepatic, renal or cardiac impairment; thromboembolic disease; undiagnosed genital bleeding; androgen-dependent tumours; porphyria (section 9.8.2)
Side-effects: nausea, dizziness, skin reactions including rashes, photosensitivity and exfoliative dermatitis, fever, backache, nervousness, mood changes, anxiety, changes in libido, vertigo, fatigue, epigastric and pleuritic pain, headache, weight gain; menstrual disturbances, vaginal dryness and irritation, flushing and reduction in breast size; musculo-skeletal spasm, joint pain and swelling, hair loss; androgenic effects including acne, oily skin, oedema, hirsutism, voice changes and rarely clitoral hypertrophy (see also Cautions); temporary alteration in lipoproteins and other metabolic changes, insulin resistance; thrombotic events; leucopenia, thrombocytopenia, eosinophilia, reversible erythrocytosis or polycythaemia reported; headache and visual disturbances may indicate benign intracranial hypertension; rarely cholestatic jaundice, pancreatitis, peliosis hepatis and benign hepatic adenomata
Dose: in women all doses should start during menstruation, preferably on the first day; usually given in up to 4 divided doses
Endometriosis, 200–800 mg daily in up to 4 divided doses, adjusted according to response, usually for 6 months (up to 9 months in some cases)
Menorrhagia (but see notes above), 200 mg daily, usually for 3 months
Severe cyclical mastalgia, 100–400 mg daily usually for 3–6 months
Benign breast cysts, 300 mg daily usually for 3–6 months
Gynaecomastia, 400 mg daily in up to 4 divided doses for 6 months (adolescents 200 mg daily, increased to 400 mg daily if no response after 2 months)
For pre-operative thinning of endometrium, 400–800 mg daily in up to 4 divided doses for 3–6 weeks

PoM **Danazol** (Non-proprietary)
Capsules, danazol 100 mg, net price 20 = £5.18; 200 mg, 20 = £9.94
Available from APS, Cox, Generics, Hillcross, Kent, Norton
PoM **Danol**® (Sanofi Winthrop)
Capsules, danazol 100 mg (grey/white), net price 100-cap pack = £29.74; 200 mg (pink/white), 56-cap pack = £32.98

GESTRINONE
Indications: endometriosis
Cautions: cardiac and renal impairment; **interactions:** Appendix 1 (gestrinone)

Contra-indications: pregnancy (use non-hormonal method of contraception) and breast-feeding; severe cardiac, renal or hepatic impairment; metabolic or vascular disorders associated with previous sex hormone treatment

Side-effects: spotting; acne, oily skin, fluid retention, weight gain, hirsutism, voice change; liver enzyme disturbances; headache; gastro-intestinal disturbances; change in libido, flushing, decrease in breast size; nervousness, depression, change in appetite; muscle cramp

Dose: 2.5 mg twice weekly starting on first day of cycle with second dose 3 days later, repeated on same two days preferably at same time each week; duration of treatment usually 6 months

MISSED DOSES. One missed dose—2.5 mg as soon as possible and maintain original sequence; two or more missed doses—discontinue, re-start on first day of new cycle (following negative pregnancy test)

PoM **Dimetriose®** (Hoechst Marion Roussel)
Capsules, gestrinone 2.5 mg, net price 8-cap pack = £73.12

GONADORELIN ANALOGUES

Administration of **gonadorelin analogues** produces an initial phase of stimulation; continued administration is followed by down-regulation of gonadotrophin-releasing hormone receptors, thereby reducing the release of gonadotrophins (follicle stimulating hormone and luteinising hormone) which in turn leads to inhibition of androgen and oestrogen production.

Gonadorelin analogues are used in the treatment of endometriosis, infertility, anaemia due to uterine fibroids (together with iron supplementation), breast cancer (section 8.3.4.1), prostate cancer (section 8.3.4.2) and before intrauterine surgery

CAUTION. Non-hormonal, barrier methods of contraception should be used during entire treatment period with gonadorelin analogues; also use with caution in patients with metabolic bone disease because decrease in bone mineral density can occur

CONTRA-INDICATIONS. Gonadorelin analogues are contra-indicated for use longer than 6 months (do not repeat), where there is undiagnosed vaginal bleeding, in pregnancy (exclude pregnancy —also barrier contraception for 1 month beforehand *or* give first injection during menstruation or shortly afterwards) and in breast-feeding

SIDE-EFFECTS. Side-effects of the gonadorelin analogues include menopausal-like symptoms (e.g. hot flushes, increased sweating, vaginal dryness, dyspareunia and loss of libido), a decrease in trabecular bone density (repeat courses not recommended), headache (rarely migraine) and hypersensitivity reactions including urticaria, pruritus, skin rashes, asthma and anaphylaxis; spray formulations can cause irritation of the nasal mucosa including nose bleeds; local reactions at injection site can occur; other side-effects also reported with some gonado-relin analogues include changes in breast size, arthralgia, visual disturbances, paraesthesia, changes in scalp and body hair, oedema of the face and extremities, weight changes, mood changes including depression

---

BUSERELIN

Indications: see under Dose; prostate cancer (section 8.3.4.2)

Cautions: see notes above; polycystic ovarian disease, depression, hypertension, diabetes

Contra-indications: see notes above; hormone-dependent tumours

Side-effects: see notes above; initially withdrawal bleeding and subsequently breakthrough bleeding, ovarian cysts (may require withdrawal), leucorrhoea; nausea, vomiting, constipation, diarrhoea; anxiety, memory and concentration disturbances, sleep disturbances, nervousness, dizziness, drowsiness; breast tenderness, lactation; abdominal pain; fatigue; increased thirst, changes in appetite, palpitations, worsening of hypertension; acne, dry skin, dry eyes; back and limb pain; altered liver function tests, altered blood lipids, leucopenia, thrombocytopenia; hearing disturbances; reduced glucose tolerance

Dose: endometriosis, *intranasally,* 300 micrograms (one 150-microgram spray in each nostril) 3 times daily (starting on 1st or 2nd day of menstruation); max. duration of treatment 6 months (do not repeat)

Pituitary desensitisation before induction of ovulation by gonadotrophins for *in vitro* fertilisation (under specialist supervision), *by subcutaneous injection,* 200–500 micrograms daily given as a single injection (occasionally up to 500 micrograms twice daily may be needed) starting in early follicular phase (day 1) *or,* after exclusion of pregnancy, in midluteal phase (day 21) and continued until down-regulation achieved (usually about 1–3 weeks) then maintained during gonadotrophin administration (stopping on administration of chorionic gonadotrophin at follicular maturity)

Intranasally, 150 micrograms (one spray in one nostril) 4 times daily during waking hours (occasionally up to 300 micrograms 4 times daily may be needed) starting in early follicular phase (day 1) *or,* after exclusion of pregnancy, in midluteal phase (day 21) and continued until down-regulation achieved (usually about 2–3 weeks) then maintained during gonadotrophin administration (stopping on administration of chorionic gonadotrophin at follicular maturity)

COUNSELLING. Avoid use of nasal decongestants before and for at least 30 minutes after treatment

PoM **Suprecur®** (Shire)
Nasal spray, buserelin (as acetate) 150 micrograms/metered spray. Net price 2 × 100-dose pack (with metered dose pumps) = £78.98. Counselling, see above

▼ *Injection,* buserelin (as acetate) 1mg/mL. Net price 5.5-mL vial = £14.81.

GOSERELIN

Indications: see under Dose; prostate cancer (section 8.3.4.2); advanced breast cancer (section 8.3.4.1)

Cautions: see notes above

Contra-indications: see notes above

Side-effects: see notes above; withdrawal bleeding, fibroid degeneration; transient changes in blood pressure

Dose: by subcutaneous injection into anterior abdominal wall, endometriosis, 3.6 mg every 28 days; max. duration of treatment 6 months (do not repeat); endometrial thinning before intrauterine surgery, 3.6 mg (may be repeated after 28 days if uterus is large or to allow flexible surgical timing); before surgery in women who have anaemia due to uterine fibroids, 3.6 mg every 28 days (with supplementary iron); max. duration of treatment 3 months

PoM **Zoladex®** (Zeneca)
Implant, goserelin 3.6 mg (as acetate) in syringe applicator. Net price each = £122.27

LEUPRORELIN ACETATE

Indications: see under Dose; prostate cancer (section 8.3.4.2)

Cautions: see notes above; family history of osteoporosis; chronic use of other drugs which reduce bone density including alcohol and tobacco

Contra-indications: see notes above

Side-effects: see notes above; breast tenderness; nausea; sleep disturbances, dizziness, fatigue

Dose: by subcutaneous or by intramuscular injection, endometriosis, 3.75 mg every 4 weeks, starting during the first 5 days of menstrual cycle; max. duration of treatment 6 months (do not repeat); endometrial thinning before intrauterine surgery, 3.75 mg given 5–6 weeks before surgery starting between days 3 and 5 of menstrual cycle

Preparations
See section 8.3.4.2

NAFARELIN

Indications: see under Dose

Cautions: see notes above

Contra-indications: see notes above

Side-effects: see notes above; ovarian cysts (may require withdrawal); myalgia; acne; palpitations; altered liver function tests

Dose: women over 18 years, endometriosis, 200 micrograms twice daily as one spray in one nostril in the morning and one spray in the other nostril in the evening (starting on 2nd, 3rd or 4th day of menstruation), max. duration of treatment 6 months (do not repeat)

Pituitary desensitisation before induction of ovulation by gonadotrophins for *in vitro* fertilisation (under specialist supervision), 400 micrograms (one spray in each nostril) twice daily starting in early follicular phase (day 2) or, after exclusion of pregnancy, in midluteal phase (day 21) and continued until down-regulation achieved (usually within 4 weeks) then maintained for few more days during gonadotrophin administration (stopping on administration of chorionic gonadotrophin at follicular maturity); discontinue if down-regulation not achieved within 12 weeks

COUNSELLING. Avoid use of nasal decongestants before and for at least 30 minutes after treatment; repeat dose if sneezing occurs during or immediately after administration

PoM **Synarel®** (Searle)
Nasal spray, nafarelin 200 micrograms (as acetate)/metered spray. Net price 30-dose unit = £30.74; 60-dose unit = £53.01. Label: 10 patient information leaflet, counselling, see above

TRIPTORELIN

Indications: see under dose; prostate cancer (section 8.3.4.2)

Cautions: see notes above

Contra-indications: see notes above

Side-effects: see notes above; myalgia; transient hypertension; asthenia

Dose: by intramuscular injection, endometriosis, 3 mg every 4 weeks starting during the first 5 days of menstrual cycle; max. duration of treatment 6 months (do not repeat)

Preparations
Section 8.3.4.2

BREAST PAIN (MASTALGIA)

Once any serious underlying cause has been ruled out, most women will respond to reassurance and reduction in dietary fat; withdrawal of an oral contraceptive or of hormone replacement therapy may help resolve the pain.

Women whose symptoms persist for longer than 6 months may require drug treatment. Danazol is the most effective but may be unacceptable owing to its unpleasant side-effects (which occur in about one-third of patients). Bromocriptine (section 6.7.1) like danazol is associated with unpleasant side-effects. Gamolenic acid can be useful and, with its lack of antioestrogenic side-effects, may be preferred particularly in younger women who wish to continue taking an oral contraceptive; whereas bromocriptine and danazol act within 2 months, gamolenic acid may require 8–12 weeks to take effect.

Symptoms recur in about 50% of women within 2 years of withdrawal of therapy but may be less severe.

GAMOLENIC ACID

Indications: see under preparation below; atopic eczema, see section 13.5.1

Cautions: history of epilepsy, concomitant treatment with epileptogenic drugs e.g. phenothiazines; pregnancy

Side-effects: occasional nausea, indigestion, headache

Dose: see under preparation below

PoM **Efamast**® (Searle)
Capsules, gamolenic acid 40 mg in evening primrose oil. Net price 224-cap pack = £23.72
Additives: include vitamin E 10 mg as *in vivo* antoxidant
Dose: symptomatic relief of cyclical and non-cyclical mastalgia, 3–4 capsules twice daily, usually for 8–12 weeks then stopped or continued at lower maintenance dose

6.7.3 Metyrapone and trilostane

Metyrapone is a competitive inhibitor of 11β-hydroxylation in the adrenal cortex; the resulting inhibition of cortisol (and to a lesser extent aldosterone) production leads to an increase in ACTH production which, in turn, leads to increased synthesis and release of cortisol precursors. It may be used as a test of anterior pituitary function.

Although most types of *Cushing's syndrome* are treated surgically, that which occasionally accompanies carcinoma of the bronchus is not usually amenable to surgery. Metyrapone has been found helpful in controlling the symptoms of the disease; it is also used in other forms of Cushing's syndrome to prepare the patient for surgery. The dosages used are either low, and tailored to cortisol production, or high, in which case corticosteroid replacement therapy is also needed.

Trilostane reversibly inhibits 3β-hydroxysteroid dehydrogenase /delta 5-4 isomerase in the adrenal cortex; the resulting inhibition of the synthesis of mineralocorticoids and glucocorticoids may be useful in *Cushing's syndrome* and *primary hyperaldosteronism*. Trilostane appears to be less effective than metyrapone for Cushing's syndrome (where it is tailored to corticosteroid production). It also has a minor role in post-menopausal breast cancer that has relapsed following initial oestrogen antagonist therapy (corticosteroid replacement therapy is also required).

See also aminoglutethimide (section 8.3.4)

METYRAPONE

Indications: see notes above and under Dose (specialist supervision in hospital)
Cautions: gross hypopituitarism (risk of precipitating acute adrenal failure); hypertension on long-term administration; hypothyroidism or hepatic impairment (delayed response); many drugs interfere with diagnostic estimation of steroids
DRIVING. Drowsiness may affect the performance of skilled tasks (e.g. driving)
Contra-indications: adrenocortical insufficiency (see Cautions); pregnancy, breast-feeding

Side-effects: occasional nausea, vomiting, dizziness, headache, hypotension, sedation; rarely abdominal pain, allergic skin reactions, hypoadrenalism, hirsutism
Dose: differential diagnosis of ACTH-dependent Cushing's syndrome, 750 mg every 4 hours for 6 doses; CHILD 15 mg/kg (minimum 250 mg) every 4 hours for 6 doses
Management of Cushing's syndrome, range 0.25–6 g daily, tailored to cortisol production; see notes above
Resistant oedema due to increased aldosterone secretion in cirrhosis, nephrosis, and congestive heart failure (with glucocorticoid replacement therapy) 3 g daily in divided doses

PoM **Metopirone**® (Novartis)
Capsules, metyrapone 250 mg. Net price 100-tab pack = £20.92. Label: 21, counselling, driving

TRILOSTANE

Indications: see notes above and under Dose (specialist supervision)
Cautions: breast cancer (concurrent corticosteroid replacement therapy needed, see under Dose), adrenal cortical hyperfunction (tailored to cortisol and electrolytes, concurrent corticosteroid therapy may be needed, see under Dose); hepatic and renal impairment; **interactions:** Appendix 1 (trilostane)
Contra-indications: pregnancy (use non-hormonal method of contraception) and breast-feeding; children
Side-effects: flushing, tingling and swelling of mouth, rhinorrhoea, nausea, vomiting, diarrhoea, and rashes reported; rarely granulocytopenia
Dose: adrenal cortical hyperfunction, 240 mg daily in divided doses for at least 3 days then tailored according to response with regular monitoring of plasma electrolytes and circulating corticosteroids (both mineralocorticoid and glucocorticoid replacement therapy may be needed); usual dose: 120–480 mg daily (may be increased to 960 mg)
Postmenopausal breast cancer (with glucocorticoid replacement therapy) following relapse to initial oestrogen receptor antagonist therapy, initially 240 mg daily increased every 3 days in steps of 240 mg to a maintenance dose of 960 mg daily (720 mg daily if not tolerated)

PoM **Modrenal**® (Wanskerne)
Capsules, trilostane 60 mg (pink/black), net price 100-cap pack = £49.50; 120 mg (pink/yellow), 100-cap pack = £98.50. Label: 21

7: Drugs used in

OBSTETRICS, GYNAECOLOGY, and URINARY-TRACT DISORDERS

In this chapter, drugs are discussed under the following headings:

For hormonal therapy of gynaecological disorders see section 6.4.1, section 6.5.1 and section 6.7.2.

7.1 Drugs used in obstetrics

Note. Because of the complexity of dosage regimens in obstetrics, in all cases **detailed specialist literature** should be consulted.

7.1.1 Prostaglandins and oxytocics

Prostaglandins and oxytocics are used to induce abortion or induce or augment labour and to minimise blood loss from the placental site. They include oxytocin, ergometrine, and the prostaglandins. All induce uterine contractions with varying degrees of pain according to the strength of contractions induced.

INDUCTION OF ABORTION. **Gemeprost**, administered vaginally, and **dinoprostone**, given by the extra-amniotic route, are the preferred prostaglandins for the *medical induction of late therapeutic abortion*. Gemeprost is a prostaglandin available in the form of pessaries to ripen and soften the cervix *before surgical abortion*, particularly in primigravida. Extra-amniotic **dinoprostone** is also of value as an adjunct in 'priming' the cervix prior to *suction termination* but is rarely used nowadays.

INDUCTION AND AUGMENTATION OF LABOUR. **Oxytocin** (*Syntocinon*®) is administered by slow intravenous infusion, using an infusion pump, to *induce or augment labour*, usually in conjunction with amniotomy. Uterine activity must be monitored carefully and hyperstimulation avoided. Large doses of oxytocin may result in excessive fluid retention.

Dinoprostone is available as vaginal tablets, pessaries and vaginal gels for the *induction of labour*. The intravenous and oral routes are rarely used.

PREVENTION AND TREATMENT OF HAEMORRHAGE. Bleeding due to *incomplete abortion* can be controlled with **ergometrine** and **oxytocin** (*Syntometrine*®) given intramuscularly, the dose being adjusted according to the patient's condition and blood loss. This is commonly used prior to surgical evacuation of the uterus, particularly when surgery is delayed. Oxytocin and ergometrine combined are more effective in early pregnancy than either drug alone.

For the routine management of the *third stage of labour* ergometrine 500 micrograms with oxytocin 5 units (*Syntometrine*® 1 mL) is given by intramuscular injection with or after delivery of the shoulders.

If ergometrine is inappropriate (e.g. in pre-eclampsia), oxytocin may be given by intramuscular injection with or after delivery of shoulder [unlicensed indication] instead of ergometrine with oxytocin.

For the prevention of postpartum haemorrhage in *high-risk cases*, intravenous injection of *either* ergometrine 125–250 micrograms alone *or* oxytocin 5–10 units is recommended, after delivery of the shoulders (repeated if necessary); alternatively intravenous infusion of oxytocin 10–20 units/ 500 mL can be given after delivery of the shoulders, particularly when the uterus is *atonic*. The use of **carboprost** now has an important role for severe events.

Provided causes such as infection or retained products of conception have been excluded, small secondary postpartum haemorrhage may be treated in domiciliary practice with **ergometrine** by mouth in a dose of 500 micrograms three times daily for 3 days.

CARBOPROST

Indications: postpartum haemorrhage due to uterine atony in patients unresponsive to ergometrine and oxytocin

Cautions: history of glaucoma or raised intra-ocular pressure, asthma, hypertension, hypotension, anaemia, jaundice, diabetes, epilepsy; uterine scars; excessive dosage may cause uterine rupture

Contra-indications: acute pelvic inflammatory disease; cardiac, renal, pulmonary, or hepatic disease

Side-effects: nausea, vomiting and diarrhoea, hyperthermia and flushing, bronchospasm; less frequent effects include raised blood pressure, dyspnoea, and pulmonary oedema; chills, headache, diaphoresis, dizziness; cardiovascular collapse also reported; erythema and pain at injection site reported

---

Dose: by deep intramuscular injection, 250 micrograms repeated if necessary at intervals of 1½ hours (in severe cases the interval may be reduced but should not be less than 15 minutes); total dose should not exceed 2 mg (8 doses)

PoM **Hemabate**® (Pharmacia & Upjohn)
Injection, carboprost as trometamol salt (tromethamine salt) 250 micrograms/mL, net price 1-mL amp = £16.50 (hosp. only)

DINOPROSTONE

Indications: see notes above and under preparations below

Cautions: history of asthma, glaucoma and raised intra-ocular pressure; cardiac, hepatic or renal impairment; hypertension; history of epilepsy; monitor uterine activity and fetal status (particular care if history of uterine hypertony); uterine rupture; see also notes above; effect of oxytocin enhanced (care needed in monitoring uterine activity when used in sequence)—see also under *Propess-RS*® and Appendix 1 (oxytocin)

Contra-indications: active cardiac, pulmonary, renal or hepatic disease; placenta praevia or unexplained vaginal bleeding during pregnancy, ruptured membranes, major cephalopelvic disproportion or fetal malpresentation, history of caesarean section or major uterine surgery, untreated pelvic infection, fetal distress, grand multiparas and multiple pregnancy, history of difficult or traumatic delivery; avoid extra-amniotic route in cervicitis or vaginitis

Side-effects: nausea, vomiting, diarrhoea; other side-effects include uterine hypertonus, severe uterine contractions, pulmonary or amniotic fluid embolism, abruptio placenta, fetal distress, maternal hypertension, bronchospasm, rapid cervical dilation, fever, backache; uterine hypercontractility with or without fetal bradycardia, low Apgar scores; cardiac arrest, uterine rupture, stillbirth or neonatal death also reported; vaginal symptoms (warmth, irritation, pain); after intravenous administration—flushing, shivering, headache, dizziness, temporary pyrexia and raised white blood cell count; also local tissue reaction and erythema after intravenous administration and possibility of infection after extra-amniotic administration

Dose: see under Preparations, below

IMPORTANT. Do not confuse dose of **Prostin E2**® vaginal **gel** with that of **Prostin E2**® vaginal **tablets**—not bioequivalent. In addition, do not confuse **Prostin E2**® vaginal gel with **Prepidil**® cervical gel—different site of administration and different indication—see under Preparations, below

PoM **Prepidil**® (Pharmacia & Upjohn)
Cervical gel, dinoprostone 200 micrograms/mL in disposable syringe. Net price 2.5-mL syringe (500 micrograms) = £14.12
Dose: by cervix, pre-induction cervical softening and dilation, inserted into cervical canal (just below level of internal cervical os), 500 micrograms [single dose gel]

▼ PoM **Propess**®-RS (Ferring)
Pessaries (within retrieval system), releasing dinoprostone approx. 5 mg over 12 hours. Net price 4-pessary pack = £173.75
Dose: by vagina, cervical ripening and induction of labour at term, 1 pessary inserted high into posterior fornix; if cervical ripening insufficient , remove pessary 8–12 hours later and replace with a second pessary (which should also be removed not more than 12 hours later); max. 2 consecutive pessaries
IMPORTANT. Effect of oxytocin enhanced—particular care needed to monitor uterine activity when oxytocin used in sequence (remove pessary beforehand)

PoM **Prostin E2**® (Pharmacia & Upjohn)
Tablets, dinoprostone 500 micrograms. Net price 10-tab pack = £14.93 (hosp. only)
Dose: by mouth, induction of labour, 500 micrograms, followed by 0.5–1 mg (max. 1.5 mg) at hourly intervals
Intravenous solution, for dilution and use as an infusion, dinoprostone 1 mg/mL, net price 0.75-mL amp = £7.43; 10 mg/mL, 0.5-mL amp = £16.05 (both hosp. only; rarely used, see product literature for dose and indications)
Extra-amniotic solution, dinoprostone 10 mg/mL. Net price 0.5-mL amp (with diluent) = £16.05 (hosp. only; less commonly used nowadays, see product literature for dose and indications)
Vaginal gel, dinoprostone 400 micrograms/mL, net price 2.5 mL (1 mg) = £14.52; 800 micrograms/mL, 2.5 mL (2 mg) = £16.00
Dose: by vagina, induction of labour, inserted high into posterior fornix (avoid administration into cervical canal), 1 mg (unfavourable primigravida 2 mg), followed after 6 hours by 1–2 mg if required; max. [gel] 3 mg (unfavourable primigravida 4 mg)
Vaginal tablets, dinoprostone 3 mg. Net price 8-vaginal tab pack = £65.04
Dose: by vagina, induction of labour, inserted high into posterior fornix, 3 mg, followed after 6–8 hours by 3 mg if labour is not established; max. 6 mg [vaginal tablets]
Note. Prostin E2 Vaginal Gel and Vaginal Tablets are **not** bioequivalent

DINOPROST

Indications: see under preparation, below
Cautions; Contra-indications; Side-effects: see under Dinoprostone

PoM **Prostin F2 alpha**® (Pharmacia & Upjohn)
Intra-amniotic injection, dinoprost 5 mg (as trometamol salt)/mL. Net price 4-mL amp = £19.71 (hosp. only; rarely used, see product literature for dose and indications)

ERGOMETRINE MALEATE

Indications: see notes above
Cautions: cardiac disease, hypertension, hepatic, and renal impairment, multiple pregnancy; porphyria (see section 9.8.2)
Contra-indications: induction of labour, first and second stages of labour, vascular disease, severe cardiac disease, impaired pulmonary function, severe hepatic and renal impairment, sepsis, severe hypertension, eclampsia
Side-effects: nausea, vomiting, headache, dizziness, tinnitus, abdominal pain, chest pain, palpitation, dyspnoea, bradycardia, transient hypertension, vasoconstriction; stroke, myo-

cardial infarction and pulmonary oedema also reported

Dose: see notes above

PoM **Ergometrine** (Non-proprietary)

Tablets, ergometrine maleate 500 micrograms. Net price 20 = £6.33
Available from Norton

Injection, ergometrine maleate 500 micrograms/mL. Net price 1-mL amp = 30p
Available from Antigen, Phoenix

With oxytocin

PoM **Syntometrine**® (Novartis)

Injection, ergometrine maleate 500 micrograms, oxytocin 5 units/mL. Net price 1-mL amp = 18p
Dose: by intramuscular injection, 1 mL; by intravenous injection, no longer recommended

GEMEPROST

Indications: see under Dose

Cautions: obstructive airways disease, cardiovascular insufficiency, raised intra-ocular pressure, cervicitis or vaginitis

IMPORTANT. For warnings relating to use of gemeprost in a patient undergoing termination with mifepristone, see under Mifepristone

Side-effects: vaginal bleeding and uterine pain; nausea, vomiting, or diarrhoea; headache, muscle weakness, dizziness, flushing, chills, backache, dyspnoea, chest pain, palpitations and mild pyrexia; uterine rupture reported (most commonly in multiparas or if history of uterine surgery or if given with intravenous oxytocics)

Dose: by vagina in pessaries, softening and dilation of the cervix to facilitate transcervical operative procedures in first trimester, inserted into posterior fornix, 1 mg 3 hours before surgery
Second trimester abortion, inserted into posterior fornix, 1 mg every 3 hours for max. of 5 administrations; second course may begin 24 hours after start of treatment (if treatment fails pregnancy should be terminated by another method)
Second trimester intra-uterine death, inserted into posterior fornix, 1 mg every 3 hours for max. of 5 administrations only; monitor for coagulopathy

PoM **Gemeprost** (Farillon)

Pessaries, gemeprost 1 mg. Net price 5-pessary pack = £121.12

OXYTOCIN

Indications: see under Dose and notes above

Cautions: particular caution needed when given for *induction or enhancement of labour* in presence of borderline cephalopelvic disproportion (avoid if significant), mild or moderate pregnancy-induced hypertension or cardiac disease, women over 35 years or with history of lower-uterine segment caesarean section (see also under contra-indications below); if fetal death in utero or meconium-stained amniotic fluid avoid tumultuous labour (may cause amniotic fluid embolism); water intoxication and hyponatraemia—avoid large infusion volumes and restrict fluid intake by mouth (see also Appendix 6); effects enhanced by concomitant prostaglandins (very careful monitoring), caudal block anaesthesia (may enhance hypertensive effects of sympathomi-

metic vasopressors), see also **interactions:** Appendix 1 (oxytocin)

Contra-indications: hypertonic uterine contractions, mechanical obstruction to delivery, fetal distress; any condition where spontaneous labour or vaginal delivery inadvisable (e.g. significant cephalopelvic disproportion, malpresentation, placenta praevia, vasa praevia, placental abruption, cord presentation or prolapse, predisposition to uterine rupture as in multiple pregnancy, polyhydramnios, grand multiparity and presence of uterine scar from major surgery—including caesarean section); avoid prolonged administration in oxytocin-resistant uterine inertia, severe pre-eclamptic toxaemia or severe cardiovascular disease

Side-effects: uterine spasm (may occur at low doses), uterine hyperstimulation (usually with excessive doses—may cause fetal distress, asphyxia and death, or may lead to hypertonicity, tetanic contractions, soft-tissue damage or uterine rupture); water intoxication and hyponatraemia associated with high doses with large infusion volumes of electrolyte-free fluid (see also under Dose below); also nausea, vomiting, arrhythmias; rashes and anaphylactoid reactions (with dyspnoea, hypotension or shock) also reported; placental abruption and amniotic fluid embolism also reported on overdose

Dose: induction of labour for medical reasons or stimulation of labour in hypotonic uterine inertia, *by intravenous infusion,* 0.001–0.004 units/minute increased at intervals of not less than 20 minutes until labour pattern established similar to normal (usually less than 0.01 units/minute for pregnancy at term); max. recommended rate 0.02 units/minute (use solution containing 10 units/500 mL if higher rate required); do not use total of more than 5 units in any one day (may be repeated the following day starting again at 0.001–0.004 units/minute)
IMPORTANT. Careful monitoring of fetal heart rate and uterine motility essential so that dosage can be adjusted to individual response (never give intravenous injection); discontinue immediately in uterine hyperactivity or fetal distress
Caesarean section, *by slow intravenous injection* immediately after delivery, 5 units
Prevention of postpartum haemorrhage, after delivery of placenta, *by slow intravenous injection,* 5 units (if infusion used for induction or enhancement of labour, increase rate during third stage and for next few hours)
Note. May be given by intramuscular injection [unlicensed route] instead of oxytocin with ergometrine (Syntometrine®), see notes above
Treatment of postpartum haemorrhage, *by slow intravenous injection,* 5 units, followed in severe cases *by intravenous infusion* of 5–20 units in 500 mL of non-hydrating diluent (e.g. glucose 5% solution) at a rate sufficient to control uterine atony
IMPORTANT. Avoid rapid intravenous injection (may cause short-lasting drop in blood pressure); prolonged administration, see warning below
Incomplete, inevitable or missed abortion, 5 units *by slow intravenous injection* followed if necessary *by intravenous infusion* at rate of 0.02–0.04 units/minute or higher
IMPORTANT. Prolonged intravenous administration at high doses with large volume of fluid (as possible in inevitable or missed abortion or postpartum haemorrhage) may cause water intoxication with hyponatraemia. To avoid: use electrolyte-containing diluent (i.e. not glucose), increase oxytocin concentration to reduce fluid, restrict fluid intake by mouth; monitor fluid and electrolytes

---

PoM **Syntocinon**® (Novartis)
Injection, oxytocin, net price 5 units/mL, 1-mL amp = 20p; 10 units/mL, 1-mL amp = 22p

With ergometrine, see Syntometrine®, p. 344

7.1.1.1 DUCTUS ARTERIOSUS

MAINTENANCE OF PATENCY
Alprostadil (prostaglandin E$_1$) is used to maintain patency of the ductus arteriosus in neonates with congenital heart defects, prior to corrective surgery in centres where intensive care is immediately available.

ALPROSTADIL
Indications: congenital heart defects in neonates prior to corrective surgery; erectile dysfunction (section 7.4.5)
Cautions: see notes above; history of haemorrhage, avoid in hyaline membrane disease, monitor arterial pressure
Side-effects: apnoea (particularly in infants under 2 kg), flushing, bradycardia, hypotension, tachycardia, cardiac arrest, oedema, diarrhoea, fever, convulsions, disseminated intravascular coagulation, hypokalaemia; cortical proliferation of long bones, weakening of the wall of the ductus arteriosus and pulmonary artery may follow prolonged use; gastric-outlet obstruction reported
Dose: by intravenous infusion, initially 50–100 nanograms/kg/minute, then decreased to lowest effective dose

PoM **Prostin VR**® (Pharmacia & Upjohn)
Intravenous solution, alprostadil 500 micrograms/mL in alcohol. For dilution and use as an infusion. Net price 1-mL amp = £62.66 (hosp. only)

CLOSURE OF DUCTUS ARTERIOSUS
Prostaglandin E$_1$ maintains patency of the ductus arteriosus; **indomethacin** is believed to close it by inhibiting prostaglandin synthesis.

INDOMETHACIN
(Indometacin)
Indications: patent ductus arteriosus in premature infants (under specialist supervision in neonatal intensive care unit); rheumatoid disease, see section 10.1.1
Cautions: may mask symptoms of infection; may reduce urine output by 50% or more (monitor carefully—see also under Anuria or Oliguria, below) and precipitate renal insufficiency especially in infants with depletion of extracellur volume (from any cause), heart failure, sepsis, or hepatic impairment, or who are receiving nephrotoxic drugs; may induce hyponatraemia; monitor renal function and electrolytes; inhibition of platelet aggregation (monitor for signs of bleeding); avoid extravasation; **interactions:** Appendix 1 (NSAIDs)
ANURIA OR OLIGURIA. If anuria or marked oliguria (urinary output of 0.6 mL/kg/hour) is evident at time of scheduled second or third dose, delay until renal function returns to normal

Contra-indications: untreated infection, bleeding (especially with active intracranial haemorrhage or gastro-intestinal bleeding), congenital heart disease where patency of ductus arteriosus necessary for satisfactory pulmonary or systemic blood flow; thrombocytopenia, coagulation defects, necrotising enterocolitis, renal impairment
Side-effects: include haemorrhagic, renal, gastro-intestinal, metabolic, and coagulation disorders; pulmonary hypertension, intracranial bleeding, fluid retention, and exacerbation of infection
Dose: by intravenous injection, over 5–10 seconds, 3 doses at intervals of 12–24 hours (provided urine output remains adequate), age less than 48 hours, 200 micrograms/kg then 100 micrograms/kg then 100 micrograms/kg; age 2–7 days, 200 micrograms/kg then 200 micrograms/kg then 200 micrograms/kg; age over 7 days, 200 micrograms/kg then 250 micrograms/kg then 250 micrograms/kg; solution prepared with 1–2 mL sodium chloride 0.9% or water for injections (not glucose and no preservatives)
If ductus arteriosus reopens a second course of 3 injections may be given

PoM **Indocid PDA**® (Morson)
Injection, powder for reconstitution, indomethacin (as sodium trihydrate). Net price 3 × 1-mg vials = £22.50 (hosp. only)

7.1.2 Mifepristone
MIFEPRISTONE
Indications: see under dose
Cautions: asthma, chronic obstructive airways disease; cardiovascular disease or risk factors; prosthetic heart valves or history of infective endocarditis (prophylaxis recommended, see section 5.1 table 2); not recommended in hepatic or renal impairment; breast-feeding (see Appendix 5); avoid aspirin and NSAIDs for at least 8–12 days after mifepristone administration; **interactions:** Appendix 1 (mifepristone)
Contra-indications: suspected ectopic pregnancy; chronic adrenal failure, long-term corticosteroid therapy, haemorrhagic disorders and anticoagulant therapy; smokers over 35 years of age when used in combination with gemeprost (smoking and alcohol must be avoided 2 days before and on the day of gemeprost administration); porphyria (section 9.8.2)
Side-effects: vaginal bleeding (sometimes severe) may occur between administration of mifepristone and surgery, and rarely abortion may occur before surgery; malaise, faintness, headache, nausea, vomiting, rashes; uterine pain after gemeprost (may be severe and require parenteral opioids); uterine and urinary-tract infections reported
Dose: therapeutic termination of intra-uterine pregnancy of up to 63 days gestation, *by mouth*, mifepristone 600 mg as a single dose in presence of doctor and observed for at least 2 hours, followed 36–48 hours later (unless abortion already complete) by gemeprost 1 mg *by vagina* and observed for at least 6 hours (or until bleeding or

---

pain at acceptable level) with follow-up visit 8–12 days later to verify complete expulsion (if treatment fails essential that pregnancy be terminated by another method)

Softening and dilatation of cervix before mechanical cervical dilatation for termination of pregnancy, 36–48 hours before procedure, *by mouth*, mifepristone 600 mg as a single dose in presence of doctor

Termination of pregnancy of 13–20 weeks gestation (in combination with gemeprost), *by mouth*, mifepristone 600 mg as a single dose (in presence of doctor and observed for at least 2 hours to ensure vomiting does not occur) followed 36–48 hours later by gemeprost 1 mg *by vagina* every 3 hours up to max. 5 mg; if abortion does not occur, 24 hours after start of treatment repeat course of gemeprost 1 mg *by vagina* up to max. 5 mg (if treatment fails pregnancy should be terminated by another method); follow-up visit after appropriate interval to assess vaginal bleeding recommended

Note. Careful monitoring essential for 6 hours after administration of gemeprost pessary (risk of profound hypotension)

▼ PoM **Mifegyne**® (Exelgyn)

Tablets, yellow, mifepristone 200 mg. Net price 3-tab pack = £41.83 (supplied to NHS hospitals and premises approved under Abortion Act 1967). Label: 10 patient information leaflet

7.1.3   Myometrial relaxants

Beta$_2$-adrenoceptor stimulants (beta$_2$-sympathomimetics) relax uterine muscle and are used in selected cases in an attempt to inhibit *premature delivery*.

Their main purpose is to permit a delay in delivery of at least 48 hours; no statistically significant effect on perinatal mortality has as yet been observed. The greatest benefit is gained by using the delay to administer corticosteroid therapy (with care to avoid fluid overload) or to implement other measures known to improve perinatal health (including transfer to a unit with neonatal intensive care facility). They are indicated for the inhibition of *uncomplicated* premature labour *between 24 and 33 weeks* of gestation. Prolonged therapy should be avoided since risks to the mother (see under Ritodrine Hydrochloride, below) increase after 48 hours and furthermore, myometrial response is reduced; oral therapy following initial parenteral treatment is not therefore recommended.

RITODRINE HYDROCHLORIDE

Indications: uncomplicated premature labour (see notes above)

Cautions: suspected cardiac disease (physician experienced in cardiology to assess), hypertension, hyperthyroidism, hypokalaemia (special risk with potassium-depleting diuretics), diabetes mellitus (closely monitor blood glucose during intravenous treatment), mild to moderate pre-eclampsia (avoid if severe—see Contra-indications), monitor blood pressure and pulse rate (should not exceed 135–140 beats per minute) and avoid over-hydration (see Appendix 6); **important:** pulmonary oedema—closely monitor state of hydration (discontinue immediately and institute diuretic therapy if pulmonary oedema occurs); beta-blockers (effect antagonised—may be used to reverse increased tendency to uterine bleeding following caesarean section); drugs likely to enhance sympathomimetic side-effects or induce arrhythmias, see also **interactions**, Appendix 1 (sympathomimetics *and* sympathomimetics, beta$_2$)

Contra-indications: cardiac disease, eclampsia and severe pre-eclampsia, intra-uterine infection, intra-uterine fetal death, antepartum haemorrhage (requires immediate delivery), placenta praevia, cord compression; not for use in first or second trimesters

Side-effects: nausea, vomiting, flushing, sweating, tremor; hypokalaemia, tachycardia, palpitations, and hypotension (left lateral position throughout infusion to minimise risk), increased tendency to uterine bleeding (see Cautions); pulmonary oedema (see below and under Cautions); chest pain or tightness (with or without ECG changes) and arrhythmias reported; salivary gland enlargement also reported; on prolonged administration (several weeks) leucopenia and agranulocytosis reported; liver function abnormalities (including increased transaminase levels and hepatitis) reported

Dose: by intravenous infusion (**important:** minimum fluid volume, see below), premature labour, initially 50 micrograms/minute, gradually increased according to response by 50 micrograms/minute every 10 minutes to 150–350 micrograms/minute and continued for 12–48 hours after contractions have ceased (max. rate of 350 micrograms/minute should not be exceeded); or *by intramuscular injection*, 10 mg every 3–8 hours continued for 12–48 hours after contractions have ceased; then *by mouth* (but see notes above), 10 mg 30 minutes before termination of intravenous infusion, repeated every 2 hours for 24 hours, followed by 10–20 mg every 4–6 hours, max. oral dose 120 mg daily

IMPORTANT. The manufacturer has issued a reminder that although *fatal pulmonary oedema* associated with ritodrine infusion is almost certainly multifactorial in origin the balance of evidence suggests that **fluid overload** is the most important single factor. The volume of infusion fluid administered should therefore be kept to a minimum (normally using dextrose 5% as the diluent), for further guidance see Appendix 6. For specific guidance on infusion rates to achieve the required dose, see product literature

PoM **Yutopar**® (Solvay)

Tablets, yellow, scored, ritodrine hydrochloride 10 mg. Net price 90-tab pack = £19.80

Injection, ritodrine hydrochloride 10 mg/mL. Net price 5-mL amp = £2.15

SALBUTAMOL

Indications: uncomplicated premature labour (see notes above); asthma, see section 3.1.1

Cautions; Contra-indications; Side-effects: see under Ritodrine Hydrochloride

Dose: by intravenous infusion, 10 micrograms/minute gradually increased to max. of 45 micrograms/minute until contractions have ceased, then gradually reduced; or *by intravenous or intramuscular injection,* 100–250 micrograms repeated according to response; then *by mouth* 4 mg every 6–8 hours

Preparations

See section 3.1.1.1

TERBUTALINE SULPHATE

Indications: uncomplicated premature labour (see notes above); asthma, see section 3.1.1

Cautions; Contra-indications; Side-effects: see under Ritodrine Hydrochloride

Dose: by intravenous infusion, 5 micrograms/minute for 20 minutes, increased every 20 minutes in steps of 2.5 micrograms/minute until contractions have ceased (more than 10 micrograms/minute should **seldom** be given—20 micrograms/minute ohould **not** be exceeded), continue for 1 hour then decrease every 20 minutes in steps of 2.5 micrograms/minute to lowest dose that maintains suppression, continue at this level for 12 hours then *by mouth* 5 mg every 8 hours for as long as is desirable to prolong pregnancy (or alternatively follow the *intravenous infusion* by *subcutaneous injection* 250 micrograms every 6 hours for a few days then *by mouth* as above)

Preparations

See section 3.1.1.1

7.2   Treatment of vaginal and vulval conditions

| 7.2.1 | Preparations for vaginal atrophy |
| 7.2.2 | Anti-infective drugs |

Symptoms are primarily referable to the vulva, but infections almost invariably involve the vagina which should also be treated. Applications to the vulva alone are likely to give only symptomatic relief without cure.

Aqueous medicated douches may disturb normal vaginal acidity and bacterial flora.

Topical anaesthetic agents give only symptomatic relief and may cause sensitivity reactions. They are indicated only in cases of pruritus where specific local causes have been excluded.

Systemic drugs are required in the treatment of infections such as gonorrhoea and syphilis (section 5.1).

7.2.1   Preparations for vaginal atrophy

TOPICAL HRT

Application of *cream* containing an oestrogen may be used on a short-term basis to improve the quality of the vaginal epithelium in *menopausal atrophic vaginitis.* It is **important** to bear in mind that topical oestrogens should be used in the **minimum effective amount** to minimise absorption of the oestrogen; if they are used on a long-term basis, some require **oral progestogen** for 10–14 days of each month to combat endometrial hyperplasia (for details see under preparations below). Modified-release vaginal tablets and an impregnated vaginal ring are now also available.

Topical oestrogens are also used prior to vaginal surgery in postmenopausal women for prolapse when there is epithelial atrophy.

For a general comment on HRT, including the role of topical oestrogens, see section 6.4.1.1.

OESTROGENS, TOPICAL

Indications: see notes above

Cautions; Contra-indications; Side-effects: see Oestrogen for HRT (section 6.4.1.1); contra-indicated in pregnancy and lactation; discontinue treatment and examine patients periodically to assess need for further treatment

PoM **Ortho® Dienoestrol** (Janssen-Cilag)

Cream, dienoestrol 0.01%. Net price 78 g with applicator = £2.61

Condoms: damages latex condoms and diaphragms

Insert 1–2 applicatorfuls daily for 1–2 weeks, then reduce to half the initial dose for 1–2 weeks; maintenance 1 applicatorful 1–3 times weekly if necessary; attempts to reduce or discontinue should be made at 3–6 month intervals with re-examination

PoM **Ortho-Gynest®** (Janssen-Cilag)

Intravaginal cream, oestriol 0.01%. Net price 80 g with applicator = £2.72

Condoms: damages latex condoms and diaphragms

Insert 1 applicatorful daily, preferably in evening; reduced to 1 applicatorful twice a week; attempts to reduce or discontinue should be made at 3–6 month intervals with re-examination

Pessaries, oestriol 500 micrograms. Net price 15 pessaries = £5.29

Condoms: damages latex condoms and diaphragms

Insert 1 pessary daily, preferably in the evening, until improvement occurs; maintenance 1 pessary twice a week; attempts to reduce or discontinue should be made at 3–6 month intervals with re-examination

PoM **Ovestin®** (Organon)

Intravaginal cream, oestriol 0.1%. Net price 15 g with applicator = £5.21

Condoms: effect on latex condoms and diaphragms not yet known

Insert 1 applicator-dose daily for 2–3 weeks, then reduce to twice a week (discontinue every 2–3 months for 4 weeks to assess need for further treatment); vaginal surgery, 1 applicator-dose daily for 2 weeks before surgery, resuming 2 weeks after surgery

---

PoM **Premarin®** (Wyeth)
Vaginal cream, conjugated oestrogens 625 micrograms/g. Net price 42.5 g with calibrated applicator = £2.19
Condoms: effect on latex condoms and diaphragms not yet known
Insert 1–2 g daily, starting on 5th day of cycle, for 3 weeks, followed by 1-week interval; if therapy long term, oral progestogen for 10–14 days at end of each cycle essential

PoM **Tampovagan®** (Co-Pharma)
Pessaries, stilboestrol 500 micrograms, lactic acid 5%. Net price 10 pessaries = £7.00
Condoms: no evidence of damage to latex condoms and diaphragms
Insert 2 pessaries at night for 2–3 weeks (short-term only, see notes above)

PoM **Vagifem®** (Novo Nordisk)
Vaginal tablets, f/c, m/r, oestradiol 25 micrograms in disposable applicators. Net price 15-applicator pack = £14.62
Condoms: no evidence of damage to latex condoms and diaphragms
Insert 1 tablet daily for 2 weeks then reduce to 1 tablet twice weekly; discontinue after 3 months to assess need for further treatment

Vaginal ring
Note. For postmenopausal urogenital conditions—not suitable for vasomotor symptoms or osteoporosis prophylaxis

PoM **Estring®** (Pharmacia & Upjohn)
Vaginal ring, releasing oestradiol approx. 7.5 micrograms/24 hours. Net price 1-ring pack = £32.90. Label: 10 patient information leaflet
To be inserted into upper third of vagina and worn continuously; replace after 3 months; max. duration of continuous treatment 2 years

NON-HORMONAL PREPARATIONS

Non-hormonal vaginal preparations include N̶H̶S̶ *Replens®* which has an acid pH and provides a high moisture content for up to 3 days, and N̶H̶S̶ *Senselle®* which is a water-based lubricant.
See section 7.2.2 for the pH-modifying preparation *Aci-jel®*.

7.2.2   Anti-infective drugs

Effective specific treatments are available for the common vaginal infections.

FUNGAL INFECTIONS

Candidal vulvitis can be treated locally with cream but is almost invariably associated with vaginal infection which should also be treated. *Vaginal candidiasis* is treated primarily with antifungal pessaries or cream inserted high into the vagina (including during menstruation).
Imidazole drugs (clotrimazole, econazole, fenticonazole, isoconazole, and miconazole) are effective in short courses of 3 to 14 days according to the preparation used; single dose preparations offer an advantage when compliance is a problem. Vaginal applications may be supplemented with antifungal cream for vulvitis and to treat other superficial sites of infection.

Nystatin is a well established treatment (but stains clothing yellow). One or two pessaries are inserted for 14 to 28 nights; they may be supplemented with cream for vulvitis and to treat other superficial sites of infection.
Recurrence is common if the full course of treatment is not completed and is also particularly likely if there are predisposing factors such as antibiotic therapy, oral contraceptive use, pregnancy, or diabetes mellitus. Possible reservoirs of infection may also lead to recontamination and should be treated. These include other skin sites such as the digits, nail beds, and umbilicus as well as the gastro-intestinal tract and the bladder. The partner may also be the source of re-infection and should be treated with cream at the same time.
Oral treatment with fluconazole or itraconazole (see section 5.2) is also effective; oral ketoconazole has been associated with fatal hepatotoxicity (see section 5.2 for CSM warning).

PREPARATIONS FOR VAGINAL AND VULVAL CANDIDIASIS
Side-effects: occasional local irritation

Canesten® (Bayer Consumer Care)
Cream (topical), clotrimazole 1%. Net price 20 g = £1.77; 50 g = £4.15
Condoms: effect on latex condoms and diaphragms not yet known
Apply to anogenital area 2–3 times daily
Vaginal cream (*10% VC®*), clotrimazole 10%. Net price 5-g applicator pack = £3.34
Condoms: effect on latex condoms and diaphragms not yet known
Insert 5 g at night as a single dose
Pessaries, clotrimazole 100 mg, net price 6 pessaries with applicator = £3.29; 200 mg, 3 pessaries with applicator = £3.29
Insert 200 mg for 3 nights *or* 100 mg for 6 nights
Pessary (Canesten 1®), clotrimazole 500 mg. Net price 1 with applicator = £3.29
Insert 1 at night as a single dose
Combi, clotrimazole 500-mg pessary and cream (topical) 1%. Net price 1 pessary and 20 g cream = £4.25
Condoms: effect on latex condoms and diaphragms not yet known

Ecostatin® (Squibb)
Cream (topical), econazole nitrate 1%. Net price 15 g = £1.49; 30 g = £2.75
Condoms: damages latex condoms and diaphragms
Apply to anogenital area twice daily
PoM[1] *Pessaries*, econazole nitrate 150 mg. Net price 3 with applicator = £3.35
Condoms: damages latex condoms and diaphragms
Insert 1 pessary for 3 nights
PoM[1] *Pessary (Ecostatin 1®)*, econazole nitrate 150 mg, formulated for single-dose therapy. Net price 1 pessary with applicator = £3.35
Condoms: damages latex condoms and diaphragms
Insert 1 pessary at night as a single dose

1. Can be sold to the public for the treatment of *vaginal candidiasis*. Unless packs labelled 'P' are available, those labelled 'PoM' can be sold providing the pharmacist *deletes* PoM from the pack and *substitutes* a capital P and provides *each purchaser* with a copy of the **patient information leaflet** supplied by the Royal Pharmaceutical Society of Great Britain.

PoM[1] *Twinpack*, econazole nitrate 150-mg pessaries and cream 1%. Net price 3 pessaries and 15 g cream = £4.35

Condoms: damages latex condoms and diaphragms

Femeron® (Janssen-Cilag)

NHS *Cream*, miconazole nitrate 2%. Net price 15g = £1.97

Condoms: damages latex condoms and diaphragms

Apply to anogenital area twice daily

Soft pessary, miconazole nitrate 1.2 g. Net price 1 = £3.55

Condoms: damages latex condoms and diaphragms

Insert 1 pessary at night as a single dose

PoM **Flagyl Compak®** see section 5.1.11

PoM [1] **Gyno-Daktarin®** (Janssen-Cilag)

Intravaginal cream, miconazole nitrate 2%. Net price 78 g with applicators = £4.95

Condoms: damages latex condoms and diaphragms

Insert 5-g applicatorful once daily for 10–14 days *or* twice daily for 7 days; *topical*, apply to anogenital area twice daily

Pessaries, miconazole nitrate 100 mg. Net price 14 = £3.35

Condoms: damages latex condoms and diaphragms

Insert 1 pessary twice daily for 7 days

Combipack, miconazole 100-mg pessaries and cream (topical) 2%. Net price 14 pessaries and 15 g cream = £4.35

Condoms: damages latex condoms and diaphragms

Ovule (= vaginal capsule) (*Gyno-Daktarin 1®*), miconazole nitrate 1.2 g in a fatty basis. Net price 1 ovule (with finger stall) = £3.35

Condoms: damages latex condoms and diaphragms

Insert 1 ovule at night as a single dose

Gyno-Pevaryl® (Janssen-Cilag)

Cream, econazole nitrate 1%. Net price 15 g = £1.50; 30 g = £3.45

Condoms: no evidence of damage to latex condoms and diaphragms

Insert 5-g applicatorful intravaginally and apply to vulva at night for at least 14 nights

Pessaries, econazole nitrate 150 mg. Net price 3 pessaries = £3.17

Condoms: damages latex condoms and diaphragms

Insert 1 pessary for 3 nights

Pessary (*Gyno-Pevaryl 1®*), econazole nitrate 150 mg, formulated for single-dose therapy. Net price 1 pessary with applicator = £3.37

Condoms: damages latex condoms and diaphragms

Insert 1 pessary at night as a single dose

Combipack, econazole nitrate 150-mg pessaries, econazole nitrate 1% cream. Net price 3 pessaries and 15 g cream = £4.35

Condoms: damages latex condoms and diaphragms

CP pack (*Gyno-Pevaryl 1®*), econazole nitrate 150-mg pessary, econazole nitrate 1% cream. Net price 1 pessary and 15 g cream = £4.35

Condoms: damages latex condoms and diaphragms

PoM **Lomexin®** (Dominion)

Pessaries, fenticonazole nitrate 200 mg, net price 3 pessaries = £2.96; 600 mg, 1 pessary = £2.96

Condoms: damages latex condoms and diaphragms

Insert 600 mg for 1 night *or* 200 mg for 3 nights

Masnoderm® (Dominion)

Cream, clotrimazole 1%. Net price 20 g = £1.54

Condoms: damages latex condoms and diaphragms

Apply to anogenital area 2–3 times daily

PoM **Nizoral®** (Janssen-Cilag)

Cream (topical), ketoconazole 2%. Net price 30 g = £3.81

Apply to anogenital area once or twice daily

PoM **Nystan®** (Squibb)

Cream and *Ointment*, see section 13.10.2

Gel (topical), nystatin 100 000 units/g. Net price 30 g = £2.66

Condoms: no evidence of damage to latex condoms and diaphragms

Apply to anogenital area 2–4 times daily

Vaginal cream, nystatin 100 000 units/4-g application. Net price 60 g with applicator = £2.77

Condoms: damages latex condoms and diaphragms

Insert 1–2 applicatorfuls at night for at least 14 nights

Pessaries, yellow, nystatin 100 000 units. Net price 28-pessary pack = £1.96

Condoms: no evidence of damage to latex condoms and diaphragms

Insert 1–2 pessaries at night for at least 14 nights

Tablets, see section 5.2

Pevaryl® (Janssen-Cilag)

Cream, econazole nitrate 1%. Net price 30 g = £2.65

Condoms: effect on latex condoms and diaphragms not yet known

Apply to anogenital area 2–3 times daily

Lotion and *Dusting powder*, see section 13.10.2

PoM [1] **Travogyn®** (Schering Health)

Vaginal tablets (= pessaries), isoconazole nitrate 300 mg. Net price 2 = £3.37

Condoms: effect on latex condoms and diaphragms not yet known

Insert 2 pessaries as a single dose preferably at night

OTHER INFECTIONS

Vaginal preparations intended to restore normal acidity (*Aci-Jel®*) may prevent recurrence of vaginal infections and permit the re-establishment of the normal vaginal flora.

Trichomonal infections commonly involve the lower urinary tract as well as the genital system and need systemic treatment with metronidazole or tinidazole (see section 5.4.2).

Bacterial infections with Gram-negative organisms are particularly common in association with gynaecological operations and trauma. Metronidazole is effective against certain Gram-negative organisms, especially *Bacteroides* spp. and may be used prophylactically in gynaecological surgery.

Topical vaginal products containing povidone–iodine can be used to treat vaginitis due to candidal, trichomonal, non-specific or mixed infections; they are also used for the pre-operative preparation of the vagina. Clindamycin cream and metronidazole gel are also indicated for bacterial vaginosis; *Sultrin®* cream is licensed for the treatment of infections due to *Haemophilus vaginalis* only.

The antiviral drugs aciclovir, famciclovir and valaciclovir may be used in the treatment of genital infection due to *herpes simplex virus*, the HSV type 2 being a major cause of genital ulceration. They have a beneficial effect on virus shedding and healing, generally giving relief from pain and other symptoms. See section 5.3 for systemic preparations, and section 13.10.3 for cream.

---

1. See footnote 1 on p. 348

PREPARATIONS FOR OTHER VAGINAL INFECTIONS

Aci-Jel® (Janssen-Cilag)

Vaginal jelly, acetic acid 0.92% in a buffered (pH 4) basis. Net price 85 g with applicator = £3.37

Condoms: effect on latex condoms and diaphragms not yet known

Non-specific infections, insert 1 applicatorful twice daily to restore vaginal acidity

Betadine® (Seton)

Cautions: avoid in pregnancy (also if planned) and in breast-feeding; renal impairment (see Appendix 3); avoid regular use in thyroid disorders

Side-effects: rarely sensitivity; may interfere with thyroid function

Vaginal Cleansing Kit, solution, povidone-iodine 10%. Net price 250 mL with measuring bottle and applicator = £2.92

Condoms: effect on latex condoms and diaphragms not yet known

To be diluted and used once daily, preferably in the morning; may be used with Betadine® pessaries or vaginal gel

Pessaries, brown, povidone-iodine 200 mg. Net price 28 pessaries with applicator = £6.34

Condoms: effect on latex condoms and diaphragms not yet known

Vaginal gel, brown, povidone-iodine 10%. Net price 80 g with applicator = £2.92

Condoms: effect on latex condoms and diaphragms not yet known

Vaginal infections or pre-operatively, insert 1 moistened pessary night and morning for up to 14 days *or* use morning pessary with 5-g gel at night *or* morning douche with pessary (or 5-g gel) at night

PoM **Dalacin®** (Pharmacia & Upjohn)

Cream, clindamycin 2% (as phosphate). Net price 40-g pack with 7 applicators = £9.05

Condoms: damages latex condoms and diaphragms

Bacterial vaginosis, insert 5-g applicatorful intravaginally at night for 7 nights

PoM **Sultrin®** (Janssen-Cilag)

Contra-indications: pregnancy; hypersensitivity to peanuts

Side-effects: sensitivity

Cream, sulphathiazole 3.42%, sulphacetamide 2.86%, sulphabenzamide 3.7%. Net price 80 g with applicator = £3.48

Condoms: damages latex condoms and diaphragms

Bacterial vaginosis, insert 1 applicatorful of cream twice daily for 10 days, then once daily if necessary (but see also notes above)

PoM **Zidoval®** (3M)

Cautions: not recommended during menstruation; manufacturer advises avoid in first trimester of pregnancy; some absorption may occur, see section 5.1.11 for systemic effects

Side-effects: local effects including irritation, candidiasis, abnormal discharge, increased pelvic pressure

Vaginal gel, metronidazole 0.75%. Net price 40-g pack with 5 applicators = £4.85

Bacterial vaginosis, insert 5-g applicatorful intravaginally at night for 5 nights

7.3   Contraceptives

7.3.1   Combined oral contraceptives
7.3.2   Progestogen-only contraceptives
7.3.3   Spermicidal contraceptives
7.3.4   Contraceptive devices

The criteria by which contraceptive methods should be judged are effectiveness, acceptability, and freedom from side-effects.

Hormonal contraception is the most effective method of fertility control, short of sterilisation, but has unwanted major and minor side-effects, especially for certain groups of women.

Intra-uterine devices have a high use-effectiveness but may produce undesirable side-effects, especially menorrhagia, or be otherwise unsuitable in a significant proportion of women; their use is generally inadvisable in nulliparous women because of the increased risk of pelvic sepsis and infertility.

Barrier methods alone (condoms, diaphragms, and caps) are less effective but can be very reliable for well-motivated couples if used in conjunction with a **spermicide**. Occasionally sensitivity reactions occur. The female condom (Femidom®) is now also available; it is prelubricated but does not contain a spermicide.

7.3.1   Combined oral contraceptives

Oral contraceptives containing an oestrogen and a progestogen are the most effective preparations for general use. Their advantages include:
  reliability;
  avoidance of dysmenorrhoea;
  less iron-deficiency anaemia;
  avoidance of pre-menstrual tension;
  less benign breast disease;
  protection against endometrial and ovarian cancer;
  protection against pelvic inflammatory disease.

CHOICE. The oestrogen content ranges from 20 to 50 micrograms and generally a preparation with the lowest oestrogen and progestogen content (but within the guidelines of the CSM advice below) which gives good cycle control and minimal side-effects in the individual woman is chosen.

Low strength preparations (containing ethinyl-oestradiol 20 micrograms) are particularly appropriate for obese or older women provided a combined oral contraceptive is otherwise suitable (but see also CSM advice below). It is recommended that the combined oral contraceptive is not continued beyond 50 years of age since there exist more suitable alternatives.

Standard strength preparations (containing ethinyl-oestradiol 30 or 35 micrograms or in 30/40 microgram *phased* preparations) are appropriate for standard use in the case of those also containing *ethynodiol* (etynodiol), *levonorgestrel* or *norethisterone*—but in the case of those also containing *desogestrel* or *gestodene*, see CSM advice below. Phased preparations are more complex to take, but provide better cycle control than the equivalent 'monophasic' levonorgestrel or norethisterone formulations.

High strength preparations (containing either ethinyloestradiol 50 micrograms or mestranol 50 micrograms) provide greater contraceptive security but with an increase in the possibility of side-effects. These are used mainly in circumstances of reduced bioavailability (e.g. during long-term use of enzyme-inducing antiepileptics, see FPA advice under Interactions below).

The progestogens desogestrel, gestodene and norgestimate in combination with ethinyloestradiol have been reported to have less adverse effects on lipids than ethynodiol, levonorgestrel and norethisterone in combination with ethinyloestradiol. However, desogestrel and gestodene have also been associated with an increased risk of *venous thromboembolism* (see CSM advice below).

CSM advice. The CSM has advised that studies in relation to venous thromboembolism have provided reassurance about thromboembolic risks associated with oral contraceptives containing *levonorgestrel, norethisterone or ethynodiol* (excess risk around 5 to 10 cases per 100 000 women per annum). The studies indicated, however, that combined oral contraceptives containing *desogestrel* and *gestodene* are associated with around a two-fold increase in the risk, compared with those containing other progestogens. There is insufficient information to know whether there is any increased risk of thromboembolism associated with combined oral contraceptives containing *norgestimate*.

The CSM has therefore advised that combined oral contraceptives containing *gestodene or desogestrel* should **not** be used by women with risk factors for venous thromboembolism, including obesity (body mass index greater than 30 kg/m²), varicose veins, or a previous history of thrombosis from any cause [it should also be noted that any personal history of venous or arterial thrombosis is already a contra-indication to any combined oral contraceptive].

Combined oral contraceptives containing *desogestrel or gestodene* should **only** be used by women who are intolerant of other combined oral contraceptives, and are prepared to accept an increased risk of thromboembolism. This advice **only** affects combined oral preparations containing *desogestrel (Marvelon®, Mercilon®)*, or *gestodene (Femodene® ED, Femodene®, Minulet®, Triadene®, Tri-Minulet®)*.

MISSED PILL. It is important to bear in mind that the critical time for loss of protection is when a pill is omitted at the *beginning* or *end* of a cycle (which lengthens the pill-free interval). The following advice is now recommended by family planning organisations:

'If you forget a pill, take it as soon as you remember, and the next one at your normal time. If you are 12 or more hours late with any pill (especially the first in the packet) the pill may not work. As soon as you remember, continue normal pill taking. However, you will not be protected for the next seven days and must either not have sex or use another method such as the sheath. If these seven days run beyond the end of your packet, start the next packet at once when you have finished the present one, i.e. do not have a gap between packets. This will mean you may not have a period until the end of two packets but this does you no harm. Nor does it matter if you see some bleeding on tablet-taking days. If you are using everyday (ED) pills—miss out the seven inactive

pills. If you are not sure which these are, ask your doctor.'

DIARRHOEA AND VOMITING. Vomiting and severe diarrhoea can interfere with absorption and limit effectiveness. Additional precautions should therefore be used during and for 7 days after recovery. If the vomiting and diarrhoea occurs during the last 7 tablets, the next pill-free interval should be omitted (in the case of ED tablets the inactive ones should be omitted).

INTERACTIONS. The effectiveness of both *combined* and *progestogen-only* oral contraceptives may be considerably reduced by interaction with drugs that induce hepatic enzyme activity [e.g. **carbamazepine, griseofulvin, phenytoin, phenobarbitone, primidone, topiramate**, and, above all, **the rifamycins (rifabutin and rifampicin)**].

Family Planning Association (FPA) advice relating to a *short-term course of an enzyme-inducing drug* (important: rifampicin. see also below) is that additional contraceptive precautions should be taken whilst taking the enzyme-inducing drug and for at least 7 days after stopping it; if these 7 days run beyond the end of a packet the new packet should be started immediately without a break (in the case of ED tablets the inactive ones should be omitted). **Important:** it should be noted that **rifampicin** is such a potent enzyme-inducing drug that even if a course lasts for less than 7 days the additional contraceptive precautions should be continued for at least 4 weeks after stopping it.

FPA advice relating to a *long-term course of an enzyme-inducing drug* (important: rifampicin, see also below) in a woman unable to use an alternative method of contraception is to take an oral contraceptive containing ethinyloestradiol 50 micrograms or more; 'tricycling' with standard ('monophasic') tablets (i.e. taking 3 packets without a break followed by a short tablet-free interval of 4 days) is recommended. **Important:** it should be noted that **rifampicin** is such a potent enzyme-inducing drug that an alternative method of contraception (such as an IUD) is **always** recommended. Since the excretory function of the liver does not return to normal for several weeks after stopping an enzyme-inducing drug, FPA advice relating to *withdrawal* is that appropriate contraceptive measures are required for 4 to 8 weeks after stopping

In the case of *combined* oral contraceptives some **broad-spectrum antibiotics** (e.g. ampicillin) may reduce their efficacy by impairing the bacterial flora responsible for recycling of ethinyloestradiol from the large bowel. FPA advice is that additional contraceptive precautions should be taken whilst taking a *short course of a broad-spectrum antibiotic* and for 7 days after stopping. If these 7 days run beyond the end of a packet the next packet should be started immediately without a break (in the case of ED tablets the inactive ones should be omitted). If the course *exceeds 2 weeks*, resistance to this interference develops, and additional precautions become unnecessary.

SURGERY. Oestrogen-containing oral contraceptives should be discontinued (and adequate alternative contraceptive arrangements made) 4 weeks before major elective surgery and all surgery to the legs; they should normally be recommenced at the first menses occurring at least 2 weeks after full mobilisation. When discontinuation is not possible, e.g. after trauma or if, by oversight, a patient admitted for an elective procedure is still on an oestrogen-containing oral contraceptive, some consideration should be given to subcutaneous heparin prophylaxis. These recommendations do not apply to minor surgery with short duration of anaesthesia, e.g. laparoscopic sterilisation or tooth extraction, or to women taking oestrogen-free hormonal contraceptives (whether by mouth or by injection).

REASON TO STOP IMMEDIATELY. Combined oral contraceptives should be stopped (pending investigation and treatment), if any of the following symptoms occur:

Sudden severe pain in chest (whether or not radiating to the left arm);

Sudden breathlessness (or cough with blood-stained sputum);

Severe pain in calf of one leg;

Severe pain in stomach;

Unusual severe, prolonged headache—especially if first time or getting progressively worse, or associated with: sudden partial or complete loss of vision; diplopia; dysphasia; vertigo; bad fainting attack or collapse (with or without focal epilepsy); weakness or very marked numbness suddenly affecting one side or one part of body; motor disturbances.

COMBINED ORAL CONTRACEPTIVES

('COC')

Indications: contraception; menstrual symptoms (section 6.4.1.2)

Cautions: risk factors for arterial disease and migraine, see below; varicose veins (avoid if associated with venous thrombosis)—see also CSM advice in notes above; hyperprolactinaemia (seek specialist advice); severe depression, long-term immobilisation, sickle-cell disease, inflammatory bowel disease including Crohn's disease; **interactions:** see above and Appendix 1 (contraceptives, oral)

RISK FACTORS FOR ARTERIAL DISEASE. Use with **caution** if any one of following factors present but **avoid** if two or more factors present:

- *family history of arterial disease* in first degree relative aged under 45 years (avoid if atherogenic lipid profile as well as family history of arterial disease);
- *diabetes mellitus* (avoid if diabetes complications present);
- *hypertension* (avoid if severe);
- *smoking* (avoid if smoking 40 or more cigarettes daily);
- *age* over 35 years (avoid if over 50 years);
- *obesity* (avoid if body mass index exceeds 39 kg/m^2— see also CSM advice in notes above);
- *migraine*—see below.

MIGRAINE. Subject should report any increase in headache frequency or onset of focal symptoms (discontinue immediately and refer urgently to neurology expert if focal neurological symptoms not typical of aura persist for more than 1 hour); **contra-indicated** in

- migraine with typical focal aura,
- severe migraine regularly lasting over 72 hours despite treatment,
- migraine without aura in subject with another risk factor for arterial disease,
- migraine treated with ergot derivatives;

use with **caution** in

- migraine without aura (and no other arterial risk factors),
- migraine controlled with 5HT$_1$ agonist (section 4.7.4.1).

Contra-indications: pregnancy; severe or multiple risk factors for arterial disease (see above), antiphospholipid antibodies (including lupus anticoagulant), history of arterial or venous thrombosis—see also CSM advice in notes above, valvular heart disease associated with pulmonary hypertension or risk of mural thrombi, ischaemic heart disease, severe hypertension, during sclerosing treatment of varicose veins—see also Cautions above; conditions where risk of arterial wall disease is higher such as an atherogenic lipid profile, or any known prothrombotic coagulation abnormality including factor V Leiden; migraine (see above), transient cerebral ischaemic attacks without headaches; liver disease including disorders of hepatic excretion (e.g. Dubin-Johnson or Rotor syndromes), infective hepatitis (until liver function returns to normal); porphyria (section 9.8.2); liver adenoma; gall-stones; after evacuation of hydatidiform mole (until return to normal of urine and plasma gonadotrophin values); history of haemolytic uraemic syndrome or history of pruritus or cholestatic jaundice during pregnancy, pemphigoid gestationis, chorea or deterioration of otosclerosis; breast or genital-tract carcinoma; undiagnosed vaginal bleeding; breast-feeding (until weaning or for 6 months after birth)

Side-effects: nausea, vomiting, headache, breast tenderness, changes in body weight, thrombosis (more common when factor V Leiden present or in blood groups A, B, and AB), changes in libido, depression, chloasma, hypertension, contact lenses may irritate, impairment of liver function, hepatic tumours, reduced menstrual loss, 'spotting' in early cycles, absence of withdrawal bleeding; rarely photosensitivity

BREAST CANCER. There is a small increase in the risk of breast cancer during use and for 10 years after stopping the combined oral contraceptive pill; this relative risk does not appear to be related to duration of use. The CSM has advised that a small increase in the risk of breast cancer is more than counterbalanced by the protective effect against cancers of the ovary and endometrium

Dose: each tablet should be taken at approximately same time each day; if delayed by longer than 12 hours contraceptive protection may be lost

21-day combined (monophasic) preparations, 1 tablet daily for 21 days; subsequent courses repeated after a 7-day interval (during which withdrawal bleeding occurs); first course usually started on 1st day of cycle—if starting on 4th day of cycle or later additional precautions (barrier methods) necessary during first 7 days

Every day (ED) combined (monophasic) preparations, 1 tablet daily starting with an *active* tablet usually on 1st day of cycle—if starting on 4th day of cycle or later additional precautions (barrier methods) necessary during first 14 days (14 rather than 7 in case course accidentally started with *inactive* tablets); withdrawal bleeding occurs when *inactive* tablets are being taken; subsequent courses repeated without interval

Biphasic and triphasic preparations, see under individual preparations below

CHANGING TO COMBINED PREPARATION CONTAINING DIFFERENT PROGESTOGEN. *21-day combined preparations:* continue current pack until last tablet and start first tablet of new brand the next day. If a 7-day break is taken before starting new brand, additional precautions (barrier methods) should be used during first 7 days of taking the new brand.

Every Day (ED) combined preparations: start the new brand (first tablet a of *21-day preparation* or the first *active* tablet of an *ED preparation* the day after taking the last *active* tablet of previous brand (omitting the *inactive* tablets). If not possible to avoid taking the *inactive* tablets of an *ED preparation*, additional precautions (barrier methods) necessary during first 14 days of taking the new brand

CHANGING FROM PROGESTOGEN-ONLY TABLET: start on 1st day of menstruation or any day if amenorrhoea present and pregnancy has been excluded

SECONDARY AMENORRHOEA (exclude pregnancy): start any day, additional precautions (barrier methods) necessary during first 7 days

AFTER CHILDBIRTH (*not* breast-feeding): start 3 weeks postpartum (increased risk of thrombosis if started earlier); later than 3 weeks postpartum additional precautions (barrier methods) necessary for first 7 days

Not recommended if woman breast-feeding—oral progestogen-only contraceptive preferred

AFTER ABORTION OR MISCARRIAGE: start same day

Low Strength

Ethinyloestradiol with Norethisterone
PoM **Loestrin 20**® (P-D)

Tablets, norethisterone acetate 1 mg, ethinyloestradiol 20 micrograms. Net price 3 × 21-tab pack = £2.58
Dose: 1 tablet daily for 21 days; subsequent courses repeated after 7-day tablet-free interval (during which withdrawal bleeding occurs); for 'starting routines' see under 'Dose' in monograph above

Ethinyloestradiol with Desogestrel
See **CSM advice** in notes above before prescribing
PoM **Mercilon**® (Organon)

Tablets, desogestrel 150 micrograms, ethinyloestradiol 20 micrograms. Net price 3 × 21-tab pack = £8.97
Dose: 1 tablet daily for 21 days; subsequent courses repeated after 7-day tablet-free interval (during which withdrawal bleeding occurs); for 'starting routines' see under 'Dose' in monograph above

---

Standard Strength

Ethinyloestradiol with Levonorgestrel
PoM **Eugynon 30**® (Schering Health)

Tablets, levonorgestrel 250 micrograms, ethinyloestradiol 30 micrograms. Net price 3 × 21-tab pack = £2.07
Dose: 1 tablet daily for 21 days; subsequent courses repeated after 7-day tablet-free interval (during which withdrawal bleeding occurs); for 'starting routines' see under 'Dose' in monograph above

PoM **Logynon**® (Schering Health)

6 *light brown tablets*, ethinyloestradiol 30 micrograms, levonorgestrel 50 micrograms;
5 *white tablets*, ethinyloestradiol 40 micrograms, levonorgestrel 75 micrograms;
10 *ochre tablets*, ethinyloestradiol 30 micrograms, levonorgestrel 125 micrograms.
Net price 3 × 21-tab pack = £3.27
Dose: 1 tablet daily for 21 days, starting with light brown tablet marked 1 on day 1 of cycle; repeat after 7-day tablet-free interval

PoM **Logynon ED**® (Schering Health)

6 *light brown tablets*, ethinyloestradiol 30 micrograms, levonorgestrel 50 micrograms;
5 *white tablets*, ethinyloestradiol 40 micrograms, levonorgestrel 75 micrograms;
10 *ochre tablets*, ethinyloestradiol 30 micrograms, levonorgestrel 125 micrograms;
7 *white, inactive tablets*.
Net price 3 × 28-tab pack = £3.27
Dose: 1 tablet daily starting in red sector on day 1 of cycle; continue in sequence without interruption

PoM **Microgynon 30**® (Schering Health)

Tablets, levonorgestrel 150 micrograms, ethinyloestradiol 30 micrograms. Net price 21-tab pack = 62p
Dose: 1 tablet daily for 21 days; subsequent courses repeated after 7-day tablet-free interval (during which withdrawal bleeding occurs); for 'starting routines' see under 'Dose' in monograph above

PoM **Microgynon 30 ED**® (Schering Health)

Tablets, beige, levonorgestrel 150 micrograms, ethinyloestradiol 30 micrograms, white inactive tablets. Net price 3 × 28-tab (7 are inactive) pack = £1.86
Dose: 1 tablet daily for 28 days (withdrawal bleeding occurs when inactive tablets being taken); subsequent courses repeated without interval; for 'starting routines' see under 'Dose' in monograph above

PoM **Ovran 30**® (Wyeth)

Tablets, levonorgestrel 250 micrograms, ethinyloestradiol 30 micrograms. Net price 21-tab pack = 57p
Dose: 1 tablet daily for 21 days; subsequent courses repeated after 7-day tablet-free interval (during which withdrawal bleeding occurs); for 'starting routines' see under 'Dose' in monograph above

PoM **Ovranette**® (Wyeth)

Tablets, levonorgestrel 150 micrograms, ethinyloestradiol 30 micrograms. Net price 3 × 21-tab pack = £1.86
Dose: 1 tablet daily for 21 days; subsequent courses repeated after 7-day tablet-free interval (during which withdrawal bleeding occurs); for 'starting routines' see under 'Dose' in monograph above

PoM **Trinordiol**® (Wyeth)

6 *light brown tablets*, ethinyloestradiol 30 micrograms, levonorgestrel 50 micrograms;
5 *white tablets*, ethinyloestradiol 40 micrograms, levonorgestrel 75 micrograms;
10 *ochre tablets*, ethinyloestradiol 30 micrograms, levonorgestrel 125 micrograms.
Net price 3 × 21-tab pack = £3.28
Dose: 1 tablet daily for 21 days, starting with light brown tablet marked 1 on day 1 of cycle; repeat after 7-day tablet-free interval

Ethinyloestradiol with Norethisterone
PoM **BiNovum**® (Janssen-Cilag)

7 *white tablets*, ethinyloestradiol 35 micrograms, norethisterone 500 micrograms;
14 *peach tablets*, ethinyloestradiol 35 micrograms, norethisterone 1 mg.
Net price 3 × 21-tab pack = £2.24
Dose: 1 tablet daily for 21 days, starting with white tablet on day 1 of cycle; repeat after 7-day tablet-free interval

---

PoM **Brevinor®** (Searle)

Tablets, norethisterone 500 micrograms, ethinyloestradiol 35 micrograms. Net price 3 × 21-tab pack = £1.67

Dose: 1 tablet daily for 21 days; subsequent courses repeated after 7-day tablet-free interval (during which withdrawal bleeding occurs); for 'starting routines' see under 'Dose' in monograph above

PoM **Loestrin 30®** (P-D)

Tablets, norethisterone acetate 1.5 mg, ethinyloestradiol 30 micrograms. Net price 3 × 21-tab pack = £3.78

Dose: 1 tablet daily for 21 days; subsequent courses repeated after 7-day tablet-free interval (during which withdrawal bleeding occurs); for 'starting routines' see under 'Dose' in monograph above

PoM **Norimin®** (Searle)

Tablets, norethisterone 1 mg, ethinyloestradiol 35 micrograms. Net price 3 × 21-tab pack = £1.90

Dose: 1 tablet daily for 21 days; subsequent courses repeated after 7-day tablet-free interval (during which withdrawal bleeding occurs); for 'starting routines' see under 'Dose' in monograph above

PoM **Ovysmen®** (Janssen-Cilag)

Tablets, norethisterone 500 micrograms, ethinyloestradiol 35 micrograms. Net price 3 × 21-tab pack = £1.70

Dose: 1 tablet daily for 21 days; subsequent courses repeated after 7-day tablet-free interval (during which withdrawal bleeding occurs); for 'starting routines' see under 'Dose' in monograph above

PoM **Synphase®** (Searle)

7 blue tablets, ethinyloestradiol 35 micrograms, norethisterone 500 micrograms;

9 white tablets, ethinyloestradiol 35 micrograms, norethisterone 1 mg;

5 blue tablets, ethinyloestradiol 35 micrograms, norethisterone 500 micrograms.

Net price 21-tab pack = £1.08

Dose: 1 tablet daily for 21 days, starting with white tablet marked 1 on day 1 of cycle; repeat after 7-day tablet-free interval

PoM **TriNovum®** (Janssen-Cilag)

7 white tablets, ethinyloestradiol 35 micrograms, norethisterone 500 micrograms;

7 light peach tablets, ethinyloestradiol 35 micrograms, norethisterone 750 micrograms;

7 peach tablets, ethinyloestradiol 35 micrograms, norethisterone 1 mg.

Net price 3 × 21-tab pack = £2.83

Dose: 1 tablet daily for 21 days, starting with white tablet on day 1 of cycle; repeat after 7-day tablet-free interval

Ethinyloestradiol with Norgestimate

PoM **Cilest®** (Janssen-Cilag)

Tablets, norgestimate 250 micrograms, ethinyloestradiol 35 micrograms. Net price 3 × 21-tab pack = £5.84

Dose: 1 tablet daily for 21 days; subsequent courses repeated after 7-day tablet-free interval (during which withdrawal bleeding occurs); for 'starting routines' see under 'Dose' in monograph above

Ethinyloestradiol with Desogestrel

See **CSM advice** in notes above before prescribing

PoM **Marvelon®** (Organon)

Tablets, desogestrel 150 micrograms, ethinyloestradiol 30 micrograms. Net price 3 × 21-tab pack = £7.02

Dose: 1 tablet daily for 21 days; subsequent courses repeated after 7-day tablet-free interval (during which withdrawal bleeding occurs); for 'starting routines' see under 'Dose' in monograph above

Ethinyloestradiol with Gestodene

See **CSM advice** in notes above before prescribing

PoM **Femodene®** (Schering Health)

Tablets, gestodene 75 micrograms, ethinyloestradiol 30 micrograms. Net price 3 × 21-tab pack = £5.70

Dose: 1 tablet daily for 21 days; subsequent courses repeated after 7-day tablet-free interval (during which withdrawal bleeding occurs); for 'starting routines' see under 'Dose' in monograph above

PoM **Femodene ED®** (Schering Health)

Tablets, gestodene 75 micrograms, ethinyloestradiol 30 micrograms. Net price 3 × 28-tab (7 are inactive) pack = £5.70

Dose: 1 tablet daily for 28 days (withdrawal bleeding occurs when inactive tablets are being taken); subsequent courses repeated without interval; for 'starting routines' see under 'Dose' in monograph above

PoM **Minulet®** (Wyeth)

Tablets, gestodene 75 micrograms, ethinyloestradiol 30 micrograms. Net price 3 × 21-tab pack = £5.70

Dose: 1 tablet daily for 21 days; subsequent courses repeated after 7-day tablet-free interval (during which withdrawal bleeding occurs); for 'starting routines' see under 'Dose' in monograph above

PoM **Triadene®** (Schering Health)

6 beige tablets, ethinyloestradiol 30 micrograms, gestodene 50 micrograms;

5 dark brown tablets, ethinyloestradiol 40 micrograms, gestodene 70 micrograms;

10 white tablets, ethinyloestradiol 30 micrograms, gestodene 100 micrograms.

Net price 3 × 21-tab pack = £7.95

Dose: 1 tablet daily for 21 days, starting with beige tablet marked 'start' on day 1 of cycle; repeat after 7-day tablet-free interval

PoM **Tri-Minulet®** (Wyeth)

6 beige tablets, ethinyloestradiol 30 micrograms, gestodene 50 micrograms;

5 dark brown tablets, ethinyloestradiol 40 micrograms, gestodene 70 micrograms;

10 white tablets, ethinyloestradiol 30 micrograms, gestodene 100 micrograms.

Net price 3 × 21-tab pack = £7.95

Dose: 1 tablet daily for 21 days, starting with beige tablet marked 1 on day 1 of the cycle; repeat after 7-day tablet-free interval

High Strength

Ethinyloestradiol with Levonorgestrel

PoM **Ovran®** (Wyeth)

Tablets, levonorgestrel 250 micrograms, ethinyloestradiol 50 micrograms. Net price 21-tab pack = 37p

Dose: 1 tablet daily for 21 days; subsequent courses repeated after 7-day tablet-free interval (during which withdrawal bleeding occurs); for 'starting routines' see under 'Dose' in monograph above

Mestranol with Norethisterone

PoM **Norinyl-1®** (Searle)

Tablets, norethisterone 1 mg, mestranol 50 micrograms. Net price 3 × 21-tab pack = £1.83

Dose: 1 tablet daily for 21 days; subsequent courses repeated after 7-day tablet-free interval (during which withdrawal bleeding occurs); for 'starting routines' see under 'Dose' in monograph above

PoM **Ortho-Novin 1/50®** (Janssen-Cilag)

Tablets, norethisterone 1 mg, mestranol 50 micrograms. Net price 3 × 21-tab pack = £2.35

Dose: 1 tablet daily for 21 days; subsequent courses repeated after 7-day tablet-free interval (during which withdrawal bleeding occurs); for 'starting routines' see under 'Dose' in monograph above

---

EMERGENCY CONTRACEPTION

HORMONAL METHOD. The hormonal (Yuzpe) method is suitable for emergency use; it is however less effective than insertion of an intra-uterine device. The hormonal method involves taking two tablets, each containing ethinyloestradiol 50 micrograms and levonorgestrel 250 micrograms, followed 12 hours later by a further two tablets. The method has only been established as effective if the first dose is taken within 72 hours (3 days) of the unprotected intercourse; it is occasionally used after 72 hours [unlicensed use] but there is no clear proof of efficacy. Providing any delay does not extend beyond 72 hours, the timing of the first dose should be such that the second dose can conveniently be taken at the correct interval *exactly 12 hours later*. It is not suitable for women with a history of thrombosis or for those with focal migraine at the time of presentation. Side-effects include nausea, vomiting, headache, dizziness, breast discomfort, and menstrual irregularities. If vomiting occurs within 2–3 hours of taking the tablets, two replacement tablets can be given with an anti-emetic (preferably not metoclopramide which is liable to cause extrapyramidal effects in young women); alternatively insertion of an intra-uterine device (see below) may be needed.

The doctor should explain to the patient:

that her next period may be *early or late:*

that she needs to use a *barrier method of contraception* until her next period;

that she should return promptly if she has any *lower abdominal pain or heavy bleeding* (and also in 3 to 4 weeks if her subsequent period is abnormally light, heavy or brief, or is absent, or she is otherwise concerned).

Pregnancy despite treatment: see Appendix 4 (contraceptives, oral)—doctor information leaflet also available

INTERACTIONS. Effectiveness of emergency contraception is reduced by enzyme-inducing drugs; the dose of emergency contraception should be increased by 50% (i.e. to 3 tablets per dose). There is no need to increase the dose for emergency contraception if the patient is taking antibiotics that are not enzyme inducers.

PoM **Schering PC4®** (Schering Health)

Tablets, s/c, norgestrel 500 micrograms (≡ levonorgestrel 250 micrograms), ethinyloestradiol 50 micrograms. Net price 4-tab pack = £1.60

For post-coital contraception as an occasional emergency measure; should not be administered if menstrual bleeding overdue or if unprotected intercourse occurred more than 72 hours previously (but see notes above)

Dose: 2 tablets as soon as possible after coitus (up to 72 hours) then 2 further tablets 12 hours later

Note. **Ovran®** also contains levonorgestrel 250 micrograms and ethinyloestradiol 50 micrograms but is not licensed or packed for post-coital contraception

IUD. An intra-uterine contraceptive device (see section 7.3.4) can be inserted up to 120 hours (5 days) after unprotected intercourse, care being taken to exclude any sexually transmitted diseases. If exposure has occurred more than 5 days previously, the device can still be inserted up to 5 days after the earliest likely calculated ovulation (i.e. within the minimum period before implantation). Insertion of an intra-uterine device is more effective than the hormonal method.

7.3.2 Progestogen-only contraceptives

7.3.2.1 Oral progestogen-only contraceptives

7.3.2.2 Parenteral progestogen-only contraceptives

7.3.2.3 Intra-uterine progestogen-only contraceptive

7.3.2.1 ORAL PROGESTOGEN-ONLY CONTRACEPTIVES

Oral progestogen-only preparations may offer a suitable alternative when oestrogens are contra-indicated (including those patients with venous thrombosis or a past history or predisposition to venous thrombosis), but have a higher failure rate than combined preparations. They are suitable for older women, for heavy smokers, and for those with hypertension, valvular heart disease, diabetes mellitus, and migraine. Menstrual irregularities (oligomenorrhoea, menorrhagia) are more common but tend to resolve on long-term treatment.

INTERACTIONS. Effectiveness of oral progestogen-only preparations is not affected by broad-spectrum antibiotics but is reduced by enzyme-inducing drugs—see p. 351 and Appendix 1 (progestogens)

SURGERY. All progestogen-only contraceptives (including those given by injection) are suitable for use as an alternative to combined oral contraceptives before major elective surgery.

STARTING ROUTINE. 1 tablet daily, on a continuous basis, starting on 1st day of cycle and taken at the same time each day (if delayed by longer than 3 hours contraceptive protection may be lost). Additional contraceptive precautions are not necessary when initiating treatment.

Changing from a combined oral contraceptive: start on the day following completion of the combined oral contraceptive course without a break (or in the case of ED tablets omitting the inactive ones).

After childbirth: start any time after 3 weeks postpartum (increased risk of breakthrough bleeding if started earlier)—lactation is not affected.

MISSED PILL. The following advice is now recommended by family planning organisations:

'If you forget a pill, take it as soon as you remember and carry on with the next pill at the right time. If the pill was more than three hours overdue you are not protected. Continue normal pill-taking but you must also use another method, such as the sheath, for the next 7 days'.

DIARRHOEA AND VOMITING. Vomiting and severe diarrhoea can interfere with absorption and limit effectiveness. Additional precautions should be used during and for 7 days after recovery.

ORAL PROGESTOGEN-ONLY CONTRACEPTIVES

(Progestogen-only pill, 'POP')

Indications: contraception

Cautions: heart disease, sex-steroid dependent cancer, past ectopic pregnancy, malabsorption syndromes, functional ovarian cysts, active liver disease, recurrent cholestatic jaundice, history of jaundice in pregnancy; **interactions:** p. 351 and Appendix 1 (progestogens)

OTHER CONDITIONS. Despite unsatisfactory evidence of hazard, product literature advises caution in history of thromboembolism, hypertension, diabetes mellitus and migraine

Contra-indications: pregnancy, undiagnosed vaginal bleeding; severe arterial disease; liver adenoma, porphyria (section 9.8.2); after evacuation of hydatidiform mole (until return to normal of urine and plasma gonadotrophin values)

Side-effects: menstrual irregularities (see also notes above); nausea, vomiting, headache, dizziness, breast discomfort, depression, skin disorders, disturbance of appetite, weight changes, changes in libido

Dose: 1 tablet daily at same time each day, starting on day 1 of cycle then continuously; if tablet delayed for 3 hours or more it should be regarded as a 'missed pill', see notes above

PoM **Femulen**® (Searle)

Tablets, ethynodiol diacetate 500 micrograms. Net price 28-tab pack = 92p

PoM **Micronor**® (Janssen-Cilag)

Tablets, norethisterone 350 micrograms. Net price 3 × 28-tab pack = £1.89

PoM **Microval**® (Wyeth)

Tablets, levonorgestrel 30 micrograms. Net price 35-tab pack = 82p

PoM **Neogest**® (Schering Health)

Tablets, brown, s/c, norgestrel 75 micrograms (≡ levonorgestrel 37.5 micrograms). Net price 35-tab pack = 82p

PoM **Norgeston**® (Schering Health)

Tablets, s/c, levonorgestrel 30 micrograms. Net price 35-tab pack = 82p

PoM **Noriday**® (Searle)

Tablets, norethisterone 350 micrograms. Net price 3 × 28-tab pack = £1.75

7.3.2.2 PARENTERAL PROGESTOGEN-ONLY CONTRACEPTIVES

Medroxyprogesterone acetate (*Depo-Provera*®) is a long-acting progestogen given by intramuscular injection; it is as effective as the combined oral preparations but because of its prolonged action should never be given without *full counselling backed by the manufacturer's approved leaflet.* It may be used as a short-term or long-term contraceptive for women who have been appropriately counselled concerning the likelihood of menstrual disturbance and the potential for a delay in return to

full fertility. Delayed return of fertility and irregular cycles may occur after discontinuation of treatment but there is no evidence of permanent infertility. Heavy bleeding has been reported in patients given medroxyprogesterone acetate in the immediate puerperium (the first dose is best delayed until 5 to 6 weeks postpartum). If the woman is not breast-feeding, the first injection may be given within 5 days postpartum (she should be warned that the risk of heavy or prolonged bleeding may be increased). Reduction in bone mineral density has also been reported. **Norethisterone enanthate** (*Noristerat*®) is a long-acting progestogen given as an oily injection which provides contraception for 8 weeks to provide short-term interim contraception e.g. before vasectomy becomes effective. The **cautions** and **contra-indications** of oral progestogen-only contraceptives apply except that since the injection also reliably inhibits ovulation, it protects against ectopic pregnancy and functional ovarian cysts.

A **levonorgestrel-releasing implant system** (*Norplant*®) is also available; it has comparable efficacy to injectable medroxyprogesterone acetate but lasts for 5 years. The **cautions** and **contra-indications** are again as for oral preparations, but irregular and prolonged bleeding and amenorrhoea are common; unlike the injectable preparations the method is almost immediately reversible on removal of the implants. The risk of ectopic pregnancy is believed to be reduced overall but the proportion of ectopic to intra-uterine pregnancies is increased among the very few pregnancies that do occur; since functional ovarian cysts may also be more common they need to be distinguished from ectopic pregnancy. *The doctor administering (or removing) the system should be fully trained in the technique and should provide full counselling backed by the manufacturer's approved leaflet.*

INTERACTIONS. Effectiveness of parenteral progestogen-only contraceptives is not affected by broad-spectrum antibiotics but may be reduced by enzyme-inducing drugs; the interval between injections of medroxyprogesterone acetate should be reduced from 12 weeks to 10 weeks—see p. 351 and Appendix 1 (progestogens)

PARENTERAL PROGESTOGEN-ONLY CONTRACEPTIVES

Indications: contraception, see also notes above and under preparations (roles vary according to preparation)

Cautions; Contra-indications; Side-effects: see notes above and under preparations; **interactions:** see notes above, p. 351 and Appendix 1 (progestogens)

COUNSELLING. Full counselling backed by *manufacturer's approved leaflet* required before administration

Dose: see under preparations

Injectable preparations

PoM **Depo-Provera**® (Pharmacia & Upjohn)

Injection (aqueous suspension), medroxyprogesterone acetate 150 mg/mL, net price 1-mL prefilled syringe = £4.55. Counselling, see patient information leaflet

Dose: by deep intramuscular injection, 150 mg within first 5 days of cycle or within first 5 days after parturition (delay until 6 weeks after parturition if breast-feeding); for long-term contraception, repeated every 12 weeks (if interval greater than 12 weeks and 5 days, exclude pregnancy before next injection and advise patient to use additional contraceptive measures (e.g. barrier) for 14 days after the injection)

Note. The 150 mg/mL strength of Depo-Provera® is also available in a 3.3-mL vial for use in cancer (see section 8.3.2)

PoM **Noristerat®** (Schering Health)

Injection (oily), norethisterone enanthate 200 mg/mL. Net price 1-mL amp = £3.00. Counselling, see patient information leaflet

Dose: by deep intramuscular injection into gluteal muscle, short-term contraception, 200 mg within first 5 days of cycle or immediately after parturition (duration 8 weeks); may be repeated once after 8 weeks (withhold breast-feeding for neonates with severe or persistent jaundice requiring medical treatment)

Implants

PoM **Norplant®** (Hoechst Marion Roussel)

Implant capsules, containing levonorgestrel 38 mg in each polydimethylsiloxane (silicone) capsule. Net price 6-implant capsule pack = £179.00. Counselling, see patient information leaflet

Dose: by subdermal implantation, set of 6 implant capsules inserted within first 5 days of cycle (preferably on 1st day—after 1st day additional precautions necessary for following 7 days) *or* on 21st day after parturition (after this day additional precautions necessary for following 7 days); remove within 5 years of insertion

---

7.3.2.3 INTRA-UTERINE PROGESTOGEN-ONLY CONTRACEPTIVE

Levonorgestrel is released directly in to the uterine cavity from an intra-uterine system (*Mirena®*). Effects are therefore mainly local and hormonal including prevention of proliferation of the endometrium, thickening of cervical mucus, and suppression of ovulation in some women (in some cycles); the physical presence of the system in the uterus may also make a minor contribution to the overall contraceptive effect. Return of fertility after removal is rapid and appears to be complete. Advantages over copper intra-uterine devices are that there may be an improvement in any dysmenorrhoea and a reduction in blood loss; there is also evidence that the frequency of pelvic inflammatory disease may be reduced (particularly in the youngest age groups who are most at risk). Generally the **cautions** and **contra-indications** are as for standard intra-uterine devices (section 7.3.4) but the risk of ectopic pregnancy is considerably reduced and pre-existing heavy menses and anaemia may be alleviated. Moreover, since the progestogen is released close to the site of the main contraceptive action (on cervical mucus and endometrium) progestogenic side-effects and **interactions** are less likely to be a problem—in particular, enzyme-inducing drugs are unlikely to have much influence on the contraceptive effect. Initially changes in the pattern and duration of menstrual bleeding (spotting or prolonged bleeding) are common and full counselling (backed by patient information leaflet) should be undertaken before insertion. Improvement usually occurs a few months after insertion and bleeding may often become scanty or absent; this may therefore be a method of choice for women who have excessively heavy menses. Functional ovarian cysts (usually asymptomatic) may occur and usually resolve spontaneously (ultrasound monitoring recommended).

INTRA-UTERINE PROGESTOGEN-ONLY CONTRACEPTIVE

Indications: contraception

Cautions; Contra-indications; Side-effects: see notes above; in case of pregnancy—remove system (teratogenicity cannot be excluded); not suitable for emergency contraception; **interactions:** see notes above and Appendix 1 (progestogens)

PoM **Mirena®** (Schering Health)

Intra-uterine system, T-shaped plastic frame (impregnated with barium sulphate and with threads attached to base) with polydimethylsiloxane reservoir releasing levonorgestrel 20 micrograms/24 hours. Net price = £99.25. Counselling, see patient information leaflet

Insert into uterine cavity within 7 days of onset of menstruation (anytime if replacement) or immediately after first-trimester termination by curettage; postpartum insertions should be delayed until 6 weeks after delivery; effective for 3 years

7.3.3 Spermicidal contraceptives

Spermicidal contraceptives are useful additional safeguards but do **not** give adequate protection if used alone; they are suitable for use with barrier methods. They have two components: a spermicide and a vehicle which itself may have some inhibiting effect on sperm activity.

> **CSM Advice.** Products such as petroleum jelly (vaseline), baby oil and oil-based vaginal and rectal preparations are likely to damage condoms and contraceptive diaphragms made from latex rubber, and may render them less effective as a barrier method of contraception and as a protection from sexually transmitted diseases (including AIDS).

Condoms: no evidence of harm to latex condoms and diaphragms with the products listed below

Delfen® (Janssen-Cilag)

Foam, nonoxinol '9' 12.5%, pressurised aerosol unit in a water-miscible basis. Net price 20 g (with applicator) = £4.65

Double Check® (FP)

Pessaries, nonoxinol '9' 6% in a water-soluble basis. Net price 10 pessaries = £1.08

Duragel® (LRC)

Gel, nonoxinol '9' 2% in a water-soluble basis. Net price 100-g tube = £3.01

Cautionary label wordings, see inside back cover   Prices are **net**, see p.1

Gynol II® (Janssen-Cilag)

Jelly, nonoxinol '9' 2% in a water-soluble basis.
Net price 81 g = £2.61; applicator = 75p

Ortho-Creme® (Janssen-Cilag)

Cream, nonoxinol '9' 2% in a water-miscible
basis. Net price 70 g = £2.44; applicator = 75p

Orthoforms® (Janssen-Cilag)

Pessaries, nonoxinol '9' 5% in a water-soluble
basis. Net price 15 pessaries = £2.40

7.3.4   Contraceptive devices

INTRA-UTERINE DEVICES

The intra-uterine device (IUD) is suitable for older
parous women but should be a last-resort contraceptive for young nulliparous women because of
the increased risk of pelvic inflammatory disease
and infertility. Inert intra-uterine devices are no
longer on the UK market but may still be worn by
some women.

Smaller devices have now been introduced in
order to minimise side-effects; these consist of a
plastic carrier wound with copper wire or fitted
with copper bands; some also have a central core of
silver with the aim of preventing fragmentation of
the copper. Family planning organisations now recommend that the replacement time for these devices
should be 5 years (8 years for Gyne-T® 380
Slimline which also has a copper collar); any copper intrauterine device licensed currently in the UK,
which is fitted in a woman over the age of 40, may
remain in the uterus until menopause.

The timing and technique of fitting an intra-
uterine device play a critical part in its subsequent
performance and call for proper training and experience. Devices should not be fitted during the heavy
days of the period; they are best fitted after the end
of menstruation and before the calculated time of
implantation. The main excess risk of infection
occurs in the first 20 days after insertion and is
believed to be related to pre-existing carriage of a
sexually transmitted disease, therefore pre-screen-
ing (at least for chlamydia) should ideally be performed. The woman should be advised to attend *as
an emergency* if she experiences sustained pain during the next 20 days.

An intra-uterine device should not be removed in
mid-cycle unless an additional contraceptive was
used for the previous 7 days. If removal is essential
(e.g. to treat severe pelvic infection) post-coital
contraception should be considered.

If an intra-uterine device fails and the woman
wishes to continue to full-term the device should be
removed in the first trimester if possible.

INTRA-UTERINE CONTRACEPTIVE DEVICES

Indications: see notes above

Cautions: anaemia, heavy menses, endometriosis,
severe primary dysmenorrhoea, history of pelvic
inflammatory disease, history of ectopic
pregnancy or tubal surgery, diabetes, fertility

problems, nulliparity and young age, severely
scarred uterus (including after endometrial resection) or severe cervical stenosis, valvular heart
disease (antibiotic cover needed)—avoid if prosthetic valve or past attack of infective endocarditis; joint and other prostheses (increased risk of
infection); epilepsy; increased risk of expulsion if
inserted before uterine involution; gynaecological
examination before insertion, 6 weeks after (or
sooner if there is a problem), then after 6 months,
then yearly; anticoagulant therapy (avoid if possible); remove if pregnancy occurs; if pregnancy
occurs, increased likelihood that it may be ectopic

Contra-indications: pregnancy, severe anaemia,
known HIV infection, recent sexually transmitted
infection (if not fully investigated and treated),
very heavy menses, unexplained uterine bleeding,
distorted or small uterine cavity, genital malignancy, trophoblastic disease, pelvic inflammatory disease, immunosuppressive therapy,
copper devices: copper allergy, Wilson's disease,
medical diathermy

Side-effects: uterine or cervical perforation, displacement, pelvic infection may be exacerbated,
heavy menses, dysmenorrhoea, allergy; *on insertion:* some pain (helped by giving an NSAID,
such as ibuprofen half-an-hour before insertion)
and bleeding, occasionally, epileptic seizure, vasovagal attack

PoM **Multiload® Cu250** (Organon)

Intra-uterine device, copper wire, surface area approx.
250 mm² wound on vertical stem of plastic carrier,
3.6 cm length, with 2 down-curving flexible arms,
monofilament thread attached to base of vertical stem;
preloaded in inserter. Net price = £6.75
For uterine length over 7 cm; replacement every 3 years
(but see notes above)

PoM **Multiload® Cu250 Short** (Organon)

Intra-uterine device, as above, with vertical stem length
2.5 cm. Net price = £6.75
For uterine length 5–7 cm; replacement every 3 years
(but see notes above)

PoM **Multiload®Cu375** (Organon)

Intra-uterine device, as above, with copper surface area
approx. 375 mm². Net price = £8.75
For uterine length over 7 cm; replacement every 5 years
(see notes above)

PoM **Novagard®** (Pharmacia & Upjohn)

Intra-uterine device, copper wire with silver core, surface
area approx. 200 mm² wound on vertical stem of T-
shaped plastic carrier, impregnated with barium sulphate
for radio-opacity, monofilament thread attached to base
of vertical stem; partially preloaded in inserter. Dimen-
sions: transverse arms, vertical stem, both 3.2 cm. Net
price = £9.90
For uterine length over 5.5 cm; replacement every 5
years (see notes above)

PoM **Nova-T®** (Schering Health)

Intra-uterine device, copper wire with silver core, surface
area approx. 200 mm² wound on vertical stem of T-
shaped plastic carrier, impregnated with barium sulphate
for radio-opacity, threads attached to base of vertical
stem. Net price = £9.90
For uterine length over 6.5 cm; replacement every 5
years (see notes above)

PoM **Ortho Gyne-T® 380 Slimline** (Janssen-Cilag)

Intra-uterine device, copper wire surface area 320 mm²
wound on vertical stem of T-shaped plastic carrier
(impregnated with radiopaque substance), plastic thread

---

attached to base of vertical stem, and copper collar surface 30 mm² on distal portion of each arm. Net price = £9.40

For uterine length over 6.5 cm; replacement every 8 years (see notes above)

OTHER CONTRACEPTIVE DEVICES

Contraceptive caps

Type A contraceptive pessary. Opaque rubber, sizes 1 to 5 (55–75 mm rising in steps of 5 mm), net price = £6.40
Available from Lamberts (Dumas Vault Cap®)
Type B contraceptive pessary Opaque rubber, sizes 22 to 31 mm (rising in steps of 3 mm), net price = £7.45
Available from Lamberts (Prentif Cavity Rim Cervical Cap®)
Type C contraceptive pessary Opaque rubber, sizes 1 to 3 (42, 48 and 54 mm), net price = £6.40
Available from Lamberts (Vimule Cap®)

Contraceptive diaphragms

Type A Diaphragm with flat metal spring. Transparent rubber with flat metal spring, sizes 55–95 mm (rising in steps of 5 mm), net price = £5.49
Available from Lamberts (Reflexions®)
Type B Diaphragm with coiled metal rim. Opaque rubber with coiled metal rim, sizes 55–95 mm (rising in steps of 5 mm), net price = £5.53
Available from Janssen-Cilag (Ortho®)
Type C Arcing Spring Diaphragm. Opaque rubber with arcing spring, sizes 55–95 mm (rising in steps of 5 mm), net price = £6.29
Available from Janssen-Cilag (All-Flex®)

Fertility thermometer
Fertility (Ovulation) Thermometer (Zeal)
Mercury in glass thermometer, range 35 to 39°C (graduated in 0.1°C). Net price = £1.59
For monitoring ovulation for the fertility awareness method of contraception

---

7.4   Drugs for genito-urinary disorders

7.4.1	Drugs for urinary retention
7.4.2	Drugs for urinary frequency, enuresis, and incontinence
7.4.3	Drugs used in urological pain
7.4.4	Bladder instillations and urological surgery
7.4.5	Drugs for impotence

For drugs used in the treatment of urinary-tract infections see section 5.1.13.

7.4.1   Drugs for urinary retention

Acute retention is painful and is treated by catheterisation.

Chronic retention is painless and often longstanding. Catheterisation is unnecessary unless there is deterioration of renal function. After the cause has initially been established and treated, drugs may be required to increase detrusor muscle tone.

Benign prostatic hyperplasia is treated either surgically or medically with alpha-blockers (see below) or with the anti-androgen finasteride (section 6.4.2).

ALPHA-BLOCKERS

The selective alpha-blockers, **alfuzosin, doxazosin, indoramin, prazosin, tamsulosin** and **terazosin** relax smooth muscle in benign prostatic hyperplasia producing an increase in urinary flow-rate and an improvement in obstructive symptoms. Side-effects of selective alpha-blockers include sedation, dizziness and hypotension (notably postural hypotension, particularly after the first dose); other side-effects associated with this group of drugs include drowsiness, weakness and lack of energy, depression, headache, dry mouth, nausea, urinary frequency and incontinence, and tachycardia and palpitations. They should be avoided in patients with a history of orthostatic hypotension and micturition syncope; special care (and reduced dosage) is needed when initiating them in the elderly, and in renal and possibly hepatic impairment. Since selective alpha-blockers are also antihypertensive, patients receiving antihypertensive treatment require reduced dosage and specialist supervision (as do those with cardiac disorders). **Interactions:** see Appendix 1 (alpha-blockers).

DRIVING. Selective alpha-blockers may cause drowsiness and so affect ability to drive or operate machinery.

ALFUZOSIN HYDROCHLORIDE
Indications; Cautions; Contra-indications; Side-effects: see notes above; avoid in severe liver impairment
Dose: 2.5 mg 3 times daily, max.10 mg daily; ELDERLY initially 2.5 mg twice daily
FIRST DOSE EFFECT. First dose may cause collapse due to hypotensive effect (therefore should be taken on retiring to bed). Patient should be warned to lie down if symptoms such as dizziness, fatigue or sweating develop, and to remain lying down until they abate completely

PoM **Xatral®** (Lorex)
Tablets, f/c, alfuzosin hydrochloride 2.5 mg. Net price 60-tab pack = £19.00; 90-tab pack = £25.00. Label: 3, counselling, see dose above

Modified release
PoM **Xatral® SR** (Lorex)
Tablets, m/r, yellow, f/c, alfuzosin hydrochloride 5 mg. Net price 60-tab pack = £23.80. Label: 3, 25, counselling, see dose above
Dose: 5 mg twice daily; ELDERLY initially 5 mg in the evening

---

DOXAZOSIN
Indications; Cautions; Contra-indications; Side-effects: see notes above and section 2.5.4
Dose: initially 1 mg daily; increased if necessary at intervals of 1–2 weeks to max. 8 mg daily; usual maintenance 2–4 mg daily

---

PoM **Cardura®** (Invicta)

Tablets, doxazosin (as mesylate) 1 mg, net price 28-tab pack = £10.56; 2 mg, 28-tab pack = £14.08; 4 mg, 28-tab pack = £17.60

INDORAMIN

Indications; Cautions; Contra-indications; Side-effects: see notes above and section 2.5.4

Dose: 20 mg twice daily; increased if necessary by 20 mg every 2 weeks to max. 100 mg daily in divided doses; ELDERLY, 20 mg at night may be adequate

PoM **Doralese®** (Bencard)

Tablets, yellow, f/c, indoramin 20 mg. net price 60-tab pack = £12.30. Label: 2

PRAZOSIN HYDROCHLORIDE

Indications; Cautions; Contra-indications; Side-effects: see notes above and section 2.5.4

Dose: initially 500 micrograms twice daily for 3–7 days, subsequently adjusted according to response; usual maintenance (and max.) 2 mg twice daily; ELDERLY initiate with lowest possible dose

FIRST DOSE EFFECT. First dose may cause collapse due to hypotensive effect (therefore should be taken on retiring to bed). Patient should be warned to lie down if symptoms such as dizziness, fatigue or sweating develop, and to remain lying down until they abate completely

PoM **Hypovase®** (Invicta)

Tablets, prazosin hydrochloride 500 micrograms, net price 56-tab pack = £2.09; 1 mg (orange, scored), 56-tab pack = £2.69; 2 mg (scored), 56-tab pack = £3.66; starter pack of 8 × 500-microgram tabs with 32 × 1-mg tabs = £2.52. Label: 3, counselling, see dose above

TAMSULOSIN HYDROCHLORIDE

Indications; Cautions; Contra-indications; Side-effects: see notes above; avoid in severe liver impairment

Dose: 400 micrograms daily after breakfast

▼ PoM **Flomax® MR** (Yamanouchi)

Capsules, m/r, tamsulosin hydrochloride 400 micrograms. Net price 30-cap pack = £23.90. Label: 25

TERAZOSIN

Indications; Cautions; Contra-indications; Side-effects: see notes above and section 2.5.4

Dose: initially 1 mg at bedtime; dose may be doubled at weekly intervals according to response, to max. 10 mg once daily; usual maintenance 5–10 mg daily

FIRST DOSE EFFECT. First dose may cause collapse due to hypotensive effect (therefore should be taken on retiring to bed). Patient should be warned to lie down if symptoms such as dizziness, fatigue or sweating develop, and to remain lying down until they abate completely

PoM **Hytrin BPH®** (Abbott)

Tablets, terazosin (as hydrochloride) 2 mg (yellow), net price 28-tab pack = £12.55; 5 mg (tan), 28-tab pack = £18.89; 10 mg (blue), 28-tab pack = £26.59; starter pack of 7 × 1-mg tab with 14 × 2-mg tab and 7 × 5-mg tab = £14.25. Label: 3, counselling, see dose above

PARASYMPATHOMIMETICS

Parasympathomimetics produce the effects of parasympathetic nerve stimulation; they possess the muscarinic rather than the nicotinic effects of acetylcholine and improve voiding efficiency by increasing detrusor muscle contraction. In the absence of obstruction to the bladder outlet they have a limited role in the relief of urinary retention. Generalised parasympathomimetic side-effects such as sweating, bradycardia, and intestinal colic may occur, particularly in the elderly.

Carbachol and **bethanechol** are choline esters that have been used in postoperative urinary retention. Bethanechol has a more selective action on the bladder than carbachol but the use of both has now been superseded by catheterisation.

Distigmine inhibits the breakdown of acetylcholine. It may help patients with an upper motor neurone neurogenic bladder.

BETHANECHOL CHLORIDE

Indications: urinary retention, but see notes above

Contra-indications: intestinal or urinary obstruction or where increased muscular activity of urinary or gastro-intestinal tract harmful; asthma, bradycardia, hyperthyroidism, recent myocardial infarction, epilepsy, hypotension, parkinsonism, vagotonia, peptic ulceration, pregnancy; **interactions**: Appendix 1 (parasympathomimetics)

Side-effects: parasympathomimetic effects such as nausea, vomiting, sweating, blurred vision, bradycardia, and intestinal colic

Dose: 10–25 mg 3–4 times daily half an hour before food

PoM **Myotonine®** (Glenwood)

Tablets, both scored, bethanechol chloride 10 mg, net price 20 = 90p; 25 mg, 20 = £1.15. Label: 22

CARBACHOL

Indications: urinary retention, but see notes above

Contra-indications; Side-effects: see under Bethanechol Chloride but side-effects more acute

Dose: by mouth, 2 mg 3 times daily half an hour before food

By subcutaneous injection (acute symptoms, postoperative urinary retention) 250 micrograms, repeated twice if necessary at 30-minute intervals

Note. Inadvertent intravenous administration of carbachol is **extremely hazardous** and calls for emergency treatment with atropine

PoM **Carbachol** (Non-proprietary)

Tablets, carbachol 2 mg. Net price 20 = £2.56. Label: 22

Note. Supplies may be difficult to obtain

Injection, carbachol 250 micrograms/mL

DISTIGMINE BROMIDE

Indications: urinary retention (see notes above); myasthenia gravis, see section 10.2.1

Cautions: asthma, bradycardia, hyperthyroidism, recent myocardial infarction, epilepsy, hypotension, parkinsonism, vagotonia, peptic ulceration, pregnancy; **interactions:** Appendix 1 (parasympathomimetics)

Contra-indications: intestinal or urinary obstruction or where increased muscular activity of urinary or gastro-intestinal tract harmful

Side-effects: see under Bethanechol Chloride, but action slower therefore side-effects less acute; see also Neostigmine (section 10.2.1)

Dose: 5 mg daily or on alternate days, half an hour before breakfast

PoM **Ubretid**® (Rhône-Poulenc Rorer)

Tablets, scored, distigmine bromide 5 mg. Net price 30-tab pack = £24.05. Label: 22

7.4.2 Drugs for urinary frequency, enuresis, and incontinence

URINARY INCONTINENCE

Antimuscarinic drugs such as **oxybutynin** and **flavoxate** are used to treat *urinary frequency*; they increase bladder capacity by diminishing unstable detrusor contractions. Both drugs may cause dry mouth and blurred vision and may precipitate glaucoma. Oxybutynin has a high level of side-effects which limits its use; the dosage needs to be carefully assessed, particularly in the elderly. Flavoxate has less marked side-effects but is also less effective. **Propantheline** was formerly widely used in urinary incontinence but had a low response rate with a high incidence of side-effects; it is now primarily indicated in adult enuresis. The **tricyclic antidepressants** imipramine, amitriptyline, and nortriptyline (see section 4.3.1) are sometimes effective in the management of the unstable bladder because of their antimuscarinic properties.

Purified bovine collagen implant (Contigen®, Bard) is indicated for *urinary incontinence* caused by intrinsic sphincter deficiency (poor or non-functioning bladder outlet mechanism). The implant is injected (with the aid of a cystoscope) in the tissues around the neck of the bladder creating increased tissue bulk so that resistance to urine outflow is achieved. It should only be used by surgeons or physicians familiar with the use of a cystoscope and trained in the technique for injection of the implant.

FLAVOXATE HYDROCHLORIDE

Indications: urinary frequency and incontinence, dysuria, urgency; bladder spasms due to catheterisation

Cautions; Contra-indications: see under Oxybutynin Hydrochloride (antimuscarinic effect considerably less marked)

Side-effects: antimuscarinic side-effects (see Atropine Sulphate, section 1.2); see also notes above

Dose: 200 mg 3 times daily; CHILD under 12 years not recommended

PoM **Urispas 200**® (Shire)

Tablets, s/c, flavoxate hydrochloride 200 mg, net price 90-tab pack = £10.79

OXYBUTYNIN HYDROCHLORIDE

Indications: urinary frequency, urgency and incontinence, neurogenic bladder instability and nocturnal enuresis

Cautions: frail elderly; hepatic or renal impairment; neuropathy; hyperthyroidism; cardiac disease where increase in rate undesirable; prostatic hypertrophy; hiatus hernia with reflux oesophagitis; pregnancy and breast-feeding; porphyria (see section 9.8.2); **interactions:** Appendix 1 (antimuscarinics)

Contra-indications: intestinal obstruction or atony, severe ulcerative colitis or toxic megacolon; significant bladder outflow obstruction; glaucoma; myasthenia gravis

Side-effects: include dry mouth, constipation, blurred vision, nausea, abdominal discomfort, facial flushing (more marked in children), difficulty in micturition (less commonly urinary retention); also headache, dizziness, drowsiness, dry skin, rash, angioedema, photosensitivity, diarrhoea, arrhythmia, restlessness, disorientation, hallucination (children at higher risk of excitatory effects); convulsions; see also notes above

Dose: 5 mg 2–3 times daily increased if necessary to max. 5 mg 4 times daily

ELDERLY 2.5–3 mg twice daily initially, increased to 5 mg twice daily according to response and tolerance

CHILD over 5 years, neurogenic bladder instability, 2.5–3 mg twice daily increased to 5 mg twice daily (max. 5 mg 3 times daily); nocturnal enuresis (preferably over 7 years, see notes below), 2.5–3 mg twice daily increased to 5 mg 2–3 times daily (last dose before bedtime)

PoM **Oxybutynin Hydrochloride** (Nonproprietary)

Tablets, oxybutynin hydrochloride 2.5 mg, net price 56-tab pack = £6.87, 84-tab pack = £10.80; 5 mg, 84-tab pack = £20.86. Label: 3

Available from APS, Berk (*Contimin*®), Dominion, Generics, Pharmacia & Upjohn

PoM **Cystrin**® (Pharmacia & Upjohn)

Tablets, oxybutynin hydrochloride 3 mg, net price 56-tab pack = £9.15; 5 mg (scored), 84-tab pack = £22.88. Label: 3

PoM **Ditropan**® (Lorex)

Tablets, both blue, scored, oxybutynin hydrochloride 2.5 mg, net price 21-tab pack = £2.93, 84-tab pack = £10.80; 5 mg, 21-tab pack = £5.72, 84-tab pack = £21.05. Label: 3

Elixir, oxybutynin hydrochloride 2.5 mg/5 mL. Net price 150-mL pack = £4.78. Label: 3.

PROPANTHELINE BROMIDE

Indications: adult enuresis, see notes above

Cautions; Contra-indications: see under Oxybutynin Hydrochloride

Side-effects: antimuscarinic side-effects (see Atropine Sulphate, section 1.2); see also notes above

Dose: 15–30 mg 2–3 times daily one hour before meals

Preparations
See section 1.2

NOCTURNAL ENURESIS

Nocturnal enuresis is a normal occurrence in young children but persists in as many as 5% by 10 years of age. In the absence of urinary-tract infection simple measures such as *bladder training* or the use of an *alarm system* may be successful. Drug therapy is not appropriate for children under 7 years of age and should be reserved for when alternative measures have failed preferably on a short-term basis to cover periods away from home. The possible side-effects and the **toxicity** of these drugs if taken in **overdose** should be borne in mind when they are prescribed.

Desmopressin (see section 6.5.2), an analogue of vasopressin, is used for nocturnal enuresis; particular care is needed to avoid fluid overload and treatment should not be continued for longer than 3 months without stopping for a week for full reassessment.

Tricyclics (see section 4.3.1) such as **amitriptyline**, **imipramine**, and less often **nortriptyline** are also used but behaviour disturbances may occur and relapse is common after withdrawal. Treatment should not normally exceed 3 months unless a full physical examination (including ECG) is given and the child is fully re-assessed.

7.4.3   Drugs used in urological pain

The acute pain of *ureteric colic* may be relieved with **pethidine** (section 4.7.2). **Diclofenac** by injection or as suppositories (section 10.1.1) is also effective and compares favourably with pethidine; other non-steroidal anti-inflammatory drugs are occasionally given by injection.

Lignocaine gel is a useful topical application in *urethral pain* or to relieve the discomfort of catheterisation (see section 15.2).

ALKALINISATION OF URINE

Alkalinisation of urine may be undertaken with **potassium citrate**. The alkalinising action may relieve the discomfort of *cystitis* caused by lower urinary tract infections. **Sodium bicarbonate** is used as a urinary alkalinising agent in some metabolic and renal disorders (see section 9.2.1.3).

POTASSIUM CITRATE

Indications: relief of discomfort in mild urinary-tract infections; alkalinisation of urine

Cautions: renal impairment, cardiac disease; elderly; **interactions:** Appendix 1 (potassium salts)

Side-effects: hyperkalaemia on prolonged high dosage, mild diuresis

Potassium Citrate Mixture (BP)

(Potassium Citrate Oral Solution)

Oral solution, potassium citrate 30%, citric acid monohydrate 5% in a suitable vehicle with a lemon flavour. Extemporaneous preparations should be recently prepared according to the following formula: potassium citrate 3 g, citric acid monohydrate 500 mg, syrup 2.5 mL, quillaia tincture 0.1 mL, lemon spirit 0.05 mL, double-strength chloroform water 3 mL, water to 10 mL. Contains about 28 mmol K^+/10 mL. Label: 27

Dose: 10 mL 3 times daily well diluted with water

Note. Concentrates for preparation of Potassium Citrate Mixture BP are available from Hillcross

Proprietary brands of potassium citrate on sale to the public for the relief of discomfort in mild urinary-tract infections include Cystopurin® (Roche Consumer Health) and Effercitrate® (Typharm)

SODIUM BICARBONATE

Indications: relief of discomfort in mild urinary-tract infections; alkalinisation of urine

Cautions; Side-effects: see section 1.1.2; also caution in elderly

Dose: 3 g in water every 2 hours until urinary pH exceeds 7; maintenance of alkaline urine 5–10 g daily

Preparations See section 9.2.1.3

SODIUM CITRATE

Indications: relief of discomfort in mild urinary-tract infections

Cautions: renal impairment, cardiac disease, pregnancy, patients on a sodium-restricted diet; elderly

Side-effects: mild diuresis

Note. Proprietary brands of Sodium Citrate on sale to the public for the relief of discomfort in mild urinary-tract infections include *Boots Cystitis Relief Sachets and Tablets,* Cymalon® (Seton), Cystemme® (Abbott), and Cystoleve® (Seton)

ACIDIFICATION OF URINE

Acidification of urine has been undertaken with **ascorbic acid** but it is not always reliable. Large doses may cause gastro-intestinal disturbances including diarrhoea; renal stones have also been reported in patients with hyperoxaluria.

For pH-modifying solutions for the maintenance of indwelling urinary catheters, see section 7.4.4.

ASCORBIC ACID

Indications: acidification of urine but see notes above

Dose: by mouth, 4 g daily in divided doses

Preparations
See section 9.6.3

OTHER PREPARATIONS FOR URINARY DISORDERS

A terpene mixture (Rowatinex®) is claimed to be of benefit in *urolithiasis* for the expulsion of calculi.

PoM **Rowatinex®** (Rowa)

Capsules, yellow, e/c, anethol 4 mg, borneol 10 mg, camphene 15 mg, cineole 3 mg, fenchone 4 mg, pinene 31 mg. Net price 50 = £7.35. Label: 25

Dose: 1–2 capsules 3–4 times daily before food; CHILD not recommended

7.4.4 Bladder instillations and urological surgery

INFECTED BLADDERS. Various solutions are available as irrigations or washouts.

Aqueous **chlorhexidine** (section 13.11.2) may be used in the management of common infections of the bladder but it is ineffective against most *Pseudomonas* spp. Solutions containing 1 in 5000 (0.02%) are used but they may irritate the mucosa and cause burning and haematuria (in which case they should be discontinued); sterile **sodium chloride solution 0.9%** (physiological saline) is usually adequate and is preferred as a mechanical irrigant.

Bladder irrigations of **amphotericin** 100 micrograms/mL (section 5.2) may be of value in mycotic infections.

DISSOLUTION OF BLOOD CLOTS. Clot retention is usually treated by irrigation with sterile **sodium chloride solution 0.9%** but sterile **sodium citrate solution for bladder irrigation 3%** may also be helpful. **Streptokinase-streptodornase** (Varidase Topical®, section 13.11.7) is an alternative.

LOCALLY ACTING CYTOTOXIC DRUGS. Bladder instillations of **doxorubicin** (section 8.1.2), **mitomycin** (section 8.1.2), and **thiotepa** (section 8.1.1) are used for recurrent superficial bladder tumours. Such instillations reduce systemic side-effects; adverse effects on the bladder (e.g. micturition disorders and reduction in bladder capacity) may occur.

Instillation of **epirubicin** (section 8.1.2) is used for treatment and prophylaxis of certain forms of superficial bladder cancer; instillation of **doxorubicin** (section 8.1.2) is also used for some papillary tumours.

INTERSTITIAL CYSTITIS. **Dimethyl sulphoxide** (dimethyl sulfoxide) may be used for symptomatic relief in patients with interstitial cystitis (Hunner's ulcer). 50 mL of a 50% solution (Rimso-50®) is instilled into the bladder, retained for 15 minutes, and voided by the patient. Treatment is repeated at intervals of 2 weeks. Bladder spasm and hypersensitivity reactions may occur and long-term use requires ophthalmic, renal, and hepatic assessment at intervals of 6 months.

DIMETHYL SULPHOXIDE

(Dimethyl Sulfoxide)
Indications: bladder washouts, see notes above

PoM **Rimso-50®** (Britannia)
Bladder instillation, sterile, dimethyl sulphoxide 50%, in aqueous solution. Net price 50 mL = £19.31

SODIUM CITRATE

Indications: bladder washouts, see notes above

Sterile Sodium Citrate Solution for Bladder Irrigation, sodium citrate 3%, dilute hydrochloric acid 0.2%, in purified water, freshly boiled and cooled, and sterilised

UROLOGICAL SURGERY

Endoscopic surgery within the urinary tract requires an isotonic irrigant since there is a high risk of fluid absorption; if this occurs in excess, hypervolaemia, haemolysis, and renal failure may result. **Glycine irrigation solution 1.5%** is the irrigant of choice for transurethral resection of the prostate gland and bladder tumours; **sterile sodium chloride solution 0.9%** (physiological saline) is used for percutaneous renal surgery.

GLYCINE

Indications: bladder irrigation during urological surgery; see notes above
Cautions; Side-effects: see notes above

Glycine Irrigation Solution (Non-proprietary)
Irrigation solution, glycine 1.5% in water for injections
Available from Baxter, Kendall

MAINTENANCE OF INDWELLING URINARY CATHETERS

The deposition which occurs in catheterised patients is usually chiefly composed of phosphate and to minimise this the catheter (if latex) should be changed at least as often as every 6 weeks. If the catheter is to be left for longer periods a silicone catheter should be used together with the appropriate use of catheter maintenance solutions. Repeated blockage usually indicates that the catheter needs to be changed.

CATHETER PATENCY SOLUTIONS

Chlorhexidine 0.02%. Available from Braun (Uro-Tainer Chlorhexidine®, 100-mL sachet = £2.41), Seton (Uriflex C®, 100-mL sachet = £2.13)
Mandelic acid 1% Available from Braun (Uro-Tainer Mandelic Acid®, 100-mL sachet = £2.41)
Sodium chloride 0.9%. Available from Braun (Uro-Tainer Sodium Chloride®, 100-mL sachet = £2.29, Uro-Tainer M®, with integral drug additive

---

Cautionary label wordings, see inside back cover

Prices are **net**, see p.1

port, 50- and 100-mL sachets = £2.71), Seton (Uriflex S®, 100-mL sachet = £2.00, Uriflex SP® with integral drug additive port, 100-mL sachet = £2.06)

Solution G, citric acid 3.23%, magnesium oxide 0.38%, sodium bicarbonate 0.7%, disodium edetate 0.01%. Available from Braun (Uro-Tainer Suby G®, 100-mL sachet = £2.41), Seton (Uriflex G®, 100-mL sachet = £2.13)

Solution R, citric acid 6%, gluconolactone 0.6%, magnesium carbonate 2.8%, disodium edetate 0.01%. Available from Braun (Uro-Tainer Solution R®, 100-mL sachet = £2.41), Seton (Uriflex R®, 100-mL sachet = £2.13)

7.4.5   Drugs for impotence

Reasons for failure to produce a satisfactory erection include *psychogenic, vascular, neurogenic,* and *endocrine abnormalities*; *many drugs* are also liable to induce impotence. Intracavernosal injection of vasoactive drugs under careful medical supervision is used for both diagnostic and therapeutic purposes.

ALPROSTADIL

Alprostadil (prostaglandin E_1) is given by intracavernosal injection or intraurethral application for the management of erectile dysfunction (after exclusion of treatable medical causes); it is also used as a diagnostic test.

ALPROSTADIL

Indications: erectile dysfunction (including aid to diagnosis); neonatal congenital heart defects (section 7.1.1.1)

Cautions: priapism—patients should be instructed to report any erection lasting 4 hours or longer—for recommendations, see below; anatomical deformations of penis (painful erection more likely)—follow up regularly to detect signs of penile fibrosis (consider discontinuation if angulation, cavernosal fibrosis or Peyronie's disease develop)

Contra-indications: predisposition to prolonged erection (as in sickle cell anaemia, multiple myeloma or leukaemia); not for use with other agents for erectile dysfunction, in patients with penile implants or when sexual activity medically inadvisable; urethral application also contra-indicated in urethral stricture, severe hypospadia, severe curvature, balanitis, urethritis

Side-effects: penile pain, priaprism (see below and under Cautions); reactions at injection site include haematoma, haemosiderin deposits, ecchymosis, penile rash, penile oedema, penile fibrosis, haemorrhage, inflammation, swelling; other local reactions include balanitis, urethral burning, urethral bleeding, penile warmth, numbness, penile infection, irritation, sensitivity, phimosis, pruritus, erythema, venous leak, abnormal ejaculation; systemic effects reported include testicular pain and swelling, scrotal disorders, changes in micturition (including haematuria),

nausea, dry mouth, hypotension (very rarely circulatory collapse) or hypertension, fainting, rapid pulse, vasodilatation, chest pain, supraventricular extrasystole, peripheral vascular disorder, dizziness, weakness, localised pain (buttocks, legs, genital, perineal, abdominal), headache, pelvic pain, back pain, influenza-like syndrome, swelling of the leg veins

PRIAPISM. If priapism should occur treatment should not be delayed more than 6 hours and is as follows:

Initial therapy by penile aspiration—using aseptic technique a 19–21 gauge butterfly needle inserted into the corpus cavernosum and 20–50 mL of blood aspirated; if necessary the procedure may be repeated on the opposite side.

If aspiration unsuccessful, *cautious* intracavernosal injection of a sympathomimetic with action on alpha-adrenergic receptors, continuously monitoring blood pressure and pulse (*extreme caution:* coronary heart disease, hypertension, cerebral ischaemia or if taking antidepressant) as follows:

—intracavernosal injections of phenylephrine 100–200 micrograms (0.5–1 mL of a 200 microgram/mL solution) every 5–10 minutes; max. total dose 1 mg [unlicensed indication][*important:* if suitable strength of phenylephrine injection not available may be specially prepared by diluting 0.1 mL of the phenylephrine 1% (10 mg/mL) injection to 5 mL with sodium chloride 0.9%];
alternatively

—intracavernosal injections of adrenaline 10–20 micrograms (0.5–1mL of a 20 microgram/mL solution) every 5–10 minutes; max. total dose 100 micrograms [*important:* if suitable strength of adrenaline not available may be specially prepared by diluting 0.1 mL of the adrenaline 1 in 1000 (1mg/mL) injection to 5 mL with sodium chloride 0.9%];
alternatively

—intracavernosal injection of metaraminol (*caution: has been associated with fatal hypertensive crises*) [see notes below for a suggested dilution and dose];

If necessary the sympathomimetic injections can be followed by further aspiration of blood through the same butterfly needle.

If sympathomimetics unsuccessful, urgent surgical referral for management (possibly including shunt procedure).

Dose: see under preparations below

Intracavernosal injection

PoM **Caverject®** (Pharmacia & Upjohn)

Injection, powder for reconstitution, alprostadil, net price 5-microgram vial = £6.74; 10-microgram vial = £7.70; 20-microgram vial = £9.95 (all with diluent-filled syringe, needles and swabs)

Dose: by direct intracavernosal injection, erectile dysfunction, first dose 2.5 micrograms, second dose 5 micrograms (if some response to first dose) *or* 7.5 micrograms (if no response to first dose), increasing in steps of 5–10 micrograms to obtain dose suitable for producing erection not lasting more than 1 hour (neurological dysfunction, first dose 1.25 micrograms, second dose 2.5 micrograms, third dose 5 micrograms, increasing in steps of 5 micrograms to obtain suitable dose); if no response to dose then next higher dose can be given within 1 hour, if there is a response the next dose should not be given for at least 24 hours; usual range 5–20 micrograms; max. 60 micrograms (max. frequency of

---

injection not more than once daily and not more than 3 times in any 1 week)

Note. The first dose must be given by medically trained personnel; self-administration may only be undertaken after proper training

Aid to diagnosis, 20 micrograms as a single dose (where evidence of neurological dysfunction, initially 5 micrograms and max. 10 micrograms)—consult product literature for details

PoM **Viridal®** (Schwarz)

Injection, powder for reconstitution, alprostadil. Net price 5-microgram vial = £6.74; 10-microgram vial = £7.70; 20-microgram vial = £9.95 (all with diluent-filled syringe)

Viridal® Starter Pack (hosp. only), contents as for *Continuation Pack* below plus *Duoject* applicator, 10-microgram starter pack = £22.67, 20-microgram starter pack = £27.63; *Viridal® Continuation Pack,* 2 double-chamber cartridges (containing alprostadil and diluent), 2 needles, swabs, 10-microgram continuation pack = £16.94, 20-microgram continuation pack = £21.90; *Duoject®* applicator available free of charge from Schwarz

Dose: by direct intracavernosal injection, erectile dysfunction, initially 5 micrograms (2.5 micrograms in primary psychogenic or neurogenic erectile dysfunction) increasing in steps of 2.5–5 micrograms to obtain dose suitable for producing erection not lasting more than 1 hour; usual range 10–20 micrograms; max. 40 micrograms (max. frequency of injection not more than once in any 1 day and not more than 2–3 times in any 1 week); erection lasting longer than 2 hours but less than 4 hours—retitrate dose

Note. The first dose must be given by medically trained personnel; self-administration may only be undertaken after proper training

Urethral application

COUNSELLING. If partner pregnant barrier contraception should be used

▼ PoM **MUSE®** (Astra)

Urethral application, alprostadil, net price 125-microgram single-use applicator = £9.14, 250-microgram single-use applicator = £9.95, 500-microgram single-use applicator = £9.95, 1-mg single-use applicator = £10.18

Condoms: no evidence of harm to latex condoms and diaphragms

Dose: by direct urethral application, erectile dysfunction, initially 250 micrograms increased or decreased in steps according to response (max. frequency of application not more than twice in 24 hours)

Note. The first dose must be given by medically trained personnel; self-administration may only be undertaken after proper training

Aid to diagnosis, 500 micrograms as a single dose

PAPAVERINE and PHENTOLAMINE

Although not licensed the smooth muscle relaxant **papaverine** is also given by intracavernosal injection for impotence. The usual dose of papaverine by intracavernosal injection is 7.5 mg initially increased according to response to a range of 30–60 mg. Patients with neurological or psychogenic impotence are more sensitive to the effect of papaverine than those with vascular abnormalities. **Phentolamine** (0.25–1.25 mg) is added if the response is inadequate [unlicensed indication].

Persistence of the erection for longer than 4 hours is an emergency requiring aspiration of the corpora; if aspiration fails, 1 mg of metaraminol [0.1 mL of 10 mg/mL metaraminol injection] can be diluted to 5 mL with sodium chloride injection 0.9% and given by careful slow injection into the corpora [unlicensed indication] [*caution:* has been associated with fatal hypertensive crisis—consider also advice under Alprostadil, above].

Other side-effects include vasovagal attacks and syncope; caution is needed in patients with cardiovascular disease and ischaemic attacks; predisposition to prolonged erection is a contra-indication.

Local side-effects include haematoma and burning pain at the site of injection and fibrotic changes in the corpora cavernosa (which may lead to Peyronie-like erectile distortion).

PAPAVERINE

Indications; Cautions; Side-effects: see notes above

Note. Papaverine is available as a 'special order' [unlicensed] product, contact BCM Specials, Martindale, or regional hospital manufacturing unit

---

PHENTOLAMINE

Indications; Cautions; Side-effects: see notes above; phaeochromocytoma, see section 2.5.4

Note. Phentolamine is not licensed for use in erectile dysfunction

---

THYMOXAMINE

Thymoxamine (moxisylyte) is a selective alpha-blocker used for erectile dysfunction; it is given by intracavernosal injection.

THYMOXAMINE HYDROCHLORIDE

(Moxisylyte Hydrochloride)

Indications: erectile dysfunction; primary Raynaud's syndrome (section 2.6.4.1)

Cautions: instruct patients to report any erection lasting 3 hours or longer—for treatment of prolonged erection see under Alprostadil; patients should remain lying down for up to 30 minutes after injection due to risk of transient hypotension; anatomical deformations of penis such as angulation, cavernosal fibrosis or Peyronie's disease (painful erection more likely); follow up after first 10 injections and regularly thereafter to assess dose requirements and adverse effects

Contra-indications: predisposition to prolonged erection (as in sickle cell anaemia, multiple myeloma or leukaemia); systolic blood pressure less than 100 mmHg; history of unstable angina, myocardial infarction or stroke within previous 3 months; not for use with other agents for erectile dysfunction or in patients with penile implants

Side-effects: penile pain, prolonged erection (see Cautions); haematoma at injection site; systemic effects reported include tiredness, nausea, dizziness (associated with transient hypotension

---

drowsiness, headache, flushing, dry mouth, sinus congestion and rhinorrhoea

Dose: *by direct intracavernosal injection,* initially 10 mg increasing according to response to max. 20 mg (max. frequency of injection not more than once daily and not more than 3 times in any 1 week with an interval of at least 48 hours between doses)

Note. The first dose must be given by medically trained personnel; self-administration may only be undertaken after proper training

▼ PoM **Erecnos®** (Fournier)

Injection, powder for reconstitution, thymoxamine hydrochloride, net price (both with diluent in double-chamber, pre-filled syringe) 10 mg/mL when reconstituted, 1-mL (10-mg) syringe = £7.70, 20 mg/mL when reconstituted, 1-mL (20-mg) syringe = £9.95

7.5   Appliances for urinary disorders

For details of **appliances for urinary disorders**, see Appendix 8.

8: Drugs used in the treatment of
MALIGNANT DISEASE and for IMMUNOSUPPRESSION

In this chapter, drug treatment is discussed under the following headings:

8.1   Cytotoxic drugs
8.2   Drugs affecting the immune response
8.3   Sex hormones and hormone antagonists in malignant disease

Malignant disease may be treated by surgery, radiotherapy, and chemotherapy. Certain tumours are highly sensitive to chemotherapy but many are not, and inappropriate drug administration in these circumstances can only increase morbidity or mortality.

8.1   Cytotoxic drugs

8.1.1   Alkylating drugs
8.1.2   Cytotoxic antibiotics
8.1.3   Antimetabolites
8.1.4   Vinca alkaloids and etoposide
8.1.5   Other antineoplastic drugs

The chemotherapy of cancer is complex and should be confined to specialists in oncology. Cytotoxic drugs have both anti-cancer activity and the potential for damage to normal tissue. Chemotherapy may be given with a curative intent or it may aim to prolong life or to palliate symptoms. In an increasing number of cases chemotherapy may be combined with radiotherapy or surgery or both as either neoadjuvant treatment (initial chemotherapy aimed at shrinking the primary tumour, thereby rendering local therapy less destructive or more effective) or as adjuvant treatment (which follows definitive treatment of the primary disease, when the risk of sub-clinical metastatic disease is known to be high). All chemotherapy drugs cause side-effects and a balance has to be struck between likely benefit and acceptable toxicity.

> **CRM guidelines on cytotoxic drug handling:**
>
> 1. Trained personnel should reconstitute cytotoxics;
>
> 2. Reconstitution should be carried out in designated areas;
>
> 3. Protective clothing (including gloves) should be worn;
>
> 4. The eyes should be protected and means of first aid should be specified;
>
> 5. Pregnant staff should not handle cytotoxics;
>
> 6. Adequate care should be taken in the disposal of waste material, including syringes, containers, and absorbent material.

Cytotoxic drugs may be used either singly, or in combination. In the latter case, the initial letters of the approved or proprietary names of the drugs, identify the regimen used. Drug combinations are frequently more toxic than single drugs but may have the advantage in certain tumours of enhanced response and increased survival. However for some tumours, single-agent chemotherapy remains the treatment of choice.

> Most cytotoxic drugs are teratogenic, and all may cause life-threatening toxicity; administration should, where possible, be confined to those experienced in their use.
>
> Because of the complexity of dosage regimens in the treatment of malignant disease, dose statements have been omitted from some of the drug entries in this chapter. *In all cases detailed specialist literature should be consulted.*
>
> Prescriptions should **not** be repeated except on the instructions of a specialist.

Cytotoxic drugs fall naturally into a number of classes, each with characteristic antitumour activity, sites of action, and toxicity. A knowledge of sites of metabolism and excretion is important because impaired drug handling as a result of disease is not uncommon and may result in enhanced toxic effects. A number of side-effects are characteristic of particular agents or groups of drugs, e.g. neurotoxicity of vinca alkaloids, and details will be provided in the appropriate sections. Most toxic effects are, however, common to many of these drugs and will be briefly outlined here.

EXTRAVASATION OF INTRAVENOUS DRUGS. A number of drugs will cause severe local tissue necrosis if leakage into the extravascular compartment occurs. Recommended modes of administration must be adhered to. Infusion of vesicant drugs should be stopped immediately if local pain is experienced. Where doubt exists as to whether significant leakage has occurred, the infusion should be discontinued and the cannula resited in another vein. There are no proven antidotes for extravasation, but general recommendations include elevation of the limb and application of ice packs three or four times daily until pain and swelling settle; if ulceration occurs plastic surgery may be required.

HYPERURICAEMIA. Hyperuricaemia, which can result in uric acid crystal formation in the urinary tract with associated renal dysfunction is a complication of the treatment of non-Hodgkin's lymphoma and leukaemia. Allopurinol (see section 10.1.4) should be started 24 hours before treating such tumours, and should be continued for 7 to 10 days (it is not required again unless further therapy is given for tumour relapse); patients should be adequately hydrated. The dose of mercaptopurine or azathioprine should be reduced if allopurinol needs to be given concomitantly (see Appendix 1).

NAUSEA AND VOMITING. Nausea and vomiting cause considerable distress to many patients who receive chemotherapy, and to a lesser extent abdominal radiotherapy, and may lead to refusal of further treatment. They may be acute (occurring within 24 hours of treatment), delayed (first occurring more than 24 hours after treatment) or anticipatory (occurring prior to subsequent doses). Delayed and anticipatory symptoms are more difficult to control than acute symptoms and require different management.

Patients vary in their susceptibility to drug-induced nausea and vomiting; those affected more often include women, patients under 50 years of age, anxious patients, and those who experience motion sickness. Susceptibility also increases with repeated exposure to the drug.

Drugs may be divided according to their emetogenic potential and some examples are given below, but the symptoms vary according to the dose, to other drugs administered and to individual susceptibility.

Mildly emetogenic treatment—fluorouracil, etoposide, methotrexate (less than $0.1\,g/m^2$), the vinca alkaloids, and abdominal radiotherapy.

Moderately emetogenic treatment—doxorubicin, intermediate and low doses of cyclophosphamide, mitozantrone, and high doses of methotrexate (0.1 to $1.2\,g/m^2$).

Highly emetogenic treatment—cisplatin, dacarbazine, and high doses of cyclophosphamide.

Prevention of acute symptoms. For patients at a low risk of emesis, pretreatment with oral phenothiazines (e.g. prochlorperazine) or with domperidone, continued for up to 24 hours after chemotherapy, is often effective (section 4.6). For patients at a higher risk dexamethasone (6 to 10 mg by mouth) and lorazepam (1 to 2 mg by mouth) may be added prior to chemotherapy.

For patients at a high risk of emesis or when other therapies are ineffective, a specific ($5HT_3$) serotonin antagonist (section 4.6) is used, often with dexamethasone (section 4.6). The $5HT_3$ antagonists are highly effective in controlling early emesis and have largely replaced the use of high-dose intravenous metoclopramide (section 4.6).

Prevention of delayed symptoms. Dexamethasone is the drug of choice for the prevention of delayed symptoms; it is used alone or with metoclopramide or prochlorperazine. The $5HT_3$ antagonists may be less effective for delayed symptoms.

Prevention of anticipatory symptoms. Good symptom control is the best way to prevent anticipatory symptoms. The addition of lorazepam to antiemetic therapy is helpful because of its amnesic, sedative and anxiolytic effects.

BONE-MARROW SUPPRESSION. All cytotoxic drugs except vincristine and bleomycin cause marrow depression. This commonly occurs 7 to 10 days after administration, but is delayed for certain drugs, such as carmustine, lomustine, and melphalan. Peripheral blood counts must be checked prior to each treatment, and doses should be reduced or therapy delayed if marrow recovery has not occurred. Fever occurring in a neutropenic patient (neutrophil count less than 0.8×10^9/litre) is an indication for immediate parenteral broad-spectrum antibiotic therapy (see section 5.1, table 1), once appropriate bacteriological investigations have taken place.

It is now possible, in selected patients, to lessen both the duration and the depth of neutropenia by the use of parenterally administered bone marrow growth factors known as colony stimulating factors (section 9.1.6) or (in patients with ovarian carcinoma receiving cisplatin and cyclophosphamide) by the use of amifostine (section 9.1.6); these tend to be used on an individual basis.

IMPAIRED IMMUNE RESPONSIVENESS. Modification of tissue reactions caused by corticosteroids and other immunosuppressive drugs may result in the rapid *spread of infection*. Suppression of clinical signs may allow diseases such as septicaemia or tuberculosis to reach an advanced stage before being recognised—**important:** for advice relating to measles and chickenpox (varicella) exposure, see p. 531 (measles) and p. 532 (varicella).

ALOPECIA. Reversible hair loss is a common complication, although it varies in degree between drugs and individual patients. No pharmacological methods of preventing this are available.

REPRODUCTIVE FUNCTION. Most cytotoxic drugs are teratogenic and should not be administered during pregnancy, especially during the first trimester (but for transplant therapy, see below).

Contraceptive advice should be offered where appropriate before cytotoxic therapy begins (and should cover the duration of contraception required after therapy has ended). Regimens that do not contain an alkylating drug may have less effect on fertility, but those with an alkylating drug carry the risk of causing permanent male sterility (there is no effect on potency). Pre-treatment counselling and consideration of sperm storage may be appropriate. Females are less severely affected, though the span of reproductive life may be shortened by the onset of a premature menopause. No increase in fetal abnormalities or abortion-rate has been recorded in patients who remain fertile after cytotoxic chemotherapy.

Transplant therapy. Female transplanted patients immunosuppressed with azathioprine should not discontinue it on becoming pregnant; there is no evidence that azathioprine used properly is teratogenic. There is some experience of cyclosporin in pregnancy but it does not appear to be any more harmful than azathioprine. Any risk to the offspring of azathioprine-treated men is small. Tacrolimus and mycophenolate mofetil have been introduced recently and are contra-indicated by the manufacturers in pregnancy.

8.1.1 Alkylating drugs

Extensive experience is available with these drugs, which are among the most widely used in cancer chemotherapy. They act by damaging DNA, thus interfering with cell replication. In addition to the side-effects common to many cytotoxic drugs (section 8.1), there are two problems associated with prolonged usage. Firstly, gametogenesis is often severely affected (see above). Secondly, prolonged use of these drugs, particularly when combined with extensive irradiation, is associated with a marked increase in the incidence of acute non-lymphocytic leukaemia.

Cyclophosphamide is widely used in the treatment of chronic lymphocytic leukaemia, the lymphomas, and solid tumours. It is given by mouth or intravenously and is inactive until metabolised by the liver. A urinary metabolite of cyclophosphamide, acrolein, may cause haemorrhagic cystitis; this is a rare but very serious complication; if it occurs cyclophosphamide is not normally used again. An increased fluid intake, for 24–48 hours after intravenous injection, will help avoid this complication. When high-dose therapy (e.g. more than 2 g intravenously) is used or when the patient is considered to be at high risk of cystitis (e.g. previous pelvic irradiation) mesna (given initially intravenously then by mouth) will also help prevent this.

Ifosfamide is related to cyclophosphamide and is given intravenously; mesna is routinely given with it to reduce urothelial toxicity.

Chlorambucil is commonly used to treat chronic lymphocytic leukaemia, the indolent non-Hodgkin's lymphomas, Hodgkin's disease, and ovarian cancer. It is given by mouth. Side-effects, apart from marrow suppression, are uncommon. However occasional patients develop severe widespread rashes which can progress to Stevens-Johnson syndrome or to toxic epidermal necrolysis. If a rash occurs further chlorambucil is contra-indicated and cyclophosphamide is substituted.

Melphalan is used to treat myeloma and occasionally solid tumours and lymphomas. It is usually given by mouth, but may also be given intravenously. Because bone marrow toxicity is delayed the drug is usually given at intervals of 4–6 weeks.

Busulphan (busulfan) is used almost exclusively to treat chronic myeloid leukaemia and is given by mouth. Frequent blood counts are necessary because excessive myelosuppression may result in irreversible bone-marrow aplasia. Hyperpigmentation of the skin is a common side-effect and, rarely, progressive pulmonary fibrosis may occur.

Lomustine is a lipid-soluble nitrosourea and is given by mouth. It is mainly used to treat Hodgkin's disease and certain solid tumours. Bone marrow toxicity is delayed, and the drug is therefore given at intervals of 4 to 6 weeks. Permanent bone marrow damage may occur with prolonged use. Nausea and vomiting are common and moderately severe.

Carmustine is given intravenously. It has similar activity and toxicity to lomustine and is most commonly given to patients with myeloma, lymphoma, and brain tumours. Cumulative renal damage and delayed pulmonary fibrosis may occur.

Mustine (chlormethine) is now much less commonly used. It is a very toxic drug which causes severe vomiting. The freshly prepared injection must be given into a fast-running intravenous infusion. Local extravasation causes severe tissue necrosis.

Estramustine is a combination of an oestrogen and mustine used predominantly in prostate cancer. It is given by mouth and has both an antimitotic effect and (by reducing testosterone concentration) a hormonal effect.

Treosulfan is given by mouth or intravenously and is used to treat ovarian cancer.

Thiotepa is usually used as an intracavitary drug for the treatment of malignant effusions or bladder cancer (section 7.4.4). It is also occasionally used to treat breast cancer, but requires parenteral administration.

Mitobronitol is occasionally used to treat chronic myeloid leukaemia; it is available on a named-patient basis only (as *Myelobromol®*, Sinclair).

BUSULPHAN

(Busulfan)

Indications: chronic myeloid leukaemia

Cautions; Side-effects: see section 8.1 and notes above; avoid in porphyria (see section 9.8.2)

Dose: induction of remission, 60 micrograms/kg to max. 4 mg daily; maintenance, 0.5–2 mg daily

PoM **Myleran®** (GlaxoWellcome)

Tablets, busulphan 500 micrograms, net price 25 = £3.53; 2 mg, 25 = £5.32

CARMUSTINE

Indications: see notes above

Cautions; Side-effects: see section 8.1 and notes above; irritant to tissues

PoM **BiCNU®** (Bristol-Myers)

Injection, powder for reconstitution, carmustine. Net price 100-mg vial (with diluent) = £12.50

CHLORAMBUCIL

Indications: see notes above (for use as an immunosuppressant see section 8.2.1)

Cautions; Side-effects: see section 8.1 and notes above; caution in renal impairment; avoid in porphyria (see section 9.8.2)

Dose: used alone, usually 100–200 micrograms/kg daily for 4–8 weeks

PoM **Leukeran®** (GlaxoWellcome)

Tablets, both yellow, chlorambucil 2 mg, net price 25 = £8.55; 5 mg, 25 = £13.04

CYCLOPHOSPHAMIDE

Indications: see notes above
Cautions; Side-effects: see section 8.1 and notes above; reduce dose in renal impairment; avoid in porphyria (see section 9.8.2); **interactions:** Appendix 1 (cyclophosphamide)

PoM **Cyclophosphamide** (Pharmacia & Upjohn)
Tablets, pink, s/c, cyclophosphamide (anhydrous) 50 mg. Net price 20 = £2.10. Label: 27
Injection, powder for reconstitution, cyclophosphamide. Net price 200-mg vial = £1.65; 500-mg vial = £2.88; 1-g vial = £5.04

PoM **Endoxana®** (ASTA Medica)
Tablets, s/c, cyclophosphamide 50 mg, net price 100-tab pack = £10.50 Label: 27
Injection, powder for reconstitution, cyclophosphamide. Net price 200-mg vial = £1.61; 500-mg vial = £2.81; 1-g vial = £4.90

ESTRAMUSTINE PHOSPHATE

Indications: prostate cancer
Cautions: see section 8.1
Contra-indications: peptic ulceration, severe liver or cardiac disease
Side-effects: see section 8.1; also gynaecomastia, altered liver function, cardiovascular disorders (angina and rare reports of myocardial infarction)
Dose: 0.14–1.4 g daily in divided doses (usual initial dose 560 mg daily)
COUNSELLING. Each dose should be taken not less than 1 hour before or 2 hours after meals and should not be taken with dairy products

PoM **Estracyt®** (Pharmacia & Upjohn)
Capsules, estramustine phosphate 140 mg (as disodium salt). Net price 100-cap pack = £149.46. Label: 23 counselling, see above

IFOSFAMIDE

Indications: see notes above
Cautions; Side-effects: see section 8.1 and notes under Cyclophosphamide; reduce dose in renal impairment; **interactions:** Appendix 1 (cyclophosphamide and ifosfamide)

PoM **Mitoxana®** (ASTA Medica)
Injection, powder for reconstitution, ifosfamide. Net price 1-g vial = £21.27; 2-g vial = £39.36 (hosp. only)

LOMUSTINE

Indications: see notes above
Cautions; Side-effects: see section 8.1 and notes above
Dose: used alone, 120–130 mg/m² body-surface every 6–8 weeks

PoM **CCNU®** (Medac)
Capsules, blue/clear, lomustine 40 mg. Net price 20-cap pack = £112.20

MELPHALAN

Indications: myelomatosis; see also notes above
Cautions; Side-effects: see section 8.1 and notes above; reduce dose in renal impairment; **interactions:** Appendix 1 (melphalan)
*Dose: by mouth,*150–300 micrograms/kg daily for 4–6 days, repeated after 4–8 weeks

PoM **Alkeran®** (GlaxoWellcome)
Tablets, melphalan 2 mg, net price 25 = £11.73; 5 mg, 25 = £20.75
Injection, powder for reconstitution, melphalan 50 mg (as hydrochloride). Net price 50-mg vial (with solvent-diluent) = £28.26

MUSTINE HYDROCHLORIDE
(Chlormethine Hydrochloride)
Indications: Hodgkin's disease—see notes above
Cautions; Side-effects: see section 8.1 and notes above; irritant to tissues (also caution in handling—vesicant and a nasal irritant)

PoM **Mustine Hydrochloride** (Knoll)
Injection, powder for reconstitution, mustine hydrochloride. Net price 10-mg vial = £15.00

THIOTEPA
Indications: see notes above and section 7.4.4
Cautions; Side-effects: see section 8.1; **interactions:** Appendix 1 (thiotepa)

PoM **Thiotepa** (Lederle)
Injection, powder for reconstitution, thiotepa, net price 15-mg vial = £4.73

TREOSULFAN
Indications: see notes above
Cautions; Side-effects: see section 8.1
Dose: by mouth, courses of 1–2 g daily in 4 divided doses to provide total dose of 21–28 g over initial 8 weeks

PoM **Treosulfan** (Medac)
Capsules, treosulfan 250 mg. Net price 20 = £28.48. Label: 25
Also Available from Farillon
Injection, powder for reconstitution, treosulfan. Net price 1 g = £15.20; 5 g = £59.60 (both in infusion bottle with transfer needle)
Also available from Farillon

UROTHELIAL TOXICITY

Urothelial toxicity, commonly manifest by haemorrhagic cystitis, is a problem peculiar to the use of cyclophosphamide or ifosfamide and is caused by a metabolite (acrolein). **Mesna** reacts specifically with this metabolite in the urinary tract, preventing toxicity. Mesna is used routinely (preferably by mouth) in patients receiving ifosfamide, and in patients receiving cyclophosphamide by the intravenous route at a high dose (e.g. more than 2 g) or in patients with previous urothelial toxicity from cyclophosphamide.

MESNA

Indications: see notes above
Contra-indications: hypersensitivity to thiol-containing compounds
Side-effects: above max. therapeutic doses, nausea, vomiting (use intravenous route), colic, diarrhoea, fatigue, headache, limb and joint pains, depression, irritability, lack of energy, rash, hypotension and tachycardia; rarely hypersensitivity reactions (more common in patients with auto-immune disorders)
Dose: calculated according to oxazaphosphorine (cyclophosphamide or ifosfamide) treatment—for details see data sheet; when given *by mouth*, dose is given 2 hours *before* oxazaphosphorine treatment and repeated 2 and 6 hours *after* treatment; when given *by intravenous injection*, dose is given *with* oxazaphosphorine treatment and repeated 4 and 8 hours *after* treatment

PoM **Uromitexan®** (ASTA Medica)
Tablets, f/c, mesna 400 mg, net price 10-tab pack = £18.25; 600 mg, 10-tab pack = £23.70
Injection, mesna 100 mg/mL. Net price 4-mL amp = £1.69; 10-mL amp = £3.79
Note. For oral administration contents of ampoule are taken in a flavoured drink such as orange juice or cola which may be stored in a refrigerator for up to 24 hours in a sealed container

8.1.2 Cytotoxic antibiotics

Drugs within this group are widely used. Many cytotoxic antibiotics act as radiomimetics and simultaneous use of radiotherapy should be **avoided** as it may result in markedly enhanced normal tissue toxicity.

Aclarubicin, daunorubicin, doxorubicin, epirubicin and idarubicin are anthracycline antibiotics. Mitozantrone is an anthracycline derivative.

Doxorubicin is one of the most successful and widely used antitumour drugs, and is used to treat the acute leukaemias, lymphomas, and a variety of solid tumours. It is given by fast running infusion, commonly at 21-day intervals. Local extravasation will cause severe tissue necrosis. Common toxic effects include nausea and vomiting, myelosuppression, alopecia, and mucositis. This drug is largely excreted by the biliary tract, and an elevated bilirubin concentration is an indication for reducing the dose. Supraventricular tachycardia related to drug administration is an uncommon complication. Higher cumulative doses are associated with development of a cardiomyopathy. It is customary to limit total cumulative doses to 450 mg/m^2 body-surface area as symptomatic and potentially fatal heart failure is increasingly common above this level. Patients with pre-existing cardiac disease, the elderly, and those who have received myocardial irradiation should be treated cautiously. Cardiac monitoring, for example by sequential radionuclide ejection fraction measurement, may assist in safely limiting total dosage. Evidence is available to suggest that weekly low-dose administration may be associated with less cardiac damage. Doxorubicin is also given by bladder instillation. A liposomal formulation for intravenous use has recently been licensed for Kaposi's sarcoma in AIDS patients.

Epirubicin is structurally related to doxorubicin and clinical trials suggest that it is as effective in the treatment of breast cancer. A maximum cumulative dose of 0.9–1 g/m^2 is recommended to help avoid cardiotoxicity. Like doxorubicin it is given intravenously and by bladder instillation.

Aclarubicin and **idarubicin** are newly introduced anthracyclines with general properties similar to those of doxorubicin. They are both given intravenously. Idarubicin may also be given by mouth.

Daunorubicin also has general properties similar to those of doxorubicin. It should be given by intravenous infusion and is indicated for acute leukaemias. A liposomal formulation for intravenous use has recently been licensed for AIDS-related Kaposi's sarcoma.

Mitozantrone (mitoxantrone) is structurally related to doxorubicin; it is used in breast cancer. It is given intravenously and is well tolerated apart from myelosuppression and dose-related cardiotoxicity; cardiac examinations are recommended after a cumulative dose of 160 mg/m^2 if this complication is to be avoided.

Bleomycin is given intravenously or intramuscularly to treat the lymphomas and certain solid tumours; it is given by the intracavitary route for malignant effusions. It causes little bone-marrow suppression but dermatological toxicity is common and increased pigmentation particularly affecting the flexures and subcutaneous sclerotic plaques may occur. Mucositis is also relatively common and an association with Raynaud's phenomenon is reported. Hypersensitivity reactions manifest by chills and fevers commonly occur a few hours after drug administration and may be prevented by simultaneous administration of a corticosteroid, for example hydrocortisone intravenously. The principal problem associated with the use of bleomycin is progressive pulmonary fibrosis. This is dose related, occurring more commonly at cumulative doses greater than 300 units and in the elderly. Basal lung crepitations or suspicious chest X-ray changes are an indication to stop therapy with this drug. Patients who have received extensive treatment with bleomycin (e.g. cumulative dose more than 100 units) may be at risk of developing respiratory failure if a general anaesthetic is given with high inspired oxygen concentrations. Anaesthetists should be warned of this.

Dactinomycin is principally used to treat paediatric cancers; it is given intravenously. Its side-effects are similar to those of doxorubicin, except that cardiac toxicity is not a problem.

Mitomycin is given intravenously to treat upper gastro-intestinal and breast cancers. It causes delayed marrow toxicity and is usually administered at 6-weekly intervals. Prolonged use may result in permanent marrow damage. It is a relatively toxic drug and may cause lung fibrosis and renal damage. It is also given by bladder instillation.

ACLARUBICIN

Indications: acute non-lymphocytic leukaemia in patients who have relapsed or are resistant or refractory to first-line chemotherapy

Cautions; Side-effects: see section 8.1 and notes above; caution in hepatic and renal impairment; irritant to tissues

PoM **Aclacin®** (Medac)

Injection, powder for reconstitution, aclarubicin 20 mg (as hydrochloride). Net price 20-mg vial = £29.20

BLEOMYCIN

Indications: squamous cell carcinoma; see also notes above

Cautions; Side-effects: see section 8.1 and notes above; reduce dose in renal impairment; also caution in handling—irritant to skin

PoM **Bleomycin** (Medac)

Injection, powder for reconstitution, bleomycin (as sulphate). Net price 15 000-unit amp = £16.29

Note. To conform to the European Pharmacopoeia ampoules previously labelled as containing '15 units' of bleomycin are now labelled as containing 15 000 units. The amount of bleomycin in the ampoule has not changed.

DACTINOMYCIN

(Actinomycin D)

Indications: see notes above

Cautions; Side-effects: see section 8.1 and notes above; irritant to tissues

PoM **Cosmegen Lyovac®** (MSD)

Injection, powder for reconstitution, dactinomycin, net price 500-microgram vial = £1.50

DAUNORUBICIN

Indications: see notes above

Cautions; Side-effects: see section 8.1 and notes above

PoM **Cerubidin®** (Rhône-Poulenc Rorer)

Injection, powder for reconstitution, daunorubicin (as hydrochloride). Net price 20-mg vial = £24.42

Lipid formulation

▼ PoM **DaunoXome®** (NeXstar)

Concentrate for intravenous infusion, daunorubicin encapsulated in liposomes. For dilution before use. Net price 50-mg vial = £155.00

For advanced AIDS-related Kaposi's sarcoma

DOXORUBICIN HYDROCHLORIDE

Indications: see notes above and section 7.4.4

Cautions; Side-effects: see section 8.1 and notes above; reduce dose in hepatic impairment; also caution in handling—irritant to skin and tissues; **interactions:** see Appendix 1 (doxorubicin)

PoM **Doxorubicin Rapid Dissolution**

(Pharmacia & Upjohn)

Injection, powder for reconstitution, doxorubicin hydrochloride, net price 10-mg vial = £18.72; 50-mg vial = £93.60

*Note.*This preparation has replaced Adriamycin®

PoM **Doxorubicin Solution for Injection**

(Pharmacia & Upjohn)

Injection, doxorubicin hydrochloride 2 mg/mL, net price 5-ml vial = £20.60; 25-mL vial = £103.00

Various strengths and sizes also available from Faulding DBL

Lipid formulation

▼ PoM **Caelyx®** (Schering-Plough)

Concentrate for intravenous infusion, doxorubicin hydrochloride 2 mg/mL encapsulated in liposomes. For dilution before use. Net price 10-mL vial = £457.00

For AIDS-related Kaposi's sarcoma in patients with low CD4 counts and extensive mucocutaneous or visceral disease

EPIRUBICIN HYDROCHLORIDE

Indications: see notes above and section 7.4.4

Cautions; Side-effects: see section 8.1 and notes above; reduce dose in hepatic impairment; irritant to tissues

PoM **Pharmorubicin® Rapid Dissolution**

(Pharmacia & Upjohn)

Injection, powder for reconstitution, epirubicin hydrochloride. Net price 10-mg vial = £18.72; 20-mg vial = £33.70; 50-mg vial = £93.60

PoM **Pharmorubicin® Solution for Injection**

(Pharmacia & Upjohn)

Injection, epirubicin hydrochloride 2 mg/mL, net price 5-mL vial = £20.60; 25-mL vial = £103.00

IDARUBICIN HYDROCHLORIDE

Indications: advanced breast cancer after failure of frontline chemotherapy (not including anthracyclines); acute leukaemias—see notes above

Cautions; Side-effects: see section 8.1 and notes above; caution in hepatic and renal impairment; also caution in handling—irritant to skin and tissues

PoM **Zavedos®** (Pharmacia & Upjohn)

Capsules, idarubicin hydrochloride, 5 mg (red), net price 1-cap pack = £28.80; 10 mg (red/white), 1-cap pack = £57.60; 25 mg (white), 1-cap pack = £144.00. Label: 25

Injection, powder for reconstitution, idarubicin hydrochloride, net price 5-mg vial = £72.80; 10-mg vial = £145.60

MITOMYCIN

Indications: see notes above and section 7.4.4

Cautions; Side-effects: see section 8.1 and notes above; irritant to tissues

PoM **Mitomycin** (Non-proprietary)
Injection, powder for reconstitution, mitomycin. Net price 10-mg vial = £20.15; 20-mg vial = £36.49
Available from Faulding DBL

PoM **Mitomycin C Kyowa®** (Kyowa Hakko)
Injection, powder for reconstitution, mitomycin. Net price 2-mg vial = £6.16; 10-mg vial = £20.28; 20-mg vial = £38.68 (hosp. only)

MITOZANTRONE
(Mitoxantrone)
Indications: see notes above
Cautions; Side-effects: see section 8.1 and notes above; intrathecal administration not recommended

PoM **Novantrone®** (Lederle)
Intravenous infusion, mitozantrone 2 mg (as hydrochloride)/mL, net price 10-mL vial = £150.43; 12.5-mL vial = £188.05; 15-mL vial = £225.60

8.1.3 Antimetabolites

Antimetabolites are incorporated into new nuclear material or combine irreversibly with vital cellular enzymes, preventing normal cellular division.

Methotrexate inhibits the enzyme dihydrofolate reductase, essential for the synthesis of purines and pyrimidines. It is given by mouth, intravenously, intramuscularly, or intrathecally.

Methotrexate is used as maintenance therapy for childhood acute lymphoblastic leukaemia. Other uses include choriocarcinoma, non-Hodgkin lymphomas, and a number of solid tumours. Intrathecal methotrexate is used in the CNS prophylaxis of childhood acute lymphoblastic leukaemia, and as a therapy for established meningeal cancer or lymphoma.

Methotrexate causes myelosuppression, mucositis, and rarely pneumonitis. It is **contra-indicated** if significant renal impairment is present, since it is excreted primarily by the kidney. It is also contra-indicated in patients with severe hepatic impairment. It should also be **avoided** if a significant pleural effusion or ascites is present as it tends to accumulate at these sites, and its subsequent return to the circulation will be associated with myelosuppression. Systemic toxicity may occur following intrathecal administration and blood counts should be carefully monitored.

Folinic acid following methotrexate administration (see Folinic Acid Rescue, below) helps to prevent methotrexate-induced mucositis or myelosuppression.

Cytarabine acts by interfering with pyrimidine synthesis. It is given subcutaneously, intravenously, or intrathecally. Its predominant use is in the induction of remission of acute myeloblastic leukaemia. It is a potent myelosuppressant and requires careful haematological monitoring.

Fludarabine is recommended for patients with B-cell chronic lymphocytic leukaemia (CLL) after initial treatment with an alkylating agent has failed; it is given intravenously daily for 5 days every 28 days. Fludarabine is generally well tolerated but does, however, cause myelosuppression (which may be cumulative), and immunosuppression (with an increased risk of opportunistic infection). Idiosyncratic CNS and pulmonary toxicity have been reported rarely. Dose reduction is recommended in renal impairment.

Cladribine is an effective but potentially toxic drug given by continuous intravenous infusion over 7 days for the treatment of hairy cell leukaemia. Myelosuppression may be severe and use is confined to experienced specialists.

Gemcitabine is given intravenously for palliative treatment in patients with locally advanced or metastatic non-small cell lung and pancreatic cancer. It is generally well tolerated but may cause mild gastro-intestinal side-effects and rashes; renal impairment and influenza-like symptoms have also been reported. Haemolytic uraemic syndrome has been reported rarely and gemcitabine should be discontinued if signs of microangiopathic haemolytic anaemia occur. Gemcitabine should not be used concurrently with radical radiotherapy.

Fluorouracil is usually given intravenously because absorption following oral administration is unpredictable. It is used to treat a number of solid tumours, including gastro-intestinal tract cancers and breast cancer. It is commonly used together with folinic acid in advanced colorectal cancer. It may also be used topically for certain malignant and pre-malignant skin lesions Toxicity is unusual, but may include myelosuppression, mucositis, and rarely a cerebellar syndrome.

Raltitrexed, a thymidylate synthase inhibitor, is given intravenously for palliation of metastatic colon cancer. It is probably of similar efficacy to fluorouracil. Raltitrexed is generally well tolerated, but may cause gastro-intestinal side-effects. Caution is advised in hepatic and renal impairment.

Mercaptopurine is used almost exclusively as maintenance therapy for the acute leukaemias. Azathioprine, a derivative of mercaptopurine, is generally used as an immunosuppressant (section 8.2.1). The dose of both drugs should be reduced if the patient is receiving allopurinol since it interferes with their metabolism.

Thioguanine (Tioguanine) is given by mouth to induce remission in acute myeloid leukaemia.

CLADRIBINE
Indications: see notes above
Cautions; Side-effects: see section 8.1 and notes above

▼ PoM **Leustat®** (Janssen-Cilag)
Injection, cladribine 1 mg/mL. For dilution and use as an infusion. Net price 10-mL vial = £364.57

CYTARABINE
Indications: acute leukaemias
Cautions; Side-effects: see section 8.1 and notes above

PoM **Cytarabine** (Non-proprietary)

Injection, cytarabine 20 mg/mL. Net price 5-mL vial = £3.84. For subcutaneous, intravenous, or intrathecal use

Injection, cytarabine 100 mg/mL. Net price 1-mL vial = £3.84; 5-mL vial = £19.00; 10-mL vial = £37.83; 20-mL vial = £71.88. **Not** for intrathecal use

All available from Faulding DBL

PoM **Cytosar®** (Pharmacia & Upjohn)

Injection, powder for reconstitution, cytarabine. Net price 100-mg vial = £3.01, 100-mg vial (with diluent) = £3.17; 500-mg vial = £14.95, 500-mg vial (with diluent) = £15.45. For intravenous injection or infusion and subcutaneous injection only; not recommended for intrathecal use

FLUDARABINE PHOSPHATE

Indications: see notes above

Cautions; Side-effects: see section 8.1 and notes above; **interactions:** Appendix 1 (Fludarabine)

PoM **Fludara®** (Schering Health)

Injection, powder for reconstitution, fludarabine phosphate. Net price 50-mg vial = £130.00

FLUOROURACIL

Indications: see notes above; genital warts, section 13.7

Cautions; Side-effects: see section 8.1; also caution in handling—irritant; **interactions:** Appendix 1 (fluorouracil)

Dose: by mouth, maintenance 15 mg/kg weekly; max. in one day 1 g

PoM **Fluorouracil** (Non-proprietary)

Capsules, fluorouracil 250 mg.

Available from Cambridge on a named patient basis

Injection, fluorouracil 25 mg/mL (as sodium salt). Net price 10-mL vial = £2.06; 20-mL vial = £3.97; 100-mL vial = £19.23

Available from Faulding DBL

PoM **Efudix®** (Roche)

Cream, fluorouracil 5%. Net price 20 g = £4.13

GEMCITABINE

Indications: see notes above

Cautions; Side-effects: see section 8.1 and notes above

▼ PoM **Gemzar®** (Lilly)

Injection, powder for reconstitution, gemcitabine (as hydrochloride), net price 200-mg vial = £32.55; 1-g vial = £162.76 (both hosp. only)

MERCAPTOPURINE

Indications: acute leukaemias

Cautions; Side-effects: see section 8.1 and notes above; reduce dose in renal impairment; avoid in porphyria (see section 9.8.2); **interactions:** Appendix 1 (mercaptopurine)

Dose: initially 2.5 mg/kg daily

PoM **Puri-Nethol®** (GlaxoWellcome)

Tablets, fawn, scored, mercaptopurine 50 mg. Net price 25 = £19.22

METHOTREXATE

Indications: see notes above and under Dose; rheumatoid arthritis, see section 10.1.3; psoriasis, see section 13.5.2

Cautions; Side-effects: see section 8.1, notes above and p. 493; reduce dose in renal impairment; dose-related toxicity in hepatic impairment; porphyria (see section 9.8.2); **interactions:** Appendix 1 (methotrexate)

Dose: by mouth, leukaemia in children (maintenance), 15 mg/m² weekly in combination with other drugs

PoM **Methotrexate** (Non-proprietary)

Tablets, yellow, methotrexate 2.5 mg. Net price 100 (Faulding DBL) = £14.19; (Lederle) = £10.59; (Pharmacia & Upjohn, Maxtrex®) = £10.43. Counselling, NSAIDs, see p. 494

Tablets, yellow, methotrexate 10 mg. Net price 100 (Faulding DBL) = £55.07; (Pharmacia & Upjohn, Maxtrex®) = £47.29. Counselling, NSAIDs, see p. 494

Injection, methotrexate 2.5 mg (as sodium salt)/mL. Net price 2-mL vial (Faulding DBL) = £1.68

Injection, methotrexate 25 mg (as sodium salt)/mL. Net price 2-mL vial (Faulding DBL) = £4.58, (Lederle) = £2.62; 8-mL vial (Lederle) = £10.02; 20-mL vial (Faulding DBL) = £39.09, (Lederle) = £25.07; 40-mL vial (Lederle) = £44.57; 200-mL vial (Lederle) = £200.57

Injection, methotrexate 100 mg/mL (not for intrathecal use). Net price 10-mL vial (Faulding DBL) = £78.33; 50-mL vial (Faulding DBL) = £380.07

RALTITREXED

Indications: see notes above

Cautions; Side-effects: see section 8.1 and notes above

PoM **Tomudex®** (Zeneca)

Injection, powder for reconstitution, raltitrexed. Net price 2-mg vial = £116.00

THIOGUANINE

(Tioguanine)

Indications: acute leukaemias

Cautions; Side-effects: see section 8.1 and notes above; reduce dose in renal impairment

Dose: initially 2–2.5 mg/kg daily

PoM **Lanvis®** (GlaxoWellcome)

Tablets, yellow, scored, thioguanine 40 mg. Net price 25-tab pack = £46.48

FOLINIC ACID RESCUE

Folinic acid (given as calcium folinate) is used to counteract the folate-antagonist action of methotrexate and thus speed recovery from methotrexate-induced mucositis or myelosuppression. It is generally given 24 hours after the methotrexate, in a dose of 15 mg by mouth every 6 hours, for 2–8 doses (depending on the dose of methotrexate). It does not counteract the antibacterial activity of folate antagonists such as trimethoprim.

Folinic acid also interacts with fluorouracil; when the two are used together in metastatic colonic cancer a favourable effect has been demonstrated on response-rate.

CALCIUM FOLINATE
(Calcium leucovorin)

Indications: see notes above

Cautions: avoid simultaneous administration of methotrexate; as for Folic Acid (section 9.1.2) **not** indicated for pernicious anaemia or other megaloblastic anaemias where vitamin B$_{12}$ deficient

Side-effects: rarely, pyrexia after parenteral administration

Dose: expressed in terms of folinic acid

As an antidote to methotrexate (started 8–24 hours after the beginning of methotrexate infusion), in general up to 120 mg in divided doses over 12–24 hours *by intramuscular or intravenous injection or infusion,* followed by 12–15 mg *intramuscularly or* 15 mg *by mouth* every 6 hours for the next 48–72 hours

Suspected methotrexate overdosage, immediate administration of folinic acid in a dose equal to (or higher than) the dose of methotrexate

PoM **Calcium Folinate** (Non-proprietary)

Tablets, scored, folinic acid (as calcium salt) 15 mg. Net price 10-tab pack (Faulding DBL) = £37.85, (Hillcross) = £27.32, (Lederle) = £41.22; 30-tab pack (Pharmacia & Upjohn, Refolinon®) = £94.50

Injection, folinic acid 3 mg (as calcium salt)/mL. Net price 1-mL amp (Faulding DBL) = £2.28; 10-mL amp (Pharmacia & Upjohn, Refolinon®) = £5.70

Injection, folinic acid 7.5 mg (as calcium salt)/mL. Net price 2-mL amp (Faulding DBL) = £7.80

Injection, folinic acid 10 mg (as calcium salt)/mL. Net price 5-mL vial (Faulding DBL) = £19.41; 10-mL vial (Faulding DBL) = £35.09; 30-mL vial (Faulding DBL) = £94.69; 35-mL vial (Lederle, Lederfolin®) = £90.98

Injection, powder for reconstitution, folinic acid (as calcium salt). Net price 15-mg vial (Lederle) = £4.46; 30-mg vial (Lederle) = £8.36

8.1.4 Vinca alkaloids and etoposide

The vinca alkaloids, **vinblastine**, **vincristine**, and **vindesine**, are used to treat the acute leukaemias, lymphomas, and some solid tumours (e.g. breast and lung cancer). **Vinorelbine**, a semi-synthetic vinca alkaloid, has recently been introduced for advanced breast cancer (where anthracycline-containing regimens have failed) and for advanced non-small cell lung cancer.

Neurological toxicity, usually manifested as peripheral or autonomic neuropathy, is a feature of treatment with all vinca alkaloids and is a limiting side-effect of vincristine; it occurs less often with vindesine, vinblastine and vinorelbine. Patients with neurological toxicity commonly experience peripheral paraesthesia, loss of deep tendon reflexes, abdominal pain, and constipation. If symptoms of neurotoxicity are severe, doses should be reduced. Motor weakness can also occur, and increasing motor weakness calls for discontinuation of treatment with these drugs. Generally recovery of the nervous system is slow but complete.

Myelosuppression is the dose-limiting side-effect of vinblastine, vindesine and vinorelbine; vincristine causes negligible myelosuppression. The vinca alkaloids may cause reversible alopecia. They cause severe local irritation and care must be taken to avoid extravasation.

Vinblastine, vincristine, vindesine and vinorelbine are for **intravenous administration only**. They are **not** for intrathecal administration because of severe neurotoxicity which is usually fatal.

Etoposide may be given orally or by slow intravenous infusion, the oral dose being double the intravenous dose. Etoposide is usually given daily for 3 5 days and courses should not be repeated more frequently than at intervals of 21 days. It has particularly useful activity in small cell carcinoma of the bronchus, the lymphomas, and testicular cancer. Toxic effects include alopecia, myelosuppression, nausea, and vomiting.

ETOPOSIDE

Indications: see notes above

Cautions: see section 8.1 and notes above; irritant to tissues

Contra-indications: see section 8.1 and notes above

Side-effects: see section 8.1 and notes above

PoM **Etoposide** (Du Pont)

Injection concentrate, etoposide 20 mg/mL. To be diluted. Net price 5-mL vial = £13.50

PoM **Vepesid**® (Bristol-Myers)

Capsules, etoposide 50 mg, net price 20 = £113.95; 100 mg, 10-cap pack = £99.57. Label: 23

Injection, etoposide 20 mg/mL. To be diluted. Net price 5-mL vial = £14.58

VINBLASTINE SULPHATE

Indications: see notes above

Cautions: see section 8.1 and notes above; caution in handling—avoid contact with eyes; irritant to tissues; hepatic impairment (Appendix 2)

Contra-indications: see section 8.1 and notes above

IMPORTANT. Intrathecal injection **contra-indicated**

Side-effects: see section 8.1 and notes above

PoM **Vinblastine** (Non-proprietary)

Injection, vinblastine sulphate 1 mg/mL. Net price 10-mL vial = £13.09

Available from Faulding DBL

PoM **Velbe**® (Lilly)

Injection, powder for reconstitution, vinblastine sulphate. Net price 10-mg amp (with diluent) = £14.15

VINCRISTINE SULPHATE

Indications: see notes above

Cautions: see section 8.1 and notes above; caution in handling—avoid contact with eyes; irritant to tissues; hepatic impairment (Appendix 2)

Contra-indications: see section 8.1 and notes above

IMPORTANT. Intrathecal injection **contra-indicated**

Side-effects: see section 8.1 and notes above

PoM **Vincristine** (Non-proprietary)

Injection, vincristine sulphate 1 mg/mL. Net price 1-mL vial = £10.92; 2-mL vial = £21.17; 5-mL vial = £44.16; 1-mL syringe = £11.34; 2-mL syringe = £20.55

Available from Faulding DBL

PoM **Oncovin**® (Lilly)

Injection, vincristine sulphate 1 mg/mL, net price 1-mL vial = £14.18; 2-mL vial = £28.05

VINDESINE SULPHATE

Indications: see notes above

Cautions: see section 8.1 and notes above; caution in handling—avoid contact with eyes; irritant to tissues; hepatic impairment (Appendix 2)

Contra-indications: see section 8.1 and notes above

IMPORTANT. Intrathecal injection **contra-indicated**

Side-effects: see section 8.1 and notes above

PoM **Eldisine**® (Lilly)

Injection, powder for reconstitution, vindesine sulphate, net price 5-mg vial (with diluent) = £78.30 (hosp. only)

VINORELBINE

Indications: see notes above

Cautions: see section 8.1 and notes above; caution in handling—avoid contact with eyes; irritant to tissues; hepatic impairment (Appendix 2)

Contra-indications: see section 8.1 and notes above

IMPORTANT. Intrathecal injection **contra-indicated**

Side-effects: see section 8.1 and notes above

▼ PoM **Navelbine**® (Fabre)

Injection concentrate, vinorelbine (as tartrate) 10 mg/mL. Net price 1-mL vial = £31.26; 5-mL vial = £147.06

8.1.5   Other antineoplastic drugs

AMSACRINE

Amsacrine has an action and toxic effects similar to those of doxorubicin (section 8.1.2) and is given *intravenously*. It is used in acute myeloid leukaemia. Side-effects include myelosuppression and mucositis; electrolytes should be monitored as fatal arrhythmias have occurred in association with hypokalaemia.

AMSACRINE

Indications: see notes above

Cautions; Side-effects: see section 8.1 and notes above; reduce dose in renal or hepatic impairment; also caution in handling—irritant to skin and tissues

PoM **Amsidine**® (Goldshield)

Concentrate for intravenous infusion, amsacrine 5 mg (as lactate)/mL, when reconstituted by mixing two solutions. Net price 1.5-mL (75-mg) amp with 13.5-mL diluent vial = £30.90. (hosp. only)

Note. Use glass apparatus for reconstitution

ALTRETAMINE

Altretamine has recently been introduced for the treatment of advanced ovarian cancer where other regimens have failed. It is given by mouth. Prophylactic anti-emetic treatment is recommended because nausea and vomiting are common and may not respond to symptomatic management. Peripheral and central neurotoxicity has been reported and regular neurological examination is therefore recommended. Altretamine should be discontinued if dose reduction fails to stabilise symptoms of neurological toxicity. Other side-effects include renal and hepatic toxicity, rash and pruritus.

ALTRETAMINE

Indications: see notes above

Cautions: see section 8.1 and notes above; hepatic and renal impairment (Appendixes 2 and 3); **interactions:** Appendix 1 (altretamine)

Contra-indications: see section 8.1 and notes above

Side-effects: see section 8.1 and notes above

▼ PoM **Hexalen**® (Speywood)

Capsules, altretamine 50 mg. Net price 60-cap pack = £149.50. Label: 21.

CARBOPLATIN

Carboplatin, a derivative of cisplatin which has probably equivalent activity in ovarian cancer, is given *intravenously*. It is also active in small cell lung cancer and is under trial in a variety of other malignancies. Carboplatin is better tolerated than cisplatin; nausea and vomiting are reduced in severity and nephrotoxicity, neurotoxicity, and ototoxicity are much less of a problem than with cisplatin. It is, however, more myelosuppressive than cisplatin.

CARBOPLATIN

Indications: see notes above
Cautions; Side-effects: see section 8.1 and notes above; reduce dose in renal impairment

PoM **Carboplatin** (Non-proprietary)
Injection, carboplatin 10 mg/mL. Net price 15-mL vial = £65.83; 45-mL vial = £197.48
Available from Faulding DBL

PoM **Paraplatin**® (Bristol-Myers)
Injection, carboplatin 10 mg/mL. Net price 5-mL vial = £22.86; 15-mL vial = £65.83; 45-mL vial = £197.48

CISPLATIN

Cisplatin has an alkylating action and is given *intravenously*. It has useful antitumour activity in certain solid tumours including ovarian cancer and testicular teratoma. It is, however, a toxic drug. Common problems include severe nausea and vomiting, nephrotoxicity (pretreatment hydration mandatory and renal function should be closely monitored), myelotoxicity, ototoxicity (high tone hearing loss and tinnitus), peripheral neuropathy, and hypomagnesaemia. These toxic effects commonly necessitate dose reduction or drug withdrawal. It is preferable that treatment with this drug be supervised by specialists familiar with its use.

CISPLATIN

Indications: see notes above
Cautions; Side-effects: see section 8.1 and notes above; reduce dose in renal impairment; **interactions:** Appendix 1 (cisplatin)

PoM **Cisplatin** (Non-proprietary)
Injection, cisplatin 1 mg/mL. Net price 10-mL vial = £5.85; 50-mL vial = £28.11; 100-mL vial = £55.64
Available from Faulding DBL
Injection, powder for reconstitution, cisplatin. Net price 50-mg vial = £17.00
Available from Pharmacia & Upjohn

CRISANTASPASE

Crisantaspase is the enzyme asparaginase produced by *Erwinia chrysanthemi.* It is given *intramuscularly* or *subcutaneously* almost exclusively in acute lymphoblastic leukaemia. Facilities for the management of anaphylaxis should be available. Side-effects also include nausea, vomiting, CNS depression, and liver function and blood lipid changes; careful monitoring is therefore necessary and the urine is tested for glucose to exclude hyperglycaemia.

CRISANTASPASE

Indications; Cautions; Side-effects: see notes above

PoM **Erwinase**® (Speywood)
Injection, powder for reconstitution, crisantaspase. Net price 20 × 10 000-unit vial = £858.00

DACARBAZINE

Dacarbazine is not commonly used on account of its toxicity. It has been used to treat melanoma and, in combination therapy, the soft tissue sarcomas. It is also a component of a commonly used combination for Hodgkin's disease (ABVD—doxorubicin [*Adriamycin*®], bleomycin, vinblastine, and dacarbazine). It is given *intravenously.* The predominant side-effects are myelosuppression and intense nausea and vomiting.

DACARBAZINE

Indications: see notes above
Cautions; Side-effects: see section 8.1; also caution in handling—irritant to skin and tissues

PoM **DTIC-Dome**® (Bayer)
Injection, powder for reconstitution, dacarbazine. Net price 200-mg vial = £7.40

HYDROXYUREA

Hydroxyurea (hydroxycarbamide) is an orally active drug used mainly in the treatment of chronic myeloid leukaemia. It is occasionally used for polycythaemia (the usual treatment is venesection). Myelosuppression, nausea, and skin reactions are the most common toxic effects

HYDROXYUREA
(Hydroxycarbamide)

Indications: see notes above
Cautions; Side-effects: see section 8.1 and notes above
Dose: 20–30 mg/kg daily *or* 80 mg/kg every third day

PoM **Hydrea**® (Squibb)
Capsules, pink/green, hydroxyurea 500 mg. Net price 20 = £2.39

PENTOSTATIN

Pentostatin is highly active in hairy cell leukaemia. It is given *intravenously* on alternate weeks and is capable of inducing prolonged complete remission. It is potentially toxic, causing myelosuppression, immunosuppression and a number of other side-effects which may be severe. Its use is probably best confined to specialist centres.

PENTOSTATIN

Indications: see notes above
Cautions; Contra-indications; Side-effects: see section 8.1 and notes above; **interactions:** Appendix 1 (pentostatin)

▼ PoM **Nipent**® (Lederle)
Injection, powder for reconstitution, pentostatin. Net price 10-mg vial = £774.00

PROCARBAZINE

Procarbazine is most often used in Hodgkin's disease, for example in MOPP (mustine, vincristine [*Oncovin*®], procarbazine, and prednisolone) chemotherapy. It is given *by mouth*. Toxic effects include nausea, myelosuppression, and a hypersensitivity rash preventing further use of this drug. It is a mild monoamine-oxidase inhibitor but dietary restriction is not considered necessary. Alcohol ingestion may cause a disulfiram-like reaction.

PROCARBAZINE
Indications: see notes above
Cautions; Side-effects: see section 8.1 and notes above; reduce dose in renal impairment; **interactions:** Appendix 1 (procarbazine)
Dose: initially 50 mg daily, increased by 50 mg daily to 250–300 mg daily in divided doses; maintenance (on remission) 50–150 mg daily to cumulative total of at least 6 g

PoM **Procarbazine** (Cambridge)
Capsules, ivory, procarbazine 50 mg (as hydrochloride). Net price 50-cap pack = £32.00. Label: 4
Note. The brand name *Natulan*® was formerly used for procarbazine capsules

RAZOXANE

Razoxane has limited activity in the leukaemias, and is little used.

RAZOXANE
Indications: see notes above
Cautions; Side-effects: see section 8.1
Dose: acute leukaemias, 150–500 mg/m² daily for 3–5 days

PoM **Razoxane** (Cambridge)
Tablets, scored, razoxane 125 mg. Net price 30-tab pack = £68.28

TAXANES

Paclitaxel is the first of a new group of drugs termed the taxanes. It is given *intravenously*. It is licensed for primary and secondary treatment of advanced ovarian cancer and for secondary treatment of breast cancer. Paclitaxel is relatively toxic and it is recommended that its use be confined to experienced specialists. Routine premedication with a corticosteroid, an antihistamine and a histamine H₂-receptor antagonist is recommended to prevent severe hypersensitivity reactions; despite premedication these reactions may still rarely occur, more commonly only bradycardia or asymptomatic hypotension occur.

In addition to hypersensitivity, side-effects of paclitaxel include myelosuppression, peripheral neuropathy, and cardiac conduction defects with arrhythmias (which are nearly always asympto-

matic). It also causes alopecia and muscle pain; nausea and vomiting is mild to moderate.

Only a minority of patients respond to paclitaxel, but the responses are sometimes prolonged.

Docetaxel is licensed for use in anthracycline-resistant breast cancer. The side-effects are similar to those for paclitaxel but persistent fluid retention (commonly seen as leg oedema which worsens during treatment) can be resistant to treatment; hypersensitivity reactions also occur. Dexamethasone by mouth for five days, starting on the day before each course of docetaxel, is recommended for reducing fluid retention and hypersensitivity reactions. Caution is advised in hepatic impairment.

DOCETAXEL
Indications: advanced breast cancer where adjuvant cytotoxic chemotherapy (including anthracycline) has failed
Cautions; Contra-indications; Side-effects: see section 8.1 and notes above; **interactions:** Appendix 1 (docetaxel)

▼ PoM **Taxotere**® (Rhône-Poulenc Rorer)
Concentrate for intravenous infusion, docetaxel 40 mg/mL. Net price 0.5-mL vial = £175.00, 2-mL vial = £575.00 (both with diluent). Hosp. only

PACLITAXEL
Indications: primary ovarian cancer (advanced or residual disease following laparotomy) in combination with cisplatin; metastatic ovarian cancer where standard platinum-containing therapy has failed; metastatic breast carcinoma where standard anthracycline-containing therapy has failed or is inappropriate
Cautions; Contra-indications; Side-effects: see section 8.1 and notes above; **interactions:** Appendix 1 (paclitaxel)

▼ PoM **Taxol**® (Bristol-Myers, Squibb)
Concentrate for intravenous infusion, paclitaxel 6 mg/mL. Net price 5-mL vial = £124.79 (hosp. only)
Note. Contains polyethoxylated castor oil which has been associated with anaphylaxis

TOPOISOMERASE I INHIBITORS

Irinotecan and topotecan are recently introduced drugs which inhibit topoisomerase I, an enzyme involved in DNA replication.

Irinotecan is given by intravenous infusion in metastatic colorectal cancer when treatment containing fluorouracil has failed.

Topotecan is given by intravenous infusion in metastatic ovarian cancer when first-line or subsequent therapy has failed.

In addition to dose-limiting myelosuppression, side-effects of irinotecan and topotecan include gastro-intestinal effects (delayed diarrhoea requiring prompt treatment may follow irinotecan treatment), asthenia, alopecia, and anorexia.

IRINOTECAN HYDROCHLORIDE

Indications: metastatic colorectal cancer where treatment with fluorouracil has failed

Cautions: see section 8.1 and notes above

Contra-indications: see section 8.1 and notes above; also chronic inflammatory bowel disease, bowel obstruction; plasma bilirubin concentration more than 1.5 times the upper limit of reference range; avoid conception for at least 3 months after cessation of treatment

Side-effects: see section 8.1 and notes above; also acute cholinergic syndrome (with early diarrhoea) and delayed diarrhoea (consult product literature)

▼ PoM **Campto**® (Rhône-Poulenc Rorer)

Concentrate for intravenous infusion, irinotecan hydrochloride 20 mg/mL, net price 2-mL vial = £53.00; 5-mL vial = £130.00

TOPOTECAN

Indications: metastatic ovarian cancer where first-line or subsequent therapy has failed

Cautions; Contra-indications; Side-effects: see section 8.1 and notes above

▼ PoM **Hycamtin**® (SmithKline Beecham)

Intravenous infusion, powder for reconstitution, topotecan (as hydrochloride). Net price 4-mg vial = £312.50

TRETINOIN

Tretinoin has recently been introduced for the induction of remission in acute promyelocytic leukaemia. It is used in previously untreated patients as well as in those who have relapsed after standard chemotherapy or who are refractory to it.

TRETINOIN

Note. Tretinoin is the acid form of vitamin A

Indications: see notes above; acne (section 13.6.1); photodamage (section 13.8.1)

Cautions: exclude pregnancy before starting treatment and avoid pregnancy during and for at least 1 month after treatment; monitor haematological profile, liver function and plasma lipids before and during treatment; increased risk of thrombo-embolism during first month of treatment; hepatic and renal impairment (Appendixes 2 and 3); **interactions:** Appendix 1 (retinoids)

Contra-indications: pregnancy (**important teratogenic risk:** see Cautions and Appendix 4) and breast-feeding

Side-effects: retinoic acid syndrome (fever, dyspnoea, acute respiratory distress, pulmonary infiltrates, pleural effusion, hyperleukocytosis, hypotension, oedema, weight gain, hepatic, renal and multi-organ failure) requires immediate treatment—consult product literature; gastro-intestinal disturbances, pancreatitis; arrhythmias, flushing, oedema; headache, benign intracranial hypertension (mainly in children), shivering, dizziness, confusion, anxiety, depression, insomnia, paraesthesia, visual and hearing disturbances; raised liver enzymes, serum creatinine and lipids; bone and chest pain, alopecia, rash, pruritus, sweating, dry skin, dryness of mucous membranes, cheilitis; thrombo-embolism reported

▼ PoM **Vesanoid**® (Roche)

Capsules, yellow/brown, tretinoin 10 mg. Net price 100-cap pack = £192.00. Label: 21.

8.2 Drugs affecting the immune response

8.2.1	Cytotoxic immunosuppressants
8.2.2	Corticosteroids and other immunosuppressants
8.2.3	Immunostimulants
8.2.4	Interferons
8.2.5	Aldesleukin

8.2.1 Cytotoxic immunosuppressants

These drugs are used to suppress rejection in organ transplant recipients and are also used to treat a variety of auto-immune and collagen diseases (see section 10.1.3). They are non-specific in their action and careful monitoring of peripheral blood counts is required, with dose adjustments for marrow toxicity. Patients receiving these drugs will be prone to atypical infections.

Azathioprine is widely used for transplant recipients and is also used to treat a number of auto-immune conditions, usually when corticosteroid therapy alone has provided inadequate control. This drug is metabolised to mercaptopurine, and doses should be reduced when concurrent therapy with allopurinol is given. The predominant toxic effect is myelosuppression, although hepatic toxicity is also well recognised.

Mycophenolate mofetil is metabolised to mycophenolic acid which has a more selective mode of action than that of azathioprine. It is licensed for the prophylaxis of acute renal transplant rejection when used in combination with cyclosporin and corticosteroids. There is evidence that compared with similar regimens incorporating azathioprine, mycophenolate mofetil reduces the risk of acute rejection episodes; the risk of opportunistic infections (particularly due to tissue-invasive cytomegalovirus) and the occurrence of blood disorders such as leucopenia may be higher.

Cyclophosphamide and chlorambucil (section 8.1.1) are less commonly prescribed as immunosuppressants.

IMPAIRED IMMUNE RESPONSIVENESS. For general comments and warnings relating to immunosuppression see p. 368 (Impaired Immune Responsiveness)

AZATHIOPRINE

Indications: see notes above

Cautions: should not be prescribed unless adequate monitoring available throughout duration of treatment; monitoring required includes full blood counts carried out at least weekly for the first 8 weeks (more frequently with higher doses or if hepatic or renal impairment) then at least every 3 months thereafter; reduce dose in severe hepatic and renal impairment and in elderly; **interactions:** Appendix 1 (azathioprine)

BONE MARROW SUPPRESSION. Patients should be warned to report immediately any evidence of infection, unexpected bruising or bleeding, or other manifestations of bone marrow suppression

Contra-indications: hypersensitivity to azathioprine or mercaptopurine (see also under Side-effects); decision to maintain or discontinue in pregnancy depends on condition being treated (see also p. 368) but as general rule should not be initiated during pregnancy

Side-effects: hypersensitivity reactions (including malaise, dizziness, vomiting, fever, rigors, muscular pains, arthralgia, disturbed liver function, cholestatic jaundice, arrhythmias, hypotension and interstitial nephritis—calling for immediate and permanent withdrawal); dose-related bone marrow suppression (see also Cautions); hair loss and increased susceptibility to infections in transplant recipients also receiving corticosteroids; nausea; rarely pancreatitis and pneumonitis

Dose: by mouth or intravenously, initially, rarely more than 3 mg/kg daily, reduced according to response; maintenance 1–3 mg/kg daily; consider withdrawal if no improvement in 3 months

Suppression of transplant rejection, loading dose, by mouth or intravenously up to 5 mg/kg; maintenance 1–4 mg/kg daily

Note. Intravenous injection is alkaline and very irritant, intravenous route should therefore be used **only** if oral route not feasible, see also Appendix 6

PoM **Azathioprine** (Non-proprietary)

Tablets, azathioprine 25 mg, net price 20 = £7.00; 50 mg, 20 = £3.84. Label: 21

Available from APS, Ashbourne (Immunoprin®), Berk, Cox, Hillcross, Lagap, Lennon (Oprisine®), Norton, Penn (Azamune®)

PoM **Imuran®** (GlaxoWellcome)

Tablets, both f/c, azathioprine 25 mg (orange), net price 100-tab pack = £39.35; 50 mg (yellow), 100-tab pack = £65.61. Label: 21

Injection, powder for reconstitution, azathioprine (as sodium salt). Net price 50-mg vial = £16.54

MYCOPHENOLATE MOFETIL

Indications: prophylaxis of acute renal transplant rejection (in combination with cyclosporin and corticosteroids) under specialist supervision

Cautions: full blood counts every week for 4 weeks then twice a month for 2 months then every month in the first year (possibly interrupt treatment if neutropenia develops); elderly (increased risk of infection, gastro-intestinal haemorrhage and pulmonary oedema); active serious gastro-intestinal disease (risk of haemorr-

hage, ulceration and perforation); delayed graft function; **interactions:** Appendix 1 (mycophenolate mofetil)

Contra-indications: pregnancy (exclude before starting and avoid for 6 weeks after discontinuation); breast-feeding

Side-effects: diarrhoea, vomiting, constipation, nausea, abdominal pain; hypertension, oedema, chest pain; dyspnoea, cough; dizziness, insomnia, headache, tremor; infection (including cytomegalovirus viraemia, herpes simplex, candidiasis, aspergillosis, urinary-tract infection and pneumonia); leucopenia (see also Cautions), anaemia, thrombocytopenia, leucocytosis, polycythaemia; electrolyte disturbances, hyperglycaemia, hypercholesterolaemia; asthenia; renal damage, haematuria; acne; lymphoproliferative disease; less frequently, gastro-intestinal perforation, abnormal liver-function tests, hepatitis, gingivitis, mouth ulceration, haemorrhage, influenza-like syndrome, hypotension, tachycardia, hypoglycaemia, weight gain; allergic reactions reported

Dose: 1 g twice daily starting within 72 hours of transplantation

▼ PoM **CellCept®** (Roche)

Capsules, blue/brown, mycophenolate mofetil 250 mg, net price 300-cap pack = £356.25. Label: 23

Tablets, lavender, mycophenolate mofetil 500 mg, net price 50-tab pack = £118.75. Label: 23

8.2.2 Corticosteroids and other immunosuppressants

Prednisolone (section 6.3.2) is widely used in oncology. It has a marked antitumour effect in acute lymphoblastic leukaemia, Hodgkin's disease, and the non-Hodgkin lymphomas. It is also active in hormone-sensitive breast cancer and may cause useful disease regression. Finally, it has a role in the palliation of symptomatic end-stage malignant disease when it may produce a sense of well-being.

The corticosteroids are also powerful immunosuppressants. They are used to prevent organ transplant rejection, and in high dose to treat rejection episodes.

Cyclosporin is a fungal metabolite and potent immunosuppressant which is virtually non-myelotoxic but markedly nephrotoxic. It has found particular use in the field of organ and tissue transplantation, for prevention of graft rejection following bone marrow, kidney, liver, pancreas, heart, and heart-lung transplantation, and for prophylaxis of graft-versus-host disease.

Tacrolimus is a macrolide immunosuppressant. Although not chemically related to cyclosporin it has a similar mode of action and side-effects, but the incidence of neurotoxicity and nephrotoxicity appears to be greater; cardiomyopathy has also been reported. Disturbance of glucose metabolism also appears to be significant; hypertrichosis appears to be less of a problem than with cyclosporin.

IMPAIRED IMMUNE RESPONSIVENESS. For general comments and warnings relating to corticosteroids and immunosuppressants see section 6.3.2 (under Prednisolone) and p. 368 (Impaired Immune Responsiveness).

CYCLOSPORIN
(Ciclosporin)

Indications: see notes above, and under Dose; atopic dermatitis and psoriasis (section 13.5.2); rheumatoid arthritis (section 10.1.3)

Cautions: monitor kidney function—dose dependent increase in serum creatinine and urea during first few weeks may necessitate dose reduction in transplant patients (exclude rejection if kidney transplant) or discontinuation in non-transplant patients; monitor liver function (dosage adjustment based on bilirubin and liver enzymes may be needed); monitor blood pressure—discontinue if hypertension develops that cannot be controlled by antihypertensives; hyperuricaemia; monitor serum potassium especially in marked renal dysfunction (and avoid high dietary potassium); measure blood lipids before treatment and thereafter as appropriate; pregnancy (see p. 368) and breast-feeding (Appendix 5); porphyria (section 9.8.2); apart from specialist use in transplant patients preferably avoid other immunosuppressants with the exception of corticosteroids (oversuppression may increase susceptibility to infection and lymphoma); **interactions:** Appendix 1 (cyclosporin)

ADDITIONAL CAUTIONS. Atopic Dermatitis and Psoriasis, section 13.5.2; Rheumatoid Arthritis, section 10.1.3

Side-effects: commonly dose-dependent increase in serum creatinine and urea during first few weeks (see also under Cautions), and less commonly renal structural changes on long-term administration; also hypertrichosis, tremor, hypertension (especially in heart transplant patients) hepatic dysfunction, fatigue, gingival hypertrophy, gastro-intestinal disturbances, and burning sensation in hands and feet (usually during first week); *occasionally* headache, rash (possibly allergic); mild anaemia, hyperkalaemia, hyperuricaemia, gout, hypomagnesaemia, hypercholesterolaemia, weight increase, oedema, pancreatitis, neuropathy, confusion, paraesthesia, convulsions, dysmenorrhoea or amenorrhoea; muscle weakness, cramps, myopathy, gynaecomastia (in patients receiving concomitant spironolactone), colitis also reported; thrombocytopenia (sometimes with haemolytic uraemic syndrome) also reported; incidence of malignancies and lymphoproliferative disorders similar to that with conventional immunosuppressive therapy

Dose: organ transplantation, used alone, 10–15 mg/kg *by mouth* 4–12 hours before transplantation followed by 10–15 mg/kg daily for 1–2 weeks post-operatively then reduced to 2–6 mg/kg daily for maintenance (dose should be adjusted by monitoring blood concentrations and renal function); dose lower if given concomitantly with

other immunosuppressant therapy (e.g. corticosteroids); if necessary one-third oral dose can be given *by intravenous infusion* over 2–6 hours

Bone-marrow transplantation, prevention and treatment of graft-versus-host disease, 3–5 mg/kg daily *by intravenous infusion* over 2–6 hours from day before transplantation to 2 weeks post-operatively (or 12.5–15 mg/kg daily *by mouth*) then 12.5 mg/kg daily *by mouth* for 3–6 months then tailed off (may take up to a year after transplantation)

CONVERSION (from oral *Sandimmun*® to *Neoral*®). Measure trough blood-cyclosporin concentration, serum creatinine and blood pressure then give same dose (mg for mg) of *Neoral*® as previous oral *Sandimmun*®; repeat measurements 4–7 days after conversion (further measurements may be needed in first 2 months, e.g. week 2 and week 4) and adjust dose accordingly. Unlike oral *Sandimmun*® which may be taken either as a single daily dose (transplant recipients) or in 2 divided doses, the daily dose of *Neoral*® is always taken in 2 divided doses.

> Because of differences in bioavailability, the brand to be dispensed should be specified by the prescriber

PoM **Neoral**® (Novartis)

Capsules, cyclosporin 25 mg (blue/grey), net price 30-cap pack = £20.54; 50 mg (yellow/white), 30-cap pack = £40.22; 100 mg (blue/grey), 30-cap pack = £76.33. Counselling, administration

Oral solution, yellow, sugar-free, cyclosporin 100 mg/mL. Net price 50 mL = £114.38. Counselling, administration

COUNSELLING. Total daily dose should be taken in 2 divided doses. Avoid grapefruit or grapefruit juice for 1 hour before dose.

Mix solution with orange juice (or squash) or apple juice (to improve taste) or with water immediately before taking (and rinse with more to ensure total dose). Do not mix with grapefruit juice. Keep medicine measure away from other liquids (including water)

PoM **Sandimmun**® (Novartis)

[1]*Capsules,* cyclosporin 25 mg (pale pink), 30-cap pack; 50 mg (yellow), 30-cap pack; 100 mg (dusky pink), 30-cap pack. Counselling, administration

[1]*Oral solution,* oily, yellow, sugar-free, cyclosporin 100 mg/mL; 50 mL. Counselling, administration

COUNSELLING. Total daily dose may be taken as a single dose (transplant recipients) or in 2 divided doses. Avoid grapefruit or grapefruit juice for 1 hour before dose

To mask taste, mix solution with cold milk, cold chocolate drink, cola, or orange juice immediately before taking (and rinse with more to ensure total dose). Do not mix with grapefruit juice. Do not use plastic cup. Keep medicine measure away from other liquids (including water)

1. *Sandimmun*® capsules and oral solution available only on named-patient basis for patients who cannot be transferred to *Neoral*®

Concentrate for intravenous infusion (oily), cyclosporin 50 mg/mL. To be diluted before use. Net price 1-mL amp = £1.77; 5-mL amp = £8.38

Note. Contains polyethoxylated castor oil which has been associated with anaphylaxis—observe for at least 30 minutes after starting infusion and at frequent intervals thereafter

TACROLIMUS

Indications: primary immunosuppression in liver and kidney allograft recipients and allograft rejection resistant to conventional immunosuppressive regimens; see also notes above

Cautions: see under Cyclosporin; also monitor ECG (**important:** also echocardiography, see CSM warning below), visual status, blood glucose, haematological and neurological parameters; **interactions:** Appendix 1 (tacrolimus)

DRIVING. May affect performance of skilled tasks (e.g. driving)

Contra-indications: hypersensitivity to macrolides; pregnancy (exclude before starting—if contraception needed non-hormonal methods should be used), breast-feeding; avoid concurrent administration with cyclosporin (care if patient has previously received cyclosporin)

Side-effects: include gastro-intestinal disturbances such as nausea, dyspepsia and ulceration; hypertension, angina, tachycardia, pleural and pericardial effusion, less frequently hypotension, arrhythmias, rarely ventricular or septal hypertrophy, cardiomyopathy (**important:** see CSM warning below) and pericarditis; tremor, headache, insomnia, anxiety, depression, encephalopathy and rarely agitation, somnolence, hallucinations, dizziness, decreased reflexes, migraine, convulsions, confusion, amblyopia, cataract, retinopathy, photophobia, deafness and tinnitus; haematological effects including leucocytosis, leucopenia, aplastic and haemolytic anaemia and rarely thrombocytopaenia; increased serum creatinine and urea, less frequently kidney damage and renal failure; electrolyte disturbances including hypercalcaemia, hypokalaemia, hyperuricaemia, thyroid disorders, altered acid-base balance and glucose metabolism; pruritus, erythema, alopecia, sweating, hirsutism, photosensitivity; allergic reactions including anaphylaxis; gynaecomastia, oedema, hepatic dysfunction, cirrhosis, pancreatitis, weight and appetite changes, isolated cases of respiratory failure and pulmonary fibrosis

CSM Warning. Cardiomyopathy has been reported in children given tacrolimus after transplantation. Patients using the drug should be monitored carefully by echocardiography for hypertrophic changes; dose reduction or discontinuation should be considered if these occur

Dose: liver transplantation, starting 6 hours after transplantation, *by mouth,* 100–200 micrograms/kg daily in 2 divided doses *or by intravenous infusion* over 24 hours, 10–50 micrograms/kg; CHILD *by mouth,* 300 micrograms/kg daily in 2 divided doses *or by intravenous infusion* over 24 hours, 50 micrograms/kg

Renal transplantation, starting within 24 hours of transplantation, *by mouth,* 150–300 micrograms/kg daily in 2 divided doses *or by intravenous infusion* over 24 hours, 50–100 micrograms/kg; CHILD *by mouth,* 300 micrograms/kg daily in 2 divided doses *or by intravenous infusion* over 24 hours, 100 micrograms/kg

Maintenance treatment, dose adjusted according to response

PoM **Prograf®** (Fujisawa)

Capsules, tacrolimus 1 mg (white), net price 50-cap pack = £89.44; 5 mg (greyish-red), 50-cap pack = £447.20. Label: 23, counselling, driving

Concentrate for intravenous infusion, tacrolimus 5 mg/mL. To be diluted before use. Net price 1-mL amp = £67.67

Note. Contains polyethoxylated castor oil which has been associated with anaphylaxis

8.2.3   Immunostimulants

A suspension of inactivated *Corynebacterium parvum* organisms (Coparvax®) was formerly used by the intracavitary route to treat malignant effusions. It has now been discontinued.

8.2.4   Interferons

Interferons are naturally occurring proteins with complex effects on immunity and cell function.

INTERFERON ALFA

Interferon alfa (formerly called leucocyte interferon or lymphoblastoid interferon) has shown some antitumour effect in certain lymphomas and solid tumours. The precise role of interferons in cancer treatment is controversial and often ill-defined. They are toxic and their use is often best confined to trials designed to evaluate their antitumour efficacy. Side-effects are dose-related, but commonly include nausea, influenza-like symptoms, lethargy, ocular side-effects and depression (suicidal behaviour reported). Myelosuppression may also occur, particularly affecting granulocyte counts. Cardiovascular problems (hypotension, hypertension, and arrhythmias), nephrotoxicity and hepatotoxicity have been reported. Other side-effects include hypersensitivity reactions, thyroid abnormalities, hyperglycaemia, psoriasiform rash, confusion, and coma and seizures (usually with high doses in the elderly).

INTERFERON ALFA

Indications: see under preparations

Cautions; Contra-indications; Side-effects: see notes above—but for full details (including monitoring and dosage details) consult product literature; pregnancy (Appendix 4); **interactions:** Appendix 1 (interferons)

PoM **Intron A®** (Schering-Plough)

Injection, interferon alfa-2b (rbe) 5-million units/mL, net price 2-mL vial = £56.52; 5-mL vial = £141.30 (all with injection equipment). For subcutaneous and intramuscular injection

Injection, powder for reconstitution, interferon alfa-2b (rbe). Net price 1-million unit vial = £5.65; 3-million unit vial = £16.96; 5-million unit vial = £28.26; 10-million unit vial = £56.52; 18-million unit vial = £101.74 (all with injection equipment and water for injection). For subcutaneous and intramuscular injection

Both for use in AIDS-related Kaposi's sarcoma, hairy cell leukaemia, follicular lymphoma, chronic myelogenous leukaemia, lymph or liver metastases of carcinoid tumour, chronic active hepatitis B, chronic hepatitis C, adjunct in malignant melanoma and maintenance of remission in multiple myeloma

PoM **Roferon-A®** (Roche)

Injection, interferon alfa-2a (rbe). Net price 3-million units/mL, 1-mL vial = £16.96; 4.5-million units/mL, 1-mL vial = £25.44; 6-million units/mL, 0.5-mL prefilled syringe = £16.96, 3-mL vial = £101.77; 9-million units/mL, 0.5-mL prefilled syringe = £25.44; 12-million units/mL, 0.5-mL prefilled syringe = £33.92; 18-million units/mL, 0.5-mL prefilled syringe = £50.88. For subcutaneous injection (vials and prefilled syringes) and intramuscular injection (vials)

For AIDS-related Kaposi's sarcoma, hairy cell leukaemia, chronic myelogenous leukaemia, recurrent or metastatic renal cell carcinoma, progressive cutaneous T-cell lymphoma, chronic active hepatitis B and chronic hepatitis C; follicular non-Hodgkins lymphoma

PoM **Viraferon®** (Schering-Plough)

Injection, interferon alfa-2b (rbe) 6-million units/mL, net price 3-mL vial = £101.74. For subcutaneous injection

For chronic active hepatitis B and chronic hepatitis C

PoM **Wellferon®** (GlaxoWellcome)

Injection, interferon alfa-N1 (lns) 3 million units/mL, net price 1-mL vial = £16.96; 5 million units/mL, 1-mL vial = £28.26; 10 million units/mL, 1-mL vial = £56.52. For subcutaneous and intramuscular injection

For hairy cell leukaemia, chronic myeloid leukaemia, chronic active hepatitis B and chronic hepatitis C

INTERFERON BETA

Interferon beta (formerly called fibroblast interferon) is licensed for use in patients with relapsing, remitting *multiple sclerosis* (characterised by at least two attacks of neurological dysfunction over the previous two-year period, followed by complete or incomplete recovery) who are able to walk unaided. It is indicated for the reduction of frequency and degree of severity of clinical relapses. There is no evidence of an effect on the progression of the disease, on duration of exacerbations (or on symptoms between exacerbations), or on disability. Not all patients respond and a deterioration in the bouts has been observed in some.

Interferon beta should not be used in those with a history of severe depressive illness (or of suicidal ideation). It should also not be used in those with inadequately controlled epilepsy, or decompensated hepatic impairment; caution is advised in those with a history of these conditions or with cardiac disorders or myelosuppression. Most frequently reported side-effects include irritation at injection site (including inflammation, pain, hypersensitivity, necrosis) and flu-like symptoms (fever, chills, myalgia, malaise or sweating) but these decrease over time. Other side-effects include hypersensitivity reactions (including bronchospasm, anaphylaxis and urticaria), menstrual disorders, depression, anxiety, emotional lability, depersonalisation, convulsions, suicide attempts and confusion.

It is recommended that patients should be referred to a neurologist for a decision on whether treatment with interferon beta is indicated (see also Note below).

INTERFERON BETA

Indications: see notes above

Note. The Standing Medical Advisory Committee on the use of Interferon Beta-1b in Relapsing-Remitting Multiple Sclerosis in Adults has recommended that patients who apparently fulfil the indications for treatment should be referred to a neurologist for a decision on whether treatment in indicated

Cautions; Contra-indications; Side-effects: see notes above—but for full details (including monitoring and dosage details consult product literature; pregnancy (Appendix 4—advise contraceptive measures if appropriate), breast-feeding (Appendix 5); **interactions:** Appendix 1 (interferons)

Interferon beta-1a

▼ PoM **Avonex®** (Biogen)

Injection, powder for reconstitution, interferon beta-1a. Net price 30-microgram (6 million unit) vial with diluent = £182.50. For intramuscular injection

Interferon beta-1b

▼ PoM **Betaferon®** (Schering Health)

Injection, powder for reconstitution, interferon beta-1b. Net price 300-microgram (9.6 million unit) vial with diluent = £53.75. For subcutaneous injection

8.2.5   Aldesleukin

Aldesleukin (recombinant interleukin-2) is licensed for use by intravenous infusion in metastatic renal cell carcinoma. This is a very toxic drug which, although responsible for tumour shrinkage in a small proportion of patients, has not been shown to increase survival. Toxicity is universal and often severe. A common acute problem is the development of a capillary leak syndrome causing pulmonary oedema and hypotension. Bone marrow, hepatic, renal, thyroid, and CNS toxicity is also common. It is for use in **specialist units only**. **Interactions:** Appendix 1 (aldesleukin).

PoM **Proleukin®** (Chiron)

Injection, powder for reconstitution, aldesleukin. Net price 18-million unit vial = £140.00

For metastatic renal cell carcinoma, **excluding** patients in whom all three of the following prognostic factors are present; performance status of Eastern Co-operative Oncology Group of 1 or greater, more than one organ with metastatic disease sites, and a period of less than 24 months between initial diagnosis of primary tumour and date of evaluation of treatment.

8.3 Sex hormones and hormone antagonists in malignant disease

8.3.1   Oestrogens
8.3.2   Progestogens
8.3.3   Androgens
8.3.4   Hormone antagonists

Hormonal manipulation has an important role in the treatment of metastatic breast, prostate, and endometrial cancer, and a more marginal role in the treatment of hypernephroma. These treatments are not curative, but may provide excellent palliation of symptoms in selected patients, sometimes for a period of years. Tumour response, and treatment toxicity should be carefully monitored and treatment changed if progression occurs or side-effects exceed benefit.

8.3.1   Oestrogens
Stilboestrol is now rarely used to treat prostate cancer because of its side-effects. It is also occasionally used in postmenopausal women with breast cancer. Toxicity is common and dose-related side-effects include nausea, fluid retention, and venous and arterial thrombosis. Impotence and gynaecomastia always occur in men, and withdrawal bleeding may be a problem in women. Hypercalcaemia and bone pain may also occur in breast cancer.

Fosfestrol is also used for prostate cancer; it is activated by the enzyme acid phosphatase to produce stilboestrol. Side-effects are as for stilboestrol; in addition, perineal pain may complicate intravenous use.

Ethinyloestradiol is the most potent oestrogen available; unlike other oestrogens it is only slowly metabolised in the liver. It is used in breast cancer.

Polyestradiol is a long-acting oestrogen.

STILBOESTROL
(Diethylstilbestrol)
Indications: see notes above
Cautions; Side-effects: cardiovascular disease (sodium retention with oedema, thromboembolism), hepatic impairment (jaundice), feminising effects in men; see also notes above
Dose: breast cancer, 10–20 mg daily
Prostate cancer, 1–3 mg daily

PoM **Stilboestrol** (Non-proprietary)
Tablets, stilboestrol 1 mg, net price 56 = £8.33;
5 mg, 28 = £7.08
Available from APS (Apstil®)

ETHINYLOESTRADIOL
Indications: see notes above; other indications, see section 6.4.1.1
Cautions; Side-effects: see under Stilboestrol and notes above
Dose: breast cancer, 1–3 mg daily

Preparations
See section 6.4.1.1

FOSFESTROL TETRASODIUM
Indications: prostate cancer
Cautions; Contra-indications; Side-effects: see under Stilboestrol and notes above; nausea and vomiting; after intravenous injection, perineal irritation and pain in bony metastases
Dose: by slow intravenous injection, 600–1200 mg daily for at least 5 days; maintenance 300 mg 1–4 times weekly
By mouth, maintenance, initially up to 240 mg 3 times daily for 7 days then reducing over 14 days to 120–360 mg daily in divided doses

PoM **Honvan®** (ASTA Medica)
Tablets, f/c, fosfestrol tetrasodium 120 mg. Net price 100-tab pack = £15.51
Note. Fosfestrol tetrasodium 100 mg tablets have now been replaced by 120 mg tablets
Injection, fosfestrol tetrasodium 60 mg/mL. Net price 5-mL amp = £1.50

POLYESTRADIOL PHOSPHATE
Indications: prostate cancer
Cautions; Side-effects: see under Stilboestrol and notes above
Dose: by deep intramuscular injection, 80–160 mg every 4 weeks; maintenance 40–80 mg

PoM **Estradurin®** (Pharmacia & Upjohn)
Injection, powder for reconstitution, polyestradiol phosphate (with mepivacaine and nicotinamide). Net price 80-mg vial (with diluent) = £3.86

8.3.2   Progestogens

Progestogens are used largely as second- or third-line therapy in breast cancer. They are also used to treat endometrial cancer and hypernephroma, but are little used for prostate cancer. **Medroxyprogesterone** or **megestrol** are usually chosen and can be given orally; high-dose or parenteral treatment cannot be recommended. Side-effects are mild but may include nausea, fluid retention, and weight gain.

GESTRONOL HEXANOATE
(Gestonorone Caproate)
Indications: see notes above; benign prostatic hypertrophy
Cautions; Contra-indications; Side-effects: see under Medroxyprogesterone acetate (section 6.4.1.2) and notes above
Dose: endometrial cancer, *by intramuscular injection,* 200–400 mg every 5–7 days
Benign prostatic hypertrophy, *by intramuscular injection,* 200 mg every week, increased to 300–400 mg every week if necessary

PoM **Depostat®** (Cambridge)
Injection (oily), gestronol hexanoate 100 mg/mL. Net price 2-mL amp = £4.28

MEDROXYPROGESTERONE ACETATE

Indications: see notes above; other indications, see section 6.4.1.2

Cautions; Contra-indications; Side-effects: see section 6.4.1.2 and notes above; glucocorticoid effects at high dose may lead to a cushingoid syndrome; **interactions:** see Appendix 1 (progestogens)

Dose: by mouth, endometrial, prostate, and renal cancer, 100–500 mg daily; breast cancer, various doses in range 0.4–1.5 g daily

By deep intramuscular injection into the gluteal muscle, various doses in range 1 g daily down to 250 mg weekly

PoM **Depo-Provera®** (Pharmacia & Upjohn)

Injection, medroxyprogesterone acetate 150 mg/mL. Net price 3.3-mL (500-mg) vial = £12.49

PoM **Farlutal®** (Pharmacia & Upjohn)

Tablets, both scored, medroxyprogesterone acetate 100 mg, net price 20 = £8.12; 250 mg, 50 = £50.73

Tablets, scored, medroxyprogesterone acetate 500 mg. Net price 56 = £113.63. Label: 27

Injection, medroxyprogesterone acetate 200 mg/mL. Net price 2.5-mL vial = £13.88; 5-mL vial = £23.14

PoM **Provera®** (Pharmacia & Upjohn)

Tablets, medroxyprogesterone acetate 100 mg (scored), net price 60-tab pack = £24.98; 200 mg (scored), 30-tab pack = £24.71; 400 mg, 30-tab pack = £48.89

Tablets, medroxyprogesterone acetate 2.5 mg, 5 mg and 10 mg, see section 6.4.1.2

MEGESTROL ACETATE

Indications: see notes above

Cautions; Contra-indications; Side-effects: see under Medroxyprogesterone acetate (section 6.4.1.2) and notes above

Dose: breast cancer, 160 mg daily in single or divided doses; endometrial cancer, 40–320 mg daily in divided doses

PoM **Megace®** (Bristol-Myers)

Tablets, both scored, megestrol acetate 40 mg, net price 20 = £5.08; 160 mg (off-white), 30-tab pack = £29.30

NORETHISTERONE

Indications: see notes above; other indications, see section 6.4.1.2

Cautions; Contra-indications; Side-effects: see section 6.4.1.2 and notes above; **interactions:** see Appendix 1 (progestogens)

Dose: breast cancer, 40 mg daily, increased to 60 mg daily if required

Preparations

See section 6.4.1.2

8.3.3 Androgens

The androgens are given parenterally and are occasionally still used as second- or third-line therapy for metastatic breast cancer.

TESTOSTERONE ESTERS

Indications: see notes above; other indications, see section 6.4.2

Cautions; Contra-indications; Side-effects: see under Testosterone and Esters (section 6.4.2)

Dose: see under Preparations

PoM **Primoteston Depot®** (Schering Health)
See section 6.4.2

PoM **Virormone®** (Paines & Byrne)
See section 6.4.2

8.3.4 Hormone antagonists

8.3.4.1 BREAST CANCER

Tamoxifen is an oestrogen receptor antagonist and at a dose of 20 mg daily is the hormonal treatment of choice for breast cancer in postmenopausal women with metastatic disease; it is also increasingly commonly used as a first-line treatment for premenopausal women. Overall, approximately 30% of patients with metastatic breast cancer respond to hormonal manipulation. This figure is increased to 60% in patients with oestrogen receptor positive tumours; receptor negative tumours respond in less than 10%.

Adjuvant hormonal treatment with tamoxifen 20 mg daily is also the treatment of choice in postmenopausal patients with high-risk breast cancer after treatment of the primary. Such treatment has consistently prolonged the period between diagnosis and the development of metastases and has also clearly increased survival. Tamoxifen is also increasingly commonly used as adjuvant treatment for premenopausal women with early breast cancer.

Side-effects are unusual with tamoxifen but patients with bony metastases may experience an exacerbation of pain, sometimes associated with hypercalcaemia. This reaction commonly precedes tumour response. Amenorrhoea commonly develops in premenopausal women. For details of endometrial changes see under Cautions (below) and for CSM advice see under Dose (below)

Patients with non-threatening metastases unresponsive to tamoxifen may still respond to a secondary hormonal treatment. Certainly patients who initially respond to tamoxifen should receive second-line hormone treatment. No clear guidelines are available; for premenopausal patients oophorectomy or a progestogen (section 8.3.2) may be used; for postmenopausal patients a progestogen or an aromatase inhibitor (see below) may be used. Patients who respond can be given further hormones on relapse; refractory patients are better treated with chemotherapy or palliative therapy.

Toremifene, also an oestrogen receptor antagonist, is licensed for hormone-dependent metastatic breast cancer in postmenopausal women.

Aminoglutethimide acts predominantly by inhibiting the conversion of androgens to oestrogens in the peripheral tissues; in breast cancer it has largely been replaced by the newer aromatase inhibitors which are better tolerated. Corticosteroid replacement therapy is necessary (section 6.3.1). Aminoglutethimide is also used as second-line treatment for prostate cancer (section 8.3.4.2). Early toxicity is common and may include drowsiness, drug fever, and a morbilliform eruption; these side-effects generally settle spontaneously. Hepatic enzyme induction occurs, and may require modification of the doses of other drugs (e.g. oral anticoagulants).

Trilostane (section 6.7.3) is also indicated for postmenopausal breast cancer. It is quite well tolerated but diarrhoea and abdominal discomfort may be a problem. Like aminoglutethimide, trilostane is an adrenal antagonist therefore corticosteroid replacement therapy is needed.

Formestane, an inhibitor of the enzyme aromatase (which metabolises androgens to oestrogens) is indicated for breast cancer in women with natural or artificial postmenopausal status.

Anastrozole is a selective non-steroidal aromatase inhibitor used to treat advanced postmenopausal breast cancer; steroid replacement therapy is not necessary.

Letrozole is another selective non-steroidal aromatase inhibitor indicated for postmenopausal women with advanced breast cancer in whom tamoxifen has failed; steroid replacement therapy is not necessary.

Goserelin (section 8.3.4.2), a gonadorelin analogue is now also indicated for management of advanced breast cancer in premenopausal women.

TAMOXIFEN

Indications: see under Dose and notes above

Cautions: occasional cystic ovarian swellings in premenopausal women, occasional hypercalcaemia if bony metastases; increased risk of thromboembolic events when used with cytotoxics; porphyria (section 9.8.2); **interactions:** Appendix 1 (tamoxifen)

ENDOMETRIAL CHANGES. An increased incidence of endometrial changes, including hyperplasia, polyps and cancer, has been reported in association with tamoxifen. Abnormal vaginal bleeding including menstrual irregularities, vaginal discharge and symptoms such as pelvic pain or pressure in those receiving (or who have previously received) tamoxifen should be promptly investigated.

Contra-indications: pregnancy (exclude before commencing and advise non-hormonal contraception if appropriate) and breast-feeding

Side-effects: hot flushes, vaginal bleeding (**important:** see also Cautions) or suppression of menstruation in some pre-menopausal women, vaginal discharge (**important:** see also Cautions), pruritus vulvae, gastro-intestinal disturbances, light-headedness, tumour flare, falls in platelet counts; occasionally fluid retention, alopecia, rashes, uterine fibroids; also visual disturbances (including corneal changes, cataracts, retinopathy—usually with very high doses); leucopenia (sometimes with anaemia and thrombocytope-

nia), rarely neutropenia; liver enzyme changes (rarely fatty liver, cholestasis, hepatitis); see also notes above

Dose: breast cancer, 20 mg daily

CSM ADVICE. The CSM has advised that tamoxifen in a dose of 20 mg daily substantially increases survival in early breast cancer, and that no further benefit has been demonstrated with higher doses. Patients should be told of the small risk of endometrial cancer (see under Cautions above) and encouraged to report relevant symptoms early. They can, however, be reassured that the benefits of treatment far outweigh the risks

Anovulatory infertility, 20 mg daily on second, third, fourth and fifth days of cycle; if necessary the daily dose may be increased to 40 mg then 80 mg for subsequent courses; if cycles irregular, start initial course on any day, with subsequent course starting 45 days later *or* on second day of cycle if menstruation occurs

PoM **Tamoxifen** (Non-proprietary)

Tablets, tamoxifen (as citrate) 10 mg, net price 30-tab pack = £2.59; 20 mg, 30-tab pack = £1.99; 40 mg, 30-tab pack = £13.32

Various strengths available from APS, Ashbourne (Oestrifen®), Berk (Emblon®), Cox, CP, Hillcross, Kent, Lagap, Lennon, Norton, Opus (Fentamox®), Pharmacia & Upjohn (Tamofen®)

PoM **Nolvadex®** (Zeneca)

Tablets, tamoxifen (as citrate) 10 mg, net price 30-tab pack = £6.05; 20 mg (Nolvadex-D®), 30-tab pack = £9.12; 40 mg (scored, Nolvadex-Forte®), 30-tab pack = £21.45

AMINOGLUTETHIMIDE

Indications: see notes above and under Dose

Cautions: see notes above; adrenal hypofunction (see below); monitor blood pressure, plasma electrolytes, blood counts, and thyroid function; **interactions:** Appendix 1 (aminoglutethimide)

ADRENAL HYPOFUNCTION. May cause adrenal hypofunction especially under conditions of stress (such as surgery, trauma, or acute illness), therefore corticosteroid replacement therapy is necessary (see section 6.3.1). If a synthetic glucocorticoid such as dexamethasone is used instead of hydrocortisone a relatively high dose may be needed (metabolism of synthetic corticosteroids accelerated)

Contra-indications: pregnancy (advise non-hormonal contraceptive methods if appropriate) and breast-feeding; porphyria (see section 9.8.2)

Side-effects: see notes above; drowsiness, lethargy, rash (sometimes with fever—usually in first 2 weeks and resolves despite continued administration); occasionally dizziness, nausea; other side-effects reported include ataxia, headache, depression, insomnia, pruritus, urticaria, diarrhoea, vomiting, constipation, anorexia, sweating, hypotension, adrenal insufficiency, hyponatraemia, hypoglycaemia, agranulocytosis, leucopenia, thrombocytopenia, hyperkalaemia, exfoliaive dermatitis, Stevens-Johnson syndrome, hypothyroidism, inappropriate ADH-secretion, masculinisation and hirsuitism in females, renal impairment, pancytopenia, anaemia, allergy, anaphylactic reactions, allergic alveolitis (withdraw immediately if suspected), cholestatic hepatitis, confusion

Dose: advanced breast or prostate cancer, 250 mg daily, increased once a week to max. 250 mg 4 times daily (in breast cancer 250 mg twice daily has proved sufficient in some patients; in prostate cancer up to 750 mg daily is usually satisfactory); given with a glucocorticoid (and sometimes with a mineralocorticoid as well)

Cushing's syndrome due to malignant disease, 250 mg daily, increased gradually to 1 g daily in divided doses (occasionally 1.5–2 g daily); glucocorticoid given only if necessary

PoM **Orimeten**® (Novartis)

Tablets, scored, aminoglutethimide 250 mg. Net price 56-tab pack = £20.22. Label: 2

Note. Tablets containing aminoglutethimide 250 mg are also available from Pharmacia & Upjohn

ANASTROZOLE

Indications: advanced breast cancer in postmenopausal women

Cautions: laboratory test for menopause if doubt

Contra-indications: pregnancy and breast-feeding; moderate or severe hepatic disease, moderate or severe renal impairment; not for premenopausal women

Side-effects: hot flushes, vaginal dryness, hair thinning, anorexia, nausea, vomiting, diarrhoea, headache, rash; asthenia and somnolence—may initially affect ability to drive or operate machinery; slight increases in total cholesterol levels reported

Dose: 1 mg daily

▼ PoM **Arimidex**® (Zeneca)

Tablets, f/c, anastrozole 1 mg. Net price 28-tab pack = £83.16 (also 84-tab pack, hosp. only)

FORMESTANE

Indications: advanced breast cancer in women with natural or artificial postmenopausal status

Cautions: no studies performed in diabetes mellitus (monitor blood glucose)

DRIVING. Drowsiness may affect performance of skilled tasks (e.g. driving)

Contra-indications: not indicated for premenopausal women; pregnancy and breast-feeding

Side-effects: nausea, vomiting, rash, pruritus, exanthema, hot flushes; rarely, facial hypertrichosis, alopecia, lethargy, drowsiness, emotional lability, headache, dizziness, oedema of lower leg, thrombophlebitis, vaginal bleeding and inflammation, pelvic cramps, constipation, diarrhoea, arthralgia and exacerbation of bone pain, muscle cramps, sore throat, and anaphylactoid reaction; pain and irritation common at injection site (with occasional sterile abscess and rarely haematoma)

Dose: by deep intramuscular injection in the gluteal muscle, 250 mg every 2 weeks (alternate sites)

PoM **Lentaron**® (Novartis)

Injection, powder for reconstitution, formestane 250 mg. Net price 250-mg vial (with diluent) = £72.73. Counselling, driving

LETROZOLE

Indications: advanced breast cancer in postmenopausal women in whom other anti-oestrogen therapy has failed

Cautions: severe renal impairment

Contra-indications: severe hepatic impairment; not indicated for premenopausal women; pregnancy and breast-feeding

Side-effects: hot flushes, nausea, vomiting, dyspepsia, constipation, diarrhoea, abdominal pain, anorexia (and weight gain), dyspnoea, chest pain, coughing, dizziness, fatigue, headache, infection, musculoskeletal pain, peripheral oedema, rash, pruritus

Dose: 2.5 mg daily until tumour progression is evident

▼ PoM **Femara**® (Novartis)

Tablets, f/c, letrozole 2.5 mg. Net price 14-tab pack = £41.58, 28-tab pack = £83.16

TOREMIFENE

Indications: hormone-dependent metastatic breast cancer in postmenopausal women

Cautions: hypercalcaemia may occur (especially if bone metastases and usually at beginning of treatment); **interactions:** Appendix 1 (toremifene)

ENDOMETRIAL CHANGES. There is a risk of increased endometrial changes including hyperplasia, polyps and cancer. Abnormal vaginal bleeding including menstrual irregularities, vaginal discharge and symptoms such as pelvic pain or pressure should be promptly investigated

Contra-indications: endometrial hyperplasia, severe hepatic impairment, history of severe thromboembolic disease; pregnancy and breast-feeding

Side-effects: hot flushes, vaginal bleeding or discharge (**important:** see also Cautions), dizziness, oedema, sweating, nausea, vomiting, chest or back pain, fatigue, headache, skin discoloration, weight increase, insomnia, constipation, dyspnoea, paresis, tremor, vertigo, pruritus, anorexia, corneal opacity (reversible), asthenia; thromboembolic events reported; rarely dermatitis, alopecia, emotional lability, depression, jaundice, stiffness

Dose: 60 mg daily

▼ PoM **Fareston**® (Orion)

Tablets, toremifene (as citrate) 60 mg. Net price 30-tab pack = £31.80

8.3.4.2 PROSTATE CANCER

Metastatic cancer of the prostate is commonly responsive to hormonal treatment designed to deprive the cancer of androgen. Treatment is probably best reserved for symptomatic metastatic disease. The standard treatment is bilateral subcapsular orchidectomy, which commonly results in responses lasting 12–18 months. Alternatively, a gonadorelin analogue such as **buserelin**, **goserelin**, **leuprorelin**, or **triptorelin** may be given. These are as effective as orchidectomy or **stilboestrol** (section 8.3.1) but are expensive and require parenteral administration, at least initially. They cause initial stimulation of luteinising hormone release by the pituitary, which in turn causes testosterone secretion by the testis; this is followed by inhibition of luteinising hormone release with achievement of an anorchic state. During the first 1 to 2 weeks of treatment a number of patients develop a tumour 'flare' which may cause spinal cord compression or increased bone pain. When such problems are anticipated, alternative treatments (e.g. orchidectomy) or the additional use of an anti-androgen such as cyproterone acetate or flutamide (see below) are recommended; anti-androgen treatment should be started 3 days before the gonadorelin analogue and continued for 3 weeks. Other side-effects of gonadorelin analogues are similar to those of orchidectomy.

Cyproterone acetate, **flutamide** and **bicalutamide** are anti-androgens which can be used to cover the tumour 'flare' which may occur after commencing gonadorelin analogue administration.

Alternative therapies if disease progression occurs despite orchidectomy or administration of gonadorelin analogue, include the use of radiotherapy, strontium, aminoglutethimide (section 8.3.4.1) or prednisolone (see section 6.3.2). Such second-line treatment may palliate symptoms well, but rarely results in appreciable disease regression.

BICALUTAMIDE

Indications: advanced prostate cancer, see also notes above

Cautions: hepatic impairment (monitor hepatic function); **interactions:** Appendix 1 (bicalutamide)

Side-effects: hot flushes, pruritus, breast tenderness, gynaecomastia, asthenia, somnolence; transient elevation of transaminase levels, cholestasis and jaundice (rarely hepatic failure); rarely thrombocytopenia, cardiovascular disorders (including angina, heart failure, conduction defects, arrhythmias and ECG changes); other effects (more common in elderly) include anorexia, dry mouth, dyspepsia, constipation, flatulence, dizziness, insomnia, decreased libido, impotence, dyspnoea, nocturia, alopecia, rashes, sweating, hyperglycaemia, peripheral oedema, weight changes, chest and abdominal pain

Dose: 50 mg daily (see also notes above)

PoM **Casodex**® (Zeneca)
Tablets, f/c, bicalutamide 50 mg. Net price 28-tab pack = £128.00

BUSERELIN

Indications: advanced prostate cancer; other indications, see section 6.7.2

Cautions: during first month monitor patients at risk of ureteric obstruction or spinal cord compression, see notes above

Side-effects: initial increase in bone pain (due to transient increases in plasma testosterone); hot flushes, decreased libido, depression, headache, dizziness, nausea, vomiting, and diarrhoea, infrequent gynaecomastia, urticaria; irritation of nasal mucosa (spray formulation only)

Dose: by subcutaneous injection, 500 micrograms every 8 hours for 7 days, then *intranasally,* 1 spray into each nostril 6 times daily (see also notes above)

COUNSELLING. Avoid use of nasal decongestants before and for at least 30 minutes after treatment.

PoM **Suprefact**® (Shire)
Injection, buserelin 1 mg (as acetate)/mL. Net price 2 × 5.5-mL vial = £29.61
Nasal spray, buserelin 100 micrograms (as acetate)/metered spray. Net price treatment pack of 4 × 10-g bottle with spray pump = £97.42. Counselling, see above

CYPROTERONE ACETATE

Indications: prostate cancer, see also notes above and for CSM advice see below; other indications, see section 6.4.2

RESTRICTION ON USE. The CSM has advised that in view of the hepatotoxicity associated with long-term doses of 300 mg daily the use of cyproterone acetate in prostate cancer should be restricted to short courses to cover testosterone flare associated with gonadorelin analogues, treatment of hot flushes after orchidectomy or gonadorelin analogues and for patients who have not responded to (or are intolerant of) other treatments

Cautions: in prostate cancer, blood counts initially and throughout treatment, monitor hepatic function (liver function tests should be performed before treatment, see also under Side-effects below); monitor adrenocortical function regularly; risk of recurrence of thromboembolic disease; diabetes mellitus, sickle-cell anaemia, severe depression (in other indications some of these are contra-indicated, see section 6.4.2)

Contra-indications: none in prostate cancer; for contra-indications relating to other indications see section 6.4.2

Side-effects: see section 6.4.2

HEPATOTOXICITY. Direct hepatic toxicity including jaundice, hepatitis and hepatic failure have been reported (usually after several months) in patients treated with cyproterone acetate 200–300 mg daily. Liver function tests should be performed before treatment and whenever symptoms suggestive of hepatotoxicity occur—if confirmed cyproterone should normally be withdrawn unless the hepatotoxicity can be explained by another cause such as metastatic disease (in which case cyproterone should be continued only if the perceived benefit exceeds the risk)

Dose: flare with initial gonadorelin therapy, 300 mg daily in 2–3 divided doses, reduced to 200 mg daily if necesssary

Long-term palliative therapy where gonadorelin analogues or orchidectomy contra-indicated, not tolerated, or where oral therapy preferred, 200–300 mg daily

Hot flushes with gonadorelin therapy or after orchidectomy, 50 mg daily; usual range 50–150 mg daily in 1–3 divided doses

PoM **Cyprostat®** (Schering Health)

Tablets, scored, cyproterone acetate 50 mg net price 168-tab pack = £96.70; 100 mg, 84-tab pack = £96.70. Label: 3, 21

Note. Tablets containing cyproterone acetate 50 mg are also available from Cox, Generics, Hillcross, Lagap

FLUTAMIDE

Indications: advanced prostate cancer, see also notes above

Cautions: cardiac disease (sodium retention with oedema); monitor hepatic function (hepatotoxic); **interactions:** Appendix 1 (flutamide)

Side-effects: gynaecomastia (sometimes with galactorrhoea); nausea, vomiting, diarrhoea, increased appetite, insomnia, tiredness; other side-effects reported include decreased libido, inhibition of spermatogenesis, gastric and chest pain, headache, dizziness, oedema, blurred vision, thirst, rashes, pruritus, haemolytic anaemia, systemic lupus erythematosus-like syndrome, and lymphoedema; hepatic injury (with transaminase abnormalities, cholestatic jaundice, hepatic necrosis, encephalopathy and occasional fatality) reported

Dose: 250 mg 3 times daily (see also notes above)

PoM **Flutamide** (Non-proprietary)

Tablets, flutamide 250 mg. Net price 84-tab pack = £96.12

Available from Boehringer Mannheim, Chiron (*Chimax®*), Cox, Hillcross, Orion

PoM **Drogenil®** (Schering-Plough)

Tablets, yellow, scored, flutamide 250 mg, net price 84-tab pack = £110.00

GOSERELIN

Indications: prostate cancer; advanced breast cancer; other indications, see section 6.7.2

Cautions: see under Buserelin

Contra-indications: pregnancy (use non-hormonal method of contraception), breast-feeding; undiagnosed vaginal bleeding

Side-effects: see under Buserelin; also rashes (reversible without stopping therapy); bruising at injection site; rotate injection site periodically; rarely hypercalcaemia in breast cancer patients

Dose: see under individual preparations

PoM **Zoladex®** (Zeneca)

Implant, goserelin 3.6 mg (as acetate) in syringe applicator. Net price each = £122.27

Dose: advanced breast cancer and prostate cancer *by subcutaneous injection* into anterior abdominal wall, 3.6 mg every 28 days (see also notes above)

PoM **Zoladex® LA** (Zeneca)

Implant, goserelin 10.8 mg (as acetate) in syringe applicator. Net price each = £366.81

Dose: prostate cancer, *by subcutaneous injection* into anterior abdominal wall, 10.8 mg every 12 weeks (see also notes above)

LEUPRORELIN ACETATE

Indications: advanced prostate cancer; other indications, see section 6.7.2

Cautions; Side-effects: see under Buserelin; also, infrequently, peripheral oedema, fatigue, nausea, irritation at injection site; rotate injection site periodically

Dose: see under individual preparations

PoM **Prostap SR®** (Wyeth)

Injection (powder for reconstitution), leuprorelin acetate, net price 3.75-mg vial with 1 mL vehicle-filled syringe = £125.40

Dose: advanced prostate cancer and endometriosis, *by subcutaneous or by intramuscular injection*, 3.75 mg every 4 weeks (see also notes above)

PoM **Prostap® 3** (Wyeth)

Injection (powder for reconstitution), leuprorelin acetate, net price 11.25-mg vial with 2 mL vehicle-filled syringe = £376.20

Dose: advanced prostate cancer, *by subcutaneous injection*, 11.25 mg every three months (see also notes above)

TRIPTORELIN

Indications: advanced prostate cancer; endometriosis, section 6.7.2

Cautions; Side-effects: see under Buserelin; also phlebitis, transient hypertension; rarely gastric pain, dry mouth, recurrence af asthma, dysuria, fever, pruritus, sweating, paraesthesia, insomnia, excessive salivation, vertigo, slight hair loss; pain, erythema and induration at injection site also reported

Dose: by intramuscular injection, 3 mg every 4 weeks (see also notes above)

▼ PoM **De-capeptyl® sr** (Speywood)

Injection (copolymer microsphere powder for aqueous suspension), triptorelin. Net price 4.2-mg vial (with diluent) = £110.00

8.3.4.3 GASTRO-ENTEROPANCREATIC TUMOURS

Octreotide is a long-acting analogue of the hypothalamic release-inhibiting hormone somatostatin; it is indicated for the relief of symptoms associated with gastro-enteropancreatic endocrine tumours and acromegaly.

OCTREOTIDE

Indications: see under Dose

Cautions: occasional sudden escape from symptomatic control with rapid recurrence of severe symptoms; in insulinoma may increase depth and duration of hypoglycaemia (close observation initially and with dose changes; marked fluctuations may be reduced by increasing administration frequency); in diabetes mellitus may reduce insulin or oral antidiabetic requirements; monitor thyroid function on long-term therapy; inhibits gallbladder motility, bile secretion and flow—ultrasonic examination of gall bladder before and at intervals of 6–12 months during treatment; avoid abrupt withdrawal (see side-effects below); **interactions:** Appendix 1 (octreotide)

Contra-indications: pregnancy (unless compelling reasons) and breast-feeding

Side-effects: gastro-intestinal disturbances including anorexia, nausea, vomiting, abdominal pain and bloating, flatulence, diarrhoea, and steatorrhoea; symptoms may be reduced by injecting between meals or at bedtime; impairment of postprandial glucose tolerance (rarely persistent hyperglycaemia on chronic administration); hepatic disturbance reported; gall stone formation reported after long-term treatment (abrupt withdrawal may result in biliary hypercontractility with associated biliary colic and pancreatitis); pain and irritation at injection site (rotate sites)

Dose: symptoms associated with carcinoid tumours with features of carcinoid syndrome, VIPomas, glucagonomas, *by subcutaneous injection,* initially 50 micrograms once or twice daily, gradually increased according to response to 200 micrograms 3 times daily (higher doses required exceptionally); maintenance doses variable; in carcinoid tumours discontinue after 1 week if no effect; if rapid response required, initial dose *by intravenous injection* (with ECG monitoring and after dilution to a concentration of 10–50% with sodium chloride 0.9% injection)

Acromegaly, short-term treatment before pituitary surgery *or* long-term treatment in those inadequately controlled by other treatment *or* until radiotherapy becomes fully effective *by subcutaneous injection,* 100–200 micrograms 3 times daily; discontinue if no improvement within 3 months

PoM **Sandostatin**® (Novartis)

Injection, octreotide (as acetate)
50 micrograms/mL, 1-mL amp = £2.90;
100 micrograms/mL, 1-mL amp = £5.46;
200 micrograms/mL 5-mL vial = £54.39;
500 micrograms/mL, 1-mL amp = £26.45

9: Drugs affecting
NUTRITION and BLOOD

In this chapter drugs and preparations are discussed under the following headings:

- **9.1** Anaemias and some other blood disorders
- **9.2** Fluids and electrolytes
- **9.3** Intravenous nutrition
- **9.4** Oral nutrition
- **9.5** Minerals
- **9.6** Vitamins
- **9.7** Bitters and tonics
- **9.8** Metabolic disorders

9.1 Anaemias and some other blood disorders

- **9.1.1** Iron-deficiency anaemias
- **9.1.2** Megaloblastic anaemias
- **9.1.3** Hypoplastic and haemolytic anaemias
- **9.1.4** Autoimmune thrombocytopenic purpura
- **9.1.5** G6PD deficiency
- **9.1.6** Drugs used in neutropenia

Before initiating treatment for anaemia it is essential to determine which type is present. Iron salts may be harmful and result in iron overload if given alone to patients with anaemias other than those due to iron deficiency.

9.1.1 Iron-deficiency anaemias

- **9.1.1.1** Oral iron
- **9.1.1.2** Parenteral iron

Treatment is only justified in the presence of a demonstrable iron-deficiency state. Before starting treatment, it is important to exclude any serious underlying cause of the anaemia (e.g. gastric erosion, colonic carcinoma).

Prophylaxis is justifiable in pregnancy for women who have additional risk factors for iron deficiency (e.g. poor diet), menorrhagia, after subtotal or total gastrectomy, and in the management of low birth-weight infants such as premature babies, twins, and in infants delivered by caesarean section.

9.1.1.1 ORAL IRON

Iron salts should be given by mouth unless there are good reasons for using another route.

Ferrous salts show only marginal differences between one another in efficiency of absorption of iron, but ferric salts are much less well absorbed. Haemoglobin regeneration rate is little affected by the type of salt used provided sufficient iron is given, and in most patients the time factor is not critical. Choice of preparation is thus usually decided by incidence of side-effects and cost.

The oral dose of elemental iron for deficiency should be 100 to 200 mg daily. It is customary to give this as dried **ferrous sulphate**, 200 mg (≡ 65 mg elemental iron) three times daily; a dose of ferrous sulphate 200 mg once or twice daily may be effective for prophylaxis or for mild iron deficiency. If side-effects arise, dosage can be reduced or a change made to an alternative iron salt. It should be remembered, however, that an apparent improvement in tolerance on changing to another salt may be due to its lower content of elemental iron. The incidence of side-effects due to ferrous sulphate is no greater than with other iron salts when compared on the basis of equivalent amounts of elemental iron.

Iron content of different iron salts

Iron salt	Amount	Content of ferrous iron
Ferrous fumarate	200 mg	65 mg
Ferrous gluconate	300 mg	35 mg
Ferrous succinate	100 mg	35 mg
Ferrous sulphate	300 mg	60 mg
Ferrous sulphate, dried	200 mg	65 mg

THERAPEUTIC RESPONSE. The haemoglobin concentration should rise by about 100–200 mg per 100 mL (1–2 g per litre) per day *or* 2 g/100 mL (20 g/litre) over 3–4 weeks. After the haemoglobin has risen to normal, treatment should be continued for a further three months in an attempt to replenish the iron stores. Epithelial tissue changes such as atrophic glossitis and koilonychia are usually improved although the response is often slow.

COMPOUND PREPARATIONS. Some oral preparations contain ascorbic acid to aid absorption, or the iron is in the form of a chelate, which can be shown experimentally to produce a modest increase in absorption of iron. However, the therapeutic advantage is minimal and cost may be increased.

There is neither theoretical nor clinical justification for the inclusion of other therapeutically active ingredients, such as the B group of vitamins (except folic acid for pregnant women, see Iron and Folic Acid below and p. 395).

MODIFIED-RELEASE CAPSULES AND TABLETS. These are designed to release iron gradually as the capsule or tablet passes along the gut so that a smaller amount of iron is present in the lumen at any one time. It is claimed that each dose unit contains enough iron for 24 hours, thus permitting once daily dosage.

These preparations are likely to carry the iron past the first part of the duodenum into an area of the gut where conditions for iron absorption are poor. The low incidence of side-effects may well be because of the small amounts of iron available under these conditions and so the preparations have no therapeutic advantage and should not be used.

SIDE-EFFECTS. Because iron salts are astringent, gastro-intestinal irritation may occur. Nausea and epigastric pain are dose-related but the relationship between dose and altered bowel habit (constipation or diarrhoea) is less clear. Oral iron, particularly modified-release preparations, may exacerbate diarrhoea in patients with inflammatory bowel disease; care is also needed in patients with intestinal strictures and diverticulae.

Iron preparations taken orally may have a constipating effect particularly in older patients, occasionally leading to faecal impaction.

FERROUS SULPHATE

Indications: iron-deficiency anaemia

Cautions: pregnancy; **interactions:** Appendix 1 (iron)

Side-effects: see notes above

Dose: see under preparations below

COUNSELLING. Although iron preparations are best absorbed on an empty stomach they may be taken after food to reduce gastro-intestinal side-effects; they may discolour stools

Ferrous Sulphate (Non-proprietary)

Tablets, coated, dried ferrous sulphate 200 mg (65 mg iron), net price 20 = 11p

Dose: prophylactic, 1 tablet daily; therapeutic, 1 tablet 2–3 times daily

Ferrous Sulphate Oral Solution, Paediatric, BP

(Paediatric Ferrous Sulphate Mixture)

Mixture, ferrous sulphate 1.2% and a suitable antioxidant in a suitable vehicle with an orange flavour. Extemporaneous preparations should be recently prepared according to the following formula: ferrous sulphate 60 mg, ascorbic acid 10 mg, orange syrup 0.5 mL, double-strength chloroform water 2.5 mL, water to 5 mL

Dose: therapeutic, CHILD up to 1 year, 5 mL 3 times daily; 1–5 years, 10 mL 3 times daily; 6–12 years, 15 mL 3 times daily *or* 25 mL twice daily. To be taken well diluted with water

Note. Orange syrup may be difficult to obtain; Paediatric Ferrous Sulphate Oral Solution, BP available from Martindale (special order)

Modified-release preparations

~~NHS~~ **Feospan®** (Evans)

Spansule® (= capsules m/r), clear/red, enclosing green and brown pellets, dried ferrous sulphate 150 mg (47 mg iron). Net price 30-cap pack = £1.11. Label: 25

Dose: 1–2 capsules daily; CHILD over 1 year 1 capsule daily; can be opened and sprinkled on food

Ferrograd® (Abbott)

Filmtabs® (= tablets f/c), m/r, red, dried ferrous sulphate 325 mg (105 mg iron). Net price 30-tab pack = 54p. Label: 25

Dose: 1 tablet daily before food

Slow-Fe® (Novartis)

Tablets, m/r, dried ferrous sulphate 160 mg (50 mg iron). Net price 28-tab pack = 25p. Label: 25

Dose: prophylactic, 1 tablet daily; therapeutic, 2 tablets daily; CHILD over 6 years, 1 tablet daily

FERROUS FUMARATE

Indications; Cautions; Side-effects: see under Ferrous Sulphate

Dose: see under preparations below

Fersaday® (Goldshield)

Tablets, brown, f/c, ferrous fumarate 322 mg (100 mg iron). Net price 28-tab pack = 50p

Dose: prophylactic, 1 tablet daily; therapeutic, 1 tablet twice daily

Fersamal® (Goldshield)

Tablets, brown, ferrous fumarate 200 mg (65 mg iron). Net price 20 = 23p

Dose: 1–2 tablets 3 times daily

Syrup, brown, ferrous fumarate 140 mg (45 mg iron)/5 mL. Net price 200 mL = £2.35

Dose: 10–20 mL twice daily; PREMATURE INFANT 0.6–2.4 mL/kg daily; CHILD up to 6 years 2.5–5 mL twice daily

Galfer® (Galen)

Capsules, red/green, ferrous fumarate 305 mg (100 mg iron). Net price 20 = 36p

Dose: 1 capsule 1–2 times daily before food

Syrup, brown, sugar-free ferrous fumarate 140 mg (45 mg iron)/5 mL. Net price 300 mL = £4.86

Dose: 10 mL 1–2 times daily before food; CHILD (full-term infant and young child) 2.5–5 mL 1–2 times daily

FERROUS GLUCONATE

Indications; Cautions; Side-effects: see under Ferrous Sulphate

Dose: see under preparations below

Ferrous Gluconate (Non-proprietary)

Tablets, red, coated, ferrous gluconate 300 mg (35 mg iron). Net price 20 = 10p

Dose: prophylactic, 2 tablets daily before food; therapeutic, 4–6 tablets daily in divided doses before food; CHILD 6–12 years, prophylactic and therapeutic, 1–3 tablets daily

FERROUS GLYCINE SULPHATE

Indications; Cautions; Side-effects: see under Ferrous Sulphate

Dose: see under preparation below

Plesmet® (Link)

Syrup, ferrous glycine sulphate equivalent to 25 mg iron/5 mL. Net price 100 mL = 65p

Dose: 5–10 mL 3 times daily; CHILD 2.5–5 mL 1–3 times daily, according to age

POLYSACCHARIDE-IRON COMPLEX

Indications; Cautions; Side-effects: see under Ferrous Sulphate

Dose: see under preparations below

Niferex® (Tillomed)

Elixir, brown, sugar-free, polysaccharide-iron complex equivalent to 100 mg of iron/5 mL. Net price 240-mL pack = £6.06; ~~NHS~~* 30-mL dropper bottle for paediatric use = £2.16. Counselling, use of dropper

Dose: prophylactic, 2.5 mL daily; therapeutic, 5 mL 1–2 times daily (once daily if required during second and third trimester of pregnancy); INFANT, (from dropper bottle) 1 drop (approx. 500 micrograms) per pound (450 g) body-weight 3 times daily; CHILD 2–6 years, 2.5 mL daily, 6–12 years 5 mL daily

* except 30 mL paediatric dropper bottle for prophylaxis and treatment of iron deficiency in infants born prematurely and endorsed 'SLS'

NHS **Niferex-150®** (Tillomed)
Capsules, brown/orange, polysaccharide-iron complex equivalent to 150 mg of iron. Net price 20 = £2.74
Dose: 1 capsule daily

SODIUM IRONEDETATE
(Sodium feredetate)
Indications; Cautions; Side-effects: see under Ferrous Sulphate
Dose: see under preparations below

Sytron® (Link)
Elixir, sugar-free, sodium ironedetate 190 mg equivalent to 27.5 mg of iron/5 mL. Net price 100 mL = 99p
Dose: 5 mL increasing gradually to 10 mL 3 times daily; INFANT and PREMATURE INFANT 2.5 mL twice daily (smaller doses should be used initially); CHILD 1–5 years 2.5 mL 3 times daily, 6–12 years 5 mL 3 times daily

IRON AND FOLIC ACID

These preparations are used for the prevention of iron and folic acid deficiencies in pregnancy; they should be distinguished from those used for the prevention of neural tube defects in women planning a pregnancy (see p. 395).

It is important to note that the small doses of folic acid contained in these preparations are inadequate for the treatment of megaloblastic anaemias.

NHS **Fefol®** (Evans)
Spansule® (=capsules m/r), clear/green, enclosing brown, yellow, and white pellets, dried ferrous sulphate 150 mg (47 mg iron), folic acid 500 micrograms. Net price 30-cap pack = £1.18. Label: 25
Dose: 1 capsule daily
Ferrograd Folic® (Abbott)
Filmtabs® (= tablets f/c), red/yellow, dried ferrous sulphate 325 mg (105 mg iron) for sustained release, folic acid 350 micrograms. Net price 30-tab pack = 60p. Label: 25
Dose: 1 tablet daily before food
NHS **Folex-350®** (Rybar)
Tablets, pink, s/c, ferrous fumarate 308 mg (100 mg iron), folic acid 350 micrograms. Net price 30-tab pack = £2.00
Dose: 1 tablet daily
NHS **Fortespan®** (SmithKline Beecham)
Spansule® (= capsules m/r), clear/green, enclosing red, yellow, and white pellets, dried ferrous sulphate 150 mg (47 mg iron), folic acid 500 micrograms. Net price 30-cap pack = £2.64. Label: 25
Dose: 1 capsule daily
Galfer FA® (Galen)
Capsules, red/yellow, ferrous fumarate 305 mg (100 mg iron), folic acid 350 micrograms. Net price 20 = 40p
Dose: 1 capsule daily before food
PoM **Lexpec with Iron-M®** (Rosemont)
Syrup, brown, sugar-free, ferric ammonium citrate equivalent to 80 mg iron, folic acid 500 micrograms/5 mL. Net price 125 mL = £3.80
Dose: 5–10 mL daily before food
Note. Lexpec with Iron-M® contains five times less folic acid than Lexpec with Iron®

Meterfolic® (Sinclair)
Tablets, grey, f/c, ferrous fumarate equivalent to 100 mg iron, folic acid 400 micrograms. Net price 30-tab pack = 60p
Dose: 1 tablet 1–2 times daily
Prevention of neural tube defects, 1 tablet daily started before conception and continued for at least first trimester
Pregaday® (Evans)
Tablets, brown, f/c, ferrous fumarate equivalent to 100 mg iron, folic acid 350 micrograms. Net price 28-tab pack = 51p
Dose: 1 tablet daily
PoM **Slow-Fe Folic®** (Novartis)
Tablets, m/r, ivory, f/c, dried ferrous sulphate 160 mg (50 mg iron), folic acid 400 micrograms. Net price 28-tab pack = 28p. Label: 25
Dose: 1–2 tablets daily

Higher folic acid content

Appropriate in context of prevention of *recurrence of neural tube defects*, see recommendations on p. 395. *Cautions:* have the theoretical disadvantage of masking anaemia due to vitamin-B_{12} deficiency (which could allow vitamin-B_{12} neuropathy to develop).

NHS PoM **Ferfolic SV®** (Sinclair)
Tablets, pink, ferrous gluconate 250 mg (30 mg iron), folic acid 4 mg, ascorbic acid 10 mg. Net price 20 = 40p
Dose: anaemia, 1–3 tablets daily after food
Prophylaxis of neural tube defects in women known to be at risk, 1 tablet daily started before conception and continued for at least first trimester; see also recommendations on p. 395
PoM **Lexpec with Iron®** (Rosemont)
Syrup, brown, sugar-free, ferric ammonium citrate equivalent to 80 mg iron, folic acid 2.5 mg/5 mL. Net price 125 mL = £3.80
Dose: 5–10 mL daily before food
Note. Lexpec with Iron® contains five times as much folic acid as Lexpec with Iron-M®

COMPOUND IRON PREPARATIONS

There is no justification for prescribing compound iron preparations, except for preparations of iron and folic acid for prophylactic use in pregnancy (see above).

NHS **Ferrous Sulphate Tablets, Compound,** green, s/c, dried ferrous sulphate equivalent to 170 mg of $FeSO_4$, copper sulphate 2.5 mg, manganese sulphate 2.5 mg. Net price 20 tabs = 48p
Dose: 1–2 tablets daily
NHS **Dencyl®** (SmithKline Beecham)
Spansule® (= capsules m/r), blue/clear, enclosing red, yellow, and white pellets, dried ferrous sulphate 150 mg (47 mg iron), folic acid 500 micrograms, zinc sulphate monohydrate 61.8 mg (22.5 mg zinc). Net price 30-cap pack = £4.74. Label: 25
Dose: 1 capsule daily during pregnancy
NHS **Ditemic®** (SmithKline Beecham)
Spansule® (= capsules m/r), orange/clear, enclosing red, orange, and white pellets, dried ferrous sulphate 150 mg (47 mg iron), zinc sulphate monohydrate 61.8 mg (22.5 mg zinc) with vitamins B group and C. Net price 30-cap pack = £7.40. Label: 25
Dose: 1–2 capsules daily; CHILD over 1 year 1 capsule daily

NHS **Ferrograd C**® (Abbott)

Filmtabs® (= tablets f/c), red, dried ferrous sulphate 325 mg (105 mg iron) for sustained release, ascorbic acid 500 mg (as sodium salt). Net price 30-tab pack = £1.62. Label: 25

Dose: 1 tablet daily before food

NHS **Fesovit Z**® (Evans)

Spansule® (= capsules m/r), orange/clear, enclosing brown, orange, and white pellets, dried ferrous sulphate 150 mg (47 mg iron), zinc sulphate monohydrate 61.8 mg (22.5 mg zinc) with vitamins B group and C. Net price 30-cap pack = £2.80. Label: 25

Dose: 1–2 capsules daily; CHILD over 1 year 1 capsule daily

NHS **Givitol**® (Galen)

Capsules, red/maroon, ferrous fumarate 305 mg (100 mg iron) with vitamins B group and C. Net price 20 = 82p

Dose: 1 capsule daily before food

9.1.1.2 PARENTERAL IRON

The only valid reason for administering iron **parenterally** is failure of oral therapy due to lack of patient cooperation, severe gastro-intestinal side-effects, continuing severe blood loss or malabsorption. Provided that the oral iron preparation is taken reliably and is absorbed, then the haemoglobin response is not significantly faster with the parenteral route. The need for a more rapid cure of the anaemia is therefore not met by parenteral administration of iron.

A suitable parenteral preparation contains a complex of iron, sorbitol and citric acid as **iron sorbitol injection**. It is **not** suitable for intravenous injection and, although the low mean molecular weight allows rapid absorption from the injection site, excretion in the saliva and substantial urinary losses also occur.

It is usual to give a course of *deep intramuscular* injections. The manufacturer's dosage schedules should be consulted; these usually include a supplement for reconstitution of iron stores.

To prevent leakage along the needle track with subsequent staining of the skin, intramuscular injections should be deep with suitable technique.

IRON SORBITOL

Colloidal solution of a complex of iron, sorbitol and citric acid, stabilised with dextrin and sorbitol; contains 5% (50 mg/mL) of iron

Indications: iron-deficiency anaemia

Cautions: oral iron should be stopped at least 24 hours before; other injectable iron preparations should be stopped a week before; urine may darken on standing

Contra-indications: liver disease, kidney disease (particularly pyelonephritis), untreated urinary-tract infections; early pregnancy; preferably avoid in patients with pre-existing cardiac abnormalities (e.g. angina or arrhythmias)

Side-effects: nausea, vomiting, taste disturbances, dizziness, flushing, occasionally severe arrhythmias

Dose: by deep intramuscular injection, calculated according to weight and iron deficit, see notes above and manufacturer's literature

PoM **Jectofer**® (Astra)

Injection, iron sorbitol (iron 50 mg/mL). Net price 2-mL amp = 45p

9.1.2   Drugs used in megaloblastic anaemias

Most megaloblastic anaemias are due to lack of either vitamin B_{12} or folate and it is essential to establish in every case which deficiency is present and the underlying cause. In emergencies, where delay might be dangerous, it is sometimes necessary to administer both substances after the bone marrow test while plasma assay results are awaited. Normally, however, appropriate treatment should be instituted only when the results of tests are available.

The most common cause of megaloblastic anaemia in the UK is *pernicious anaemia* in which lack of gastric intrinsic factor due to an auto-immune gastritis causes malabsorption of vitamin B_{12}.

Vitamin B_{12} is also needed in the treatment of megaloblastosis due to *prolonged nitrous oxide anaesthesia,* which inactivates the vitamin, and in the rare syndrome of *congenital transcobalamin II deficiency.*

Vitamin B_{12} should be given prophylactically after *total gastrectomy* or *total ileal resection* (or after *partial gastrectomy* if a vitamin B_{12} absorption test shows vitamin B_{12} malabsorption).

Apart from dietary deficiency, all other causes of vitamin-B_{12} deficiency are attributable to *malabsorption* so there is little place for the use of vitamin B_{12} orally and none for vitamin B_{12} intrinsic factor complexes given by mouth.

Hydroxocobalamin has completely replaced cyanocobalamin as the form of vitamin B_{12} of choice for therapy; it is retained in the body longer than cyanocobalamin and thus for maintenance therapy can be given at intervals of up to 3 months. Treatment is generally initiated with frequent administration of intramuscular injections to replenish the depleted body stores. Thereafter, maintenance treatment, which is usually for life, can be instituted. There is no evidence that doses larger than those recommended provide any additional benefit in vitamin-B_{12} neuropathy.

Folic acid has few indications for long-term therapy since most causes of folate deficiency are self-limiting or will yield to a short course of treatment. It should not be used in undiagnosed megaloblastic anaemia unless vitamin B_{12} is administered concurrently otherwise neuropathy may be precipitated (see above).

In *folate-deficient megaloblastic anaemia* (e.g. due to poor nutrition, pregnancy, or antiepileptics), standard treatment to bring about a haematological remission and replenish body stores, is oral administration of folic acid 5 mg daily for 4 months; up to 15 mg daily may be necessary in malabsorption states.

For *prophylaxis in chronic haemolytic states or in renal dialysis,* it is sufficient to give folic acid 5 mg daily or even weekly, depending on the diet and the rate of haemolysis.

For *prophylaxis in pregnancy* the dose of folic acid is 200–500 micrograms daily (see Iron and Folic Acid, section 9.1.1.1). See also Prevention of Neural Tube Defects below.

Folinic acid is also effective in the treatment of folate-deficient megaloblastic anaemia but it is generally used in association with cytotoxic drugs (see section 8.1.3); it is given as calcium folinate.

PREVENTION OF NEURAL TUBE DEFECTS. Recommendations of an expert advisory group of the Department of Health include the advice that:

To prevent *recurrence of neural tube defect* women who wish to become pregnant (or who are at risk of becoming pregnant) should be advised to take folic acid supplements at a dose of 5 mg daily (reduced to 4 mg daily if a suitable preparation becomes available); supplementation should continue until the twelfth week of pregnancy. Women receiving antiepileptic therapy need individual counselling by their doctor before starting folic acid.

To prevent *first occurrence of neural tube defect* women who are planning a pregnancy should be advised to take folic acid as a medicinal or food supplement at a dose of 400 micrograms daily before conception and during the first 12 weeks of pregnancy. Women who have not been supplementing and who suspect they are pregnant should start at once and continue until the twelfth week of pregnancy.

There is **no** justification for prescribing multiple-ingredient vitamin preparations containing vitamin B₁₂ or folic acid.

HYDROXOCOBALAMIN

Indications: see under dose below
Cautions: should not be given before diagnosis fully established but see also notes above; arrhythmias secondary to hypokalaemia can occur at the beginning of treatment
Contra-indications: megaloblastic anaemia of pregnancy
Side-effects: itching, exanthema; fever, chills, hot flushes; nausea, dizziness; rarely acneiform and bullous eruptions; anaphylaxis
Dose: by intramuscular injection, pernicious anaemia and other macrocytic anaemias without neurological involvement, initially 0.25–1 mg on alternate days for 1–2 weeks, then 250 micrograms weekly until blood count within the normal range, thereafter 1 mg every 2–3 months
Pernicious anaemia and other macrocytic anaemias with neurological involvement, initially 1 mg on alternate days until no further improvement occurs, then 1 mg every 2 months
Prophylaxis of macrocytic anaemias associated with vitamin-B₁₂ deficiency, 1 mg every 2–3 months
Tobacco amblyopia and Leber's optic atrophy, initially 1 mg daily for 2 weeks, then 1 mg twice weekly until no further improvement occurs, thereafter 1 mg every 1–3 months
CHILD, dosages as for adult

PoM **Hydroxocobalamin** (Non-proprietary)
Injection, hydroxocobalamin 1 mg/mL. Net price 1-mL amp = £2.50
Note. The BP directs that when vitamin B₁₂ injection is prescribed or demanded hydroxocobalamin injection shall be dispensed or supplied
The brand names NHS Cobalin-H® (Link) and NHS Neo-Cytamen® (Evans) are used for hydroxocobalamin injection

CYANOCOBALAMIN

Indications: see notes above
Dose: by mouth, vitamin-B₁₂ deficiency of dietary origin, 50–150 micrograms or more daily taken between meals; CHILD 35–50 micrograms twice daily
By intramuscular injection, initially 1 mg repeated 10 times at intervals of 2–3 days, maintenance 1 mg every month, but see notes above

Cyanocobalamin (Non-proprietary)
NHS **Tablets*, cyanocobalamin 50 micrograms. Net price 50-tab pack = £2.52
* except to treat or prevent vitamin-B₁₂ deficiency in a patient who is a vegan or who has a proven vitamin-B₁₂ deficiency of dietary origin and endorsed 'SLS'
Note. The brand name NHS Cytacon® (Goldshield) is used for cyanocobalamin tablets
NHS *Liquid*, cyanocobalamin 35 micrograms/5 mL. Net price 200 mL = £2.36
Note. The brand name NHS Cytacon® (Goldshield) is used for cyanocobalamin liquid
PoM *Injection*, cyanocobalamin 1 mg/mL. Net price 1-mL amp = £1.67
Note. The BP directs that when vitamin B₁₂ injection is prescribed or demanded hydroxocobalamin injection shall be dispensed or supplied
The brand name NHS Cytamen® (Evans) is used for cyanocobalamin injection

FOLIC ACID

Indications: see notes above
Cautions: should never be given alone in the treatment of Addisonian pernicious anaemia and other vitamin B₁₂-deficiency states because it may precipitate the onset of subacute combined degeneration of the spinal cord. Do not use in malignant disease unless megaloblastic anaemia due to folate deficiency is an important complication (some malignant tumours are folate-dependent); **interactions:** Appendix 1 (vitamins)
Dose: initially, 5 mg daily for 4 months (see notes above); maintenance, 5 mg every 1–7 days depending on underlying disease; CHILD up to 1 year, 500 micrograms/kg daily; over 1 year, as adult dose
Prevention of neural tube defects, see notes above

PoM ¹ **Folic Acid** (Non-proprietary)
Tablets, folic acid 400 micrograms, net price = 90-tab pack = £2.13; 5 mg, 20 = 7p
Note. 400-microgram tablets available from Lane (Preconceive®), 5-mg tablets available from various suppliers
1. Can be sold to the public provided daily doses do not exceed 500 micrograms
Syrup, folic acid 2.5 mg/5 mL. Net price 125 mL = £7.80
Available from Hillcross, Rosemont (Lexpec®, sugar-free)

9.1.3   Drugs used in hypoplastic, haemolytic, and renal anaemias

Anabolic steroids, pyridoxine, antilymphocyte immunoglobulin, and various corticosteroids are used in hypoplastic and haemolytic anaemias.

The place of **anabolic steroids** in the therapy of *aplastic anaemia* remains somewhat controversial and their effectiveness is unclear. There is a wide variation in the reported successful responses. Occasional patients, however, do seem to derive benefit. Since nandrolone decanoate requires intramuscular injection it is unsuitable in aplastic anaemia or cytotoxic aplasia because of the low platelet count. Oxymetholone tablets (available only on named-patient basis) may alternatively be used in aplastic anaemia. Controlled trials have shown that antilymphocyte globulin produces a response in 50% of acquired cases; higher response rates have been reported when cyclosporin is given as well.

It is unlikely that dietary deprivation of **pyridoxine** (section 9.6.2) produces haematological effects in man. However, certain forms of *sideroblastic anaemia* respond to pharmacological doses, possibly reflecting its role as a co-enzyme during haemoglobin synthesis. Pyridoxine is indicated in both *idiopathic acquired* and *hereditary sideroblastic anaemias*. Although complete cures have not been reported, some increase in haemoglobin may occur; the dose required is usually high, up to 400 mg daily. *Reversible sideroblastic anaemias* respond to treatment of the underlying cause but in pregnancy, haemolytic anaemias, and alcohol dependence, or during isoniazid treatment, pyridoxine is also indicated.

Corticosteroids (see section 6.3) have an important place in the management of a wide variety of haematological disorders. They include conditions with an immune basis such as *auto-immune haemolytic anaemia*, *immune thrombocytopenias* and *neutropenias*, and *major transfusion reactions*. They are also used in chemotherapy schedules for many types of *lymphoma*, *lymphoid leukaemias*, and *paraproteinaemias*, including *myelomatosis*. Corticosteroids are used in *aplastic anaemias*, where their value is more debatable.

NANDROLONE

Indications: aplastic anaemia but see notes above; postmenopausal osteoporosis, see section 6.4.3

Cautions; Contra-indications; Side-effects: see section 6.4.3

Dose: by *deep intramuscular injection*, aplastic anaemia (but not recommended, see notes above), nandrolone decanoate 50–100 mg weekly

PoM **Deca-Durabolin 100**® (Organon)

Injection (oily), nandrolone decanoate 100 mg/mL. Net price 1-mL amp = £7.34

Note. Contains arachis (peanut) oil

ERYTHROPOIETIN

Epoetin (recombinant human erythropoietin) is used for the anaemia associated with erythropoietin deficiency in chronic renal failure, to increase the yield of autologous blood in normal individuals and to shorten the period of anaemia in patients receiving platinum-containing chemotherapy. The clinical efficacy of epoetin alfa and epoetin beta is similar. Epoetin beta is also used for the prevention of anaemia in premature infants of low birth-weight.

Other factors which contribute to the anaemia of chronic renal failure such as iron or folate deficiency should be corrected before treatment and monitored during therapy. Parenteral iron has been recommended to improve the response in resistant patients. Aluminium toxicity, concurrent infection or other inflammatory disease may impair the response to epoetin.

EPOETIN ALFA and BETA

(Recombinant human erythropoietins)

Indications: see under preparations, below

Cautions: inadequately treated or poorly controlled blood pressure (monitor closely blood pressure, haemoglobin, and electrolytes), interrupt treatment if blood pressure uncontrolled; exclude other causes of anaemia (e.g. folic acid or vitamin B_{12} deficiency) and give iron supplements if necessary (see also notes above); ischaemic vascular disease; thrombocytosis (monitor platelet count for first 8 weeks); history of convulsions; malignant disease; chronic liver failure; sudden stabbing migraine-like pain is warning of hypertensive crisis; increase in heparin dose may be needed; pregnancy and breast-feeding; **interactions:** Appendix 1 (epoetin)

Contra-indications: uncontrolled hypertension

Side-effects: dose-dependent increase in blood pressure or aggravation of hypertension; in isolated patients with normal or low blood pressure, hypertensive crisis with encephalopathy-like symptoms and generalised tonic-clonic seizures requiring immediate medical attention; dose-dependent increase in platelet count (but thrombocytosis rare) regressing during treatment; influenza-like symptoms (may be reduced if intravenous injection given over 5 minutes); shunt thrombosis especially if tendency to hypotension or arteriovenous shunt complications; isolated reports of hyperkalaemia, increase in plasma creatinine, urea and phosphate, convulsions, skin reactions, palpebral oedema, anaphylaxis

Dose: aimed at increasing haemoglobin concentration at rate not exceeding 2 g/100 mL/month to stable level of 10–12 g/100 mL (9.5–11 g/100 mL in children); see under preparations, below

Note. Although epoetin alfa and beta are clinically indistinguishable the prescriber must specify which is required

---

Epoetin alfa

PoM **Eprex**® (Janssen-Cilag)

Injection, epoetin alfa 2000 units/mL, net price 0.5-mL (1000-unit) vial = £8.78, 0.5-mL (1000-unit) prefilled syringe = £9.23, 1-mL (2000-unit) vial = £17.55; 4000 units/mL, 0.5-mL (2000-unit) prefilled syringe = £18.00, 1-mL (4000-unit) vial = £35.10; 10 000 units/mL, 0.3-mL (3000-unit) prefilled syringe = £26.78, 0.4-mL (4000-unit) prefilled syringe = £35.55, 1-mL (10 000-unit) vial = £87.75, 1-mL (10 000-unit) prefilled syringe = £88.20. An auto-injector device is available for use with 1-mL prefilled syringes

Dose: anaemia associated with chronic renal failure in patients on haemodialysis, *by subcutaneous injection* (max. 1 mL per injection site) or *by intravenous injection* over 1–5 minutes, initially 50 units/kg 3 times weekly adjusted according to response in steps of 25 units/kg at intervals of 4 weeks; max. 600 units/kg weekly in 3 divided doses; maintenance dose (when haemoglobin concentration of 10–12 g/100 mL achieved), usually 30–100 units/kg 3 times weekly; CHILD (intravenous route only) initially as for adults; maintenance dose (when haemoglobin concentration of 9.5–11 g/ 100 mL achieved), under 10 kg usually 75–150 units/kg 3 times weekly, 10–30 kg usually 60–150 units/kg 3 times weekly, over 30 kg usually 30–100 units/kg 3 times weekly

Anaemia associated with chronic renal failure in adults on peritoneal dialysis, *by subcutaneous injection* (max. 1 mL per injection site), initially 50 units/kg twice weekly; maintenance dose (when haemoglobin concentration of 10–12 g/100 mL achieved), 25–50 units/kg twice weekly

Severe symptomatic anaemia of renal origin in adults with renal insufficiency not yet on dialysis, preferably *by subcutaneous injection* (max. 1 mL per injection site), initially 50 units/kg 3 times weekly increased according to response in steps of 25 units/kg at intervals of 4 weeks; maintenance dose (when haemoglobin concentration of 10–12 g/100 mL achieved), 17–33 units/kg 3 times weekly; max. 600 units/kg weekly in 3 divided doses;

Anaemia in adults receiving platinum-containing chemotherapy, *by subcutaneous injection* (max. 1 mL per injection site), initially 150 units/kg 3 times weekly, increased if appropriate rise in haemoglobin (or reticulocyte count) not achieved after 4 weeks to 300 units/kg 3 times weekly; discontinue if inadequate response after 4 weeks at higher dose; reduce dose by 25–50% if haemoglobin rise exceeds 2 g/100 mL per month; suspend if haemoglobin exceeds 14 g/100 mL until it falls below 12 g/100 mL and reinstate with dose at 25% below previous dose; continue epoetin for 1 month after end of chemotherapy

To increase yield of autologous blood (to avoid homologous blood) in predonation programme in moderate anaemia *either* when large volume of blood required for elective major surgery *or* if insufficient period to obtain required volume of blood, *by intravenous injection* over 1–5 minutes, 600 units/kg twice weekly for 3 weeks before surgery; consult product literature for details and advice on ensuring high iron stores

Note. Subcutaneous dose generally about 20–30% lower than intravenous; when changing route give same dose then adjust according to weekly haemoglobin measurements

Epoetin beta

▼ PoM **NeoRecormon**® (Boehringer Mannheim)

Injection, powder for reconstitution, epoetin beta, net price 500-unit vial = £4.39 (available with water for injection in ampoule or syringe)

Note. Avoid contact of reconstituted injection with glass; use only plastic materials

NeoRecormon® *Multidose injection*, powder for reconstitution, epoetin beta, net price 50 000-unit vial = £438.75; 100 000-unit vial = £877.50 (both with solvent)

Contra-indications: not for use in neonates owing to presence of benzyl alcohol as additive

Note. Avoid contact of reconstituted injection with glass; use only plastic materials

NeoRecormon® *Reco-Pen*, (for subcutaneous use), double-chamber cartridges (containing epoetin beta and solvent), net price 10 000-unit cartridge = £87.75; 20 000-unit cartridge = £175.50; for use with *Reco-Pen* injection device, available free from Boehringer Mannheim

Contra-indications: not for use in neonates owing to presence of benzyl alcohol as additive

Dose: anaemia associated with chronic renal failure in dialysis patients, symptomatic anaemia of renal origin in patients not yet on dialysis, ADULT and CHILD

By subcutaneous injection, initially 60 units/kg weekly (in 1–7 divided doses) for 4 weeks, increased according to response at intervals of 4 weeks in steps of 60 units/kg; maintenance dose (when haemoglobin concentration of 10–12 g/100 mL achieved), initially reduce dose by half then adjust according to response at intervals of 1–2 weeks; max. 720 units/kg weekly

By intravenous injection over 2 minutes (or *Recormon*® only, *by short-term intravenous infusion*) initially 40 units/kg 3 times weekly for 4 weeks, increased according to response to 80 units/kg 3 times weekly with further increases if needed at intervals of 4 weeks in steps of 20 units/kg; maintenance dose (when haemoglobin concentration of 10–12 g/100 mL achieved), initially reduce dose by half then adjust according to response at intervals of 1–2 weeks; max. 720 units/kg weekly

Prevention of anaemias of prematurity in infants with birth-weight of 750–1500 g and gestational age of less than 34 weeks, *by subcutaneous injection* (of single dose, unpreserved injection), 250 units/kg 3 times weekly preferably starting within 3 days of birth and continued for 6 weeks

Anaemia in adults with solid tumours receiving platinum-containing chemotherapy, *by subcutaneous injection*, initially 450 units/kg weekly (in 3–7 divided doses), increased if appropriate rise in haemoglobin not achieved after 4 weeks to 900 units/kg weekly (in 3–7 divided doses); reduce dose by half if haemoglobin rise exceeds 2 g/100 mL per month; suspend if haemoglobin exceeds 14 g/100 mL until concentration falls below 12 g/100 mL and reinstate at 50% of the previous weekly dose; continue for up to 3 weeks after end of chemotherapy

Note. If haemoglobin concentration falls by more than 1 g/100 mL in the first cycle of chemotherapy despite treatment with epoetin beta, further treatment may not be effective

To increase yield of autologous blood (to avoid homologous blood) in predonation programme in moderate anaemia when blood conserving procedures are insufficient or unavailable, consult product literature

---

PoM **Recormon®** (Boehringer Mannheim)
Injection, powder for reconstitution, epoetin beta.
Net price 1000-unit vial = £8.78; 2000-unit vial =
£17.55; 5000-unit vial = £43.88; 10 000-unit vial
= £87.75 (all with water for injections)
Note. Avoid contact of reconstituted injection with glass;
use only plastic materials
Recormon® S *injection* (for subcutaneous use),
powder for reconstitution, epoetin beta. Net price
1000-unit vial = £8.78; 2000-unit vial = £17.55;
5000-unit vial = £43.88; 10 000-unit vial =
£87.75 (all with syringe and water for injections)
Dose: see under *NeoRecormon®*

___

IRON OVERLOAD

Severe tissue iron overload may occur in aplastic
and other refractory anaemias, mainly as the result
of repeated blood transfusions. It is a particular
problem in refractory anaemias with hyperplastic
bone marrow, especially *thalassaemia major*, where
excessive iron absorption from the gut and inappropriate iron therapy may add to the tissue siderosis.

Iron overload associated with haemochromatosis
may be treated with repeated venesection. Venesection may also be used for patients who have
received multiple transfusions and whose bone marrow has recovered. Where venesection is contra-
indicated, the long-term administration of the iron
chelating compound **desferrioxamine mesylate** is
useful. Subcutaneous infusions of desferrioxamine
(20–40 mg/kg over 8–12 hours) are given on 3 to 7
nights each week. Desferrioxamine (up to 2 g per
unit of blood) may also be given through the infusion line at the time of blood transfusion.

Iron excretion induced by desferrioxamine is
enhanced by administration of vitamin C (section
9.6.3) in a dose of 200 mg daily (100 mg in infants);
it should be given separately from food since it also
enhances iron absorption. Vitamin C should be
avoided for 1–2 weeks after starting desferrioxamine treatment.

Infusion of desferrioxamine may be used to treat
aluminium overload in dialysis patients; theoretically 100 mg of desferrioxamine binds with 4.1 mg
of aluminium.

Orally active iron chelators are under clinical
study but are not available for general use.

___

DESFERRIOXAMINE MESYLATE
(Deferoxamine Mesilate)
 Indications: see notes above; iron poisoning, see
 Emergency Treatment of Poisoning
 Cautions: renal impairment; eye and ear examinations before treatment and at 3-month intervals
 during treatment; aluminium-related encephalopathy (may exacerbate neurological dysfunction);
 pregnancy, breast-feeding; **interactions:** Appendix 1 (desferrioxamine)
 Side-effects: gastro-intestinal   disturbances;
 hepatic and renal impairment; arrhythmias, hypotension (especially when given too rapidly by
 intravenous injection); anaphylaxis; dizziness;
 convulsions; Yersinia infection more frequent;
 disturbances of hearing and vision (including lens

opacity and retinopathy); skin reactions; pain on
intramuscular injection; local irritation on subcutaneous infusion (usually if infusion concentration or dose too high)
 Dose: see notes above; iron poisoning, see Emergency Treatment of Poisoning
 Note. For full details and warnings relating to administration, consult product literature

Preparations
See under Emergency Treatment of Poisoning

___

9.1.4   Drugs used in autoimmune thrombocytopenic purpura

It is usual to commence the treatment of autoimmune (idiopathic) thrombocytopenic purpura with
corticosteroids, e.g. prednisolone 1 mg/kg daily,
gradually reducing the dosage over the subsequent
weeks. In patients who fail to achieve a satisfactory
platelet count or relapse when corticosteroid dosage
is reduced or withdrawn, splenectomy is considered.

Other therapy that has been tried in refractory
cases includes azathioprine (section 8.2.1), cyclophosphamide (section 8.1.1), vincristine (section
8.1.4), cyclosporin (section 8.2.2), and danazol
(section 6.7.3). Intravenous immunoglobulins (section 14.5), have also been used in refractory cases
or where a temporary rapid rise in platelets is
needed, as in pregnancy or pre-operatively. For
patients with chronic severe thrombocytopenia
refractory to other therapy, tranexamic acid (section
2.11) may be given to reduce the severity of
haemorrhage.

___

9.1.5   G6PD deficiency

Glucose 6-phosphate dehydrogenase (G6PD) deficiency is highly prevalent in populations originating
from most parts of Africa, from most parts of Asia,
from Oceania, and from Southern Europe; it can
also be encountered, rarely, in any other population.

Subjects with G6PD deficiency are susceptible to
developing acute haemolytic anaemia on taking a
number of common drugs. They are also susceptible to developing acute haemolytic anaemia upon
ingestion of fava beans (broad beans, *Vicia faba*);
this is termed *favism* and tends to be more severe in
children or when the fresh fava beans are eaten raw.

When prescribing drugs for patients who are
G6PD deficient, the following three points should
be kept in mind:

1. G6PD deficiency is genetically heterogeneous; different genetic variants entail different susceptibility to the
haemolytic risk from drugs; thus, a drug found to be safe
in some G6PD-deficient subjects may not be equally
safe in others;
2. no test specifically designed to identify potential risk in
G6PD-deficient subjects is currently carried out by manufacturers;
3. the risk and severity of haemolysis is almost always
dose-related.

The table below should be read with these points
in mind. Whenever possible, a test for G6PD deficiency should be done before prescribing a drug in

___

the list, especially if the patient belongs to a population group in which G6PD deficiency is common.

A very small group of G6PD-deficient individuals, with chronic non-spherocytic haemolytic anaemia, have haemolysis even in the absence of an exogenous trigger. These patients must be regarded as being at high risk of severe exacerbation of haemolysis following administration of any of the drugs listed below.

Drugs with definite risk of haemolysis in most G6PD-deficient subjects

Dapsone and other sulphones (higher doses for dermatitis herpetiformis more likely to cause problems)
Methylene blue
Niridazole [not on UK market]
Nitrofurantoin
Pamaquin [not on UK market]
Primaquine (30 mg weekly for 8 weeks has been found to be without undue harmful effects in African and Asian people, see section 5.4.1)
4-Quinolones (including ciprofloxacin, nalidixic acid, norfloxacin, and ofloxacin)
Sulphonamides (including co-trimoxazole; some sulphonamides, e.g. sulphadiazine, have been tested and found not to be haemolytic in many G6PD-deficient subjects)

Drugs with possible risk of haemolysis in some G6PD-deficient subjects

Aspirin (acceptable in a dose of at least 1 g daily in most G6PD-deficient subjects)
Chloroquine (acceptable in acute malaria)
Menadione, water-soluble derivatives (e.g. menadiol sodium phosphate)
Probenecid
Quinidine (acceptable in acute malaria)
Quinine (acceptable in acute malaria)

Note. Mothballs may contain naphthalene which also causes haemolysis in subjects with G6PD-deficiency.

9.1.6 Drugs used in neutropenia

Recombinant human granulocyte-colony stimulating factor (rhG-CSF) stimulates the production of neutrophils and may reduce the duration of chemotherapy-induced neutropenia and thereby reduce the incidence of associated sepsis; there is as yet no evidence that it improves overall survival. **Filgrastim** (unglycosylated rhG-CSF) and **lenograstim** (glycosylated rhG-CSF) have similar effects; both have been used in a variety of clinical settings but they do not have any clear-cut routine indications. In congenital neutropenia filgrastim usually elevates the neutrophil count with appropriate clinical response. Prolonged use may be associated with an increased risk of myeloid malignancy.

Molgramostim (recombinant human granulocyte macrophage-colony stimulating factor) stimulates the production of all granulocytes and monocytes. It has more side-effects than granulocyte-colony stimulating factor and is ineffective in congenital neutropenia.

Treatment with recombinant human growth factors should only be administered by those experienced in their use.

FILGRASTIM

(Recombinant human granulocyte-colony stimulating factor, G-CSF)

Indications: (specialist use only) reduction in duration of neutropenia and incidence of febrile neutropenia in cytotoxic chemotherapy of non-myeloid malignancy; reduction in duration of neutropenia (and associated sequelae) in myeloablative therapy followed by bone-marrow transplantation; mobilisation of peripheral blood progenitor cells for harvesting and subsequent autologous infusion; severe congenital neutropenia, cyclic neutropenia, or idiopathic neutropenia and history of severe or recurrent infections (distinguish carefully from other haematological disorders, consult product literature)

Cautions: tumours with myeloid characteristics (risk of tumour growth), pre-malignant myeloid conditions; reduced myeloid precursors; monitor leucocyte count (discontinue treatment if leucocytosis, consult product literature); monitor platelet count and haemoglobin; regular morphological and cytogenetic bone marrow examinations recommended in severe congenital neutropenia (possible risk of myelodysplastic syndromes or leukaemia); monitor spleen size; osteoporotic bone disease (monitor bone density if given for more than 6 months); does not prevent other toxic effects of high-dose chemotherapy; pregnancy; breast-feeding; **interactions:** Appendix 1 (filgrastim)

Contra-indications: severe congenital neutropenia (Kostman's syndrome) with abnormal cytogenetics

Side-effects: musculoskeletal pain, transient hypotension, disturbances in liver enzymes and serum uric acid; thrombocytopenia; urinary abnormalities including dysuria; allergic reactions (more common after intravenous infusion), proteinuria, haematuria, and transient decrease in blood glucose reported; on long-term use cutaneous vasculitis also reported, also splenic enlargement, hepatomegaly, headache, diarrhoea, anaemia, epistaxis, alopecia, osteoporosis, and rash, reactions at injection site

Dose: cytotoxic-induced neutropenia, preferably *by subcutaneous injection or by intravenous infusion* (over 30 minutes), ADULT and CHILD, 500 000 units/kg daily started not less than 24 hours after cytotoxic chemotherapy, continued until neutrophil count in normal range, usually for up to 14 days
Myeloablative therapy followed by bone-marrow transplantation, *by intravenous infusion* over 30 minutes or over 24 hours *or by subcutaneous infusion* over 24 hours, 1 million units/kg daily, started not less than 24 hours following cytotoxic chemotherapy (and within 24 hours of bone-marrow infusion), then adjusted according to absolute neutrophil count (consult product literature)
Mobilisation of peripheral blood progenitor cells, used alone, *by subcutaneous injection or by subcutaneous infusion* over 24 hours, 1 million units/kg daily for 6 days; used following adjunctive myelosuppressive chemotherapy (to improve yield), *by subcutaneous injection*, 500 000 units/kg daily, started the day after completion of chemotherapy and continued until neutrophil count in normal range; for timing of leukapheresis consult product literature
Severe chronic neutropenia, *by subcutaneous injection*, ADULT and CHILD, in severe congenital neutropenia, initially 1.2 million units/kg daily in single or divided doses (initially 500 000 units/kg daily in idiopathic or cyclic neutropenia), adjusted according to response (consult product literature)

▼ PoM **Neupogen**® (Amgen)
Injection, filgrastim 30 million units (300 micrograms)/mL; net price 1-mL vial or pre-filled syringe = £77.03, 1.6-mL (48 million-unit) vial or pre-filled syringe = £122.85

LENOGRASTIM

(Recombinant human granulocyte-colony stimulating factor, rHuG-CSF)

Indications: (specialist use only) reduction in the duration of neutropenia and associated complications following bone-marrow transplantation for non-myeloid malignancy or following treatment with cytotoxic chemotherapy associated with a significant incidence of febrile neutropenia; mobilisation of peripheral blood progenitor cells for harvesting and subsequent autologous infusion

Cautions: see under Filgrastim; **interactions:** Appendix 1 (lenograstim)

Side-effects: see under Filgrastim

Dose: following bone-marrow transplantation, *by intravenous infusion,* ADULT and CHILD over 2 years 19.2 million units/m² daily started the day after transplantation, continued until neutrophil count stable in acceptable range (max. 28 days)

Cytotoxic-induced neutropenia, *by subcutaneous injection,* ADULT and CHILD over 2 years 19.2 million units/m² daily started the day after completion of chemotherapy, continued until neutrophil count stable in acceptable range (max. 28 days)

Mobilisation of peripheral blood progenitor cells, used alone, *by subcutaneous injection,* 1.28 million units/kg daily for 4–6 days; used following adjunctive myelosuppressive chemotherapy (to improve yield), *by subcutaneous injection,* 19.2 million units/m² daily, started the day after completion of chemotherapy and continued until neutrophil count in acceptable range; for timing of leukapheresis consult product literature

▼ PoM **Granocyte**® (Chugai)
Injection, powder for reconstitution, lenograstim, net price 13.4 million-unit (105-microgram) vial (with 1-mL amp water for injections) = £42.00; 33.6 million-unit (263-microgram) vial (with 1-mL amp water for injections) = £77.03

MOLGRAMOSTIM

(Recombinant human granulocyte macrophage-colony stimulating factor, GM-CSF)

Indications: (specialist use only) reduction of severity of neutropenia (and risk of infection) in cytotoxic chemotherapy; acceleration of myeloid recovery following bone-marrow transplantation; neutropenia in patients treated with ganciclovir in AIDS-related cytomegalovirus retinitis

Cautions: monitor serum albumin concentration and full blood count including differential white cell, platelet and haemoglobin; monitor closely patients with pulmonary disease; history of or predisposition to autoimmune disease; pregnancy and breast-feeding; not recommended for patients under 18 years

Contra-indications: myeloid malignancies

Side-effects: nausea, diarrhoea, vomiting, anorexia; dyspnoea, asthenia, fatigue; rash, fever, rigors, flushing, musculoskeletal pain; local reaction following subcutaneous injection; also reported, non-specific chest pain, stomatitis, headache, increased sweating, abdominal pain, pruritus, peripheral oedema, dizziness, paraesthesia, and myalgia; serious reactions

reported include anaphylaxis, cardiac failure, capillary leak syndrome, cerebrovascular disorders, confusion, convulsions, hypotension, cardiac rhythm abnormalities, intracranial hypertension, pericardial effusion, pericarditis, pleural effusion, pulmonary oedema, syncope

Dose: (first dose under medical supervision)

Cytotoxic chemotherapy, *by subcutaneous injection,* 60 000–110 000 units/kg daily, starting 24 hours after last dose of chemotherapy, continued for 7–10 days

Bone-marrow transplantation, *by intravenous infusion,* 110 000 units/kg daily, starting day after transplantation, continued until absolute neutrophil count in desirable range (see product literature); max. duration of treatment 30 days

Adjunct in ganciclovir treatment, *by subcutaneous injection,* 60 000 units/kg daily for 5 days then adjusted to maintain desirable absolute neutrophil count and white blood cell count

▼ PoM **Leucomax**® (Novartis, Schering-Plough)
Injection, powder for reconstitution, molgramostim, net price 1.67 million-unit (150-microgram) vial = £38.51; 3.33 million-unit (300-microgram) vial = £77.02; 4.44 million-unit (400 microgram) vial = £102.69

CYTOTOXIC-INDUCED NEUTROPENIC INFECTION

Amifostine is specifically licensed for the reduction of risk of infection related to neutropenia in patients undergoing treatment with cisplatin and cyclophosphamide for advanced ovarian carcinoma; it should be given within 30 minutes before chemotherapy.

Other drugs for the reduction of risk of infection associated with neutropenia include granulocyte-colony stimulating factor and granulocyte macrophage-colony stimulating factor.

AMIFOSTINE

Indications: (specialist use only) reduction of neutropenia-related risk of infection due to cyclophosphamide and cisplatin treatment in patients with advanced ovarian carcinoma

Cautions: ensure adequate hydration before treatment; infuse with patient supine and monitor arterial blood pressure (interrupt infusion if blood pressure decreases significantly, see product literature); interrupt antihypertensive therapy 24 hours beforehand and monitor patients closely; infuse over 15 minutes (longer infusion associated with higher incidence of side-effects); administer anti-emetic drugs with amifostine and before highly emetogenic chemotherapy; monitor serum calcium in patients at risk of hypocalcaemia; not recommended in renal and hepatic impairment; pregnancy and breast-feeding; **interactions:** Appendix 1 (amifostine)

Side-effects: hypotension (reversed by infusion of physiological saline and postural management), nausea, vomiting, flushing, chills, dizziness, somnolence, hiccups, sneezing; rarely clinical hypocalcaemia; allergic reactions

---

Dose: by *intravenous infusion* over 15 minutes, 910 mg/m^2 once daily started within 30 minutes before chemotherapy (reduced to 740 mg/m^2 for subsequent cycles if full dose could not be given first time due to hypotension lasting more than 5 minutes after interruption, see product literature); CHILD and ELDERLY (over 70 years) not recommended

▼ PoM **Ethyol**® (Schering-Plough)
Intravenous infusion, powder for reconstitution, amifostine. Net price 500-mg vial = £160.00

9.2   Fluids and electrolytes

9.2.1   Oral administration
9.2.2   Intravenous administration
9.2.3   Plasma and plasma substitutes

The following tables give a selection of useful electrolyte values:

Electrolyte concentrations—intravenous fluids

Intravenous infusion	Millimoles per litre				
	Na$^+$	K$^+$	HCO$_3^-$	Cl$^-$	Ca^{2+}
Normal Plasma Values	142	4.5	26	103	2.5
Sodium Chloride 0.9%	150	—	—	150	—
Compound Sodium Lactate (Hartmann's)	131	5	29	111	2
Sodium Chloride 0.18% and Glucose 4%	30	—	—	30	—
Potassium Chloride 0.3% and Glucose 5%	—	40	—	40	—
Potassium Chloride 0.3% and Sodium Chloride 0.9%	150	40	—	190	—
To correct metabolic acidosis					
Sodium Bicarbonate 1.26%	150	—	150	—	—
Sodium Bicarbonate 8.4% for cardiac arrest	1000	—	1000	—	—
Sodium Lactate (M/6)	167	—	167	—	—

Electrolyte content—gastro-intestinal secretions

Type of fluid	Millimoles per litre				
	H$^+$	Na$^+$	K$^+$	HCO$_3^-$	Cl$^-$
Gastric	40–60	20–80	5–20	—	100–150
Biliary	—	120–140	5–15	30–50	80–120
Pancreatic	—	120–140	5–15	70–110	40–80
Small bowel	—	120–140	5–15	20–40	90–130

Faeces, vomit, or aspiration should be saved and analysed where possible if abnormal losses are suspected; where this is impracticable the approximations above may be helpful in planning replacement therapy

9.2.1   Oral administration

9.2.1.1   Oral potassium
9.2.1.2   Oral sodium and water
9.2.1.3   Oral bicarbonate

Sodium and potassium salts, which may be given by mouth to prevent deficiencies or to treat established deficiencies of mild or moderate degree, are discussed in this section. Oral preparations for removing excess potassium and preparations for oral rehydration therapy are also included here. Oral bicarbonate, for metabolic acidosis, is also described in this section.

For reference to calcium, magnesium, and phosphate, see section 9.5.

9.2.1.1 ORAL POTASSIUM

Compensation for potassium loss is especially necessary:
1. in those taking digoxin or anti-arrhythmic drugs, where potassium depletion may induce arrhythmias;
2. in patients in whom secondary hyperaldosteronism occurs, e.g. renal artery stenosis, cirrhosis of the liver, the nephrotic syndrome, and severe heart failure;
3. in patients with excessive losses of potassium in the faeces, e.g. chronic diarrhoea associated with intestinal malabsorption or laxative abuse.

Measures to compensate for potassium loss may also be required in the elderly since they frequently take inadequate amounts of potassium in the diet (but see below for **warning** on **renal insufficiency**). Measures may also be required during long-term administration of drugs known to induce potassium loss (e.g. corticosteroids). Potassium supplements are **seldom required** with the small doses of diuretics given to treat hypertension; **potassium-sparing diuretics** (rather than potassium supplements) are recommended for prevention of hypokalaemia due to diuretics such as frusemide or the thiazides when these are given to eliminate oedema.

DOSAGE. If potassium salts are used for the *prevention of hypokalaemia*, then doses of potassium chloride 2 to 4 g (approx. 25 to 50 mmol) daily by mouth are suitable in patients taking a normal diet. *Smaller doses* must be used if there is *renal insufficiency (common in the elderly)* otherwise there is **danger of hyperkalaemia**. Potassium salts cause nausea and vomiting therefore poor compliance is a major limitation to their effectiveness; where appropriate, potassium-sparing diuretics are preferable (see also above). When there is *established potassium depletion* larger doses may be necessary, the quantity depending on the severity of any continuing potassium loss (monitoring of plasma-potassium concentration and specialist advice would be required). Potassium depletion is frequently associated with chloride depletion and with metabolic alkalosis, and these disorders require correction.

ADMINISTRATION. Potassium salts are preferably given as a liquid (or effervescent) preparation, rather than modified-release tablets; they should be given as the chloride (the use of effervescent potassium tablets BPC 1968 should be restricted to *hyperchloraemic states*, section 9.2.1.3).

Salt substitutes. A number of salt substitutes which contain significant amounts of potassium chloride are readily available as health food products (e.g. *Losalt*® and *Ruthmol*®). These should not be used by patients with renal failure as potassium intoxication may result.

POTASSIUM CHLORIDE

Indications: potassium depletion (see notes above)

Cautions: elderly, mild to moderate renal impairment (close monitoring required), intestinal stricture, history of peptic ulcer, hiatus hernia (for sustained-release preparations); **important:** special hazard if given with drugs liable to raise plasma potassium concentration such as potassium-sparing diuretics, ACE inhibitors, or cyclosporin, for other **interactions:** Appendix 1 (potassium salts)

Contra-indications: severe renal impairment, plasma potassium concentrations above 5 mmol/litre

Side-effects: nausea and vomiting (severe symptoms may indicate obstruction), oesophageal or small bowel ulceration

Dose: see notes above

Note. Do not confuse Effervescent Potassium Tablets BPC 1968 (section 9.2.1.3) with effervescent potassium chloride tablets. Effervescent Potassium Tablets BPC 1968 do not contain chloride ions and their use should be restricted to hyperchloraemic states (section 9.2.1.3). Effervescent Potassium Chloride Tablets BP are usually available in two strengths, one containing 6.7 mmol each of K⁺ and Cl⁻ (corresponding to Kloref®), the other containing 12 mmol K⁺ and 8 mmol Cl⁻ (corresponding to Sando-K®). Generic prescriptions must specify the strength required.

Kay-Cee-L® (Geistlich)
Syrup, red, sugar-free, potassium chloride 7.5% (1 mmol/mL each of K⁺ and Cl⁻). Net price 500 mL = £3.00. Label: 21

Kloref® (Cox)
Tablets, effervescent, betaine hydrochloride, potassium benzoate, bicarbonate, and chloride, equivalent to potassium chloride 500 mg (6.7 mmol each of K⁺ and Cl⁻). Net price 50 = £1.66. Label: 13, 21

Kloref-S® (Cox)
Granules, effervescent, sugar-free, betaine hydrochloride, potassium bicarbonate and chloride equivalent to potassium chloride 1.5 g (20 mmol each of K⁺ and Cl⁻)/sachet. Net price 30 sachets = £3.30. Label: 13, 21

Sando-K® (Novartis)
Tablets, effervescent, potassium bicarbonate and chloride equivalent to potassium 470 mg (12 mmol of K⁺) and chloride 285 mg (8 mmol of Cl⁻). Net price 20 = 34p. Label: 13, 21

Modified-release preparations
Avoid unless effervescent tablets or liquid preparations inappropriate

Slow-K® (Novartis)
Tablets, m/r, orange, s/c, potassium chloride 600 mg (8 mmol each of K⁺ and Cl⁻). Net price 20 = 10p. Label: 25, 27, counselling, swallow whole with fluid during meals while sitting or standing

POTASSIUM REMOVAL

Ion-exchange resins may be used to remove excess potassium in *mild hyperkalaemia* or in *moderate hyperkalaemia* when there are not ECG changes; intravenous therapy is required in emergencies (section 9.2.2).

POLYSTYRENE SULPHONATE RESINS

Indications: hyperkalaemia associated with anuria or severe oliguria, and in dialysis patients

Cautions: children (impaction of resin with excessive dosage or inadequate dilution); monitor for electrolyte disturbances (stop if plasma-potassium concentration below 5 mmol/litre); pregnancy and breast-feeding; sodium-containing resin in congestive heart failure, hypertension, renal impairment, and oedema

Contra-indications: obstructive bowel disease; oral administration or reduced gut motility in neonates; avoid calcium-containing resin in hyperparathyroidism, multiple myeloma, sarcoidosis, or metastatic carcinoma

Side-effects: rectal ulceration following rectal administration; colonic necrosis reported following enemas containing sorbitol; sodium retention, hypercalcaemia, gastric irritation, anorexia, nausea and vomiting, constipation (discontinue treatment—avoid magnesium-containing laxatives), diarrhoea; calcium-containing resin may cause hypercalcaemia (in dialysed patients and occasionally in those with renal impairment), hypomagnesaemia

Dose: by mouth, 15 g 3–4 times daily in water (not fruit squash which has a high potassium content) or as a paste; CHILD 0.5–1 g/kg daily in divided doses

By rectum, as an enema, 30 g in methylcellulose solution, retained for 9 hours followed by irrigation to remove resin from colon; NEONATE and CHILD, 0.5–1 g/kg daily

Calcium Resonium® (Sanofi Winthrop)
Powder, buff, calcium polystyrene sulphonate. Net price 300 g = £43.23. Label: 13

Resonium A® (Sanofi Winthrop)
Powder, buff, sodium polystyrene sulphonate. Net price 454 g = £58.53. Label: 13

9.2.1.2 ORAL SODIUM AND WATER

Sodium chloride is indicated in states of sodium depletion and usually needs to be given intravenously (section 9.2.2). In chronic conditions associated with mild or moderate degrees of sodium depletion, e.g. in salt-losing bowel or renal disease, oral supplements of sodium chloride or sodium bicarbonate (section 9.2.1.3), according to the acid-base status of the patient, may be sufficient.

SODIUM CHLORIDE

Indications: sodium depletion; see also section 9.2.2.

Slow Sodium® (Novartis)

Tablets, m/r, sodium chloride 600 mg (approx. 10 mmol each of Na⁺ and Cl⁻). Net price 100-tab pack = 55p. Label: 25

> *Dose:* prophylaxis of sodium chloride deficiency 4–8 tablets daily with water (in severe depletion up to max. 20 tablets daily)
>
> Chronic renal salt wasting, up to 20 tablets daily with appropriate fluid intake
>
> CHILD, according to requirements

ORAL REHYDRATION THERAPY (ORT)

As a worldwide problem *diarrhoea* is by far the most important indication for fluid and electrolyte replacement. Intestinal absorption of sodium and water is enhanced by glucose (and other carbohydrates). Replacement of fluid and electrolytes lost through diarrhoea can therefore be achieved by giving solutions containing sodium, potassium, and glucose or another carbohydrate such as rice starch.

Oral rehydration solutions should:

enhance the absorption of water and electrolytes;
replace the electrolyte deficit adequately and safely;
contain an alkalising agent to counter acidosis;
be slightly hypo-osmolar (about 250 mmol/litre);
be simple to use in hospital and at home;
be palatable and acceptable, especially to children;
be readily available.

It is the policy of the World Health Organization (WHO) to promote a single oral rehydration solution but use it flexibly (e.g. by giving extra water between drinks of oral rehydration solution to moderately dehydrated infants).

Oral rehydration solutions used in the UK are lower in sodium (35–60 mmol/litre) and higher in glucose (up to 200 mmol/litre) than the WHO formulation. They are of benefit for *mild to moderate diarrhoea,* when the body's homoeostatic mechanisms are still working and will not be harmful, but they may be suboptimal in correction of fluid loss and electrolyte imbalance. In the *more severe diarrhoeas* the WHO formulation is marginally more effective in correcting dehydration; it carries no danger of hypernatraemia if used correctly. In acute diarrhoea normal feeding can continue as soon as the fluid deficit has been corrected; breast-feeding in particular should be offered between oral rehydration drinks.

For intravenous rehydration see section 9.2.2.

ORAL REHYDRATION SALTS (ORS)

Indications: fluid and electrolyte loss in diarrhoea, see notes above

Dose: according to fluid loss, usually 200–400 mL solution after every loose motion; INFANT 1–1½ times usual feed volume; CHILD 200 mL after every loose motion

UK formulations

Note. After reconstitution any unused solution should be discarded no later than 1 hour after preparation unless stored in a refrigerator when it may be kept for up to 24 hours.

Proprietary brands of oral rehydration salts on sale to the public include *Boots Diareze Oral rehydration treatment.*

Diocalm Junior® (SmithKline Beecham Healthcare)

Oral powder, sodium chloride 350 mg, potassium chloride 300 mg, sodium citrate 590 mg, anhydrous glucose 4 g/sachet. Net price 5-sachet pack (orange-flavoured) = £1.29

Reconstitute one sachet with 200 mL of water (freshly boiled and cooled for infants)

> *Note.* Five sachets reconstituted with 1 litre of water provide Na⁺ 60 mmol, K⁺ 20 mmol, Cl⁻ 50 mmol, citrate 10 mmol, and glucose 111 mmol

Dioralyte® (Rhône-Poulenc Rorer)

Effervescent tablets, sodium chloride 117 mg, sodium bicarbonate 336 mg, potassium chloride 186 mg, citric acid anhydrous 384 mg, anhydrous glucose 1.62 g. Net price 10-tab pack (blackcurrant- or citrus-flavoured) = £1.29

Reconstitute 2 tablets with 200 mL of water (only for adults and for children over 1 year)

> *Note.* Ten tablets when reconstituted with 1 litre of water provide Na⁺ 60 mmol, K⁺ 25 mmol, Cl⁻ 45 mmol, citrate 20 mmol, and glucose 90 mmol

Oral powder, sodium chloride 470 mg, potassium chloride 300 mg, disodium hydrogen citrate 530 mg, glucose 3.56 g/sachet. Net price 20 sachet-pack (blackcurrant- or citrus-flavoured or natural) = £4.69

Reconstitute one sachet with 200 mL of water (freshly boiled and cooled for infants).

> *Note.* Five sachets reconstituted with 1 litre of water provide Na⁺ 60 mmol, K⁺ 20 mmol, Cl⁻ 60 mmol, citrate 10 mmol, and glucose 90 mmol

Dioralyte® Relief (Rhône-Poulenc Rorer)

Oral powder, sodium chloride 350 mg, potassium chloride 300 mg, sodium citrate 580 mg, cooked rice powder 6 g/sachet, net price 20 sachet-pack (apricot-flavoured) = £5.63

Reconstitute one sachet with 200 mL of water (freshly boiled and cooled for infants)

> *Note.* 5 sachets when reconstitued with 1 litre of water provide Na⁺ 60 mmol, K⁺ 20 mmol, Cl⁻ 50 mmol and citrate 10 mmol; contains aspartame (section 9.4.1)

Electrolade® (Eastern)

Oral powder, sodium chloride 236 mg, potassium chloride 300 mg, sodium bicarbonate 500 mg, anhydrous glucose 4 g/sachet (banana-, blackcurrant-, melon-, or orange-flavoured). Net price 6-sachet (plain or multiflavoured) pack = £1.33, 20-sachet (single- or multiflavoured) pack = £4.25

Reconstitute one sachet with 200 mL of water (freshly boiled and cooled for infants)

> *Note.* Five sachets when reconstituted with 1 litre of water provide Na⁺ 50 mmol, K⁺ 20 mmol, Cl⁻ 40 mmol, HCO₃⁻ 30 mmol, and glucose 111 mmol

Rehidrat® (Searle)

Oral powder, sodium chloride 440 mg, potassium chloride 380 mg, sodium bicarbonate 420 mg, citric acid 440 mg, glucose 4.09 g, sucrose 8.07 g, fructose 70 mg/sachet. Net price 24-sachet pack

---

(orange, blackcurrant or lemon and lime flavour) = £6.44; 16-sachet pack (mixed flavours) = £4.29

Note. Lemon and lime version stains vomit green; blackcurrant version contains greater amounts of glucose (4.13 g) and sucrose (8.17 g), and less fructose (10 mg)

Reconstitute one sachet with 250 mL of water (freshly boiled and cooled for infants)

Note. Four sachets when reconstituted with 1 litre of water provide Na$^+$ 50 mmol, K$^+$ 20 mmol, Cl$^-$ 50 mmol, HCO$_3^-$ 20 mmol, citrate 9 mmol, glucose approx. 91 mmol, sucrose approx. 94 mmol, and fructose approx. 1–2 mmol

WHO formulations

WHO Oral Rehydration Salts

Oral powder, sodium chloride 3.5 g, potassium chloride 1.5 g, sodium citrate 2.9 g, anhydrous glucose 20 g. To be dissolved in sufficient water to produce 1 litre (providing Na$^+$ 90 mmol, K$^+$ 20 mmol, Cl$^-$ 80 mmol, citrate 10 mmol, glucose 111 mmol/litre)

Note. Recommended by the WHO and the United Nations Childrens Fund but not commonly used in the UK. Corresponds to Oral Rehydration Salts—Citrate (Formula C) BP; the alternative WHO formulation corresponds to Oral Rehydration Salts—Bicarbonate (Formula B) BP and is less stable

9.2.1.3 ORAL BICARBONATE

Sodium bicarbonate is given by mouth for *chronic acidotic states* such as uraemic acidosis or renal tubular acidosis. The dose for correction of metabolic acidosis is not predictable and the response must be assessed; 4.8 g daily (57 mmol each of Na$^+$ and HCO$_3^-$) or more may be required. For severe metabolic acidosis, sodium bicarbonate can be given intravenously (section 9.2.2).

Sodium bicarbonate may also be used to make the pH of the urine alkaline (see section 7.4.3); for use in dyspepsia see section 1.1.2.

Sodium supplements may increase blood pressure or cause fluid retention and pulmonary oedema in those at risk; hypokalaemia may be exacerbated.

Where *hyperchloraemic acidosis* is associated with potassium deficiency, as in some renal tubular and gastro-intestinal disorders it may be appropriate to give oral **potassium bicarbonate**, although acute or severe deficiency should be managed by intravenous therapy.

SODIUM BICARBONATE

Indications: see notes above
Cautions: see notes above; avoid in respiratory acidosis; **interactions:** Appendix 1 (antacids and adsorbents)
Dose: see notes above

Sodium Bicarbonate (Non-proprietary)

Capsules, sodium bicarbonate 500 mg (approx. 6 mmol each of Na$^+$ and HCO$_3^-$). Net price 20 = 44p

Available from Norton

Tablets, sodium bicarbonate 600 mg, net price 20 tabs = 50p

POTASSIUM BICARBONATE

Indications: see notes above
Cautions: cardiac disease, renal impairment; **interactions:** Appendix 1 (potassium salts)
Contra-indications: hypochloraemia; plasma potassium concentration above 5 mmol/litre
Side-effects: nausea and vomiting
Dose: see notes above

Potassium Tablets, Effervescent, potassium

bicarbonate 500 mg, potassium acid tartrate 300 mg, each tablet providing 6.5 mmol of K$^+$. To be dissolved in water before administration. Net price 100 = £3.90. Label: 13, 21

Available from APS, Cox, Hillcross

Note. These tablets do not contain chloride; for effervescent tablets containing potassium and chloride, see under Potassium Chloride, section 9.2.1.1

WATER

The term water used without qualification means either potable water freshly drawn direct from the public supply and suitable for drinking or freshly boiled and cooled purified water. The latter should be used if the public supply is from a local storage tank or if the potable water is unsuitable for a particular preparation. (Water for injections, section 9.2.2.)

9.2.2   Intravenous administration

Solutions of electrolytes are given intravenously, to meet normal fluid and electrolyte requirements or to replenish substantial deficits or continuing losses, when the patient is nauseated or vomiting and is unable to take adequate amounts by mouth. When intravenous administration is not possible large volumes of fluid can also be given subcutaneously by hypodermoclysis.

In an individual patient the nature and severity of the electrolyte imbalance must be assessed from the history and clinical and biochemical examination. Sodium, potassium, chloride, magnesium, phosphate, and water depletion can occur singly and in combination with or without disturbances of acid-base balance; for reference to the use of magnesium and phosphates, see section 9.5.

Isotonic solutions may be infused safely into a peripheral vein. Solutions more concentrated than plasma, for example 20% glucose are best given through an indwelling catheter positioned in a large vein.

INTRAVENOUS SODIUM

Sodium chloride in isotonic solution provides the most important extracellular ions in near physiological concentration and is indicated in *sodium depletion* which may arise from such conditions as gastro-enteritis, diabetic ketoacidosis, ileus, and ascites. In a severe deficit of from 4 to 8 litres, 2 to 3 litres of isotonic sodium chloride may be given over 2 to 3 hours; thereafter infusion can usually be at a slower rate.

Excessive administration should be avoided; the jugular venous pressure should be assessed, the bases of the lungs should be examined for crepitations, and in elderly or seriously ill patients it is often helpful to monitor the right atrial (central) venous pressure.

Compound sodium lactate (Hartmann's solution) can be used instead of isotonic sodium chloride solution during surgery or in the initial management of the injured or wounded.

Sodium chloride and glucose solutions are indicated when there is combined *water and sodium depletion*. A 1:1 mixture of isotonic sodium chloride and 5% glucose allows some of the water (free of sodium) to enter body cells which suffer most from dehydration while the sodium salt with a volume of water determined by the normal plasma Na⁺ remains extracellular. Combined sodium, potassium, chloride, and water depletion may occur, for example, with severe diarrhoea or persistent vomiting; replacement is carried out with sodium chloride intravenous infusion 0.9% and glucose intravenous infusion 5% with potassium as appropriate.

SODIUM CHLORIDE

Indications: electrolyte imbalance, also section 9.2.1.2

Cautions: restrict intake in impaired renal function, cardiac failure, hypertension, peripheral and pulmonary oedema, toxaemia of pregnancy

Side-effects: administration of large doses may give rise to sodium accumulation and oedema

Dose: see notes above

PoM Sodium Chloride Intravenous Infusion, usual strength sodium chloride 0.9% (9 g, 150 mmol each of Na⁺ and Cl⁻/litre), this strength being supplied when normal saline for injection is requested. Net price 2-mL amp = 23p; 5-mL amp = 28p; 10-mL amp = 32p; 20-mL amp = 87p; 50-mL amp = £1.85

In hospitals, 500- and 1000-mL packs, and sometimes other sizes, are available

Note. The term 'normal saline' should **not** be used to describe sodium chloride intravenous infusion 0.9%; the term 'physiological saline' is acceptable but it is preferable to give the composition (i.e. sodium chloride intravenous infusion 0.9%).

With other ingredients

PoM Sodium Chloride and Glucose Intravenous Infusion, usual strength sodium chloride 0.18% (1.8 g, 30 mmol each of Na⁺ and Cl⁻/litre) and 4% of anhydrous glucose

In hospitals, 500- and 1000-mL packs, and sometimes other sizes are available

PoM Ringer's Solution for Injection, calcium chloride (dihydrate) 322 micrograms, potassium chloride 300 micrograms, sodium chloride 8.6 mg/mL, providing the following ions (in mmol/litre), Ca²⁺ 2.2, K⁺ 4, Na⁺ 147, Cl⁻ 156

In hospitals, 500- and 1000-mL packs, and sometimes other sizes, are available

PoM Sodium Lactate Intravenous Infusion, Compound (Hartmann's Solution for Injection; Ringer-Lactate Solution for Injection), sodium chloride 0.6%, sodium lactate 0.25%, potassium chloride 0.04%, calcium chloride 0.027% (containing Na⁺ 131 mmol, K⁺ 5 mmol, Ca²⁺ 2 mmol, HCO₃⁻ (as lactate) 29 mmol, Cl⁻ 111 mmol/litre)

In hospitals, 500- and 1000-mL packs, and sometimes other sizes, are available

INTRAVENOUS GLUCOSE

Glucose solutions (5%) are mainly used to replace water deficits and should be given alone when there is no significant loss of electrolytes. Average water requirements in a healthy adult are 1.5 to 2.5 litres daily and this is needed to balance unavoidable losses of water through the skin and lungs and to provide sufficient for urinary excretion. Water depletion (dehydration) tends to occur when these losses are not matched by a comparable intake, as for example may occur in coma or dysphagia or in the aged or apathetic who may not drink water in sufficient amount on their own initiative.

Excessive loss of water without loss of electrolytes is uncommon, occurring in fevers, hyperthyroidism, and in uncommon water-losing renal states such as diabetes insipidus or hypercalcaemia. The volume of glucose solution needed to replace deficits varies with the severity of the disorder, but usually lies within the range of 2 to 6 litres.

Glucose solutions are also given in regimens with calcium, bicarbonate, and insulin for the emergency management of *hyperkalaemia*. They are also given, after correction of hyperglycaemia, during treatment of diabetic ketoacidosis, when they must be accompanied by continuing insulin infusion.

GLUCOSE

(Dextrose Monohydrate)

Note. Glucose BP is the monohydrate but Glucose Intravenous Infusion BP is a sterile solution of anhydrous glucose or glucose monohydrate, potency being expressed in terms of anhydrous glucose

Indications: fluid replacement (see notes above), provision of energy (section 9.3)

Side-effects: glucose injections especially if hypertonic may have a low pH and may cause venous irritation and thrombophlebitis

Dose: water replacement, see notes above; energy source, 1–3 litres daily of 20–50% solution

PoM Glucose Intravenous Infusion, glucose or anhydrous glucose (potency expressed in terms of anhydrous glucose), usual strength 5% (50 mg/mL). 25% solution, net price 25-mL amp = £2.21; 50% solution, 25-mL amp = £3.11, 50-mL amp = £1.26

In hospitals, 500- and 1000-mL packs, and sometimes other sizes, are available; also available from IMS (Min-I-Jet® Glucose, 50% in 50-ml disposable syringe).

Cautionary label wordings, see inside back cover | Prices are **net**, see p.1

INTRAVENOUS POTASSIUM

Potassium chloride and sodium chloride intravenous infusion and **potassium chloride and glucose** intravenous infusion are used to correct severe *hypokalaemia* and depletion and when sufficient potassium cannot be taken by mouth. Potassium chloride, as ampoules containing 1.5 g (20 mmol K⁺) in 10 mL[1], may be added to 500 mL of sodium chloride or glucose intravenous infusion and given slowly over 2 to 3 hours with specialist advice and ECG monitoring in difficult cases[2]. Repeated measurements of plasma potassium are necessary to determine whether further infusions are required and to avoid the development of hyperkalaemia; this is *especially liable to occur* in renal impairment.

1. **Important**: mix infusion solution **thoroughly** after adding potassium chloride; use ready-prepared solutions when possible
2. Higher concentrations may be given in severe cases but require infusion pump control

POTASSIUM CHLORIDE

Indications: electrolyte imbalance; see also oral potassium supplements, section 9.2.1.1
Cautions: for intravenous infusion the concentration of solution should not usually exceed 3.2 g (43 mmol)/litre; specialist advice and ECG monitoring (see notes above)
Side-effects: rapid infusion toxic to heart
Dose: by slow intravenous infusion, depending on the deficit or the daily maintenance requirements, see also notes above

PoM **Potassium Chloride and Glucose Intravenous Infusion,** usual strength potassium chloride 0.3% (3 g, 40 mmol each of K⁺ and Cl⁻/litre) with 5% of anhydrous glucose
In hospitals, 500- and 1000-mL packs, and sometimes other sizes, are available

PoM **Potassium Chloride and Sodium Chloride Intravenous Infusion,** usual strength potassium chloride 0.3% (3 g/litre) and sodium chloride 0.9% (9 g/litre), containing 40 mmol of K⁺, 150 mmol of Na⁺, and 190 mmol of Cl⁻/litre
In hospitals, 500- and 1000-mL packs, and sometimes other sizes, are available

PoM **Potassium Chloride, Sodium Chloride, and Glucose Intravenous Infusion,** sodium chloride 0.18% (1.8 g, 30 mmol of Na⁺/litre) with 4% of anhydrous glucose and usually sufficient potassium chloride to provide 10–40 mmol of K⁺/litre (to be specified by the prescriber)
In hospitals, 500- and 1000-mL packs, and sometimes other sizes, are available

PoM **Potassium Chloride Solution, Strong,** (sterile), potassium chloride 15% (150 mg, approximately 2 mmol each of K⁺ and Cl⁻/mL). Net price 10-mL amp = 40p
IMPORTANT. Must be diluted with **not less** than 50 times its volume of sodium chloride intravenous infusion 0.9% or other suitable diluent and **mixed well**
Solutions containing 10 and 20% of potassium chloride are also available in both 5- and 10-mL ampoules

BICARBONATE AND LACTATE

Sodium bicarbonate is used to control severe *metabolic acidosis* (as in renal failure). Since this condition is usually attended by sodium depletion, it is reasonable to correct this first by the administration of isotonic sodium chloride intravenous infusion, provided the kidneys are not primarily affected and the degree of acidosis is not so severe as to impair renal function. In these circumstances, isotonic sodium chloride alone is usually effective as it restores the ability of the kidneys to generate bicarbonate. In renal acidosis or in severe metabolic acidosis of any origin (for example blood pH < 7.1) sodium bicarbonate (1.26%) may be infused with isotonic sodium chloride when the acidosis remains unresponsive to correction of anoxia or fluid depletion; a total volume of up to 6 litres (4 litres of sodium chloride and 2 litres of sodium bicarbonate) may be necessary in the adult. In severe shock due for example to cardiac arrest (see section 2.7), metabolic acidosis may develop without sodium depletion; in these circumstances sodium bicarbonate is best given in a small volume of hypertonic solution, such as 50 mL of 8.4% solution intravenously; plasma pH should be monitored.

Sodium bicarbonate infusion is also used in the emergency management of *hyperkalaemia* (see also under Glucose).

Sodium lactate intravenous infusion is obsolete in metabolic acidosis, and carries the risk of producing lactic acidosis, particularly in seriously ill patients with poor tissue perfusion or impaired hepatic function.

SODIUM BICARBONATE

Indications: metabolic acidosis
Dose: by slow intravenous injection, a strong solution (up to 8.4%), or by continuous intravenous infusion, a weaker solution (usually 1.26%), an amount appropriate to the body base deficit (see notes above)

PoM **Sodium Bicarbonate Intravenous Infusion,** usual strength sodium bicarbonate 1.26% (12.6 g, 150 mmol each of Na⁺ and HCO₃⁻/litre); various other strengths available
In hospitals, 500- and 1000-mL packs, and sometimes other sizes, are available

PoM **Min-I-Jet® Sodium Bicarbonate** (IMS)
Intravenous injection, sodium bicarbonate in disposable syringe, net price 4.2%, 10 mL = £4.81; 8.4%, 10 mL = £5.19, 50 mL = £7.75

SODIUM LACTATE

Indications: see notes above

PoM **Sodium Lactate Intravenous Infusion,** sodium lactate M/6, contains the following ions (in mmol/litre), Na⁺ 167, HCO₃⁻ (as lactate) 167

WATER

PoM **Water for Injections.** Net price 1-mL amp = 15p; 2-mL amp = 14p; 5-mL amp = 21p; 10-mL amp = 25p; 20-mL amp = 53p; 50-mL amp = £1.50

9.2.3 Plasma and plasma substitutes

Albumin solutions, prepared from whole blood, contain soluble proteins and electrolytes but no clotting factors, blood group antibodies, or plasma cholinesterases; they may be given without regard to the recipient's blood group.

Albumin solutions are used for the treatment of severe hypoproteinaemia, particularly when associated with a low plasma volume. The use of these solutions in acute plasma or blood loss may be wasteful; plasma substitutes are more appropriate. Concentrated albumin solutions may also be used to obtain a diuresis in hypoalbuminaemic patients (e.g. in hepatic cirrhosis).

ALBUMIN SOLUTION
(Human Albumin Solution)

A solution containing protein derived from plasma, serum, or normal placentas; at least 95% of the protein is albumin. The solution may be isotonic (containing 4–5% protein) or concentrated (containing 15–25% protein).

Indications: see under preparations, below

Cautions: history of cardiac or circulatory disease (administer slowly to avoid rapid rise in blood pressure and cardiac failure, and monitor cardiovascular and respiratory function); correct dehydration when administering concentrated solution

Contra-indications: cardiac failure; severe anaemia

Side-effects: allergic reactions with nausea, vomiting, increased salivation, fever, and chills reported

Isotonic solutions

Indications: acute or sub-acute loss of plasma volume e.g. in burns, pancreatitis, trauma, and complications of surgery; plasma exchange

Available as: *Human Albumin Solution 4.5%* (50-, 100-, and 400-mL bottles—Immuno); *Alba®* *4.5%* (100- and 400-mL bottles—SNBTS); *Albuminar-5®* (500-mL vials—Centeon); *Albutein® 5%* (250- and 500-mL vials—Alpha); *Zenalb® 4.5* (50-, 100-, 250-, and 500-mL bottles—BPL)

Concentrated solutions (20–25%)

Indications: severe hypoalbuminaemia associated with low plasma volume and generalised oedema where salt and water restriction with plasma volume expansion are required; adjunct in the treatment of hyperbilirubinaemia by exchange transfusion in the newborn

Available as: *Albumin Solution 20%* (100-mL vials—SNBTS); *Human Albumin Solution 20%* (10-, 50-, and 100-mL vials—Immuno); *Albutein® 20%* (50- and 100-mL vials—Alpha); *Albutein® 25%* (20-, 50-, and 100-mL vials—Alpha); *Zenalb® 20* (5-, 50-, and 100-mL bottles—BPL)

PLASMA SUBSTITUTES

Dextrans, **gelatin**, and the etherified starches, **hetastarch** and **pentastarch** are macromolecular substances which are slowly metabolised; they may be used at the outset to expand and maintain blood volume in shock arising from conditions such as burns or septicaemia. They are rarely needed when shock is due to sodium and water depletion as, in these circumstances, the shock responds to water and electrolyte repletion. They should not be used to maintain plasma volume in conditions such as burns or peritonitis where there is loss of plasma protein, water and electrolytes over periods of several days or weeks. In these situations, plasma or plasma protein fractions containing large amounts of albumin should be given. Plasma substitutes may be used as an immediate short-term measure to treat haemorrhage until blood is available.

Dextrans may interfere with blood group cross-matching or biochemical measurements and these should be carried out before infusion is begun. Dextran 70 by intravenous infusion is used predominantly for volume expansion. Dextran 40 intravenous infusion is used in an attempt to improve peripheral blood flow in ischaemic disease of the limbs. Dextrans 40 and 70 have also been used in the prophylaxis of thromboembolism but are now rarely used for this purpose.

> **Dosage.** Because of the complex requirements relating to blood volume expansion and the primary significance of blood, plasma protein, and electrolyte replacement, detailed dose statements have been omitted. *In all cases product literature and other specialist literature should be consulted.*

DEXTRAN 40

Dextrans of weight average molecular weight about '40 000' 10% in glucose intravenous infusion 5% or in sodium chloride intravenous infusion 0.9%

Indications: conditions associated with peripheral local slowing of the blood flow; prophylaxis of post-surgical thromboembolic disease (but see notes above)

Cautions; Contra-indications; Side-effects: see under Dextran 70 Intravenous Infusion; correct dehydration before infusion and give adequate fluids during therapy; very special care in those at risk of vascular overloading

Dose: by intravenous infusion, initially 500–1000 mL; further doses are given according to the patient's condition (see notes above)

PoM **Gentran 40®** (Baxter)

Intravenous infusion, dextran 40 intravenous infusion in glucose intravenous infusion 5% or in sodium chloride intravenous infusion 0.9%. Net price 500-mL bottle (both) = £4.78

PoM **Rheomacrodex®** (Cambridge)

Intravenous infusion, dextran 40 intravenous infusion in glucose intravenous infusion 5% or in sodium chloride intravenous infusion 0.9%. Net price 500-mL bottle (both) = £6.35

DEXTRAN 70

Dextrans of weight average molecular weight about '70 000' 6% in glucose intravenous infusion 5% or in sodium chloride intravenous infusion 0.9%

Indications: short-term blood volume expansion; prophylaxis of post-surgical thromboembolic disease (but see notes above)

Cautions: congestive heart failure, renal impairment; blood samples for cross-matching should ideally be taken before infusion; see also notes above

Contra-indications: severe congestive heart failure; renal failure; bleeding disorders such as thrombocytopenia and hypofibrinogenaemia

Side-effects: urticarial and other hypersensitivity reactions—rarely severe anaphylactoid reactions

Dose: *by intravenous infusion,* after moderate to severe haemorrhage or in the shock phase of burn injury (initial 48 hours), 500–1000 mL rapidly initially followed by 500 mL later if necessary (see also notes above); total dosage should not exceed 20 mL/kg during initial 24 hours; CHILD total dosage should not exceed 20 mL/kg

PoM **Gentran 70**® (Baxter)

Intravenous infusion, dextran 70 intravenous infusion in glucose intravenous infusion 5% or in sodium chloride intravenous infusion 0.9%. Net price 500-mL bottle (both) = £4.78

GELATIN

Note. The gelatin is partially degraded

Indications: low blood volume

Cautions: congestive heart failure, renal impairment; blood samples for cross-matching should ideally be taken before infusion; haemorrhagic diasthesis

Contra-indications: severe congestive heart failure; renal failure

Side-effects: urticarial and other hypersensitivity reactions—rarely severe anaphylactoid reactions

Dose: *by intravenous infusion,* initially 500–1000 mL of a 3.5–4% solution (see notes above)

PoM **Gelofusine**® (Braun)

Intravenous infusion, succinylated gelatin (modified fluid gelatin, average molecular weight 30 000) 4%, sodium chloride 0.9%. Net price 500-mL bottle = £4.50

PoM **Haemaccel**® (Hoechst Marion Roussel)

Intravenous infusion, polygeline (degraded and modified gelatin, average molecular weight 30 000) 35 g, Na⁺ 145 mmol, K⁺ 5.1 mmol, Ca²⁺ 6.25 mmol, Cl⁻ 145 mmol/litre. Net price 500-mL bottle = £3.71

ETHERIFIED STARCH

A starch composed of more than 90% of amylopectin that has been etherified with hydroxyethyl groups; hetastarch has a higher degree of etherification than pentastarch

Indications: low blood volume

Cautions; Contra-indications; Side-effects: see under Dextran 70 Intravenous Infusion; pruritus reported

Dose: see under preparations below

Hetastarch
PoM **Hespan**® (Geistlich)

Intravenous infusion, hetastarch (weight average molecular weight 450 000) 6% in sodium chloride intravenous infusion 0.9%. Net price 500-mL Steriflex® bag = £16.30

Dose: by intravenous infusion, 500–1000 mL; usual daily max. 1500 mL (see notes above)

Hexastarch
PoM **eloHAES**® (Fresenius)

Intravenous infusion, hexastarch (weight average molecular weight 200 000) 6% in sodium chloride intravenous infusion 0.9%. Net price 500-mL Steriflex® bag = £12.50

Dose: by intravenous infusion, 500–1000 mL; usual daily max. 1500 mL (see notes above)

Pentastarch
PoM **HAES-steril**® (Fresenius)

Intravenous infusion, pentastarch (weight average molecular weight 200 000), net price (both in sodium chloride intravenous infusion 0.9%) 6%, 500 mL = £10.50; 10%, 500 mL = £16.50

Dose: by intravenous infusion, pentastarch 6%, up to 2500 mL daily; pentastarch 10%, up to 1500 mL daily (see notes above)

PoM **Pentaspan**® (Geistlich)

Intravenous infusion, pentastarch (weight average molecular weight 250 000) 10% in sodium chloride intravenous infusion 0.9%. Net price 500-mL Intraflex bag = £11.25

Dose: by intravenous infusion, 500–2000 mL; usual daily max. 2000 mL (see notes above)

9.3   Intravenous nutrition

When adequate feeding through the alimentary tract is not possible, nutrients may be given by intravenous infusion. This may be in addition to ordinary oral or tube feeding—**supplemental parenteral nutrition**, or may be the sole source of nutrition—**total parenteral nutrition** (TPN). Indications for this method include preparation of undernourished patients for surgery, chemotherapy, or radiation therapy; severe or prolonged disorders of the gastro-intestinal tract; major surgery, trauma, or burns; prolonged coma or refusal to eat; and some patients with renal or hepatic failure. The composition of proprietary preparations available is given in the table below.

Total parenteral nutrition requires the use of a solution containing amino acids, glucose, fat, electrolytes, trace elements, and vitamins. This is now commonly provided by the pharmacy in the form of the 3-litre bag. Loading doses of vitamin B_{12} and folic acid are advised and other vitamins are given parenterally twice weekly.

The nutrition solution is infused through a central venous catheter inserted under full surgical precautions. Alternatively infusion through a peripheral vein is used for supplementary as well as total parenteral nutrition for periods of up to a month, depending on the availability of peripheral veins; factors prolonging cannula life and preventing thrombophlebitis include the use of soft polyurethane paediatric cannulae and use of feeds of low osmolality and neutral pH. Only nutritional fluids should be given by the dedicated intravenous line.

Before starting, the patient should be well oxygenated with a near normal circulating blood volume and attention should be given to renal function and acid-base status. Appropriate biochemical tests should have been carried out beforehand and serious deficits corrected. Nutritional and electrolyte status must be monitored throughout treatment.

Complications of long-term TPN include gall bladder sludging, gall stones, cholestasis and abnormal liver function tests. For details of the prevention and management of TPN complications, specialist literature should be consulted.

Protein is given as mixtures of essential and non-essential synthetic L-amino acids. Ideally, all essential amino acids should be included with a wide variety of non-essential ones to provide sufficient nitrogen together with electrolytes (see also section 9.2.2). Solutions vary in their composition of amino acids; they often contain an energy source (usually glucose) and electrolytes.

Energy is provided in a ratio of 0.6 to 1.1 megajoules (150–250 kcals) per gram of protein nitrogen. Energy requirements must be met if amino acids are to be utilised for tissue maintenance. A mixture of carbohydrate and fat energy sources (usually 30–50% as fat) gives better utilisation of amino acids than glucose alone.

Glucose is the preferred source of carbohydrate, but if more than 180 g is given per day frequent monitoring of blood glucose is required, and insulin may be necessary. Glucose in various strengths from 10 to 50% must be infused through a central venous catheter to avoid thrombosis.

In total parenteral nutrition regimens, it is necessary to provide adequate phosphate in order to allow phosphorylation of the glucose; between 20 and 30 mmol of phosphate is required daily.

Fructose and sorbitol have been used in an attempt to avoid the problem of hyperosmolar hyperglycaemic non-ketotic acidosis but other metabolic problems may occur, as with xylitol and ethanol which are now rarely used.

Fat emulsions have the advantages of a high energy to fluid volume ratio, neutral pH, and iso-osmolarity with plasma, and provide essential fatty acids. Several days of adaptation may be required to attain maximal utilisation. Reactions include occasional febrile episodes (usually only with 20% emulsions) and rare anaphylactic responses. Interference with biochemical measurements such as those for blood gases and calcium may occur if samples are taken before fat has been cleared. Daily checks are necessary to ensure complete clearance from the plasma in conditions where fat metabolism may be disturbed. **Additives may only be mixed with fat emulsions where compatibility is known.**

SUPPLEMENTARY PREPARATIONS

PoM **Addiphos®** (Pharmacia & Upjohn)
Solution, sterile, phosphate 40 mmol, K+ 30 mmol, Na+ 30 mmol/20 mL. For addition to *Vamin®* solutions and glucose intravenous infusions. Net price 20-mL vial = £1.15

PoM **Additrace®** (Pharmacia & Upjohn)
Solution, trace elements for addition to *Vamin®* solutions, traces of Fe^{3+}, Zn^{2+}, Mn^{2+}, Cu^{2+}, Cr^{3+}, Se^{4+}, Mo^{6+}, F-, I-. For adults and children over 40 kg. Net price 10-mL amp = £1.75

PoM **Cernevit®** (Nestlé Clinical)
Solution, dl-alpha tocopherol 11.2 units, ascorbic acid 125 mg, biotin 69 micrograms, cholecalciferol 220 units, cyanocobalamin 6 micrograms, folic acid 414 micrograms, glycine 250 mg, nicotinamide 46 mg, pantothenic acid (as dexpanthenol) 17.25 mg, pyridoxine hydrochloride 5.5 mg, retinol (as palmitate) 3500 units, riboflavine (as dihydrated sodium phosphate) 4.14 mg, thiamine (as cocarboxylase tetrahydrate) 3.51 mg. Dissolve in 5 mL water for injections. Net price per vial = £2.90

▼ PoM **Dipeptiven®** (Fresenius)
Solution, N(2)-L-alanyl-L-glutamine 200 mg/mL (providing L-alanine 82 mg, L-glutamine 134.6 mg). For addition to infusion solutions containing amino acids. Net price 50 mL = £25.00, 100 mL = £29.60
Dose: amino acid supplement for hypercatabolic or hypermetabolic states, 300–400 mg/kg daily; max. 400 mg/kg daily, dose not to exceed 20% of total amino acid intake

PoM **Multibionta®** (Merck)
Solution, ascorbic acid 500 mg, dexpanthenol 25 mg, nicotinamide 100 mg, pyridoxine hydrochloride 15 mg, riboflavine sodium phosphate 10 mg, thiamine hydrochloride 50 mg, tocopheryl acetate 5 mg, vitamin A 10 000 units. For addition to infusion solutions. Net price 10-mL amp = £1.61
Contra-indications: not for use in neonates owing to presence of benzyl alcohol as additive

PoM **Peditrace®** (Pharmacia & Upjohn)
Solution, trace elements for addition to *Vaminolact®*, *Vamin® 14 Electrolyte-Free* solutions and glucose intravenous infusions, traces of Zn^{2+}, Cu^{2+}, Mn^{2+}, Se^{4+}, F-, I-. For use in infants (when kidney function established, usually second day of life) and children. Net price 10-mL vial = £3.10
Cautions: reduced biliary excretion especially in cholestatic liver disease or in markedly reduced urinary excretion (careful biochemical monitoring required); total parenteral nutrition exceeding 1 month (measure serum manganese concentration and check liver function before commencing treatment and regularly during treatment)—discontinue if manganese concentration raised or if cholestasis develops

PoM **Solivito N®** (Pharmacia & Upjohn)
Solution, powder for reconstitution, biotin 60 micrograms, cyanocobalamin 5 micrograms, folic acid 400 micrograms, glycine 300 mg, nicotinamide 40 mg, pyridoxine hydrochloride 4.9 mg, riboflavine sodium phosphate 4.9 mg, sodium ascorbate 113 mg, sodium pantothenate 16.5 mg, thiamine mononitrate 3.1 mg. Dissolve in water for injections or glucose intravenous infusion for adding to glucose intravenous infusion or *Intralipid®*; dissolve in *Vitlipid N®* or *Intralipid®* for adding to *Intralipid®* only. Net price per vial = £1.75

Proprietary Infusion Fluids for Parenteral Feeding

Preparation	Nitrogen g/litre	[1]Energy kJ/litre	K+	Mg2+	Na+	Acet-	Cl-	Other components/litre
Aminoplex 12 (Geistlich) Net price 500 mL = £11.31; 1000 mL = £19.07	12.44		30	2.5	35	5	67	malic acid 4.6 g
Aminoplex 24 (Geistlich) Net price 250 mL = £9.79; 500 mL = £17.28	24.9		30	2.5	35	5	67	malic acid 4.5 g
Aminosteril 8 (Fresenius) Net price 500 mL = £7.95	7.95				55			
Aminosteril 14 (Fresenius) Net price 500 mL = £9.90; 1000 mL = £16.00	13.52				93			
Aminosteril 16 (Fresenius) Net price 500 mL = £10.90	15.9				109			
Clinimix N9G20E (Baxter) Net price (dual compartment bag of amino acids with electrolytes 1000 mL and glucose 20% with calcium 1000 mL) = £29.00	4.55	1680	30	2.5	35	50	40	Ca2+ 2.25 mmol, phosphate 15 mmol, anhydrous glucose 100 g
Clinimix N14G30E (Baxter) Net price (dual compartment bag of amino acids with electrolytes 1000 mL and glucose 30% with calcium 1000 mL) = £33.00	7	2520	30	2.5	35	70	40	Ca2+ 2.25 mmol, phosphate 15 mmol, anhydrous glucose 150 g
FreAmine III 8.5% (Fresenius) Net price 500 mL = £14.39; 1000 mL = £21.06	13.0				10	72	<3	phosphate 10 mmol
FreAmine III 10% (Fresenius) Net price 500 mL = £13.60; 1000 mL = £23.50	15.3				10	89	<3	phosphate 10 mmol
FreAmine HBC 6.9% (Fresenius) Net price 750 mL = £14.43	9.73				10	57	<3	
Glamin (Pharmacia & Upjohn) Net price 250 mL = £14.16; 500 mL = £26.38; 1000 mL = £52.76	22.4				62			
Glucoplex 1000 (Geistlich) Net price 500 mL = £3.30; 1000 mL = £4.71		4200	30	2.5	50		67	acid phosphate 18 mmol, Zn2+ 0.046 mmol, anhydrous glucose 240 g
Glucoplex 1600 (Geistlich) Net price 500 mL = £3.64; 1000 mL = £4.88		6720	30	2.5	50		67	acid phosphate 18 mmol, Zn2+ 0.046 mmol, anhydrous glucose 400 g
Hepanutrin (Geistlich) Net price 500 mL = £15.74	15.6							
HeplexAmine 8% (Fresenius) Net price 500 mL = £16.31	12				10	61	<3	phosphate 10 mmol
Hyperamine 30 (Braun) Net price 500 mL = £23.67	30				5			
Intrafusin 22 (Pharmacia & Upjohn) Net price 500 mL = £14.38	22.8							
Intralipid 10% (Pharmacia & Upjohn) Net price 100 mL = £3.90; 500 mL = £8.58		4600						soya oil 100 g, glycerol 22 g, purified egg phospholipids 12 g, phosphate 15 mmol
Intralipid 20% (Pharmacia & Upjohn) Net price 100 mL = £5.85; 250 mL = £9.65; 500 mL = £12.87		8400						soya oil 200 g, glycerol 22 g, purified egg phospholipids 12 g, phosphate 15 mmol
Intralipid 30% (Pharmacia & Upjohn) Net price 333 mL = £14.40		12600						soya oil 300 g, glycerol 16.7 g, purified egg phospholipids 12 g, phosphate 15 mmol
Ivelip 10% (Baxter) Net price 100 mL = £4.78; 500 mL = £9.51		4600						soya oil 100 g, glycerol 25 g
Ivelip 20% (Baxter) Net price 100 mL = £6.58; 500 mL = £14.53; 1000 mL = £25.84		8400						soya oil 200 g, glycerol 25 g
KabiMix 9 (Pharmacia & Upjohn) Net price 2580 mL = £64.00	3.49	2600	23	1.9	31	55	31	Ca2+ 1.9 mmol, anhydrous glucose 58.14 g, phosphate 10.9 mmol, soya oil 38.76 g, glycerol 4.26 g, purified egg phospholipids 2.33 g
KabiMix 14 (Pharmacia & Upjohn) Net price 2580 mL = £70.00	5.23	3570	23	1.9	31	90	31	Ca2+ 1.9 mmol, anhydrous glucose 116.28 g, phosphate 10.9 mmol, soya oil 38.76 g, glycerol 4.26 g, purified egg phospholipids 2.33 g
Lipofundin MCT/LCT 10% (Braun) Net price 100 mL = £7.70; 500 mL = £12.90		4430						soya oil 50 g, medium chain triglycerides 50 g

1. Excludes protein- or amino acid-derived energy
2. For use in neonates and children only

Note. 1000 kcal = 4200 kJ; 1000 kJ = 238.8 kcal. All entries are PoM

Proprietary Infusion Fluids for Parenteral Feeding

Preparation	Nitrogen g/litre	[1]Energy kJ/litre	K+	Mg2+	Na+	Acet-	Cl-	Other components/litre
Lipofundin MCT/LCT 20% (Braun) Net price 100 mL = £8.79; 250 mL = £11.30; 500 mL = £19.18		8000						soya oil 100 g, medium chain triglycerides 100 g
Lipofundin S 10% (Braun) Net price 100 mL = £6.00; 500 mL = £9.80		4470						soya oil 100 g, glycerol 25 g
Lipofundin S 20% (Braun) Net price 100 mL = £7.00; 500 mL = £15.30		8520						soya oil 200 g, glycerol 25 g
Lipovenos 10% (Fresenius) Net price 500 mL = £9.50		4600						fractionated soya oil 100 g, egg lecithin 12 g, glycerol 25 g
Lipovenos 20% (Fresenius) Net price 100 mL = £4.90; 250 mL = £5.60; 500 mL = £14.50		8400						fractionated soya oil 200 g, egg lecithin 12 g, glycerol 25 g
Nephramine 5.4% (Fresenius) Net price 250 mL = £14.72	6.4				5	44	<3	essential amino acids only
Nutracel 400 (Baxter) Net price 500 mL = £2.54		3400		18		0.16	66	Ca2+ 15 mmol, Mn2+ 0.01 mmol, Zn2+ 0.08 mmol, anhydrous glucose 200 g
Nutracel 800 (Baxter) Net price 1000 mL = £4.39		3400		9		0.08	33	Ca2+ 7.5 mmol, Mn2+ 0.005 mmol, Zn2+ 0.04 mmol, anhydrous glucose 200 g
Nutriflex Basal (Braun) Net price (dual compartment bag of 800 mL and 1200 mL) = £28.35	4.6	2095	30	5.7	49.9	35	50	Ca2+ 3.6 mmol, phosphate 12.8 mmol, anhydrous glucose 125 g
Nutriflex Peri 40/80 (Braun) Net price (dual compartment bag of 800 mL and 1200 mL) = £33.00	5.7	1340	15	4	27	19.5	31.6	Ca2+ 2.5 mmol, phosphate 5.7 mmol, anhydrous glucose 80 g
Nutriflex Plus (Braun) Net price (dual compartment bag of 800 mL and 1200 mL) = £39.18	6.8	2510	25	5.7	37.2	22.9	35.5	Ca2+ 3.6 mmol, phosphate 20 mmol, anhydrous glucose 150 g
Nutriflex Special (Braun) Net price (dual compartment bag of 750 mL and 750 mL) = £43.30	10	4020	25.7	5	40.5	22	49.5	Ca2+ 4.1 mmol, phosphate 15 mmol, anhydrous glucose 240 g
Plasma-Lyte 148 (water) (Baxter) Net price 1000 mL = £1.59			5	1.5	140	27	98	gluconate 23 mmol
Plasma-Lyte 148 (dextrose 5%) (Baxter) Net price 1000 mL = £1.59		840	5	1.5	140	27	98	gluconate 23 mmol, anhydrous glucose 50 g
Plasma-Lyte M (dextrose 5%) (Baxter) Net price 1000 mL = £1.33		840	16	1.5	40	12	40	Ca2+ 2.5 mmol, lactate 12 mmol, anhydrous glucose 50 g
[2]Primene 10% (Baxter) Net price 100 mL = £6.05; 250 mL = £8.29	15						15.6	
Synthamin 9 (Baxter) Net price 500 mL = £6.97; 1000 mL = £12.92	9.1		60	5	70	100	70	acid phosphate 30 mmol
Synthamin 14 (Baxter) Net price 500 mL = £10.09; 1000 mL = £17.94; 3000 mL = £51.29	14.0		60	5	70	140	70	acid phosphate 30 mmol
Synthamin 14 without electrolytes (Baxter) Net price 500 mL = £10.34; 1000 mL = £18.33	14.0					68	34	
Synthamin 17 (Baxter) Net price 500 mL = £13.26; 1000 mL = £24.08	16.5		60	5	70	150	70	acid phosphate 30 mmol
Synthamin 17 without electrolytes (Baxter) Net price 500 mL = £13.26	16.5					82	40	
Vamin 9 (Pharmacia & Upjohn) Net price 500 mL = £5.85; 1000 mL = £10.04	9.4		20	1.5	50		50	Ca2+ 2.5 mmol
Vamin 9 Glucose (Pharmacia & Upjohn) Net price 100 mL = £3.02; 500 mL = £6.14; 1000 mL = £11.02	9.4	1700	20	1.5	50		50	Ca2+ 2.5 mmol, anhydrous glucose 100 g
Vamin 14 (Pharmacia & Upjohn) Net price 500 mL = £8.63; 1000 mL = £14.67	13.5		50	8	100	135	100	Ca2+ 5 mmol, SO4 2- 8 mmol
Vamin 14 (Electrolyte-Free) (Pharmacia & Upjohn) Net price 500 mL = £8.63; 1000 mL = £14.67	13.5				90			
Vamin 18 (Electrolyte-Free) (Pharmacia & Upjohn) Net price 500 mL = £10.97; 1000 mL = £19.74	18				110			
Vaminolact (Pharmacia & Upjohn) Net price 100 mL = £3.36; 500 mL = £7.75	9.3							
Vitrimix KV (Pharmacia & Upjohn) Net price (combined pack of Intralipid 20% 250 mL and Vamin 9 glucose 750 mL) = £19.90	7.0	3340	15	1.1	38		38	Ca2+ 1.9 mmol, anhydrous glucose 75 g, soya oil 50 g, purified egg phospholipids 3 g, glycerol 5.5 g, phosphate 3.75 g

PoM **Vitlipid N®** (Pharmacia & Upjohn)
Emulsion, adult, vitamin A 330 units, ergocalciferol 20 units, *dl*-alpha tocopherol 1 unit, phytomenadione 15 micrograms/mL. For addition to *Intralipid®*. For adults and children over 11 years. Net price 10-mL amp = £1.71
Emulsion, infant, vitamin A 230 units, ergocalciferol 40 units, *dl*-alpha tocopherol 0.7 unit, phytomenadione 20 micrograms/mL. For addition to *Intralipid®*. Net price 10-mL amp = £1.71

Administration. Because of the complex requirements relating to parenteral nutrition full details relating to administration have been omitted. In all cases *product literature and other specialist literature should be consulted.*

9.4   Oral nutrition

9.4.1   Foods for special diets
9.4.2   Enteral nutrition

9.4.1   Foods for special diets

These are preparations that have been modified to eliminate a particular constituent from a food or are nutrient mixtures formulated as substitutes for the food. They are for patients who either cannot tolerate or cannot metabolise certain common constituents of food.

PHENYLKETONURIA. Phenylketonuria (phenylalaninaemia), which results from the inability to metabolise phenylalanine, is managed by restricting its dietary intake to a small amount sufficient for tissue building and repair. Aspartame (as a sweetener in some foods and medicines) contributes to the phenylalanine intake and may affect control of phenylketonuria. Where the presence of aspartame is specified in the product literature this is indicated in the BNF against the preparation.

COELIAC DISEASE. Coeliac disease, which results from an intolerance to gluten, is managed by completely eliminating gluten from the diet.

ACBS. In certain clinical conditions some foods may have the characteristics of drugs and the Advisory Committee on Borderline Substances advises as to the circumstances in which such foods may be regarded as drugs and so can be prescribed in the NHS. Prescriptions for these foods issued in accordance with the advice of this committee and endorsed 'ACBS' will normally not be investigated. See Appendix 7 for details of these foods and a listing by clinical condition (consult Drug Tariff for late amendments).

Preparations
See Appendix 7

9.4.2   Enteral nutrition

The body's reserves of protein rapidly become exhausted in severely ill patients, especially during chronic illness or in those with severe burns, extensive trauma, pancreatitis, or intestinal fistula. Much

can be achieved by frequent meals and by persuading the patient to take supplementary snacks of ordinary food between the meals.

However, extra calories, protein, other nutrients, and vitamins are often best given by supplementing ordinary meals with sip or tube feeds of one of the nutritionally complete foods.

When patients cannot feed normally at all, for example patients with severe facial injury, oesophageal obstruction, or coma, a diet composed solely of nutritionally complete foods must be given. This is planned by a dietitian who will take into account the protein and total energy requirement of the patient and decide on the form and relative contribution of carbohydrate and fat to the energy requirements.

There are a number of nutritionally complete foods available and their use reduces an otherwise heavy workload in hospital or in the home. Most contain protein derived from milk or soya. Some contain protein hydrolysates or free amino acids and are only appropriate for patients who have diminished ability to break down protein, as may be the case in inflammatory bowel disease or pancreatic insufficiency.

Even when nutritionally complete feeds are being given it may be important to monitor water and electrolyte balance. Extra minerals (e.g. magnesium and zinc) may be needed in patients where gastrointestinal secretions are being lost. Additional vitamins may also be needed. Regular haematological and biochemical tests may be needed particularly in the unstable patient.

Some feeds are supplemented with vitamin K; for drug interactions of vitamin K see Appendix 1 (vitamins).

CHILDREN. Infants and young children have special requirements and in most situations liquid feeds prepared for adults are totally unsuitable and should not be given. Expert advice should be sought.

Preparations
See Appendix 7

9.5   Minerals

9.5.1   Calcium and magnesium
9.5.2   Phosphorus
9.5.3   Fluoride
9.5.4   Zinc

See section 9.1.1 for iron salts.

9.5.1   Calcium and magnesium

9.5.1.1   Calcium supplements
9.5.1.2   Hypercalcaemia
9.5.1.3   Magnesium

9.5.1.1 CALCIUM SUPPLEMENTS

Calcium supplements are usually only required where dietary calcium intake is deficient. This dietary requirement varies with age and is relatively greater in childhood, pregnancy, and lactation, due to an increased demand, and in old age, due to impaired absorption. In osteoporosis, a calcium intake which is double the recommended daily amount (RDA) reduces the rate of bone loss. If the actual dietary intake is less than the RDA, a supplement of as much as 40 mmol is appropriate.

In hypocalcaemic tetany an initial intravenous injection of 10 mL (2.25 mmol) of calcium gluconate injection 10% should be followed by the continuous infusion of about 40 mL (9 mmol) daily, but plasma calcium should be monitored. This regimen can also be used, immediately but temporarily, to reduce the toxic effects of hyperkalaemia.

Calcium may also be used in cardiac resuscitation (see section 2.7.3).

CALCIUM SALTS

Indications: see notes above; calcium deficiency

Cautions: renal impairment; sarcoidosis; **interactions:** Appendix 1 (calcium salts)

Contra-indications: conditions associated with hypercalcaemia and hypercalciuria (eg. some forms of malignant disease)

Side-effects: mild gastro-intestinal disturbances; bradycardia, arrhythmias, and irritation after intravenous injection

Dose: by mouth, daily in divided doses, see notes above

By slow intravenous injection, acute hypocalcaemia, calcium gluconate 1–2 g (2.25–4.5 mmol of Ca²⁺)

CHILD obtain paediatric advice

Oral preparations

Calcium Gluconate (Non-proprietary)

Tablets, calcium gluconate 600 mg (53.4 mg calcium or 1.35 mmol Ca²⁺). Net price 20 = 49p. Label: 24

Effervescent tablets, calcium gluconate 1 g (89 mg calcium or 2.25 mmol Ca²⁺). Net price 100 = £9.26. Label: 13

Note. Each tablet usually contains 4.46 mmol Na⁺

Calcium Lactate (Non-proprietary)

Tablets, calcium lactate 300 mg (39 mg calcium or 1 mmol Ca²⁺). Net price 20 = 21p

Cacit® (Procter & Gamble Pharm.)

Tablets, effervescent, pink, calcium carbonate 1.25 g, providing calcium citrate when dispersed in water (500 mg calcium or 12.6 mmol Ca²⁺). Net price 76-tab pack = £16.72. Label: 13

Calcichew® (Shire)

Tablets (both chewable), calcium carbonate 1.25 g (500 mg calcium or 12.6 mmol Ca²⁺), net price 100-tab pack = £10.97; 2.5 g (*Calcichew Forte*®, 1 g calcium or 25 mmol Ca²⁺), 100-tab pack = £21.94. Label: 24

Additives: include aspartame

Calcidrink® (Shire)

Granules, effervescent, calcium carbonate 2.52 g (1 g calcium or 25 mmol Ca²⁺). Net price 30-sachet pack = £8.48. Label: 13

Calcium-500 (Martindale)

Tablets, pink, f/c, calcium carbonate 1.25 g (500 mg calcium or 12.5 mmol Ca²⁺). Net price 100-tab pack = £10.32. Label: 25

Calcium-Sandoz® (Novartis)

Syrup, calcium glubionate 1.09 g, calcium lactobionate 723 mg (108.3 mg calcium or 2.7 mmol Ca²⁺)/5 mL. Net price 500 mL = £2.41

Citrical® (Shire)

Granules, calcium carbonate 1.26 g (500 mg calcium or 12.6 mmol Ca²⁺)/sachet. Net price 90-sachet pack = £23.40. Label: 13

Ossopan® (Sanofi Winthrop)

Tablets, buff, f/c, hydroxyapatite 830 mg (calcium 178 mg or 4.4 mmol Ca²⁺). Net price 50 = £10.09

Granules, brown, hydroxyapatite 3.32 g (calcium 712 mg or 17.8 mmol Ca²⁺)/sachet. Net price 28-sachet pack = £18.04

Ostram® (Merck)

Powder, calcium phosphate 3.3 g (1.2 g calcium or 29.9 mmol Ca²⁺)/sachet. Net price 30-sachet pack = £5.95. Label: 13

Sandocal® (Novartis)

Sandocal-400 tablets, effervescent, calcium lactate gluconate 930 mg, calcium carbonate 700 mg, anhydrous citric acid 1.189 g, providing calcium 400 mg (10 mmol Ca²⁺). Net price 5 × 20-tab pack = £7.20. Label: 13

Sandocal-1000 tablets, effervescent, calcium lactate gluconate 2.327 g, calcium carbonate 1.75 g, anhydrous citric acid 2.973 g providing 1 g calcium (25 mmol Ca²⁺). Net price 3 × 10-tab pack = £6.45. Label: 13

Titralac®, section 9.5.2.2

Parenteral preparations

PoM **Calcium Gluconate** (Non-proprietary)

Injection, calcium gluconate 10% (8.9 mg calcium or 220 micromol Ca²⁺/mL. Net price 10-ml amp = 48p

Available from Antigen, Phoenix

PoM **Min-I-Jet**® **Calcium Chloride 10%** (IMS)

Injection, calcium chloride 100 mg/mL (27.3 mg calcium or 680 micromol Ca²⁺/mL). Net price 10-mL disposable syringe = £4.02

With vitamin D
See section 9.6.4

9.5.1.2 HYPERCALCAEMIA

Severe hypercalcaemia calls for urgent treatment before detailed investigation of the cause. Dehydration should be corrected first, if necessary with intravenous infusion of **sodium chloride 0.9%**. Drugs (such as thiazides and vitamin D compounds) which promote hypercalcaemia, should be discontinued and dietary calcium should be restricted.

If *severe hypercalcaemia persists* drugs which inhibit mobilisation of calcium from the skeleton may be required. The **bisphosphonates** are useful and disodium pamidronate (see section 6.6.2) is probably the most effective.

Corticosteroids (see section 6.3) are widely given, but may only be useful where hypercalcaemia is due to sarcoidosis or vitamin D intoxication; they often take several days to achieve the desired effect.

Calcitonin (see section 6.6.1) is relatively non-toxic but is expensive and its effect can wear off after a few days despite continued use; it is rarely effective where bisphosphonates have failed to reduce serum calcium adequately.

Intravenous chelating drugs such as **trisodium edetate** are rarely used; they usually cause pain in the limb receiving the infusion and may cause renal damage.

After treatment of severe hypercalcaemia the underlying cause must be established. *Further treatment* is governed by the same principles as for initial therapy. Salt and water depletion and drugs promoting hypercalcaemia should be avoided; oral administration of a bisphosphonate may be useful. **Sodium cellulose phosphate**, which binds calcium in the gut, is rarely helpful, and any associated increase in serum phosphate may be harmful. Similarly, oral and intravenous phosphate may only achieve a reduction in serum calcium by precipitating calcium phosphate in the tissues, resulting in nephrocalcinosis and impairment of renal function. Parathyroidectomy may be indicated for hyperparathyroidism.

SODIUM CELLULOSE PHOSPHATE

Indications: reduction of calcium absorption from food in conditions such as hypercalciuria and hypercalcaemia (but see also notes above)

Cautions: renal impairment (avoid if severe); pregnancy and breast-feeding; growing children

Contra-indications: congestive heart failure and other conditions in which low sodium intake essential, severe renal impairment

Side-effects: occasional diarrhoea; magnesium deficiency reported

Dose: 5 g 3 times daily with meals; CHILD 10 g daily in 3 divided doses with meals

Calcisorb® (3M)
Sachets, sodium cellulose phosphate 5 g. Net price 90-sachet pack = £18.72. Label: 13, 21, counselling, may be sprinkled on food

TRISODIUM EDETATE

Indications: hypercalcaemia (but see notes above); lime burns in the eye (see under Preparations)

Cautions: repeated plasma-calcium determinations important; caution in tuberculosis; avoid rapid infusion, see under Dose

Contra-indications: impaired renal function

Side-effects: nausea, diarrhoea, cramp; in overdosage renal damage

Dose: hypercalcaemia, *by intravenous infusion* over 2–3 hours, up to 70 mg/kg daily; CHILD up to 60 mg/kg daily

IMPORTANT. Ensure rate of infusion and concentration correct (see Appendix 6); too rapid a rate or too high a concentration is extremely hazardous and repeated measurements of plasma calcium concentrations are important for control and maintenance of near normal ionised calcium concentrations. Decrease infusion rate on signs of increased muscle reactivity; discontinue if tetany occurs and restart cautiously only after plasma ionised and total calcium concentrations indicate need for further treatment (and tetany has stopped)

PoM Limclair® (Sinclair)
Injection, trisodium edetate 200 mg/mL. For dilution and use as an intravenous infusion. Net price 5-mL amp = £4.76
Note. For topical use in the eye, dilute 1 mL to 50 mL with sterile purified water

9.5.1.3 MAGNESIUM

Magnesium is an essential constituent of many enzyme systems, particularly those involved in energy generation; the largest stores are in the skeleton.

Magnesium salts are not well absorbed from the gastro-intestinal tract which explains the use of magnesium sulphate (section 1.6.4) as an osmotic laxative.

Magnesium is mainly excreted by the kidneys and is therefore retained in renal failure although significant *hypermagnesaemia* (causing muscle weakness and arrhythmias) is rare.

HYPOMAGNESAEMIA. Since magnesium is secreted in large amounts in the gastro-intestinal fluid, excessive losses in diarrhoea, stoma or fistula are the most common of the causes of *hypomagnesaemia*; deficiency may also occur in alcoholism or diuretic therapy and it has been reported after prolonged treatment with aminoglycosides. Hypomagnesaemia often causes secondary hypocalcaemia (with which it may be confused) and also hypokalaemia and hyponatraemia.

Symptomatic *hypomagnesaemia* is associated with a deficit of 0.5–1 mmol/kg; up to 160 mmol Mg^{2+} over up to 5 days may be required to replace the deficit (allowing for urinary losses). Magnesium is given initially by intravenous infusion or by intramuscular injection of **magnesium sulphate**; the intramuscular injection is painful. Plasma magnesium concentrations should be measured to determine the rate and duration of infusion and the dose should be reduced in renal impairment. To prevent *recurrence of the deficit*, magnesium may be given by mouth in a dose of 24 mmol Mg^{2+} daily in divided doses; a suitable preparation is magnesium glycerophosphate tablets [not licensed, available from IDIS]. For maintenance (e.g. in intravenous nutrition), parenteral doses of magnesium are of the order of 10–20 mmol Mg^{2+} daily (often about 12 mmol Mg^{2+} daily).

ARRHYTHMIAS. Magnesium sulphate has also been recommended for the emergency treatment of *serious arrhythmias*, especially in the presence of hypokalaemia (when hypomagnesaemia may also be present) and when salvos of rapid ventricular tachycardia show the characteristic twisting wave front known as *torsades de pointes*. The usual dose of magnesium sulphate is intravenous injection of 8 mmol Mg^{2+} over 10–15 minutes (repeated once if necessary).

MYOCARDIAL INFARCTION. Evidence suggesting a sustained reduction in mortality in patients with *suspected myocardial infarction* given an initial intravenous injection of magnesium sulphate 8 mmol Mg²⁺ over 20 minutes followed by an intravenous infusion of 65–72 mmol Mg²⁺ over the following 24 hours, has not been borne out by a larger study. Some workers, however, continue to hold the view that magnesium is beneficial if given immediately (and for as long as there is a likelihood of reperfusion taking place).

ECLAMPSIA. Magnesium sulphate has been shown to have a major role in *eclampsia* for the prevention of recurrent seizures. Regimens in the UK may vary between hospitals but typically involve initial intravenous administration of magnesium sulphate 4 g (approx. 16 mmol Mg²⁺) over up to 20 minutes followed by intravenous infusion at a rate of 1 g (approx. 4 mmol Mg²⁺) every hour; recurrence of seizures may require an additional intravenous bolus of 2–4 g (approx. 8–16 mmol Mg²⁺). ECG monitoring is carried out as is monitoring of blood pressure and of clinical signs of overdosage (loss of patellar reflexes, weakness, nausea, sensation of warmth, flushing, drowsiness, double vision, and slurred speech—calcium gluconate injection is used for the management of magnesium toxicity); plasma-magnesium concentration is monitored where it is considered necessary. It is also essential to monitor the fetal heart rate continuously.

MAGNESIUM SULPHATE

Indications: see notes above; constipation, section 1.6.4; paste for boils, section 13.10.5
Cautions: hepatic impairment (see Appendix 2); renal impairment (risk of accumulation); monitor magnesium and other electrolytes closely; in severe hypomagnesaemia administer initially via controlled infusion device (preferably syringe pump); **interactions:** Appendix 1 (magnesium salts)
Side-effects: generally associated with hypermagnesaemia, nausea, vomiting, thirst, flushing of skin, hypotension, arrhythmias, coma, respiratory depression, drowsiness, confusion, loss of tendon reflexes, muscle weakness, colic and diarrhoea following oral administration
Dose: see notes above

PoM **Magnesium Sulphate** (Non-proprietary)
Injection, magnesium sulphate 50% (approx. 2 mmol Mg²⁺/mL), net price 2-mL (1-g) amp = £4.18; 10 mL (5-g) amp = £1.57
Available from Aurum, Evans

9.5.2   Phosphorus

9.5.2.1   Phosphate supplements
9.5.2.2   Phosphate-binding agents

9.5.2.1 PHOSPHATE SUPPLEMENTS

Oral phosphate supplements may be required in addition to vitamin D in a small minority of patients with hypophosphataemic vitamin D-resistant rickets. Diarrhoea is a common side-effect and should prompt a reduction in dosage.

Phosphate infusion is occasionally needed in alcohol dependence or in phosphate deficiency arising from use of parenteral nutrition deficient in phosphate supplements; phosphate depletion also occurs in severe diabetic ketoacidosis. For *established hypophosphataemia*, monobasic potassium phosphate may be infused at a maximum rate of 9 mmol every 12 hours. Excessive doses of phosphates may cause hypocalcaemia and metastatic calcification; it is **essential** to monitor closely plasma concentrations of calcium, phosphate, potassium, and other electrolytes.

For phosphate requirements in *total parenteral nutrition* regimens, see section 9.3.

Phosphate-Sandoz® (Novartis)

Tablets, effervescent, anhydrous sodium acid phosphate 1.936 g, sodium bicarbonate 350 mg, potassium bicarbonate 315 mg, equivalent to phosphorus 500 mg (16.1 mmol phosphate), sodium 468.8 mg (20.4 mmol Na⁺), potassium 123 mg (3.1 mmol K⁺). Net price 20 = 73p. Label: 13
Dose: hypercalcaemia, up to 6 tablets daily adjusted according to response; CHILD under 5 years up to 3 tablets daily
Vitamin D-resistant hypophosphataemic osteomalacia, 4–6 tablets daily; CHILD under 5 years 2–3 tablets daily

9.5.2.2 PHOSPHATE-BINDING AGENTS

Aluminium-containing and calcium-containing antacids are used as phosphate-binding agents in the management of hyperphosphataemia complicating renal failure. Calcium-containing phosphate-binding agents are contra-indicated in hypercalcaemia or hypercalciuria. Phosphate binding agents which contain aluminium may increase plasma aluminium in dialysis patients.

ALUMINIUM HYDROXIDE

Indications: hyperphosphataemia
Cautions: hyperaluminaemia; porphyria (see section 9.8.2); see also notes above; **interactions:** Appendix 1 (antacids and adsorbents)

Aluminium Hydroxide (Non-proprietary)

Mixture (gel), about 4% w/w Al₂O₃ in water. Net price 200 mL = 41p
Dose: hyperphosphataemia, 20–100 mL according to requirements of patient; antacid, see section 1.1.1
Note. The brand name NHS *Aludrox®* (Pfizer Consumer) is used for aluminium hydroxide mixture, net price 200 mL = £1.18. For NHS *Aludrox®* tablets see preparations with magnesium, section 1.1.1

Alu-Cap® (3M)

Capsules, green/red, dried aluminium hydroxide 475 mg (low Na⁺). Net price 120-cap pack = £4.22
Dose: phosphate-binding agent in renal failure, 4–20 capsules daily in divided doses with meals; antacid, see section 1.1.1

CALCIUM CARBONATE

Indications: hyperphosphataemia
Cautions: see notes above; **interactions:** Appendix 1 (calcium salts)
Side-effects: hypercalcaemia

Calcichew®, section 9.5.1.1
Calcium-500, section 9.5.1.1
Titralac® (3M)

Tablets, calcium carbonate 420 mg (168 mg calcium or 4.2 mmol Ca²⁺), glycine 180 mg. Net price 180-tab pack = £2.94

COUNSELLING. May be chewed, crushed or swallowed whole

Dose: calcium supplement, or phosphate-binding agent (with meals) in renal failure, according to the requirements of the patient

---

9.5.3 Fluoride

Availability of adequate fluoride confers significant resistance to dental caries. It is now considered that the topical action of fluoride on enamel and plaque is more important than the systemic effect.

Where the natural fluoride content of the drinking water is significantly less than 1 mg per litre (one part per million) artificial fluoridation is the most economical method of supplementing fluoride intake.

Daily administration of tablets or drops is a suitable alternative, but systemic fluoride supplements should not be prescribed without reference to the fluoride content of the local water supply; they are not advisable when the water contains more than 700 micrograms per litre (0.7 parts per million). In addition, infants need not receive fluoride supplements until the age of 6 months.

Use of dentifrices which incorporate sodium fluoride or monofluorophosphate is also a convenient source of fluoride.

Individuals who are either particularly caries prone or medically compromised may be given additional protection by use of fluoride rinses or by application of fluoride gels. Rinses may be used daily or weekly; daily use of a less concentrated rinse is more effective than weekly use of a more concentrated one. Gels must be applied on a regular basis under professional supervision; extreme caution is necessary to prevent the child from swallowing any excess. Less concentrated gels have recently become available for home use. Varnishes are also available and are particularly valuable for young or handicapped children since they adhere to the teeth and set in the presence of moisture.

SODIUM FLUORIDE

Note. Sodium fluoride 2.2 mg provides approx. 1 mg fluoride ion

Indications: prophylaxis of dental caries—see notes above

Contra-indications: not for areas where drinking water is fluoridated

Side-effects: occasional white flecks on teeth with recommended doses; rarely yellowish-brown discoloration if recommended doses are exceeded

Dose: expressed as fluoride ion (F⁻):

Water content less than 300 micrograms F⁻/litre (0.3 parts per million), CHILD up to 6 months none; 6 months–3 years 250 micrograms F⁻ daily, 3–6 years 500 micrograms F⁻ daily, over 6 years 1 mg F⁻ daily

Water content between 300 and 700 micrograms F⁻/litre (0.3–0.7 parts per million), CHILD up to 3 years none, 3–6 years 250 micrograms F⁻ daily, over 6 years 500 micrograms F⁻ daily

Water content above 700 micrograms F⁻/litre (0.7 parts per million), supplements not advised

Note. These doses reflect the recommendations of the British Dental Association, the British Society of Paediatric Dentistry and the British Association for the Study of Community Dentistry (*Br Dent J* 1997; **182:** 6–7)

Tablets

COUNSELLING. Tablets should be sucked or dissolved in the mouth and taken preferably in the evening

There are arrangements for health authorities to supply fluoride tablets in the course of pre-school dental schemes, and they may also be supplied in school dental schemes.

En-De-Kay® (Stafford-Miller)

Fluotabs 2–4 years, natural orange-flavoured, scored, sodium fluoride 1.1 mg (500 micrograms F⁻). Net price 200-tab pack = £1.83

Fluotabs 4+ years, natural orange-flavoured, scored, sodium fluoride 2.2 mg (1 mg F⁻). Net price 200-tab pack = £1.83

Fluor-a-day® (Dental Health)

Tablets, buff, sodium fluoride 1.1 mg (500 micrograms F⁻), net price 200-tab pack = £1.77; 2.2 mg (1 mg F⁻), 200-tab pack = £1.77

FluoriGard® (Colgate-Palmolive)

Tablets 0.5, purple, grape-flavoured, scored, sodium fluoride 1.1 mg (500 micrograms F⁻). Net price 200-tab pack = £1.82

Tablets 1.0, orange, orange-flavoured, scored, sodium fluoride 2.2 mg (1 mg F⁻). Net price 200-tab pack = £1.82

Oral drops

Note. Fluoride supplements not considered necessary below 6 months of age (see notes above)

En-De-Kay® (Stafford-Miller)

Fluodrops® (= paediatric drops), sugar-free, sodium fluoride 550 micrograms (250 micrograms F⁻)/0.15 mL. Net price 60 mL = £1.36

Note. Corresponds to Sodium Fluoride Oral Drops DPF 0.37% equivalent to sodium fluoride 80 micrograms (F⁻ 36 micrograms)/drop

FluoriGard® (Colgate-Palmolive)

Drops, sugar-free, sodium fluoride 275 micrograms (125 micrograms F⁻)/drop. Net price 30 mL = £1.62

Note. Corresponds to Sodium Fluoride Oral Drops DPF 0.84% equivalent to sodium fluoride 275 micrograms (F⁻ 125 micrograms)/drop

Mouthwashes

Rinse mouth for 1 minute and spit out

COUNSELLING. Avoid eating, drinking, or rinsing mouth for 15 minutes after use

En-De-Kay® (Stafford-Miller)

Daily fluoride mouthrinse (= mouthwash), blue, sodium fluoride 0.05%. Net price 250 mL = £1.51

CHILD 6 years and over, for *daily* use, rinse with 10 mL

PoM *Fluorinse* (= mouthwash), red, sodium fluoride 2%. Net price 100 mL = £3.20. Counselling, see above

CHILD 8 years and over, for *daily* use, dilute 5 drops to 10 mL of water; for *weekly* use, dilute 20 drops to 10 mL

FluoriGard® (Colgate-Palmolive)
Daily dental rinse (= mouthwash), blue, sodium
fluoride 0.05%. Net price 500 mL = £2.73. Counselling, see above
CHILD 6 years and over, for *daily* use, rinse with 10 mL
Weekly dental rinse (= mouthwash), blue, sodium
fluoride 0.2%. Net price 150 mL = £2.22. Counselling, see above
CHILD 6 years and over, for *weekly* use, rinse with
10 mL

9.5.4   Zinc

Oral zinc therapy should only be given when there
is good evidence of deficiency (hypoproteinaemia
spuriously lowers plasma-zinc concentrations).
Zinc deficiency can occur in individuals on inadequate diets, in malabsorption, with increased body
loss due to trauma, burns and protein-losing conditions, and during intravenous feeding. Therapy
should continue until clinical improvement occurs
and be replaced by dietary measures unless there is
severe malabsorption, metabolic disease, or continuing zinc loss. Side-effects of zinc salts are abdominal pain and dyspepsia.

ZINC SALTS
Indications; Cautions; Side-effects: see notes
above; **interactions:** Appendix 1 (zinc)

Solvazinc® (Thames)
Effervescent tablets, yellow-white, zinc sulphate
monohydrate 125 mg (45 mg zinc). Net price 30 =
£4.32. Label: 13, 21
Dose: ADULT and CHILD over 30 kg, 1 tablet in water
1–3 times daily after food; CHILD under 10 kg, ½ tablet
daily; 10–30 kg, ½ tablet 1–3 times daily

Z Span® (Goldshield)
Spansule® (= capsules m/r), blue/clear, enclosing
white and grey pellets, zinc sulphate monohydrate
61.8 mg (22.5 mg zinc). Net price 30-cap pack =
£3.16
Dose: ADULT and CHILD over 12 years, supplement, 1
capsule daily; deficiency (short-term treatment only) 1
capsule 3 times daily then adjusted according to
response; can be opened and pellets sprinkled on cool
food; not to be chewed

9.6   Vitamins

9.6.1	Vitamin A
9.6.2	Vitamin B group
9.6.3	Vitamin C
9.6.4	Vitamin D
9.6.5	Vitamin E
9.6.6	Vitamin K
9.6.7	Multivitamin preparations

Vitamins are used for the prevention and treatment
of specific deficiency states or where the diet is
known to be inadequate; they may be prescribed in
the NHS to prevent or treat deficiency but not as
dietary supplements.
Their use as general 'pick-me-ups' is of unproven
value and, in the case of preparations containing
vitamin A or D, may actually be harmful if patients
take more than the prescribed dose. The 'fad' for
mega-vitamin therapy with water-soluble vitamins,
such as ascorbic acid and pyridoxine, is unscientific
and can be harmful.
Dietary reference values for vitamins are available in the Department of Health publication:
Dietary Reference Values for Food Energy and Nutrients
for the United Kingdom: Report of the Panel on Dietary
Reference Values of the Committee on Medical Aspects
of Food Policy. *Report on Health and Social Subjects
41.* London: HMSO, 1991

9.6.1   Vitamin A

Deficiency of vitamin A (retinol) is associated with
ocular defects (particularly xerophthalmia) and an
increased susceptibility to infections, but deficiency
is rare in Britain (even in disorders of fat absorption). Despite initial epidemiological evidence suggesting that vitamin A or carotene may have a
protective effect against some epithelial cancers, the
claims have not been substantiated.
Massive overdose can cause rough skin, dry hair,
an enlarged liver, and a raised erythrocyte sedimentation rate and raised serum calcium and serum
alkaline phosphatase concentrations.
In view of evidence suggesting that high levels of
vitamin A may cause birth defects, women who are
(or may become) pregnant are advised not to take
vitamin A supplements (including tablets and fish-
liver oil drops), except on the advice of a doctor or
an antenatal clinic; nor should they eat liver or
products such as liver paté or liver sausage.

VITAMIN A
(Retinol)
Indications; Cautions; Side-effects: see notes
above
Dose: see notes above and under preparations

Vitamins A and D
Halibut-liver Oil (Non-proprietary)
Capsules, vitamin A 4000 units [also contains vit-
amin D]. Net price 20 = 18p
Available from Thornton & Ross
Vitamins A and D (Non-proprietary)
Capsules, vitamin A 4000 units, vitamin D
400 units. Net price 20 = 54p
Available from CP
NHS **Halycitrol®** (LAB)
Emulsion, vitamin A 4600 units, vitamin D
380 units/5 mL. Net price 114 mL = £1.50
Dose: 5 mL daily but see notes above

Vitamins A, D, and C for children
Children's Vitamin Drops (Houghs)
Oral drops, ascorbic acid (as sodium ascorbate)
20 mg, vitamin A 700 units, vitamin D 300 units/5
drops.
Recommended by Department of Health for routine supplementation in young children. Available direct to public under the Welfare Food Scheme from maternity and
child health clinics and welfare food distribution centres; not available on prescription
Dose: CHILD 1 month–5 years, 5 drops daily
Note. The Department of Health recommends these
drops for children aged 6 months to 2 years (preferably
5 years particularly in winter and early spring); some

infants from 1 month of age may also benefit (for details see *Present Day Practice in Infant Feeding* 3rd Report)
Minadex® (Seven Seas)

Oral drops, ascorbic acid 15 mg, vitamin A 750 units, vitamin D 200 units/0.14 mL. Net price 25-mL pack with pipette = £1.45

Note. May contain arachis (peanut) oil

Dose: INFANT and CHILD under 5 years, 0.28 mL (upper level on graduated pipette) daily; INFANT fed on vitamin D-fortified milk, CHILD over 5 years and ADULT, 0.14 mL (lower level on graduated pipette) daily

Vitamin A injection
PoM **Vitamin A Palmitate** (Cambridge)

Injection, vitamin A (retinol) 50 000 units (as palmitate)/mL. Net price 2-mL amp = £2.28

Dose: by deep intramuscular injection, deficiency, 100 000 units monthly, increased to weekly in acute deficiency states; courses no longer than 6 weeks with 2-week interval

Liver disease, 100 000 units every 2–4 months

INFANT under 1 year and CHILD 50 000 units monthly

Note. Contains polyethoxylated castor oil which has been associated with anaphylaxis; do **not** mix or dilute

Cautions: children, liver disease (specialist use), see also notes above

9.6.2   Vitamin B group

Deficiency of the B vitamins, other than deficiency of vitamin B_{12} (section 9.1.2) is rare in Britain and is usually treated by preparations containing thiamine (B_1), riboflavine (B_2), and nicotinamide, which is used in preference to nicotinic acid, as it does not cause vasodilatation. Other members (or substances traditionally classified as members) of the vitamin B complex such as aminobenzoic acid, biotin, choline, inositol, and pantothenic acid or panthenol may be included in vitamin B preparations but there is no evidence of their value.

The severe deficiency states Wernicke's encephalopathy and Korsakoff's psychosis, especially as seen in chronic alcoholism, are best treated by the parenteral administration of B vitamins (*Pabrinex®*); anaphylaxis has been reported with these preparations (see CSM advice, below).

As with other vitamins of the B group, pyridoxine (B_6) deficiency is rare, but it may occur during isoniazid therapy and is characterised by peripheral neuritis. High doses of pyridoxine are given in some metabolic disorders, such as hyperoxaluria, and it is also used in sideroblastic anaemia (section 9.1.3). Pyridoxine has been tried in a wide variety of other disorders, including the premenstrual syndrome, but there is little sound evidence to support the claims, and overdosage induces toxic effects.

Nicotinic acid inhibits the synthesis of cholesterol and triglyceride (see section 2.12). Folic acid and vitamin B_{12} are used in the treatment of megaloblastic anaemia (section 9.1.2). Folinic acid (available as calcium folinate) is used in association with cytotoxic therapy (section 8.1.3).

RIBOFLAVINE

(Riboflavin, vitamin B_2)
Indications: see notes above

Preparations

Injections of vitamins B and C, see under Thiamine

Oral vitamin B complex preparations, see below

THIAMINE

(Vitamin B_1)
Indications: see notes above

Cautions: anaphylactic shock may occasionally follow injection (see CSM advice below)

Dose: mild chronic deficiency, 10–25 mg daily; severe deficiency, 200–300 mg daily

> **CSM advice**
>
> Since potentially serious allergic adverse reactions may occur during, or shortly after, administration, the CSM has recommended that:
>
> 1. Use be restricted to patients in whom parenteral treatment is essential;
>
> 2. Intravenous injections should be administered slowly (over 10 minutes);
>
> 3. Facilities for treating anaphylaxis should be available when administered.

Thiamine (Non-proprietary)

Tablets, thiamine hydrochloride 25 mg, net price 20 = 18p; 50 mg, 20 = 30p; 100 mg, 20 = 51p; 300 mg, 20 = 79p

Available from Roche Consumer Health (~~NHS~~ Benerva®)

PoM **Pabrinex®** (Link)

Parenteral vitamins B and C for rapid correction of severe depletion or malabsorption (e.g in alcoholism, after acute infections, postoperatively, or in psychiatric states), maintenance of vitamins B and C in chronic intermittent haemodialysis

Dose: see CSM advice above

Coma or delirium from alcohol, from opioids, or from barbiturates, collapse following narcosis, by intravenous injection or infusion of *I/V High potency*, 2-3 pairs every 8 hours

Psychosis following narcosis or electroconvulsive therapy, toxicity from acute infections, by intravenous injection or infusion of *I/V High potency* or by deep intramuscular injection into the gluteal muscle of *I/M High potency*, 1 pair twice daily for up to 7 days

Haemodialysis, by intravenous infusion of *I/V High potency* (in sodium chloride intravenous infusion 0.9%) 1 pair every 2 weeks

I/M High potency injection, for intramuscular use only, ascorbic acid 500 mg, nicotinamide 160 mg, pyridoxine hydrochloride 50 mg, riboflavine 4 mg, thiamine hydrochloride 250 mg/7 mL. Net price 7 mL (in 2 amps) = £1.94

I/V High potency injection, for intravenous use only, ascorbic acid 500 mg, anhydrous glucose 1 g, nicotinamide 160 mg, pyridoxine hydrochloride 50 mg, riboflavine 4 mg, thiamine hydrochloride 250 mg/10 mL. Net price 10 mL (in 2 amps) = £1.74

Oral vitamin B complex preparations, see below

PYRIDOXINE HYDROCHLORIDE
(Vitamin B$_6$)

Indications: see under Dose

Cautions: **interactions:** Appendix 1 (vitamins)

Dose: deficiency states, 20–50 mg up to 3 times daily

Isoniazid neuropathy, prophylaxis 10 mg daily; therapeutic, 50 mg three times daily

Idiopathic sideroblastic anaemia, 100–400 mg daily in divided doses

Premenstrual syndrome, 50–100 mg daily (but notes above)

> **Important**. Following reports of peripheral neuropathy, the Royal Pharmaceutical Society of Great Britain has advised that pharmacists should treat products containing more than 10 mg per daily dose of pyridoxine (vitamin B$_6$) as pharmacy medicines; this should also apply to supplements sold under food law. Until labelling of food supplements has been revised, purchasers of supplements containing a daily dose of 10 mg or less should be advised not to exceed the recommended dose.

Pyridoxine (Non-proprietary)

Tablets, pyridoxine hydrochloride 20 mg, net price 20 = 32p; 50 mg, 20 = 30p

Available from Cox, Hillcross, Roche Consumer Health (NHS Benadon®)

NHS Orovite Complement B6® (Seton)

Tablets, m/r, yellow, pyridoxine hydrochloride 100 mg. Net price 28-tab pack = £2.16. Label: 25

Injections of vitamins B and C, see under Thiamine

NICOTINAMIDE

Indications: see notes above; acne vulgaris, see section 13.6.1

Nicotinamide (Non-proprietary)

Tablets, nicotinamide 50 mg. Net price 20 = £1.24

Injections of vitamins B and C, see under Thiamine

ORAL VITAMIN B COMPLEX PREPARATIONS

Note. Other multivitamin preparations are in section 9.6.7.

Vitamin B Tablets, Compound, nicotinamide 15 mg, riboflavine 1 mg, thiamine hydrochloride 1 mg. Net price 20 = 7p

Dose: prophylactic, 1–2 tablets daily

Vitamin B Tablets, Compound, Strong, brown, f/c or s/c, nicotinamide 20 mg, pyridoxine hydrochloride 2 mg, riboflavine 2 mg, thiamine hydrochloride 5 mg. Net price 20 = 11p

Dose: treatment of vitamin-B deficiency, 1–2 tablets 3 times daily

NHS Vigranon B® (Wallace Mfg)

Syrup, thiamine hydrochloride 5 mg, riboflavine 2 mg, nicotinamide 20 mg, pyridoxine hydrochloride 2 mg, panthenol 3 mg/5 mL. Net price 150 mL = £1.85

OTHER COMPOUNDS

Potassium aminobenzoate has been used in the treatment of various disorders associated with excessive fibrosis such as scleroderma but its therapeutic value is **doubtful**.

Potaba® (Glenwood)

Capsules, red/white, potassium aminobenzoate 500 mg. Net price 20 = £1.42. Label: 21

Tablets, potassium aminobenzoate 500 mg. Net price 20 = £1.00. Label: 21

Envules® (= powder in sachets), potassium aminobenzoate 3 g. Net price 40 sachets = £15.37. Label: 13, 21

Dose: Peyronie's disease, scleroderma, 12 g daily in divided doses after food

9.6.3   Vitamin C
(Ascorbic acid)

Vitamin C therapy is essential in scurvy, but less florid manifestations of vitamin C deficiency are commonly found, especially in the elderly. It is rarely necessary to prescribe more than 100 mg daily except early in the treatment of scurvy.

Claims that vitamin C ameliorates colds or promotes wound healing have not been proved.

ASCORBIC ACID

Indications: prevention and treatment of scurvy

Dose: prophylactic, 25–75 mg daily; therapeutic, not less than 250 mg daily in divided doses

Ascorbic Acid (Non-proprietary)

Tablets, ascorbic acid 50 mg, net price 20 = 8p; 100 mg, 20 = 23p; 200 mg, 20 = 34p; 500 mg (label: 24), 20 = 59p

Available from APS, Cox, Roche Consumer Health (NHS Redoxon®)

NHS *Tablets*, effervescent, ascorbic acid 1 g. Net price 10-tab pack = £1.14. Label: 13

Available from Roche Consumer Health (NHS Redoxon®)

Injection, ascorbic acid 100 mg/mL. Net price 5-mL amp = £2.28

For children's welfare vitamin drops containing vitamin C with A and D, see vitamin A

9.6.4   Vitamin D

Note. The term Vitamin D is used for a range of compounds which possess the property of preventing or curing rickets. They include ergocalciferol (calciferol, vitamin D$_2$), cholecalciferol (vitamin D$_3$), dihydrotachysterol, alfacalcidol (1α-hydroxycholecalciferol), and calcitriol (1,25-dihydroxycholecalciferol).

Simple vitamin D *deficiency*, which is not uncommon in Asians consuming unleavened bread and in the elderly living alone, can be prevented by taking an oral supplement of only 10 micrograms (400 units) of **ergocalciferol** (calciferol, vitamin D$_2$) daily. Since there is no plain tablet of this strength available **calcium and ergocalciferol tablets** can be given (although the calcium is unnecessary).

Vitamin D deficiency caused by *intestinal malabsorption* or *chronic liver disease* usually requires vitamin D in pharmacological doses, such as **calciferol tablets** up to 1 mg (40 000 units) daily; the hypocalcaemia of *hypoparathyroidism* often requires doses of up to 2.5 mg (100 000 units) daily in order to achieve normocalcaemia. The newer vitamin D derivatives, **alfacalcidol** and **calcitriol**, have a shorter duration of action, and therefore have the advantage that problems associated with hypercalcaemia due to excessive dosage are shorter lasting and easier to treat.

Vitamin D requires hydroxylation by the kidney to its active form therefore the hydroxylated derivatives **alfacalcidol** or **calcitriol** should be prescribed if patients with *severe renal impairment* require vitamin D therapy. Calcitriol is also licensed for the management of postmenopausal osteoporosis.

Important. All patients receiving pharmacological doses of vitamin D should have the plasma calcium concentration checked at intervals (initially weekly) and whenever nausea or vomiting are present. Breast milk from women taking pharmacological doses of vitamin D may cause hypercalcaemia if given to an infant.

ERGOCALCIFEROL
(Calciferol, Vitamin D₂)

Indications: see notes above

Cautions: take care to ensure correct dose in infants; monitor plasma calcium in patients receiving high doses and in renal impairment

Contra-indications: hypercalcaemia; metastatic calcification

Side-effects: symptoms of overdosage include anorexia, lassitude, nausea and vomiting, diarrhoea, weight loss, polyuria, sweating, headache, thirst, vertigo, and raised concentrations of calcium and phosphate in plasma and urine

Dose: see notes above

Daily supplements

Note. There is no plain vitamin D tablet available for treating simple deficiency (see notes above). Alternatives include vitamins capsules (see 9.6.7), preparations of vitamins A and D (see 9.6.1), and calcium and ergocalciferol tablets (see below).

Calcium and Ergocalciferol (Non-proprietary)
(Calcium and Vitamin D)

Tablets, calcium lactate 300 mg, calcium phosphate 150 mg (97 mg calcium or 2.4 mmol Ca²⁺), ergocalciferol 10 micrograms (400 units). Net price 20 = 24p. Counselling, crush before administration or may be chewed

Cacit® D3 (Procter & Gamble Pharm.)

Granules, effervescent, calcium carbonate 1.25 g (500 mg calcium or 12.6 mmol Ca²⁺), cholecalciferol 11 micrograms (440 units)/sachet. Net price 30-sachet pack = £8.10. Label: 13

Calceos® (Thames)

Tablets (chewable), calcium carbonate 1.25 g (500 mg calcium or 12.6 mmol Ca ²⁺), cholecalciferol 10 micrograms (400 units). Net price 60-tab pack = £8.18. Label: 24

Calcichew® D3 (Shire)

Tablets (chewable), calcium carbonate 1.25 g (500 mg calcium or 12.6 mmol Ca²⁺), cholecalciferol 5 micrograms (200 units). Net price 100-tab pack = £13.65. Label: 24

Additives: include aspartame

Calcichew® D3 Forte (Shire)

Tablets (chewable), calcium carbonate 1.25 g (500 mg calcium or 12.6 mmol Ca²⁺), cholecalciferol 10 micrograms (400 units). Net price 100-tab pack = £16.50. Label: 24

Additives: include aspartame

Pharmacological strengths (see notes above)

Calciferol (Non-proprietary)

Tablets, cholecalciferol or ergocalciferol 250 micrograms (10 000 units), net price 20 = £2.67; 1.25 mg (50 000 units) may also be available

Available from Norton

Note. The BP directs that when calciferol tablets qualified by a descriptor relating to strength (such as 'high strength') are prescribed or demanded, the intention of the prescriber or purchaser with respect to the strength expressed in micrograms or milligrams per tablet should be ascertained. To avoid **errors** arising from the use of such titles prescribers are required to **abandon** them and **specify strength required**

PoM *Injection,* cholecalciferol or ergocalciferol, 7.5 mg (300 000 units)/mL in oil. Net price 1-mL amp = £5.92, 2-mL amp = £7.07

ALFACALCIDOL
(1α-Hydroxycholecalciferol)

Indications: see notes above

Cautions; Contra-indications; Side-effects: see under Ergocalciferol

Dose: by mouth or by intravenous injection over 30 seconds, ADULT and CHILD over 20 kg, initially 1 microgram daily (elderly 500 nanograms), adjusted to avoid hypercalcaemia; maintenance, usually 0.25–1 microgram daily; NEONATE and PREMATURE INFANT initially 50–100 nanograms/kg daily, CHILD under 20 kg initially 50 nanograms/kg daily

PoM **AlfaD®** (Berk)

Capsules, alfacalcidol 250 nanograms (pink), net price 100-cap pack = £11.78; 1 microgram (orange), 30-cap pack = £10.53

Ingredients: include arachis (peanut) oil

PoM **One-Alpha®** (Leo)

Capsules, alfacalcidol 250 nanograms, net price 20 = £2.36; 1 microgram (brown), 20 = £7.02

Note. Contains sesame oil

Solution, sugar-free, alfacalcidol 200 nanograms/mL. Net price 60 mL = £15.19 (with oral syringe)

Injection, alfacalcidol 2 micrograms/mL, net price 0.5-mL amp = £2.43, 1-mL amp = £4.63

Note. Contains propylene glycol and should be used with caution in small premature infants

---

CALCITRIOL
(1,25-Dihydroxycholecalciferol)

Indications: see notes above

Cautions; Contra-indications; Side-effects: see under Ergocalciferol

Dose: see under preparations below

PoM **Calcijex®** (Abbott)

Injection, calcitriol 1 microgram/mL, net price 1-mL amp = £5.71; 2 micrograms/mL, 1-mL amp = £11.42

Dose: hypocalcaemia in dialysis patients with chronic renal failure, by intravenous injection (or injection through catheter) after haemodialysis, initially 500 nanograms (approx. 10 nanograms/kg) 3 times a week, increased if necessary in steps of 250–500 nanograms at intervals of 2–4 weeks; usual dose 0.5–3 micrograms 3 times a week; CHILD not established

PoM **Rocaltrol®** (Roche)

Capsules, calcitriol 250 nanograms (red/white), net price 20 = £4.31; 500 nanograms (red), 20 = £7.71

Dose: renal osteodystrophy, ADULT, initially 250 nanograms daily or on alternate days, increased if necessary in steps of 250 nanograms at intervals of 2–4 weeks; usual dose 0.5–1 micrograms daily; CHILD not established

Established postmenopausal osteoporosis, 250 nanograms twice daily (monitor plasma calcium and creatinine, see product literature)

CHOLECALCIFEROL
(Colecalciferol, vitamin D₃)

Indications; Cautions; Contra-indications; Side-effects: see under Ergocalciferol—alternative to ergocalciferol in calciferol tablets and injection

DIHYDROTACHYSTEROL
Indications; Cautions; Contra-indications; Side-effects: see under Ergocalciferol

AT 10® (Sanofi Winthrop)

Oral solution, dihydrotachysterol 250 micrograms/mL. Net price 15-mL dropper bottle = £21.27

Note. Contains arachis (peanut) oil

Dose: acute, chronic, and latent forms of hypocalcaemic tetany due to hypoparathyroidism, consult product literature

9.6.5   Vitamin E
(Tocopherols)

The daily requirement of vitamin E has not been well defined but is probably about 3 to 15 mg daily. There is little evidence that oral supplements of vitamin E are essential in adults, even where there is fat malabsorption secondary to cholestasis. In young children with congenital cholestasis, abnormally low vitamin E concentrations may be found in association with neuromuscular abnormalities, which usually respond only to the parenteral administration of vitamin E.

Vitamin E has been tried for various other conditions but there is little scientific evidence of its value.

ALPHA TOCOPHERYL ACETATE
Indications: see notes above

Cautions: predisposition to thrombosis; increased risk of necrotising enterocolitis in premature infants weighing less than 1.5 g

Side-effects: diarrhoea and abdominal pain with doses more than 1 g daily

Vitamin E Suspension (Cambridge)

Suspension, alpha tocopheryl acetate 500 mg/5 mL. Net price 100 mL = £10.74

Dose: malabsorption in cystic fibrosis, 100–200 mg daily; CHILD under 1 year 50 mg daily; 1 year and over, 100 mg daily

Malabsorption in abetalipoproteinaemia, ADULT and CHILD 50–100 mg/kg daily

Malabsorption in chronic cholestasis, INFANT 150–200 mg/kg daily

Note. Tablets containing tocopheryl acetate 50 mg and 200 mg available from Roche Consumer Health (Ephynal®)

9.6.6   Vitamin K

Vitamin K is necessary for the production of blood clotting factors and proteins necessary for the normal calcification of bone.

Because vitamin K is fat soluble, patients with fat malabsorption, especially in biliary obstruction or hepatic disease, may become deficient. For oral administration to prevent vitamin-K deficiency in malabsorption syndromes, a water-soluble preparation, **menadiol sodium phosphate** must be used; the usual dose is about 10 mg daily.

Vitamin K is used for prophylaxis against haemorrhagic disease of the newborn. Fears about the safety of parenteral vitamin K appear to be unfounded; uncertainties remain regarding the relative efficacy of prophylaxis with oral vitamin K.

Oral coumarin anticoagulants act by interfering with vitamin K metabolism in the hepatic cells and their effects can be antagonised by giving vitamin K; for British Society for Haematology Guidelines, see section 2.8.2.

MENADIOL SODIUM PHOSPHATE
Indications; Dose: see notes above

Cautions: G6PD deficiency (see section 9.1.5) and vitamin E deficiency (risk of haemolysis); **interactions:** Appendix 1 (vitamins)

Contra-indications: neonates and infants, late pregnancy

Menadiol Phosphate (Non-proprietary)

Tablets, scored, menadiol sodium phosphate equivalent to 10 mg of menadiol phosphate. Net price 100-tab pack = £9.28

Available from Cambridge

PHYTOMENADIONE
(Vitamin K₁)

Indications; Dose: see notes above

Cautions: intravenous injections should be given very slowly (see also below); **interactions:** Appendix 1 (vitamins)

Konakion® (Roche)

Tablets, s/c, phytomenadione 10 mg. Net price 25-tab pack = £4.62. To be chewed or allowed to dissolve slowly in the mouth (Label: 24)

PoM *Injection*, phytomenadione 2 mg/mL, net price 0.5-mL amp = 24p

Note. Contains polyethoxylated castor oil which has been associated with anaphylaxis; should not be diluted therefore **not** for intravenous infusion—for intramuscular or slow intravenous injection

Colloidal formulation
PoM **Konakion® MM** (Roche)
Injection, phytomenadione 10 mg/mL in a mixed micelles vehicle. Net price 1-mL amp = 45p

Additives: include glycocholic acid 54.6 mg/amp, lecithin

Cautions: reduce dose in elderly; liver impairment (glycocholic acid may displace bilirubin); reports of anaphylactoid reactions

Note. Konakion® MM may be administered by slow intravenous injection or by intravenous infusion in glucose 5% (see Appendix 6); **not** for intramuscular injection

PoM **Konakion® MM Paediatric** (Roche)
Injection, phytomenadione 10 mg/mL. Net price 0.2-mL amp = £1.62

Additives: include glycocholic acid 10.9 mg/amp, lecithin

Cautions: parenteral administration in premature infants of less than 2.5 kg (increased risk of kernicterus)

Note. Konakion® MM Paediatric may be administered *by mouth* or *by intramuscular injection* or *by intravenous injection*

9.6.7   Multivitamin preparations

Vitamins Capsules, ascorbic acid 15 mg, nicotinamide 7.5 mg, riboflavine 500 micrograms, thiamine hydrochloride 1 mg, vitamin A 2500 units, vitamin D 300 units. Net price 20 = 20p

Abidec® (W-L)
Drops, vitamins A, B group, C, and D. Net price 25 mL (with dropper) = £1.78

Dalivit® (Eastern)
Oral drops, vitamins A, B group, C, and D, net price 25 mL = £1.60, 50 mL = £2.86

VITAMIN AND MINERAL SUPPLEMENTS
AND ADJUNCTS TO SYNTHETIC DIETS

Forceval® (Unigreg)
Capsules, brown/red, vitamins (ascorbic acid 60 mg, biotin 100 micrograms, cyanocobalamin 3 micrograms, folic acid 400 micrograms, nicotinamide 18 mg, pantothenic acid 4 mg, pyridoxine 2 mg, riboflavine 1.6 mg, thiamine 1.2 mg, vitamin A 2500 units, vitamin D_2 400 units, vitamin E 10 mg, minerals and trace elements (calcium 100 mg, chromium 200 micrograms, copper 2 mg, iodine 140 micrograms, iron 12 mg, magnesium 30 mg, manganese 3 mg, molybdenum 250 micrograms, phosphorus 77 mg, potassium 4 mg, selenium 50 micrograms, zinc 15 mg). Net price 30-cap pack = £5.39, 45-cap pack = £7.70; 90-cap pack = £14.70

Dose: vitamin and mineral deficiency and as adjunct in synthetic diets, 1 capsule daily

Junior capsules, brown, vitamins (ascorbic acid 25 mg, biotin 50 micrograms, cyanocobalamin 2 micrograms, folic acid 100 micrograms, nicotinamide 7.5 mg, pantothenic acid 2 mg, pyridoxine 1 mg, riboflavine 1 mg, thiamine 1.5 mg, vitamin A 1250 units, vitamin D_2 200 units, vitamin E 5 mg, vitamin K_1 25 micrograms),

minerals and trace elements (chromium 50 micrograms, copper 1 mg, iodine 75 micrograms, iron 5 mg, magnesium 1 mg, manganese 1.25 mg, molybdenum 50 micrograms, selenium 25 micrograms, zinc 5 mg). Net price 30-cap pack = £4.05, 60-cap pack = £7.70

Dose: vitamin and mineral deficiency and as adjunct in synthetic diets, CHILD over 5 years, 2 capsules daily

Ketovite® (Paines & Byrne)
PoM *Tablets*, yellow, ascorbic acid 16.6 mg, riboflavine 1 mg, thiamine hydrochloride 1 mg, pyridoxine hydrochloride 330 micrograms, nicotinamide 3.3 mg, calcium pantothenate 1.16 mg, alpha tocopheryl acetate 5 mg, inositol 50 mg, biotin 170 micrograms, folic acid 250 micrograms, acetomenaphthone 500 micrograms. Net price 100-tab pack = £4.17

Dose: prevention of deficiency in disorders of carbohydrate or amino acid metabolism, 1 tablet 3 times daily; with Ketovite® Liquid as vitamin supplement with synthetic diets

Liquid, pink, sugar-free, vitamin A 2500 units, ergocalciferol 400 units, choline chloride 150 mg, cyanocobalamin 12.5 micrograms/5 mL. Net price 150-mL pack = £2.70

Dose: prevention of deficiency in disorders of carbohydrate or amino acid metabolism, 5 mL daily; with Ketovite® Tablets as vitamin supplement with synthetic diets

9.7   Bitters and tonics

Mixtures containing simple and aromatic bitters, such as alkaline gentian mixture, are traditional remedies for loss of appetite. All depend on suggestion.

Gentian Mixture, Acid, BP

Mixture, concentrated compound gentian infusion 10%, dilute hydrochloric acid 5% in a suitable vehicle. Extemporaneous preparations should be recently prepared according to the following formula: concentrated compound gentian infusion 1 mL, dilute hydrochloric acid 0.5 mL, double-strength chloroform water 5 mL, water to 10 mL

Dose: 10 mL 3 times daily in water before meals

Gentian Mixture, Alkaline, BP

(Alkaline Gentian Oral Solution)
Mixture, concentrated compound gentian infusion 10%, sodium bicarbonate 5% in a suitable vehicle. Extemporaneous preparations should be recently prepared according to the following formula: concentrated compound gentian infusion 1 mL, sodium bicarbonate 500 mg, double-strength chloroform water 5 mL, water to 10 mL

Dose: 10 mL 3 times daily in water before meals

NHS **Effico®** (Pharmax)
Tonic, green, thiamine hydrochloride 180 micrograms, nicotinamide 2.1 mg, caffeine 20.2 mg, compound gentian infusion 0.31 mL/5 mL. Net price 300-mL pack = £1.91, 500-mL pack = £2.59

NHS **Labiton®** (LAB)
Tonic, brown, thiamine hydrochloride 375 micrograms, caffeine 3.5 mg, kola nut dried extract 3.025 mg, alcohol 1.4 mL/5 mL. Net price 200 mL = £2.22

NHS **Metatone**® (W-L)
Tonic, thiamine hydrochloride 500 micrograms, calcium glycerophosphate 45.6 mg, manganese glycerophosphate 5.7 mg, potassium glycerophosphate 45.6 mg, sodium glycerophosphate 22.8 mg/5 mL. Net price 300 mL = £2.32

9.8 Metabolic disorders

9.8.1 Wilson's disease, carnitine deficiency, and Gaucher's disease

9.8.2 Acute porphyrias

This section covers drugs used in metabolic disorders and not readily classified elsewhere.

9.8.1 Wilson's disease, carnitine deficiency, and Gaucher's disease

WILSON'S DISEASE

Penicillamine (see also section 10.1.3) is used in Wilson's disease (hepatolenticular degeneration) to aid the elimination of copper ions. See below for other indications.

Trientine is used for the treatment of Wilson's disease only, in patients intolerant of penicillamine; it is **not** an alternative to penicillamine for rheumatoid arthritis or cystinuria.

PENICILLAMINE

Indications: see under Dose below
Cautions; Contra-indications; Side-effects: see section 10.1.3
Dose: Wilson's disease, 1.5–2 g daily in divided doses before food; max. 2 g daily for 1 year; maintenance 0.75–1 g daily; ELDERLY, 20 mg/kg daily in divided doses; CHILD, up to 20 mg/kg daily in divided doses, minimum 500 mg daily
Chronic active hepatitis (after disease controlled with corticosteroids), initially 500 mg daily in divided doses slowly increased over 3 months; usual maintenance dose 1.25 g daily; ELDERLY not recommended
Cystinuria, therapeutic, 1–3 g daily in divided doses before food, adjusted to maintain urinary cystine below 200 mg/litre. Prophylactic (maintain urinary cystine below 300 mg/litre) 0.5–1 g at bedtime; maintain adequate fluid intake (at least 3 litres daily); CHILD and ELDERLY minimum dose to maintain urinary cystine below 200 mg/litre
Severe active rheumatoid arthiritis, see section 10.1.3
Copper and lead poisioning, see Emergency Treatment of Poisoning

Preparations
See section 10.1.3

TRIENTINE DIHYDROCHLORIDE

Indications: Wilson's disease in patients intolerant of penicillamine

Cautions: see notes above; pregnancy; **interactions:** Appendix 1 (trientine)
Side-effects: nausea; penicillamine-induced systemic lupus erythematosus may not resolve on transfer to trientine
Dose: 1.2–2.4 g daily in 2–4 divided doses before food

▼ PoM **Trientine Dihydrochloride Capsules,**
trientine dihydrochloride 300 mg. Label: 6, 22
Available from K & K-Greeff
Note. The CSM has requested that in addition to the usual CSM reporting request special records should also be kept by the pharmacist

CARNITINE DEFICIENCY

Carnitine is available for the management of primary carnitine deficiency due to inborn errors of metabolism or of secondary deficiency in haemodialysis patients.

CARNITINE

Indications: primary and secondary carnitine deficiency
Cautions: renal impairment; monitoring of free and acyl carnitine in blood and urine recommended; pregnancy (but appropriate to use) and breast-feeding
Side-effects: nausea, vomiting, abdominal pain, diarrhoea, body odour; side-effects may be dose-related—monitor tolerance during first week and after any dose increase
Dose: primary deficiency, *by mouth*, up to 200 mg/kg daily in 2–4 divided doses; higher doses of up to 400 mg/kg daily occasionally required; *by intravenous injection*, up to 100 mg/kg daily in 3–4 divided doses
Secondary deficiency, *by intravenous injection*, 20 mg/kg after each dialysis session (dosage adjusted according to carnitine concentration); maintenance, *by mouth*, 1 g daily

PoM **Carnitor**® (Shire)
Chewable tablets, L-carnitine 1 g. Net price 10-tab pack = £35.00
Oral liquid, L-carnitine 1 g/10-mL single-dose bottle. Net price 10 × 10-mL single-dose bottle = £35.00
Paediatric solution, L-carnitine 30%. Net price 20 mL = £21.00
Injection, L-carnitine 200 mg/mL. Net price 5-mL amp = £11.90

GAUCHER'S DISEASE

Alglucerase is administered as enzyme replacement therapy in Gaucher's disease, a familial disorder affecting principally the liver, spleen, bone marrow, and lymph nodes.

ALGLUCERASE

Indications: (specialist use only) type I Gaucher's disease
Cautions: pregnancy and breast-feeding; monitor for alglucerase antibodies
Contra-indications: androgen-sensitive tumours
Side-effects: abdominal pain, diarrhoea, nausea, vomiting, pain and irritation at injection site, hypersensitivity reactions reported

Dose: *by intravenous infusion,* initially up to 60 units/kg usually every 14 days (frequency adjusted in the range every 2 days to every 4 weeks according to response and patient convenience); lower initial dose of 2.3 units/kg 3 times weekly improves haematological parameters and organomegaly; maintenance, reduce dose at intervals of 6–12 months

▼ PoM **Ceredase**® (Genzyme)

Concentrate for intravenous infusion, alglucerase 10 units/mL. To be diluted before use. Net price 5-mL vial = £154.50; 80 units/mL, 5-mL vial = £1236.00

Note. Contains traces of chorionic gonadotrophin: may interfere with pregnancy test (false positive; delay test for 48 hours after infusion); increases testosterone production (may cause early virilisation in boys especially at high doses)

9.8.2   Acute porphyrias

The acute porphyrias (acute intermittent porphyria, variegate porphyria, hereditary coproporphyria and 5-aminolaevulinic dehydratase deficiency porphyria) are hereditary disorders of haem biosynthesis; they have a prevalence of about 1 in 10 000 of the population.

Great care must be taken when prescribing for patients with acute porphyria since many drugs can induce acute porphyric crises. Since acute porphyrias are hereditary, relatives of affected individuals should be screened and advised about the potential danger of certain drugs.

Haem arginate (*Normosang*®, not on UK market) is administered by short intravenous infusion as haem replacement in moderate, severe or unremitting acute porphyria crises. It is available from Orphan Europe or Farillon. Supplies may be obtained outside office hours from the on-call pharmacist at:

University Hospital of Wales, Cardiff	(01222) 747747
St. James's University Hospital, Leeds	(0113) 243 3134
or	(0113) 283 7010
King's College Hospital, London	0171-737 4000
or	0171-346 3347

Further information may be obtained from:
Welsh Drug Information Centre
University Hospital of Wales
Cardiff CF4 4XW
Telephone (01222) 742979

> See next page for a list of drugs unsafe for use in acute porphyrias

---

Drugs unsafe for use in acute porphyrias

The following list contains drugs on the UK market that have been classified as 'unsafe' in porphyria because they have been shown to be porphyrinogenic in animals or *in vitro*, or have been associated with acute attacks in patients.

Note. Quite modest changes in chemical structure can lead to changes in porphyrinogenicity but where possible general statements have been made about groups of drugs; these should be checked first

Drug groups (please check **first**)

Amphetamines	Benzodiazepines[4]	Gold Salts	Sulphonamides[8]
Anabolic Steroids	Cephalosporins	Hormone Replacement	Sulphonylureas[9]
Antidepressants[1]	Contraceptives, steroid[5]	Therapy[5]	
Antihistamines[2]	Diuretics[6]	Menopausal Steroids[5]	
Barbiturates[3]	Ergot Derivatives[7]	Progestogens	

Individual Drugs (please check groups above **first**)

Alcohol	Danazol	Lignocaine[14]	Phenoxybenzamine
Alcuronium	Dapsone	Lisinopril	Phenylbutazone
Aluminium-containing	Dexfenfluramine	Loxapine	Phenytoin
Antacids[10]	Dextropropoxyphene[13]	Mebeverine	Piroxicam
Aminoglutethimide	Diclofenac	Mefenamic Acid	Pivampicillin[16]
Amiodarone	Doxycycline	Meprobamate	Prilocaine
Azapropazone	Econazole	Methotrexate	Probenecid
Baclofen	Enflurane	Methyldopa	Pyrazinamide
Bromocriptine	Erythromycin	Metoclopramide[15]	Pyrazinamide
Busulphan	Ethamsylate	Metyrapone	Ranitidine
Captopril	Ethionamide	Miconazole	Rifampicin
Carbamazepine	Ethosuximide	Mifepristone	Simvastatin
Carisoprodol	Etomidate	Minoxidil[15]	Sulphinpyrazone
Chloral Hydrate[11]	Fenfluramine	Nalidixic Acid	Sulpiride
Chlorambucil	Flucloxacillin	Nifedipine	Tamoxifen
Chloramphenicol	Flupenthixol	Nitrofurantoin	Theophylline[17]
Chloroform[12]	Griseofulvin	Orphenadrine	Thioridazine
Clonidine	Halothane	Oxybutynin	Tinidazole
Cocaine	Hydralazine	Oxycodone	Triclofos[11]
Colistin	Hyoscine	Oxymetazoline	Trimethoprim
Cyclophosphamide	Isometheptene Mucate	Oxytetracycline	Valproate[4]
Cycloserine	Isoniazid	Pentazocine[13]	Verapamil
Cyclosporin	Ketoconazole		Zuclopenthixol

1. Includes tricyclic (and related) and MAOIs.
2. Most antihistamines should be avoided but cetirizine, chlorpheniramine, cyclizine, diphenhydramine, doxylamine, ketotifen, loratadine, and trimeprazine thought to be safe.
3. Includes methohexitone, primidone, and thiopentone.
4. Status epilepticus has been treated successfully with intravenous diazepam; temazepam is thought to be safe; where essential, seizure prophylaxis has been undertaken with clonazepam or valproate.
5. Includes both progestogen-only and combined (progestogen content more hazardous than oestrogen).
6. Acetazolamide, amiloride, bumetanide, cyclopenthiazide, ethacrynic acid, and triamterene have been used.
7. Includes ergometrine (oxytocin probably safe), lysuride and pergolide.

8. Includes co-trimoxazole and sulphasalazine.
9. Glipizide is thought to be safe
10. Absorption limited but magnesium-containing antacids preferable.
11. Although evidence of hazard is uncertain, manufacturer advises avoid
12. Small amounts in medicines probably safe.
13. Morphine, diamorphine, codeine, dihydrocodeine, and pethidine are thought to be safe.
14. Bupivacaine is thought to be safe.
15. May be used with caution if safer alternative not available.
16. Ampicillin and amoxicillin probably safe.
17. Includes aminophylline.

10: Drugs used in the treatment of
MUSCULOSKELETAL and JOINT DISEASES

In this chapter, drug treatment is discussed under the following headings:

10.1 Drugs used in rheumatic diseases and gout

10.2 Drugs used in neuromuscular disorders

10.3 Drugs for the relief of soft-tissue inflammation

For treatment of septic arthritis see section 5.1, table 1.

10.1 Drugs used in rheumatic diseases and gout

10.1.1 Non-steroidal anti-inflammatory drugs

10.1.2 Corticosteroids

10.1.3 Drugs which suppress the rheumatic disease process

10.1.4 Drugs for treatment of gout

Most rheumatic diseases require symptomatic treatment to relieve pain. In *osteoarthritis* (degenerative joint disease) or for *soft-tissue lesions*, paracetamol (alone or with a low dose of an opioid analgesic—as in co-codamol 8/500 or co-dydramol 10/500) should be used first and can often give adequate pain relief. If a non-steroidal anti-inflammatory drug (NSAID) is required in patients whose symptoms vary, it can be given intermittently (for a few months at a time) and an analgesic such as paracetamol is used during periods of remission. When pain and stiffness are due to *inflammatory rheumatic disease* treatment with an NSAID is indicated.

Drugs are also available which may affect the disease process itself and favourably influence the outcome. For *rheumatoid arthritis* these include penicillamine, gold salts, antimalarials (chloroquine and hydroxychloroquine), immunosuppressants (azathioprine, cyclophosphamide, and methotrexate), and sulphasalazine—they are sometimes known as second-line or disease-modifying antirheumatic drugs; recent evidence has suggested that corticosteroids may also be able to reduce the rate of joint destruction. Drugs which may affect the disease process in *psoriatic arthritis* include gold salts, azathioprine, and methotrexate, and for *gout* they include uricosuric drugs and allopurinol.

10.1.1 Non-steroidal anti-inflammatory drugs (NSAIDs)

In *single doses* NSAIDs have analgesic activity comparable to that of paracetamol (section 4.7.1), but paracetamol is preferred, particularly in the elderly (see also Prescribing for the Elderly, p. 16).

In regular *full dosage* NSAIDs have both a lasting analgesic and an anti-inflammatory effect which makes them particularly useful for the treatment of continuous or regular pain associated with inflammation. Therefore, although paracetamol often gives adequate pain control in osteoarthritis (osteoarthrosis), NSAIDs are more appropriate than paracetamol or the opioid analgesics in the *inflammatory arthritides* (e.g. rheumatoid arthritis) and in some cases of *advanced osteoarthritis*. They may also be of benefit in the less well defined conditions of *back pain* and *soft-tissue disorders*.

CHOICE. Differences in anti-inflammatory activity between different NSAIDs are small, but there is considerable variation in individual patient tolerance and response. About 60% of patients will respond to any NSAID; of the others, those who do not respond to one may well respond to another. A full analgesic effect should normally be obtained within a week, whereas an anti-inflammatory effect may not be achieved (or may not be clinically assessable) for up to three weeks. If appropriate responses are not obtained within these times, another NSAID should be tried.

The main differences between NSAIDs are in the incidence and type of side-effects. Before treatment is started the prescriber should weigh efficacy against possible side-effects.

Ibuprofen is a propionic acid derivative with anti-inflammatory, analgesic, and antipyretic properties. It has fewer side-effects than other NSAIDs but its anti-inflammatory properties are weaker. Doses of 1.6 to 2.4 g daily are needed for rheumatoid arthritis and it is unsuitable for conditions where inflammation is prominent such as acute gout.

Other propionic acid derivatives:

Naproxen has emerged as one of the first choices as it combines good efficacy with a low incidence of side-effects (but more than ibuprofen, see CSM comment below) and administration is only twice daily.

Fenbufen is claimed to be associated with less gastro-intestinal bleeding, but there is a high risk of rashes (see p. 430).

Fenoprofen is as effective as naproxen, and **flurbiprofen** may be slightly more effective. Both are associated with slightly more gastro-intestinal side-effects than ibuprofen.

Ketoprofen has anti-inflammatory properties similar to ibuprofen and has more side-effects (see also CSM comment below).

Tiaprofenic acid is as effective as naproxen; it has more side-effects than ibuprofen (**important:** reports of severe cystitis, see CSM advice on p. 434).

Drugs with properties similar to those of propionic acid derivatives:

Azapropazone is similar in effect to naproxen; it has a tendency to cause rashes and is associated with an increased risk of severe gastro-intestinal toxicity (**important:** see CSM restrictions on p. 429).

Diclofenac and **aceclofenac** have actions similar to that of naproxen; their side-effects are also similar to naproxen.

Diflunisal is an aspirin derivative but its clinical effect more closely resembles that of the propionic acid derivatives than that of its parent compound. Its long duration of action allows twice-daily administration.

Etodolac is comparable in effect to naproxen; side-effects appear to be comparable to those of ibuprofen but long-term data are awaited.

Indomethacin (Indometacin) has an action equal to or superior to that of naproxen, but with a high incidence of side-effects including headaches, dizziness, and gastro-intestinal disturbances (see also CSM comment below).

Ketorolac is used in the short-term management of moderate to severe postoperative pain (section 15.1.4.2)

Mefenamic acid is a related analgesic but its anti-inflammatory properties are minor and side-effects differ in that diarrhoea and occasionally haemolytic anaemia may occur which necessitate discontinuation of treatment.

Meloxicam has recently been introduced for the short-term treatment of osteoarthritis and long-term treatment of rheumatoid arthritis.

Nabumetone is comparable in effect to naproxen.

Phenylbutazone is a potent anti-inflammatory drug but because of occasional serious side-effects its use is limited to the hospital treatment of ankylosing spondylitis; prolonged administration may be necessary but it should not be used unless other drugs have failed.

Piroxicam is as effective as naproxen and has a prolonged duration of action which permits once-daily administration. It has more gastro-intestinal side-effects than ibuprofen, especially in the elderly (see also CSM comment below).

Sulindac is similar in tolerance to naproxen.

Tenoxicam is similar in activity and tolerance to naproxen. Its long half-life allows once-daily administration.

Tolfenamic acid is indicated for the treatment of migraine (section 4.7.4.1)

CAUTIONS and CONTRA-INDICATIONS. NSAIDs should be used with caution in the elderly (risk of serious side-effects and fatalities, see also Prescribing for the Elderly p. 16), in allergic disorders (they are **contra-indicated** in patients with a history of hypersensitivity to aspirin or any other NSAID—which includes those in whom attacks of asthma, angioedema, urticaria or rhinitis have been precipitated by aspirin or any other NSAID), during pregnancy and breast-feeding (see Appendixes 4 and 5), and in coagulation defects.

In patients with renal, cardiac, or hepatic impairment caution is required since the use of NSAIDs may result in deterioration of renal function (see also under Side-effects, below and Appendixes 2 and 3); the dose should be kept as **low as possible** and renal function should be **monitored**.

NSAIDs should not be given to patients with active peptic ulceration (see also **CSM advice** below). While it is preferable to avoid them in patients with current or previous gastro-intestinal ulceration or bleeding, and to withdraw them if gastro-intestinal lesions develop, nevertheless patients with serious rheumatic diseases (e.g. rheumatoid arthritis) are usually dependent on NSAIDs for effective relief of pain and stiffness. For advice on the management of NSAID-associated peptic ulcers, see section 1.3.

For **interactions** of NSAIDs, see Appendix 1 (NSAIDs)

CSM warning (asthma)

Any degree of worsening of asthma may be related to the ingestion of NSAIDs, either prescribed or (in the case of ibuprofen and others) purchased over the counter.

CSM advice (g.i. side-effects)

Recent evidence on the relative safety of 7 oral NSAIDs has indicated differences in the risks of serious upper gastro-intestinal side-effects. **Azapropazone** is associated with the *highest risk* (**important:** see also restrictions on p. 429) and **ibuprofen** with the *lowest*; **piroxicam, ketoprofen, indomethacin, naproxen** and **diclofenac** are associated with *intermediate risks* (possibly higher in the case of piroxicam). There are insufficient data to reach clear conclusions on other available oral NSAIDs.

Recommendations are that NSAIDs associated with low risk *should generally be preferred*, to start at the *lowest recommended dose, not to use more than one* oral NSAID at a time, and to remember that all NSAIDs are *contra-indicated* in patients with peptic ulceration.

Previous recommendations of the CSM have included the advice that in patients with a history of peptic ulcer disease and in the elderly, NSAIDs should be given only after other forms of treatment have been carefully considered.

SIDE-EFFECTS. The side-effects of NSAIDs vary in severity and frequency. Gastro-intestinal discomfort, nausea, diarrhoea, and occasionally bleeding and ulceration occur (see also CSM advice above); dyspepsia may be minimised by taking these drugs with food or milk. Other side-effects include hypersensitivity reactions (particularly rashes, angioedema, and bronchospasm—see CSM advice above), headache, dizziness, vertigo, hearing disturbances such as tinnitus, photosensitivity, and haematuria. Blood disorders have also occurred. Fluid retention may occur (rarely precipitating congestive heart failure in elderly patients). Renal failure may be provoked by NSAIDs especially in patients with pre-existing renal impairment (**important**, see also under Cautions above). Rarely, papillary necrosis or interstitial fibrosis associated with NSAIDs may lead to renal failure. Hepatic damage, alveolitis, pulmonary eosinophilia, pancreatitis, eye changes, Stevens-Johnson syndrome and toxic epidermal necrolysis are other rare side-effects. Induction of or exacerbation of colitis has been reported. Aseptic meningitis has been reported rarely with NSAIDs; patients with connective tissue disorders such as systemic lupus erythematosus may be especially susceptible.

Overdosage: see Emergency Treatment of Poisoning, p. 20.

IBUPROFEN

Indications: pain and inflammation in rheumatic disease (including juvenile arthritis) and other musculoskeletal disorders; mild to moderate pain including dysmenorrhoea; postoperative analgesia; fever and pain in children see section 4.7.1

Cautions; Contra-indications; Side-effects: see notes above; **interactions:** Appendix 1 (NSAIDs); **overdosage:** see Emergency Treatment of Poisoning, p. 20

Dose: initially 1.2–1.8 g daily in 3–4 divided doses preferably after food; increased if necessary to max. of 2.4 g daily; maintenance dose of 0.6–1.2 g daily may be adequate; CHILD 20 mg/kg daily in divided doses (juvenile arthritis, up to 40 mg/kg daily), not recommended for children under 7 kg

PoM **Ibuprofen** (Non-proprietary)

Tablets, coated, ibuprofen 200 mg, net price 20 = 14p; 400 mg, 20 = 29p; 600 mg, 20 = 44p. Label: 21

Various strengths available from APS (*Apsifen®*), Ashbourne (*Arthrofen®*), Berk (*Lidifen®*), Cox, CP, DDSA (*Ebufac®*), Isis (*Isisfen®*), Kent, Lagap (*Ibular®*), Norton, Rima (*Rimafen®*), Pharmacia & Upjohn (*Motrin®*, including an 800-mg strength)

Note. Proprietary brands of ibuprofen preparations are on sale to the public; brand names include, Advil®, Anadin Ibuprofen®, Boots Fever & Pain Relief®, Cuprofen®, Galprofen®, Hedex® Ibuprofen, Ibrufhalal®, Ibufem®, Inoven®, Junifen®, Librofem®, Migrafen®, Novaprin®, Nurofen®, Pacifene®, PhorPain®, Proflex®, Relcofen®; compound proprietary preparations containing ibuprofen include Advil® Cold and Sinus (ibuprofen, pseudoephedrine), Lemsip® Power + (ibuprofen, pseudoephedrine), Nurofen® Cold & Flu (ibuprofen, pseudoephedrine), Nurofen® Plus (ibuprofen, codeine), Solpaflex® (ibuprofen, codeine), Vicks Action® (ibuprofen, pseudoephedrine),

PoM **Brufen®** (Knoll)

Tablets, all magenta, ibuprofen 200 mg (s/c), net price 20 = 62p; 400 mg (s/c), 20 = £1.17; 600 mg (f/c), 20 = £1.85. Label: 21

Syrup, orange, ibuprofen 100 mg/5 mL. Net price 500 mL = £7.34. Label: 21

Dose: 20 mg/kg daily in divided doses *or* 1–2 years 2.5 mL 3–4 times daily, 3–7 years 5 mL 3–4 times daily, 8–12 years 10 mL 3–4 times daily; not recommended for children weighing less than 7 kg; juvenile rheumatoid arthritis up to 40 mg/kg daily in divided doses

Granules, effervescent, ibuprofen 600 mg/sachet. Net price 20-sachet pack = £5.15. Label: 13, 21

Note. Contains sodium approx. 9 mmol/sachet

Junifen Sugar-Free® : see section 4.7.1
Topical preparations : section 10.3.2

Modified release

PoM **Brufen Retard®** (Knoll)

Tablets, m/r, f/c, ibuprofen 800 mg, net price 56-tab pack = £10.10. Label: 25, 27

Dose: 2 tablets daily as a single dose, preferably in the early evening, increased in severe cases to 3 tablets daily in 2 divided doses; CHILD not recommended

PoM **Fenbid®** (Goldshield)

Spansule® (= capsule m/r), maroon/pink, enclosing off-white pellets, ibuprofen 300 mg. Net price 120-cap pack = £9.64. Label: 25

Dose: 1–3 capsules every 12 hours; CHILD not recommended

With codeine

For an adverse comment on compound analgesic preparations, see p. 195. For details of the **side-effects, cautions,** and **contra-indications** of opioid analgesics, see p. 200 (**important:** the elderly are particularly susceptible to opioid side-effects).

PoM **Codafen Continus®** (Napp)

Tablets, white/pink, ibuprofen 300 mg (m/r), codeine phosphate 20 mg (m/r). Net price 112-tab pack = £12.57. Label: 2, 21, 25

Dose: 1–2 tablets every 12 hours; max. 3 tablets every 12 hours; CHILD not recommended

---

ACECLOFENAC

Indications: pain and inflammation in rheumatoid arthritis, osteoarthritis and ankylosing spondylitis

Cautions; Contra-indications; Side-effects: see notes above; avoid in porphyria (see section 9.8.2); **interactions:** Appendix 1 (NSAIDs)

Dose: 100 mg twice daily (reduce to 100 mg daily initially in hepatic impairment); CHILD not recommended

▼ PoM **Preservex®** (UCB Pharma)

Tablets, f/c, aceclofenac 100 mg, net price 60-tab pack = £14.95. Label: 21

ACEMETACIN

(Glycolic acid ester of indomethacin)

Indications: pain and inflammation in rheumatic disease and other musculoskeletal disorders; postoperative analgesia

Cautions; Contra-indications; Side-effects: see under Indomethacin and notes above

DRIVING. Dizziness may affect performance of skilled tasks (e.g. driving)

Dose: 120 mg daily in divided doses with food, increased if necessary to 180 mg daily; CHILD not recommended

PoM **Emflex®** (Merck)

Capsules, yellow/orange, acemetacin 60 mg, net price 90-cap pack = £21.36. Label: 21, counselling, driving

---

AZAPROPAZONE

Indications: see under CSM restrictions, below

CSM RESTRICTIONS. CSM *has restricted* azapropazone to use in rheumatoid arthritis, ankylosing spondylitis and acute gout only when other NSAIDs have been tried and failed, *has* **contra-indicated** it in patients with a history of peptic ulceration, and *has reduced* the maximum daily dose to 600 mg for rheumatoid arthritis and ankylosing spondylitis in patients over 60 years

Cautions; Contra-indications; Side-effects: see notes above; also specifically contra-indicated if history of peptic ulceration, inflammatory bowel disease or blood disorder; for specific restrictions and contra-indications relating to renal impairment see under Dose; photosensitivity, see CSM advice below; avoid in porphyria (see section 9.8.2); **important:** reports of serious enhancement of effect of warfarin; other **interactions:** Appendix 1 (NSAIDs)

PHOTOSENSITIVITY. CSM has reminded of need to advise patients taking azapropazone to avoid direct exposure to sunlight (or to use sunblock preparations)

Dose:

Rheumatoid arthritis and ankylosing spondylitis, 1.2 g daily in 2 or 4 divided doses; in renal impairment or in elderly 300 mg twice daily, avoid altogether in severe renal impairment; CHILD not recommended

Acute gout (always ensure increased fluid intake), 1.8 g daily in divided doses until acute symptoms subside (usually by day 4) *then* 1.2 g daily in divided doses until symptoms resolve—consider appropriate alternative therapy if they persist; in mild renal impairment or in elderly, 1.8 g daily for first 24 hours then 1.2 g daily in divided doses reducing to max. 600 mg daily in divided doses as soon as possible (preferably by day 4) then continuing only until acute symptoms resolve—consider appropriate alternative therapy if they persist, and *avoid altogether for gout* in moderate to severe renal impairment and *avoid for gout in elderly* even in mild renal impairment; CHILD not recommended

PoM **Rheumox**® (Wyeth)

Capsules, orange, azapropazone 300 mg. Net price 20 = £2.86. Label: 11 (also photosensitivity counselling, see above), 21

Tablets, orange, f/c, scored, azapropazone 600 mg. Net price 20 = £4.98. Label: 11 (also photosensitivity counselling, see above), 21

DICLOFENAC SODIUM

Indications: pain and inflammation in rheumatic disease (including juvenile arthritis) and other musculoskeletal disorders; acute gout; postoperative pain

Cautions; Contra-indications; Side-effects: see notes above; porphyria (see section 9.8.2); suppositories may cause rectal irritation; **interactions:** Appendix 1 (NSAIDs)

INTRAVENOUS USE. Additional contra-indications include concomitant NSAID or anticoagulant use (including low-dose heparin), history of haemorrhagic diathesis, history of confirmed or suspected cerebrovascular bleeding, operations with high risk of haemorrhage, history of asthma, moderate or severe renal impairment, hypovolaemia, dehydration

Dose: by mouth, 75–150 mg daily in 2–3 divided doses, preferably after food

By *deep intramuscular injection* into the gluteal muscle, acute exacerbations and post-operative, 75 mg once daily (twice daily in severe cases) for max. of 2 days

Ureteric colic, 75 mg then a further 75 mg after 30 minutes if necessary

By *intravenous infusion* (in hospital setting), 75 mg over 30–120 minutes repeated if necessary after 4–6 hours for max. 2 days

Prevention of postoperative pain, initially after surgery 25–50 mg over 15–60 minutes then 5 mg/hour for max. 2 days

By *rectum* in suppositories, 75–150 mg daily in divided doses

Max. total daily dose by any route 150 mg

CHILD 1–12 years, juvenile arthritis, *by mouth or by rectum,* 1–3 mg/kg daily in divided doses (25 mg e/c tablets, 12.5 mg and 25 mg suppositories only)

PoM **Diclofenac Sodium** (Non-proprietary)

Tablets, both e/c, diclofenac sodium 25 mg, net price 20 = 88p; 50 mg, 20 = £1.67. Label: 5, 25

Available from APS, Ashbourne (Diclozip®), Berk (Flamrase®), Cox, Dexcel Pharma (Dicloflex®), Eastern (Volraman®), Isis (Isclofen®, 50 mg), Kent (Enzed®), Lagap (Rhumalgan®), Norton, Opus (Lofensaid®), 3link (Valenac®), Sterwin

Injection, diclofenac sodium 25 mg/mL. Net price 3-mL amp = 83p

Available from Antigen

Note. Licensed for intramuscular use

PoM **Voltarol**® (Novartis)

Tablets, both e/c, diclofenac sodium 25 mg (yellow), net price 84-tab pack = £7.88; 50 mg (brown), 84-tab pack = £15.32. Label: 5, 25

Dispersible tablets, pink, diclofenac, equivalent to diclofenac sodium 50 mg, net price 21-tab pack = £5.15. Label: 13, 21

Note. Voltarol Dispersible tablets are more suitable for **short-term** use in acute conditions for which treatment required for no more than 3 months (no information on use beyond 3 months)

Injection, diclofenac sodium 25 mg/mL. Net price 3-mL amp = 83p

Suppositories, diclofenac sodium 12.5 mg, net price 10 = 72p; 25 mg, 10 = £1.28; 50 mg, 10 = £2.10; 100 mg, 10 = £3.76

Emulgel® gel, section 10.3.2

Modified release

PoM **Diclomax SR**® (P-D)

Capsules, m/r, yellow, diclofenac sodium 75 mg. Net price 56-cap pack = £13.01. Label: 21, 25

Dose: 1 capsule 1–2 times daily *or* 2 capsules once daily, preferably with food; CHILD not recommended

PoM **Diclomax Retard**® (P-D)

Capsules, m/r, diclofenac sodium 100 mg. Net price 28-tab pack = £9.36. Label: 21, 25

Dose: 1 capsule daily preferably with food; CHILD not recommended

PoM **Motifene®** 75 mg (Sankyo)

Capsules, e/c, m/r, diclofenac sodium 75 mg (enclosing e/c pellets containing diclofenac sodium 25 mg and m/r pellets containing diclofenac sodium 50 mg). Net price 56-cap pack = £14.99. Label: 25

Dose: 1 capsule 1-2 times daily; CHILD not recommended

PoM **Voltarol® 75 mg SR** (Geigy)

Tablets, m/r, pink, diclofenac sodium 75 mg. Net price 28-tab pack = £8.68; 56-tab pack = £17.35. Label: 21, 25

Dose: 75 mg 1–2 times daily preferably with food; CHILD not recommended

Note. Modified-release tablets containing diclofenac sodium 75 mg available from Bartholomew Rhodes (*Diclotard® 75 MR*), Dexcel Pharma (*Dicloflex® SR*), Hillcross (*Dexomon® SR*), Lagap (*Rhumalgan® CR*), Norton, Opus (*Lofensaid® Retard 75*), Sterwin (*Slofenac® SR*), Trinity (*Volsaid® Retard*)

PoM **Voltarol® Retard** (Novartis)

Tablets, m/r, red, diclofenac sodium 100 mg. Net price 28-tab pack = £12.72. Label: 21, 25

Dose: 1 tablet daily preferably with food; CHILD not recommended

Note. Modified-release tablets containing diclofenac sodium 100 mg available from APS, Bartholomew Rhodes (*Diclotard® 100 MR*), Berk (*Flamrase® SR[1]*), Cox (*Flamatak® MR*), Dexcel Pharma (*Dicloflex® Retard*), Ethical Generics Ltd (*Digenac® XL[1]*), Hillcross (*Dexomon® Retard 100*), Lagap (*Rhumalgan® CR*), Norton, Opus (*Lofensaid® Retard 100*), Pharmacia & Upjohn (*Flexotard® MR*), Sterwin (*Slofenac® SR*), Trinity (*Volsaid® Retard*)

1. Also licensed for dysmenorrhoea and associated menorrhagia

With misoprostol

For prophylaxis against NSAID-induced gastroduodenal ulceration in patients requiring diclofenac for rheumatoid arthritis or osteoarthritis; cautions, contra-indications, and side-effects of misoprostol, see section 1.3.4

PoM **Arthrotec®** (Searle)

Arthrotec® 50 tablets, diclofenac sodium (in e/c core) 50 mg, misoprostol 200 micrograms. Net price 60-tab pack = £14.98; 140-tab pack = £34.94 (hosp. only). Label: 21, 25

Dose: 1 tablet 2–3 times daily with food; CHILD not recommended

Arthrotec® 75 tablets, diclofenac sodium (in e/c core) 75 mg, misoprostol 200 micrograms. Net price 60-tab pack = £17.59. Label: 21, 25

Dose: 1 tablet twice daily with food; CHILD not recommended

DIFLUNISAL

Indications: pain and inflammation in rheumatic disease and other musculoskeletal disorders; mild to moderate pain including dysmenorrhoea

Cautions; Contra-indications; Side-effects: see notes above; **interactions:** Appendix 1 (NSAIDs)

Dose: mild to moderate pain, initially 1 g, then 500 mg every 12 hours (increased to max. 500 mg every 8 hours if necessary)

Osteoarthritis, rheumatoid arthritis, 0.5–1 g daily as a single daily dose *or* in 2 divided doses

Dysmenorrhoea, initially 1 g, then 500 mg every 12 hours

CHILD not recommended

PoM **Diflunisal** (Non-proprietary)

Tablets, coated, diflunisal 250 mg, net price 20 = £1.80; 500 mg, 20 = £3.61. Label: 21, 25, counselling, avoid aluminium hydroxide

Available from APS

PoM **Dolobid®** (Morson)

Tablets, both f/c, diflunisal 250 mg (peach), net price 20 = £1.80; 500 mg (orange), 20 = £3.61. Label: 21, 25, counselling, avoid aluminium hydroxide

ETODOLAC

Indications: pain and inflammation in rheumatoid arthritis and osteoarthritis

Cautions; Contra-indications; Side-effects: see notes above; **interactions:** Appendix 1 (NSAIDs)

Dose: 200 mg or 300 mg twice daily *or* 400 mg or 600 mg once daily; max. 600 mg daily; CHILD not recommended

PoM **Lodine®** (Monmouth)

Capsules, etodolac 200 mg (light- and dark-grey), net price 60-cap pack = £10.55; 300 mg (light-grey), 60-cap pack = £14.65. Label: 21

Tablets, brown, f/c, etodolac 200 mg. Net price 60-tab pack = £10.55. Label: 21

Modified release
PoM **Lodine SR®** (Monmouth)

Tablets, m/r, light-grey, etodolac 600 mg. Net price 30-tab pack = £15.50. Label : 25

Dose: 1 tablet daily; CHILD not recommended

FENBUFEN

Indications: pain and inflammation in rheumatic disease and other musculoskeletal disorders

Cautions; Contra-indications; Side-effects: see notes above, but also high risk of rashes (discontinue immediately); erythema multiforme and Stevens-Johnson syndrome reported; also allergic interstitial lung disorders (may follow rashes); **interactions:** Appendix 1 (NSAIDs)

Dose: 300 mg in the morning and 600 mg at bedtime *or* 450 mg twice daily; CHILD under 14 years not recommended

PoM **Lederfen®** (Lederle)

Capsules, dark blue, fenbufen 300 mg. Net price 84-cap pack = £18.83. Label: 21

Note. Fenbufen capsules also available from APS, Ashbourne (Fenbuzip®), Cox, Hillcross, Norton

Tablets, both light blue, f/c, fenbufen 300 mg, net price 84-tab pack = £18.83; 450 mg, 56-tab pack = £18.83. Label: 21

Note. Fenbufen tablets also available from APS, Ashbourne (*Fenbuzip®*), Cox (450 mg), Hillcross, Kent, Norton

FENOPROFEN

Indications: pain and inflammation in rheumatic disease and other musculoskeletal disorders; mild to moderate pain

Cautions; Contra-indications; Side-effects: see notes above; upper respiratory infection, nasopharyngitis, and cystitis also reported; **interactions:** Appendix 1 (NSAIDs)

Dose: 200–600 mg 3–4 times daily with food; max. 3 g daily; CHILD not recommended

PoM **Fenopron®** (Novex)

Tablets, both orange, fenoprofen (as calcium salt) 300 mg (*Fenopron®* 300), net price 100-tab pack = £9.45; 600 mg (*Fenopron®* 600, scored), 100-tab pack = £18.29. Label: 21

FLURBIPROFEN

Indications: pain and inflammation in rheumatic disease and other musculoskeletal disorders; mild to moderate pain including dysmenorrhoea; postoperative analgesia

Cautions; Contra-indications; Side-effects: see notes above; suppositories may cause rectal irritation; **interactions:** Appendix 1 (NSAIDs)

Dose: by mouth or by rectum in suppositories, 150–200 mg, daily in divided doses, increased in acute conditions to 300 mg daily

Dysmenorrhoea, initially 100 mg, then 50–100 mg every 4–6 hours; max. 300 mg daily CHILD not recommended

PoM **Froben®** (Knoll)

Tablets, both yellow, s/c, flurbiprofen 50 mg, net price 20 = £1.65; 100 mg, 20 = £3.13. Label: 21

Note. Flurbiprofen tablets also available from APS, Cox, Du Pont, Kent, Lagap, Norton

Suppositories, flurbiprofen 100 mg. Net price 12 = £2.90

Modified release
PoM **Froben SR®** (Knoll)

Capsules, m/r, yellow, enclosing off-white beads, flurbiprofen 200 mg. Net price 30-cap pack = £10.88. Label: 21, 25

Dose: rheumatic disease, 1 capsule daily, preferably in the evening; CHILD not recommended

INDOMETHACIN

(Indometacin)

Indications: pain and moderate to severe inflammation in rheumatic disease and other acute musculoskeletal disorders; acute gout; dysmenorrhoea; closure of ductus arteriosus (section 7.1.1.1)

Cautions; Contra-indications: see notes above; caution also in epilepsy, parkinsonism, psychiatric disturbances; during prolonged therapy ophthalmic and blood examinations particularly advisable; avoid rectal administration in proctitis and haemorrhoids; **interactions:** Appendix 1 (NSAIDs)

DRIVING. Dizziness may affect performance of skilled tasks (e.g. driving)

Side-effects: see notes above; frequently gastro-intestinal disturbances (including diarrhoea), headache, dizziness, and light-headedness; gastro-intestinal ulceration and bleeding; rarely, drowsiness, confusion, insomnia, convulsions, psychiatric disturbances, depression, syncope, blood disorders (particularly thrombocytopenia), hypertension, hyperglycaemia, blurred vision, corneal deposits, peripheral neuropathy, and intestinal strictures; suppositories may cause rectal irritation and occasional bleeding

Dose: by mouth, rheumatic disease, 50–200 mg daily in divided doses, with food; CHILD not recommended

Acute gout, 150–200 mg daily in divided doses

Dysmenorrhoea, up to 75 mg daily

By rectum in suppositories, 100 mg at night and in the morning if required; CHILD not recommended

Combined oral and rectal treatment, max. total daily dose 150–200 mg

PoM **Indomethacin** (Non-proprietary)

Capsules, indomethacin 25 mg, net price 20 = 24p; 50 mg, 20 = 49p. Label: 21, counselling, driving, see above

Available from APS, Ashbourne (*Indomax®*), Berk (*Imbrilon®*), Cox, Galen (*Mobilan®*), Kent, Morson (*Indocid®*), Norton, Rima (*Rimacid®*)

Suspension, sugar-free, indomethacin 25 mg/5 mL. Net price 200 mL = £3.12. Label: 21, counselling, driving, see above

Available from Morson (Indocid®)

Suppositories, indomethacin 100 mg. Net price 10 = £1.09. Counselling, driving, see above

Available from Berk (*Imbrilon®*), Cox, Morson (*Indocid®*), Norton

Modified release
PoM **Indomethacin m/r preparations**

Capsules, m/r, indomethacin 75 mg. Net price 20 = £1.40. Label: 21, 25, counselling, driving, see above

Dose: 1 capsule 1–2 times daily; CHILD not recommended

Available from Ashbourne (*Indomax 75 SR®*), Bartholomew Rhodes (*Indotard®*), Cox (*Pardelprin®*), Generics (*Slo-Indo®*), Hillcross (*Rheumacin LA®*), Lagap (*Indolar SR®*), Morson (*Indocid-R®*), Opus (*Maximet SR®*), Pharmacia & Upjohn (*Indomod®*; also 25- mg strength), Trinity (*Artracin SR®*)

Tablets, m/r, indomethacin 25 mg (*Flexin-25 Continus®*, green), net price 56-tab pack = £7.15; 50 mg (*Flexin-LS Continus®*, red), 28-tab pack = £7.15; 75 mg (*Flexin Continus®*, yellow), 28-tab pack = £10.21. Label: 21, 25, counselling, driving, see above

Dose: initially 75 mg daily, adjusted in steps of 25–50 mg; range 25–200 mg daily in 1–2 divided doses; dysmenorrhoea, up to 75 mg daily; CHILD not recommended

Available from Napp

KETOPROFEN

Indications: pain and mild inflammation in rheumatic disease and other musculoskeletal disorders, and after orthopaedic surgery; acute gout; dysmenorrhoea

Cautions; Contra-indications; Side-effects: see notes above; pain may occur at injection site (occasionally tissue damage); suppositories may cause rectal irritation; **interactions:** Appendix 1 (NSAIDs)

Dose: by mouth, rheumatic disease, 100–200 mg daily in 2–4 divided doses with food; CHILD not recommended

Pain and dysmenorrhoea, 50 mg up to 3 times daily; CHILD not recommended

By rectum in suppositories, rheumatic disease, 100 mg at bedtime; CHILD not recommended

Combined oral and rectal treatment, max. total daily dose 200 mg

By deep intramuscular injection into the gluteal muscle, 50–100 mg every 4 hours (max. 200 mg in 24 hours) for up to 3 days; CHILD not recommended

PoM **Orudis®** (Rhône-Poulenc Rorer)
Capsules, ketoprofen 50 mg (green/purple), net price 112-cap pack = £9.52; 100 mg (pink), 56-cap pack = £9.55. Label: 21
Suppositories, ketoprofen 100 mg. Net price 10 = £4.10
PoM **Oruvail®** (Rhône-Poulenc Rorer)
Injection, ketoprofen 50 mg/mL. Net price 2-mL amp = 73p
Gel, section 10.3.2

Modified release
PoM **Oruvail®** (Rhône-Poulenc Rorer)
Capsules, all m/r, enclosing white pellets, ketoprofen 100 mg (pink/purple), net price 56-cap pack = £17.52; 150 mg (pink), 28-cap pack = £10.00; 200 mg (pink/white), 28-cap pack = £17.47. Label: 21, 25
Dose: 100–200 mg once daily with food; CHILD not recommended
Note. Modified-release capsules containing ketoprofen 100 mg and 200 mg also available from APS (Ketovail®), Ashbourne (Ketozip XL®-200 mg), Bartholomew Rhodes (Ketotard® 200XL), Cox (Jomethid XL®-200 mg), Du Pont (Ketoprofen CR®), Lagap (Larafen CR®-200 mg), Opus (Fenoket®-200 mg), Trinity (Ketocid®-200 mg)

MEFENAMIC ACID

Indications: mild to moderate pain in rheumatoid arthritis (including juvenile arthritis), osteoarthritis, and related conditions; dysmenorrhoea and menorrhagia

Cautions; Contra-indications: see notes above; also specifically contra-indicated in inflammatory bowel disease; blood tests required during long-term treatment; porphyria (see section 9.8.2); **interactions:** Appendix 1 (NSAIDs)

Side-effects: see notes above; drowsiness; diarrhoea or rashes (withdraw treatment); thrombocytopenia, haemolytic anaemia and aplastic anaemia reported; convulsions in overdosage

Dose: 500 mg 3 times daily preferably after food; CHILD over 6 months, 25 mg/kg daily in divided doses for not longer than 7 days, except in juvenile arthritis

PoM **Mefenamic Acid** (Non-proprietary)
Capsules, mefenamic acid 250 mg. Net price 20 = 58p. Label: 21
Available from APS, Ashbourne (*Dysman 250®*), Berk (*Contraflam®*), Cox, Kent, Lagap, Norton, Opus (*Opustan 250®*), P-D (*Ponstan®*), Sterwin, Trinity (*Meflam 250®*)
Tablets, mefenamic acid 500 mg, net price 20 = £1.56. Label: 21
Available from APS, Ashbourne (*Dysman 500®*), Berk, Cox, Norton, Opus (*Opustan 500®*), P-D (*Ponstan Forte®*), Trinity (*Meflam 500®*)
Paediatric oral suspension, mefenamic acid 50 mg/5 mL. Net price 125 mL = £3.37. Label: 21
Available from P-D (*Ponstan®*)

MELOXICAM

Indications: pain and inflammation in rheumatic disease; exacerbation of osteoarthritis (short-term)

Cautions; Contra-indications; Side-effects: see notes above; contra-indicated in renal failure (unless receiving dialysis); avoid rectal administration in proctitis or haemorrhoids; **interactions:** Appendix 1 (NSAIDs)

Dose: by mouth, osteoarthritis, 7.5 mg daily with food, increased if necessary to max. 15 mg once daily

Rheumatoid arthritis, 15 mg once daily with food (reduced to 7.5 mg daily in elderly and in dialysis patients)

By rectum, in suppositories, rheumatoid arthritis, 15 mg once daily

CHILD under 15 years not recommended

▼ PoM **Mobic®** (Boehringer Ingelheim)
Tablets, both yellow, scored, meloxicam 7.5 mg, net price 30-tab pack = £10.00; 15 mg, 30-tab pack = £13.90. Label: 21
Suppositories, meloxicam 15 mg. Net price 12 = £6.00

NABUMETONE

Indications: pain and inflammation in osteoarthritis and rheumatoid arthritis

Cautions; Contra-indications; Side-effects: see notes above; **interactions:** Appendix 1 (NSAIDs)

Dose: 1 g at night, in severe conditions 0.5–1 g in morning as well; elderly 0.5–1 g daily; CHILD not recommended

PoM **Relifex®** (Bencard)
Tablets, red, f/c, nabumetone 500 mg. Net price 56-tab pack = £18.11. Label: 21, 25
Suspension, sugar-free, nabumetone 500 mg/ 5 mL. Net price 300-mL pack = £25.22. Label: 21

NAPROXEN

Indications: pain and inflammation in rheumatic disease (including juvenile arthritis) and other musculoskeletal disorders; dysmenorrhoea; acute gout

---

Abbreviations and symbols, see inside front cover   Prices are **net**, see p. 1

Cautions; Contra-indications; Side-effects: see notes above; suppositories may cause rectal irritation and occasional bleeding; **interactions:** Appendix 1 (NSAIDs)

Dose: by mouth, 0.5–1 g daily in 2 divided doses *or* 1 g once daily; CHILD (over 5 years), juvenile arthritis, 10 mg/kg daily in 2 divided doses

Acute musculoskeletal disorders and dysmenorrhoea, 500 mg initially, then 250 mg every 6–8 hours as required; max. dose after first day 1.25 g daily; CHILD under 16 years not recommended

Acute gout, 750 mg initially, then 250 mg every 8 hours until attack has passed; CHILD under 16 years not recommended

By rectum in suppositories, 500 mg at bedtime; if necessary 500 mg in morning as well; CHILD under 16 years not recommended

PoM **Naproxen** (Non-proprietary)

Tablets, naproxen 250 mg, net price 20 = £1.55; 500 mg, 20 = £3.22. Label: 21

Available from APS, Ashbourne (*Arthrosin®*), Berk (Timpron®), BHR (*Prosaid®*), Cox, CP (*Arthroxen®*), Lagap (*Laraflex®*), Norton, Shire (*Valrox®*), Sterwin

PoM **Naprosyn®** (Roche)

Tablets, all scored, naproxen 250 mg (buff), net price 56-tab pack = £5.12; 500 mg (buff), 56-tab pack = £10.23. Label: 21

Tablets, all e/c, (*Naprosyn EC®*), naproxen 250 mg, net price 56-tab pack = £5.12; 375 mg, 56 tab pack = £7.68; 500 mg, 56-tab pack = £10.23. Label: 5, 25

Suspension, orange, naproxen 125 mg/5 mL. Contains about 1.7 mmol Na⁺/5 mL. Net price 240 mL = £3.82. Label: 21

Suppositories, naproxen 500 mg. Net price 10 = £2.39

PoM **Nycopren®** (Ardern)

Tablets, both e/c, naproxen 250 mg, net price 56-tab pack = £5.79; 500 mg, 56-tab pack = £11.58. Label: 5, 25

PoM **Synflex®** (Roche)

Tablets, blue, naproxen sodium 275 mg. Net price 60-tab pack = £8.49. Label: 21

Note. 275 mg naproxen sodium ≡ 250 mg naproxen

Dose: musculoskeletal disorders, postoperative analgesia, 550 mg twice daily when necessary, preferably after food; max. 1.1 g daily; CHILD under 16 years not recommended

Dysmenorrhoea, initially 550 mg then 275 mg every 6–8 hours as required; max. of 1.375 g on first day and 1.1 g daily thereafter; CHILD under 16 years not recommended

Modified release

PoM **Naprosyn® S/R** (Roche)

Tablets, m/r, f/c, scored, naproxen 500 mg (as sodium salt), net price 56-tab pack = £15.29. Label: 25

Dose: rheumatic and musculoskeletal disorders, 1–2 tablets once daily; CHILD under 16 years not recommended

With misoprostol

For cautions, contra-indications, and side-effects of misoprostol, see section 1.3.4

PoM **Napratec®** (Searle)

Combination pack, 56 yellow scored tablets, naproxen 500 mg; 56 white scored tablets, misoprostol 200 micrograms. Net price = £19.80. Label: 21

Dose: patients requiring naproxen for rheumatoid arthritis, osteoarthritis, or ankylosing spondylitis, with prophylaxis against NSAID-induced gastroduodenal ulceration, 1 naproxen 500-mg tablet and 1 misoprostol 200-microgram tablet taken together twice daily with food; CHILD not recommended

PHENYLBUTAZONE

Indications: ankylosing spondylitis when other therapy is unsuitable

Cautions: blood counts before and during treatment if for more than 7 days; elderly (reduce dose); breast-feeding; allergic disorders (see also under Contra-indications, below), withdraw treatment if acute pulmonary syndrome including fever and dyspnoea occurs; see also notes above; **interactions:** Appendix 1 (NSAIDs)

COUNSELLING. Warn patient to tell doctor immediately if sore throat, mouth ulcers, bruising, fever, malaise, rash, or non-specific illness develops.

Contra-indications: cardiovascular disease, pulmonary, renal and hepatic impairment; pregnancy; history of peptic ulceration, gastro-intestinal haemorrhage, inflammatory bowel disease, or blood disorders (including coagulation defects); history of hypersensitivity precipitated by aspirin or other NSAIDs (see also below); porphyria (see section 9.8.2); Sjögren's syndrome; thyroid disease; children under 14

HYPERSENSITIVITY. NSAIDs are **contra-indicated** in patients with a history of hypersensitivity to aspirin or any other NSAID—*which includes those* in whom attacks of *asthma, angioedema, urticaria or rhinitis* have been precipitated by aspirin or any other NSAID

Side-effects: see notes above; parotitis, stomatitis, goitre, pancreatitis, hepatitis, nephritis, visual disturbances; rarely leucopenia, thrombocytopenia, agranulocytosis, aplastic anaemia, erythema multiforme (Stevens-Johnson syndrome), toxic epidermal necrolysis (Lyell's syndrome), pulmonary toxicity

Dose: initially 200 mg 2–3 times daily for 2 days, with or after food, then reduced to minimum effective, usually 100 mg 2–3 times daily; CHILD under 14 years not recommended

PoM **Butacote®** (Novartis)

Tablets, pale blue, e/c, s/c, phenylbutazone 100 mg, net price 20 = 40p (hosp. only). Label: 5, 21, 25, counselling, blood disorder symptoms (see above)

PIROXICAM

Indications: pain and inflammation in rheumatic disease (including juvenile arthritis) and other musculoskeletal disorders; acute gout

Cautions; Contra-indications: see notes above; porphyria (see section 9.8.2); **interactions:** Appendix 1 (NSAIDs)

Side-effects: see notes above; pain may occur at injection site (occasionally tissue damage); suppositories may cause rectal irritation and occasional bleeding

Dose: *by mouth or by rectum*, rheumatic disease, initially 20 mg daily, maintenance 10–30 mg daily, in single or divided doses

CHILD (over 6 years) *by mouth*, juvenile arthritis, less than 15 kg, 5 mg daily; 16–25 kg, 10 mg; 26–45 kg, 15 mg; over 46 kg, 20 mg

Acute musculoskeletal disorders, 40 mg daily in single or divided doses for 2 days, then 20 mg daily for 7–14 days; CHILD not recommended

Acute gout, 40 mg initially, then 40 mg daily in single or divided doses for 4–6 days; CHILD not recommended

By deep intramuscular injection into gluteal muscle, for initial treatment of acute conditions, as dose by mouth (on short-term basis); CHILD not recommended

PoM **Piroxicam** (Non-proprietary)
Capsules, piroxicam 10 mg, net price 20 = £1.38; 20 mg, 20 = £2.74. Label: 21
Available from APS, Ashbourne (*Pirozip*®), Berk (*Flamatrol*®), Cox, Hillcross, Kent (*Kentene*®), Lagap (*Larapam*®), Norton, Opus (*Piroflam*®)

PoM **Feldene**® (Pfizer)
Capsules, piroxicam 10 mg (maroon/blue), net price 56-cap pack = £6.00; 20 mg (maroon), 28-cap pack = £6.00. Label: 21
Tablets, (*Feldene Melt*®), piroxicam 20 mg, net price 28-tab pack = £9.83. Label: 10 patient information leaflet, 21
Note. Feldene Melt® tablets can be taken by placing on tongue or by swallowing; contain aspartame equivalent to phenylalanine 140 micrograms/tablet (see section 9.4.1)
Dispersible tablets, piroxicam 10 mg (scored), net price 56-tab pack = £9.75; 20 mg, 28-tab pack = £9.75. Label: 13, 21
Note. Piroxicam dispersible tablets also available from Hillcross
Injection, piroxicam 20 mg/mL. Net price 1-mL amp = 70p
Suppositories, piroxicam 20 mg. Net price 10 = £5.20
Gel, section 10.3.2

SULINDAC

Indications: pain and inflammation in rheumatic disease and other musculoskeletal disorders; acute gout

Cautions; Contra-indications; Side-effects: see notes above; also caution if history of renal stones and ensure adequate hydration; urine discoloration occasionally reported; **interactions:** Appendix 1 (NSAIDs)

Dose: 200 mg twice daily with food (may be reduced according to response); max. 400 mg daily; acute gout should respond within 7 days; limit treatment of peri-articular disorders to 7–10 days; CHILD not recommended

PoM **Clinoril**® (MSD)
Tablets, both yellow, scored, sulindac 100 mg, net price 20 = £2.24; 200 mg, 20 = £4.32. Label: 21
Note. Sulindac tablets also available from APS, Generics

TENOXICAM

Indications: pain and inflammation in rheumatic disease and other musculoskeletal disorders

Cautions; Contra-indications; Side-effects: see notes above; **interactions:** Appendix 1 (NSAIDs)

Dose: *by mouth*, rheumatic disease, 20 mg daily; CHILD not recommended

Acute musculoskeletal disorders, 20 mg daily for 7 days; max. 14 days; CHILD not recommended

By intravenous or intramuscular injection, for initial treatment for 1–2 days, as dose by mouth; CHILD not recommended

PoM **Mobiflex**® (Roche)
Tablets, red-brown, f/c, tenoxicam 20 mg. Net price 28-tab pack = £14.10. Label: 21
Injection, powder for reconstitution, tenoxicam 20 mg. Net price per amp (with solvent) = 93p

TIAPROFENIC ACID

Indications: pain and inflammation in rheumatic disease and other musculoskeletal disorders

Cautions; Contra-indications; Side-effects: see notes above; also contra-indicated in active bladder or prostate disease (or symptoms) and history of recurrent urinary-tract disorders—if urinary symptoms develop discontinue immediately and perform urine tests and culture; see also CSM advice below; **interactions:** Appendix 1 (NSAIDs)

CSM ADVICE. Following reports of **severe cystitis** associated with tiaprofenic acid the CSM has recommended that tiaprofenic acid *should not be given* to patients with pre-existing urinary-tract disorders and *should be stopped* if urinary symptoms develop. Patients *should be advised* to stop taking tiaprofenic acid and to report to their doctor promptly if they develop urinary-tract symptoms (such as increased frequency, nocturia, urgency, pain on urinating, or blood in urine)

Dose: 600 mg daily in 2–3 divided doses; CHILD not recommended

PoM **Surgam**® (Hoechst Marion Roussel)
Tablets, tiaprofenic acid 200 mg, net price 84-tab pack = £15.89; 300 mg, 56-tab pack = £15.89. Label: 21
Note. Tiaprofenic acid tablets also available from Cox

Modified release
PoM **Surgam SA**® (Hoechst Marion Roussel)
Capsules, m/r, maroon/pink enclosing white pellets, tiaprofenic acid 300 mg. Net price 56-cap pack = £15.89. Label: 25
Dose: 2 capsules once daily; CHILD not recommended

ASPIRIN AND THE SALICYLATES

Aspirin was the traditional first choice anti-inflammatory analgesic but most physicians now prefer to start treatment with another NSAID which may be better tolerated and more convenient for the patient.

In regular high dosage aspirin has about the same anti-inflammatory effect as other NSAIDs. The required dose for active inflammatory joint disease is at least 3.6 g daily. There is little anti-inflammatory effect with less than 3 g daily. Gastro-intestinal side-effects such as nausea, dyspepsia, and gastro-intestinal bleeding may occur with any dosage of aspirin but anti-inflammatory doses are associated with a much higher incidence of side-effects. Anti-inflammatory doses of aspirin may also cause mild chronic salicylate intoxication (salicylism) characterised by dizziness, tinnitus, and deafness; these symptoms may be controlled by reducing the dosage.

ASPIRIN
(Acetylsalicylic Acid)

Indications: pain and inflammation in rheumatic disease and other musculoskeletal disorders (including juvenile arthritis); see also section 4.7.1; antiplatelet, see section 2.9

Cautions: asthma, allergic disease, uncontrolled hypertension, hepatic or renal impairment (avoid if severe), dehydration, pregnancy (particularly at term) (see also Appendix 4), elderly; G6PD-deficiency (see section 9.1.5); **interactions:** Appendix 1 (aspirin)

REYE'S SYNDROME. Owing to an association with Reye's syndrome the CSM has recommended that aspirin-containing preparations should no longer be given to children under the age of 12 years, unless specifically indicated, e.g. for juvenile arthritis (Still's disease). It is **important** to advise families that aspirin is not a suitable medicine for children with minor illnesses.

Contra-indications: gastro-intestinal ulceration; children under 12 years (except for juvenile arthritis) and breast-feeding (association with Reye's syndrome, see above); haemophilia and other bleeding disorders; not for treatment of gout

HYPERSENSITIVITY. Aspirin and other NSAIDs are **contra-indicated** in patients with a history of hypersensitivity to aspirin or any other NSAID—*which includes those* in whom attacks of *asthma, angioedema, urticaria or rhinitis* have been precipitated by aspirin or any other NSAID

Side-effects: common with anti-inflammatory doses; gastro-intestinal discomfort or nausea, ulceration with occult bleeding (but occasionally major haemorrhage); also other haemorrhage (e.g. subconjunctival); hearing disturbances such as tinnitus (leading rarely to deafness), vertigo, mental confusion, hypersensitivity reactions (angioedema, bronchospasm and rashes); increased bleeding time; rarely oedema, myocarditis, blood disorders, particularly thrombocytopenia; **overdosage:** see Emergency Treatment of Poisoning, p. 20

Dose: 0.3–1 g every 4 hours; max. in acute conditions 8 g daily; CHILD, juvenile arthritis, up to 80 mg/kg daily in 5–6 divided doses, increased in acute exacerbations to 130 mg/kg. Doses should be taken after food

Note. High doses of aspirin are very rarely required and are now given under specialist supervision only, and with plasma monitoring (especially in children)

Preparations
See section 4.7.1

BENORYLATE
(Benorilate)

(Aspirin-paracetamol ester; 2 g benorylate is equivalent to approximately 1.15 g aspirin and 970 mg paracetamol)

Indications: pain and inflammation in rheumatic disease and other musculoskeletal disorders; mild to moderate pain; pyrexia

Cautions; Contra-indications; Side-effects: see under Aspirin (above) and Paracetamol (section 4.7.1)

Dose: rheumatic disease, 4–8 g daily divided into 2–3 doses; max. 6 g daily for elderly; CHILD not recommended

Mild to moderate pain, 2 g twice daily preferably after food; CHILD not recommended

Benoral® (Sanofi Winthrop)
Tablets, benorylate 750 mg. Net price 100-tab pack = £8.67. Label: 21, 31
Granules, benorylate 2 g/sachet. Net price 60 sachet-pack = £13.77. Label: 13, 21, 31
Suspension, sugar-free, benorylate 2 g/5 mL. Net price 300 mL = £11.86. Label: 21, 31
Note. Generic versions of benorylate tablets and suspension are available from various manufacturers

10.1.2 Corticosteroids

10.1.2.1 SYSTEMIC CORTICOSTEROIDS

The general actions and uses of the corticosteroids are described in section 6.3. Treatment with corticosteroids in rheumatic diseases should be reserved for specific indications, e.g. when other anti-inflammatory drugs are unsuccessful.

In severe, possibly life-threatening, situations a high initial dose of corticosteroid is given to induce remission and the dose then gradually reduced to the lowest maintenance dose that will control the disease or, if possible, discontinued altogether. A major problem is that relapse may occur as dosage reduction is made, particularly if this is carried out too rapidly. The tendency is therefore to increase and maintain dosage and consequently the patient becomes dependent on corticosteroids. For this reason pulse doses of corticosteroids (e.g. methylprednisolone (as sodium succinate) up to 1 g intravenously on three consecutive days) is in current use to suppress highly active inflammatory disease while longer term and slower acting medication is being commenced.

Prednisolone is used for most purposes; it has the advantage over the more potent corticosteroids (see section 6.3.2) of permitting finer dosage adjustments. To minimise side-effects the maintenance dose of prednisolone should be kept as low as possible, usually 7.5 mg daily. Recent evidence has suggested that prednisolone 7.5 mg daily may substantially reduce the rate of joint destruction in moderate to severe *rheumatoid arthritis* of less than 2 years duration. The reduction in joint destruction must be distinguished from mere symptomatic improvement (which lasts only 6 to 12 months at this dose) and care should be taken to avoid increas-

---

ing the dosage which should not exceed the equivalent of prednisolone 7.5 mg daily. Current evidence supports maintenance of this anti-erosive dose for 2–4 years only, after which, treatment should be tapered off to avoid possible long-term adverse effects.

Polymyalgia rheumatica and *giant cell (temporal) arteritis* are always treated with corticosteroids. The usual initial dose of prednisolone in polymyalgia rheumatica is 10 to 15 mg daily and in giant cell arteritis 40 to 60 mg daily (the higher dose being used if visual symptoms occur). Treatment should be continued until remission of disease activity and doses then gradually reduced to a maintenance level of about 7.5–10 mg daily. Relapse is common if therapy is stopped within 3 years but most patients can discontinue treatment after approximately 3 to 6 years after which recurrences become rare.

Polyarteritis nodosa and *polymyositis* are usually treated with corticosteroids. An initial dose of 60 mg of prednisolone daily is often used and reduced to a maintenance dose of 10 to 15 mg daily.

Systemic lupus erythematosus is treated with corticosteroids when necessary using a similar dosage regimen to that for polyarteritis nodosa and polymyositis (above). Patients with pleurisy, pericarditis, or other systemic manifestations will respond to corticosteroids. It may then be possible to reduce the dosage; alternate-day treatment is sometimes adequate, and the drug may be gradually withdrawn. In some mild cases corticosteroid treatment may be stopped after a few months. Many mild cases of systemic lupus erythematosus do not require corticosteroid treatment. Alternative treatment with anti-inflammatory analgesics, and possibly chloroquine, should be considered.

Ankylosing spondylitis should not be treated with long-term corticosteroids; rarely, pulse doses may be needed and may be useful in extremely active disease that does not respond to conventional treatment.

10.1.2.2 LOCAL CORTICOSTEROID INJECTIONS

Corticosteroids are injected locally for an anti-inflammatory effect. In inflammatory conditions of the joints, particularly in rheumatoid arthritis, they are given by *intra-articular injection* to relieve pain, increase mobility, and reduce deformity in one or a few joints. Full aseptic precautions are essential; infected areas should be avoided. Occasionally an acute inflammatory reaction develops after an intra-articular or soft-tissue injection of a corticosteroid. This may be a reaction to the microcrystalline suspension of the corticosteroid used, but must be distinguished from sepsis introduced into the injection site. An almost insoluble compound such as triamcinolone hexacetonide has a long-acting (depot) effect and is preferred for intra-articular injection.

Smaller amounts of corticosteroids may also be injected directly into soft tissues for the relief of inflammation in conditions such as *tennis* or *golfer's elbow* or *compression neuropathies*. In *tendinitis*, injections should be made into the tendon sheath and not directly into the tendon (due to the absence of a true tendon sheath, the Achilles tendon should not be injected). A soluble preparation (e.g. containing betamethasone or dexamethasone sodium phosphate) is preferred for injection into the carpal tunnel.

Hydrocortisone acetate or one of the synthetic analogues such as triamcinolone hexacetonide is generally used for local injection. The risk of necrosis and muscle wasting may be slightly increased with triamcinolone; flushing has been reported with intra-articular corticosteroid injections. Charcot-like arthropathies have also been reported (particularly following repeated intra-articular injections).

Corticosteroid injections are also injected into soft tissues for the treatment of skin lesions (see section 13.4).

LOCAL CORTICOSTEROID INJECTIONS

Indications: local inflammation of joints and soft tissues (for details, see product literature)

Cautions; Contra-indications; Side-effects: see notes above (for details see also product literature)

Dose: see under preparations

Dose calculated as dexamethasone sodium phosphate

PoM **Dexamethasone** (Organon)

Injection, dexamethasone sodium phosphate 5 mg/mL (≡ dexamethasone 4 mg/mL ≡ dexamethasone phosphate 4.8 mg/mL). Net price 1-mL amp = 83p; 2-mL vial = £1.27

Dose: by intra-articular or intrasynovial injection (for details see product literature), 0.4–4 mg (calculated as dexamethasone sodium phosphate) according to size; where appropriate may be repeated at intervals of 3–21 days according to response

Dose calculated as dexamethasone phosphate

PoM **Decadron®** (MSD)

Injection, dexamethasone phosphate 4 mg/mL (≡ dexamethasone 3.33 mg/mL ≡ dexamethasone sodium phosphate 4.17 mg/mL). Net price 2-mL vial = £1.76

Dose: by intra-articular or intrasynovial injection (for details see product literature), 0.4–4 mg (calculated as dexamethasone phosphate) according to size (*soft-tissue infiltration* 2–6 mg); where appropriate may be repeated at intervals of 3–21 days; also for *intralesional injection*

Note. Injection containing Dexamethasone phosphate 4 mg/mL (as sodium phosphate) is also available from Faulding DBL

Hydrocortisone acetate

PoM **Hydrocortistab®** (Knoll)

Injection, (aqueous suspension), hydrocortisone acetate 25 mg/mL. Net price 1-mL amp = £1.05

Dose: by intra-articular or intrasynovial injection (for details see product literature), 5–50 mg according to size; where appropriate may be repeated at intervals of 21 days; not more than 3 joints should be treated on any one day; CHILD 5–30 mg (divided)

Methylprednisolone acetate
PoM **Depo-Medrone®** (Pharmacia & Upjohn)
Injection (aqueous suspension), methylprednisolone acetate 40 mg/mL. Net price 1-mL vial = £2.70; 2-mL vial = £4.87; 3-mL vial = £7.05

Dose: by intra-articular or intrasynovial injection (for details see product literature), 4–80 mg, according to size; where appropriate may be repeated at intervals of 7–35 days; also for *intralesional injection*

PoM **Depo-Medrone® with Lidocaine**
(Pharmacia & Upjohn)
Injection (aqueous suspension), methylprednisolone acetate 40 mg, lignocaine hydrochloride 10 mg/mL. Net price 1-mL vial = £2.70; 2-mL vial = £4.87

Dose: by intra-articular or intrasynovial injection (for details see product literature), 4–80 mg, according to size; where appropriate may be repeated at intervals of 7–35 days

Prednisolone acetate
PoM **Deltastab®** (Knoll)
Injection (aqueous suspension), prednisolone acetate 25 mg/mL. Net price 1-mL amp = £1.05

Dose: by intra-articular or intrasynovial injection (for details see product literature), 5–25 mg according to size; not more than 3 joints should be treated on any one day; where appropriate may be repeated when relapse occurs

For *intramuscular injection*, see section 6.3.2

Triamcinolone acetonide
PoM **Adcortyl® Intra-articular/Intradermal**
(Squibb)
Injection (aqueous suspension), triamcinolone acetonide 10 mg/mL. Net price 1-mL amp = £1.02; 5-mL vial = £4.14

Dose: by intra-articular injection or intrasynovial injection (for details see product literature), 2.5–15 mg according to size (for larger doses use *Kenalog®*); where appropriate may be repeated when relapse occurs

By intradermal injection, (for details see product literature): 2–3 mg; max. 5 mg at any one site (total max. 30 mg); where appropriate may be repeated at intervals of 1–2 weeks

CHILD under 6 years not recommended

PoM **Kenalog® Intra-articular/Intramuscular**
(Squibb)
Injection (aqueous suspension), triamcinolone acetonide 40 mg/mL. Net price 1-mL vial = £1.70

Dose: by intra-articular or intrasynovial injection (for details see product literature), 5–40 mg according to size; total max. 80 mg (for doses below 5 mg use *Adcortyl® Intra-articular/Intradermal*); where appropriate may be repeated when relapse occurs; CHILD under 6 years not recommended

For *intramuscular injection*, see section 6.3.2

Triamcinolone hexacetonide
PoM **Lederspan®** (Lederle)
Injection (aqueous suspension), triamcinolone hexacetonide 5 mg/mL. Net price 5-mL vial = £2.85

Dose: by intralesional injection (for details see product literature), up to 500 micrograms/square inch of affected skin

Injection (aqueous suspension), triamcinolone hexacetonide 20 mg/mL. Net price 1-mL vial = £2.48; 5 mL vial = £9.65

Dose: by intra-articular or intrasynovial injection (for details see product literature), 2–30 mg according to size; where appropriate may be repeated at intervals of 21–28 days; for *intralesional injection*, see above

10.1.3   Drugs which suppress the rheumatic disease process

Certain drugs such as gold, penicillamine, hydroxychloroquine, chloroquine, immunosuppressants, and sulphasalazine may suppress the disease process in *rheumatoid arthritis*, as may gold and immunosuppressants in *psoriatic arthritis*. They are sometimes known as second-line or disease-modifying antirheumatic drugs (DMARDs). Unlike NSAIDs they do not produce an immediate therapeutic effect but require 4 to 6 months of treatment for a full response. If one of these drugs does not lead to objective benefit within 6 months, it should be discontinued.

These drugs may improve not only the symptoms and signs of inflammatory joint disease but also extra-articular manifestations such as vasculitis. They reduce the erythrocyte sedimentation rate and sometimes the titre of rheumatoid factor. Some (e.g. cyclosporin) may retard erosive damage as judged radiologically.

These drugs are used in rheumatoid arthritis where treatment with NSAIDs alone provides inadequate control. Since, in the first few months, the course of rheumatoid arthritis is unpredictable, it is usual to delay treatment for about 6 months depending on the progress of the disease, but treatment should be initiated if severe symptoms persist.

Penicillamine and immunosuppressants are also sometimes used in rheumatoid arthritis where there are troublesome extra-articular features such as vasculitis, and in patients who are taking excessive doses of corticosteroids. Where the response is satisfactory there is often a striking reduction in requirements of both corticosteroids and other drugs. Gold and penicillamine are effective in *palindromic rheumatism* and chloroquine is sometimes used to treat *systemic* and *discoid lupus erythematosus*.

JUVENILE CHRONIC ARTHRITIS. Gold, penicillamine, and related drugs may also be used to treat *juvenile chronic arthritis* when indications are similar.

GOLD

Gold may be given by intramuscular injection as sodium aurothiomalate or by mouth as auranofin.

Sodium aurothiomalate must be given by deep intramuscular injection and the area gently massaged. A test dose of 10 mg must be given followed by doses of 50 mg at weekly intervals until there is definite evidence of remission. Benefit is not to be expected until about 300 to 500 mg has been given; if there is no remission after 1 g has been given it should be discontinued. In patients who do respond, the interval between injections is then gradually increased to 4 weeks and treatment is continued for up to 5 years after complete remission. If relapse occurs the dosage frequency may be immediately increased to 50 mg weekly and only once control has been obtained again should the dosage frequency be decreased; if no response is seen within 2 months, alternative treatment should be sought. It is important to avoid complete relapse since second courses of gold are not usually effective. Children may be given 1 mg/kg weekly to a maximum of 50 mg weekly, the intervals being gradually increased to 4 weeks according to response; an initial test dose is given corresponding to one-tenth to one-fifth of the calculated dose.

Auranofin is given by mouth. If there is no response after 9 months treatment should be discontinued.

Gold therapy should be discontinued in the presence of blood disorders or proteinuria (associated with immune complex nephritis) which is repeatedly above 300 mg/litre without other cause (such as urinary-tract infection). Urine tests and full blood counts (including total and differential white cell and platelet counts) must therefore be performed before each intramuscular injection; in the case of oral treatment the urine and blood tests should be carried out monthly. Rashes with pruritus often occur after 2 to 6 months of intramuscular treatment and may necessitate discontinuation of treatment; the most common side-effect of oral therapy, diarrhoea with or without nausea or abdominal pain, may respond to bulking agents (such as bran) or temporary reduction in dosage.

SODIUM AUROTHIOMALATE

Indications: active progressive rheumatoid arthritis, juvenile arthritis

Cautions: see notes above; patients should report pruritus, metallic taste, fever, sore throat or tongue, buccal ulceration, purpura, epistaxis, bleeding gums, bruising, menorrhagia, diarrhoea; renal and hepatic impairment, elderly, history of urticaria, eczema, colitis, drugs which cause blood disorders; annual chest X-ray; **interactions:** Appendix 1 (gold)

Contra-indications: severe renal and hepatic disease (see notes above); history of blood disorders or bone marrow aplasia, exfoliative dermatitis, systemic lupus erythematosus, necrotising enterocolitis, pulmonary fibrosis; pregnancy and breast-feeding (see Appendixes 4 and 5); porphyria (see section 9.8.2)

Side-effects: severe reactions (occasionally fatal) in up to 5% of patients; mouth ulcers, skin reactions (including, on prolonged parenteral treatment, irreversible pigmentation in sun-exposed areas), proteinuria, blood disorders (sometimes sudden and fatal); rarely colitis, peripheral neuritis, pulmonary fibrosis, hepatotoxicity with cholestatic jaundice, nephrotic syndrome, alopecia

Dose: by deep intramuscular injection, administered on expert advice, see notes above

PoM **Myocrisin**® (JHC)
Injection, sodium aurothiomalate 20 mg/mL, net price 0.5-mL (10-mg) amp = £3.31; 40 mg/mL, 0.5-mL (20-mg) amp = £4.82; 100 mg/mL, 0.5-mL (50-mg) amp = £9.80

AURANOFIN

Indications: active progressive rheumatoid arthritis when NSAIDs inadequate alone

Cautions; Contra-indications: see under Sodium Aurothiomalate; also caution in inflammatory bowel disease

BLOOD COUNTS. Withdraw if platelets fall below 100 000/mm³ or if signs and symptoms suggestive of thrombocytopenia occur, see also notes above

Side-effects: diarrhoea most common (reduced by bulking agents such as bran); see also under Sodium Aurothiomalate

Dose: administered on expert advice, 6 mg daily (initially in 2 divided doses then if tolerated as single dose), if response inadequate after 6 months, increase to 9 mg daily (in 3 divided doses), discontinue if no response after a further 3 months; CHILD not recommended

COUNSELLING. Warn patient to tell doctor immediately if sore throat, mouth ulcers, bruising, fever, malaise, rash, diarrhoea or non-specific illness develops

PoM **Ridaura**® (Yamanouchi)
Tablets, pale yellow, f/c, auranofin 3 mg. Net price 60-tab pack = £28.00. Label: 21, counselling, blood disorder symptoms (see above)

PENICILLAMINE

Penicillamine has a similar action to gold, and more patients are able to continue treatment than with gold but side-effects occur frequently. Penicillamine should be discontinued if there is no improvement within 1 year.

Patients should be warned not to expect improvement for at least 6 to 12 weeks after treatment is initiated. If remission has been sustained for 6 months, reduction of dosage by 125 to 250 mg every 12 weeks may be attempted.

Blood counts, including platelets, and urine examinations should be carried out every 1 or 2 weeks for the first 2 months then every 4 weeks to detect blood disorders and proteinuria (they should also be carried out in the week after any dose increase). A reduction in platelet count calls for discontinuation with subsequent re-introduction at a lower dosage and then, if possible, gradual increase. Proteinuria, associated with immune complex nephritis, occurs in up to 30% of patients, but may resolve despite continuation of treatment; treatment may be continued provided that renal function tests remain normal, oedema is absent, and the 24-hour urinary excretion of protein does not exceed 2 g.

Nausea may occur but is not usually a problem provided that penicillamine is taken before food or on retiring and that low initial doses are used and only gradually increased. Loss of taste may occur about 6 weeks after treatment is started but usually returns 6 weeks later irrespective of whether or not treatment is discontinued; mineral supplements are not recommended. Rashes are a common side-effect. Those which occur in the first few months of treatment disappear when the drug is stopped and treatment may then be re-introduced at a lower dose level and gradually increased. Late rashes are more resistant and often necessitate discontinuation of treatment.

Patients who are hypersensitive to penicillin may react rarely to penicillamine.

PENICILLAMINE

Indications: see notes above and under Dose

Cautions: see notes above; renal impairment (see Appendix 3), pregnancy (see Appendix 4); avoid concurrent gold, chloroquine, hydroxychloroquine, or immunosuppressive treatment; avoid oral iron within 2 hours of a dose; **interactions:** Appendix 1 (penicillamine)

BLOOD COUNTS and URINE TESTS. See notes above. Longer intervals may be adequate in cystinuria and Wilson's disease. Consider withdrawal if platelets fall below 120 000/mm³ or white blood cells below 2500/mm³ or if 3 successive falls within normal range (can restart at reduced dose when counts return to normal but permanent withdrawal necessary if recurrence of neutropenia or thrombocytopenia)

COUNSELLING. Warn patient to tell doctor immediately if sore throat, mouth ulcers, bruising, fever, malaise, rash, or non-specific illness develops.

Contra-indications: hypersensitivity (except in life-threatening situation when desensitisation may be attempted—see product literature); lupus erythematosus

Side-effects: (see also notes above) initially nausea, anorexia, fever, and skin reactions, taste loss (mineral supplements not recommended); blood disorders including thrombocytopenia, neutropenia, agranulocytosis and aplastic anaemia; proteinuria, rarely haematuria (withdraw immediately); haemolytic anaemia, nephrotic syndrome, lupus erythematosus-like syndrome, polymyositis (rarely with cardiac involvement), dermatomyositis, mouth ulcers, stomatitis, alopecia, brochiolitis and pneumonitis, myasthenia gravis-like syndrome, pemphigus, Goodpasture's syndrome, and Stevens-Johnson syndrome also reported; in non-rheumatoid conditions rheumatoid arthritis-like syndrome also reported; late rashes (reduce dose or withdraw treatment)

Dose: severe active rheumatoid arthritis, administered on expert advice, ADULT initially 125–250 mg daily before food for 1 month increased by similar amounts at intervals of not less than 4 weeks to usual maintenance of 500–750 mg daily in divided doses; max. 1.5 g daily; ELDERLY initially up to 125 mg daily before food for 1 month increased by similar amounts at intervals of not less than 4 weeks; max. 1 g daily; CHILD maintenance of 15–20 mg/kg daily (initial dose lower and increased at intervals of 4 weeks over a period of 3-6 months)

Wilson's disease, chronic active hepatitis, and cystinuria, see section 9.8

Copper and lead poisoning, see Emergency Treatment of Poisoning, p. 24

PoM **Penicillamine** (Non-proprietary)

Tablets, penicillamine 125 mg, net price 20 = £1.71; 250 mg, 20 = £3.16. Label: 6, 22, counselling, blood disorder symptoms (see above)

Available from APS, Cox, Hillcross, Norton

PoM **Distamine®** (Dista)

Tablets, all f/c, penicillamine 125 mg, net price 20 = £2.17; 250 mg, 20 = £3.74. Label: 6, 22, counselling, blood disorder symptoms (see above)

PoM **Pendramine®** (ASTA Medica)

Tablets, both scored, f/c, penicillamine 125 mg, net price 20 = £1.80; 250 mg, 20 = £3.27. Label: 6, 22, counselling, blood disorder symptoms (see above)

ANTIMALARIALS

Chloroquine and **hydroxychloroquine** have a similar action to, and are better tolerated than, gold or penicillamine; retinopathy is rare provided the doses given below are not exceeded.

These drugs should not be used for psoriatic arthritis. It should also be noted that it is difficult to distinguish ageing changes from drug-induced retinopathy in the elderly.

Mepacrine (see section 5.4.4) is sometimes used in discoid lupus erythematosus.

CHLOROQUINE

Indications: active rheumatoid arthritis (including juvenile arthritis), systemic and discoid lupus erythematosus; malaria, see section 5.4.1

Cautions: hepatic and renal impairment, pregnancy (but for malaria benefit outweighs risk, see Appendix 4, Antimalarials) porphyria, may exacerbate psoriasis, neurological disorders (especially history of epilepsy), may aggravate myasthenia gravis, severe gastro-intestinal disorders, G6PD deficiency (see section 9.1.5); elderly (see notes above); avoid concurrent hepatotoxic drugs—other **interactions:** Appendix 1 (chloroquine)

Advice of College of Ophthalmologists on long-term therapy.

1. Eye examination before long-term chloroquine or hydroxychloroquine to establish baseline;
2. Patient to stop taking and seek immediate advice from prescribing medical practitioner or general practitioner or ophthalmologist if any disturbance of vision noted;
3. Prescribing medical practitioner to be responsible for monitoring if considered necessary;
4. If monitoring considered necessary, *once monthly Amsler testing by patient* may detect premaculopathy (visual disturbance in absence of ophthalmoscopically visible macular changes—which is frequently reversible).

Ocular toxicity very unlikely with chloroquine phosphate not exceeding 4 mg/kg daily (= chloroquine base approx. 2.5 mg/kg daily) or hydroxychloroquine sulphate not exceeding 6.5 mg/kg daily.

To avoid excessive dosage in obese patients special care needed to *calculate on basis of lean body-weight.*

Side-effects: gastro-intestinal disturbances, headache; also convulsions, visual disturbances, irreversible retinal damage, corneal opacities, depigmentation or loss of hair, skin reactions (rashes, pruritus), ECG changes; rarely blood disorders (thrombocytopenia, agranulocytosis and aplastic anaemia), psychosis, erythema multiforme reported; **important:** very toxic in **overdosage**—immediate advice from poisons centres essential (see also p. 22)

Dose: administered on expert advice, chloroquine (base) 150 mg daily; max. 2.5 mg/kg daily, see recommendations above; CHILD, up to 3 mg/kg daily

Note. Chloroquine base 150 mg ≡ chloroquine sulphate 200 mg ≡ chloroquine phosphate 250 mg (approx.).

Preparations
See section 5.4.1

HYDROXYCHLOROQUINE SULPHATE

Indications: active rheumatoid arthritis (including juvenile arthritis), systemic and discoid lupus erythematosus

Cautions; Side-effects: see under Chloroquine and notes (above); avoid in breast-feeding

Dose: administered on expert advice, initially 400 mg daily in divided doses; maintenance 200–400 mg daily; max. 6.5 mg/kg daily (but not exceeding 400 mg daily), see recommendations under Chloroquine, above; CHILD, up to 6.5 mg/kg daily (max. 400 mg daily)

PoM **Plaquenil**® (Sanofi Winthrop)
Tablets, orange, s/c, hydroxychloroquine sulphate 200 mg. Net price 56-tab pack = £18.88. Label: 5, 21

IMMUNOSUPPRESSANTS

When used in *rheumatoid arthritis* **immunosuppressants** have a similar action to gold and are useful alternatives in cases that have failed to respond to gold, penicillamine, chloroquine, or hydroxychloroquine.

Azathioprine (see section 8.2.1) is usually chosen and is usually given in a dose of 1.5 to 2.5 mg/kg daily in divided doses. Blood counts are needed to detect possible neutropenia and/or thrombocytopenia which is usually resolved by reducing the dose. Nausea, vomiting, and diarrhoea may occur, usually starting early during the course of treatment, and may necessitate withdrawal of the drug; herpes zoster infection may also occur.

Methotrexate has also been shown to be effective. It is usually given in an initial dose of 2.5 mg by mouth once a week, increased slowly to a maximum of 15 mg once a week (occasionally 20 mg), subject to regular full blood counts (including differential white cell count and platelet count), renal and liver-function tests.

Cyclosporin (Ciclosporin) has also been shown to be effective and is now also licensed for severe active rheumatoid arthritis when conventional therapy is inappropriate or ineffective. There is some evidence that cyclosporin may retard the rate of erosive progression and improve symptom control in patients only partially responsive to methotrexate.

Cyclophosphamide (see section 8.1.1) may be used at a dose of 1 to 1.5 mg/kg daily by mouth for rheumatoid arthritis with severe systemic manifestations [unlicensed indication]; it is toxic and regular blood counts (including platelet count) should be carried out. Cyclophosphamide may also be given intravenously in a dose of 0.5 to 1 g (with prophylactic mesna) for *severe systemic rheumatoid arthritis* and for other connective tissue diseases (especially with active vasculitis), repeated initially at fortnightly then at monthly intervals (according to clinical response and haematological monitoring).

Immunosuppressants are also used in the management of severe cases of *systemic lupus erythematosus* and other connective tissue disorders. They are often given in conjunction with corticosteroids for patients with severe or progressive renal disease though the evidence for their benefit is doubtful. They may be used in cases of *polymyositis* which are resistant to corticosteroids. They are used for their corticosteroid-sparing effect in patients whose corticosteroid requirements are excessive. **Azathioprine** is usually used.

Azathioprine and methotrexate are used in the treatment of *psoriatic arthropathy* [unlicensed indication] for severe or progressive cases which are not controlled with anti-inflammatory drugs.

AZATHIOPRINE

Indications: see notes above; transplantation rejection, see section 8.2.1

Cautions; Contra-indications; Side-effects: see under Azathioprine, section 8.2.1

Dose: by mouth, initially, rarely more than 3 mg/kg daily, reduced according to response; maintenance 1–3 mg/kg daily; consider withdrawal if no improvement within 3 months

Preparations
See section 8.2.1

CYCLOSPORIN
(Ciclosporin)

Indications: severe active rheumatoid arthritis when conventional therapy inappropriate or ineffective; graft-versus-host disease, see section 8.2.2; atopic dermatitis and psoriasis, see section 13.5.2.

Cautions; Side-effects: see section 8.2.2
ADDITIONAL CAUTIONS IN RHEUMATOID ARTHRITIS. **Contra-indicated** in abnormal renal function, uncontrolled hypertension (see also below), uncontrolled infections, and malignancy. Measure serum creatinine at least twice before treatment and monitor every 2 weeks for first 3 months, then every 4 weeks (or more frequently if dose increased or concomitant NSAIDs introduced or increased (see also *interactions:* Appendix 1 (cyclosporin)), reducing dose if serum creatinine increases more than 30% above baseline in more than 1 measurement; if above 50%, reducing dose by 50% (even if within normal range) and discontinuing if reduction not successful within 1 month; monitor blood pressure (discontinue if hypertension develops that cannot be controlled by antihypertensive therapy); monitor hepatic function if concomitant NSAIDs given.

Dose: ADULT over 18 years *by mouth*, administered in accordance with expert advice initially, 2.5 mg/kg daily in 2 divided doses, if necessary increased gradually after 6 weeks to max. 4 mg/kg daily (discontinue if response insufficient after 3 months); dose adjusted according to response for maintenance and treatment reviewed after 6 months (continue only if benefits outweigh risks); CHILD and under 18 years, not recommended

IMPORTANT. For preparations and counselling and for advice on conversion between the preparations, see section 8.2.2

Preparations
See section 8.2.2

METHOTREXATE
Indications: severe active rheumatoid arthritis unresponsive to conventional therapy; malignant disease, see section 8.1.3; psoriasis, see section 13.5.2

Cautions; Contra-indications; Side-effects: see Methotrexate, section 13.5.2

PULMONARY TOXICITY. Pulmonary toxicity may be a special problem in rheumatoid arthritis (patient to contact doctor immediately if dyspnoea or cough). For other special warnings, including CSM advice and counselling advice relating to interaction with aspirin and NSAIDs, see Methotrexate, section 13.5.2.

Dose: by mouth, 7.5 mg once weekly (as a single dose or divided into 3 doses of 2.5 mg given at intervals of 12 hours), adjusted according to response; max. total weekly dose 20 mg

Preparations
See section 8.1.3

SULPHASALAZINE

Sulphasalazine (Sulfasalazine) has a beneficial effect in suppressing the inflammatory activity of rheumatoid arthritis. Side-effects include rashes, gastro-intestinal intolerance and, especially in patients with rheumatoid arthritis, occasional leucopenia, neutropenia, and thrombocytopenia. These haematological abnormalities occur usually in the first 3 to 6 months of treatment and are reversible on cessation of treatment. Close monitoring of full blood counts (including differential white cell count and platelet count) is necessary initially, and at monthly intervals during the first 3 months (liver function tests also being performed at monthly intervals for the first 3 months). Although the manufacturer recommends renal function tests, evidence of practical value is unsatisfactory.

SULPHASALAZINE
(Sulfasalazine)

Indications: active rheumatoid arthritis; ulcerative colitis, see section 1.5 and notes above

Cautions; Contra-indications; Side-effects: see section 1.5 and notes above

The CSM has recommended that patients receiving sulphasalazine should be advised to report any unexplained bleeding, bruising, purpura, sore throat, fever or malaise that occurs during treatment. A blood count should be performed and the drug stopped immediately if there is suspicion of a blood dyscrasia.

Dose: by mouth, administered on expert advice, as enteric-coated tablets, initially 500 mg daily, increased by 500 mg at intervals of 1 week to a max. of 2–3 g daily in divided doses

PoM **Sulphasalazine** (Non-proprietary)
Tablets, e/c, sulphasalazine 500 mg. Net price 112-tab pack = £12.11. Label: 5, 14, 25, counselling, blood disorder symptoms (see CSM recommendation above), contact lenses may be stained
Available from Cox (*Sulazine EC*®)

PoM **Salazopyrin EN-Tabs**® (Pharmacia & Upjohn)
Tablets, e/c, yellow, f/c, sulphasalazine 500 mg. Net price 112-tab pack = £12.11. Label: 5, 14, 21, 25, counselling, blood disorder symptoms (see CSM recommendation above), contact lenses may be stained

10.1.4   Drugs for treatment of gout

It is important to distinguish drugs used for the treatment of acute attacks of gout from those used in the long-term control of the disease. The latter exacerbate and prolong the acute manifestations if started during an attack.

ACUTE ATTACKS

Acute attacks of gout are usually treated with high doses of **NSAIDs** such as diclofenac, indomethacin, ketoprofen, naproxen, piroxicam, or sulindac (section 10.1.1). The use of azapropazone should be restricted to patients in whom less toxic drugs have been ineffective (**important:** see CSM restrictions on p. 429). Colchicine is an alternative. Aspirin is *not* indicated in gout. Allopurinol and uricosurics are not effective in treating an acute attack and may prolong it indefinitely if started during the acute episode.

Colchicine is probably as effective as NSAIDs. Its use is limited by the development of toxicity at higher doses, but it is of value in patients with heart failure since, unlike NSAIDs, it does not induce fluid retention; moreover it can be given to patients receiving anticoagulants.

COLCHICINE
Indications: acute gout, short-term prophylaxis during initial therapy with allopurinol and uricosuric drugs; familial Mediterranean fever (recurrent polyserositis)

Cautions: elderly, gastro-intestinal disease, cardiac, hepatic and renal impairment; **interactions:** Appendix 1 (colchicine)

Contra-indications: pregnancy and breast-feeding

Side-effects: most common are nausea, vomiting, and abdominal pain; excessive doses may also cause profuse diarrhoea, gastro-intestinal haemorrhage, rashes, renal and hepatic damage. Rarely peripheral neuritis, myopathy, alopecia, and with prolonged treatment blood disorders

---

Dose: treatment of gout, 1 mg initially, followed by 500 micrograms every 2–3 hours until relief of pain is obtained or vomiting or diarrhoea occurs, or until a total dose of 10 mg has been reached. The course should not be repeated within 3 days

Prevention of gout attacks during initial treatment with allopurinol or uricosuric drugs, 500 micrograms 2–3 times daily

Prophylaxis of familial Mediterranean fever, 0.5–2 mg daily

PoM **Colchicine** (Non-proprietary)
Tablets, colchicine 500 micrograms, net price 20 = £3.03
Available from CP, Hillcross, Kent, Norton

INTERVAL TREATMENT

For long-term ('interval') control of gout the formation of uric acid from purines may be reduced with the **xanthine-oxidase inhibitor** allopurinol, or the **uricosuric drugs** probenecid or sulphinpyrazone may be used to increase the excretion of uric acid in the urine. Treatment should be continued indefinitely to prevent further attacks of gout by correcting the hyperuricaemia. These drugs should never be started during an acute attack. The initiation of treatment may precipitate an acute attack therefore colchicine or an anti-inflammatory analgesic should be used as a prophylactic and continued for at least one month after the hyperuricaemia has been corrected (usually about 3 months of prophylaxis). However, if an acute attack develops during treatment, then the treatment should continue at the same dosage and the acute attack treated in its own right.

Allopurinol is a well tolerated drug which is widely used. It is especially useful in patients with renal impairment or urate stones where uricosuric drugs cannot be used; it is *not* indicated for the treatment of asymptomatic hyperuricaemia. It is usually given once daily, since the active metabolite of allopurinol has a long half-life, but doses over 300 mg daily should be divided. It may occasionally cause rashes.

Probenecid and **sulphinpyrazone** (sulfinpyrazone) can be used instead of allopurinol, or in conjunction with it in cases that are resistant to treatment.

Aspirin and salicylates antagonise the uricosuric drugs; they do not antagonise allopurinol but are nevertheless *not* indicated in gout.

Crystallisation of urate in the urine may occur with the uricosuric drugs and it is important to ensure an adequate urine output especially in the first few weeks of treatment. As an additional precaution the urine may be rendered alkaline.

ALLOPURINOL

Indications: prophylaxis of gout and of uric acid and calcium oxalate renal stones

Cautions: administer prophylactic colchicine or NSAID (*not* aspirin or salicylates) until at least 1 month after hyperuricaemia corrected; ensure adequate fluid intake (2 litres/day); hepatic and renal impairment (see Appendix 3); in neoplastic conditions treatment with allopurinol (if required) should be commenced before cytotoxic drugs are given; pregnancy and breast-feeding; **interactions:** Appendix 1 (allopurinol)

Contra-indications: not a treatment for acute gout but continue if attack develops when already receiving allopurinol, and treat attack separately (see notes above)

Side-effects: rashes (**withdraw** therapy; if rash mild re-introduce cautiously but **discontinue** immediately if recurrence—hypersensitivity reactions occur rarely and include exfoliation, fever, lymphadenopathy, arthralgia, and eosinophilia resembling Stevens-Johnson or Lyell's syndrome, vasculitis, hepatitis, interstitial nephritis and very rarely epilepsy); gastro-intestinal disorders; rarely malaise, headache, vertigo, drowsiness, visual and taste disturbances, hypertension, symptomless xanthine deposits in muscle, alopecia, hepatotoxicity, paraesthesia and neuropathy, blood disorders (including leucopenia, thrombocytopenia, haemoytic anaemia and aplastic anaemia)

Dose: initially 100–300 mg daily as a single dose, preferably after food, then adjusted according to plasma or urinary uric acid concentration; usual maintenance dose in mild conditions 100–200 mg daily, in moderately severe conditions 300–600 mg daily, in severe conditions 700–900 mg daily; doses over 300 mg daily given in divided doses; CHILD (in neoplastic conditions, enzyme disorders) 10–20 mg/kg daily *or* 100–400 mg daily

PoM **Allopurinol** (Non-proprietary)
Tablets, allopurinol 100 mg, net price 20 = 24p; 300 mg, 20 = 59p. Label: 8, 21, 27
Available from APS, Ashbourne (Xanthomax®), Berk (Caplenal®), Cox, CP, DDSA (Cosuric®), Kent, Norton, Rima (Rimapurinol®)

PoM **Zyloric®** (GlaxoWellcome)
Tablets, allopurinol 100 mg, net price 100-tab pack = £10.96; 300 mg, 28-tab pack = £7.86. Label: 8, 21, 27

PROBENECID

Indications: gout prophylaxis (to correct hyperuricaemia); reduction of tubular excretion of penicillins and certain cephalosporins, see section 5.1

Cautions: see notes above; during initial gout therapy administer prophylactic colchicine or NSAID (*not* aspirin or salicylates), ensure adequate fluid intake (about 2 litres daily) and render urine alkaline if uric acid overload is high; peptic ulceration, renal impairment (avoid if severe); transient false-positive Benedict's test; G6PD-deficiency (see section 9.1.5); **interactions:** Appendix 1 (probenecid)

Contra-indications: history of blood disorders, nephrolithiasis, porphyria (see section 9.8.2), acute gout attack; avoid aspirin and salicylates

Side-effects: gastro-intestinal disturbances, urinary frequency, headache, flushing, dizziness, alopecia, anaemia, haemolytic anaemia, sore

---

gums; hypersensitivity reactions including anaphylaxis, dermatitis, pruritus, urticaria, fever and Stevens-Johnson syndrome; rarely nephrotic syndrome, hepatic necrosis, leucopenia, aplastic anaemia; toxic epidermal necrolysis reported with concurrent colchicine

Dose: uricosuric therapy, initially 250 mg twice daily after food, increased after a week to 500 mg twice daily then up to 2 g daily in 2–4 divided doses according to plasma-uric acid concentration and reduced for maintenance

PoM **Benemid**® (MSD)
Tablets, scored, probenecid 500 mg. Net price 20 = 66p. Label: 12, 21, 27

SULPHINPYRAZONE
(Sulfinpyrazone)
Indications: gout prophylaxis, hyperuricaemia
Cautions; Contra-indications: see under Probenecid; regular blood counts advisable; avoid in hypersensitivity to NSAIDs; cardiac disease (may cause salt and water retention); **interactions:** Appendix 1 (sulphinpyrazone)
Side-effects: gastro-intestinal disturbances, occasionally allergic skin reactions, salt and water retention; rarely blood disorders, gastro-intestinal ulceration and bleeding, acute renal failure, raised liver enzymes, jaundice and hepatitis
Dose: initially 100–200 mg daily with food (or milk) increasing over 2–3 weeks to 600 mg daily (rarely 800 mg daily), continued until serum uric acid concentration normal then reduced for maintenance (maintenance dose may be as low as 200 mg daily)

PoM **Anturan**® (Novartis)
Tablets, both yellow, s/c, sulphinpyrazone 100 mg, net price 20 = 94p; 200 mg, 84-tab pack = £7.82. Label: 12, 21

10.2 Drugs used in neuromuscular disorders

10.2.1 Drugs which enhance neuromuscular transmission

Anticholinesterases are used as first-line treatment in *myasthenia gravis.*

Corticosteroids are only given concomitantly if anticholinesterase treatment is failing.

Plasmapheresis may produce temporary remission in otherwise unresponsive patients.

ANTICHOLINESTERASES

Anticholinesterase drugs enhance neuromuscular transmission in voluntary and involuntary muscle in myasthenia gravis. They prolong the action of acetylcholine by inhibiting the action of the enzyme acetylcholinesterase. Excessive dosage of these drugs may impair neuromuscular transmission and precipitate 'cholinergic crises' by causing a depolarising block. This may be difficult to distinguish from a worsening myasthenic state.

Muscarinic side-effects of anticholinesterases include increased sweating, salivary, and gastric secretion, also increased gastro-intestinal and uterine motility, and bradycardia. These parasympathomimetic effects are antagonised by atropine.

Edrophonium has a very brief action and is therefore used mainly for the diagnosis of myasthenia gravis. A single test-dose usually causes substantial improvement in muscle power (lasting about 5 minutes) in patients with the disease (if respiration already impaired, *only* in conjunction with someone skilled at intubation).

Edrophonium can also be used to determine whether a patient with myasthenia is receiving inadequate or excessive treatment with cholinergic drugs. If treatment is excessive an injection of edrophonium will either have no effect or will intensify symptoms (if respiration already impaired, *only* in conjunction with someone skilled at intubation). Conversely, transient improvement may be seen if the patient is being inadequately treated. The test is best performed just before the next dose of anticholinesterase.

Neostigmine produces a therapeutic effect for up to 4 hours. Its pronounced muscarinic action is a disadvantage, and simultaneous administration of an antimuscarinic drug such as atropine or propantheline may be required to prevent colic, excessive salivation, or diarrhoea. In severe disease neostigmine may be given every 2 hours. The maximum that most patients can tolerate is 180 mg daily.

Pyridostigmine is less powerful and slower in action than neostigmine but it has a longer duration of action. It is preferable to neostigmine because of its smoother action and the need for less frequent dosage. It is particularly preferred in patients whose muscles are weak on wakening. It has a comparatively mild gastro-intestinal effect but an antimuscarinic drug may still be required. It is inadvisable to exceed a daily dose of 720 mg.

Distigmine has the longest action but the danger of a 'cholinergic crisis' caused by accumulation of the drug is greater than with shorter-acting drugs.

Neostigmine and edrophonium are also used to reverse the actions of the non-depolarising muscle relaxants (see section 15.1.6).

NEOSTIGMINE
Indications: myasthenia gravis; other indications, see section 15.1.6
Cautions: asthma (*extreme* caution), bradycardia, recent myocardial infarction, epilepsy, hypotension, parkinsonism, vagotonia, peptic ulceration, renal impairment, pregnancy and breastfeeding. Atropine or other antidote to muscarinic effects may be necessary (particularly when neostigmine is given by injection), but it should not be given routinely as it may mask signs of overdosage; **interactions:** Appendix 1 (parasympathomimetics)
Contra-indications: intestinal or urinary obstruction
Side-effects: nausea, vomiting, increased salivation, diarrhoea, abdominal cramps (more marked

with higher doses). Signs of overdosage are increased gastro-intestinal discomfort, bronchial secretions, and sweating, involuntary defaecation and micturition, miosis, nystagmus, bradycardia, hypotension, agitation, excessive dreaming, and weakness eventually leading to fasciculation and paralysis

Dose: by *mouth*, neostigmine bromide 15–30 mg at suitable intervals throughout day, total daily dose 75–300 mg (but see also notes above); NEONATE 1–5 mg every 4 hours, half an hour before feeds; CHILD up to 6 years initially 7.5 mg, 6–12 years initially 15 mg, usual total daily dose 15–90 mg

By subcutaneous or intramuscular injection, neostigmine methylsulphate 1–2.5 mg at suitable intervals throughout day (usual total daily dose 5–20 mg); NEONATE 50–250 micrograms every 4 hours half an hour before feeds; CHILD 200–500 micrograms as required

PoM **Neostigmine** (Non-proprietary)
Tablets, scored, neostigmine bromide 15 mg. Net price 20 = £2.40
Available from Cambridge
Injection, neostigmine methylsulphate 2.5 mg/mL. Net price 1-mL amp = 28p
Available from Antigen, Phoenix

DISTIGMINE BROMIDE

Indications: myasthenia gravis; urinary retention and other indications, see section 7.4.1

Cautions; Contra-indications; Side-effects: see under Neostigmine

Dose: initially 5 mg daily half an hour before breakfast, increased at intervals of 3–4 days if necessary to a max. of 20 mg daily; CHILD up to 10 mg daily according to age

Preparations
See section 7.4.1

EDROPHONIUM CHLORIDE

Indications: see under Dose and notes above; surgery, see section 15.1.6

Cautions; Contra-indications; Side-effects: see under Neostigmine; have resuscitation facilities; *extreme* caution in respiratory distress (see notes above) and in asthma

Note. Severe cholinergic reactions can be counteracted by injection of atropine sulphate (which should always be available)

Dose: diagnosis of myasthenia gravis, *by intravenous injection*, 2 mg followed after 30 seconds (if no adverse reaction has occurred) by 8 mg; in adults without suitable veins, *by intramuscular injection*, 10 mg

Detection of overdosage or underdosage of cholinergic drugs, *by intravenous injection*, 2 mg (best before next dose of anticholinesterase, see notes above)

CHILD *by intravenous injection*, 20 micrograms/kg followed after 30 seconds (if no adverse reaction has occurred) by 80 micrograms/kg

PoM **Edrophonium** (Non-proprietary)
Injection, edrophonium chloride 10 mg/mL. Net price 1-mL amp = £3.31
Available from Cambridge

PYRIDOSTIGMINE BROMIDE

Indications: myasthenia gravis

Cautions; Contra-indications; Side-effects: see under Neostigmine; weaker muscarinic action

Dose: by *mouth*, 30–120 mg at suitable intervals throughout day, total daily dose 0.3–1.2 g (but see also notes above); NEONATE 5–10 mg every 4 hours, ½–1 hour before feeds; CHILD up to 6 years initially 30 mg, 6–12 years initially 60 mg, usual total daily dose 30–360 mg

PoM **Mestinon**® (Roche)
Tablets, scored, pyridostigmine bromide 60 mg. Net price 20 = £1.11

IMMUNOSUPPRESSANT THERAPY

Corticosteroids (see section 6.3) are established as treatment for myasthenia gravis where *thymectomy* is inadvisable or to reduce the risk of surgery beforehand. The initial dose may be high (up to 100 mg **prednisolone** daily) but most advise starting with a smaller dose (20 mg prednisolone daily) and gradually increasing it. There is grave risk of exacerbation of the myasthenia during the initial stages of therapy, particularly in the first 2-3 weeks, therefore inpatient supervision is essential. Improvement usually begins after about 2 weeks on the high-dose regimen. In some patients a prolonged remission may be induced, but often patients need a maintenance dose of 10–40 mg of prednisolone daily; alternate-day therapy is popular. Patients who need a corticosteroid may benefit from the addition of **azathioprine** (see section 8.2.1) in a dose of 2 mg/kg daily which may allow a reduction in corticosteroid dosage.

10.2.2   Skeletal muscle relaxants

Drugs described below are used for the relief of chronic muscle spasm or spasticity; they are not indicated for spasm associated with minor injuries. They act principally on the central nervous system with the exception of dantrolene which has a peripheral site of action. They differ in action from the muscle relaxants used in anaesthesia (see section 15.1.5) which block transmission at the neuro-muscular junction.

The underlying cause of spasticity should be treated and any aggravating factors (e.g. pressure sores, infection) remedied. Skeletal muscle relaxants are effective in most forms of spasticity except the rare alpha variety. The major disadvantage of treatment with these drugs is that reduction in muscle tone can cause a loss of splinting action of the spastic leg and trunk muscles and sometimes lead to an increase in disability.

Dantrolene acts directly on skeletal muscle and produces fewer central adverse effects making it a

---

drug of choice. The dose should be increased slowly.

Baclofen inhibits transmission at spinal level and also depresses the central nervous system. The dose should be increased slowly to avoid the major side-effects of sedation and hypotonia (other adverse events are uncommon).

Diazepam may also be used. Sedation and, occasionally, extensor hypotonus are disadvantages. Other benzodiazepines also have muscle-relaxant properties. Muscle-relaxant doses of benzodiazepines are similar to anxiolytic doses (see section 4.1.2).

Tizanidine is a newly introduced alpha$_2$-adrenoceptor agonist indicated for spasticity associated with multiple sclerosis or spinal cord injury.

BACLOFEN

Indications: chronic severe spasticity resulting from disorders such as multiple sclerosis or traumatic partial section of spinal cord

Cautions: psychiatric illness, cerebrovascular disease, elderly; diabetes mellitus; respiratory, hepatic or renal impairment, epilepsy ; history of peptic ulcer; hypertonic bladder sphincter; pregnancy (see Appendix 4); avoid abrupt withdrawal (may precipitate autonomic dysreflexia, see also CSM advice below); porphyria (see section 9.8.2); **interactions:** Appendix 1 (muscle relaxants)

WITHDRAWAL. The CSM has advised that serious side-effects can occur with abrupt withdrawal; to minimise risk, therapy should be discontinued by gradual dose reduction over at least 1–2 weeks (longer if symptoms occur)

DRIVING. Drowsiness may affect performance of skilled tasks (e.g. driving); effects of alcohol enhanced

Contra-indications: peptic ulceration

Side-effects: frequently sedation, drowsiness, nausea; occasionally lightheadedness, lassitude, confusion, dizziness, ataxia, hallucinations, headache, euphoria, insomnia, depression, tremor, nystagmus, paraesthesias, convulsions, muscular pain and weakness, respiratory or cardiovascular depression, hypotension, dry mouth, gastro-intestinal and urinary disturbances; rarely visual disorders, taste alterations, increased sweating, rash, blood sugar changes, altered liver function tests, and paradoxical increase in spasticity

Dose: by mouth, 5 mg 3 times daily, preferably after food, gradually increased; max. 100 mg daily; CHILD 0.75–2 mg/kg daily (over 10 years, max. 2.5 mg/kg daily) *or* 2.5 mg 4 times daily increased gradually according to age to maintenance: 1–2 years 10–20 mg daily, 2–6 years 20–30 mg daily, 6–10 years 30–60 mg daily

By intrathecal injection, see preparation below

PoM **Baclofen** (Non-proprietary)

Tablets, baclofen 10 mg. Net price 20 = £1.08. Label: 2, 8

Available from APS, Ashbourne (Baclospas®), Berk (Balgifen®), Cox, Lagap, Norton

PoM **Lioresal®** (Novartis)

Tablets, scored, baclofen 10 mg. Net price 84-tab pack = £9.03. Label: 2, 8

Additives: include gluten

Liquid, sugar-free, baclofen 5 mg/5 mL. Net price 300 mL = £7.46. Label: 2, 8

By intrathecal injection

PoM **Lioresal®**

Intrathecal injection, baclofen, 50 micrograms/mL, net price 1-mL amp (for test dose) = £2.50; 500 micrograms/mL, 20-mL amp (for use with implantable pump) = £55.55; 2 mg/mL, 5-mL amp (for use with implantable pump) = £55.55

Important: consult product literature for full instructions on dose testing and titration–it is important that patients are monitored closely in an appropriately equipped and staffed environment during screening and immediately following pump implantation, and that resuscitation equipment is available for immediate use

Dose: by intrathecal injection, specialist use only, for ADULT over 18 years with severe chronic spasticity unresponsive to oral antispastic drugs (or where side-effects of oral therapy unacceptable), initial *test dose* (with resuscitation equipment to hand, see also above) 25–50 micrograms over at least 1 minute via catheter or lumbar puncture, increased in steps to max. 100 micrograms to determine appropriate dose *then dose-titration phase,* most often using infusion pump (implanted into chest wall or abdominal wall tissues in experienced centres only) to establish *appropriate maintenance dose* (ranging from 10 to 1200 micrograms daily; usual range 300–800 micrograms daily) retaining some spasticity to avoid sensation of paralysis; CHILD under 18 years, not recommended

DANTROLENE SODIUM

Indications: chronic severe spasticity of voluntary muscle

Cautions: impaired cardiac and pulmonary function; test liver function before and at intervals during therapy; therapeutic effect may take a few weeks to develop but if treatment is ineffective it should be discontinued after 4–6 weeks. Avoid when spasticity is useful, for example, locomotion; **interactions:** Appendix 1 (muscle relaxants).

DRIVING. Drowsiness may affect performance of skilled tasks (e.g. driving); effects of alcohol enhanced

Contra-indications: hepatic impairment (may cause severe liver damage); acute muscle spasm

Side-effects: transient drowsiness, dizziness, weakness, malaise, fatigue, diarrhoea (withdraw if severe, discontinue treatment if recurs on re-introduction), anorexia, nausea, headache, rash; less frequently constipation, dysphagia, speech and visual disturbances, confusion, nervousness, insomnia, depression, seizures, chills, fever, increased urinary frequency; rarely, tachycardia, erratic blood pressure, dyspnoea, haematuria, possible crystalluria, urinary incontinence or retention, pleural effusion, pericarditis, dose-related hepatotoxicity (occasionally fatal) may be more common in women over 30 especially those taking oestrogens

Dose: initially 25 mg daily, may be increased at weekly intervals to max. of 100 mg 4 times daily; usual dose 75 mg 3 times daily; CHILD not recommended

---

Cautionary label wordings, see inside back cover

PoM **Dantrium®** (Procter & Gamble Pharm.)

Capsules, both orange/brown, dantrolene sodium 25 mg, net price 20 = £3.42; 100 mg, 20 = £11.97. Label: 2

Injection—see section 15.1.8

DIAZEPAM

Indications: muscle spasm of varied aetiology, including tetanus; other indications, see sections 4.1.2, 4.8, 15.1.4.1

Cautions; Contra-indications; Side-effects: see section 4.1.2; also hypotonia; special precautions for intravenous injection (see section 4.8.2)

Dose: by mouth, 2–15 mg daily in divided doses, increased if necessary in spastic conditions to 60 mg daily according to response

Cerebral spasticity in selected cases, CHILD 2–40 mg daily in divided doses

By intramuscular or by slow intravenous injection (into a large vein at a rate of not more than 5 mg/minute), in acute muscle spasm, 10 mg repeated if necessary after 4 hours

Note. Only use intramuscular route when oral and intravenous routes not possible; special precautions for intravenous injection see section 4.8.2

Tetanus, ADULT and CHILD, *by intravenous injection*, 100–300 micrograms/kg repeated every 1–4 hours; *by intravenous infusion* (*or by nasoduodenal tube*), 3–10 mg/kg over 24 hours, adjusted according to response

Preparations

See section 4.1.2

TIZANIDINE

Indications: spasticity associated with multiple sclerosis or spinal cord injury or disease

Cautions: elderly, renal impairment (Appendix 3), pregnancy and breast-feeding, monitor liver function monthly for first 4 months and in those who develop unexplained nausea, anorexia or fatigue; **interactions:** Appendix 1 (tizanidine)

DRIVING Drowsiness may affect performance of skilled tasks (e.g. driving); effects of alcohol enhanced

Contra-indications: severe hepatic impairment

Side-effects: drowsiness, fatigue, dizziness, dry mouth, nausea, gastro-intestinal disturbances, hypotension; also reported, bradycardia, insomnia, hallucinations and altered liver enzymes (discontinue if persistently raised—consult product literature); rarely acute hepatitis

Dose: initially 2 mg daily as a single dose increased according to response at intervals of at least 3–4 days in steps of 2 mg daily (and given in divided doses) usually up to 24 mg daily in 3–4 divided doses; max. 36 mg daily; CHILD not recommended

▼ PoM **Zanaflex®** (Athena)

Tablets, scored, tizanidine (as hydrochloride) 2 mg, net price 120-tab pack = £71.76; 4 mg, 120-tab pack = £89.70. Label: 2

OTHER MUSCLE RELAXANTS

The clinical efficacy of carisoprodol, meprobamate (section 4.1.2), and methocarbamol as muscle relaxants is **not** well established although they have been included in compound analgesic preparations.

CARISOPRODOL

Indications: short-term symptomatic relief of muscle spasm (but see notes above)

Cautions; Contra-indications; Side-effects: see under Meprobamate, section 4.1.2. Drowsiness is common; avoid in porphyria (see section 9.8.2)

Dose: 350 mg 3 times daily; ELDERLY half adult dose or less

PoM **Carisoma®** (Pharmax)

Tablets, carisoprodol 125 mg, net price 100 = £7.43; 350 mg, 100 = £8.32. Label: 2

METHOCARBAMOL

Indications: short-term symptomatic relief of muscle spasm (but see notes above)

Cautions: hepatic and renal impairment (avoid injection in renal impairment); **interactions:** Appendix 1 (as for Anxiolytics and Hypnotics)

DRIVING. Drowsiness may affect performance of skilled tasks (e.g. driving); effects of alcohol enhanced

Contra-indications: coma or pre-coma, brain damage, epilepsy, myasthenia gravis

Side-effects: lassitude, light-headedness, dizziness, restlessness, anxiety, confusion, drowsiness, nausea, allergic rash or angioedema, convulsions

Dose: by mouth, 1.5 g 4 times daily (elderly 750 mg or less); may be reduced to 750 mg 3 times daily

By slow intravenous injection or by infusion, 1–3 g (max. rate 300 mg/min.); max. dose 3 g (elderly, 1.5 g) daily for 3 days

PoM **Robaxin®** (Shire)

750 Tablets, scored, methocarbamol 750 mg. Net price 20 = £2.30. Label: 2

Injection, methocarbamol 100 mg/mL in aqueous macrogol '300'. Net price 10-mL amp = £2.33

NOCTURNAL LEG CRAMPS

Quinine salts (section 5.4.1) 200 mg to 300 mg at bedtime are effective in reducing the frequency of nocturnal leg cramps by about 25% in ambulatory patients. It may take up to 4 weeks for improvement to become apparent and it is then given on a continuous basis if there is benefit. Patients should be monitored closely during the early stages for adverse effects as well as for benefit. Treatment should be interrupted at intervals of approximately 3 months to assess the need for further quinine treatment. Quinine is very toxic in overdosage and accidental fatalities have occurred in children (see also below).

QUININE

Indications; Dose: see notes above; malaria, see section 5.4.1

Cautions; Contra-indications; Side-effects: see section 5.4.1; **important:** very toxic in **overdosage**—immediate advice from poison centres essential (see also p. 22)

Preparations

See section 5.4.1

10.3   Drugs for the relief of soft-tissue inflammation

10.3.1   Enzymes
10.3.2   Rubefacients and other topical antirheumatics

10.3.1   Enzymes

Hyaluronidase is used to render the tissues more easily permeable to injected fluids, e.g. for introduction of fluids by subcutaneous infusion (termed hypodermoclysis).

HYALURONIDASE

Indications: enhance permeation of subcutaneous or intramuscular injections, local anaesthetics and subcutaneous infusions; promote resorption of excess fluids and blood

Cautions: infants or elderly (control speed and total volume and avoid overhydration especially in renal impairment)

Contra-indications: do not apply direct to cornea; avoid sites where infection or malignancy; not for anaesthesia in unexplained premature labour; not to be used to reduce swelling of bites or stings; not for intravenous administration

Side-effects: occasional severe allergy

Dose: With subcutaneous or intramuscular injection, 1500 units dissolved directly in solution to be injected (ensure compatibility)

With local anaesthetics, 1500 units mixed with local anaesthetic solution (ophthalmology, 15 units/mL)

Hypodermoclysis, 1500 units dissolved in 1 mL water for injections or 0.9% sodium chloride injection, administered before start of 500–1000 mL infusion fluid

Extravasation or haematoma, 1500 units dissolved in 1 mL water for injections or 0.9% sodium chloride injection, infiltrated into affected area (as soon as possible after extravasation)

PoM **Hyalase**® (CP)

Injection, powder for reconstitution, hyaluronidase (ovine). Net price 1500-unit amp = £6.91

10.3.2   Rubefacients and other topical antirheumatics

Rubefacients act by counter-irritation. Pain, whether superficial or deep-seated, is relieved by any method which itself produces irritation of the skin. Counter-irritation is comforting in painful lesions of the muscles, tendons, and joints, and in

non-articular rheumatism. Rubefacients probably all act through the same essential mechanism and differ mainly in intensity and duration of action.

Topical **NSAIDs** (e.g. benzydamine, felbinac, ibuprofen, salicylamide) may provide some slight relief of pain in musculoskeletal conditions.

TOPICAL NSAIDs AND COUNTER-IRRITANTS

CAUTIONS. Apply with gentle massage only. Avoid contact with eyes, mucous membranes, and inflamed or broken skin; discontinue if rash develops. Hands should be washed immediately after use. Not for use with occlusive dressings. Topical application of large amounts may result in systemic effects including hypersensitivity and asthma (renal disease has also been reported). Not generally suitable for children. Patient packs carry a **warning** to avoid during **pregnancy** or **breast-feeding**.

HYPERSENSITIVITY. For NSAID hypersensitivity and asthma warning, see p. 427

PHOTOSENSITIVITY. Patients should be advised against excessive exposure to sunlight of area treated in order to avoid possibility of photosensitivity

Algesal® (Solvay)
Cream, diethylamine salicylate 10%. Net price 50 g = 75p. Apply three times daily
Balmosa® (Pharmax)
Cream, camphor 4%, capsicum oleoresin 0.035%, menthol 2%, methyl salicylate 4%. Net price 40 g = 68p
Difflam® (3M)
Cream, benzydamine hydrochloride 3%. Net price 100 g = £7.00. Apply 3–6 times daily for up to 10 days
PoM **Feldene**® (Pfizer)
Gel, piroxicam 0.5%. Net price 60 g = £5.00; 112 g = £7.84 (also 7.5 g starter pack, hosp. only)
Apply 3–4 times daily; therapy should be reviewed after 4 weeks
Ibugel® (Dermal)
Gel, ibuprofen 5%. Net price 100 g = £6.53
Apply up to 3 times daily
Ibuspray® (Dermal)
Spray application, ibuprofen 5%. Net price 100-mL = £6.95. Label: 15.
Apply 3-4 times daily
Intralgin® (3M)
Gel, benzocaine 2%, salicylamide 5% in an alcoholic vehicle. Net price 50 g = 49p
Movelat® (Sankyo)
Cream, mucopolysaccharide polysulphate (heparinoid) 0.2%, salicylic acid 2%, thymol 0.1%. Net price 100 g = £4.14. Apply up to 4 times daily
Gel, mucopolysaccharide polysulphate (heparinoid) 0.2%, salicylic acid 2%. Net price 100 g = £4.14. Apply up to 4 times daily
PoM **Oruvail**® (Rhône-Poulenc Rorer)
Gel, ketoprofen 2.5%. Net price 100 g = £6.78
Apply 2–4 times daily for up to 7 days (usual recommended dose 15 g daily)
PoM **Powergel**® (Searle)
Gel, ketoprofen 2.5%. Net price 50 g = £3.25; 100 g = £6.25; Twinpack (2 × 50-g pack) = £6.50
Apply 2–3 times daily for up to max. 10 days
Proflex® (Novartis Consumer Health)
Cream, ibuprofen 5%. Net price 100 g = £6.50
Apply 3–4 times daily
Transvasin® (Seton)
Cream, ethyl nicotinate 2%, hexyl nicotinate 2%, thurfyl salicylate 14%. Net price 40 g = 89p; 80 g = £1.51
Apply at least twice daily

Cautionary label wordings, see inside back cover   Prices are **net**, see p.1

Spray application, hydroxyethyl salicylate 5%, diethyl-amine salicylate 5%, methyl nicotinate 1%. Net price 125 mL = £1.52

PoM **Traxam®** (Lederle)
Foam, felbinac 3.17%. Net price 100 g = £7.00. Label:15
Gel, felbinac 3%. Net price 100 g = £7.00
Apply 2–4 times daily; max. 25 g daily; therapy should be reviewed after 14 days
Note. Felbinac is an active metabolite of the NSAID fenbufen

PoM **Voltarol Emulgel®** (Novartis)
Gel, diclofenac diethylammonium salt 1.16% (equivalent to diclofenac sodium 1%). Net price 20 g (hosp. only) = £1.55; 100 g = £7.00. Apply 3–4 times daily; therapy should be reviewed after 14 days (or after 28 days for osteoarthritis)

Topical NSAIDs and counter–irritants on sale to the public together with their significant ingredients include:

Algesal® (diethylamine salicylate), **Algipan Rub®** (capsicin, glycol salicylate, methyl nicotinate), **Balmosa®** (camphor, capsicum oleoresin, menthol, methyl salicylate), **Bengués Balsam®** (menthol, methyl salicylate), **BN Liniment®** (turpentine oil, strong ammonia solution, ammonium chloride), **Boots Muscular Pain Relief Gel®** (ketoprofen), **Boots Pain Relief Balm®** (ethyl nicotinate, glycol monosalicylate, nonylic acid vanillylamide), **Boots Pain Relief Embrocation®** (camphor, turpentine oil), **Boots Pain Relief Warming Spray®** (camphor, ethyl nicotinate, methyl salicylate), **Cremalgin®** (capsicin, glycol salicylate, methyl nicotinate) **Deep Freeze Cold Gel®** (menthol), **Deep Freeze Pain Relief Spray®** (dichlorodifluoromethane, trichlorofluoromethane), **Deep Heat Extra Strength®**, **Deep Heat Massage Liniment®**, **Deep Heat Maximum®**, **Deep Heat Pre–Sport Rub®** (menthol, methyl salicylate), **Deep Heat Rub®** (eucalyptus oil, menthol, methyl salicylate, turpentine oil), **Deep Heat Spray Relief®** (glycol salicylate, ethyl salicylate, methyl salicylate, methyl nicotinate), **Deep Relief®** (ibuprofen, menthol), **Difflam® Cream** (benzydamine), **Dubam Cream®** (methyl salicylate, menthol, cineole), **Dubam Spray®** (ethyl salicylate, methyl salicylate, glycol salicylate, methyl nicotinate), **Elliman's Universal Embrocation®** (acetic acid, turpentine oil) **Feldene P® Gel** (piroxicam), **Fenbid® Gel** (ibuprofen), **Fiery Jack Cream®** (capsicum oleoresin, diethylamine salicylate, glycol salicylate, methyl nicotinate), **Fiery Jack Ointment®** (capsicum oleoresin) **Goddard's White Oil Embrocation®** (dilute acetic acid, dilute ammonia solution, turpentine oil) **Ibuleve®**, **Ibuleve Sports Gel®** (ibuprofen), **Intralgin®** (benzocaine, salicylamide) **Lloyds Cream®** (diethyl salicylate) **Movelat® Relief Cream** (mucopolysaccharide polysulphate, salicylic acid, thymol), **Movelat® Relief Gel** (mucopolysaccharide polysulphate, salicylic acid) **Nasciodine®** (camphor, iodine, menthol, methyl salicylate, turpentine oil), **Nella Red Oil®** (clove oil, mustard oil, methyl nicotinate) **Oruvail® Gel** (ketoprofen 30-g tube; 100-g tube prescribable on NHS (PoM)) **PR Freeze Spray®** (dimethylether, dimethoxymethane), **PR Heat Spray®** (ethyl nicotinate, methyl salicylate, camphor); **Proflex Cream®** (ibuprofen), **Proflex Pain Relief Gel®** (ibuprofen)

Radian®-B Ibuprofen Gel (ibuprofen), **Radian®-B Muscle Lotion**, **Radian®-B Heat Spray** (ammonium salicylate, camphor, menthol, salicylic acid), **Radian®-B Muscle Rub** (camphor, capsicin, menthol, methyl salicylate), **Ralgex Cream®** (capsicin, glycol monosalicylate, methyl nicotinate), **Ralgex Freeze Spray®** (methoxymethane, glycol monosalicylate, isopentane), **Ralgex Low Odour Spray®** (glycol monosalicylate, methyl nicotinate), **Ralgex Spray®** (ethyl salicylate, methyl salicylate, glycol monosalicylate, methyl nicotinate), **Ralgex Stick®** (capsicin, ethyl salicylate, methyl salicylate, glycol salicylate, menthol) **Salonair®** (benzyl nicotinate, camphor, glycol salicylate, menthol, methyl salicylate, squalane), **Salonpas Plasters®** (glycol salicylate, methyl salicylate), **Solpaflex® Gel** (ketoprofen) **Tiger Balm Red Extra Strength®** (camphor, clove oil, cajuput oil, cinnamon oil, menthol, peppermint oil), **Tiger Balm®** (cajuput oil, camphor, clove oil, menthol, peppermint oil), **Transvasin Cream®** (ethyl nicotinate, hexyl nicotinate, thurfyl salicylate), **Transvasin Spray®** (diethylamine salicylate, hydroxyethyl salicylate, methyl salicylate), **Traxam Pain Relief®** (felbinac) **Zam–Buk®** (camphor, eucalyptus oil, thyme oil, colophony)

TOPICAL ANALGESIC FOR POST-HERPETIC NEURALGIA AND DIABETIC NEUROPATHY

PoM **Axsain®** (Bioglan)
Cream, capsaicin 0.075%. Net price 45 g = £15.04. For post-herpetic neuralgia (**important: after** lesions have healed), apply up to 3–4 times daily; for painful diabetic neuropathy, under supervision of hospital consultant, apply 3–4 times daily for 8 weeks then review

POULTICES

Kaolin Poultice, heavy kaolin 52.7%, thymol 0.05%, boric acid 4.5%, peppermint oil 0.05%, methyl salicylate 0.2%, glycerol 42.5%. Net price 200 g = £1.91
Warm and apply directly or between layers of muslin; avoid application of overheated poultice
Kaolin Poultice K/L Pack® (K/L)
Kaolin poultice. Net price 4 × 100-g pouches = £5.19

11: Drugs acting on the
EYE

In this chapter, drug treatment is discussed under the following headings:

The entries in this chapter generally relate only to local eye treatment. Systemic indications and side effects of many of the drugs are given elsewhere (see index).

11.1   Administration of drugs to the eye

EYE DROPS AND EYE OINTMENTS. When administered in the form of eye drops, drugs penetrate the globe, probably through the cornea. However, systemic effects, which are usually undesirable, may well arise from absorption of drugs into the general circulation via conjunctival vessels or from the nasal mucosa after the excess of the preparation has drained down through the tear ducts; nasal drainage of drugs is much more often associated with eye drops than with eye ointments. For example, timolol (a beta-blocker), administered as eye drops may induce bronchospasm or bradycardia in susceptible individuals. The extent of systemic absorption following ocular administration is highly variable.

Eye drops are generally instilled into the pocket formed by gently pulling the lower eyelid, one drop is all that is needed. An eye ointment is generally applied by squeezing a short length in the lower fornix, with the eyelid pulled down gently; the ointment melts rapidly and blinking helps to spread it.

When two different preparations in the form of eye drops are required at the same time of day, for example pilocarpine and timolol in glaucoma, dilution and overflow may occur when one immediately follows the other. The patient should therefore leave an interval of 5 minutes.

Generally it is inadvisable for patients to continue to wear contact lenses, particularly hydrophilic (soft) contact lenses, when receiving eye drops. For warnings relating to eye drops and contact lenses, see section 11.9.

EYE LOTIONS. These are solutions for the irrigation of the conjunctival sac. They act mechanically to flush out irritants or foreign bodies as a first-aid treatment. Sterile sodium chloride 0.9% solution (section 11.8.1) is usually used. In emergency, tap water drawn freshly from the main (not stored water) will suffice.

OTHER PREPARATIONS. Subconjunctival injection may be used to administer anti-infective drugs, mydriatics, or corticosteroids for conditions not responding to topical therapy. The drug diffuses through the cornea and sclera to the anterior and posterior chambers and vitreous humour in higher concentration than can be achieved by absorption from eye drops. However, because the dose-volume is limited (usually not more than 1 mL), this route is suitable only for drugs which are readily soluble.

Drugs such as antibiotics and corticosteroids may be administered systemically to treat an eye condition.

Suitable plastic devices which gradually release a specified amount of drug over a period of, say, 1 week are also used (e.g. *Ocuserts®*).

11.2   Control of microbial contamination

Preparations for the eye should be sterile when issued. Eye drops in multiple-application containers are suitably preserved but care should be taken to avoid contamination of the contents during use.

Eye drops in multiple-application containers for *domiciliary use* should not be used for more than 4 weeks after first opening (unless otherwise stated).

Eye drops for use in *hospital wards* should be discarded 1 week after opening. Individual containers should be provided for each patient. Containers used before an operation should be discarded at the time of the operation and fresh containers supplied. A fresh supply should also be provided upon discharge from hospital; it may be acceptable in specialist ophthalmology units to issue on discharge eye drop bottles that have been in use for the patient for less than 36 hours.

Eye drops used in *out-patient departments* should be discarded at the end of each day. In clinics for eye diseases and in accident and emergency departments, where the dangers of infection are high, single-application packs should be used; if a multiple-application pack is used, it should be discarded after single use.

Diagnostic dyes (e.g. fluorescein) should be used only from single-application packs.

In *eye surgery* it is wise to use single-application containers. Preparations used during intra-ocular procedures and others that may penetrate into the anterior chamber must be isotonic and without preservatives and buffered if necessary to a neutral pH. Large volume intravenous infusion preparations are not suitable for this purpose. For all surgical procedures, a previously unopened container is used for each patient.

11.3   Anti-infective eye preparations

11.3.1   Antibacterials
11.3.2   Antifungals
11.3.3   Antivirals

EYE INFECTIONS. Most acute superficial eye infections can be treated topically. Blepharitis and conjunctivitis are often caused by staphylococci; keratitis and endophthalmitis may be bacterial, viral, or fungal.

Bacterial *blepharitis* is treated by application of an antibacterial eye ointment to the conjunctival sac or to the lid margins. Systemic treatment may occasionally be required and is usually undertaken after culturing organisms from the lid margin and determining their antibiotic sensitivity; antibiotics such as the tetracyclines given for 3 months or longer may be appropriate.

Acute *infective conjunctivitis* is treated with antibacterial eye drops and eye ointment. A poor response might indicate viral or allergic conjunctivitis. *Gonococcal conjunctivitis* is treated with systemic and topical antibiotics.

Corneal ulcer and *keratitis* require specialist treatment and may call for subconjunctival or systemic administration of antibiotics.

Endophthalmitis is a medical emergency which also calls for specialist management and often requires parenteral, subconjunctival, or intra-ocular administration of antibiotics.

For reference to the treatment of *crab lice of the eyelashes*, see section 13.10.4

11.3.1   Antibacterials

Bacterial infections are generally treated topically with eye drops and eye ointments. Systemic administration is sometimes appropriate in blepharitis. In intra-ocular infection, a variety of routes (intracorneal, intravitreal and systemic) may be used.

Chloramphenicol has a broad spectrum of activity and is the drug of choice for *superficial eye infections*. Other antibiotics with a broad spectrum of activity include **framycetin**, **gentamicin**, and **neomycin**, and also **ciprofloxacin** and **ofloxacin**. Gentamicin and possibly ciprofloxacin and ofloxacin are effective for infections caused by *Pseudomonas aeruginosa*.

Ciprofloxacin eye drops are licensed for *corneal ulcers*; intensive application (especially in the first 2 days) is required throughout the day and night.

Chlortetracycline is used in the treatment of *chlamydial infections* including *trachoma* (consult World Health Organization guidelines).

Fusidic acid is useful for staphylococcal infections.

Propamidine isethionate is of little value in bacterial infections but is specific for the rare but devastating condition of *acanthamoeba keratitis* (neomycin may be used as an adjunct; see also section 11.9).

WITH CORTICOSTEROIDS. Many antibiotic preparations also incorporate a corticosteroid but such mixtures should **not** be used unless a patient is under close specialist supervision. In particular they should not be prescribed for undiagnosed 'red eye' which is sometimes caused by the herpes simplex virus and may be difficult to diagnose (section 11.4).

ADMINISTRATION
Eye drops. Apply 1 drop at least every 2 hours then reduce frequency as infection is controlled and continue for 48 hours after healing.
Eye ointment. Apply *either* at night (if eye drops used during the day) *or* 3–4 times daily (if eye ointment used alone).

CHLORAMPHENICOL

Indications: see notes above
Side-effects: transient stinging; rare reports of aplastic anaemia
Administration: see notes above

PoM **Chloramphenicol** (Non-proprietary)
Eye drops, chloramphenicol 0.5%. Net price 10 mL = 51p
Eye ointment, chloramphenicol 1%. Net price 4 g = 88p
PoM **Chloromycetin®** (Forley)
Ophthalmic ointment (= eye ointment), chloramphenicol 1%. Net price 4 g = £2.01
Redidrops (= eye drops), chloramphenicol 0.5%. Net price 5 mL = £1.65; 10 mL = £2.01
   Additives: include phenylmercuric acetate
PoM **Sno Phenicol®** (Chauvin)
Eye drops, chloramphenicol 0.5%, in a viscous vehicle. Net price 10 mL = £1.08
   Additives: include chlorhexidine acetate

Single use
PoM **Minims® Chloramphenicol** (Chauvin)
Eye drops, chloramphenicol 0.5%. Net price 20 × 0.5 mL = £4.92

CHLORTETRACYCLINE

Indications: local treatment of infections, including trachoma (see notes above)
Administration: see notes above

PoM **Aureomycin®** (Lederle)
Ophthalmic ointment (= eye ointment), chlortetracycline hydrochloride 1%. Net price 3.5 g = 92p

---

CIPROFLOXACIN

Indications: superficial bacterial infections, see notes above; corneal ulcers
Cautions: not recommended for children under 1 year; pregnancy and breast-feeding
Side-effects: local burning and itching; lid margin crusting; hyperaemia; bad taste; corneal staining, keratitis, lid oedema, tearing, photophobia, corneal infiltrates; nausea and visual disturbances reported

---

Administration: superficial bacterial infection, see notes above

Corneal ulcer, apply throughout day and night, first day 2 drops every 15 minutes for 6 hours then every 30 minutes for the rest of the day, second day apply 2 drops every hour, third to fourteenth days apply 2 drops every 4 hours; if longer treatment required physician to decide frequency (max. duration of treatment 21 days)

PoM **Ciloxan®** (Alcon)
Ophthalmic solution (= eye drops), ciprofloxacin (as hydrochloride) 0.3%. Net price 5 mL = £4.94
Additives: include benzalkonium chloride

FRAMYCETIN SULPHATE
Indications: see notes above
Administration: see notes above

PoM **Soframycin®** (Hoechst Marion Roussel)
Eye drops, framycetin sulphate 0.5%. Net price 10 mL = £4.84
Additives: include benzalkonium chloride
Eye ointment, framycetin sulphate 0.5%. Net price 5 g = 2.64

FUSIDIC ACID
Indications: see notes above
Administration: see under preparation below

PoM **Fucithalmic®** (Leo)
Eye drops, m/r, fusidic acid 1% in gel basis (liquifies on contact with eye). Net price 5 g = £2.19
Additives: include benzalkonium chloride, disodium edetate
Apply twice daily

GENTAMICIN
Indications: see notes above
Administration: see notes above

PoM **Cidomycin®** (Hoechst Marion Roussel)
Drops (for ear or eye), gentamicin 0.3% (as sulphate). Net price 8 mL = £1.31
Additives: include benzalkonium chloride, disodium edetate
Eye ointment, gentamicin 0.3% (as sulphate), net price 5 g = £1.97
PoM **Garamycin®** (Schering-Plough)
Drops (for ear or eye), gentamicin 0.3% (as sulphate). Net price 10 mL = £1.79
Additives: include benzalkonium chloride
PoM **Genticin®** (Roche)
Drops (for ear or eye), gentamicin 0.3% (as sulphate). Net price 10 mL = £2.00
Additives: include benzalkonium chloride

Single use
PoM **Minims® Gentamicin** (Chauvin)
Eye drops, gentamicin 0.3% (as sulphate). Net price 20 × 0.5 mL = £5.75

NEOMYCIN SULPHATE
Indications: see notes above
Administration: see notes above

PoM **Neomycin** (Non-proprietary)
Eye drops, neomycin sulphate 0.5% (3500 units/mL). Net price 10 mL = £2.54
Available from Martindale
Eye ointment, neomycin sulphate 0.5% (3500 units/g). Net price 3 g = £1.05
Available from Martindale
PoM **Neosporin®** (Dominion)
Eye drops, gramicidin 25 units, neomycin sulphate 1700 units, polymyxin B sulphate 5000 units/mL. Net price 5 mL = £5.36
Additives: include thiomersal
Apply 2–4 times daily or more frequently if required

Single use
PoM **Minims® Neomycin Sulphate** (Chauvin)
Eye drops, neomycin sulphate 0.5%. Net price 20 × 0.5 mL = £5.75
Additives: include disodium edetate

OFLOXACIN
Indications; Administration: see notes above
Cautions: pregnancy and breast-feeding; not to be used for more than 10 days
Side-effects: local irritation including photophobia; dizziness, numbness, nausea and headache reported

PoM **Exocin®** (Allergan)
Ophthalmic solution (= eye drops), ofloxacin 0.3%. Net price 5 mL = £2.27
Additives: include benzalkonium chloride

POLYMYXIN B SULPHATE
Indications; Administration: see notes above

PoM **Polyfax®** (Dominion)
Eye ointment, polymyxin B sulphate 10 000 units, bacitracin zinc 500 units/g. Net price 4 g = £3.41
PoM **Polytrim®** (Dominion)
Eye drops, trimethoprim 0.1%, polymyxin B sulphate 10 000 units/mL. Net price 5 mL = £3.19
Additives: include thiomersal
Eye ointment, trimethoprim 0.5%, polymyxin B sulphate 10 000 units/g. Net price 4 g = £3.19

PROPAMIDINE ISETHIONATE
Indications: local treatment of infections (but see notes above)

Brolene® (Rhône-Poulenc Rorer)
Eye drops, propamidine isethionate 0.1%. Net price 10 mL = £2.23
Apply 4 times daily
Additives: include benzalkonium chloride
Note. Eye drops containing propamidine isethionate 0.1% also available from Typharm (*Golden Eye Drops*)
Eye ointment, dibromopropamidine isethionate 0.15%. Net price 5 g = £2.35
Apply 1–2 times daily
Note. Eye ointment containing dibromopropamidine isethionate 0.15% also available from Typharm (*Golden Eye Ointment*)

11.3.2　Antifungals

Fungal infections of the cornea are rare but can occur after agricultural injuries, especially in hot and humid climates. Orbital mycosis is rare, and when it occurs is usually due to direct spread of infection from the paranasal sinuses. Increasing age, debility, or immunosuppression may encourage fungal proliferation. The spread of infection via the bloodstream occasionally produces a metastatic endophthalmitis.

Many different fungi are capable of producing ocular infection; they may be identified by appropriate laboratory procedures.

Antifungal preparations for the eye are not generally available. Treatment will normally be carried out at specialist centres, but requests for information about supplies of preparations not available commercially should be addressed to the local Health Authority (or equivalent in Scotland or Northern Ireland), or to the nearest hospital ophthalmology unit, or to Moorfields Eye Hospital, City Road, London EC1V 2PD (tel. 0171-253 3411).

11.3.3　Antivirals

Herpes simplex infections producing, for example, dendritic corneal ulcer can be treated with **aciclovir**.

ACICLOVIR
(Acyclovir)

Indications: local treatment of herpes simplex infections
Side-effects: mild stinging and local inflammation reported
Administration: apply 5 times daily (continue for at least 3 days after complete healing)

PoM **Zovirax®** (GlaxoWellcome)
Eye ointment, aciclovir 3%. Net price 4.5 g = £10.67
Tablets and *injection*, see section 5.3
Cream, see section 13.10.3

11.4　Corticosteroids and other anti-inflammatory preparations

　11.4.1　Corticosteroids
　11.4.2　Other anti-inflammatory preparations

11.4.1　Corticosteroids

Corticosteroids administered topically, by subconjunctival injection, and systemically have an important place in treating uveitis and scleritis; they are also used to reduce post-operative inflammation following eye operations.

Topical corticosteroids should normally only be used under expert supervision; they should not be prescribed for undiagnosed 'red eye'. There are two main dangers from topical corticosteroids. First the 'red eye' may be caused by herpes simplex virus

which produces a dendritic ulcer; corticosteroids aggravate the condition which may lead to loss of vision or even loss of the eye. Second, again arising from the use of eye drop formulations, a 'steroid glaucoma' may be produced, after a few weeks treatment, in patients predisposed to chronic simple glaucoma. Other side-effects include delayed hypersensitivity reactions and, in susceptible patients, thinning of the cornea and sclera (with perforation). Use of a combination product containing a corticosteroid with an anti-infective is rarely justified.

Systemic corticosteroids (section 6.3.2) may be useful for ocular conditions. The risk of producing glaucoma is not great, but 'steroid cataract' is a very high risk (75%) if more than 15 mg of prednisolone or equivalent is given daily for several years. The longer the duration, the greater is the risk.

BETAMETHASONE
Indications: local treatment of inflammation (short-term)
Cautions; Side-effects: see notes above
Administration: apply eye drops every 1–2 hours until controlled then reduce frequency, eye ointment 2–4 times daily or at night when used with eye drops

PoM **Betnesol®** (Evans)
Drops (for ear, eye, or nose), betamethasone sodium phosphate 0.1%. Net price 10 mL = £1.31
　Additives: include benzalkonium chloride
Eye ointment, betamethasone sodium phosphate 0.1%. Net price 3 g = 56p
PoM **Betnesol-N®** (Evans)
Drops (for ear, eye, or nose), see section 12.1.1
Eye ointment, betamethasone sodium phosphate 0.1%, neomycin sulphate 0.5%. Net price 3 g = 64p
PoM **Vista-Methasone®** (Martindale)
Drops (for ear, eye, or nose), betamethasone sodium phosphate 0.1%. Net price 5 mL = £1.15; 10 mL = £1.31
　Additives: include benzalkonium chloride
PoM **Vista-Methasone N®** (Martindale)
Drops (for ear, eye, or nose), see section 12.1.1

CLOBETASONE BUTYRATE
Indications: local treatment of inflammation (short-term)
Cautions; Side-effects: see notes above; reduced tendency to raise intra-ocular pressure
Administration: apply eye drops 4 times daily; severe conditions every 1–2 hours until controlled then reduce frequency

PoM **Cloburate®** (Dominion)
Eye drops, clobetasone butyrate 0.1%. Net price 10 mL = £2.85
　Additives: include benzalkonium chloride
PoM **Cloburate-N®** (Dominion)
Eye drops, clobetasone butyrate 0.1%, neomycin sulphate 0.5%. Net price 10 mL = £3.20
　Additives: include benzalkonium chloride

DEXAMETHASONE

Indications: local treatment of inflammation (short-term)

Cautions; Side-effects: see notes above

Administration: apply eye drops 4–6 times daily; severe conditions every 30–60 minutes until controlled then reduce frequency

PoM **Maxidex®** (Alcon)

Eye drops, dexamethasone 0.1%, hypromellose 0.5%. Net price 5 mL = £1.49; 10 mL = £2.95

Additives: include benzalkonium chloride

PoM **Maxitrol®** (Alcon)

Eye drops, dexamethasone 0.1%, hypromellose 0.5%, neomycin 0.35% (as sulphate), polymyxin B sulphate 6000 units/mL. Net price 5 mL = £1.77

Additives: include benzalkonium chloride

Eye ointment, dexamethasone 0.1%, neomycin 0.35% (as sulphate), polymyxin B sulphate 6000 units/g. Net price 3.5 g = £1.52

Additives: include hydroxybenzoates

PoM **Sofradex®** (Hoechst Marion Roussel)

Drops and ointment (for ear or eye), see section 12.1.1

FLUOROMETHOLONE

Indications: local treatment of inflammation (short-term)

Cautions; Side-effects: see notes above; reduced tendency to raise intra-ocular pressure

Administration: apply eye drops 2–4 times daily (initially every hour for 24–48 hours then reduce frequency)

PoM **FML®** (Allergan)

Ophthalmic suspension (= eye drops), fluorometholone 0.1%, polyvinyl alcohol (Liquifilm®) 1.4%. Net price 5 mL = £1.79; 10 mL = £3.09

Additives: include benzalkonium chloride, disodium edetate, polysorbate 80

PoM **FML-Neo®** (Allergan)

Eye drops, fluorometholone 0.1%, neomycin sulphate 0.5%, polyvinyl alcohol (Liquifilm®) 1.4%. Net price 5 mL = £2.08

Additives: include benzalkonium chloride, disodium edetate, polysorbate 80

HYDROCORTISONE ACETATE

Indications: local treatment of inflammation (short-term)

Cautions; Side-effects: see notes above

PoM **Hydrocortisone** (Non-proprietary)

Eye drops, hydrocortisone acetate 1%. Net price 10 mL = £3.13

Available from Martindale

Eye ointment, hydrocortisone acetate 0.5%, net price 3 g = £1.67; 1%, 3 g = £1.70; 2.5%, 3 g = £1.42

Available from Martindale

PoM **Neo-Cortef®** (Dominion)

Drops and *ointment* (for ear or eye), see section 12.1.1

Note. Eye drops containing hydrocortisone acetate 1.5% and neomycin sulphate 0.5% also available from Martindale

PREDNISOLONE

Indications: local treatment of inflammation (short-term)

Cautions; Side-effects: see notes above

Administration: apply eye drops every 1–2 hours until controlled then reduce frequency

PoM **Pred Forte®** (Allergan)

Eye drops, prednisolone acetate 1%. Net price 5 mL = £1.59; 10 mL = £3.19

Additives: include benzalkonium chloride, disodium edetate, polysorbate 80

Apply 2–4 times daily

PoM **Predsol®** (Evans)

Drops (for ear or eye), prednisolone sodium phosphate 0.5%. Net price 10 mL = £1.31

Additives: include benzalkonium chloride

PoM **Predsol-N®** (Evans)

Drops (for ear or eye), see section 12.1.1

Single use

PoM **Minims® Prednisolone** (Chauvin)

Eye drops, prednisolone sodium phosphate 0.5%. Net price 20 × 0.5 mL = £5.75

11.4.2 Other anti-inflammatory preparations

Other preparations used for the topical treatment of inflammation and allergic conjunctivitis include antihistamines, lodoxamide, and sodium cromoglycate.

Topical preparations of **antihistamines** such as eye drops containing antazoline sulphate (with xylometazoline hydrochloride as *Otrivine-Antistin®*) or the recently introduced **levocabastine** may be used for short-term treatment of allergic conjunctivitis.

Sodium cromoglycate eye drops may be useful for vernal keratoconjunctivitis and other allergic forms of conjunctivitis. **Nedocromil sodium** eye drops have recently been introduced for allergic conjunctivitis.

Lodoxamide eye drops have been introduced for allergic conjunctival conditions including seasonal allergic conjunctivitis.

ANTAZOLINE

Indications: allergic conjunctivitis

Otrivine-Antistin® (CIBA Vision)

Eye drops, antazoline sulphate 0.5%, xylometazoline hydrochloride 0.05%. Net price 10 mL = £2.13

Additives: include benzalkonium chloride, disodium edetate

Apply 2–3 times daily

Note. Xylometazoline is a sympathomimetic; it should be avoided in angle-closure glaucoma and absorption may result in systemic side-effects and the possibility of interaction with other drugs

LEVOCABASTINE

Indications: seasonal allergic conjunctivitis

Side-effects: local irritation, blurred vision, local oedema, urticaria, dyspnoea, headache, drowsiness

Administration: ADULT and CHILD over 9 years, apply twice daily, increased if necessary to 3–4 times daily, discontinue if no improvement within 3 days; max. 4 weeks treatment per year

▼ PoM **Livostin®** (CIBA Vision)
Eye drops, levocabastine 0.05% (as hydrochloride). Net price 4 mL = £8.49
<small>Additives: include benzalkonium chloride disodium edetate, polysorbate 80</small>

LODOXAMIDE
Indications: allergic conjunctivitis
Side-effects: mild transient burning, stinging, itching, and lacrimation; flushing and dizziness reported
Administration: ADULT and CHILD over 4 years, apply eye drops 4 times daily

PoM **Alomide®** (Alcon)
Ophthalmic solution (= eye drops), lodoxamide 0.1% (as trometamol). Net price 10 mL = £5.48
<small>Additives: include benzalkonium chloride, disodium edetate</small>

NEDOCROMIL SODIUM
Indications: allergic conjunctivitis
Side-effects: transient burning and stinging; distinctive taste reported
Administration: seasonal and perennial conjunctivitis, ADULT and CHILD over 6 years, apply twice daily increased if necessary to 4 times daily; max. 12 weeks treatment for seasonal allergic conjunctivitis
Vernal keratoconjunctivitis, ADULT and CHILD over 6 years, apply 4 times daily

PoM **Rapitil®** (Fisons)
Eye drops, nedocromil sodium 2%. Net price 5 mL = £8.24
<small>Additives: include benzalkonium chloride, disodium edetate</small>

SODIUM CROMOGLYCATE
Indications: allergic conjunctivitis
Side-effects: transient burning and stinging
Administration: apply eye drops 4 times daily, eye ointment 2–3 times daily

PoM ¹**Sodium Cromoglycate** (Non-proprietary)
Eye drops, sodium cromoglycate 2%. Net price 13.5 mL = £2.29
<small>Available from Baker Norton (*Hay-Crom®* Aqueous), Fisons (*Opticrom® Aqueous*), Genus, Lennon, Opus (*Viz-on®*), Pharma-Global (*Vividrin®*)</small>
Eye ointment, sodium cromoglycate 4%. Net price 5 g = £8.28
<small>Available from Fisons (*Opticrom®*)</small>
<small>1. Sodium cromoglycate 2% eye drops and 4% eye ointment can be sold to the public (in max. pack sizes of 10 mL for eye drops and 5 g for eye ointment) for treatment of acute seasonal (allergic) conjunctivitis; proprietary brands of eye drops on sale to the public include *Boots Hayfever Relief*, *Clariteyes®*, *Hay-Crom®* Hay Fever, *Opticrom® Allergy*, and *Optrex® Hayfever Allergy*</small>

11.5 Mydriatics and cycloplegics

Antimuscarinics dilate the pupil and paralyse the ciliary muscle; they vary in potency and duration of action.

Short-acting, relatively weak mydriatics, such as **tropicamide 0.5%**, facilitate the examination of the fundus of the eye. **Cyclopentolate** 1% or **atropine** are preferable for producing cycloplegia for refraction in young children. Atropine 1% (in ointment form) is sometimes preferred for children under 5 years of age. Atropine, which has a longer duration of action, is also used for the treatment of anterior uveitis mainly to prevent posterior synechiae, often with phenylephrine 10% eye drops (2.5% in children, the elderly, and those with cardiac disease).

CAUTIONS. Darkly pigmented iris is more resistant to pupillary dilatation and caution should be exercised to avoid overdosage. Mydriasis may precipitate acute angle-closure glaucoma in a very few patients, usually aged over 60 years and hypermetropic (long-sighted), who are predisposed to the condition because of a shallow anterior chamber. Phenylephrine may interact with systemically administered monoamine-oxidase inhibitors; other **interactions**: Appendix 1 (sympathomimetics).
DRIVING. Patients should be warned not to drive for 1 to 2 hours after mydriasis.

SIDE-EFFECTS. Ocular side-effects of mydriatics and cycloplegics include transient stinging and raised intra-ocular pressure; on prolonged administration, local irritation, hyperaemia, oedema and conjunctivitis may occur. Contact dermatitis is not uncommon with the antimuscarinic mydriatic drugs, especially atropine.

Toxic systemic reactions to atropine and cyclopentolate may occur in the very young and the very old; see under Atropine Sulphate and Belladonna Alkaloids (section 1.2) for systemic side-effects of antimuscarinic drugs.

ANTIMUSCARINICS

ATROPINE SULPHATE
Indications: refraction procedures in young children; see also notes above
Cautions: see notes above; risk of systemic effects with eye drops in infants under 3 months—eye ointment preferred
Side-effects: see notes above

PoM **Atropine** (Non-proprietary)
Eye drops, atropine sulphate 0.5%, net price 10 mL = £1.91; 1%, 10 mL = 78p
<small>Available from Martindale</small>
Eye ointment, atropine sulphate 1%. Net price 3 g = £1.88
<small>Available from Martindale</small>
PoM **Isopto Atropine®** (Alcon)
Eye drops, atropine sulphate 1%, hypromellose 0.5%. Net price 5 mL = 99p
<small>Additives: include benzalkonium chloride</small>

Single use
PoM **Minims® Atropine Sulphate** (Chauvin)
Eye drops, atropine sulphate 1%. Net price 20 ×
0.5 mL = £4.92

CYCLOPENTOLATE HYDROCHLORIDE
Indications: see notes above
Cautions: see notes above
Side-effects: see notes above

PoM **Mydrilate®** (Boehringer Ingelheim)
Eye drops, cyclopentolate hydrochloride 0.5%, net
price 5 mL = 73p; 1%, 5 mL = 98p
Additives: include benzalkonium chloride

Single use
PoM **Minims® Cyclopentolate** (Chauvin)
Eye drops, cyclopentolate hydrochloride 0.5 and
1%. Net price 20 × 0.5 mL (both) = £4.92

HOMATROPINE HYDROBROMIDE
Indications: see notes above
Cautions: see notes above
Side-effects: see notes above

PoM **Homatropine** (Non-proprietary)
Eye drops, homatropine hydrobromide 1%, net
price 10 mL = £1.36; 2%, 10 mL = £1.58
Available from Martindale

Single use
PoM **Minims® Homatropine Hydrobromide**
(Chauvin)
Eye drops, homatropine hydrobromide 2%. Net
price 20 × 0.5 mL = £5.75

TROPICAMIDE
Indications: see notes above
Cautions: see notes above
Side-effects: see notes above

PoM **Mydriacyl®** (Alcon)
Eye drops, tropicamide 0.5%, net price 5 mL =
£1.36; 1%, 5 mL = £1.68
Additives: include benzalkonium chloride

Single use
PoM **Minims® Tropicamide** (Chauvin)
Eye drops, tropicamide 0.5 and 1%. Net price 20 ×
0.5 mL (both) = £5.75

SYMPATHOMIMETICS

PHENYLEPHRINE HYDROCHLORIDE
Indications: mydriasis; see also notes above
Cautions: children and elderly (avoid 10%
strength); cardiovascular disease (avoid or use
2.5% strength only); tachycardia; hyperthyroidism; diabetes
Contra-indications: angle-closure glaucoma
Side-effects: eye pain and stinging (may require
local anaesthetic a few minutes beforehand);

blurred vision, photophobia; systemic effects
include arrhythmias, hypertension, coronary
artery spasm

Phenylephrine (Non-proprietary)
Eye drops, phenylephrine hydrochloride 10%. Net
price 10 mL = £2.78
Available from Martindale
See also under Hypromellose (section 11.8.1)

Single use
Minims® Phenylephrine Hydrochloride
(Chauvin)
Eye drops, phenylephrine hydrochloride 2.5%, net
price 20 × 0.5 mL = £5.75; 10%, 20 × 0.5 mL =
£5.75

11.6 Treatment of glaucoma

Glaucoma is usually associated with an abnormally
high intra-ocular pressure; it may result in blindness. The rise in pressure is almost always due to
reduced outflow of aqueous humour, the inflow
remaining constant.

Probably the commonest condition is *chronic
simple glaucoma* where the obstruction is in the
trabecular meshwork. It is commonly first treated
with a topical beta-blocker and other drugs added as
necessary to control the intra-ocular pressure e.g.
adrenaline or pilocarpine.

Dorzolamide, a topical carbonic anhydrase inhibitor, can be used as an alternative to topical beta-
blockers or as an adjunct to them. Acetazolamide is
a carbonic anhydrase inhibitor which is given by
mouth.

Latanoprost is a prostaglandin analogue which
increases the uveoscleral outflow of aqueous
humour. It is indicated for open-angle glaucoma
and ocular hypertension in patients for whom other
drugs are inappropriate.

Brimonidine, a selective alpha$_2$ adrenoceptor
stimulant, has recently been introduced for open-
angle glaucoma and ocular hypertension when
other drugs are inappropriate.

Apraclonidine (section 11.8.2) is an alpha$_2$-
adrenoceptor stimulant which reduces the rate of
production of aqueous humour.

In emergency or before surgery, mannitol 20%
(up to max. of 500 mL) should be given by slow
intravenous infusion until the intra-ocular pressure
has been satisfactorily reduced. Acetazolamide by
intravenous injection may also be used for the
emergency management of raised intra-ocular pressure.

If supplementary topical treatment is required
after *iridectomy* or a drainage operation in either
open-angle or angle-closure glaucoma, a beta-
blocker is preferred to pilocarpine. This is because
of the risk that posterior synechiae will be formed
as a result of the miotic effect of pilocarpine, especially in angle-closure glaucoma. It is then also
advantageous to utilise the mydriatic side-effect of
adrenaline.

MIOTICS

The small pupil is an unfortunate side-effect of these drugs (except when pilocarpine is used temporarily prior to operation for *angle-closure glaucoma*). The key factor is the opening up of the inefficient drainage channels in the trabecular meshwork resulting from contraction or spasm of the ciliary muscle. This also produces accommodation spasm that may result in blurring of vision and browache (a particular disadvantage in patients under 40 years of age).

Pilocarpine has a duration of action of 3 to 4 hours. **Carbachol** is sometimes used to lower intra-ocular pressure, usually in conjunction with other miotics.

Ecothiopate iodide (as *Phospholine Iodide®*, Dominion) is no longer on the UK market but is still available on a named-patient basis for use under expert supervision.

Generalised parasympathomimetic side effects such as sweating, bradycardia and intestinal colic may follow systemic absorption of these eye drops; other effects may include hypersalivation and bronchospasm.

CARBACHOL

Indications: see notes above

Administration: apply eye drops up to 4 times daily

PoM **Isopto Carbachol®** (Alcon)

Eye drops, carbachol 3%, hypromellose 1%. Net price 10 mL = £1.76

Additives: include benzalkonium chloride

PILOCARPINE

Indications; Side-effects: see notes above

Administration: apply eye drops 3–6 times daily; long acting preparations, see under preparations below

PoM **Pilocarpine Hydrochloride** (Non-proprietary)

Eye drops, pilocarpine hydrochloride 0.5%, net price 10 mL = £1.21; 1%, 10 mL = 96p; 2%, 10 mL = £1.07; 3%, 10 mL = £1.30; 4%, 10 mL = £1.47

Available from APS, Cox, Martindale

PoM **Isopto Carpine®** (Alcon)

Eye drops, all with hypromellose 0.5%; pilocarpine hydrochloride 0.5%, net price 10 mL = 73p; 1%, 10 mL = 81p; 2%, 10 mL = 90p; 3%, 10 mL = 97p; 4%, 10 mL = £1.04

Additives: include benzalkonium chloride

PoM **Sno Pilo®** (Chauvin)

Eye drops, in a viscous vehicle, pilocarpine hydrochloride 1%, net price 10 mL = £1.04; 2%, 10 mL = £1.14; 4%, 10 mL = £1.36

Additives: include benzalkonium chloride

Single use

PoM **Minims® Pilocarpine Nitrate** (Chauvin)

Eye drops, pilocarpine nitrate 1, 2, and 4%. Net price 20 × 0.5 mL (all) = £4.92

Long acting

PoM **Ocusert®** (Dominion)

Pilo-20 ocular insert, pilocarpine 20 micrograms released per hour for 1 week. Net price pack of 2 inserts = £9.64; 8 inserts = £35.08. Counselling, method of use

Pilo-40 ocular insert, pilocarpine 40 micrograms released per hour for 1 week. Net price pack of 2 inserts = £11.24; 8 inserts = £40.90. Counselling, method of use

PoM **Pilogel®** (Alcon)

Ophthalmic gel, pilocarpine hydrochloride 4%, carbomer 940 (polyacrylic acid) 3.5%. Net price 5 g = £6.86

Additives: include benzalkonium chloride, disodium edetate

Apply 1–1.5 cm gel once daily at bedtime

SYMPATHOMIMETICS

Adrenaline probably acts both by reducing the rate of production of aqueous humour and by increasing the outflow through the trabecular meshwork. It is contra-indicated in angle-closure glaucoma because it is a mydriatic, unless an iridectomy has been carried out. Side-effects include severe smarting and redness of the eye; adrenaline should be used with caution in patients with hypertension and heart disease.

Dipivefrine is a prodrug of adrenaline. It is stated to pass more rapidly through the cornea and is then converted to the active form.

Guanethidine enhances and prolongs the effects of adrenaline. Prolonged use, particularly of the higher strengths may result in conjunctival fibrosis with secondary corneal changes; the conjunctiva and cornea should be examined at least every six months.

Brimonidine, a selective alpha$_2$-adrenoceptor stimulant has been introduced recently for the reduction of intra-ocular pressure in open-angle glaucoma or ocular hypertension in patients for whom beta-blockers are inappropriate; it may also be used as adjunctive therapy when intra-ocular pressure is inadequately controlled by a beta-blocker alone.

Apraclonidine (section 11.8.2) is another alpha$_2$-adrenoceptor stimulant. Eye drops containing apraclonidine 0.5% are used for a short term to delay laser treatment or surgery for glaucoma in patients not adequately controlled by another drug; eye drops containing 1% are used for post-operative control of intra-ocular pressure after anterior segment laser surgery.

ADRENALINE

Indications; Contra-indications; Side-effects: see notes above

Administration: apply eye drops 1–2 times daily

PoM **Eppy®** (Chauvin)
Eye drops, adrenaline 1%. Net price 7.5 mL = £4.06
Additives: include benzalkonium chloride, also acetylcysteine as antoxidant

PoM **Simplene®** (Chauvin)
Eye drops, adrenaline, in a viscous vehicle, 0.5%, net price 7.5 mL = £3.45; 1%, 7.5 mL = £3.79
Additives: include benzalkonium chloride, also acetylcysteine as antoxidant

BRIMONIDINE TARTRATE

Indications: adjunct to beta-blockers or used alone in raised intra-ocular pressure in ocular hypertension or open-angle glaucoma in patients unresponsive to beta-blockers or if beta-blockers contra-indicated

Cautions: severe cardiovascular disease; cerebral or coronary insufficiency, Raynaud's syndrome, postural hypotension, depression, hepatic or renal impairment; pregnancy, breast-feeding; **interactions:** Appendix 1 (alpha$_2$-adrenoceptor stimulants)

DRIVING. Drowsiness may affect performance of skilled tasks (e.g. driving)

Side-effects: ocular reactions include hyperaemia, burning, stinging, blurring, pruritus, allergy, and conjunctival follicles; occasionally corneal erosion and staining, photophobia, eyelid inflammation, conjunctivitis; headache, dry mouth, taste alteration, fatigue, dizziness, drowsiness reported; rarely depression, nasal dryness, palpitations, and hypersensitivity reactions

Administration: apply one drop twice daily

▼ PoM **Alphagan®** (Allergan)
Eye drops, brimonidine tartrate 0.2%, net price 5 mL = £10.80
Additives: include benzalkonium chloride

DIPIVEFRINE HYDROCHLORIDE

Indications; Contra-indications; Side-effects: as for Adrenaline, see notes above
Administration: apply 1 drop twice daily

PoM **Dipivefrine Hydrochloride** (Non-proprietary)
Eye drops, dipivefrine hydrochloride 0.1%. Net price 5 mL = £3.33
Additives: include benzalkonium chloride, disodium edetate
Available fom Dominion

PoM **Propine®** (Allergan)
Eye drops, dipivefrine hydrochloride 0.1%. Net price 5 mL = £3.99, 10 mL = £4.99, triple pack (3 × 5 mL) = £10.47
Additives: include benzalkonium chloride, disodium edetate

GUANETHIDINE MONOSULPHATE

Indications; Cautions: see notes above
Administration: apply eye drops 1–2 times daily

PoM **Ganda®** (Chauvin)
Eye drops '1+0.2', guanethidine monosulphate 1%, adrenaline 0.2% in a viscous vehicle. Net price 7.5 mL = £4.49
Additives: include benzalkonium chloride

Eye drops '3 + 0.5', guanethidine monosulphate 3%, adrenaline 0.5% in a viscous vehicle. Net price 7.5 mL = £5.86
Additives: include benzalkonium chloride

BETA-BLOCKERS

Topical application of a beta-blocker to the eye reduces intra-ocular pressure effectively in *chronic simple glaucoma*, probably by reducing the rate of production of aqueous humour. Administration by mouth also reduces intra-ocular pressure but this route is not used since side-effects may be troublesome.

Beta-blockers used as eye drops include **timolol** and, more recently, **betaxolol, carteolol, levobunolol**, and **metipranolol**.

CAUTIONS, CONTRA-INDICATIONS AND SIDE-EFFECTS. Systemic absorption may follow topical application therefore eye drops containing a beta-blocker are contra-indicated in patients with bradycardia, heart block, or heart failure. **Important:** for a warning to avoid in asthma see CSM advice below. Consider also other cautions, contra-indications and side-effects of beta-blockers (p. 75). Local side-effects of eye drops include transitory dry eyes and allergic blepharoconjunctivitis.

CSM advice. The CSM has advised that beta-blockers, even those with apparent cardioselectivity, should not be used in patients with asthma or a history of obstructive airways disease, unless no alternative treatment is available. In such cases the risk of inducing bronchospasm should be appreciated and appropriate precautions taken.

INTERACTIONS. Since systemic absorption may follow topical application the possibility of interactions, in particular, with drugs such as verapamil should be borne in mind. See also Appendix 1 (beta-blockers).

BETAXOLOL HYDROCHLORIDE

Indications; Cautions; Contra-indications; Side-effects: see notes above
Administration: apply eye drops twice daily

PoM **Betoptic®** (Alcon)
Eye drops, betaxolol (as hydrochloride) 0.25%, net price 5 mL = £4.77; 0.5%, 5 mL = £5.17
Additives: include benzalkonium chloride

CARTEOLOL HYDROCHLORIDE

Indications; Cautions; Contra-indications; Side-effects: see notes above
Administration: apply eye drops twice daily

PoM **Teoptic®** (CIBA Vision)
Eye drops, carteolol hydrochloride 1%, net price 5 mL = £4.83; 3 × 5 mL = £12.32; 2%, 5 mL = £5.67; 3 × 5 mL = £14.46
Additives: include benzalkonium chloride

LEVOBUNOLOL HYDROCHLORIDE

Indications; Cautions; Contra-indications; Side-effects: see notes above

Administration: apply eye drops once or twice daily

PoM **Betagan®** (Allergan)

Eye drops, levobunolol hydrochloride 0.5%, polyvinyl alcohol (Liquifilm®) 1.4%. Net price 5-mL bottle with C Cap® = £4.88, triple pack (3 × 5 mL) = £12.45

Additives: include benzalkonium chloride, disodium edetate

Unit dose eye drops, levobunolol hydrochloride 0.5%, polyvinyl alcohol (Liquifilm®) 1.4%. Net price 30 × 0.4 mL = £10.45

Additives: include disodium edetate

METIPRANOLOL

Indications; Cautions; Contra-indications; Side-effects: see notes above but in chronic open angle glaucoma **restricted** to patients allergic to preservatives or to those wearing soft contact lenses (in whom benzalkonium chloride should be avoided); granulomatous anterior uveitis reported (discontinue treatment)

Administration: apply eye drops twice daily

PoM **Minims® Metipranolol** (Chauvin)

Eye drops, metipranolol 0.1%, net price 20 × 0.5 mL = £10.19; 0.3%, 20 × 0.5 mL = £11.09

TIMOLOL MALEATE

Indications; Cautions; Contra-indications; Side-effects: see notes above

Administration: apply eye drops twice daily; long acting preparations, see under preparations below

PoM **Timolol** (Non-proprietary)

Eye drops, timolol (as maleate) 0.25%, net price 5 mL = £5.18; 0.5%, 5 mL = £5.82

Available from APS, Bioglan, Cox, Hillcross, Lennon, Norton, Opus (*Glau-opt®*)

PoM **Timoptol®** (MSD)

Eye drops, in Ocumeter® metered-dose unit, timolol (as maleate) 0.25%, net price 5 mL = £5.18; 0.5%, 5 mL = £5.82

Additives: include benzalkonium chloride

Unit dose eye drops, timolol (as maleate) 0.25%, net price 30 × 0.25 mL = £9.60; 0.5%, 30 × 0.25 mL = £10.97

Long acting

▼ PoM **Timoptol®–LA** (MSD)

Ophthalmic gel-forming solution (= eye drops), timolol (as maleate) 0.25%, net price 2.5 mL = £5.18; 0.5%, 2.5 mL = £5.82

Additives: include benzododecinium bromide

Apply eye drops once daily

CARBONIC ANHYDRASE INHIBITORS AND SYSTEMIC DRUGS

The **carbonic anhydrase inhibitors**, acetazolamide and dorzolamide, reduce intra-ocular pressure by reducing aqueous humour secretion. Systemic use also produces weak diuresis.

Acetazolamide is given by mouth or by intravenous injection (intramuscular injections are painful because of the alkaline pH of the solution). Acetazolamide is a sulphonamide; blood disorders, rashes and other sulphonamide-related side-effects occur occasionally. It is not generally recommended for long-term use but electrolyte disturbances and metabolic acidosis that occur may be corrected by administering potassium bicarbonate (as effervescent potassium tablets, section 9.2.1.3).

Dorzolamide, a topical carbonic anhydrase inhibitor, is licensed for use in patients resistant to beta-blockers or those in whom beta-blockers are contra-indicated. It is used alone or as an adjunct to a topical beta-blocker. Systemic absorption may rarely give rise to sulphonamide-like side-effects and may require discontinuation if severe.

The **osmotic diuretics**, intravenous hypertonic **mannitol,** or **glycerol** by mouth, are useful short-term ocular hypotensive drugs.

ACETAZOLAMIDE

Indications: reduction of intra-ocular pressure in open-angle glaucoma, secondary glaucoma, and peri-operatively in angle-closure glaucoma; diuresis (section 2.2.7); epilepsy (section 4.8.1)

Cautions: not generally recommended for prolonged use but if given monitor blood count and plasma electrolyte concentration; pulmonary obstruction (risk of acidosis); elderly; pregnancy and breast-feeding; avoid extravasation at injection site (risk of necrosis); **interactions:** Appendix 1 (diuretics)

Contra-indications: hypokalaemia, hyponatraemia, hyperchloraemic acidosis; severe hepatic impairment; renal impairment; sulphonamide hypersensitivity

Side-effects: nausea, vomiting, diarrhoea, taste disturbance; loss of appetite, paraesthesia, flushing, headache, dizziness, fatigue, irritability, depression; thirst, polyuria; reduced libido; metabolic acidosis and electrolyte disturbances on long-term therapy; occasionally, drowsiness, confusion, hearing disturbances, urticaria, malaena, glycosuria, haematuria, abnormal liver function, renal calculi, blood disorders including agranulocytosis and thrombocytopenia, rashes including Stevens-Johnson syndrome and toxic epidermal necrolysis; rarely, photosensitivity, liver damage, flaccid paralysis, convulsions; transient myopia reported

Dose: *by mouth or by intravenous injection,* 0.25–1 g daily in divided doses

By intramuscular injection, as for intravenous injection but preferably avoided because of alkaline pH

PoM **Diamox®** (Storz)

Tablets, acetazolamide 250 mg. Net price 112-tab pack = £11.53. Label: 3

Sodium Parenteral (= injection), powder for reconstitution, acetazolamide (as sodium salt). Net price 500-mg vial = £14.76

PoM **Diamox®** **SR** (Storz)

Capsules, m/r, two-tone orange, enclosing orange f/c pellets, acetazolamide 250 mg. Net price 28-cap pack = £10.50. Label: 3, 25
Dose: 1–2 capsules daily

DORZOLAMIDE

Indications: adjunct to beta-blockers or used alone in raised intra-ocular pressure in ocular hypertension, open-angle glaucoma, or pseudoexfoliative glaucoma in patients unresponsive to beta-blockers or if beta-blockers contra-indicated

Cautions: hepatic impairment; systemic absorption follows topical application; **interactions:** Appendix 1 (dorzolamide)

Contra-indications: severe renal impairment or hyperchloraemic acidosis; pregnancy and breast-feeding

Side-effects: burning, stinging and itching of the eye, bitter taste, blurred vision, tearing, conjunctivitis, superficial punctate keratitis, eyelid inflammation, anterior uveitis, transient myopia; headache, dizziness, paraesthesia, asthenia, nausea; rash and allergic reactions (including urticaria, angioedema, bronchosopasm); urolithiasis

Administration: used alone, apply 3 times daily; with topical beta-blocker, apply twice daily

▼ PoM **Trusopt®** (MSD)

Ophthalmic solution (= eye drops), dorzolamide (as hydrochloride) 2%. Net price 5 mL = £9.31
Additives: include benzalkonium chloride

PROSTAGLANDIN ANALOGUE

Latanoprost, a recently introduced prostaglandin analogue, increases uveoscleral outflow. It is indicated for open-angle glaucoma and ocular hypertension when other drugs are inappropriate; there is little experience of its use in other variants of glaucoma. Patients should be monitored for any changes to eye coloration since latanoprost may increase the brown pigment in the iris; particular care is required in those with mixed coloured irides and those receiving treatment to one eye only.

LATANOPROST

Indications: intra-ocular pressure in open-angle glaucoma and ocular hypertension in patients intolerant or unresponsive to other drugs

Cautions: before initiating treatment, advise patients of possible change in eye colour; monitor for eye colour change; brittle or severe asthma; not to be used within 5 minutes of use of thiomersal-containing preparations; manufacturer advises avoid in pregnancy and in breast-feeding

Side-effects: brown pigmentation particularly in those with mixed coloured irides (withdraw treatment if possible); ocular irritation; conjunctival hyperaemia; transient punctate epithelial erosions; macular oedema reported rarely

Administration: apply 1 drop once daily, preferably in the evening

▼ PoM **Xalatan®** (Pharmacia & Upjohn)

Eye-drops, latanoprost 50 micrograms/mL, net price 2.5 mL = £16.00
Additives: include benzalkonium chloride

11.7 Local anaesthetics

Oxybuprocaine and amethocaine are probably the most widely used topical local anaesthetics. Proxymetacaine causes less initial stinging and is useful for children. Oxybuprocaine or a combined preparation of lignocaine and fluorescein is used for tonometry. Amethocaine produces a more profound anaesthesia and is suitable for use before minor surgical procedures, such as the removal of corneal sutures. It has a temporary disruptive effect on the corneal epithelium. Lignocaine, with or without adrenaline, is injected into the eyelids for minor surgery, while retrobulbar or peribulbar injections are used for surgery of the globe itself. Local anaesthetics should never be used for the management of ocular symptoms.

AMETHOCAINE HYDROCHLORIDE
Indications: local anaesthetic

PoM **Amethocaine** (Non-proprietary)

Eye drops, amethocaine hydrochloride 0.5%, net price, 10 mL = £3.22; 1%, 10 mL = £3.61
Available from Martindale

Single use
PoM **Minims® Amethocaine Hydrochloride** (Chauvin)

Eye drops, amethocaine hydrochloride 0.5 and 1%. Net price 20 × 0.5 mL (both) = £5.75

LIGNOCAINE HYDROCHLORIDE
Indications: local anaesthetic

PoM **Minims® Lignocaine and Fluorescein** (Chauvin)

Eye drops, lignocaine hydrochloride 4%, fluorescein sodium 0.25%. Net price 20 × 0.5 mL = £6.93

OXYBUPROCAINE HYDROCHLORIDE
Indications: local anaesthetic

PoM **Minims® Benoxinate (Oxybuprocaine) Hydrochloride** (Chauvin)

Eye drops, oxybuprocaine hydrochloride 0.4%. Net price 20 × 0.5 mL = £4.92

PROXYMETACAINE HYDROCHLORIDE
Indications: local anaesthetic

PoM **Ophthaine®** (Squibb)

Eye drops, proxymetacaine hydrochloride 0.5%. Net price 15 mL = £4.49
Additives: include benzalkonium chloride, chlorbutol

Cautionary label wordings, see inside back cover

Prices are **net**, see p.1

Single use
PoM **Minims® Proxymetacaine Hydrochloride** (Chauvin)
Eye drops, proxymetacaine hydrochloride 0.5%. Net price 20 × 0.5 mL = £6.95

With fluorescein
PoM **Minims® Proxymetacaine and Fluorescein** (Chauvin)
Eye drops, proxymetacaine hydrochloride 0.5%, fluorescein sodium 0.25%. Net price 20 × 0.5 mL = £7.95

11.8   Miscellaneous ophthalmic preparations

11.8.1   Tear deficiency, ocular lubricants and astringents
11.8.2   Ocular diagnostic and peri-operative preparations

Certain eye drops, e.g. amphotericin, ceftazidime, cefuroxime, colistin, desferrioxamine, dexamethasone, gentamicin and vancomycin may be prepared aseptically from material supplied for injection; for details on preparation of trisodium edetate eye drops see section 9.5.1.2.

11.8.1   Tear deficiency, ocular lubricants and astringents

Chronically sore eyes associated with reduced tear secretion, usually in cases of rheumatoid arthritis (Sjögren's syndrome), often respond to hypromellose eye drops and mucolytic agents.

Sodium chloride 0.9% drops are sometimes used for relieving symptoms due to tear film deficiency and as 'comfort drops' by contact lens wearers to facilitate lens removal.

Simple eye ointment is a bland sterile preparation which may be used to soften crusts in blepharitis or as a bland lubricant at night; it is also used to protect the ocular surface.

Zinc sulphate is a traditional astringent which has been used in eye drops for treatment of excessive lacrimation.

ACETYLCYSTEINE
Indications: tear deficiency, impaired or abnormal mucus production
Administration: apply eye drops 3–4 times daily

PoM **Ilube®** (Alcon)
Eye drops, acetylcysteine 5%, hypromellose 0.35%. Net price 10 mL = £4.63
Additives: include benzalkonium chloride, disodium edetate

CARBOMERS
(Polyacrylic acid)
Synthetic high molecular weight polymers of acrylic acid cross-linked with either allyl ethers of sucrose or allyl ethers of pentaerythritol

Indications: dry eyes including keratoconjunctivitis sicca, unstable tear film
Administration: apply 3–4 times daily or as required

GelTears (Chauvin)
Gel (= eye drops), carbomer 940 (polyacrylic acid) 0.2%. Net price 10 g = £2.90
Additives: include benzalkonium chloride
Viscotears® (CIBA Vision)
Liquid gel (= eye drops), carbomer 940 (polyacrylic acid) 0.2%. Net price 10 g = £2.95
Additives: include cetrimide, disodium edetate

HYDROXYETHYLCELLULOSE
Indications: tear deficiency

Minims® Artificial Tears (Chauvin)
Eye drops, hydroxyethylcellulose 0.44%. Net price 20 × 0.5 mL = £5.75

HYPROMELLOSE
Indications: tear deficiency

Hypromellose (Non-proprietary)
Eye drops, hypromellose 0.3%. Net price 10 mL = 54p
Available from Cox, Martindale, Norton
Isopto Alkaline® (Alcon)
Eye drops, hypromellose 1%. Net price 10 mL = 99p
Additives: include benzalkonium chloride
Isopto Plain® (Alcon)
Eye drops, hypromellose 0.5%. Net price 10 mL = 85p
Additives: include benzalkonium chloride
Moisture-eyes® (Co-Pharma)
Eye drops, hypromellose 0.3% (buffered). Net price 10 mL = £1.13
Additives: include benzalkonium chloride
Tears Naturale® (Alcon)
Eye drops, dextran '70' 0.1%, hypromellose 0.3%. Net price 15 mL = £1.68
Additives: include benzalkonium chloride, disodium edetate

With phenylephrine
Isopto Frin® (Alcon)
Eye drops, phenylephrine hydrochloride 0.12%, hypromellose 0.5%. Net price 10 mL = £1.14
Additives: include benzethonium chloride

LIQUID PARAFFIN
Indications: dry eye conditions

Lacri-Lube® (Allergan)
Eye ointment, white soft paraffin 57.3%, liquid paraffin 42.5%, wool alcohols 0.2%. Net price 3.5 g = £1.99, 5 g = £2.59
Lubri-Tears® (Alcon)
Eye ointment, white soft paraffin 60%, liquid paraffin 30%, wool fat 10%. Net price 5 g = £2.29

PARAFFIN, YELLOW, SOFT
Indications: see notes above

Simple Eye Ointment, liquid paraffin 10%, wool fat 10%, in yellow soft paraffin. Net price 4 g = £1.99
Available from Martindale

POLYVINYL ALCOHOL
Indications: tear deficiency

Hypotears® (CIBA Vision)
Eye drops, macrogol '8000' 2%, polyvinyl alcohol 1%. Net price 15 mL = £1.09
Additives: include benzalkonium chloride, disodium edetate
Liquifilm Tears® (Allergan)
Ophthalmic solution (= eye drops), polyvinyl alcohol 1.4%. Net price 15 mL = £1.69
Additives: include benzalkonium chloride, disodium edetate
Preservative-free ophthalmic solution (= eye drops), polyvinyl alcohol 1.4%, povidone 0.6%. Net price 30 × 0.4 mL = £5.60
Sno Tears® (Chauvin)
Eye drops, polyvinyl alcohol 1.4%. Net price 10 mL = £1.10
Additives: include benzalkonium chloride, disodium edetate

SODIUM CHLORIDE
Indications: irrigation, including first-aid removal of harmful substances; intra-ocular or topical irrigation during surgical procedures

Sodium Chloride 0.9% Solutions
See section 13.11.1
Balanced Salt Solution
Solution (sterile), sodium chloride 0.64%, sodium acetate 0.39%, sodium citrate 0.17%, calcium chloride 0.048%, magnesium chloride 0.03%, potassium chloride 0.075%.
Available from Alcon (15 mL and 30 mL) and from CIBA Vision (*Iocare®,* 15 mL and 500 mL)

Single use
Minims® Sodium Chloride (Chauvin)
Eye drops, sodium chloride 0.9%. Net price 20 × 0.5 mL = £4.92

ZINC SULPHATE
Indications; Cautions: see notes above

Zinc Sulphate (Non-proprietary)
Eye drops, zinc sulphate 0.25%. Net price 10 mL = £2.43
Available from Martindale

11.8.2 Ocular diagnostic and peri-operative preparations

OCULAR DIAGNOSTIC PREPARATIONS

Fluorescein sodium and **rose bengal** are used in diagnostic procedures and for locating damaged areas of the cornea due to injury or disease. Rose bengal is much more efficient for the diagnosis of conjunctival epithelial damage but it stings excessively unless a local anaesthetic is instilled beforehand.

FLUORESCEIN SODIUM
Indications: detection of lesions and foreign bodies

Minims® Fluorescein Sodium (Chauvin)
Eye drops, fluorescein sodium 1 or 2%. Net price 20 × 0.5 mL (both) = £4.92

With local anaesthetic
Section 11.7

ROSE BENGAL
Indications: detection of lesions and foreign bodies

Minims® Rose Bengal (Chauvin)
Eye drops, rose bengal 1%. Net price 20 × 0.5 mL = £5.75

OCULAR PERI-OPERATIVE DRUGS

Drugs used to prepare the eye for surgery and drugs that are injected into the anterior chamber at the time of surgery are included here.
Special presentations of **sodium chloride 0.9%** solution are used routinely in intra-ocular surgery (section 11.8.1).

ACETYLCHOLINE CHLORIDE
Indications: cataract surgery, penetrating keratoplasty, iridectomy, and other anterior segment surgery requiring rapid complete miosis

PoM **Miochol®** (CIBA Vision)
Solution for intra-ocular irrigation, acetylcholine chloride 1%, mannitol 3% when reconstituted. Net price 2 mL-vial = £8.32

APRACLONIDINE
Note. Apraclonidine is a derivative of clonidine
Indications; Administration: control of intra-ocular pressure, see under preparations below
Cautions: history of angina, severe coronary insufficiency, recent myocardial infarction, cardiac failure, cerebrovascular disease, vasovagal attack, chronic renal failure; depression; pregnancy and breast-feeding; monitor intra-ocular pressure and visual fields; loss of effect may occur over time; suspend treatment if reduction in vision occurs in end-stage glaucoma; exaggerated reduction in intra-ocular pressure following peri-operative use should be closely monitored; **interactions:** Appendix 1 (alpha$_2$-adrenoceptor stimulants)
DRIVING. Drowsiness may affect performance of skilled tasks (e.g. driving)
Contra-indications: history of severe or unstable and uncontrolled cardiovascular disease

Side-effects: dry mouth, taste disturbance; hyperaemia, ocular pruritus, discomfort and tearing (withdraw if ocular intolerance including oedema of lids and conjunctiva); headache, asthenia, dry nose; lid retraction, conjunctival blanching and mydriasis reported after peri-operative use; since absorption may follow topical application systemic effects (see Clonidine Hydrochloride, section 2.5.2) may occur

PoM **Iopidine®** (Alcon)
Ophthalmic solution (= eye drops), apraclonidine 1% (as hydrochloride). Net price 12 × 2 single use 0.25-mL units = £81.90
Administration: control or prevention of postoperative elevation of intra-ocular pressure after anterior segment laser surgery, apply 1 drop 1 hour before laser procedure then 1 drop immediately after completion of procedure; CHILD not recommended
Iopidine 0.5% ophthalmic solution (= eye drops), apraclonidine 0.5% (as hydrochloride). Net price 5 mL = £11.45
Administration: short-term adjunctive treatment of chronic glaucoma in patients not adequately controlled by another drug (see note below), apply 1 drop 3 times daily usually for max. 1 month; CHILD not recommended
Note. May not provide additional benefit if patient already using two drugs that suppress the production of aqueous humour

CHYMOTRYPSIN
Indications: zonulolysis in intracapsular cataract extraction

PoM **Zonulysin®** (Henleys)
Injection, powder for reconstitution, alphachymotrypsin 300 USP units (≡ 1.5 microkatals). Net price per vial (with diluent) = £9.47

DICLOFENAC SODIUM
Indications: inhibition of intraoperative miosis during cataract surgery (but does not possess intrinsic mydriatic properties); postoperative inflammation in cataract surgery; pain in corneal epithelial defects after photorefractive keratectomy

PoM **Voltarol® Ophtha** (CIBA Vision)
Eye drops, diclofenac sodium 0.1%. Net price pack of 5 single-dose units = £4.99, 40 single-dose units = £39.90

FLURBIPROFEN SODIUM
Indications: inhibition of intraoperative miosis (but does not possess intrinsic mydriatic properties); anterior segment inflammation following postoperative and post-laser trabeculoplasty when corticosteroids contra-indicated

PoM **Ocufen®** (Allergan)
Ophthalmic solution (= eye drops), flurbiprofen sodium 0.03%, polyvinyl alcohol (Liquifilm®) 1.4%. Net price 40 × 0.4 mL = £38.90

KETOROLAC TROMETAMOL
Indications: prophylaxis and reduction of inflammation and associated symptoms following ocular surgery

▼ PoM **Acular®** (Allergan)
Eye drops, ketorolac trometamol 0.5%. Net price 5 mL = £6.99
Additives: include benzalkonium chloride, disodium edetate

SODIUM HYALURONATE
A visco-elastic polymer normally present in the aqueous and vitreous humour
Indications: used during surgical procedures on the eye
Side-effects: occasional hypersensitivity (avian origin); occasional transient rise in intra-ocular pressure

PoM **Healonid®** (Pharmacia & Upjohn)
Injection, sodium hyaluronate 10 mg/mL in disposable syringes, net price 0.5 mL = £44.87, 0.85 mL = £67.24; 14 mg/mL (Healonid® GV), 0.55 mL = £71.70
PoM **Ophthalin®** (CIBA Vision)
Injection, sodium hyaluronate 1% (10 mg/mL) in disposable syringe, net price 1 mL = £57.00; 1.5% (15 mg/mL) (Ophthalin® Plus), 1 mL = £65.00

11.9   Contact lenses

Note. Some recommendations in this section involve non-licensed indications.

For cosmetic reasons many people prefer to wear contact lenses rather than spectacles; contact lenses are also sometimes required for medical indications. Visual defects are corrected by either rigid ('hard' or gas permeable) lenses or soft (hydrogel) lenses; soft lenses are the most popular type, because they are the most comfortable, though they may not give the best vision. Lenses should usually be worn for a specified number of hours each day. Continuous (extended) wear involves much greater risks to eye health and is not recommended except where medically indicated.

Contact lenses require meticulous care. Poor compliance with directions for use, and with daily cleaning and disinfection, may result in complications which include ulcerative keratitis, conjunctival problems (such as purulent or papillary conjunctivitis).

Acanthamoeba keratitis, a sight-threatening condition, is associated with ineffective lens cleaning and disinfection or the use of contaminated lens cases. The condition is especially associated with the use of soft lenses (including disposable lenses). Acanthamoeba keratitis is treated by specialists with intensive use of polyhexanide (polyhexamethylene biguanide), propamidine isethionate, chlorhexidine and neomycin drops, sometimes in combination.

CONTACT LENSES AND DRUG TREATMENT. Special care is required in prescribing eye preparations for contact lens users. Some drugs and preservatives in eye preparations can accumulate in hydrogel lenses and may induce toxic reactions. Therefore, unless medically indicated, the lenses should be removed before instillation and not worn during the period of treatment. Alternatively, unpreserved drops can be used. Ointment preparations should never be used in conjunction with contact lens wear.

Many drugs given systemically can also have adverse effects on contact lens wear. These include oral contraceptives (particularly those with a higher oestrogen content), drugs which reduce blink rate (e.g. anxiolytics, hypnotics, antihistamines, and muscle relaxants), drugs which reduce tear production (e.g. antihistamines, antimuscarinics, phenothiazines and related drugs, some beta-blockers, diuretics, and tricyclic antidepressants), and drugs which increase lacrimation (including ephedrine and hydralazine). Other drugs that may affect contact lens wear are isotretinoin (may cause conjunctival inflammation), primidone (may cause ocular or eyelid oedema), aspirin (salicylic acid appears in tears and may be absorbed by contact lenses—leading to irritation), and rifampicin and sulphasalazine (may discolour lenses).

 Prices are **net**, see p.1

12: Drugs used in the treatment of diseases of the
EAR, NOSE, and OROPHARYNX

In this chapter, drug treatment is discussed under the following headings:

12.1   Drugs acting on the ear
12.2   Drugs acting on the nose
12.3   Drugs acting on the oropharynx

12.1   Drugs acting on the ear

12.1.1 Otitis externa
12.1.2 Otitis media
12.1.3 Removal of ear wax

12.1.1   Otitis externa

Otitis externa is an inflammatory reaction of the meatal skin. It is important to exclude an underlying chronic otitis media before treatment is commenced. Many cases recover after thorough cleansing of the external ear canal by suction, dry mopping, or gentle syringing. A frequent problem in resistant cases is the difficulty in applying lotions and ointments satisfactorily to the relatively inaccessible affected skin. The most effective method is to introduce a ribbon gauze dressing soaked with **corticosteroid** ear drops or with an astringent such as **aluminium acetate** solution. When this is not practical, the ear should be gently cleansed with a probe covered in cotton wool and the patient encouraged to lie with the affected ear uppermost for ten minutes after the canal has been filled with a liberal quantity of the appropriate solution.

If infection is present, a topical anti-infective which is not used systemically (such as **neomycin** or **clioquinol**) may be used, but for only about a week as excessive use may result in fungal infections; these may be difficult to treat and require expert advice. Sensitivity to the anti-infective or solvent may occur and resistance to antibacterials is a possibility with prolonged use. **Chloramphenicol** may also be used but the ear drops contain propylene glycol and cause sensitivity in about 10% of patients (the eye ointment can be used instead [unlicensed indication]). Solutions containing an anti-infective and a corticosteroid (such as *Locorten-Vioform®*) are used for treating cases where infection is present with inflammation and eczema. In view of reports of ototoxicity in patients with a perforated tympanic membrane (eardrum), the CSM has issued a reminder that treatment with a topical aminoglycoside antibiotic is contra-indicated in those with a tympanic perforation. However, many specialists do use these drops cautiously in patients with a perforation (section 12.1.2).

An acute infection may cause severe pain and a systemic antibiotic is required with a simple analgesic such as paracetamol. When a resistant staphylococcal infection (a boil) is present in the external auditory meatus, **flucloxacillin** is the drug of choice (section 5.1, table 1).

The skin of the pinna adjacent to the ear canal is often affected by eczema. Topical corticosteroid creams and ointments (see section 13.4) are then required, but prolonged use should be avoided.

ASTRINGENT PREPARATIONS

ALUMINIUM ACETATE

Indications: inflammation in otitis externa (see notes above)

Aluminium Acetate Ear drops (13%) consists of aluminium acetate solution, BP.

Insert into the meatus or apply on a gauze wick which should be kept saturated with the ear drops

Available from manufacturers of 'special order' products

Aluminium Acetate Ear drops (8%)

Prepared by diluting 8 parts of aluminium acetate solution, BP, with 5 parts of purified water, freshly boiled and cooled; it must be freshly prepared. Directions as above

ANTI-INFLAMMATORY PREPARATIONS

BETAMETHASONE SODIUM PHOSPHATE

Indications: eczematous inflammation in otitis externa (see notes above)

Cautions: avoid prolonged use

Contra-indications: untreated infection

Side-effects: local sensitivity reactions

PoM **Betnesol®** (Evans)

Drops (for ear, eye, or nose), betamethasone sodium phosphate 0.1%. Net price 10 mL = £1.31

Additives: include benzalkonium chloride

Ear, apply 2–3 drops every 2–3 hours; reduce frequency when relief obtained; *eye,* see section 11.4.1; *nose,* see section 12.2.1

PoM **Vista-Methasone®** (Martindale)

Drops (for ear, eye, or nose), betamethasone sodium phosphate 0.1%. Net price 5 mL = £1.15; 10 mL = £1.31

Additives: include benzalkonium chloride

Ear, apply 2–3 drops every 3–4 hours; reduce frequency when relief obtained; *eye,* see section 11.4.1; *nose,* see section 12.2.1

With antibacterial

PoM **Betnesol-N®** (Evans)

Drops (for ear, eye, or nose), betamethasone sodium phosphate 0.1%, neomycin sulphate 0.5%. Net price 10 mL = £1.35

Additives: include benzalkonium chloride

Ear, apply 2–3 drops 3–4 times daily; *eye,* see section 11.4.1; *nose,* section 12.2.3

PoM **Vista-Methasone N®** (Martindale)

Drops (for ear, eye, or nose), betamethasone sodium phosphate 0.1%, neomycin sulphate 0.5%. Net price 5 mL = £1.23; 10 mL = £1.35

Additives: include thiomersal

Ear, apply 2–3 drops every 3–4 hours; reduce frequency when relief obtained; *eye,* see section 11.4.1; *nose,* section 12.2.3

DEXAMETHASONE

Indications: eczematous inflammation in otitis externa (see notes above)

Cautions: avoid prolonged use

Contra-indications: untreated infection

Side-effects: local sensitivity reactions

With antibacterial

PoM **Otomize®** (Stafford-Miller)

Ear spray, dexamethasone 0.1%, neomycin sulphate 3250 units/mL, glacial acetic acid 2%. Net price 5-mL pump-action aerosol unit = £3.85

Apply 1 metered spray into the ear 3 times daily

PoM **Sofradex®** (Hoechst Marion Roussel)

Drops (for ear or eye), dexamethasone (as sodium metasulphobenzoate) 0.05%, framycetin sulphate 0.5%, gramicidin 0.005%. Net price 10 mL = £5.46

Ear, apply 2–3 drops 3–4 times daily; *eye,* see section 11.4.1

Ointment (for ear or eye), dexamethasone 0.05%, framycetin sulphate 0.5%, gramicidin 0.005%. Net price 5 g = £3.90

Ear, apply 1–2 times daily; *eye,* see section 11.4.1

FLUMETHASONE PIVALATE

(Flumetasone Pivalate)

Indications: eczematous inflammation in otitis externa (see notes above)

Cautions: avoid prolonged use

Contra-indications: untreated infection

Side-effects: local sensitivity reactions

With antibacterial

PoM **Locorten-Vioform®** (Novartis Consumer Health)

Ear drops, flumethasone pivalate 0.02%, clioquinol 1%. Net price 7.5 mL = £1.02

Apply 2–3 drops into the ear twice daily for up to 7–10 days; not recommended for child under 2 years

HYDROCORTISONE

Indications: eczematous inflammation in otitis externa (see notes above)

Cautions: avoid prolonged use

Contra-indications: untreated infection

Side-effects: local sensitivity reactions

With antibacterial

PoM **Gentisone HC®** (Roche)

Ear drops, hydrocortisone acetate 1%, gentamicin 0.3% (as sulphate). Net price 10 mL = £4.16

Additives: include benzalkonium chloride

Apply 2–4 drops into the ear 3–4 times daily and at night

PoM **Neo-Cortef®** (Dominion)

Drops (for ear or eye), hydrocortisone acetate 1.5%, neomycin sulphate 0.5%. Net price 10 mL = £4.30

Additives: include miripirium chloride (myristyl-gamma-picolinium chloride)

Ear, apply 2–3 drops 3–4 times daily; *eye,* see section 11.4.1

Ointment (for ear or eye), hydrocortisone acetate 1.5%, neomycin sulphate 0.5%. Net price 3.9 g = £1.60

Ear, apply 1–2 times daily; *eye,* see section 11.4.1

PoM **Otosporin®** (GlaxoWellcome)

Ear drops, hydrocortisone 1%, neomycin sulphate 3400 units, polymyxin B sulphate 10 000 units/mL. Net price 5 mL = £2.15; 10 mL = £4.30

Apply 3 drops into the ear 3–4 times daily

PREDNISOLONE SODIUM PHOSPHATE

Indications: eczematous inflammation in otitis externa (see notes above)

Cautions: avoid prolonged use

Contra-indications: untreated infection

Side-effects: local sensitivity reactions

PoM **Predsol®** (Evans)

Drops (for ear or eye), prednisolone sodium phosphate 0.5%. Net price 10 mL = £1.31

Additives: include benzalkonium chloride

Ear, apply 2–3 drops every 2–3 hours; reduce frequency when relief obtained; *eye,* see section 11.4.1

With antibacterial

PoM **Predsol-N®** (Evans)

Drops (for ear or eye), prednisolone sodium phosphate 0.5%, neomycin sulphate 0.5%. Net price 10 mL = £1.20

Additives: include benzalkonium chloride

Ear, apply 2–3 drops 3–4 times daily; *eye,* see section 11.4.1

TRIAMCINOLONE ACETONIDE

Indications: eczematous inflammation in otitis externa (see notes above)

Cautions: avoid prolonged use

Contra-indications: untreated infection

Side-effects: local sensitivity reactions

With antibacterial

PoM **Audicort®** (Wyeth)

Ear drops, triamcinolone acetonide 0.1%, neomycin (as neomycin undecenoate) 0.35%. Net price 10 mL = £4.30

Apply 2–5 drops into the ear 3–4 times daily; CHILD not recommended

PoM **Tri-Adcortyl Otic®** (Squibb)

Ear ointment, triamcinolone acetonide 0.1%, gramicidin 0.025%, neomycin 0.25% (as sulphate), nystatin 100 000 units/g in *Plastibase®*. Net price 10 g = £1.58

Apply into the ear 2–4 times daily

ANTI-INFECTIVE PREPARATIONS

CHLORAMPHENICOL

Indications: bacterial infection in otitis externa (but see notes above)
Cautions: avoid prolonged use (see notes above)
Side-effects: high incidence of sensitivity reactions to vehicle

PoM **Chloramphenicol** (Non-proprietary)
Ear drops, chloramphenicol 5% in propylene glycol. Net price 10 mL = £1.33
Apply 2–3 drops into the ear 2–3 times daily

CLIOQUINOL

Indications: mild bacterial or fungal infections in otitis externa (see notes above)
Cautions: avoid prolonged use (see notes above)
Contra-indications: perforated tympanic membrane
Side-effects: local sensitivity; stains skin and clothing

With corticosteroid
PoM **Locorten-Vioform®,** see Flumethasone (p. 465)

CLOTRIMAZOLE

Indications: fungal infection in otitis externa (see notes above)
Side-effects: occasional local irritation or sensitivity

Canesten® (Baypharm)
Solution, clotrimazole 1% in polyethylene glycol (macrogol 400). Net price 20 mL = £2.32
Ear, apply 2–3 times daily continuing for at least 14 days after disappearance of infection; *skin,* see section 13.10.2

FRAMYCETIN SULPHATE

Indications; Cautions; Side-effects: see under Gentamicin

With corticosteroid
PoM **Sofradex®,** see Dexamethasone (p. 465)

GENTAMICIN

Indications: bacterial infection in otitis externa (see notes above)
Cautions; Contra-indications: avoid prolonged use; slight risk of ototoxicity increased if perforated eardrum (see notes above); pregnancy and breast-feeding
Side-effects: local sensitivity

PoM **Cidomycin®** (Hoechst Marion Roussel)
Drops (for ear or eye), gentamicin 0.3% (as sulphate). Net price 8 mL = £1.31
Additives: include benzalkonium chloride, disodium edetate
Ear, apply 2–4 drops 3–4 times daily and at night; *eye,* see section 11.3.1

PoM **Garamycin®** (Schering-Plough)
Drops (for ear or eye), gentamicin 0.3% (as sulphate). Net price 10 mL = £1.79
Additives: include benzalkonium chloride
Ear, apply 3–4 drops 3–4 times daily; reduce frequency when relief obtained; *eye,* see section 11.3.1
PoM **Genticin®** (Roche)
Drops (for ear or eye), gentamicin 0.3% (as sulphate). Net price 10 mL = £2.00
Additives: include benzalkonium chloride
Ear, apply 2–3 drops 3–4 times daily and at night; *eye,* see section 11.3.1

With corticosteroid
PoM **Gentisone HC®,** see Hydrocortisone (p. 465)

NEOMYCIN SULPHATE

Indications: bacterial infection in otitis externa (see notes above)
Cautions; Contra-indications: avoid prolonged use (see notes above); slight risk of ototoxicity increased if perforated eardrum (see notes above)
Side-effects: local sensitivity

With corticosteroid
PoM **Audicort®,** see Triamcinolone (p. 465)
PoM **Betnesol-N®,** see Betamethasone (p. 464)
PoM **Neo-Cortef®,** see Hydrocortisone (p. 465)
PoM **Otomize®,** see Dexamethasone (p. 465)
PoM **Otosporin®,** see Hydrocortisone (p. 465)
PoM **Predsol-N®,** see Prednisolone (p. 465)
PoM **Tri-Adcortyl Otic®,** see Triamcinolone (p. 465)
PoM **Vista-Methasone N®,** see Betamethasone (p. 464)

OTHER AURAL PREPARATIONS

Choline salicylate is a mild analgesic but it is of doubtful value when applied topically. There is no place for the use of local anaesthetics in ear drops.

NHS **Audax®** (Seton)
Ear drops, choline salicylate 20%, glycerol 12.6%. Net price 10 mL = £2.10

12.1.2   Otitis media

Acute otitis media is the commonest cause of severe pain in small children and recurrent attacks, especially in infants, are particularly distressing. *Otitis media with effusion* ('glue ear') is present in about 10% of the child population and in 90% of children with cleft palates; this condition should be referred to hospital because of the risk of permanent damage to middle ear function and impaired language development. Chronic otitis media is thought to be a legacy of untreated or resistant cases of otitis media with effusion.

Local treatment of *acute otitis media* is ineffective and there is no place for drops containing a local anaesthetic. Many attacks are viral in origin and need only treatment with a **simple analgesic** such as paracetamol for pain. Severe attacks of bacterial origin should be treated with **systemic antibiotics**; bacterial examination of any discharge is helpful in selecting the appropriate treatment (section 5.1, table 1). Again, simple analgesics such as paracetamol are used to relieve pain. In *recurrent* *acute otitis media* a daily dose of a prophylactic antibiotic (trimethoprim or erythromycin) during the winter months can be tried.

The organisms recovered from patients with *chronic otitis media* are often opportunists living in the debris, keratin, and necrotic bone present in the middle ear and mastoid. Thorough cleansing with an aural suction tube may completely control infection of many years duration. Acute exacerbations of chronic infection may require systemic antibiotics (section 5.1, table 1). A swab should be taken to determine the organism present and its antibiotic sensitivity. Unfortunately the culture often produces *Pseudomonas aeruginosa* and *Proteus* spp, sensitive only to parenteral antibiotics. Local debridement of the meatal and middle ear contents may then be followed by topical treatment with ribbon gauze dressings as for otitis externa (section 12.1.1). This is particularly true with infections in mastoid cavities when dusting powders can also be tried.

The CSM has issued a reminder (section 12.1.1) that topical treatment with ototoxic antibiotics is contra-indicated in the presence of a perforation. However, many specialists use ear drops containing **aminoglycosides** (e.g. neomycin) or **polymyxins** if the otitis media has failed to settle with systemic antibiotics; it is considered that the pus in the middle ear associated with otitis media carries a higher risk of ototoxicity than the drops themselves.

12.1.3   Removal of ear wax

Wax is a normal bodily secretion which provides a protective film on the meatal skin and need only be removed if it causes deafness or interferes with a proper view of the ear drum. As a general rule syringing is best avoided in patients with a history of recurring otitis externa, a perforated ear drum, or previous ear surgery. A person who has hearing only in one ear should not have that ear syringed because even a very slight risk of damage is unacceptable in this situation.

Wax may be removed by syringing with warm water. If necessary, wax can be softened with simple remedies such as **olive oil** or **almond oil** before syringing. The patient should lie with the affected ear uppermost for 5 to 10 minutes after a generous amount of the solution has been introduced into the ear. Some proprietary preparations containing organic solvents can cause irritation of the meatal skin, and in most cases the simple remedies which are indicated above are just as effective and less likely to cause irritation. **Docusate sodium** is an ingredient in a number of proprietary preparations.

Almond Oil
Allow to warm to room temperature before use
Olive Oil
Allow to warm to room temperature before use
Sodium Bicarbonate Ear Drops, BP
Ear drops, sodium bicarbonate 5%
  Extemporaneous preparations should be recently prepared according to the following formula: sodium bicarbonate 500 mg, glycerol 3 mL, freshly boiled and cooled purified water to 10 mL

Cerumol® (LAB)
Ear drops, chlorbutol 5%, paradichlorobenzene 2%, arachis (peanut) oil 57.3%. Net price 11 mL = £1.35
Exterol® (Dermal)
Ear drops, urea-hydrogen peroxide complex 5% in glycerol. Net price 8 mL = £1.97
Molcer® (Wallace Mfg)
Ear drops, docusate sodium 5%. Net price 15 mL = £1.32
Otex® (DDD)
Ear drops, urea hydrogen peroxide 5%. Net price 8 mL = £2.45
Waxsol® (Norgine)
Ear drops, docusate sodium 0.5%. Net price 10 mL = 95p

12.2   Drugs acting on the nose

12.2.1   Drugs used in nasal allergy
12.2.2   Topical nasal decongestants
12.2.3   Anti-infective nasal preparations

Rhinitis is often self-limiting and sinusitis is best treated with systemic antibiotics (section 5.1, table 1). There are few indications for nasal sprays and drops except in allergic rhinitis (section 12.2.1). Many nasal preparations contain sympathomimetic drugs which may damage the nasal cilia (section 12.2.2). Douching the nose with salt and water is **not** recommended for the treatment of chronic rhinitis. However some ENT departments use saline sniffs for a short period after endonasal surgery.

NASAL POLYPS. Short-term use of corticosteroid nasal drops helps to produce significant shrinkage of nasal polyps; to be effective, the drops must be administered with the patient in the 'head down' position. The reduction in swelling can be maintained by continuing treatment with a corticosteroid nasal spray.

12.2.1   Drugs used in nasal allergy

Mild cases of allergic rhinitis are controlled by **oral antihistamines** (section 3.4.1), **systemic nasal decongestants** are of doubtful value (section 3.10).

More persistent symptoms and nasal congestion can be relieved by topical preparations of **corticosteroids** (beclometasone, betamethasone, budesonide, flunisolide, fluticasone, mometasone and triamcinolone) and **cromoglycate** and **nedocromil**; topical antihistamines (azelastine and levocabastine) are also used in allergic rhinitis. In seasonal allergic rhinitis (e.g. hay fever), treatment should begin 2 to 3 weeks before the season commences and may have to be continued for several months; treatment may be required for years in perennial rhinitis.

In allergic rhinitis, topical preparations of corticosteroids and cromoglycate have a well-established role; although it may be less effective, cromoglycate is often the first choice in children. Topical antihistamines are considered less effective than topical corticosteroids but probably more effective than cromoglycate.

Very disabling symptoms occasionally justify the use of **systemic corticosteroids** for short periods (section 6.3), for example in students taking important examinations. They may also be used at the beginning of a course of treatment with a corticosteroid spray to relieve severe mucosal oedema and allow the spray to penetrate the nasal cavity.

ANTIHISTAMINES

AZELASTINE HYDROCHLORIDE

Indications: allergic rhinitis
Side-effects: irritation of nasal mucosa; taste disturbance

PoM ¹**Rhinolast**® (ASTA Medica)

Aqueous nasal spray, azelastine hydrochloride 140 micrograms (0.14 mL)/metered spray. Net price 20 mL (with metered pump) = £12.48

ADULT and CHILD over 5 years, apply 140 micrograms (1 spray) into each nostril twice daily

1. Can be sold to the public for nasal administration in aqueous form (other than by aerosol) if supplied for the treatment of seasonal allergic rhinitis in adults and children over 12 years, subject to max. single dose of 140 micrograms per nostril, max. daily dose of 280 micrograms per nostril, and a pack size limit of 36 doses; a proprietary brand (*Rhinolast*® *Hayfever*) is on sale to the public

LEVOCABASTINE

Indications: treatment of allergic rhinitis
Cautions: renal impairment (see Appendix 3)
Side-effects: nasal irritation; headache, fatigue, somnolence reported

▼ PoM **Livostin**® (CIBA Vision)

Aqueous nasal spray, levocabastine (as hydrochloride) 0.05%. Net price 10-mL spray pump = £8.90

ADULT and CHILD over 9 years, apply 2 sprays into each nostril twice daily for no more than 4 weeks, increased if necessary to 3–4 times daily

CORTICOSTEROIDS

Nasal sprays containing corticosteroids have a useful role in the prophylaxis and treatment of allergic rhinitis (see notes above).

CAUTIONS. Corticosteroid nasal sprays should be avoided in the presence of untreated nasal infections, and also after nasal surgery (until healing has occurred); they should also be avoided in pulmonary tuberculosis. Patients transferred from systemic corticosteroids may experience exacerbation of some symptoms.

SIDE-EFFECTS. Local side-effects include dryness, irritation of nose and throat, epistaxis and rarely ulceration; rarely, nasal septal perforation (usually following nasal surgery) and raised intra-ocular pressure may occur. Taste disturbance may also occur, particularly if the nasal spray is swallowed. Hypersensitivity reactions, including bronchospasm, have been reported.

BECLOMETHASONE DIPROPIONATE

(Beclometasone Dipropionate)
Indications: prophylaxis and treatment of allergic and vasomotor rhinitis
Cautions: see notes above
Side-effects: see notes above

PoM ¹**Beclomethasone** (Non-proprietary)

Nasal spray, beclomethasone dipropionate 50 micrograms/metered spray. Net price 200-spray unit = £4.56

Available from Ashbourne (*Zonivent*®), Baker Norton (*Nasobec Aqueous*®), Bartholomew Rhodes

1. Can be sold to the public for nasal administration (other than by aerosol) if supplied for the prevention and treatment of seasonal allergic rhinitis in adults and children over 12 years subject to max. single dose of 100 micrograms per nostril, max. daily dose of 200 micrograms per nostril, and a pack size limit of 200 doses; proprietary brands on sale to the public include *Beconase*® *Hayfever,* *Boots Hayfever Relief*®, *Nasobec*® *Hayfever*

PoM **Beconase**® (A&H)

Nasal spray (aqueous suspension), beclomethasone dipropionate 50 micrograms/metered spray. Net price 200-spray unit with applicator = £5.01

ADULT and CHILD over 6 years, apply 100 micrograms (2 sprays) into each nostril twice daily *or* 50 micrograms (1 spray) into each nostril 3–4 times daily; max. total 400 micrograms (8 sprays) daily

BETAMETHASONE SODIUM PHOSPHATE

Indications: non-infected inflammatory conditions of nose
Cautions: see notes above
Side-effects: see notes above

PoM **Betnesol**® (Evans)

Drops (for ear, eye, or nose), betamethasone sodium phosphate 0.1%. Net price 10 mL = £1.31
Additives: include benzalkonium chloride
Nose, apply 2–3 drops into each nostril 2–3 times daily; *ear,* section 12.1.1; *eye,* see section 11.4.1

PoM **Vista-Methasone**® (Martindale)

Drops (for ear, eye, or nose), betamethasone sodium phosphate 0.1%. Net price 5 mL = £1.15, 10 mL = £1.31
Additives: include benzalkonium chloride
Nose, apply 2–3 drops into each nostril twice daily; *ear,* section 12.1.1; *eye,* see section 11.4.1

BUDESONIDE

Indications: prophylaxis and treatment of allergic and vasomotor rhinitis; nasal polyps
Cautions: see notes above
Side-effects: see notes above

PoM **Rhinocort Aqua**® (Astra)

Nasal spray, budesonide 100 micrograms/metered spray. Net price 100-spray unit = £5.85
Rhinitis, ADULT and CHILD over 12 years, apply 200 micrograms (2 sprays) into each nostril once daily in the morning *or* 100 micrograms (1 spray) into each nostril twice daily; when control achieved reduce to 100 micrograms (1 spray) into each nostril once daily
Nasal polyps, ADULT and CHILD over 12 years, 100 micrograms (1 spray) into each nostril twice daily for up to 3 months

---

FLUNISOLIDE

Indications: prophylaxis and treatment of allergic rhinitis
Cautions: see notes above
Side-effects: see notes above

PoM **¹Syntaris®** (Roche)

Aqueous nasal spray, flunisolide 25 micrograms/metered spray. Net price 240-spray unit with pump and applicator = £5.50

ADULT, apply 50 micrograms (2 sprays) into each nostril twice daily, increased if necessary to max. 3 times daily then reduced for maintenance; CHILD over 5 years initially 25 micrograms (1 spray) into each nostril up to 3 times daily for no longer than 4 weeks of continuous treatment

1. Flunisolide non-pressurised nasal spray can be sold to the public (in max. pack size of 240 metered units) for the prevention and treatment (in adults and children of not less than 12 years) of seasonal allergic rhinitis, including hayfever; max. adult dose 50 micrograms per nostril and max. daily dose 100 micrograms per nostril (children 12–16 years max. 25 micrograms per nostril and max, daily dose 75 micrograms per nostril)

FLUTICASONE PROPIONATE

Indications: prophylaxis and treatment of allergic rhinitis
Cautions: see notes above
Side-effects: see notes above

PoM **Flixonase®** (A&H)

Aqueous nasal spray, fluticasone propionate 50 micrograms/metered spray. Net price 120-spray unit with applicator = £11.43

ADULT and CHILD over 12 years, apply 100 micrograms (2 sprays) into each nostril once daily, preferably in the morning, increased to twice daily if required; max. total 8 sprays daily; CHILD 4–11 years, 50 micrograms (1 spray) into each nostril once daily, increased to twice daily if required; max. total 4 sprays daily

MOMETASONE FUROATE

Indications: prophylaxis and treatment of allergic rhinitis
Cautions: see notes above
Side-effects: see notes above

▼ PoM **Nasonex®** (Schering-Plough)

Aqueous nasal spray, mometasone furoate 50 micrograms/metered spray. Net price 120-spray unit = £11.43

ADULT and CHILD over 12 years, apply 100 micrograms (2 sprays) into each nostril once daily, increased if necessary to max. 200 micrograms (4 sprays) into each nostril once daily; when control achieved reduce to 50 micrograms (1 spray) into each nostril once daily

TRIAMCINOLONE ACETONIDE

Indications: prophylaxis and treatment of allergic rhinitis
Cautions: see notes above
Side-effects: see notes above

▼ PoM **Nasacort®** (Rhône-Poulenc Rorer)

Aqueous nasal spray, triamcinolone acetonide 55 micrograms/metered spray. Net price 120-spray unit = £8.00

ADULT and CHILD over 12 years apply 110 micrograms (2 sprays) into each nostril once daily; when control achieved, reduce to 55 micrograms (1 spray) into each nostril once daily; CHILD 6–12 years, 55 micrograms (1 spray) into each nostril once daily

CROMOGLYCATE AND NEDOCROMIL

NEDOCROMIL SODIUM

Indications: prophylaxis and treatment of seasonal allergic rhinitis
Side-effects: mild nasal irritation; taste disturbance

PoM **Tilarin®** (Fisons)

Aqueous nasal spray, nedocromil sodium 1%. Net price 15 mL = £7.90

ADULT and CHILD over 12 years, apply 1 spray into each nostril 4 times daily; CHILD under 12 years not recommended

SODIUM CROMOGLYCATE

(Sodium Cromoglicate)
Indications: prophylaxis of allergic rhinitis
Side-effects: local irritation; rarely transient bronchospasm

Rynacrom® (Fisons)

4% aqueous nasal spray, sodium cromoglycate 4% (5.2 mg/squeeze). Net price 22 mL with pump = £10.13

Additives: include benzalkonium chloride
ADULT and CHILD, apply 1 squeeze into each nostril 3–4 times daily

Vividrin® (Pharma-Global)

Nasal spray, sodium cromoglycate 2%. Net price 15 mL = £5.45

Additives: include benzalkonium chloride
ADULT and CHILD, apply 1 spray into each nostril 4–6 times daily

With sympathomimetic
Rynacrom Compound® (Fisons)

Nasal spray, sodium cromoglycate 2% (2.6 mg/metered spray) and xylometazoline hydrochloride 0.025% (32.5 micrograms/metered spray). Net price 26 mL with pump = £7.51

Additives: include benzalkonium chloride
Apply 1 spray into each nostril 4 times daily
Note. A proprietary brand of sodium cromoglycate 2% and xylometazoline hydrochloride 0.025% (*Resiston One®*) is on sale to the public

12.2.2   Topical nasal decongestants

The nasal mucosa is sensitive to changes in atmospheric temperature and humidity and these alone may cause slight nasal congestion. The nose and nasal sinuses produce a litre of mucus in 24 hours and much of this finds its way silently into the stomach via the nasopharynx. Slight changes in the nasal airway, accompanied by an awareness of mucus passing along the nasopharynx causes some patients to be inaccurately diagnosed as suffering from chronic sinusitis. These symptoms are particularly noticeable in the later stages of the common cold. **Sodium chloride** 0.9% given as nasal drops may relieve nasal congestion by helping to liquefy mucous secretions. Corticosteroid nasal drops produce shrinkage of nasal polyps (section 12.2).

Symptomatic relief from the nasal congestion associated with vasomotor rhinitis and the common cold can be obtained by the short-term use (usually not longer than 7 days) of decongestant nasal drops and sprays. These all contain sympathomimetic drugs which exert their effect by vasoconstriction of the mucosal blood vessels which in turn reduces the thickness of the nasal mucosa. They are of limited value as they can give rise to a rebound phenomenon (rhinitis medicamentosa) as their effects wear off, due to a secondary vasodilatation with a subsequent temporary increase in nasal congestion. This in turn tempts the further use of the decongestant, leading to a vicious circle of events. **Ephedrine nasal drops** is the safest sympathomimetic preparation and can give relief for several hours. The more potent sympathomimetic drugs oxymetazoline, phenylephrine, and xylometazoline are more likely to cause a rebound effect. **All** of these preparations may cause a hypertensive crisis if used during treatment with a monoamine-oxidase inhibitor.

Non-allergic watery rhinorrhoea often responds well to treatment with **ipratropium bromide**.

Inhalations of **warm moist air** are useful in the treatment of symptoms of acute infective conditions, and the use of compounds containing volatile substances such as menthol and eucalyptus may encourage their use (section 3.8). There is no evidence that nasal preparations containing antihistamines and anti-infective agents have any therapeutic effect.

Systemic nasal decongestants—see section 3.10.

SYMPATHOMIMETICS

EPHEDRINE HYDROCHLORIDE

Indications: nasal congestion

Cautions: avoid excessive or prolonged use; caution in infants under 3 months (no good evidence of value—if irritation occurs might narrow nasal passage); **interactions:** Appendix 1 (sympathomimetics)

Side-effects: local irritation; after excessive use tolerance with diminished effect, rebound congestion

Administration: see below

Ephedrine Nasal Drops, BP

Nasal drops, ephedrine hydrochloride in a suitable aqueous vehicle
Note. The BP directs that if no strength is specified 0.5% drops should be supplied; net price 10 mL = £1.05
Instil 1–2 drops into each nostril up to 3 or 4 times daily when required

XYLOMETAZOLINE HYDROCHLORIDE

Indications: nasal congestion

Cautions; Side-effects: see under Ephedrine Hydrochloride

Xylometazoline Nasal Drops, xylometazoline hydrochloride 0.1%, net price 10 mL = £1.46
Instil 2–3 drops into each nostril 2–3 times daily when required; max. duration 7 days; not recommended for children under 12 years

Xylometazoline Nasal Drops, Paediatric, xylometazoline hydrochloride 0.05%, net price 10 mL = £1.46
CHILD over 3 months instil 1–2 drops into each nostril 1–2 times daily when required (not recommended for infants under 3 months of age, doctor's advice only under 2 years); max. duration 7 days
Note. The brand name NHS*Otrivine®* is used for xylometazoline adult nasal drops 0.1%, children's nasal drops 0.05%, and adult nasal spray 0.1%

Sympathomimetic nasal preparations on sale to the public (not prescribable on the NHS) include: **Afrazine®** (oxymetazoline), **Dristan®** (oxymetazoline), **Fenox®** (phenylephrine), **Nazo-Mist®** (xylometazoline), **Otrivine®** (xylometazoline—prescribable in non-proprietary form as nasal drops, see above), **Sudafed®** nasal spray (oxymetazoline), **Vicks Sinex®** (oxymetazoline)

ANTIMUSCARINIC

IPRATROPIUM BROMIDE

Indications: rhinorrhoea associated with allergic and non-allergic rhinitis

Cautions: see section 3.1.2; avoid spraying near eyes

Side-effects: nasal dryness and epistaxis

Administration: apply 42 micrograms (2 sprays) into each nostril 2–3 times daily; CHILD under 12 years not recommended

PoM **Rinatec®** (Boehringer Ingelheim)
Nasal spray 0.03%, ipratropium bromide 21 micrograms/metered spray. Net price 180-dose unit = £4.55
Additives: include benzalkonium chloride

12.2.3   Nasal preparations for infection and epistaxis

There is **no** evidence that topical anti-infective nasal preparations have any therapeutic value; for elimination of nasal staphylococci, see below.

Systemic treatment of sinusitis—see section 5.1, table 1.

PoM **Betnesol-N®** (Evans)
Drops (for ear, eye, or nose), betamethasone sodium phosphate 0.1%, neomycin sulphate 0.5%. Net price 10 mL = £1.35
Additives: include benzalkonium chloride
Nose, apply 2–3 drops into nostril 2–3 times daily; *eye,* see section 11.4.1; *ear,* see section 12.1.1

PoM **Dexa-Rhinaspray®** (Boehringer Ingelheim)
Nasal spray, dexamethasone 21-isonicotinate 20 micrograms, neomycin sulphate 100 micrograms, tramazoline hydrochloride 120 micrograms/metered spray. Net price 125-dose unit = £2.15
Allergic rhinitis (but not recommended, see notes above), ADULT and CHILD over 12 years, apply 1 spray into each nostril 2-3 times daily; max. duration 14 days; CHILD 5-12 years 1 spray into each nostril up to twice daily; under 5 years not recommended

NHS [1] PoM **Locabiotal®** (Servier)

Spray, fusafungine 500 micrograms/metered spray. Net price 50-spray unit with nasal (yellow) and oral (white) adapters = £1.55

Additives: include alcohol

1. Except for treatment of infections and inflammation of the oropharynx and endorsed 'SLS'

Infection and inflammation of upper respiratory tract (but not recommended, see notes above), using nasal adapter, 1 spray into each nostril every 4 hours (withdraw if no improvement after 7 days); CHILD 1 spray into each nostril every 6 hours

Note. May also be sprayed into mouth using oral adapter

PoM **Vista-Methasone N®** (Martindale)

Drops (for ear, eye, or nose), betamethasone sodium phosphate 0.1%, neomycin sulphate 0.5%. Net price 5 mL = £1.23, 10 mL = £1.35

Additives: include thiomersal

Nose, apply 2–3 drops into each nostril twice daily; *eye,* see section 11.4.1; *ear,* see section 12.1.1

NASAL STAPHYLOCOCCI

Elimination of organisms such as staphylococci from the nasal vestibule can be achieved by the use of a cream containing **chlorhexidine and neomycin** (*Naseptin®*), but re-colonisation frequently occurs. Coagulase-positive staphylococci can be obtained from the noses of 40% of the population.

A nasal ointment containing **mupirocin** is also available; it should probably be kept in reserve for resistant cases. To avoid the development of resistance its use in hospital should, if possible, be avoided and it should not be used for longer than 10 days.

PoM **Bactroban Nasal®** (Beecham)

Nasal ointment, mupirocin 2% (as calcium salt) in white soft paraffin basis. Net price 3 g = £6.24

For eradication of nasal carriage of staphylococci, including methicillin-resistant *Staphylococcus aureus* (MRSA), apply 2–3 times daily to the inner surface of each nostril

PoM **Naseptin®** (Zeneca)

Cream, chlorhexidine hydrochloride 0.1%, neomycin sulphate 3250 units/g. Net price 15 g = 99p

Ingredients: include arachis (peanut) oil

For eradication of nasal carriage of staphylococci, apply to nostrils 4 times daily for 10 days; for preventing nasal carriage of staphylococci apply to nostrils twice daily

EPISTAXIS

Bismuth iodoform paraffin paste (BIPP) is used for packing cavities after ear, nose and oropharyngeal surgery as a mild disinfectant and astringent; it is also used to pack nasal cavities in acute epistaxis. It is available either as a paste, to be applied to ribbon gauze packing, or as BIPP-impregnated ribbon gauze.

BISMUTH SUBNITRATE AND IODOFORM

Indications: packing cavities after ear, nose or oropharyngeal surgery; epistaxis

Cautions: hyperthyroidism

Side-effects: erythematous rash (discontinue use); encephalopathy reported only with large packs or when placed directly on neural tissue

Bismuth Subnitrate and Iodoform (Non-proprietary)

Paste, 30-g sachet, net price = £14.65

Impregnated gauze, sterile, net price 1.25 cm x 100 cm, 10 = £89.70; 1.25 cm x 125 cm, 5 = £44.85; 1.25 cm x 200 cm, 5 = £62.05; 1.25 cm x 300 cm, 5 = £81.15; 2.5 cm x 100 cm, 10 = £97.20; 2.5 cm x 125 cm, 5 = £48.60; 2.5 cm x 200 cm, 5 = £70.35; 2.5 cm x 300 cm, 5 = £92.55

Available from Aurum and Trinity

12.3   Drugs acting on the oropharynx

12.3.1 Drugs for oral ulceration and inflammation
12.3.2 Oropharyngeal anti-infective drugs
12.3.3 Lozenges and sprays
12.3.4 Mouthwashes, gargles, and dentifrices
12.3.5 Treatment of dry mouth

12.3.1   Drugs for oral ulceration and inflammation

Ulceration of the oral mucosa may be caused by trauma (physical or chemical), recurrent aphthae, infections, carcinoma, dermatological disorders, nutritional deficiencies, gastro-intestinal disease, haematopoietic disorders, and drug therapy. It is important to establish the diagnosis in each case as the majority of these lesions require specific management in addition to local treatment. Patients with an unexplained mouth ulcer of more than 3 weeks' duration require urgent referral to hospital to exclude oral cancer. Local treatment aims at protecting the ulcerated area, or at relieving pain or reducing inflammation.

SIMPLE MOUTHWASHES. A **saline** or **compound thymol glycerin** mouthwash (section 12.3.4) may relieve the pain of traumatic ulceration. The mouthwash is made up with warm water and used at frequent intervals until the discomfort and swelling subsides.

ANTISEPTIC MOUTHWASHES. Secondary bacterial infection may be a feature of any mucosal ulceration; it can increase discomfort and delay healing. Use of a **chlorhexidine** or **povidone-iodine** mouthwash (section 12.3.4) is often beneficial and may accelerate healing of recurrent aphthae.

MECHANICAL PROTECTION. **Carmellose gelatin paste** may relieve some discomfort arising from ulceration by protecting the ulcer site. The paste adheres to the mucosa, but is difficult to apply effectively to some parts of the mouth.

CORTICOSTEROIDS. Topical corticosteroid therapy may be used for some forms of oral ulceration. In the case of aphthous ulcers it is most effective if applied in the 'prodromal' phase.

Thrush or other types of candidiasis are recognised complications of corticosteroid treatment.

Hydrocortisone lozenges are allowed to dissolve next to an ulcer and are useful in recurrent aphthae, erosive lichen planus, discoid lupus erythematosus, and benign mucous membrane pemphigoid.

Triamcinolone dental paste is designed to keep the corticosteroid in contact with the mucosa for long enough to permit penetration of the lesion, but is difficult for patients to apply properly.

Systemic corticosteroid therapy is reserved for severe conditions such as pemphigus vulgaris (section 6.3.4).

LOCAL ANALGESICS. Local analgesics have a limited role in the management of oral ulceration. When applied topically their action is of a relatively short duration so that analgesia cannot be maintained continuously throughout the day. The main indication for a topical local analgesic is to relieve the pain of otherwise intractable oral ulceration particularly when it is due to major aphthae. For this purpose lignocaine 5% ointment or lozenges containing a local anaesthetic are applied to the ulcer. When local anaesthetics are used in the mouth care must be taken not to produce anaesthesia of the pharynx before meals as this might lead to choking.

Benzydamine mouthwash or spray may be useful in palliating the discomfort associated with a variety of ulcerative conditions. It has also been found to be effective in reducing the discomfort of post-irradiation mucositis. Some patients find the full-strength mouthwash causes some stinging and, for them, it should be diluted with an equal volume of water.

Choline salicylate dental gel has some analgesic action and may provide relief for recurrent aphthae, but excessive application or confinement under a denture irritates the mucosa and can itself cause ulceration. Benefit in teething may merely be due to pressure of application (comparable with biting a teething ring); excessive use can lead to salicylate poisoning.

OTHER PREPARATIONS. **Carbenoxolone** gel or mouthwash may be of some value. **Tetracycline** rinsed in the mouth may also be of value.

BENZYDAMINE HYDROCHLORIDE
Indications: painful inflammatory conditions of oropharynx
Side-effects: occasional numbness or stinging

Difflam® (3M)
Oral rinse, green, benzydamine hydrochloride 0.15%. Net price 300 mL = £4.10
Rinse or gargle, using 15 mL (diluted with water if stinging occurs) every 1½–3 hours as required, usually for not more than 7 days; not suitable for children aged 12 years or under

Spray, benzydamine hydrochloride 0.15%. Net price 30-mL unit = £3.57
ADULT, 4–8 puffs onto affected area every 1½–3 hours; CHILD under 6 years 1 puff per 4 kg to max. 4 puffs every 1½–3 hours; 6–12 years 4 puffs every 1½–3 hours

CARBENOXOLONE SODIUM
Indications: mild oral and perioral lesions

Bioral Gel® (Sterling Health)
Gel, carbenoxolone sodium 2% in adhesive basis. Net price 5 g = £2.12
Apply after meals and at bedtime

PoM **Bioplex®** (Thames)
Mouthwash granules, carbenoxolone sodium 1% (20 mg/sachet). Net price 24 × 2-g sachets = £9.60
For mouth ulcers, rinse with 1 sachet in 30–50 mL of warm water 3 times daily and at bedtime

---

CARMELLOSE SODIUM
Indications: mechanical protection of oral and perioral lesions

Orabase® (ConvaTec)
Oral paste, carmellose sodium 16.58%, pectin 16.58%, gelatin 16.58%, in *Plastibase®*. Net price 30 g = £1.72; 100 g = £3.81
Apply a thin layer when necessary after meals

Orahesive® (ConvaTec)
Powder, carmellose sodium, pectin, gelatin, equal parts. Net price 25 g = £1.98
Sprinkle on the affected area

CORTICOSTEROIDS
Indications: oral and perioral lesions
Contra-indications: untreated oral infection
Side-effects: occasional exacerbation of local infection

PoM ¹**Adcortyl in Orabase®** (Squibb)
Oral paste, triamcinolone acetonide 0.1% in adhesive basis. Net price 10 g = £1.27
ADULT and CHILD, apply a thin layer 2–4 times daily; do not rub in; use limited to 5 days for children and short-term use also advised for elderly
1. A 5-g tube (*Adcortyl in Orabase®* for Mouth Ulcers) is on sale to the public for the treatment of common mouth ulcers for a treatment period not exceeding 5 days

Corlan® (Evans)
Pellets (= lozenges), hydrocortisone 2.5 mg (as sodium succinate). Net price 20 = £1.40
ADULT and CHILD, 1 lozenge 4 times daily, allowed to dissolve slowly in the mouth in contact with the ulcer; if ulcers recur rapidly treatment may be continued for a period at reduced dosage

---

LOCAL ANAESTHETICS
Indications: relief of pain in oral lesions
Cautions: avoid prolonged use; hypersensitivity

Preparations
Local anaesthetics are included in some mouth ulcer preparations, for details see below
Local anaesthetics are also included in some throat lozenges and sprays, see section 12.3.3

Teething gels
Teething gels containing local anaesthetics include: *Anbesol®*, *Calgel®*, *Dentinox®*, *Rinstead®*, *Woodward's®*, *Ulc-Aid®*

SALICYLATES

Indications: mild oral and perioral lesions
Cautions: frequent application, especially in children, may give rise to salicylate poisoning

Note. CSM warning on aspirin and Reye's syndrome does not apply to non-aspirin salicylates or to topical preparations such as teething gels

Choline salicylate
Choline Salicylate Dental Gel, BP

Oral gel, choline salicylate 8.7% in a flavoured gel basis

Available as *Bonjela®* (R&C), net price 15 g (sugar-free) = £1.53; *Dinnefords Teejel®* (Seton), 10 g = £1.02

Apply ½-inch of gel with gentle massage not more often than every 3 hours; CHILD over 4 months ¼-inch of gel not more often than every 3 hours; max. 6 applications daily

Salicylic acid
Pyralvex® (Norgine)

Oral paint, brown, rhubarb extract (anthraquinone glycosides 0.5%), salicylic acid 1%. Net price 10 mL with brush = £1.41

Apply 3–4 times daily; CHILD under 12 years not recommended

TETRACYCLINE

Indications: severe recurrent aphthous ulceration; oral herpes (section 12.3.2)
Side-effects: fungal superinfection
For side-effects, cautions and contra-indications relating to systemic administration of tetracyclines see section 5.1.3

Local application
For preparation of a mouthwash, the contents of a 250-mg tetracycline capsule (see section 5.1.3) can be stirred into a small amount of water, then held in the mouth for 2–3 minutes 3-4 times daily usually for 3 days; longer courses are sometimes used (but precautions may be required to avoid oral thrush, section 12.3.2); it should preferably not be swallowed [unlicensed indication]

Note. Tetracycline stains teeth; avoid in children under 12 years of age

The following list includes topical treatments for mouth ulcers on sale to the public, together with their significant ingredients:

Adcortyl in Orabase® for Mouth Ulcers (triamcinolone acetonide), **Anbesol®** (cetylpyridinium, chlorocresol, lignocaine), **Bansor®** (cetrimide), **Bioral Gel®** (carbenoxolone), **Bonjela gel®** (choline salicylate), **Bonjela pastilles®** (aminacrine, lignocaine), **Dinnefords Teejel®** (choline salicylate), **Frador®** (chlorbutol, menthol), **Medijel®** (aminacrine, lignocaine), **Oragard®** (cetylpyridinium, lignocaine), **Pyralvex®** (anthraquinone glycoside, salicylic acid), **Rinstead gel®** (benzocaine, chloroxylenol), **Rinstead pastilles®** (chloroxylenol, menthol).

12.3.2   Oropharyngeal anti-infective drugs

The most common cause of a sore throat is a viral infection which does not benefit from anti-infective treatment. Streptococcal sore throats require systemic **penicillin** therapy (section 5.1, table 1).

Acute ulcerative gingivitis (Vincent's infection) responds to systemic **metronidazole** 200 mg 3 times daily for 3 days (section 5.1.11).

Preparations administered in the dental surgery for the local treatment of periodontal disease include gels of metronidazole (*Elyzol®*, Dumex) and of minocycline (*Dentomycin®*, Lederle).

FUNGAL INFECTIONS

Candida albicans may cause thrush and other forms of stomatitis which are sometimes a sequel to the use of broad-spectrum antibiotics or of cytotoxics; withdrawing the causative drug may lead to rapid resolution. Otherwise, an antifungal drug may be effective.

Of the antifungal drugs used for mouth infections, **amphotericin** and **nystatin** are not absorbed from the gastro-intestinal tract and are used by local application in the mouth. **Miconazole** occupies an intermediate position since it is used by local application in the mouth but is also absorbed to the extent that potential interactions need to be considered. **Fluconazole** and **itraconazole** are absorbed when taken by mouth and are available for administration by mouth for oropharyngeal candidiasis (section 5.2).

AMPHOTERICIN

Indications: oral and perioral fungal infections
Side-effects: mild gastro-intestinal disturbances reported

PoM **Fungilin®** (Squibb)

Lozenges, yellow, amphotericin 10 mg. Net price 60-lozenge pack = £3.95. Label: 9, 24, counselling, after food

Dissolve 1 lozenge slowly in the mouth 4 times daily, may require 10–15 days' treatment (continued for 48 hours after lesions have resolved); increase to 8 daily if infection severe

Oral suspension, yellow, sugar-free, amphotericin 100 mg/mL. Net price 12 mL with pipette = £2.31. Label: 9, counselling, use of pipette, hold in mouth, after food

Place 1 mL in the mouth after food and retain near lesions 4 times daily for 14 days (continued for 48 hours after lesions have resolved)

MICONAZOLE

Indications: see under Preparations; intestinal fungal infections (section 5.2)
Cautions: pregnancy and breast-feeding; avoid in porphyria (section 9.8.2); **interactions:** Appendix 1 (antifungals, imidazole and triazole)
Contra-indications: hepatic impairment
Side-effects: nausea and vomiting, diarrhoea (with long-term treatment); rarely allergic reactions; isolated reports of hepatitis

---

PoM **¹Daktarin®** (Janssen-Cilag)

Oral gel, sugar-free, orange-flavoured, miconazole 24 mg/mL. Net price 15-g tube = £2.27, 80-g tube = £5.00. Label: 9, counselling, hold in mouth, after food

Prevention and treatment of oral fungal infections, place 5–10 mL in the mouth after food and retain near lesions 4 times daily; CHILD under 2 years 2.5 mL twice daily, 2–6 years 5 mL twice daily, over 6 years 5 mL 4 times daily; treatment continued for 48 hours after lesions have resolved

Localised lesions, smear small amount of gel on affected area with clean finger (dental prostheses should be removed at night and brushed with gel)

1. 15-g tube can be sold to the public

PoM **Dumicoat®** (Dumex)

Denture lacquer, miconazole 50 mg/g. Net price pack of 3 × 1-g bottles (with brushes and cleansing tissues) = £13.50. Label: 10 patient information leaflet

Candida-associated denture stomatitis, apply contents of 1 bottle to upper surface of upper denture after thorough cleansing, allow to dry, and replace; repeat twice at intervals of 1 week

NYSTATIN

Indications: oral and perioral fungal infections

Side-effects: oral irritation and sensitisation, nausea reported; see also section 5.2

Dose: (as pastilles or as suspension) 100 000 units 4 times daily after food, usually for 7 days (continued for 48 hours after lesions have resolved)

Note. Immunosuppressed patients may require higher doses (e.g. 500 000 units 4 times daily)

PoM **Nystatin** (Non-proprietary)

Oral suspension, nystatin 100 000 units/mL. Net price 30 mL = £1.98. Label: 9, counselling, hold in mouth, after food

Available from Hillcross, Lagap, Opus (*Infestat®*), Rosemont (*Nystamont®*, sugar-free)

PoM **Nystan®** (Squibb)

Pastilles, yellow/brown, nystatin 100 000 units. Net price 28-pastille pack = £3.24. Label: 9, 24, counselling, after food

Oral suspension, yellow, nystatin 100 000 units/mL. Net price 30 mL with pipette = £2.05. Label: 9, counselling, use of pipette, hold in mouth, after food

Oral suspension (sugar-free), nystatin 100 000 units/mL when reconstituted with water. Net price 24 mL with pipette = £1.67. Label: 9, counselling, use of pipette, hold in mouth, after food

VIRAL INFECTIONS

The management of herpes infections of the mouth is a soft diet, adequate fluid intake, analgesics as required, and the use of **chlorhexidine** mouthwash (section 12.3.4) to control plaque accumulation if toothbrushing is painful. In the case of severe herpetic stomatitis, systemic **aciclovir** is required (see section 5.3).

Herpes infections of the mouth may also respond to **tetracycline** (section 12.3.1) rinsed in the mouth.

Idoxuridine 0.1% paint has been superseded by more effective preparations.

12.3.3   Lozenges and sprays

There is no convincing evidence that antiseptic lozenges and sprays have a beneficial action and they sometimes irritate and cause sore tongue and sore lips. Some of these preparations also contain local anaesthetics which relieve pain but may cause sensitisation.

The following list includes throat lozenges and sprays on sale to the public, together with their significant ingredients.

AAA® (benzocaine), **Bradosol®** (benzalkonium), **Bradosol Plus®** (domiphen, lignocaine), **Dequacaine®** (benzocaine, dequalinium), **Dequadin®** (dequalinium), **Eludril®** spray (amethocaine, chlorhexidine), **Labosept®** (dequalinium), **Meggezones®** (menthol), **Mentholatum®** lozenges (amylmetacresol, menthol), **Merocaine®** (benzocaine, cetylpyridinium), **Merocets®** lozenges (cetylpyridinium), **Merothol®** lozenges (cetylpyridinium, menthol), **Strepsils®** lozenges (amylmetacresol, dichlorobenzyl alcohol), **Strepsils Dual Action®** lozenges (amylmetacresol, dichlorobenzyl alcohol, lignocaine), **Strepsils® spray** (lignocaine), **TCP®** pastilles (phenols), **Tyrozets®** (benzocaine, tyrothricin), **Valda®** (menthol, thymol), **Vicks Ultra Chloraseptic®** (benzocaine)

12.3.4   Mouthwashes, gargles, and dentifrices

Mouthwashes have a mechanical cleansing action and freshen the mouth. Warm **compound sodium chloride mouthwash** or **compound thymol glycerin** is as useful as any.

Mouthwashes containing an oxidising agent, such as **hydrogen peroxide**, may be useful in the treatment of acute ulcerative gingivitis (Vincent's infection) since the organisms involved are anaerobes. It also has a mechanical cleansing effect due to frothing when in contact with oral debris. **Sodium perborate** is similar in effect to hydrogen peroxide.

There is evidence that **chlorhexidine** has a specific effect in inhibiting the formation of plaque on teeth. A chlorhexidine mouthwash may be useful as an adjunct to other oral hygiene measures for oral infection or when toothbrushing is not possible.

Povidone–iodine mouthwash is useful for mucosal infections but does not inhibit plaque accumulation. It should not be used for periods longer than 14 days because a significant amount of iodine is absorbed.

There is no convincing evidence that gargles are effective.

CETYLPYRIDINIUM CHLORIDE

Indications: oral hygiene

Merocet® (Seton)

Solution (= mouthwash or gargle), yellow, cetylpyridinium chloride 0.05%. Net price 200 mL = £1.72

To be used undiluted or diluted with an equal volume of warm water

---

CHLORHEXIDINE GLUCONATE

Indications: oral hygiene; plaque inhibition
Side-effects: idiosyncratic mucosal irritation; reversible brown staining of teeth

Chlorohex 2000® (Colgate-Palmolive)
Mouthwash, chlorhexidine gluconate 0.2% (mint-flavoured). Net price 300 mL = £2.20
Rinse the mouth with 10 mL for about 1 minute twice daily

Corsodyl® (SmithKline Beecham Healthcare)
Dental gel, chlorhexidine gluconate 1%. Net price 50 g = £1.21
Brush on the teeth once or twice daily
Mouthwash, chlorhexidine gluconate 0.2%. Net price 300 mL (original or mint) = £1.93, 600 mL (mint) = £3.85
Rinse the mouth with 10 mL for about 1 minute twice daily
Oral spray, chlorhexidine gluconate 0.2% (mint-flavoured). Net price 60 mL = £4.10
Apply as required to tooth and gingival surfaces using up to max. 12 actuations (approx. 0.14 mL/actutation) twice daily

Eludril® (Chefaro)
Mouthwash, chlorhexidine gluconate 0.1%, chlorbutol 0.5%. Net price 90 mL = £1.19; 250 mL = £2.38; 500 mL = £4.38
Use 10–15 mL in a third of a tumblerful of warm water 2–3 times daily

HEXETIDINE

Indications: oral hygiene

Oraldene® (Warner Lambert)
Mouthwash or *gargle,* red, hexetidine 0.1%. Net price 100 mL = £1.13; 200 mL = £1.78
Use 15 mL undiluted 2–3 times daily

OXIDISING AGENTS

Indications: oral hygiene, see notes above

Hydrogen Peroxide Mouthwash, DPF, consists of Hydrogen Peroxide Solution 6% (≡ approx. 20 volume) BP
Rinse the mouth for 2–3 minutes with 15 mL in half a tumblerful of warm water 2–3 times daily

Bocasan® (Oral B Labs)
Mouthwash, sodium perborate 68.6% (buffered). Net price 20 × 1.7-g sachet pack = £1.75
Use 1 sachet in 30 mL of water 3 times daily after meals
Cautions: do not use for longer than 7 days because of possible absorption of borate; not recommended in renal impairment or for children under 5 years

POVIDONE–IODINE

Indications: oral hygiene
Cautions: pregnancy; breast-feeding; see also notes above
Contra-indications: avoid regular use in patients with thyroid disorders or those receiving lithium therapy
Side-effects: idiosyncratic mucosal irritation and hypersensitivity reactions; may interfere with thyroid-function tests and with tests for occult blood

Betadine® (Seton)
Mouthwash or *gargle,* amber, povidone-iodine 1%. Net price 250 mL = £1.17
Adults and children over 6 years, up to 10 mL undiluted or diluted with an equal quantity of warm water for up to 30 seconds up to 4 times daily for up to 14 days

SODIUM CHLORIDE

Indications: oral hygiene, see notes above

Sodium Chloride Mouthwash, Compound, BP

Mouthwash, sodium bicarbonate 1%, sodium chloride 1.5% in a suitable vehicle with a peppermint flavour.
Extemporaneous preparations should be prepared according to the following formula: sodium chloride 1.5 g, sodium bicarbonate 1 g, concentrated peppermint emulsion 2.5 mL, double-strength chloroform water 50 mL, water to 100 mL
To be diluted with an equal volume of warm water

THYMOL

Indications: oral hygiene, see notes above

Compound Thymol Glycerin, BP 1988, glycerol 10%, thymol 0.05% with colouring and flavouring
To be used undiluted or diluted with 3 volumes of warm water
Mouthwash Solution-tablets, consist of tablets which may contain antimicrobial, colouring, and flavouring agents in a suitable soluble effervescent basis to make a mouthwash suitable for dental purposes.
Dissolve 1 tablet in a tumblerful of warm water

12.3.5   Treatment of dry mouth

Xerostomia (dry mouth) may be caused by irradiation of the head and neck region, damage to or disease of the salivary glands, or by the administration of drugs with antimuscarinic (anticholinergic) side-effects (e.g. antispasmodics, tricyclic antidepressants, and some antipsychotics). Dry mouth may be relieved in many patients by simple measures such as frequent sips of cool drinks or sucking pieces of ice or sugar-free fruit pastilles.

An **artificial saliva** can provide useful relief of dry mouth. A properly balanced artificial saliva should be of a neutral pH and contain electrolytes (including fluoride) to correspond approximately to the composition of saliva. Of the proprietary preparations available, *Luborant®* is licensed for any condition giving rise to a dry mouth; *Saliva Orthana®, Salivace®, Saliveze®, Glandosane®* and *Oralbalance®* have ACBS approval for dry mouth associated only with radiotherapy or sicca syndrome. *Salivix®* pastilles, which act locally as salivary stimulants, are also available and have similar ACBS approval.

Pilocarpine tablets are restricted to use in xerostomia following irradiation for head and neck cancer. They are effective only in patients who have some residual salivary gland function, and therefore should be withdrawn if there is no response.

LOCAL TREATMENT

Glandosane® (Fresenius)

Aerosol spray, carmellose sodium 500 mg, sorbitol 1.5 g, potassium chloride 60 mg, sodium chloride 42.2 mg, magnesium chloride 2.6 mg, calcium chloride 7.3 mg, and dipotassium hydrogen phosphate 17.1 mg/50 g. Net price 50-mL unit (neutral, lemon or peppermint flavoured) = £3.95

ACBS: patients suffering from dry mouth as a result of having (or having undergone) radiotherapy, or sicca syndrome, spray onto oral and pharyngeal mucosa as required

Luborant® (Antigen)

Oral spray, pink, sorbitol 1.8 g, carmellose sodium (sodium carboxymethylcellulose) 390 mg, dibasic potassium phosphate 48.23 mg, potassium chloride 37.5 mg, monobasic potassium phosphate 21.97 mg, calcium chloride 9.972 mg, magnesium chloride 3.528 mg, sodium fluoride 258 micrograms/60 mL, with preservatives and colouring agents. Net price 60-mL unit = £3.96

Saliva deficiency, 2–3 sprays onto oral mucosa up to 4 times daily, or as directed

Oralbalance® (Ethical Research)

Saliva replacement gel, lactoperoxidase, glucose oxidase, xylitol in a gel basis. Net price 50-g tube = £3.60. ACBS: patients suffering from dry mouth as a result of having (or having undergone) radiotherapy, or sicca syndrome, apply to gums and tongue as required

Saliva Orthana® (Nycomed)

Oral spray, gastric mucin 3.5%, xylitol 2%, sodium fluoride 4.2 mg/litre, with preservatives and flavouring agents. Net price 50-mL bottle = £3.80; 450-mL refill = £25.10

Lozenges, mucin 65 mg, xylitol 59 mg, in a sorbitol basis. Net price 45-lozenge pack = £2.75

ACBS: patients suffering from dry mouth as a result of having (or having undergone) radiotherapy, or sicca syndrome, spray 2–3 times onto oral and pharyngeal mucosa, when required

Note. Saliva Orthana® lozenges do not contain fluoride

Salivace® (Penn)

Oral spray, carmellose sodium (sodium carboxymethylcellulose), xylitol, calcium chloride, dibasic potassium phosphate, sodium chloride, potassium chloride, and methyl hydroxybenzoate. Net price 100 mL = £4.95

ACBS: patients suffering from dry mouth as a result of having (or having undergone) radiotherapy, or sicca syndrome, 1–2 sprays onto oral mucosa as required

Saliveze® (Wyvern)

Oral spray, carmellose sodium (sodium carboxymethylcellulose), calcium chloride, magnesium chloride, potassium chloride, sodium chloride, and dibasic sodium phosphate. Net price 50-mL bottle (mint-flavoured) = £3.50

ACBS: patients suffering from dry mouth as a result of having (or having undergone) radiotherapy, or sicca syndrome, 1 spray onto oral mucosa as required

Salivix® (Thames)

Pastilles, sugar-free, reddish-amber, acacia, malic acid and other ingredients. Net price 50-pastille pack = £2.86

ACBS: patients suffering from dry mouth as a result of having (or having undergone) radiotherapy, or sicca syndrome, suck 1 pastille when required

SYSTEMIC TREATMENT

PILOCARPINE HYDROCHLORIDE

Indications: symptoms of salivary gland hypofunction in xerostomia following irradiation for head and neck cancer (see also notes above)

Cautions: close medical supervision in asthma (avoid if uncontrolled, see Contra-indications) and in cardiovascular disease; cholelithiasis or biliary tract disease, peptic ulcer, hepatic impairment (reduce initial dose), renal impairment; risk of increased urethral smooth muscle tone and renal colic; eye examinations before treatment (decreased visual acuity more likely at night and in patients with central lens changes); maintain adequate fluid intake to avoid dehydration associated with excessive sweating; cognitive or psychiatric disturbances; **interactions:** Appendix 1 (parasympathomimetics)

COUNSELLING. Blurred vision may affect ability to drive, particularly at night, and to perform hazardous activities in reduced lighting

Contra-indications: uncontrolled asthma and chronic obstructive airways disease (increased bronchial secretions and increased airways resistance); acute iritis, narrow-angle glaucoma; pregnancy and breast-feeding

Side-effects: sweating; also chills, diarrhoea, nausea, vomiting, lachrymation, abdominal pain, amblyopia, hypertension, constipation, abnormal vision (see Counselling), dizziness, rhinitis, asthenia, increased urinary frequency, headache, dyspepsia, vasodilatation, flushing; other possible side-effects include: respiratory distress, gastro-intestinal spasm, AV block, tachycardia, bradycardia, other arrhythmias, hypotension, shock, confusion, tremors

Dose: 5 mg 3 times daily with or immediately after meals (last dose always with evening meal); if dose tolerated but response not sufficient after 4-8 weeks, may be increased to max. 30 mg daily in divided doses (but associated with increased side-effects); discontinue if no improvement after 3 months; CHILD not recommended

PoM **Salagen®** (Chiron)

Tablets, f/c, pilocarpine hydrochloride 5 mg. Net price 84-tab pack = £51.43. Label: 21, 27, counselling, driving

13: Drugs acting on the
SKIN

In this chapter, drug treatment is discussed under the following headings:

Suitable quantities of dermatological preparations to be prescribed for specific areas of the body are:

	Creams and Ointments	Lotions
Face	15 to 30 g	100 mL
Both hands	25 to 50 g	200 mL
Scalp	50 to 100 g	200 mL
Both arms or both legs	100 to 200 g	200 mL
Trunk	400 g	500 mL
Groins and genitalia	15 to 25 g	100 mL

These amounts are usually suitable for an adult for twice daily application for 1 week. The recommendations do not apply to corticosteroid preparations—for suitable quantities of corticosteroid preparations see section 13.4

ADDITIVES. The following additives in topical preparations may be associated with sensitisation, particularly of eczematous skin. Details of whether they are contained in preparations listed in the BNF are given after the preparation entry.

Beeswax	Hydroxybenzoates
Benzyl alcohol	(parabens)
Butylated hydroxy-	Isopropyl palmitate
anisole	Polysorbates
Butylated hydroxy-	Propylene glycol
toluene	Sorbic acid
Chlorocresol	Wool fat and related
Edetic acid (EDTA)	substances including
Ethylenediamine	lanolin[1]
Fragrances	

1. Purified versions of wool fat have reduced the problem

13.1 Vehicles

Both vehicle and active ingredients are important in the treatment of skin conditions; it is being increasingly recognised that the vehicle alone may have more than a mere placebo effect. The vehicle affects the degree of hydration of the skin, has a mild anti-inflammatory effect, and aids the penetration of active drug in the preparation.

The vehicle may take the form of an *application, collodion, cream, dusting powder, lotion, ointment,* or *paste*:

Applications are usually viscous solutions, emulsions, or suspensions for application to the skin.

Collodions are painted on the skin and allowed to dry to leave a flexible film over the site of application.

Creams are emulsions of oil and water and are generally well absorbed into the skin. They may contain an antimicrobial preservative unless the active ingredient or basis has sufficient intrinsic bactericidal or fungicidal activity. Generally, creams are cosmetically more acceptable than ointments as they are less greasy and easier to apply.

Dusting powders are finely divided powders that contain one or more active ingredients with or without auxiliary substances. They are intended to be applied to skin for therapeutic, prophylactic or lubricant purposes. Dusting powder intended for large open wounds or severely injured skin should be sterile.

Lotions have a cooling effect and may be preferred to ointments or creams when it is intended to apply the preparation over a hairy area. *Shake lotions* (such as calamine lotion) containing insoluble powders and leave a deposit of inert powder on the skin surface.

Ointments are greasy preparations which are normally anhydrous and insoluble in water, and are more occlusive than creams. They are particularly suitable for chronic, dry lesions. The most commonly used ointment bases consist of soft paraffin or a combination of soft, liquid and hard paraffin. Some modern ointment bases have both *hydrophilic and lipophilic* properties; they may have occlusive properties on the skin surface, encourage hydration, and also be miscible with water; they often have a mild anti-inflammatory effect. *Water-soluble ointments* contain macrogols which are freely soluble in water and are therefore readily washed off; they have a limited but useful application in circumstances where ready removal is desirable.

Pastes are stiff preparations containing a high proportion of finely powdered solids such as zinc oxide and starch suspended in an ointment. They are used for circumscribed lesions such as those which occur in lichen simplex, chronic eczema, or psoriasis. They are less occlusive than ointments and can be used to protect inflamed, lichenified, or excoriated skin.

DILUTION. The BP directs that creams and ointments should **not** normally be diluted but that should dilution be necessary care should be taken, in particular, to prevent microbial contamination. The appropriate diluent should be used and heating should be avoided during mixing; excessive dilution may affect the stability of some creams. Diluted creams should normally be used within 2 weeks of their preparation.

13.2   Emollient and barrier preparations

13.2.1   Emollients
13.2.2   Barrier preparations
13.2.3 ⸱ Dusting powders

BORDERLINE SUBSTANCES. The preparations marked 'ACBS' are regarded as drugs when prescribed in accordance with the advice of the Advisory Committee on Borderline Substances for the clinical conditions listed. Prescriptions issued in accordance with this advice and endorsed 'ACBS' will normally not be investigated. See Appendix 7 for listing by clinical condition.

13.2.1   Emollients

Emollients soothe, smooth and hydrate the skin and are indicated for all dry or scaling disorders. Their effects are short-lived and they should be applied frequently even after improvement occurs. They are useful in dry and eczematous disorders, and to a lesser extent in psoriasis (section 13.5.2). Light emollients such as aqueous cream are suitable for many patients with dry skin but a wide range of more greasy preparations including white soft paraffin and emulsifying ointment are available; the severity of the condition, patient preference and site of application will often guide the choice of emollient. Some ingredients may rarely cause sensitisation (section 13.1) and this should be suspected if an eczematous reaction occurs.

Calamine and zinc oxide may be included since they are particularly useful in dry eczema. Thickening agents such as talc and kaolin may also be included. Preparations containing an antibacterial should be avoided unless infection is present (section 13.10).

Urea is employed as a hydrating agent. It is used in scaling conditions and may be useful in elderly patients. It is occasionally used with other topical agents such as corticosteroids to enhance penetration.

Aqueous Cream, BP, emulsifying ointment 30%, phenoxyethanol 1% in freshly boiled and cooled purified water. Net price 100 g = 24p
Emulsifying Ointment, BP, emulsifying wax 30%, white soft paraffin 50%, liquid paraffin 20%. Net price 100 g = 30p
Hydrous Ointment, BP (oily cream), dried magnesium sulphate 0.5%, phenoxyethanol 1%, wool alcohols ointment 50%, in freshly boiled and cooled purified water. Net price 100 g = 42p
Paraffin, White Soft, BP (white petroleum jelly). Net price 100 g = 32p

Paraffin, Yellow Soft, BP (yellow petroleum jelly). Net price 100 g = 31p
Zinc Cream, BP, zinc oxide 32%, arachis (peanut) oil 32%, calcium hydroxide 0.045%, oleic acid 0.5%, wool fat 8%, in freshly boiled and cooled purified water. Net price 50 g = 24p
For napkin and urinary rash and eczematous conditions
Zinc Ointment, BP, zinc oxide 15%, in Simple Ointment BP 1988 (which contains wool fat 5%, hard paraffin 5%, cetostearyl alcohol 5%, white soft paraffin 85%. Net price 25 g = 13p
For napkin and urinary rash and eczematous conditions
Zinc and Castor Oil Ointment, BP, zinc oxide 7.5%, castor oil 50%, arachis (peanut) oil 30.5%, white beeswax 10%, cetostearyl alcohol 2%. Net price 25 g = 14p
For napkin and urinary rash
Alcoderm® (Galderma)
Cream, containing liquid paraffin, cetyl alcohol, stearyl alcohol, sodium lauryl sulphate, carbomer, triethanolamine, sorbitan monostearate, sorbitol, spermaceti, silicone fluid. Net price 60 g = £2.40
For dry skin conditions
Additives: include hydroxybenzoates (parabens), isopropyl palmitate
Lotion, water-miscible, ingredients as above. Net price 120 mL = £2.86
For dry skin conditions
Aveeno® (Bioglan)
Cream, colloidal oatmeal, white oat fraction in emollient basis. Net price 100 mL = £3.60
ACBS: For endogenous and exogenous eczema, xeroderma, ichthyosis, and senile pruritus (pruritus of the elderly) associated with dry skin
Additives: include benzyl alcohol
Dermamist® (Yamanouchi)
Spray application, white soft paraffin 10% in a basis containing liquid paraffin, fractionated coconut oil. Net price 250-mL pressurised aerosol unit = £9.60
For dry skin conditions including eczema, ichthyosis, pruritus of the elderly
Caution: flammable
Additives: none as listed in section 13.1
Diprobase® (Schering-Plough)
Cream, cetomacrogol 2.25%, cetostearyl alcohol 7.2%, liquid paraffin 6%, white soft paraffin 15%, water-miscible basis used for Diprosone® cream. Net price 50 g = £1.61; 500-g dispenser = £6.92
For dry skin conditions
Additives: include chlorocresol
Ointment, liquid paraffin 5%, white soft paraffin 95%, basis used for Diprosone® ointment. Net price 50 g = £1.61
For dry skin conditions
Additives: none as listed in section 13.1
Dermalex® —section 13.10.5
Drapolene® —section 13.2.2
E45® (Crookes)
Cream, light liquid paraffin 12.6%, white soft paraffin 14.5%, hypoallergenic hydrous wool fat (hypoallergenic lanolin) 1% in self-emulsifying monostearin. Net price 50 g = £1.18; 125 g = £2.39; 500 g = £5.61
For dry skin conditions
Additives: include hydroxybenzoates (parabens)
Emollient Wash Cream, soap substitute, zinc oxide 5% in an emollient basis. Net price 250 mL = £2.75
ACBS: for endogenous and exogenous eczema, xeroderma, ichthyosis and senile pruritus (pruritus of the elderly) associated with dry skin
Additives: include butylated hydroxytoluene

Epaderm® (Seton)

Ointment, emulsifying wax 30%, yellow soft paraffin 30%, liquid paraffin 40%, net price 125 g = £3.84; 500 g = £6.50.

For use as an emollient or soap substitute

Additives: none as listed in section 13.1

Hewletts Cream® (Kestrel)

Cream, hydrous wool fat 4%, zinc oxide 8%, arachis (peanut) oil, oleic acid, white soft paraffin. Net price 35 g = £1.19; 400 g = £4.85

For nursing hygiene and care of skin, and chapped hands

Additives: include fragrance

Humiderm® (ConvaTec)

Cream, pyrrolidone carboxylic acid 5% (as sodium salt). Net price 60 g = £2.46

For dry skin conditions

Additives: include hydroxybenzoates (parabens), propylene glycol

Hydromol® (Quinoderm Ltd)

Cream, arachis (peanut) oil 10%, isopropyl myristate 5%, liquid paraffin 10%, sodium pyrrolidone carboxylate 2.5%, sodium lactate 1%. Net price 50 g = £2.04; 100 g = £3.40; 500 g = £10.94.

For dry skin conditions

Additives: include hydroxybenzoates (parabens)

Kamillosan® (Norgine)

Ointment, chamomile extracts 10.5% in a basis containing wool fat. Net price 30 g = £1.50

For napkin rash, sore nipples and chapped hands

Additives: include beeswax, hydroxybenzoates (parabens)

Keri® (Bristol-Myers)

Lotion, mineral oil 16%, with lanolin oil. Net price 190-mL pump pack = £3.56; 380-mL pump pack = £5.81.

For dry skin conditions and napkin rash

Additives: include hydroxybenzoates (parabens), propylene glycol, fragrance

Lacticare® (Stiefel)

Lotion, lactic acid 5%, sodium pyrrolidone carboxylate 2.5%. Net price 150 mL = £3.19.

For dry skin conditions

Additives: include isopropyl palmitate, fragrance

Lipobase® (Yamanouchi)

Cream, fatty cream basis used for Locoid Lipocream®. Net price 50 g = £2.05

Additives: include hydroxybenzoates (parabens)

Morhulin® (Seton)

Ointment, cod-liver oil 11.4%, zinc oxide 38%, in a basis containing wool fat and paraffin. Net price 50 g = £1.08; 350 g = £5.06.

For minor wounds, varicose ulcers, and pressure sores

Additives: include wool fat derivative

Neutrogena® Dermatological Cream (Neutrogena)

Cream, glycerol 40% in an emollient basis. Net price 100 g = £3.67.

For dry skin conditions

Additives: include hydroxybenzoates (parabens)

Oilatum® (Stiefel)

Cream, arachis (peanut) oil 21%. Net price 40 g = £1.79; 80 g = £2.78

For dry skin conditions

Additives: include fragrance

Shower emollient (gel), light liquid paraffin 70%. Net price 125 g = £4.84

For dry skin conditions including dermatitis

Additives: include fragrance

Sudocrem® (Tosara)

Cream, benzyl alcohol 0.39%, benzyl benzoate 1.01%, benzyl cinnamate 0.15%, wool fat 4%, zinc oxide 15.25%. Net price 30 g = 80p; 60 g = 85p; 125 g = £1.40; 250 g = £2.44; 400 g = £3.57.

For napkin rash and pressure sores

Additives: include beeswax (synthetic), polysorbates, propylene glycol, fragrance

Ultrabase® (Schering Health)

Cream, water-miscible, containing liquid paraffin and white soft paraffin. Net price 50 g = £1.05; 500-g dispenser = £6.89.

For dry skin conditions

Additives: include hydroxybenzoates (parabens), disodium edetate, fragrance

Unguentum Merck® (Merck)

Cream, cetostearyl alcohol, glyceryl monostearate, saturated neutral oil, liquid paraffin, white soft paraffin, propylene glycol, polysorbate '40', silicic acid, sorbic acid. Net price 50 g = £1.59; 100 g = £3.13; 200 mL dispenser = £6.19; 500 g = £9.55.

For dry skin conditions

Vaseline Dermacare® (Elida Gibbs)

Cream, dimethicone 1%, white soft paraffin 15%. Net price 150 mL = £2.11

ACBS: for endogenous and exogenous eczema, xeroderma, ichthyosis and senile pruritus (pruritus of the elderly) associated with dry skin

Additives: include hydroxybenzoates (parabens)

Lotion, dimethicone 1%, liquid paraffin 4%, white soft paraffin 5% in an emollient basis. Net price 75 mL = £1.18; 200 mL = £2.29

ACBS: as for Vaseline Dermacare® Cream

Additives: include disodium edetate, hydroxybenzoates (parabens), wool fat

Preparations containing urea

Aquadrate® (Procter & Gamble Pharm.)

Cream, urea 10%. Net price 30 g = £1.59; 100 g = £4.79

For dry, scaling and itching skin, apply thinly and rub into area when required

Additives: none as listed in section 13.1

Balneum® Plus (Merck)

Cream, urea 5%, lauromacrogols 3%. Net price 100 g = £5.58

For dry, scaling and itching skin, apply twice daily

Additives: include benzyl alcohol, polysorbates

Calmurid® (Galderma)

Cream, urea 10%, lactic acid 5%. Diluent aqueous cream, life of diluted cream 14 days. Net price 100 g = £4.75; 500-g dispenser = £21.48

For dry, scaling and itching skin, apply a thick layer for 3–5 minutes, massage into area, and remove excess, usually twice daily. Use half-strength cream for 1 week if stinging occurs

Additives: none as listed in section 13.1

Nutraplus® (Galderma)

Cream, urea 10%. Net price 100 g = £4.37

For dry, scaling and itching skin, apply 2–3 times daily

Additives: include hydroxybenzoates (parabens), propylene glycol

With antimicrobials

Dermol® 500 (Dermal)

Lotion, benzalkonium chloride 0.1%, chlorhexidine hydrochloride 0.1%, liquid paraffin 2.5%, isopropyl myristate 2.5%. Net price 500-mL dispenser = £6.79.

For dry and pruritic skin conditions including eczema and dermatitis used directly on the skin or as soap substitute

Additives: none as listed in section 13.1

13.2.1.1 EMOLLIENT BATH ADDITIVES

Alpha Keri Bath® (Bristol-Myers)

Bath oil, liquid paraffin 91.7%, oil-soluble fraction of wool fat 3%. Net price 240 mL = £3.45; 480 mL = £6.43

For dry skin conditions including ichthyosis and pruritus of the elderly, add 10–20 mL /bath (infants 5 mL)

Additives: include fragrance

Aveeno® (Bioglan)

Aveeno® Bath oil, colloidal oatmeal, white oat fraction in emollient basis. Net price 250 mL = £4.08

ACBS: for endogenous and exogenous eczema, xeroderma, ichthyosis, and senile pruritus (pruritus of the elderly) associated with dry skin, add 20–30 mL/bath

Additives: include beeswax, fragrance

Aveeno Oilated® Bath additive, oatmeal, white oat fraction in emollient basis. Net price 10 × 50-g sachets = £6.30

ACBS: as for Aveeno® Bath oil; add 1 sachet/bath (infants half sachet)

Additives: none as listed in section 13.1

Aveeno Regular® Bath additive, oatmeal, white oat fraction in emollient basis. Net price 10 × 50-g sachets = £6.30

ACBS: as for Aveeno® Bath oil; add 1 sachet/bath (infants half sachet)

Additives: none as listed in section 13.1

Balneum® (Merck)

Balneum® bath oil, soya oil 84.75%. Net price 200 mL = £2.79; 500 mL = £6.06; 1 litre = £11.70

For dry skin conditions including those associated with dermatitis and eczema; add 20 mL/bath (infant 5mL)

Additives: include butylated hydroxytoluene, propylene glycol, fragrance

Balneum Plus® bath oil, soya oil 82.95%, mixed lauromacrogols 15%. Net price 500 mL = £7.50

For dry skin conditions including those associated with dermatitis and eczema where pruritus also experienced; add 20 mL/bath (infant 5 mL)

Additives: include butylated hydroxytoluene, propylene glycol, fragrance

Balneum with Tar®—section 13.5.2

Diprobath® (Schering-Plough)

Bath additive, isopropyl myristate 39%, light liquid paraffin 46%. Net price 500 mL = £7.50

For dry skin conditions including dermatitis and eczema; add 25 mL/bath (infant 10 mL)

Additives: none as listed in section 13.1

E45® (Crookes)

Emollient bath oil, cetyl dimethicone 5%. Net price 250 mL = £2.75; 500 mL = £4.57

ACBS: for endogenous and exogenous eczema, xeroderma, ichthyosis, and senile pruritus (pruritus of the elderly) associated with dry skin; add 15 mL/bath

Additives: include butylated hydroxyanisole

Emmolate® (Bio-Medical)

Bath oil, acetylated wool alcohols 5%, liquid paraffin 65%. Net price 200 mL = £2.25

For contact dermatitis, dry skin conditions including ichthyosis and pruritus of the elderly; add 15–20 mL/bath (infant and child 5–10 mL)

Additives: none as listed in section 13.1

Emulsiderm® (Dermal)

Liquid emulsion, liquid paraffin 25%, isopropyl myristate 25%, benzalkonium chloride 0.5%. Net price 300 mL (with 15-mL measure) = £4.33; 1 litre (with 30-mL measure) = £13.95

For dry skin conditions including eczema and ichthyosis; add 7–30 mL/bath

Additives: include polysorbate 60

Hydromol Emollient® (Quinoderm Ltd)

Bath additive, isopropyl myristate 13%, light liquid paraffin 37.8%. Net price 150 mL = £1.72; 350 mL = £3.32; 1 litre = £7.80

For dry skin conditions including eczema, ichthyosis and pruritus of the elderly; add 1–3 capfuls/bath (infant ½–2 capfuls)

Additives: none as listed in section 13.1

Oilatum® (Stiefel)

Oilatum Emollient® bath additive (emulsion), acetylated wool alcohols 5%, liquid paraffin 63.4%. Net price 250 mL = £2.75; 500 mL = £4.57

For dry skin conditions including dermatitis, pruritus of the elderly and ichthyosis; add 5–15 mL/bath (infant 2.5–10 mL)

Additives: include isopropyl palmitate, fragrance

Oilatum Plus® bath additive, benzalkonium chloride 6%, triclosan 2%, light liquid paraffin 52.5%. Net price 500 mL = £7.86

For topical treatment of eczema including eczema at risk from infection; add 1–2 capfuls/bath (infant over 6 months 1 mL)

Additives: include wool fat, isopropyl palmitate

13.2.2   Barrier preparations

Barrier preparations often contain water-repellent substances such as **dimethicone** or other silicones. They are used for areas around stomata (see also Appendix 8), sore areas in the elderly, bedsores, etc. They are no substitute for adequate nursing care, and it is doubtful if they are any more effective than the traditional compound **zinc ointments**.

NAPKIN RASH. Barrier creams and ointments are used for protection against napkin rash which is usually a local dermatitis. The first line of treatment is to ensure that napkins are changed frequently, and that tightly fitting plastic pants are avoided. The rash may clear when left exposed to the air and a napkin rash preparation (see preparations below) may be helpful. If the rash is associated with a fungal infection, an antifungal cream such as clotrimazole cream (section 13.10.2) is useful. A mild corticosteroid such as hydrocortisone may be useful but treatment should be limited to a week or less and it should be remembered that the occlusive effect of napkins and plastic pants may increase absorption (for cautions, see Hydrocortisone p. 483).

Conotrane® (Yamanouchi)

Cream, benzalkonium chloride 0.1%, dimethicone '350' 22%. Net price 100 g = 99p; 500 g = £3.74

For napkin and urinary rash and pressure sores

Additives: include fragrance

Drapolene® (Warner Lambert)

Cream, benzalkonium chloride 0.01%, cetrimide 0.2% in a water-miscible basis. Net price 75 g = 98p; 150 g = £1.60; 350 g = £3.57; 500 g = £4.99

For napkin and urinary rash; minor wounds

Additives: include chlorocresol, wool fat

Metanium® (Roche Consumer Health)

Ointment, titanium dioxide 20%, titanium peroxide 5%, titanium salicylate 3%, titanium tannate 0.1%, in a silicone basis. Net price 30 g = £1.42

For napkin rash and related disorders

Additives: none as listed in section 13.1

Siopel® (Zeneca)

Barrier cream, dimethicone '1000' 10%, cetrimide 0.3%, arachis (peanut) oil. Net price 50 g = 62p

For dermatoses, colostomy and ileostomy care, urinary rash, and related conditions

Additives: include butylated hydroxytoluene, hydroxybenzoates (parabens)

Sprilon® (S&N Hlth.)

Spray application, dimethicone 1.04%, zinc oxide 12.5%, in a basis containing wool fat, wool alcohols, cetostearyl alcohol, dextran, white soft paraffin, liq-

---

uid paraffin, propellants. Net price 115-g pressurised aerosol unit = £3.71

For urinary rash, pressure sores, and ileostomy

Caution: flammable

Vasogen® (Pharmax)

Barrier cream, dimethicone 20%, calamine 1.5%, zinc oxide 7.5%. Net price 50 g= 70p; 100 g = £1.20

For napkin and urinary rash, pressure sores, and pruritus ani

Additives: include hydroxybenzoates (parabens), wool fat

13.2.3 Dusting powders

Dusting powders are used in folds where friction may occur between opposing skin surfaces. They should not be applied in areas that are very moist as they tend to cake and abrade the skin. **Talc** acts as a lubricant powder but does not absorb moisture whereas **starch** is less lubricant but absorbs water. Other inert powders such as kaolin or zinc oxide may also be used in the formulation of dusting powders. See also section 13.11 for antiseptic dusting powders.

Talc Dusting Powder, BP, starch 10% in sterilised purified talc. Net price 100 g = 43p

Zinc, Starch and Talc Dusting-powder, BPC, zinc oxide 25%, starch 25%, sterilised purified talc 50%. Net price 50 g = 22p

ZeaSORB® (Stiefel)

Dusting powder, aldioxa 0.2%, chloroxylenol 0.5%, pulverised maize core 45%. Net price 50 g = £2.15

Additives: include fragrance

13.3 Topical local anaesthetics and antipruritics

Pruritus may be caused by systemic disease (such as drug hypersensitivity, obstructive jaundice, endocrine disease, and certain malignant diseases) as well as by skin disease (e.g. psoriasis, eczema, urticaria, and scabies). Where possible the underlying causes should be treated. There is no really effective topical antipruritic. **Calamine** preparations are widely prescribed for pruritus, and **emollient** preparations (section 13.2.1) may also be of value. **Crotamiton** does not appear to be any more effective than calamine. An emollient may be of value where the pruritus is associated with dry skin (which is common in otherwise healthy elderly people).

Insect stings are also best treated with calamine preparations. Topical antihistamines and local anaesthetics may very occasionally cause sensitisation and are only marginally effective.

For preparations used in *pruritus ani,* see section 1.7.1.

CALAMINE

Indications: pruritus

Calamine Cream, Aqueous, BP, calamine 4%, zinc oxide 3%, liquid paraffin 20%, self-emulsifying glyceryl monostearate 5%, cetomacrogol emulsifying wax 5%, phenoxyethanol 0.5%, freshly boiled and cooled purified water 62.5%. Net price 100 mL = 53p

Calamine Lotion, BP, calamine 15%, zinc oxide 5%, glycerol 5%, bentonite 3%, sodium citrate 0.5%, liquefied phenol 0.5%, in freshly boiled and cooled purified water. Net price 200 mL = 62p

Calamine Lotion, Oily, BP1980, calamine 5%, arachis (peanut) oil 50%, oleic acid 0.5%, wool fat 1%, in calcium hydroxide solution. Net price 200 mL = £1.02

CROTAMITON

Indications: pruritus (including pruritus after scabies), but see notes above

Cautions: avoid use near eyes and broken skin

Contra-indications: acute exudative dermatoses

Eurax® (Novartis Consumer Health)

Cream, crotamiton 10%. Net price 30 g = £1.97; 100 g = £3.38

Additives: include beeswax, hydroxybenzoates (parabens), fragrance

Lotion, crotamiton 10%. Net price 100 mL = £2.55

Additives: include propylene glycol, sorbic acid, fragrance

TOPICAL LOCAL ANAESTHETICS

Indications: relief of local pain, see notes above. See section 15.2 for use in surface anaesthesia

Cautions: occasionally cause hypersensitivity

Note. Topical local anaesthetic preparations may be absorbed, especially through mucosal surfaces, therefore excessive application should be avoided and they should preferably not be used for more than about 3 days; not generally suitable for young children

The following is a list of topical local anaesthetic preparations on sale to the public, together with their significant ingredients:
Anethaine® (amethocaine), **Anthisan® Plus** (benzocaine, mepyramine), **BurnEze®** (benzocaine), **Dermidex®** (lignocaine, alcloxa, cetrimide chlorbutol), **Lanacane® cream** (benzocaine, chlorothymol, resorcinol), **Lanasting®** (lignocaine, benzyl alcohol), **Solarcaine®** (benzocaine, triclosan), **Wasp–Eze®** **spray** (benzocaine, mepyramine)

TOPICAL ANTIHISTAMINES

Indications: see notes above

Cautions: may cause hypersensitivity; avoid in eczema, photosensitivity (diphenhydramine); not recommended for longer than 3 days

The following is a list of topical antihistamine preparations on sale to the public, together with their significant ingredients:
Aller–Eze® cream (diphenhydramine), **Anthisan®** (mepyramine), **Anthisan® Plus** (mepyramine, benzocaine), **Boots Bite & Sting Antihistamine cream** (mepyramine), **Caladryl®** (diphenhydramine, calamine, camphor), **R.B.C.®** (antazoline, calamine, camphor, cetrimide, menthol), **Wasp–Eze®** **ointment** (antazoline), **Wasp–Eze®** **spray** (mepyramine, benzocaine)

13.4 Topical corticosteroids

Topical corticosteroids are used for the treatment of inflammatory conditions of the skin other than those due to an infection, in particular the *eczematous disorders* (for further details see section 13.5.1). Corticosteroids suppress various components of the inflammatory reaction while in use; they are in no sense curative, and when treatment is discontinued a rebound exacerbation of the condition may occur. They are indicated for the relief of symptoms and for the suppression of signs of the disorder when potentially less harmful measures are ineffective.

Topical corticosteroids are of no value in the treatment of *urticaria* and are **contra-indicated** in *rosacea* and in *ulcerative conditions* since they worsen the condition. They should not be used indiscriminately in *pruritus* (where they act by alleviating inflammation) and are **not** recommended for *acne vulgaris.*

Systemic or potent topical corticosteroids should be avoided or given only under specialist supervision *in psoriasis* because, although they may suppress the psoriasis in the short term, relapse or vigorous rebound occurs on withdrawal (sometimes precipitating severe pustular psoriasis). Topical use of potent corticosteroids on widespread psoriasis also leads to systemic as well as to local side-effects. It is reasonable, however, to prescribe a weaker corticosteroid (such as hydrocortisone) for short periods (perhaps up to 4 weeks) for *flexural* and *facial psoriasis* (**important:** not more potent than hydrocortisone 1% on the face). In the case of *scalp psoriasis* it is reasonable to use a more potent corticosteroid such as betamethasone or fluocinonide.

In general, the most potent topical corticosteroids should be reserved for recalcitrant dermatoses such as *chronic discoid lupus erythematosus, lichen simplex chronicus, hypertrophic lichen planus*, and *palmoplantar pustulosis*. With rare exceptions, potent corticosteroids should not be used on the face as they may precipitate a rosacea-like disorder and cause skin atrophy.

Intralesional corticosteroid injections (section 10.1.2.2) are more effective than the very potent topical corticosteroid preparations and they should be reserved for severe cases where there are localised lesions (such as *keloid scars* or *hypertrophic lichen planus*) and topical treatment has failed. Their effects may last for several weeks or even months. Particular care is needed to inject accurately into the lesion in order to avoid severe skin atrophy and loss of pigmentation.

SIDE-EFFECTS. Unlike the *potent* and *very potent* groups, the *moderate* and *mild* groups are rarely associated with side-effects. The more potent the preparation the more care is required, as absorption through the skin can cause severe pituitary-adrenal-axis suppression and Cushing's syndrome (section 6.3.2), both of which depend on the area of the body treated and the duration of the treatment. Absorption is greatest from areas of thin skin, raw surfaces, and intertriginous areas, and is increased by occlusion.

Local side-effects include:
(a) spread and worsening of untreated infection;
(b) thinning of the skin which may be restored over a period of time after stopping although the original structure may never return;
(c) irreversible striae atrophicae and telangiectasia;
(d) contact dermatitis;
(e) perioral dermatitis, an inflammatory papular disorder on the face of young women;
(f) acne at the site of application in some patients;
(g) mild depigmentation

CHOICE OF FORMULATION. *Water-miscible* creams are suitable for moist or weeping lesions whereas *ointments* are generally chosen for dry, lichenified or scaly lesions or where a more occlusive effect is required. *Lotions* may be useful when minimal application to a large area is required or for the treatment of exudative lesions. *Occlusive polythene dressings* increase absorption, but also increase the risk of side-effects; they are therefore used only under supervision on a short-term basis for very thick areas of skin (such as the palms and soles). The *inclusion of urea* or *salicylic acid* increases the penetration of the corticosteroid.

TOPICAL CORTICOSTEROID POTENCIES

Potency	Examples
Mild	Hydrocortisone 1%
Moderately potent	Clobetasone butyrate 0.05%
Potent	Betamethasone 0.1% (as valerate)
	Hydrocortisone butyrate
Very potent	Clobetasol propionate 0.05%

The preparation containing the **least potent** drug at the lowest strength which is effective is the one of choice; dilution should be avoided whenever possible.

FREQUENCY OF APPLICATION. Corticosteroid preparations should normally be applied once or twice daily. It is not necessary to apply them more frequently.

Suitable quantities of corticosteroid preparations to be prescribed for specific areas of the body are:

	Creams and Ointments
Face and neck	15 to 30 g
Both hands	15 to 30 g
Scalp	15 to 30 g
Both arms	30 to 60 g
Both legs	100 g
Trunk	100 g
Groins and genitalia	15 to 30 g

These amounts are usually suitable for an adult for twice daily application for 1 week

CHILDREN. Children, especially babies, are particularly susceptible to side-effects. The more potent corticosteroids are **contra-indicated** in infants under 1 year, and in general should be **avoided** in paediatric treatment or if necessary used with great care for short periods; a mild corticosteroid such as hydrocortisone 1% ointment or cream is useful for treating napkin rash (section 13.2.2) and for atopic eczema in childhood (but see caution below).

COMPOUND PREPARATIONS. The advantages of including other substances (such as antibacterials or antifungals) with corticosteroids in topical preparations are debatable, but they may have a place where there is associated bacterial or fungal infection.

HYDROCORTISONE

Indications: mild inflammatory skin disorders such as eczemas (but for over-the-counter preparations, see below); napkin rash, see notes above and section 13.2.2

Cautions: see notes above; also avoid prolonged use in infants and children (extreme caution in dermatoses of infancy including napkin rash—where possible treatment should be limited to 5–7 days), avoid prolonged use on the face (and keep away from eyes); more potent corticosteroids **contra-indicated** in infants under 1 year (see also notes above)

PSORIASIS. Risks of more potent corticosteroids in psoriasis include possibility of rebound relapse, development of generalised pustular psoriasis, and local and systemic toxicity, see also section 13.5.2; they are specifically **contra-indicated** in widespread plaque psoriasis

Contra-indications: untreated bacterial, fungal, or viral skin lesions; rosacea (acne rosacea), perioral dermatitis; not recommended for acne vulgaris (more potent corticosteroids specifically **contra-indicated**)

Side-effects: see notes above

Administration: apply thinly 1–2 times daily

PoM **Hydrocortisone** (Non-proprietary)

Cream, hydrocortisone 0.5%, net price, 15 g = 34p; 30 g = 60p; 1%, 15 g = 42p. Label: 28. Potency: mild

Ointment, hydrocortisone 0.5%, net price 15 g = 39p; 30 g = 60p; 1%, 15 g = 38p. Label: 28. Potency: mild

When hydrocortisone cream or ointment is prescribed and no strength is stated, the 1% strength should be supplied

Over–the–counter products. The following is a list of skin creams and ointments that contain hydrocortisone (alone or with other ingredients) that can be sold to the public: **Dermacort**® (hydrocortisone 0.1%, cream), **Eurax Hc**® (hydrocortisone 0.25%; crotamiton 10%, cream), **Hc45**® (hydrocortisone acetate 1%, cream), **Lanacort**® (hydrocortisone acetate 1%, cream and ointment), **Zenoxone**® (hydrocortisone 1%, cream). They can be sold to the public for treatment of allergic contact dermatitis, irritant dermatitis, insect bite reactions and mild to moderate eczema

Cautions: not for children under 10 years or in pregnancy, without medical advice

Contra-indications: eyes/face, anogenital region, broken or infected skin (including cold sores, acne, and athlete's foot)

Administration: apply sparingly over small area 1–2 times daily for max. of 1 week

Proprietary hydrocortisone preparations

Note. The following preparations are PoM; those on sale to the public (with restrictions) are specified above.

PoM **Cobadex**® (Cox)

Cream, hydrocortisone 1%, dimethicone '350' 20%. Net price 20 g = £1.00. Label: 28. Potency: mild

Additives: include hydroxybenzoates (parabens), polysorbate 80, propylene glycol

PoM **Dioderm**® (Dermal)

Cream, hydrocortisone 0.1%. Net price 30 g = £2.69. Label: 28. Potency: mild

Additives: include propylene glycol

Note. Although this contains only 0.1% hydrocortisone, the formulation is designed to provide a clinical activity comparable to that of Hydrocortisone Cream 1% BP

PoM **Efcortelan**® (GlaxoWellcome)

Cream, hydrocortisone 0.5%, net price, 30 g = 60p; 1%, 30 g = 74p; 2.5%, 30 g = £1.66. Label: 28. Potency: mild

Additives: include chlorocresol

Ointment, hydrocortisone 0.5%, net price, 30 g = 60p; 1%, 30 g = 74p; 2.5%, 30 g = £1.66. Label: 28. Potency: mild

Additives: none as listed in section 13.1

PoM **Hydrocortisyl**® (Hoechst Marion Roussel)

Cream, hydrocortisone 1%. Net price 15 g = 27p. Label: 28. Potency: mild

Additives: include chlorocresol

Ointment, hydrocortisone 1%. Net price 15 g = 27p. Label: 28. Potency: mild

Additives: include wool fat

PoM **Mildison**® (Yamanouchi)

Lipocream, hydrocortisone 1%. Net price 30 g = £2.19. Label: 28. Potency: mild

Additives: include hydroxybenzoates (parabens)

Compound preparations

Note. Compound preparations with coal tar, section 13.5.2

PoM **Alphaderm**® (Procter & Gamble Pharm.)

Cream, hydrocortisone 1%, urea 10%. Net price 30 g = £2.36; 100 g = £7.32. Label: 28. Potency: moderate

Additives: none as listed in section 13.1

PoM **Calmurid HC**® (Galderma)

Cream, hydrocortisone 1%, urea 10%, lactic acid 5%. Net price 30 g = £2.33; 100 g = £7.30. Label: 28. Potency: moderate

Additives: none as listed in section 13.1

Note. Manufacturer advises dilute to half-strength with aqueous cream for 1 week if stinging occurs then transfer to undiluted preparation (but see section 13.1 for advice to avoid dilution where possible)

PoM **Eurax-Hydrocortisone**® (Novartis Consumer Health)

Cream, hydrocortisone 0.25%, crotamiton 10%. Net price 30 g = 91p. Label: 28. Potency: mild

Additives: include hydroxybenzoates (parabens), propylene glycol, fragrance

Note. A 15-g tube is on sale to the public for treatment of contact dermatitis and insect bites (Eurax Hc®)

PoM **Hydrocal**® (Bioglan)

Cream, hydrocortisone acetate 1%, in a basis containing calamine. Net price 100 g = £3.10. Label: 28. Potency: mild

Additives: include hydroxybenzoates (parabens), polysorbates

With antimicrobials

See notes above for comment on compound preparations

PoM **Canesten HC**® (Baypharm)

Cream, hydrocortisone 1%, clotrimazole 1%. Net price 30 g = £2.25. Label: 28. Potency: mild

Additives: include benzyl alcohol

Note. A 15-g tube is on sale to the public for the treatment of athlete's foot and fungal infection of skin folds with associated inflammation (Canesten® Hydrocortisone)

Cautionary label wordings, see inside back cover

Prices are **net**, see p.1

PoM **Daktacort®** (Janssen-Cilag)

Cream, hydrocortisone 1%, miconazole nitrate 2%. Net price 30 g = £2.24. Label: 28. Potency: mild

Additives: include butylated hydroxyanisole, disodium edetate

Ointment, hydrocortisone 1%, miconazole nitrate 2%. Net price 30 g = £2.25. Label: 28. Potency: mild

Additives: none as listed in section 13.1

PoM **Econacort®** (Squibb)

Cream, hydrocortisone 1%, econazole nitrate 1%. Net price 30 g = £2.25. Label: 28. Potency: mild

Additives: include butylated hydroxyanisole

PoM **Fucidin H®** (Leo)

Cream, hydrocortisone acetate 1%, fusidic acid 2%. Net price 15 g = £3.22; 30 g = £5.55. Label: 28. Potency: mild

Additives: include butylated hydroxyanisole, potassium sorbate

Gel, hydrocortisone acetate 1%, fusidic acid 2%. Net price 15 g = £2.84; 30 g = £4.93. Label: 28. Potency: mild

Additives: include hydroxybenzoates (parabens), polysorbate 80

Ointment, hydrocortisone acetate 1%, sodium fusidate 2%. Net price 15 g = £2.63; 30 g = £4.56. Label: 28. Potency: mild

Additives: include wool fat

PoM **Gregoderm®** (Unigreg)

Ointment, hydrocortisone 1%, neomycin sulphate 0.4%, nystatin 100 000 units/g, polymyxin B sulphate 7250 units/g. Net price 15 g = £2.51. Label: 28. Potency: mild

Additives: none as listed in section 13.1

PoM **Nystaform-HC®** (Bayer)

Cream,   hydrocortisone   0.5%,   nystatin 100 000 units/g, chlorhexidine hydrochloride 1%. Net price 30 g = £2.66. Label: 28. Potency: mild

Additives: include benzyl alcohol, polysorbate '60'

Ointment,   hydrocortisone   1%,   nystatin 100 000 units/g, chlorhexidine acetate 1%. Net price 30 g = £2.66. Label: 28. Potency: mild

Additives: none as listed in section 13.1

PoM **Quinocort®** (Quinoderm Ltd)

Cream, hydrocortisone 1%, potassium hydroxyquinoline sulphate 0.5%. Net price 30 g = £1.56. Label: 28. Potency: mild

Additives: include edetic acid (EDTA), chlorocresol

PoM **Terra-Cortril®** (Pfizer)

Topical ointment, hydrocortisone 1%, oxytetracycline 3% (as hydrochloride). Net price 15 g = £1.01; 30 g = £1.82. Label: 28. Potency: mild

Additives: none as listed in section 13.1

PoM **Terra-Cortril Nystatin®** (Pfizer)

Cream, hydrocortisone 1%, nystatin 100 000 units/g, oxytetracycline 3% (as calcium salt). Net price 30 g = £2.01. Label: 28. Potency: mild

Additives: include hydroxybenzoates (parabens), polysorbate, propylene glycol, fragrance

PoM **Timodine®** (R&C)

Cream,   hydrocortisone   0.5%,   nystatin 100 000 units/g, benzalkonium chloride solution 0.2%, dimethicone '350' 10%. Net price 30 g = £2.38. Label: 28. Potency: mild

Additives: include butylated hydroxyanisole, hydroxybenzoates (parabens), sorbic acid

PoM **Vioform-Hydrocortisone®** (Novartis Consumer Health)

Cream, hydrocortisone 1%, clioquinol 3%. Net price 30 g = £1.53. Label: 28. Potency: mild

Additives: none as listed in section 13.1

Ointment, hydrocortisone 1%, clioquinol 3%. Net price 30 g = £1.53. Label:28. Potency: mild

Additives: none as listed in section 13.1

Caution: stains clothing

HYDROCORTISONE BUTYRATE

Indications: severe inflammatory skin disorders such as eczemas unresponsive to less potent corticosteroids; psoriasis, see notes above

Cautions; Contra-indications; Side-effects: see under Hydrocortisone and notes above

Administration: apply thinly 1–2 times daily

PoM **Locoid®** (Yamanouchi)

Cream, hydrocortisone butyrate 0.1%. Net price 30 g = £2.27; 100 g = £6.95. Label: 28. Potency: potent

Additives: include hydroxybenzoates (parabens)

Lipocream, hydrocortisone butyrate 0.1%. Net price 30 g = £2.38; 100 g = £7.29. Label: 28. Potency: potent

Additives: include hydroxybenzoates (parabens)

Note. For bland cream basis see Lipobase®, section 13.2.1

Ointment, hydrocortisone butyrate 0.1%. Net price 30 g = £2.27; 100 g = £6.95. Label: 28. Potency: potent

Additives: none as listed in section 13.1

Scalp lotion, hydrocortisone butyrate 0.1%, in an aqueous isopropyl alcohol basis. Net price 30 mL = £3.20; 100 mL = £9.81. Label: 15, 28. Potency: potent

Additives: none as listed in section 13.1

PoM **Locoid Crelo®** (Yamanouchi)

Lotion (topical emulsion), hydrocortisone butyrate 0.1% in a water-miscible basis. Net price 100 g (with applicator nozzle) = £8.33. Label: 28. Potency: potent

Additives: include hydroxybenzoates (parabens), propylene glycol

With antimicrobials

See notes above for comment on compound preparations

PoM **Locoid C®** (Yamanouchi)

Cream, hydrocortisone butyrate 0.1%, chlorquinaldol 3%. Net price 30 g = £2.97. Label: 28. Potency: potent

Additives: none as listed in section 13.1

Caution: causes staining

Ointment, ingredients as for cream, in a greasy basis. Net price 30 g = £2.97. Label: 28. Potency: potent

Additives: none as listed in section 13.1

Caution: causes staining

ALCLOMETASONE DIPROPIONATE

Indications: inflammatory skin disorders such as eczemas

Cautions; Contra-indications; Side-effects: see under Hydrocortisone and notes above

Administration: apply thinly 1–2 times daily

PoM **Modrasone®** (Dominion)

Cream, alclometasone dipropionate 0.05%. Net price 50 g = £2.95. Label: 28. Potency: moderate

Additives: include chlorocresol, propylene glycol

Ointment, alclometasone dipropionate 0.05%. Net price 50 g = £2.95. Label: 28. Potency: moderate

Additives: include beeswax, propylene glycol

BECLOMETHASONE DIPROPIONATE

Indications: severe inflammatory skin disorders such as eczemas unresponsive to less potent corticosteroids; psoriasis, see notes above
Cautions; Contra-indications; Side-effects: see under Hydrocortisone and notes above
Administration: apply thinly 1–2 times daily

PoM **Propaderm®** (GlaxoWellcome)
Cream, beclomethasone dipropionate 0.025%. Net price 30 g = £1.58. Label: 28. Potency: potent
Additives: include propylene glycol
Ointment, beclomethasone dipropionate 0.025%. Net price 30 g = £1.58. Label: 28. Potency: potent
Additives: include propylene glycol

BETAMETHASONE ESTERS

Indications: severe inflammatory skin disorders such as eczemas unresponsive to less potent corticosteroids; psoriasis, see notes above
Cautions; Contra-indications; Side-effects: see under Hydrocortisone and notes above. Application of more than 100 g per week of 0.1% preparation is likely to cause adrenal suppression
Administration: apply thinly 1–2 times daily

PoM **Betamethasone Valerate** (Non-proprietary)
Cream, betamethasone 0.1% (as valerate). Net price 30 g = £1.40. Label: 28. Potency: potent
Ointment, betamethasone 0.1% (as valerate) Net price 30 g = £1.40. Label: 28. Potency: potent
PoM **Betacap®** (Dermal)
Scalp application, betamethasone 0.1% (as valerate) in a water-miscible basis containing coconut oil derivative. Net price 100 mL = £4.42. Label: 15, 28. Potency: potent
Additives: none as listed in section 13.1
PoM **Betnovate®** (GlaxoWellcome)
Cream, betamethasone 0.1% (as valerate), in a water-miscible basis. Net price 30 g = £1.40; 100 g = £3.95. Label: 28. Potency: potent
Additives: include chlorocresol
Ointment, betamethasone 0.1% (as valerate), in an anhydrous paraffin basis. Net price 30 g = £1.40; 100 g = £3.95. Label: 28. Potency: potent
Additives: none as listed in section 13.1
Lotion, betamethasone 0.1% (as valerate). Net price 100 mL = £4.75. Label: 28. Potency: potent
Additives: include hydroxybenzoates (parabens)
Scalp application, betamethasone 0.1% (as valerate) in a water-miscible basis. Net price 100 mL = £5.18. Label: 15, 28. Potency: potent
Additives: none as listed in section 13.1
PoM **Betnovate-RD®** (GlaxoWellcome)
Cream, betamethasone 0.025% (as valerate) in a water-miscible basis (1 in 4 dilution of Betnovate® cream). Net price 100 g = £3.26. Label: 28. Potency: moderate
Additives: include chlorocresol
Ointment, betamethasone 0.025% (as valerate) in an anhydrous paraffin basis (1 in 4 dilution of Betnovate® ointment). Net price 100 g = £3.26. Label: 28. Potency: moderate
Additives: none as listed in section 13.1

PoM **Bettamousse®** (Evans)
Foam (= scalp application), betamethasone valerate 0.12% (≡ betamethasone 0.1%). Net price 100 g = £7.50. Label: 28. Potency: potent
Additives: include polysorbate 60, propylene glycol
Caution: flammable
PoM **Diprosone®** (Schering-Plough)
Cream, betamethasone 0.05% (as dipropionate). Net price 30 g = £2.51; 100 g = £7.12. Label: 28. Potency: potent
Additives: include chlorocresol
Ointment, betamethasone 0.05% (as dipropionate). Net price 30 g = £2.51; 100 g = £7.12. Label: 28. Potency: potent
Additives: none as listed in section 13.1
Lotion, betamethasone 0.05% (as dipropionate). Net price 30 mL = £3.17; 100 mL = £9.07. Label: 28. Potency: potent
Additives: none as listed in section 13.1

With salicylic acid
See notes above for comment on compound preparations
PoM **Diprosalic®** (Schering-Plough)
Ointment, betamethasone 0.05% (as dipropionate), salicylic acid 3%. Net price 30 g = £3.30; 100 g = £9.50. Label: 28. Potency: potent
Additives: none as listed in section 13.1
Apply thinly 1–2 times daily; max. 60 g per week
Scalp application, betamethasone 0.05% (as dipropionate), salicylic acid 2%, in an alcoholic basis. Net price 100 mL = £10.50. Label: 28. Potency: potent
Additives: include disodium edetate
Apply a few drops 1–2 times daily

With antimicrobials
See notes above for comment on compound preparations
PoM **Betnovate-C®** (GlaxoWellcome)
Cream, betamethasone 0.1% (as valerate), clioquinol 3%. Net price 30 g = £1.72. Label: 28. Potency: potent
Additives: include chlorocresol
Caution: stains clothing
Ointment, betamethasone 0.1% (as valerate), clioquinol 3%. Net price 30 g = £1.72. Label: 28. Potency: potent
Additives: none as listed in section 13.1
Caution: stains clothing
PoM **Betnovate-N®** (GlaxoWellcome)
Cream, betamethasone 0.1% (as valerate), neomycin sulphate 0.5%. Net price 30 g = £1.72; 100 g = £4.77. Label: 28. Potency: potent
Additives: include chlorocresol
Ointment, betamethasone 0.1% (as valerate), neomycin sulphate 0.5%. Net price 30 g = £1.72; 100 g = £4.77. Label: 28. Potency: potent
Additives: none as listed in section 13.1
PoM **Fucibet®** (Leo)
Cream, betamethasone 0.1% (as valerate), fusidic acid 2%. Net price 15 g = £3.74; 30 g = £6.32; 60 g = £12.64. Label: 28. Potency: potent
Additives: include chlorocresol
PoM **Lotriderm®** (Dominion)
Cream, betamethasone 0.05% (as dipropionate), clotrimazole 1%. Net price 15 g = £3.40. Label: 28. Potency: potent
Additives: include benzyl alcohol, propylene glycol

CLOBETASOL PROPIONATE

Indications: short-term treatment only of severe resistant inflammatory skin disorders such as recalcitrant eczemas unresponsive to less potent corticosteroids; psoriasis, see notes above

Cautions; Contra-indications; Side-effects: see under Hydrocortisone and notes above. Not more than 50 g of 0.05% preparation should be applied per week

Administration: apply thinly 1–2 times daily for up to 4 weeks

PoM **Dermovate®** (GlaxoWellcome)

Cream, clobetasol propionate 0.05%. Net price 30 g = £2.56; 100 g = £7.52. Label: 28. Potency: very potent

Additives: include beeswax (or beeswax substitute), chlorocresol, propylene glycol

Ointment, clobetasol propionate 0.05%. Net price 30 g = £2.56; 100 g = £7.52. Label: 28. Potency: very potent

Additives: include propylene glycol

Scalp application, clobetasol propionate 0.05%, in a thickened alcoholic basis. Net price 30 mL = £2.93; 100 mL = £9.91. Label: 15, 28. Potency: very potent

Additives: none as listed insection 13.1

With antimicrobials

See notes above for comment on compound preparations

PoM **Dermovate-NN®** (GlaxoWellcome)

Cream, clobetasol propionate 0.05%, neomycin sulphate 0.5%, nystatin 100 000 units/g. Net price 30 g = £3.50. Label: 28. Potency: very potent

Additives: include beeswax substitute

Ointment, ingredients as for cream, in a paraffin basis. Net price 30 g = £3.50. Label: 28. Potency: very potent

Additives: none as listed in section 13.1

CLOBETASONE BUTYRATE

Indications: eczemas and dermatitis of all types; maintenance between courses of more potent corticosteroids

Cautions; Contra-indications; Side-effects: see under Hydrocortisone and notes above

Administration: apply thinly 1–2 times daily

PoM **Eumovate®** (GlaxoWellcome)

Cream, clobetasone butyrate 0.05%. Net price 30 g = £1.76; 100 g = £5.16. Label: 28. Potency: moderate

Additives: include beeswax substitute, chlorocresol

Ointment, clobetasone butyrate 0.05%. Net price 30 g = £1.76; 100 g = £5.16. Label: 28. Potency: moderate

Additives: none as listed in section 13.1

With antimicrobials

See notes above for comment on compound preparations

PoM **Trimovate®** (GlaxoWellcome)

Cream, clobetasone butyrate 0.05%, oxytetracycline 3% (as calcium salt), nystatin 100 000 units/g. Net price 30 g = £3.13. Label: 28. Potency: moderate

Additives: include chlorocresol

Caution: stains clothing

DESOXYMETHASONE

(Desoximetasone)

Indications: severe acute inflammatory, allergic, and chronic skin disorders; psoriasis, see notes above

Cautions; Contra-indications; Side-effects: see under Hydrocortisone and notes above

Administration: apply thinly 1–2 times daily

PoM **Stiedex®** (Stiefel)

LP Oily cream, desoxymethasone 0.05%. Net price 30 g = £2.86; 100 g = £8.58. Label:28. Potency: moderate

Additives: include edetic acid (EDTA), wool fat

Lotion, desoxymethasone 0.25%, salicylic acid 1%. Net price 50 mL = £8.05. Label: 28. Potency: potent

Additives: include disodium edetate, propylene glycol

DIFLUCORTOLONE VALERATE

Indications: severe inflammatory skin disorders such as eczemas unresponsive to less potent corticosteroids; high strength (0.3%), short-term treatment of severe exacerbations; psoriasis, see notes above

Cautions; Contra-indications; Side-effects: see under Hydrocortisone and notes above; not more than 60 g of 0.3% applied per week

Administration: apply thinly 1–2 times daily for up to 4 weeks (0.1% preparations) or 2 weeks (0.3% preparations), reducing strength as condition responds

PoM **Nerisone®** (Schering Health)

Cream, diflucortolone valerate 0.1%. Net price 30 g = £1.59. Label: 28. Potency: potent

Additives: include disodium edetate, hydroxybenzoates (parabens)

Oily cream, diflucortolone valerate 0.1%. Net price 30 g = £2.56. Label: 28. Potency: potent

Additives: none as listed in section 13.1

Ointment, diflucortolone valerate 0.1%. Net price 30 g = £1.59. Label: 28. Potency: potent

Additives: none as listed in section 13.1

PoM **Nerisone Forte®** (Schering Health)

Oily cream, diflucortolone valerate 0.3%. Net price 15 g = £2.09. Label: 28. Potency: very potent

Additives: none as listed in section 13.1

Ointment, diflucortolone valerate 0.3%. Net price 15 g = £2.09. Label: 28. Potency: very potent

Additives: none as listed in section 13.1

FLUOCINOLONE ACETONIDE

Indications: inflammatory skin disorders such as eczemas; psoriasis, see notes above

Cautions; Contra-indications; Side-effects: see under Hydrocortisone and notes above

Administration: apply thinly 1–2 times daily, reducing strength as condition responds

PoM **Synalar®** (Zeneca)

Cream, fluocinolone acetonide 0.025%. Net price 30 g = £1.37. Label: 28. Potency: potent

Additives: include benzyl alcohol, polysorbates, propylene glycol

---

Gel, fluocinolone acetonide 0.025%. Net price 30 g = £1.45. For use on scalp and other hairy areas. Label: 28. Potency: potent
Additives: include hydroxybenzoates (parabens), propylene glycol

Ointment, fluocinolone acetonide 0.025%. Net price 30 g = £1.37. Label: 28. Potency: potent
Additives: include propylene glycol, wool fat

PoM **Synalar 1 in 4 Dilution**® (Zeneca)
Cream, fluocinolone acetonide 0.00625%. Net price 50 g = £1.56. Label: 28. Potency: moderate
Additives: include benzyl alcohol, polysorbates, propylene glycol

Ointment, fluocinolone acetonide 0.00625%. Net price 50 g = £1.83. Label: 28. Potency: moderate
Additives: include propylene glycol, wool fat

PoM **Synalar 1 in 10 Dilution**® (Zeneca)
Cream, fluocinolone acetonide 0.0025%. Net price 50 g = £1.48. Label: 28. Potency: mild
Additives: include benzyl alcohol, polysorbates, propylene glycol

With antibacterials
See notes above for comment on compound preparations
PoM **Synalar C**® (Zeneca)
Cream, fluocinolone acetonide 0.025%, clioquinol 3%. Net price 15 g = 94p. Label: 28. Potency: potent
Additives: include disodium edetate, hydroxybenzoates (parabens), polysorbates, propylene glycol

Ointment, ingredients as for cream. Net price 15 g = 94p. Label: 28. Potency: potent.
Caution: stains clothing
Additives: include propylene glycol, wool fat

PoM **Synalar N**® (Zeneca)
Cream, fluocinolone acetonide 0.025%, neomycin sulphate 0.5%. Net price 30 g = £1.41. Label: 28. Potency: potent
Additives: include hydroxybenzoates (parabens), polysorbates, propylene glycol

Ointment, ingredients as for cream, in a greasy basis. Net price 30 g = £1.41. Label: 28. Potency: potent
Additives: include propylene glycol, wool fat

FLUOCINONIDE
Indications: severe inflammatory skin disorders such as eczemas unresponsive to less potent corticosteroids; psoriasis, see notes above
Cautions; Contra-indications; Side-effects: see under Hydrocortisone and notes above
Administration: apply thinly 1–2 times daily

PoM **Metosyn**® (Zeneca)
FAPG cream, fluocinonide 0.05%. Net price 25 g = £1.22; 100 g = £4.59. Label: 28. Potency: potent
Additives: include propylene glycol

Ointment, fluocinonide 0.05%. Net price 25 g = £1.22; 100 g = £4.59. Label: 28. Potency: potent
Additives: include propylene glycol

Scalp lotion, fluocinonide 0.05% in a propylene glycol-alcohol basis. Net price 30 mL (with applicator) = £1.56. Label: 15, 28. Potency: potent
Additives: include propylene glycol

FLUOCORTOLONE
Indications: severe inflammatory skin disorders such as eczemas unresponsive to less potent corticosteroids; psoriasis, see notes above
Cautions; Contra-indications; Side-effects: see under Hydrocortisone and notes above

Administration: apply thinly 1–2 times daily, reducing strength as condition responds

PoM **Ultralanum Plain**® (Schering Health)
Cream, fluocortolone hexanoate 0.25%, fluocortolone pivalate 0.25%. Net price 50 g = £2.95. Label: 28. Potency: moderate
Additives: include disodium edetate, hydroxybenzoates (parabens), fragrance

Ointment, fluocortolone 0.25%, fluocortolone hexanoate 0.25%. Net price 50 g = £2.95. Label: 28. Potency: moderate
Additives: include wool fat, fragrance

FLURANDRENOLONE
(Fludroxycortide)
Indications: inflammatory skin disorders such as eczemas
Cautions; Contra-indications; Side-effects: see under Hydrocortisone and notes above
Administration: apply thinly 1–2 times daily, reducing strength as condition responds

PoM **Haelan**® (Novex)
Cream, flurandrenolone 0.0125%. Net price 60 g = £3.26. Label: 28. Potency: moderate
Additives: include propylene glycol

Ointment, flurandrenolone 0.0125%. Net price 60 g = £3.26. Label: 28. Potency: moderate
Additives: include beeswax, polysorbate

Tape, polythene adhesive film impregnated with flurandrenolone 4 micrograms/cm². Net price 7.5 cm × 50 cm – £4.05; 7.5 cm × 200 cm = £13.62
For chronic localised recalcitrant dermatoses (but not acute or weeping), cut tape to fit lesion, apply to clean, dry skin shorn of hair, usually for 12 of each 24 hours
Note. Haelan® Tape cannot be prescribed on form FP10 (GP10 in Scotland) since it is not reimbursable

FLUTICASONE PROPIONATE
Indications: inflammatory skin disorders such as dermatitis and eczemas unresponsive to less potent corticosteroids
Cautions; Contra-indications; Side-effects: see under Hydrocortisone and notes above
Administration: apply cream thinly once daily *or* ointment twice daily

PoM **Cutivate**® (GlaxoWellcome)
Cream, fluticasone propionate 0.05%. Net price 15 g = £2.35; 50 g = £6.95. Label: 28. Potency: potent
Additives: include propylene glycol

Ointment, fluticasone propionate 0.005%. Net price 15 g = £2.35, 50 g = £6.95. Label: 28. Potency: potent

HALCINONIDE
Indications: short-term treatment only of severe resistant inflammatory skin disorders such as recalcitrant eczemas unresponsive to less potent corticosteroids; psoriasis, see notes above
Cautions; Contra-indications; Side-effects: see under Hydrocortisone and notes above
Administration: apply thinly 1–2 times daily

PoM **Halciderm Topical®** (Squibb)
Cream, halcinonide 0.1%. Net price 30 g = £3.40.
Label: 28. Potency: very potent
Additives: include propylene glycol

MOMETASONE FUROATE

Indications: severe inflammatory skin disorders
such as eczemas unresponsive to less potent corticosteroids; psoriasis, see notes above
Cautions; Contra-indications; Side-effects: see
under Hydrocortisone and notes above
Administration: apply thinly once daily (to scalp
in case of lotion)

PoM **Elocon®** (Schering-Plough)
Cream, mometasone furoate 0.1%. Net price 30 g
= £4.88; 100 g = £14.05. Label: 28. Potency:
potent
Additives: none as listed in section 13.1
Ointment, mometasone furoate 0.1%. Net price
30 g = £4.88; 100 g = £14.05. Label: 28. Potency:
potent
Additives: none as listed in section 13.1
Lotion, mometasone furoate 0.1% in an aqueous
isopropyl alcohol basis. Net price 30 mL = £4.88.
Label: 28. Potency: potent
Additives: include propylene glycol

TRIAMCINOLONE ACETONIDE

Indications: severe inflammatory skin disorders
such as eczemas unresponsive to less potent corticosteroids; psoriasis, see notes above
Cautions; Contra-indications; Side-effects: see
under Hydrocortisone and notes above
Administration: apply thinly 1–2 times daily

PoM **Adcortyl®** (Squibb)
Cream, triamcinolone acetonide 0.1%. Net price
30 g = £1.59. Label: 28. Potency: potent
Additives: include benzyl alcohol, propylene glycol
Ointment, triamcinolone acetonide 0.1%. Net price
30 g = £1.59. Label: 28. Potency: potent
Additives: none as listed in section 13.1

With antimicrobials
See notes above for comment on compound preparations
PoM **Adcortyl with Graneodin®** (Squibb)
Cream, triamcinolone acetonide 0.1%, gramicidin
0.025%, neomycin 0.25% (as sulphate). Net price
25 g = £3.00. Label: 28. Potency: potent
Additives: include benzyl alcohol, propylene glycol
PoM **Aureocort®** (Lederle)
Ointment, triamcinolone acetonide 0.1%, chlor-
tetracycline hydrochloride 3%, in an anhydrous
greasy basis containing wool fat and white soft
paraffin. Net price 15 g = £2.70. Label: 28.
Potency: potent
Additives: include hydroxybenzoates (parabens), wool fat
Caution: stains clothing
PoM **Nystadermal®** (Squibb)
Cream, triamcinolone acetonide 0.1%, nystatin
100 000 units/g. Net price 15 g = £2.27. Label: 28.
Potency: potent
Additives: include benzyl alcohol, propylene glycol, fragrance

PoM **Pevaryl TC®** (Janssen-Cilag)
Cream, triamcinolone 0.1%, econazole nitrate 1%.
Net price 15 g = £4.00. Label: 28. Potency: potent
Additives: include butylated hydroxyanisole, disodium edetate,
benzoic acid
PoM **Tri-Adcortyl®** (Squibb)
Cream, triamcinolone acetonide 0.1%, gramicidin
0.025%, neomycin 0.25% (as sulphate), nystatin
100 000 units/g. Net price 30 g = £3.15. Label: 28.
Potency: potent
Additives: include benzyl alcohol, ethylenediamine, propylene
glycol, fragrance
Ointment, ingredients as for cream, in an ointment basis.
Net price 30 g = £3.15. Label: 28. Potency: potent
Additives: none as listed in section 13.1
Note. Not recommended owing to presence of ethylenedi-
amine in the cream and also because combination of
antibiotic with antifungal not considered useful in either
the cream or ointment

13.5 Preparations for eczema and psoriasis

13.5.1 Preparations for eczema
13.5.2 Preparations for psoriasis

13.5.1 Preparations for eczema

An eczematous disorder (dermatitis) is a cutaneous
reaction characterised by inflammation and itching.
Where possible, the cause (e.g. household detergent) should be established and removed; a patient
with suspected contact dermatitis should be patch
tested to establish the diagnosis. *Atopic eczema* is
the most common form of eczema and usually
requires regular application of an **emollient** (section 13.2.1) with short courses of a **mild to moderate topical corticosteroid** (section 13.4); the
topical corticosteroid chosen should always be the
least potent that is effective. In *mild to moderate
atopic eczema* use of the topical corticosteroid
should be restricted to periods of one to two weeks,
in conjunction with regular use of an **emollient**
(section 13.2.1). *Severe atopic eczema* on the limbs
or body (or a flare-up of mild to moderate eczema)
may require application of a **potent or moderately
potent corticosteroid** for the first one to two
weeks, followed by a **weaker preparation** as the
condition improves; an **emollient** should also be
used and, if itching is a major problem, consideration should be given to administration of an **antihistamine** by mouth and possibly of an **antibiotic**
by mouth.

Dry, fissured, scaly lesions are treated with bland
emollients (section 13.2.1) which are often all that
is necessary to allay irritation and permit healing.
Preparations such as **aqueous cream** or **emulsifying ointment** are used as soap substitutes and in
the bath; addition of a bath oil may also be helpful.

Weeping eczemas may be treated with topical
corticosteroid creams (section 13.4) ; they are, however, commonly secondarily infected. Wet dressings
of **potassium permanganate** (0.01%) (section
13.11.6) are applied; if a large area is involved,
potassium permanganate baths are taken. When
necessary **topical antibacterials** are used (section
13.10.1) but those which are not given systemically
should usually be chosen.

Coal tar (section 13.5.2) is used occasionally in chronic atopic eczema.

Ichthammol has a milder action than coal tar and is usually used in chronic lichenified forms of eczema. It can be applied conveniently to flexures of the limbs as **zinc paste and ichthammol bandage** (Appendix 9).

Cyclosporin (section 13.5.2) is now available for *severe resistant atopic dermatitis*; its use calls for specialist care in a hospital context.

Gamolenic acid has been claimed to improve atopic eczema. However, the evidence in favour of a useful therapeutic effect is poor.

For comment on the role of **corticosteroids** in eczema see section 13.4.

ICHTHAMMOL
Indications: chronic lichenified eczema
Side-effects: skin irritation
Administration: apply 1–3 times daily

Ichthammol Ointment, BP 1980, ichthammol 10%, yellow soft paraffin 45%, wool fat 45%. Net price 25 g = 21p
Zinc and Ichthammol Cream, BP, ichthammol 5%, cetostearyl alcohol 3%, wool fat 10%, in zinc cream. Net price 100 g = 73p
Zinc Paste and Ichthammol Bandage, BP (Ichthopaste®, Icthaband®), see Appendix 9

GAMOLENIC ACID
Indications: see under preparation below; mastalgia, section 6.7.2
Cautions: history of epilepsy, concomitant treatment with epileptogenic drugs e.g. phenothiazines; pregnancy
Side-effects: occasional nausea, indigestion, headache; rarely hypersensitivity reactions including rash, urticaria, pruritus and abdominal pain
Dose: see under preparation below

PoM **Epogam®** (Searle)
Capsules, gamolenic acid 40 mg in evening primrose oil. Net price 240-cap pack = £24.41. Counselling, see below
Additives: include vitamin E 10 mg as *in vivo* antioxidant
Dose: symptomatic relief of atopic eczema (but see notes above), 4–6 capsules twice daily; CHILD 1–12 years, 2–4 capsules twice daily
Paediatric capsules, gamolenic acid 80 mg in evening primrose oil. Net price 60-cap pack = £15.41. Counselling, see below
Additives: include vitamin E 20 mg as *in vivo* antioxidant
Dose: symptomatic relief of atopic eczema (but see notes above), CHILD 1–12 years, 1–2 capsules twice daily
COUNSELLING. Capsules may be cut open and contents swallowed or taken on bread; paediatric capsules have 'snip-off' neck for convenience of administration

SEBORRHOEIC DERMATITIS

Seborrhoeic dermatitis (seborrhoeic eczema) is often associated with malassezia (pityrosporum) infection. Seborrhoeic dermatitis may respond *either* to a **mild topical corticosteroid** (section 13.4), *or* to a **topical antifungal** such as ketoconazole cream (section 13.10.2) *or* to a combination of both. Topical application of **lithium succinate and zinc sulphate** ointment has also been shown to

be effective. **Coal tar, salicylic acid,** and **sulphur** preparations (section 13.5.2) are also used for seborrhoeic dermatitis usually of the scalp.

Seborrhoeic dermatitis of the scalp (including dandruff) is managed with topical scalp preparations, see section 13.9

LITHIUM SUCCINATE
Indications: seborrhoeic dermatitis
Cautions: may exacerbate psoriasis; avoid eyes, mucous membranes
Side-effects: occasional skin irritation
Administration: ADULT and CHILD over 12 years, initially apply thinly twice daily, then reduce

PoM **Efalith®** (Searle)
Ointment, lithium succinate 8%, zinc sulphate 0.05%. Net price 20 g = £3.00
Additives: include wool fat derivative

13.5.2 Preparations for psoriasis

Psoriasis is characterised by epidermal thickening and scaling. It commonly affects extensor surfaces and the scalp. For mild conditions, treatment, other than reassurance and an **emollient**, may be unnecessary.

In more troublesome cases of psoriasis, local application of salicylic acid, coal tar, calcipotriol, or dithranol may have a beneficial effect.

Salicylic acid may be used in all hyperkeratotic and scaling conditions to enhance the rate of loss of surface scale. Preparations containing salicylic acid 2% are used initially and then gradually increased to concentrations of 3 to 6%. Side-effects are few but include irritation, or, when large areas are treated, salicylate toxicity.

Coal tar is more active than salicylic acid and has anti-inflammatory and antiscaling properties. It is used in psoriasis and occasionally in *chronic atopic eczema*. The formulation and strength chosen depends on patient acceptability and severity of the condition; the 'thicker' the patch of eczema or psoriasis the stronger the concentration of coal tar required. **Coal tar paste** or **zinc and coal tar paste** are generally suitable for most cases but are limited by their unpleasant appearance and smell and they may not be used on the face. Some of the newer preparations are more acceptable. Preparations such as *Carbo-Dome®* are suitable for treating the scalp. **Zinc paste and coal tar bandage** (Appendix 9) is useful for treating the limbs. **Tar shampoos** are described in section 13.9. When lesions are extensive coal tar baths are useful. Combinations of coal tar with zinc or salicylic acid have no advantage over the simpler preparations. Preparations containing hydrocortisone and coal tar are useful in eczemas.

Dithranol is very effective in psoriasis. The preparation is applied carefully to the lesion. Usual concentrations are 0.1–3.0%; applications of lower concentrations are preferably left on the skin overnight but higher concentrations (1.0–3.0%) should normally only be applied for short contact periods of 30–60 minutes (**important:** if using above 0.1% the sensitivity of the skin must first be tested—further increases must be gradual). Dithranol must be used with caution as it can cause quite severe skin irritation (especially to perilesional skin). For this reason it must be applied only to the lesions and it is customary to start with low concentrations (e.g. 0.1%) and gradually build up (e.g. every 7 days) to the maximum concentration which produces a therapeutic effect without irritation. It should not be applied to flexural areas since burning may occur. Hands should be washed thoroughly after use. Some patients are intolerant to dithranol even in low concentrations; it is important to recognise them early in treatment because continued use can result in their psoriasis becoming unstable. Fair skin is more sensitive than dark skin. Proprietary preparations may be more convenient as they may cause less staining than dithranol paste. *Ingram's method* of applying dithranol is sometimes used in hospital. The patient soaks in a warm bath containing coal tar solution 1 in 800 and after drying is exposed to ultraviolet radiation B (UVB) to produce a slight erythema. **Dithranol paste** is applied to the lesions and the normal skin protected by applying talc and stockinette dressings. The procedure is repeated daily.

UVB phototherapy is also effective by itself in mild to moderate, guttate or chronic plaque psoriasis.

Calcipotriol is a vitamin D derivative that is now widely used for topical application for mild to moderate psoriasis affecting up to 40% of skin area; a scalp solution is now also available. Advantages are that it does not have an unpleasant smell and does not stain clothing. **Tacalcitol**, another vitamin D analogue, has been introduced recently for once-daily application in the treatment of plaque psoriasis.

Tazarotene is a retinoid introduced recently for topical use in mild to moderate plaque psoriasis affecting up to 10% of skin area.

PUVA, photochemotherapy using psoralens with long-wave ultraviolet irradiation (UVA), is effective in some patients with psoriasis. Special lamps are required, and a psoralen, generally methoxsalen [unlicensed] is given by mouth to sensitise the skin to the effects of irradiation. Treatment is only available in specialist centres; it has to be carefully regulated, owing to the short-term hazard of severe burning and the long-term hazards of cataract formation, accelerated ageing of the skin, and the development of skin cancer.

Acitretin is a retinoid given by mouth for the treatment of *severe resistant or complicated psoriasis* and some of the *congenital disorders of keratinisation* including Darier's disease (keratosis follicularis). It is a metabolite of **etretinate** (which it has replaced). It should be prescribed **only** by, or under the supervision of, a consultant dermatologist and is available to hospitals (or specified retail pharmacies) **only**. It is a retinoid (a vitamin A derivative) with marked effects on keratinising epithelia. A therapeutic effect occurs after 2 to 4 weeks with maximum benefit after 4 to 6 weeks. Acitretin treats only manifestations not the ultimate causes of these diseases, but treatment should be limited to a period

of 6 to 9 months with a 3- to 4-month rest period before repeating treatment. Most patients suffer from dryness and cracking of the lips. Other side-effects include a mild transient increase in the rate of hair fall (reversible on withdrawal), occasional generalised pruritus, paronychia, and nose bleeds. There is a tendency for the plasma lipids to rise in some patients. Acitretin is **teratogenic** and must be **avoided** in pregnancy. Contraceptive measures must be taken at least **1 month before** and during treatment by women who may become pregnant and for at least **two years after** a course of the drug.

An antimetabolite, usually **methotrexate**, may also be used for *severe resistant psoriasis*, but this must again always be done under hospital supervision, the dose being adjusted according to severity of the condition and in accordance with haematological and biochemical measurements; the usual dose is 10 to 25 mg of methotrexate once weekly, by mouth.

Cyclosporin is now also available for *severe resistant psoriasis* and once again its use calls for specialist care in a hospital context.

For comment on the limited role of **corticosteroids** in psoriasis, see section 13.4.

TOPICAL PREPARATIONS FOR PSORIASIS

CALCIPOTRIOL

Indications: see under Administration

Cautions: pregnancy; avoid use on face and inadvertent transfer to other body areas; wash hands thoroughly after application; risk of hypercalcaemia if max. recommended weekly dose exceeded (reported with less in generalised pustular or erythrodermic exfoliative psoriasis)

Contra-indications: disorders of calcium metabolism

Side-effects: local irritation; also dermatitis, pruritus, erythema, aggravation of psoriasis, photosensitivity; rarely facial or perioral dermatitis; hypercalcaemia (see Cautions)

Administration: cream or *ointment,* mild to moderate plaque psoriasis affecting up to 40% of skin area, apply once or twice daily; max. 100 g weekly (less with *scalp solution,* see below); CHILD over 6 years, apply twice daily; 6–12 years max. 50 g weekly; over 12 years max. 75 g weekly

PoM **Dovonex®** (Leo)
Cream, calcipotriol 50 micrograms/g. Net price 30 g = £8.15; 60 g = £16.30; 120 g = £29.40
Additives: include disodium edetate
Ointment, calcipotriol 50 micrograms/g. Net price 30 g = £8.15; 60 g = £16.30; 120 g = £29.40
Additives: include disodium edetate, propylene glycol
Scalp solution, calcipotriol 50 micrograms/mL. Net price 60 mL = £22.28
Additives: include propylene glycol
Scalp psoriasis, apply to scalp twice daily; max. 60 mL weekly (may be less with cream or ointment, see below); CHILD not recommended
MAX. WHEN PREPARATIONS USED TOGETHER. Max. total calcipotriol 5 mg in any one week (e.g. *scalp solution* 60 mL with *cream* or *ointment* 30 g or *cream* or *ointment* 60 g with *scalp solution* 30 mL)

TACALCITOL

Indications: plaque psoriasis

Cautions: pregnancy; avoid use on scalp, contact with eyes and inadvertent transfer to other body areas; wash hands thoroughly after application; risk of hypercalcaemia in generalised pustular or erythrodermic exfoliative psoriasis; monitor plasma calcium if risk of hypercalcaemia or in renal impairment; may be degraded by UV light (including sunlight)

Contra-indications: disorders of calcium metabolism including hypercalcaemia (see Cautions)

Side-effects: local irritation including itching, erythema, burning, paraesthesia

Administration: apply daily preferably at bedtime; max. 5 g daily; usual max. duration 2 courses of 12 weeks per year; CHILD not recommended

▼ PoM **Curatoderm**® (Merck)

Ointment, tacalcitol (as monohydrate) 4 micrograms/g. Net price 30 g = £15.09; 60 g = £26.06

Additives: none as listed in section 13.1

TAZAROTENE

Indications: mild to moderate plaque psoriasis affecting up to 10% of skin area

Cautions: advise patients to wash hands immediately after use, avoid contact with eyes, face, intertriginous areas, hair-covered scalp, eczematous or inflamed skin avoid excessive exposure to UV light (including sunlight, solariums, PUVA or UVB treatment); do not apply emollients or cosmetics within 1 hour of application

Contra-indications: pregnancy—advise women of child-bearing age to ensure adequate contraceptive protection; breast-feeding

Side-effects: local irritation (more common with higher concentration and may require discontinuation), burning, erythema, desquamation, non-specific rash, contact dermatitis, and worsening of psoriasis; rarely stinging and inflamed, dry or painful skin

Administration: apply once daily in the evening usually for up to 12 weeks; CHILD under 18 years not recommended

▼ PoM **Zorac**® (Allergan)

Gel, tazarotene 0.05%, net price 30 g = £14.75, 60 g = £27.50; 0.1%, 30 g = £15.50, 60 g = £29.00

Additives: include benzyl alcohol, butylated hydroxyanisole, butylated hydroxytoluene, disodium edetate, polysorbate 40

COAL TAR

Indications: psoriasis and occasionally chronic atopic eczema

Cautions: avoid eyes, mucosa and broken or inflamed skin; use suitable chemical protection gloves for extemporaneous preparation

Contra-indications: not for use in sore, acute, or pustular psoriasis or in presence of infection

Side-effects: skin irritation and acne-like eruptions, photosensitivity; stains skin, hair, and fabric

Administration: apply 1–3 times daily starting with low-strength preparations

Note. For shampoo preparations see section 13.9; impregnated dressings see Appendix 9

Non-proprietary preparations

May be difficult to obtain—moreover some patients may find newer proprietary preparations more acceptable

Calamine and Coal Tar Ointment, BP, calamine 12.5 g, strong coal tar solution 2.5 g, zinc oxide 12.5 g, hydrous wool fat 25 g, white soft paraffin 47.5 g

Apply 1–2 times daily

Coal Tar and Salicylic Acid Ointment, BP, coal tar 2 g, salicylic acid 2 g, emulsifying wax 11.4 g, white soft paraffin 19 g, coconut oil 54 g, polysorbate '80' 4 g, liquid paraffin 7.6 g

Apply 1–2 times daily

Coal Tar Paste, BP, strong coal tar solution 7.5%, in compound zinc paste

Apply 1–2 times daily

Zinc and Coal Tar Paste, BP, zinc oxide 6%, coal tar 6%, emulsifying wax 5%, starch 38%, yellow soft paraffin 45%

Apply 1–2 times daily

Proprietary preparations

Alphosyl® (Stafford-Miller)

Cream, coal tar extract 5%, allantoin 2%, in a vanishing-cream basis. Net price 100 g = £2.44

Additives: include beeswax, hydroxybenzoates (parabens), isopropyl palmitate, propylene glycol

Psoriasis, apply to skin 2–4 times daily

Lotion, coal tar extract 5%, allantoin 2%. Net price 250 mL = £2.21

Additives: include isopropyl palmitate, propylene glycol

Psoriasis, apply to skin or scalp 2–4 times daily

Carbo-Dome® (Lagap)

Cream, coal tar solution 10%, in a water-miscible basis. Net price 30 g = £3.95; 100 g = £8.93

Additives: include beeswax, hydroxybenzoates (parabens)

Psoriasis, apply to skin 2–3 times daily

Clinitar® (Shire)

Cream, coal tar extract 1%. Net price 100 g = £5.37

Additives: include isopropyl palmitate, propylene glycol

Psoriasis and eczema, apply to skin 1–2 times daily

Gelcosal® (Quinoderm Ltd)

Gel, strong coal tar solution 5%, pine tar 5%, salicylic acid 2%. Net price 50 g = £3.12

Additives: none as listed in section 13.1

Psoriasis and chronic scaling dermatitis, apply to skin twice daily

Gelcotar® (Quinoderm Ltd)

Gel, strong coal tar solution 5%, pine tar 5%. Net price 50 g = £2.83; 500 g = £14.74

Additives: none as listed in section 13.1

Psoriasis and chronic dermatitis, apply to skin twice daily

Liquid, see section 13.9

Pragmatar® (Bioglan)

Cream, cetyl alcohol-coal tar distillate 4%, salicylic acid 3%, sulphur (precipitated) 3%. Net price 25 g = £3.12; 100 g = £10.07

Additives: include fragrance

Scaly skin disorders, apply thinly once daily; dandruff and other seborrhoeic conditions, apply to scalp once weekly or in severe cases daily. Dilute with a few drops of water before application to infants

Psoriderm® (Dermal)

Cream, coal tar 6%, lecithin 0.4%. Net price 225 mL = £3.55

Additives: include hydroxybenzoates (parabens), isopropyl palmitate, propylene glycol

Psoriasis, apply to skin or scalp twice daily

Scalp lotion—section 13.9

PsoriGel® (Galderma)

Gel, coal tar solution USP 7.5% in an alcoholic emollient basis. Net price 100 g = £4.23

Additives: include propylene glycol

Psoriasis and eczema, apply to skin or scalp 1–2 times daily

Bath preparations

Coal Tar Solution, BP, coal tar 20%, polysorbate '80' 5%, in alcohol (96%). Net price 100 mL = 76p

Use 100 mL in a bath

Note. Strong Coal Tar Solution BP contains coal tar 40%

Balneum with Tar® (Merck)

Bath oil, coal tar distillate 30%, soya oil 55%. Net price 200 mL = £3.23.

Additives: none as listed in section 13.1

Psoriasis, eczema, pruritic dermatoses, and ichthyosis, use 1 measure (20 mL) in bath (infants 10 mL) and soak for 20 minutes

Polytar Emollient® (Stiefel)

Bath additive, coal tar solution 2.5%, arachis (peanut) oil extract of coal tar 7.5%, tar 7.5%, cade oil 7.5%, liquid paraffin 35%. Net price 350 mL = £4.87.

Additives: include isopropyl palmitate

Psoriasis, eczema, atopic and pruritic dermatoses, use 2–4 capfuls (15–30 mL) in bath and soak for 20 minutes

Psoriderm® (Dermal)

Bath emulsion, coal tar 40%. Net price 200 mL = £3.09.

Additives: include polysorbate 20

Psoriasis, use 30 mL in a bath and soak for 5 minutes

With corticosteroids

PoM Alphosyl HC® (Stafford-Miller)

Cream, coal tar extract 5%, hydrocortisone 0.5%, allantoin 2%. Net price 30 g = £1.66; 100 g = £4.73. Label: 28. Potency: mild

Additives: include beeswax, hydroxybenzoates (parabens), isopropyl palmitate, wool fat

Psoriasis, apply thinly 1–2 times daily; CHILD under 5 years not recommended

PoM Tarcortin® (Stafford-Miller)

Cream, coal tar extract 5%, hydrocortisone 0.5%. Net price 100 g = £3.08. Label: 28. Potency: mild

Additives: include hydroxybenzoates (parabens), isopropyl palmitate, propylene glycol, fragrance

Psoriasis, eczema, seborrhoea and dermatoses, apply to skin thinly 1–2 times daily

DITHRANOL

Indications: subacute and chronic psoriasis, see notes above

Cautions: avoid use near eyes and sensitive areas of skin; see also notes above

Contra-indications: hypersensitivity; acute and pustular psoriasis

Side-effects: local burning sensation and irritation; stains skin, hair, and fabrics

Administration: see notes above and under preparations

Note. Some of these dithranol preparations also contain coal tar or salicylic acid—for cautions and side-effects see under Coal Tar (above) or under Salicylic Acid

PoM *Dithranol Ointment, BP dithranol, in yellow soft paraffin; usual strengths 0.1–2%. Part of basis may be replaced by hard paraffin if a stiffer preparation is required. Label: 28

* PoM if dithranol content more than 1%, otherwise P

Dithranol Paste, BP, dithranol in zinc and salicylic acid (Lassar's) paste. Usual strengths 0.1–1% of dithranol. Label: 28

Dithrocream® (Dermal)

Cream, dithranol 0.1%, net price 50 g = £4.24; 0.25%, 50 g = £4.55; 0.5%, 50 g = £5.24; 1%, 50 g = £6.10; PoM 2%, 50 g = £7.64. Label: 28. For application to skin or scalp; 0.1–0.5% suitable for overnight treatment, 1–2% for max. 1 hour

Additives: include chlorocresol, salicylic acid

Micanol® (Evans)

Cream, dithranol 1% in a lipid-stabilised basis, net price 50 g = £7.98; PoM 3%, 50 g = £9.94. Label: 28

For application to skin, for up to 30 minutes, if necessary 3% cream may be used under medical supervision; apply to scalp for up to 30 minutes

Note. At the end of contact time use plenty of lukewarm (not hot) water to rinse off cream; soap should not be used

Additives: none as listed in section 13.1

Psorin® (Thames)

Ointment, dithranol 0.11%, crude coal tar 1%, salicylic acid 1.6%. Net price 50 g = £5.30, 100 g = £10.50. Label: 28. For application to skin up to twice daily

Additives: include beeswax, wool fat

Scalp gel, dithranol 0.25%, salicylic acid 1.6% in gel basis contaning methyl salicylate. Net price 50 g = £3.98. Label: 28. For application to scalp, initially apply on alternate days for 10–20 minutes; may be increased to daily application for max. 1 hour and then wash off

Additives: none as listed in section 13.1

SALICYLIC ACID

For coal tar preparations containing salicylic acid, see under Coal Tar p. 491; for dithranol preparations containing salicylic acid see under Dithranol, above

Indications: hyperkeratotic skin disorders

Cautions: see notes above; avoid broken or inflamed skin

SALICYLATE TOXICITY. If large areas of skin are treated, salicylate toxicity may be a hazard

Side-effects: sensitivity, excessive drying, irritation, systemic effects after widespread use (see under Cautions)

Salicylic Acid Collodion, BP —section 13.7

Salicylic Acid Ointment, BP, salicylic acid 2%, in wool alcohols ointment. Net price 25 g = 17p

Apply twice daily

Zinc and Salicylic Acid Paste, BP (Lassar's Paste), zinc oxide 24%, salicylic acid 2%, starch 24%, white soft paraffin 50%. Net price 25 g = 14p

Apply twice daily

ORAL RETINOIDS FOR PSORIASIS

ACITRETIN

Note. Acitretin is a metabolite of etretinate

Indications: severe extensive psoriasis resistant to other forms of therapy; palmoplantar pustular psoriasis; severe congenital ichthyosis; severe Darier's disease (keratosis follicularis)

Cautions: exclude pregnancy before starting—patients should avoid pregnancy at least 1 month before, during, and for at least 2 years after treatment, should avoid tetracycline, high doses of vitamin A (more than 4000–5000 units daily) and use of keratolytics, and should not donate blood during or for at least 1 year after stopping therapy (teratogenic risk); monitor hepatic function and plasma lipids at start, 1 month after initiating treatment, and then at intervals of 3 months; diabetes (can alter glucose tolerance—initial frequent blood glucose checks); radiographic assessment on long-term treatment; investigate atypical musculoskeletal symptoms; not recommended for children except under exceptional circumstances (premature epiphyseal closure reported); patients should avoid excessive exposure to sunlight and unsupervised use of sunlamps; **interactions:** Appendix 1 (retinoids)

Contra-indications: hepatic and renal impairment; pregnancy (**important teratogenic risk:** see Cautions and Appendix 4); breast-feeding

Side-effects: (mainly dose-related) dryness of mucous membranes (sometimes erosion), of skin (sometimes scaling, thinning, erythema especially of face, and pruritus), and of conjunctiva (sometimes conjunctivitis and decreased tolerance of contact lenses); other side-effects reported include palmoplantar exfoliation, epistaxis, epidermal fragility, paronychia, granulomatous lesions, reversible hair thinning and alopecia, myalgia and arthralgia, occasional nausea, headache, malaise, drowsiness and sweating; benign intracranial hypertension (**avoid** concomitant tetracyclines); photosensitivity, mood changes and blood disorders (including thrombocytopenia and anaemia) reported for etretinate, raised liver enzymes, rarely jaundice and hepatitis (**avoid** concomitant methotrexate); raised triglycerides; decreased night vision reported; skeletal hyperostosis and extraosseous calcification reported following long-term administration of etretinate (and premature epiphyseal closure in children, see Cautions)

Dose: administered in accordance with expert advice, initially 25–30 mg daily (Darier's disease 10 mg daily) for 2–4 weeks, then adjusted according to response, usually within range 25–50 mg daily (in some cases up to max. 75 mg daily) for further 6–8 weeks (in Darier's disease and ichthyosis not more than 50 mg daily for up to 6 months); CHILD (**important:** exceptional circumstances only, see Cautions), 500 micrograms/kg daily (occasionally up to 1 mg/kg daily to max. 35 mg daily for limited periods) with careful monitoring of musculoskeletal development

PoM **Neotigason**® (Roche)

Capsules, acitretin 10 mg (brown/white), net price 56-cap pack = £26.53; 25 mg (brown/yellow), 56-cap pack = £61.57 (**hosp. or specified retail pharmacy only**—see product literature for details, specialist dermatological supervision). Label: 10 patient information leaflet, 21

ORAL IMMUNOSUPPRESSANTS FOR PSORIASIS

CYCLOSPORIN

(Ciclosporin)

Indications: see under Dose; transplantation and graft-versus-host disease, see section 8.2.2

Cautions; Side-effects: section 8.2.2

ADDITIONAL CAUTIONS IN ATOPIC DERMATITIS AND PSORIASIS. **Contra-indicated** in abnormal renal function, hypertension not under control (see also below), infections not under control, and malignancy (see also below). Dermatological and physical examination, including blood pressure and renal function measurements required at least twice before starting; discontinue if hypertension develops that cannot be controlled by dose reduction or antihypertensive therapy; avoid excessive exposure to sunlight and use of UVB or PUVA; *in atopic dermatitis*, also allow herpes simplex infections to clear before starting (if they occur during treatment withdraw if severe); *Staphylococcus aureus* skin infections not absolute contra-indication providing controlled (but avoid erythromycin unless no other alternative—see also **interactions**: Appendix 1 (cyclosporin)); monitor serum creatinine every 2 weeks throughout; *in psoriasis*, also exclude malignancies (including those of skin and cervix) before starting (biopsy any lesions not typical of psoriasis) and treat patients with malignant or pre-malignant conditions of skin only after appropriate treatment (and if no other option); monitor serum creatinine every 2 weeks for first 3 months then every 2 months (monthly if dose more than 2.5 mg/kg daily), reducing dose by 25–50% if increases more than 30% above baseline (even if within normal range) and discontinuing if reduction not successful within 1 month; also discontinue if lymphoproliferative disorder develops

Dose: ADULT over 16 years *by mouth,* administered in accordance with expert advice

Short-term treatment (max. 8 weeks) of severe atopic dermatitis where conventional therapy ineffective or inappropriate, initially 2.5 mg/kg daily in 2 divided doses, if good initial response not achieved within 2 weeks, increase rapidly to max. 5 mg/kg daily; initial dose of 5 mg/kg daily if very severe; CHILD under 16 years not recommended

Severe psoriasis where conventional therapy ineffective or inappropriate, initially 2.5 mg/kg daily in 2 divided doses, increased gradually to max. 5 mg/kg daily if no improvement within 1 month (discontinue if response still insufficient after 6 weeks); initial dose of 5 mg/kg daily justified if condition requires rapid improvement; CHILD under 16 years not recommended

IMPORTANT. For preparations and counselling and for advice on conversion between the preparations, see section 8.2.2

Preparations

Section 8.2.2

METHOTREXATE

Indications: severe uncontrolled psoriasis unresponsive to conventional therapy (specialist use only); malignant disease (section 8.1.3); rheumatoid arthritis (section 10.1.3)

Cautions; Contra-indications; Side-effects: see also notes above, section 8.1.3, and product literature; investigations required before starting include full blood count, renal function tests (**contra-indicated** if significant impairment, see section 8.1.3 and Appendix 3), liver function tests (**contra-indicated** if abnormalities, see below and Appendix 2), followed by close monitoring during treatment (see also CSM advice, below); **contra-indicated** in pregnancy (following administration to woman or man, avoid conception for **at least 6 months** after stopping) and breast-feeding (see Cytotoxic drugs, Appendixes 4 and 5) and immunodeficiency syndromes; may decrease male or female fertility (effect may be reversible); extreme caution in peptic ulceration, ulcerative colitis, diarrhoea and ulcerative stomatitis (withdraw if stomatitis develops—may be first sign of gastro-intestinal toxicity); photosensitivity—lesions of psoriasis aggravated by UV radiation (skin ulceration reported); **interactions:** see below and Appendix 1 (methotrexate)

CSM ADVICE. In view of reports of blood dyscrasias (including fatalities) and liver cirrhosis with low-dose methotrexate, the CSM has advised:

• full blood count and renal and liver function tests before starting treatment and repeated weekly until therapy stabilised, thereafter patients should be monitored every 2-3 months

• patients should report all symptoms and signs suggestive of infection, especially sore throat

Treatment with folinic acid (as calcium folinate, section 8.1.3) may be required in acute toxicity

BLOOD COUNT. Haematopoietic suppression may occur abruptly; factors likely to increase toxicity include advanced age, renal impairment and concomitant administration of another anti-folate drug. Any profound drop in white cell or platelet count calls for immediate withdrawal of methotrexate and introduction of supportive therapy

LIVER TOXICITY. Liver cirrhosis reported. Treatment should not be started or should be discontinued if any abnormality of liver function tests or liver biopsy is present or develops during therapy. Abnormalities may return to normal within 2 weeks after which treatment may be recommenced if judged appropriate

PULMONARY TOXICITY. May be special problem in rheumatoid arthritis (patient to contact doctor immediately if dyspnoea or cough)

ASPIRIN and other NSAIDs. If aspirin or other NSAIDs are given concurrently the dose of methotrexate should be carefully monitored. Patients should be advised to avoid self-medication with over-the-counter aspirin or ibuprofen

Dose: by mouth, 10–25 mg once weekly, adjusted according to response; ELDERLY consider dose reduction (extreme caution); CHILD not recommended

IMPORTANT. Note that the above dose is a **weekly** dose

Preparations

Section 8.1.3

13.6   Acne and rosacea

13.6.1 Topical preparations for acne
13.6.2 Oral preparations for acne

The treatment of acne depends on whether it is predominantly inflammatory or comedonal. If the acne proves unresponsive to topical preparations, oral preparations may be required.

ROSACEA. Rosacea is not comedonal (but may exist with acne which may be comedonal). Spots associated with rosacea are responsive to topical metronidazole (section 13.10.2) or to oral administration of tetracycline 500 mg twice daily (section 5.1.3) or of erythromycin 500 mg twice daily (section 5.1.5); courses usually last 6–12 weeks and are repeated intermittently; alternatively, doxycycline (section 5.1.3) in a dose of 50 mg twice daily for 2–4 weeks followed by 50 mg once daily for a further 8 weeks may be used if tetracycline is inappropriate. Isotretinoin is occasionally given in refractory cases [unlicensed indication]. Camouflagers (section 13.8.2) may be required for the redness.

13.6.1   Topical preparations for acne

Significant comedonal acne responds well to topical retinoids (see p. 495), whereas both comedones and inflamed lesions respond well to benzoyl peroxide or azelaic acid (see below). Alternatively, topical application of an antibiotic such as erythromycin or clindamycin may be effective for inflammatory or comedonal acne. If topical preparations prove inadequate oral preparations may be needed (section 13.6.2).

BENZOYL PEROXIDE AND AZELAIC ACID

Both comedones and inflamed lesions respond well to **benzoyl peroxide** or **azelaic acid**. Benzoyl peroxide and azelaic acid irritate the skin, but it is thought that irritation is associated with the therapeutic effect; the scaling and redness often subsides with continued treatment.

BENZOYL PEROXIDE

Indications: acne vulgaris

Cautions: avoid contact with eyes, mouth, and mucous membranes; may bleach fabrics

Side-effects: skin irritation

Administration: apply 1–2 times daily, starting treatment with lower-strength preparations

Acnecide® (Galderma)

Gel, benzoyl peroxide, in an aqueous gel basis, 5%, net price 60 g = £3.00; 10%, 60 g = £3.30
Additives: include propylene glycol

Nericur® (Schering Health)

Gel, benzoyl peroxide, in an aqueous gel basis, 5%, net price 30 g = £1.45; 10%, 30 g = £1.60
Additives: include propylene glycol

PanOxyl® (Stiefel)

Aquagel (= aqueous gel), benzoyl peroxide 2.5%, net price 40 g = £1.76; 5%, 40 g = £1.92; 10%, 40 g = £2.07.
Additives: include propylene glycol

Cream, benzoyl peroxide, in a non-greasy basis, 5%, net price 40 g = £1.51
Additives: include isopropyl palmitate, propylene glycol

Gel, benzoyl peroxide, in an aqueous alcoholic basis, 5%, net price 40 g = £1.51; 10%, 40 g = £1.69
Additives: include fragrance

Lotion, benzoyl peroxide, in a non-greasy basis, 5% , net price 30 mL = £1.51; 10%, 30 mL = £1.51
Additives: include isopropyl palmitate, propylene glycol

Wash, benzoyl peroxide, in a detergent basis, 10%, net price 150 mL = £4.00
Additives: none as listed in section 13.1

With antimicrobials
Acnidazil® (J&J MSD)

Cream, benzoyl peroxide 5%, miconazole nitrate 2%. Net price 15 g = £2.23; 30 g = £3.55
Additives: include polysorbate 20, propylene glycol

PoM **Benzamycin®** (Bioglan)

Gel, pack for reconstitution, providing erythromycin 3% and benzoyl peroxide 5% in an alcoholic basis. Net price per pack to provide 23.3 g = £8.31, 46.6 g = £15.99
Additives: none as listed in section 13.1
Apply twice daily (very fair skin, initially once daily at night)

Quinoderm® (Quinoderm Ltd)

Cream, benzoyl peroxide 5%, potassium hydroxyquinoline sulphate 0.5%, in an astringent vanishing-cream basis. Net price 50 g = £2.04
Additives: include edetic acid (EDTA)

Cream, benzoyl peroxide 10%, potassium hydroxyquinoline sulphate 0.5%, in an astringent vanishing-cream basis. Net price 25 g = £1.30; 50 g = £2.26
Additives: include edetic acid (EDTA)

Lotio-gel, benzoyl peroxide 5%, potassium hydroxyquinoline sulphate 0.5%, in an astringent creamy basis. Net price 30 mL = £1.47
Additives: include edetic acid (EDTA)

AZELAIC ACID

Indications: acne vulgaris
Cautions: pregnancy, breast-feeding; avoid contact with eyes
Side-effects: local irritation (reduce frequency or discontinue use temporarily); rarely photosensitisation

PoM **Skinoren®** (Schering Health)

Cream, azelaic acid 20%, net price 30 g = £5.00
Additives: include propylene glycol
Apply twice daily (sensitive skin, once daily for first week). Extended treatment may be required but manufacturer advises period of treatment should not exceed 6 months

TOPICAL ANTIBIOTICS FOR ACNE

Topical antibiotics are used for mild to moderately severe acne. Topical preparations of erythromycin, tetracycline, and clindamycin seem to be quite useful for many patients with the milder forms of acne; they can produce mild irritation of the skin but rarely sensitise.

Cross resistance, especially between erythromycin and clindamycin is an increasing problem. To avoid this:

when possible use non-antibiotic antimicrobials (such as benzoyl peroxide);

avoid concomitant treatment with different oral and topical antibiotics;

if a particular antibiotic is effective, use it for repeat courses.

Topical neomycin is not suitable owing to sensitisation.

ANTIBIOTICS

Indications: acne vulgaris
Cautions: some manufacturers advise preparations containing alcohol are not suitable for use with benzoyl peroxide

DURATION OF TREATMENT. Usual max. duration of treatment 10–12 weeks to minimise problems with antibiotic resistance (but course may be repeated after interval of few weeks)

PoM **Benzamycin®** see under Benzoyl Peroxide above

PoM **Dalacin T®** (Pharmacia & Upjohn)

Topical solution, clindamycin (as phosphate) 1%, in an aqueous alcoholic basis. Net price (both with applicator) 30 mL = £4.54; 50 mL = £7.57
Additives: include propylene glycol
Apply twice daily

Lotion, clindamycin (as phosphate) 1% in an aqueous basis. Net price 30 mL = £5.32; 50 mL = £8.87
Additives: include hydroxybenzoates (parabens)
Apply twice daily

PoM **Stiemycin®** (Stiefel)

Solution, erythromycin 2% in an alcoholic basis. Net price 50 mL = £9.00
Additives: include propylene glycol
Apply twice daily

PoM **Topicycline®** (Monmouth)

Solution, powder for reconstitution, tetracycline hydrochloride, 4-epitetracycline hydrochloride, providing tetracycline hydrochloride 2.2 mg/mL when reconstituted with solvent containing *n*-decyl methyl sulphoxide and citric acid in 40% alcohol. Net price per pack of powder and solvent to provide 70 mL = £7.70
Additives: none as listed in section 13.1
Apply twice daily

PoM **Zineryt®** (Yamanouchi)

Topical solution, powder for reconstitution, erythromycin 40 mg, zinc acetate 12 mg/mL when reconstituted with solvent containing ethanol. Net price per pack of powder and solvent to provide 30 mL = £8.04; 90 mL = £22.91
Additives: none as listed in section 13.1.
Apply twice daily

TOPICAL RETINOIDS AND RELATED PREPARATIONS FOR ACNE

Topical application of **tretinoin** (which is the acid form of vitamin A) or of its isomer **isotretinoin** is anticomedogenic. They are useful in treating acne but patients should be warned that some redness and skin peeling may occur after application for several days but settles with time. Isotretinoin is also given by mouth, see section 13.6.2 for **additional warnings**.

Adapalene is a recently introduced retinoid-like drug indicated for mild to moderate acne

ADAPALENE

Indications: mild to moderate acne
Cautions: see under Tretinoin
Contra-indications: pregnancy (see Appendix 4), breast-feeding, eczematous or broken skin; avoid in severe acne involving large areas
Side-effects: irritation (discontinue if severe)
Administration: apply thinly once daily before retiring

▼ PoM **Differin**® (Galderma)
Gel, adapalene 0.1%, net price 30 g = £8.00
    Additives: include disodium edetate, hydroxybenzoates (parabens), propylene glycol

TRETINOIN

Note. Tretinoin is the acid form of vitamin A
Indications: see under preparatations below; photodamage (section 13.8.1); malignant disease (section 8.1.5)
Cautions: avoid contact with eyes, nostrils, mouth, and mucous membranes; do not use simultaneously with other peeling agents (can be alternated every 12 hours with benzoyl peroxide); do not use with ultra-violet lamps (and minimise exposure to sunlight)
Contra-indications: pregnancy, eczema, broken or sunburned skin; personal or family history of cutaneous epithelioma
Side-effects: irritation, erythema, peeling; changes in pigmentation, photosensitivity
Administration: see under preparations below

PoM **Retin-A**® (Janssen-Cilag)
Cream, tretinoin 0.025%, net price 60 g = £6.03.
    Acne vulgaris, for dry or fair skin, apply thinly 1–2 times daily
    Additives: include butylated hydroxytoluene, sorbic acid
Gel, tretinoin 0.01%, net price 60 g = £6.03; 0.025%, 60 g = £6.03.
    Acne vulgaris and other keratotic conditions, apply thinly 1–2 times daily
    Additives: include butylated hydroxytoluene
Lotion, tretinoin 0.025%. Net price 100 mL = £6.94.
    Acne vulgaris, for application to large areas such as the back, apply thinly 1–2 times daily
    Additives: include butylated hydroxytoluene

ISOTRETINOIN

Note. Isotretinoin is an isomer of tretinoin
Indications; Cautions; Contra-indications; Side-effects: (*after topical application* **only**): see under Tretinoin and notes above
    IMPORTANT. For **indications, cautions, contra-indications** and **side-effects** of isotretinoin **when given by mouth**, see p. 498
Administration: apply thinly 1–2 times daily

PoM **Isotrex**® (Stiefel)
Gel, isotretinoin 0.05%. Net price 30 g = £6.96.
    Label: 10 patient information leaflet
    Additives: include butylated hydroxytoluene

With antibacterial
PoM **Isotrexin**® (Stiefel)
Gel, isotretinoin 0.05%, erythromycin 2% in ethanolic basis. Net price 30 g = £8.75. Label: 10 patient information leaflet
    Additives: include butylated hydroxytoluene

TOPICAL CORTICOSTEROIDS FOR ACNE

Topical **corticosteroids** should **not** be used in acne.

CORTICOSTEROIDS

Indications: not recommended (see notes above)
Cautions; Contra-indications; Side-effects: section 13.4 and notes above

PoM **Actinac**® (Hoechst Marion Roussel)
Lotion (powder for reconstitution with solvent), chloramphenicol 40 mg, hydrocortisone acetate 40 mg, allantoin 24 mg, butoxyethyl nicotinate 24 mg, precipitated sulphur 320 mg/g. Discard after 21 days. Net price 2 × 6.25 g bottles powder with 2 × 20-mL bottles solvent = £9.30. Label: 28. Potency: mild
    Additives: none as listed in section 13.1

OTHER TOPICAL PREPARATIONS FOR ACNE

Salicylic acid is of dubious value in acne and is no longer used although some preparations still have a role in seborrhoeic eczema. Preparations containing **sulphur** and **abrasive agents** are no longer considered beneficial in acne.

A topical preparation of **nicotinamide** has recently been made available for inflammatory acne.

ABRASIVE AGENTS

Indications: acne vulgaris (but see notes above)
Cautions: avoid contact with eyes; discontinue use temporarily if skin becomes irritated
Contra-indications: superficial venules, telangiectasia

Brasivol® (Stiefel)
Paste No. 1, aluminium oxide 38.09% in fine particles, in a soap-detergent basis; *Paste No. 2*, aluminium oxide 52.2% in medium particles, net price 75 g (both) = £2.49
    Additives: include fragrance
    Use instead of soap 1–3 times daily, starting with *No.1*
NHS **Ionax Scrub**® (Galderma)
Gel, polyethylene granules 21.9%, benzalkonium chloride 0.25% in a foaming aqueous alcoholic basis. Net price 60 g = £3.13
    Additives: include propylene glycol
    Use instead of soap 1–2 times daily

NICOTINAMIDE

Indications: see under preparation
Cautions: avoid contact with eyes and mucous membranes (including nose and mouth); reduce frequency of application if excessive dryness, irritation or peeling
Side-effects: dryness of skin; also pruritus, erythema, burning and irritation

Papulex® (Euroderma)

Gel, nicotinamide 4%. Net price 60 g = £7.98

Additives: none as listed in section 13.1

Inflammatory acne vulgaris, apply twice daily; reduce to once daily or on alternate days if irritation occurs

SALICYLIC ACID

Indications: acne vulgaris

Cautions: avoid contact with mouth, eyes, mucous membranes; systemic effects after excessive use (see section 10.1.1)

Side-effects: local irritation

Acnisal® (Euroderma)

Topical solution, salicylic acid 2% in a detergent basis. Net price 177 mL = £4.13. Use up to 3 times daily

Additives: include benzyl alcohol, hydroxybenzoates (parabens)

SULPHUR

Cautions: avoid contact with eyes, mouth, and mucous membranes; causes skin irritation

With resorcinol

Prolonged application of resorcinol may interfere with thyroid function therefore not recommended

NHS **Eskamel®** (Goldshield)

Cream, resorcinol 2%, sulphur 8%, in a non-greasy flesh-coloured basis. Net price 25 g = £2.52

Additives: include propylene glycol, fragrance

With salicylic acid

See above for cautions relating to salicylic acid

Salicylic Acid and Sulphur Cream, BP 1980, salicylic acid 2%, precipitated sulphur 2%, in aqueous cream

Salicylic Acid and Sulphur Ointment, BPC, salicylic acid 3%, precipitated sulphur 3%, in hydrous ointment (oily cream)

13.6.2   Oral preparations for acne

ORAL ANTIBIOTICS FOR ACNE

Systemic antibacterial treatment is useful. **Tetracycline** (section 5.1.3), **erythromycin** (section 5.1.5), and occasionally other antibacterials are used. The usual dosage regimen for tetracycline and erythromycin, is 500 mg twice daily for 3 months reduced to 250 mg twice daily for a further 3 months. If there is no improvement after the first 3 months the antibiotic should be changed. Maximum improvement usually occurs after 4 to 6 months but in the more severe cases treatment may need to be continued for two or more years.

As an alternative to tetracycline, **minocycline** (section 5.1.3) offers less likelihood of bacterial resistance but may sometimes cause irreversible pigmentation; it is given in a dosage of 100 mg daily. **Doxycycline** may also be used in a dosage of 50 mg daily. Although **trimethoprim** is not licensed for acne it, too, is used in a dosage of 100 mg twice daily.

Concomitant use of different topical and systemic antibiotics is undesirable owing to the increased likelihood of the development of bacterial resistance.

HORMONE TREATMENT FOR ACNE

Cyproterone acetate with **ethinyloestradiol** (*Dianette®*) contains an anti-androgen. It is no more effective than an oral broad spectrum antibiotic but is useful in women who also wish to receive oral contraception.

Improvement of acne probably occurs because of decreased sebum secretion which is under androgen control. Some women with moderately severe hirsutism may also benefit as hair growth is also androgen-dependent. Its contra-indications include pregnancy and a predisposition to thrombosis.

CYPROTERONE ACETATE

Indications: see notes above; male hypersexuality, see section 6.4.2; prostate cancer, section 8.3.4.2

Cautions; Contra-indications; Side-effects: see under Combined Oral Contraceptives (section 7.3.1)

With ethinyloestradiol

PoM **Dianette®** (Schering Health)

Tablets, beige, s/c, cyproterone acetate 2 mg, ethinyloestradiol 35 micrograms. Net price 21-tab pack = £5.52

Dose: 1 tablet daily for 21 days starting on 1st day of menstrual cycle and repeated after a 7-day interval, usually for several months; withdraw when acne or hirsutism completely resolved (repeat courses may be given if recurrence)

ORAL RETINOID FOR ACNE

Isotretinoin (*Roaccutane®*) is a retinoid used for the systemic treatment of nodulo-cystic and conglobate acne and severe acne which has failed to respond to an adequate course of a systemic antimicrobial agent. It is also useful in women with acne developing in the third or fourth decades of life, since this late onset acne is frequently resistant to antibiotics.

It acts primarily by greatly reducing sebum secretion. It should be prescribed **only** by, or under the supervision of, a consultant dermatologist, and is available to hospitals **only**. It is given in doses of 500 micrograms/kg/day for at least 16 weeks but doses may be adjusted if necessary after 4 weeks. Repeat courses are occasionally required. An exacerbation is common some 2–4 weeks after starting treatment but usually subsides after a few weeks.

Side-effects of isotretinoin include dry lips, sore eyes, nose bleeds, mild transient hair loss, and joint pains. The drug is **teratogenic** and must **not** be given to women who are pregnant or those who may become pregnant unless there is concomitant effective contraception and then only after detailed explanation by the physician. The contraceptive measures must continue for at least **one month** after ceasing treatment with the drug.

ISOTRETINOIN

Note. Isotretinoin is an isomer of tretinoin

Indications: see notes above

Cautions: exclude pregnancy before starting—pregnancy must be avoided at least 1 month before, during, and for at least 1 month after treatment; avoid donating blood during and for at least 1 month after treatment; monitor hepatic function and plasma lipids at start, 1 month after initiating treatment, then at intervals of 3 months; avoid tetracyclines, high doses of vitamin A (more than 4000–5000 units daily) and use of keratolytics during treatment; monitor blood glucose in diabetic patients, monitor for keratitis (especially in those with dry eye syndrome); **interactions:** Appendix 1 (retinoids)

WAX EPILATION. Warn patient to avoid wax epilation during treatment and for 2 months after stopping (risk of epidermal stripping)

Contra-indications: pregnancy (**important teratogenic risk:** see Cautions and Appendix 4); breast-feeding; renal or hepatic impairment; hypervitaminosis A, hyperlipidaemia

Side-effects: (mainly dose-related) dryness of skin (with scaling, thinning, erythema, pruritus), epidermal fragility (trauma may cause blistering); rarely acne fulminans, facial hyperpigmentation; dryness of nasal mucosa (with mild epistaxis), of pharyngeal mucosa (with hoarseness), of conjunctiva (sometimes conjunctivitis), decreased tolerance to contact lenses and rarely keratitis; visual disturbances (papilloedema, optic neuritis, corneal opacities, cataracts, decreased night vision, photophobia, blurred vision)—expert referral and consider withdrawal; hair thinning (reversible on withdrawal) or (rarely) hirsutism; nausea, headache, malaise, drowsiness, sweating; benign intracranial hypertension (avoid concomitant tetracyclines); myalgia and arthralgia; raised serum creatinine concentrations reported; raised liver enzymes (rarely jaundice and hepatitis); raised plasma triglycerides and cholesterol (risk of pancreatitis if triglycerides above 8 g/litre); allergic vasculitis and granulomatous lesions reported, other side-effects reported include hearing deficiency, mood changes, convulsions, menstrual irregularities, hyperuricaemia, inflammatory bowel disease, paronychia and Gram-positive infections, bone changes (including early epiphyseal closure and skeletal hyperostosis following long-term administration), thrombocytopenia, thrombocytosis, neutropenia and anaemia, lymphadenopathy, and haematuria and proteinuria

Dose: initially 500 micrograms/kg daily (in 1–2 divided doses) with food for 4 weeks; if good response continue for further 8–12 weeks; if little response, up to 1 mg/kg daily for 8–12 weeks; if intolerant, reduce dose to 100–200 micrograms/kg daily

PoM **Roaccutane®** (Roche)

Capsules, isotretinoin 5 mg (red-violet/white), net price 56-cap pack = £19.08; 20 mg (red-violet/white), 56-cap pack = £54.98 (**hosp. or specified retail pharmacy only**—consult product literature for details, specialist dermatological supervision). Label: 10, patient information card, 21

13.7   Preparations for warts and calluses

The least destructive method possible should be chosen to treat these lesions as they are self-limiting (in patients who are not immunosuppressed) and all viral warts including those on the soles of the feet (verrucas) eventually disappear spontaneously.

Salicylic acid preparations act as keratolytics; they are useful but can cause considerable irritation of the treated area. They are suitable for the removal of *warts and calluses.* An ointment containing **podophyllum resin with salicylic acid** (*Posalfilin®*) is available for treating *plantar warts* (for podophyllum preparations suitable for treating genital warts see next page).

Preparations containing **formaldehyde** and **glutaraldehyde** are also available.

SALICYLIC ACID

Indications: see under preparations

Cautions: protect surrounding skin and avoid broken skin; not suitable for application to face, anogenital region, or large areas

Contra-indications: diabetes or if peripheral blood circulation impaired

Side-effects: skin irritation, see notes above

ADMINISTRATION. Instructions in proprietary packs generally incorporate advice to remove dead skin by gentle rubbing with a pumice stone and to cover with plaster after application (unless in collodion basis)

Salicylic Acid Collodion, BP, salicylic acid 12%, in flexible collodion. Label: 15. For warts and calluses, apply daily or on alternate days

Cuplex® (S&N Hlth.)

Gel, salicylic acid 11%, lactic acid 4%, copper acetate (= Cu^{2+} 0.0011%), in a collodion basis. Net price 5 g = £2.33. Label: 15. For plantar and mosaic warts, corns, and calluses, apply twice daily

Duofilm® (Stiefel)

Paint, salicylic acid 16.7%, lactic acid 16.7%, in flexible collodion. Net price 15 mL (with applicator) = £1.95. Label: 15. For plantar and mosaic warts, apply daily

Occlusal® (Euroderma)

Application, salicylic acid 26% in polyacrylic solution. Net price 10 mL (with applicator) = £2.41. Label : 15. For common and plantar warts, apply daily

Salactol® (Dermal)

Paint, salicylic acid 16.7%, lactic acid 16.7%, in flexible collodion. Net price 10 mL (with applicator) = £1.93. Label: 15. For warts, particularly plantar warts, verrucas, corns, and calluses, apply daily

Salatac® (Dermal)

Gel, salicylic acid 12%, lactic acid 4% in a collodion basis. Net price 8 g (with applicator) =

£3.52. Label: 15. For warts, verrucas, corns, and calluses, apply daily

Verrugon® (Pickles)

Ointment, salicylic acid 50% in a paraffin basis. Net price 6 g = £1.81. For plantar warts, apply daily

With podophyllum

Posalfilin® (Norgine)

Ointment, podophyllum resin 20%, salicylic acid 25%. Net price 10 g = £3.12. For plantar warts apply daily

Note. Owing to the salicylic acid content, not suitable for anogenital warts; owing to the podophyllum content also contra-indicated in pregnancy

FORMALDEHYDE

Indications: see under preparations

Cautions; Contra-indications; Side-effects: see under Salicylic Acid

Formaldehyde Lotion, formaldehyde solution, BP, 3 mL, water to 100 mL. For plantar warts, applied at night as a soak

Veracur® (Typharm)

Gel, formaldehyde 0.75% in a water-miscible gel basis. Net price 15 g = £2.10. For warts, particularly plantar warts, apply twice daily

GLUTARALDEHYDE

Indications: see under preparations

Cautions; Contra-indications; Side-effects: see under Salicylic Acid, stains skin brown

Glutarol® (Dermal)

Solution (= application), glutaraldehyde 10%. Net price 10 mL (with applicator) = £2.33. For warts, particularly plantar warts, apply twice daily

Verucasep® (Galen)

Gel, glutaraldehyde 10%. Net price 15 g = £1.95. For warts, particularly plantar warts, apply twice daily

GENITAL WARTS

Podophyllum preparations may be useful for *genital warts* but can cause considerable irritation of the treated area and can cause **severe toxicity** on excessive application (see Cautions below). They are contra-indicated in pregnancy. Preparations containing the major active constituent **podophyllotoxin** (*Condyline®* and *Warticon®*) are now also available for genital warts.

Fluorouracil injectable gel has recently been introduced for external genital warts.

PODOPHYLLUM

Indications: see under preparations

Cautions: avoid normal skin and open wounds; keep away from face; very irritant to eyes; **important:** see also warnings below

Contra-indications: pregnancy and breast-feeding; children

Side-effects: see notes above

PoM **Podophyllin Paint, Compound, BP,** (podophyllum resin 15% in compound benzoin tincture), podophyllum resin 1.5 g, compound benzoin tincture to 10 mL; 5 mL to be dispensed unless otherwise directed. Label: 15

External genital warts, applied weekly in genitourinary clinic (or at a general practitioner's surgery by trained nurses after screening for other sexually transmitted diseases)

IMPORTANT. Should be allowed to stay on the treated area for not longer than 6 hours and then washed off. Care should be taken to avoid splashing the surrounding skin during application (which must be covered with soft paraffin as a protection). Where there are a large number of warts only a few should be treated at any one time as **severe toxicity** caused by absorption of podophyllin has been reported

Podophyllotoxin

PoM **Condyline®** (Ardern)

Solution, podophyllotoxin 0.5% in alcoholic basis. Net price 3.5 mL (with applicators) = £14.49. Label: 15

Condylomata acuminata affecting the penis or the female external genitalia, apply twice daily for 3 consecutive days; treatment may be repeated at weekly intervals if necessary for a total of five 3-day treatment courses; direct medical supervision for lesions in the female and for lesions greater than 4 cm² in the male; max. 50 single applications ('loops') per session (see product literature)

PoM **Warticon®** (Perstorp)

Cream, podophyllotoxin 0.15%. Net price 5 g (with mirror) = £17.40

Condylomata acuminata affecting the penis or the female external genitalia, apply twice daily for 3 consecutive days; treatment may be repeated at weekly intervals if necessary for a total of four 3-day treatment courses; direct medical supervision for lesions greater than 4 cm²

Solution, blue, podophyllotoxin 0.5% in alcoholic basis. Net price 3 mL (with applicators—*Warticon®*[for men]; with applicators and mirror—*Warticon Fem®* [for women]) = £14.50. Label: 15

Condylomata acuminata affecting the penis or the female external genitalia, apply twice daily for 3 consecutive days; treatment may be repeated at weekly intervals if necessary for a total of four 3-day treatment courses; max. 50 single applications ('loops') per session (see product literature)

FLUOROURACIL

Indications: external genital warts; malignant disease, section 8.1.3

Cautions: avoid prolonged exposure of treated area to sunlight or UV radiation; avoid contact with mucous membranes; use appropriate techniques in handling—CRM guidelines, section 8.1

COUNSELLING. Advise patient to use appropriate contraceptive methods to prevent pregnancy during treatment

Contra-indications: pregnancy; breast-feeding

Side-effects: local reactions including pain at injection site, swelling, bruising, erythema, burning, itching, stinging, desquamation, eschar formation, induration, pigmentation changes, infection, necrosis; treatment-associated ulceration

Dose: see under preparation

Cautionary label wordings, see inside back cover

▼ PoM **AccuSite®** (Matrix)

Injectable gel, fluorouracil 3.33% (in purified bovine collagen matrix) and adrenaline 0.1% (in aqueous solution) in separate prefilled syringes for mixing before use to provide gel containing fluorouracil 30 mg and adrenaline 100 micrograms/mL. Net price per kit = £72.18

Administration: by intradermal or intralesional injection (for details consult product literature), 0.25–1 mL per lesion (according to size of lesion) to total max. 5 mL per visit; repeat once weekly for max. 6 weeks; if response inadequate, repeat treatment cycle once only after an interval of 4 weeks

Additives: include sodium metabisulphite, disodium edetate

Note. Risk of hypersensitivity reactions to bovine collagen in patients with history of dietary beef allergy and in those with systemic connective tissue disorders, e.g. rheumatoid arthritis, progressive systemic sclerosis

13.8   Sunscreens and camouflagers

13.8.1   Sunscreening preparations
13.8.2   Camouflagers

13.8.1   Sunscreening preparations

Solar ultraviolet irradiation can be harmful to the skin. It is responsible for disorders such as *polymorphic light eruption, solar urticaria,* and the various *cutaneous porphyrias.* It also provokes (or at least aggravates) disorders such as *rosacea* and *lupus erythematosus.* It may also cause photosensitivity in patients taking some drugs such as demeclocycline, phenothiazines, or amiodarone. All these conditions (as well as *sunburn*) may occur after relatively short periods of exposure to the sun. Exposure over longer periods may cause more serious problems. Both *melanoma* and *non-melanoma skin cancer* are now thought to be caused in many instances by solar ultraviolet irradiation. It is now also believed that exposure to the sun causes the skin to wrinkle and develop other signs *associated with ageing.* Solar ultraviolet irradiation also provokes attacks of *recurrent herpes labialis* (although it is not known whether the effect of sunlight exposure is local or systemic).

Solar ultraviolet radiation is approximately 200–400 nm in wavelength. The medium wavelengths (280–310 nm, known as UVB) cause sunburn and contribute to the long-term changes responsible for skin cancer and ageing. The long wavelengths (310–400 nm, known as UVA) do not cause sunburn but are responsible for many *photosensitivity reactions* and *photodermatoses;* they also seem to contribute to long-term damage and to be involved in the pathogenesis of *skin cancer* and *photodamage.*

Sunscreen preparations contain substances that protect the skin against UVB and hence against sunburn. The sun protection factor (SPF, usually indicated in the preparation title) provides guidance on the degree of protection offered against UVB; it indicates the multiples of protection provided against burning, compared with unprotected skin;

for example, an SPF of 8 should enable a person to remain 8 times longer in the sun without burning. Such preparations, however, do not prevent long-term damage associated with UVA, which might not become apparent for 10 to 20 years. Preparations that also contain reflective substances, such as titanium dioxide, provide the most effective protection against UVA. Some products now indicate the degree of protection offered against UVA with a star rating system. This system does not refer to an absolute measure but indicates the protection against UVA relative to protection against UVB for the same product. Four stars indicate that the product offers a balanced amount of UVA and UVB protection; products with three, two, or one star rating indicate that the protection offered is greater against UVB than UVA. However the usefulness of the star rating system remains controversial.

Some sunscreens, particularly aminobenzoates, may rarely cause photosensitivity reactions. Bergamot oil (which contains 5-methoxypsoralen) occasionally causes photosensitisation with subsequent pigmentation; it is suspected of increasing the incidence of skin cancers, but this has not been established.

BORDERLINE SUBSTANCES. The preparations marked 'ACBS' are regarded as drugs when prescribed for skin protection against ultraviolet radiation in abnormal cutaneous photosensitivity resulting from genetic disorders or photodermatoses, including those resulting from radiotherapy; chronic or recurrent herpes simplex labialis. Preparations with SPF less than 15 are no longer prescribable. See also Appendix 7.

Ambre Solaire® (Garnier)

Total sunblock cream (UVA and UVB protection; UVB-SPF60), avobenzone 3.5%, 4-methylbenzylidene camphor 5%, terephthalylidene dicamphor sulphonic acid 3.25%, titanium dioxide 4.1%. Net price 50 mL = £4.12. ACBS

Additives: include hydroxybenzoates (parabens), disodium edetate

Coppertone® (Scholl)

Ultrashade 23 lotion, (UVA and UVB protection; UVB-SPF23), ethylhexyl *p*-methoxycinnamate 7.5%, oxybenzone 3%, padimate-O 2.5%. Net price 150 mL = £4.46. ACBS

Additives: include hydroxybenzoates (parabens), wool fat, fragrance

Piz Buin® (Novartis Consumer Health)

Sunblock lotion (UVA and UVB protection; UVB-SPF 20), ethylhexyl *p*-methoxycinnamate 7.5%, avobenzone 1.5%, titanium dioxide 3%. Net price 200 mL = £6.92. ACBS

Additives: include hydroxybenzoates (parabens), propylene glycol, fragrance

RoC® (RoC)

Total sunblock cream (UVA and UVB protection; UVB-SPF 25), colourless or tinted, containing avobenzone, ethylhexyl *p*-methoxycinnamate. Net price 50 mL = £4.06. ACBS

Additives: include beeswax, hydroxybenzoates (parabens)

Spectraban® (Stiefel)

Lotion (UVB protection; UVB-SPF 25), aminobenzoic acid 5%, padimate-O 3.2%, in an alcoholic basis. Net price 150 mL = £3.45. ACBS

Additives: include fragrance

Caution: flammable; stains clothing

Ultra lotion (UVA and UVB protection; UVB-SPF 28), water resistant, avobenzone 2%, oxybenzone 3%, padimate-O 8%, titanium dioxide 2%. Net price 150 mL = £5.45. ACBS

Additives: include benzyl alcohol, disodium edetate, sorbic acid, fragrance

Sun E45® (Crookes)

Lotion (UVA and UVB protection; UVB-SPF 15), water-resistant, titanium dioxide 2%, zinc oxide 13.5%. Net price 100 mL = £4.78. ACBS

Additives: include hydroxybenzoates (parabens), isopropyl palmitate

Lotion (UVA and UVB protection; UVB-SPF 25), water-resistant, titanium dioxide 3.6%, zinc oxide 14%. Net price 100 mL = £5.04. ACBS

Additives: include hydroxybenzoates (parabens), isopropyl palmitate

Sunblock lotion (UVA and UVB protection; UVB-SPF 50), water-resistant, titanium dioxide 6.4%, zinc oxide 16%. Net price 100 mL = £5.42. ACBS

Additives: include hydroxybenzoates (parabens), isopropyl palmitate

Uvistat® (Windsor)

Lipscreen (UVA and UVB protection; UVB-SPF 15), ethylhexyl *p*-methoxycinnamate 3%, avobenzone 4%. Net price 5-g stick = £1.58. ACBS

Additives: include butylated hydroxyanisole, fragrance

Babysun cream (UVA and UVB protection; UVB-SPF 22), water-resistant, ethylhexyl *p*-methoxycinnamate 7%, avobenzone 4%, titanium dioxide 4.5%. Net price 50 g = £3.63, 100 g = £5.10. ACBS

Additives: include disodium edetate, hydroxybenzoates (parabens), fragrance

Cream (UVA and UVB protection; UVB-SPF 22 but marketed as 'factor 20'), water-resistant, ethylhexyl *p*-methoxycinnamate 7%, avobenzone 4%, titanium dioxide 4.5%. Net price 50 g = £3.40, 100 g = £5.10. ACBS

Additives: include disodium edetate, hydroxybenzoates (parabens), fragrance

Lotion (UVA and UVB protection; UVB-SPF 25), tinted, water-resistant, methylbenzylidene camphor 6%, avobenzone 4%, titanium dioxide 4%. Net price 200 mL = £5.08. ACBS

Additives: include edetic acid (EDTA), hydroxybenzoates (parabens), fragrance

Ultrablock cream (UVA and UVB protection; UVB-SPF 30), ethylhexyl *p*-methoxycinnamate 7.5%, avobenzone 4%, titanium dioxide 6.5%. Net price 50 g = £4.08. ACBS

Additives: include disodium edetate, hydroxybenzoates (parabens), fragrance

---

PHOTODAMAGE

Application of tretinoin 0.05% cream is reported to be associated with gradual improvement in photodamaged skin (usually within 3–4 months of starting).

TRETINOIN

Note. Tretinoin is the acid form of vitamin A

Indications: mottled hyperpigmentation, roughness and fine wrinkling of photodamaged skin due to chronic sun exposure; acne vulgaris (section 13.6); malignant disease (section 8.1.5)

Cautions; Contra-indications; Side-effects: see section 13.6.1

Administration: apply thinly at night, then reduce to 1-3 nights weekly

NHS PoM **Retinova®** (Janssen-Cilag)

Cream, tretinoin 0.05%, net price 20 g = £13.75.

Additives: include fragrance

13.8.2   Camouflagers

Disfigurement of the skin can be very distressing to patients and have a marked psychological effect. In skilled hands, or with experience, these preparations can be very effective in concealing scars and birthmarks. The depigmented patches in vitiligo are also very disfiguring and camouflage creams are of great cosmetic value.

BORDERLINE SUBSTANCES. The preparations marked 'ACBS' are regarded as drugs when prescribed for postoperative scars and other deformities and as an adjunctive therapy in the relief of emotional disturbances due to disfiguring skin disease, such as vitiligo. See also Appendix 7.

Boots Covering Cream® (Boots)

Cream (2 shades). Net price 50 g = £3.15. ACBS

Additives:include hydroxybenzoates (parabens)

Covermark® (Epiderm)

Classic foundation (masking cream, 10 shades). Net price 30 g = £11.23. ACBS

Additives: include beeswax, hydroxybenzoates (parabens), fragrance

Finishing powder. Net price 75 g = £9.50. ACBS

Additives: include beeswax, hydroxybenzoates (parabens), fragrance

Dermablend® (Baker Norton)

Cover creme. Net price 10.7 g (10 shades) = £6.56; 28.4 g (11 shades)= £11.08. ACBS

Additives: include beeswax, hydroxybenzoates (parabens)

Leg and body cover, (7 shades). Net price 64 g = £9.82. ACBS

Additives: include beeswax, hydroxybenzoates (parabens)

Setting powder. Net price 28 g = £9.45. ACBS

Additives: include hydroxybenzoates (parabens)

Dermacolor® (Fox)

Camouflage creme, (30 shades). Net price 30 g = £7.25. ACBS

Additives: include beeswax, wool fat, fragrance

Fixing powder, (5 shades). Net price 60 g = £5.88. ACBS

Additives: include fragrance

Keromask® (Network Management)

Masking cream, (2 shades). Net price 15 mL = £4.53. ACBS

Additives: include butylated hydroxyanisole, hydroxybenzoates (parabens), wool fat

Finishing powder. Net price 25 g = £4.53. ACBS

Additives: none as listed in section 13.1

Veil® (Blake)

Cover cream, (20 shades). Net price 19 g = £5.40; 44 g = £8.80; 70 g = £12.60. ACBS

Additives: include hydroxybenzoates (parabens), wool fat derivative

---

Finishing powder, translucent. Net price 35 g = £5.40. ACBS

Additives: include butylated hydroxyanisole, hydroxybenzoates (parabens)

13.9   Shampoos and some other scalp preparations

Dandruff is considered to be a mild form of seborrhoeic dermatitis (see also section 13.5.1). The treatment of choice is the frequent use of a mild detergent shampoo generally once or twice weekly; this rids the scalp of scale but does not have a therapeutic effect in itself. Shampoos containing antimicrobial agents such as **pyrithione zinc** (which are widely available) and **selenium sulphide** may have beneficial effects. Shampoos containing **tar** extracts may be useful and they are also used in *psoriasis*. **Ketoconazole** shampoo is probably the most effective.

For more severe conditions, **ketoconazole** shampoo may be used on the scalp, alone or with **corticosteroid** gels and lotions (section 13.4).

Shampoos containing **coal tar** and **salicylic acid** may also be useful. Patients who do not respond to these treatments may need to be referred to exclude the possibility of other skin conditions.

Cradle cap in infants may be treated with **olive oil** or **arachis oil** (ground-nut oil, peanut oil) applications followed by shampooing.

See also section 13.5 (psoriasis and eczema), section 13.10.4 (lice), and section 13.10.2 (ringworm).

Alphosyl 2 in 1® (Stafford-Miller)

Shampoo, alcoholic coal tar extract 5%. Net price 125 mL = £1.81; 250 mL = £3.43.

Additives: include hydroxybenzoates (parabens), fragrance

Dandruff, use once or twice weekly as necessary; psoriasis, seborrhoeic dermatitis, scaling and itching, use every 2–3 days

Baltar® (Merck)

Shampoo, coal tar distillate 1.5% in soap-free basis. Net price 200 mL = £2.28

Additives: include fragrance

Scaly scalp disorders including psoriasis, eczema, seborrhoeic and pruritic dermatitis, and dandruff, apply 1–3 times weekly; CHILD under 2 years not recommended

Betadine® (Seton)

Scalp and skin cleanser—section 13.11.4

Shampoo solution, povidone–iodine 4%, in a surfactant solution. Net price 250 mL = £2.43.

Additives: include fragrance

Seborrhoeic scalp conditions associated with excessive dandruff, pruritus, scaling, exudation and erythema, infected scalp lesions (recurrent furunculosis, infective folliculitis, impetigo), apply 1–2 times weekly; CHILD under 2 years not recommended

Capasal® (Dermal)

Shampoo, coal tar 1%, coconut oil 1%, salicylic acid 0.5%. Net price 250 mL = £5.28

Additives: none as listed in section 13.1

Scaly scalp disorders including psoriasis, seborrhoeic dermatitis, dandruff, and cradle cap, apply daily as necessary

Ceanel Concentrate® (Quinoderm Ltd)

Shampoo, cetrimide 10%, undecenoic acid 1%, phenylethyl alcohol 7.5%. Net price 50 mL = £1.18; 150 mL = £3.11; 500 mL = £9.07

Additives: none as listed in section 13.1

Scalp psoriasis, seborrhoeic dermatitis, dandruff, apply 3 times in first week then twice weekly

Clinitar® (Shire)

Shampoo solution, coal tar extract 2%. Net price 100 g = £2.50

Additives: include polysorbates, fragrance

Scalp psoriasis, seborrhoeic dermatitis, and dandruff, apply up to 3 times weekly

Cocois® (Evans)

Scalp ointment, coal tar solution 12%, salicylic acid 2%, precipitated sulphur 4%, in a coconut oil emollient basis. Net price 40 g (with applicator nozzle) = £5.04; 100 g = £9.46

Additives: none as listed in section 13.1

Scaly scalp disorders including psoriasis, eczema, seborrhoeic dermatitis and dandruff, apply to scalp once weekly as necessary (if severe use daily for first 3–7 days), shampoo off after 1 hour; CHILD 6–12 years, medical supervision required (not recommended under 6 years)

Gelcotar® (Quinoderm Ltd)

Liquid, strong coal tar solution 1.25%, cade oil 0.5%, in a shampoo basis. Net price 150 mL = £1.53; 350 mL = £3.06

Additives: include chlorocresol

Scalp psoriasis, seborrhoeic dermatitis, and dandruff, apply twice weekly

Gel, see section 13.5.2

Ionil T® (Galderma)

Shampoo application, benzalkonium chloride 0.2%, coal tar solution 4.25%, salicylic acid 2% in an alcoholic basis. Net price 200 mL = £2.56

Additives: include disodium edetate

Scalp psoriasis, seborrhoeic dermatitis, apply 1–2 times weekly; CHILD under 12 years not recommended

Lenium® (Janssen-Cilag)

Cream, selenium sulphide 2.5%. Net price 42 g = £1.28; 100 g = £1.97

Additives: include fragrance

Seborrhoeic dermatitis and dandruff, apply twice weekly for 2 weeks then once weekly for 2 weeks and then as necessary

Caution: avoid using 48 hours before or after applying hair colouring or waving preparations

Meted® (Euroderma)

Shampoo, salicylic acid 3%, sulphur 5%. Net price 120 mL = £3.90

Additives: include fragrance

Scaly scalp disorders including psoriasis, seborrhoeic dermatitis, and dandruff, apply at least twice weekly

PoM Nizoral® (Janssen-Cilag)

Shampoo, ketoconazole 2%. Net price 120 mL = £8.75

Additives: none as listed in section 13.1

For seborrhoeic dermatitis and dandruff apply twice weekly for 2–4 weeks, for pityriasis versicolor once daily for max. 5 days

Note. Can be sold to the public for the prevention and treatment of dandruff and seborrhoeic dermatitis of the scalp as a shampoo formulation containing ketoconazole max. 2%, in a pack containing max.120 mL and labelled to show a max. frequency of application of once every 3 days; a brand on sale to the public is *Nizoral*® *Dandruff Shampoo*; *Neutrogena*® *Long Lasting Dandruff Control Shampoo* containing ketoconazole 1% is available as a cosmetic.

Pentrax® (Euroderma)
Shampoo, coal tar 4.3%. Net price 120 mL = £3.90
Additives: none as listed in section 13.1
Scaly scalp disorders including psoriasis, seborrhoeic dermatitis, and dandruff, apply at least twice weekly

Polytar® (Stiefel)
Liquid, arachis (peanut) oil extract of crude coal tar 0.3%, cade oil 0.3%, coal tar solution 0.1%, oleyl alcohol 1%, tar 0.3%. Net price 250 mL = £2.23
Additives: include polysorbate 80, fragrance
Scalp disorders including psoriasis, seborrhoea, eczema, pruritus and dandruff, apply 1–2 times weekly

Polytar AF® (Stiefel)
Shampoo, arachis (peanut) oil extract of coal tar 0.3%, cade oil 0.3%, coal tar solution 0.1%, pine tar 0.3%, pyrithione zinc 1%. Net price 150 mL = £4.40.
Additives: include fragrance
Scaly scalp disorders including psoriasis, seborrhoeic dermatitis, and dandruff, apply 2–3 times weekly for at least 3 weeks

Polytar Plus® (Stiefel)
Liquid, ingredients as Polytar® liquid with hydrolysed animal protein 3%. Net price 350 mL = £3.29
Additives: include polysorbate 80, fragrance
Scalp disorders including psoriasis, seborrhoea, eczema, pruritus and dandruff, apply 1–2 times weekly

Pragmatar® —section 13.5.2

Psoriderm® (Dermal)
Scalp lotion (= shampoo), coal tar 2.5%, lecithin 0.3%. Net price 250 mL – £5.33
Additives: include disodium edetate
Scalp psoriasis, use as necessary

Selsun® (Abbott)
Shampoo application, selenium sulphide 2.5%
Net price 50 mL = £1.39; 100 mL = £1.87; 150 mL = £2.63
Additives: include fragrance
Seborrhoeic dermatitis and dandruff, apply twice weekly for 2 weeks then once weekly for 2 weeks and then as necessary; CHILD under 5 years not recommended; pityriasis versicolor, see section 13.10.2 [unlicensed indication]
Caution: avoid using 48 hours before or after applying hair colouring or waving preparations

T/Gel® (Neutrogena)
Shampoo, coal tar extract 2%. Net price 125 mL = £2.80; 250 mL = £4.46
Additives: include hydroxybenzoates (parabens), tetrasodium edetate, fragrance
Scalp psoriasis, seborrhoeic dermatitis, dandruff, apply as necessary

MALE-PATTERN BALDNESS

Topical application of **minoxidil** may stimulate limited hair growth in a small proportion of patients but only for as long as it is used.

MINOXIDIL
Indications: male-pattern baldness (men and women)
Cautions; Contra-indications; Side-effects: see section 2.5.1 (only about 1.4% absorbed); monitor hypertensive patients closely; avoid contact with eyes, mouth and mucous membranes, broken, infected, or inflamed skin; avoid inhalation of spray mist and use with topically applied drugs

known to enhance absorption; local side-effects: irritant dermatitis, allergic contact dermatitis
Administration: ADULT aged 18–65 years, apply 1 mL twice daily to dry hair and scalp (discontinue if no improvement after 1 year)

N<del>HS</del> **Regaine®** (Pharmacia & Upjohn)
Topical solution, minoxidil 2% in an aqueous alcoholic basis. Net price 60-mL bottle with applicators = £14.16
Additives: include propylene glycol
Cautions: flammable; wash hands after application

13.10 Anti-infective skin preparations

13.10.1 Antibacterial preparations
13.10.2 Antifungal preparations
13.10.3 Antiviral preparations
13.10.4 Parasiticidal preparations
13.10.5 Preparations for minor cuts and abrasions

13.10.1 Antibacterial preparations

13.10.1.1 Antibacterial preparations only used topically
13.10.1.2 Antibacterial preparations also used systemically

For many skin infections such as *erysipelas* and *cellulitis* systemic antibacterial treatment is the method of choice because the infection is too deeply sited for adequate penetration of topical preparations. For details of suitable treatment see section 5.1.

Impetigo may be treated by topical application of **fusidic acid** or **mupirocin** or, if widespread, with oral administration of **flucloxacillin** or **erythromycin** (section 5.1, table 1). Mild antiseptics such as **povidone-iodine** (section 13.11.4) are used to soften crusts and exudate.

Although there are a great many antibacterial drugs presented in topical preparations some are potentially hazardous and frequently their use is not necessary if adequate hygienic measures can be taken. Moreover not all skin conditions that are oozing, crusted, or characterised by pustules are actually infected. Topical antibiotics should be **avoided** on *leg ulcers* unless used in short courses for defined infections; treatment of bacterial colonisation is generally inappropriate.

To minimise the development of resistant organisms it is advisable to limit the choice of antibiotics applied topically to those not used systemically. Unfortunately some of these, for example neomycin, may cause sensitisation, and there is cross-sensitivity with other aminoglycoside antibiotics, such as gentamicin. If *large areas of skin* are being treated, ototoxicity may also be a hazard with aminoglycoside antibiotics (and also with polymyxins), particularly in children, in the elderly, and in those with renal impairment. *Resistant organisms* are more common in hospitals, and whenever possible swabs for bacteriological examination should be taken before beginning treatment.

Mupirocin is not related to any other antibiotic in use; it is effective for skin infections, particularly those due to Gram positive organisms but it is not indicated for pseudomonal infection. Although *Staphylococcus aureus* strains with low level resistance to mupirocin are emerging, it is generally useful when there is resistant infection. To avoid the development of resistance it should not be used for longer than 10 days and its use in hospital should if possible be avoided.

Silver sulphadiazine is used in the treatment of infected burns.

13.10.1.1 ANTIBACTERIAL PREPARATIONS ONLY USED TOPICALLY

FRAMYCETIN SULPHATE

Indications: bacterial skin infections

Cautions; Side-effects: sensitisation (see also notes above); large areas, see below

LARGE AREAS. If large areas of skin are being treated ototoxicity may be a hazard, particularly in children, in the elderly, and in those with renal impairment

N̶H̶S̶ PoM **Soframycin**® (Hoechst Marion Roussel)
Ointment, framycetin sulphate 1.5%, gramicidin 0.005%, in a wool fat and paraffin basis. Net price 15 g = £1.68
Additives: include wool fat
Superficial bacterial infection, apply up to 3 times daily (short-term use)
Sofra-Tulle® *see* Framycetin Gauze Dressing, Appendix 9

MUPIROCIN

Indications: bacterial skin infections (see also notes above)

Administration: apply up to 3 times daily for up to 10 days

PoM **Bactroban**® (Beecham)
Ointment, mupirocin 2%. Net price 15 g = £4.71
Additives: none as listed in section 13.1
Note. Manufacturer advises: contains macrogol therefore caution in renal impairment; may sting
Nasal ointment, see section 12.2.3

NEOMYCIN SULPHATE

Indications: bacterial skin infections

Cautions; Side-effects: sensitisation (see also notes above); large areas, see below

LARGE AREAS. If large areas of skin are being treated ototoxicity may be a hazard, particularly in children, in the elderly, and in those with renal impairment

PoM **Neomycin Cream BPC**
Cream, neomycin sulphate 0.5%, cetomacrogol emulsifying ointment 30%, chlorocresol 0.1%, disodium edetate 0.01%, in freshly boiled and cooled purified water. Net price 15 g = 88p
Apply up to 3 times daily (short-term use)

PoM **Cicatrin**® (GlaxoWellcome)
Cream, neomycin sulphate 3300 units, bacitracin zinc 250 units, cysteine 2 mg, glycine 10 mg, threonine 1 mg/g. Net price 15 g = 90p; 30 g = £1.80
Additives: include wool fat derivative
Superficial bacterial infection of skin, apply up to 3 times daily; ADULT max. 60 g daily for 3 weeks; do not repeat for at least 3 months; CHILD reduced dose
Dusting powder, neomycin sulphate 3300 units, bacitracin zinc 250 units, cysteine 2 mg, glycine 10 mg, threonine 1 mg/g. Net price 15 g = 90p; 50 g = £3.00
Additives: none as listed in section 13.1
Superficial bacterial infection of skin, apply up to 3 times daily, ADULT max. 50 g daily for 4 weeks; do not repeat for at least 3 months; CHILD reduced dose
PoM **Graneodin**® (Squibb)
Ointment, neomycin sulphate 0.25%, gramicidin 0.025%. Net price 25 g = £1.47
Additives: none as listed in section 13.1
Superficial bacterial infection of skin, apply 2–4 times daily (for max. 7 days—possibly longer for sycosis barbae)

POLYMYXINS
(Includes colistin sulphate and polymyxin B sulphate)
Indications: bacterial skin infections

Cautions; Side-effects: sensitisation (see also notes above); large areas, see below

LARGE AREAS. If large areas of skin are being treated ototoxicity may be a hazard, particularly in children, in the elderly, and in those with renal impairment

PoM **Polyfax**® (Dominion)
Ointment, polymyxin B sulphate 10 000 units, bacitracin zinc 500 units/g. Net price 20 g = £4.84
Apply 3 times daily
PoM **Colomycin**® (Pharmax)
Powder, sterile, for making topical preparations (usually 1%), colistin sulphate. Net price 1 g vial = £19.24

SILVER SULPHADIAZINE

Indications: prophylaxis and treatment of infection in burn wounds; as an adjunct to short-term treatment of infection in leg ulcers and pressure sores; as an adjunct to prophylaxis of infection in skin graft donor sites and extensive abrasions; for conservative management of finger-tip injuries

Cautions: hepatic and renal impairment; G6PD deficiency; pregnancy and breast-feeding (avoid in late pregnancy and in neonate—see also Appendix 4); may inactivate enzymatic debriding agents therefore concomitant use may be inappropriate; for large amounts see also **interactions:** Appendix 1 (co-trimoxazole and sulphonamides)

LARGE AREAS. Plasma-sulphadiazine concentrations may approach therapeutic levels with *side-effects* and *interactions* as for sulphonamides (see section 5.1.8) if large areas of skin are treated. Owing to the association of sulphonamides with severe blood and skin disorders treatment should be stopped immediately if blood disorders or rashes develop—but leucopenia developing 2–3 days after starting treatment of burns patients is reported usually to be self-limiting and silver sulphadiazine need not usually be discontinued provided blood counts are monitored carefully to ensure return to normality within a few days. Argyria may also occur if large areas of skin are treated (or if application is prolonged).

Contra-indications: pregnancy and breast-feeding; sensitivity to sulphonamides; not recommended for neonates (see also Appendix 4)

Side-effects: allergic reactions including burning, itching and rashes; argyria reported following prolonged use; leucopenia reported (monitor blood levels)

PoM **Flamazine**® (S&N Hlth.)

Cream, silver sulphadiazine 1%. Net price 50 g = £4.30; 250 g = £11.52; 500 g = £20.40

Additives: include polysorbates, propylene glycol

In burns apply daily with sterile applicator or more frequently if volume of exudate large; in leg ulcers daily (or every 48 hours—not recommended for leg or pressure ulcers that are very exudative); in finger-tip injuries apply every 2–3 days—for details see product literature

---

13.10.1.2 ANTIBACTERIAL PREPARATIONS ALSO USED SYSTEMICALLY

CHLORTETRACYCLINE HYDROCHLORIDE

Indications: bacterial skin infections (see notes above)

Cautions: see notes above; overgrowth with non-susceptible organisms; stains clothing

Side-effects: rarely local hypersensitivity reactions

Administration: apply 1 to 3 times daily

PoM **Aureomycin**® (Lederle)

Ointment, chlortetracycline hydrochloride 3%. Net price 30 g = £1.77

Additives: include hydroxybenzoates (parabens), wool fat

FUSIDIC ACID

Indications: staphylococcal skin infections

Cautions: see notes above; avoid contact with eyes

Side-effects: rarely local hypersensitivity reactions

Administration: apply 3–4 times daily

PoM **Fucidin**® (Leo)

Cream, fusidic acid 2%. Net price 15 g = £2.87; 30 g = £4.84

Additives: include butylated hydroxyanisole

Gel, fusidic acid 2%. Net price 15 g = £2.48; 30 g = £4.29

Additives: include hydroxybenzoates (parabens), polysorbate 80

Ointment, sodium fusidate 2%. Net price 15 g = £2.34; 30 g = £3.97

Additives: include wool fat

PoM **Fucidin Intertulle**® *see* Appendix 9

GENTAMICIN

Indications: bacterial skin infections

Cautions; Side-effects: sensitisation (see also notes above); large areas, see below

LARGE AREAS. If large areas of skin are being treated ototoxicity may be a hazard, particularly in children, in the elderly, and in those with renal impairment

Administration: apply 3–4 times daily

PoM **Cidomycin Topical**® (Hoechst Marion Roussel)

Cream, gentamicin 0.3% (as sulphate). Net price 30 g = £3.31

Additives: include hydroxybenzoates (parabens), propylene glycol

METRONIDAZOLE

Indications: see under preparations

Cautions: avoid exposure to strong sunlight or UV light

Side-effects: local skin irritation

Rosacea (see also section 13.6)

PoM **Metrogel**® (Novartis)

Gel, metronidazole 0.75%. Net price 40 g = £17.36. Label: 10 patient information leaflet

Additives: include hydroxybenzoates (parabens), propylene glycol

Administration: acute inflammatory exacerbations of acne rosacea, apply thinly twice daily for 8–9 weeks; avoid contact with eyes

PoM **Rozex**® (Stafford-Miller)

Gel, metronidazole 0.75%. Net price 30 g = £12.00. Label: 10 patient information leaflet

Additives: include disodium edetate, hydroxybenzoates (parabens), propylene glycol

Administration: inflammatory papules, pustules and erythema of acne rosacea, apply thinly twice daily; avoid contact with eyes

Malodorous tumours

PoM **Anabact**® (ASTA Medica)

Gel, metronidazole 0.75%. Net price 15 g = £4.70; 30 g = £8.31

Additives: include hydroxybenzoates (parabens), propylene glycol

Administration: fungating malodorous tumours, apply to clean wound twice daily and cover with non-adherent dressing

PoM **Metrotop**® (Seton)

Gel, metronidazole 0.8%. Net price 15 g = £4.95; 30 g = £8.75

Additives: none as listed in section 13.1

Administration: de-odourisation of fungating malodorous tumours, apply to clean wound 1 to 2 times daily and cover (flat wounds, apply liberally; cavities, smear on paraffin gauze and pack loosely); use tube once only

---

TETRACYCLINE HYDROCHLORIDE

Indications; Cautions; Side-effects: see under Chlortetracycline Hydrochloride

PoM **Achromycin Topical**® (Lederle)

Ointment, tetracycline hydrochloride 3%. Net price 30 g = £1.44

Additives: include hydroxybenzoates (parabens), wool fat

Apply 1–3 times daily

13.10.2 Antifungal preparations

Ideally skin scrapings should be examined to confirm diagnosis before treatment is begun. Widespread or intractable fungal infections are treated systemically (see section 5.2). Most localised infections are treated with the topical preparations described below.

Most ringworm infections, including tinea pedis, can be treated adequately with topical preparations. The imidazoles **clotrimazole, econazole, miconazole** and **sulconazole** are all effective and commonly used. Nail ringworm (tinea unguium) and scalp ringworm (*T. capitis*) are treated systemically (section 5.2). **Amorolfine** is a newly introduced antifungal that differs chemically from other antifungals and has some activity against moulds. It is available as a cream for fungal skin infections and a lacquer for fungal nail infections. **Terbinafine** has also been recently introduced in the form of a cream; it is also available for systemic administration (section 5.2). Combinations of imidazoles and weak corticosteroids may be of use in the treatment of eczematous intertrigo and, in the first few days only, of a severely inflamed patch of ringworm. **Compound benzoic acid ointment** (Whitfield's ointment) was also quite effective but was cosmetically less acceptable than the proprietary preparations and is rarely used. The **undecenoates** are less effective in treating ringworm infections.

Pityriasis versicolor (tinea versicolor) may be treated topically with a 3-day course of selenium sulphide shampoo repeated after a month; it is applied to the scalp and affected areas and left on overnight. Topical imidazoles (clotrimazole, ketoconazole, and miconazole) and topical terbinafine are alternatives but large quantities may be required. Pityriasis versicolor may be treated systemically with itraconazole; fluconazole is an alternative. Relapse is common, especially in immunocompromised individuals (section 5.2)

Candidal skin infections may also be treated by topical application with the broad-spectrum antifungals, clotrimazole, econazole, and miconazole. Oral preparations of some antifungals are now also available (section 5.2), but should preferably be reserved for those who are resistant to (or intolerant of) topical preparations. **Nystatin** preparations are also equally as effective in candidiasis although they are ineffective against infections due to dermatophyte fungi (tinea).

Lotions or sprays are generally chosen for application to large and hairy areas. Ointments are best avoided on moist surfaces because of their occlusive properties. Nail lacquers and paints may be effective for early fungal dystrophy of the nails and should be considered when up to 2 nails are affected (or where systemic therapy is contra-indicated). Dusting-powders have no place in the treatment of fungal infections, except for toiletry or cosmetic purposes, as they are therapeutically ineffective and may cause skin irritation.

AMOROLFINE

Indications: see under preparations

Cautions: pregnancy, breast-feeding; avoid eyes, ears, and mucous membranes

Side-effects: occasional transient burning sensation, erythema, pruritus

PoM **Loceryl®** (Roche)
Cream, amorolfine (as hydrochloride) 0.25%. Net price 20 g = £4.83. Label: 10 patient information leaflet
Additives: include disodium edetate
Administration: fungal skin infections, apply once daily after cleansing in the evening for at least 2–3 weeks (up to 6 weeks for foot mycosis) continuing for 3–5 days after lesions have healed
Nail lacquer, amorolfine (as hydrochloride) 5%. Net price 5-mL pack (with nail files, spatulas and cleansing swabs) = £34.38. Label: 10 patient information leaflet
Administration: fungal nail infections, apply to infected nails 1–2 times weekly after filing and cleansing; allow to dry (approx. 3 minutes); treat finger nails for 6 months, toe nails for 9–12 months (review at intervals of 3 months); avoid nail varnish or artificial nails during treatment

BENZOIC ACID
Indications: ringworm (tinea), but see notes above

Benzoic Acid Ointment, Compound, BP
(Whitfield's ointment), benzoic acid 6%, salicylic acid 3%, in emulsifying ointment
Apply twice daily

BENZOYL PEROXIDE
Indications: fungal skin infections, particularly tinea pedis

Quinoped® (Quinoderm Ltd)
Cream, benzoyl peroxide 5%, potassium hydroxyquinoline sulphate 0.5%, in an astringent basis. Net price 25 g = £1.13
Additives: include edetic acid (EDTA)
Apply twice daily

CLOTRIMAZOLE
Indications: fungal skin infections
Side-effects: occasional skin irritation or sensitivity
Administration: apply 2–3 times daily continuing for 14 days after lesions have healed

Canesten® (Baypharm)
Cream, clotrimazole 1%. Net price 20 g = £1.77; 50 g = £4.15
Additives: include benzyl alcohol, polysorbate 60
Note. A generic version of clotrimazole 1% cream is available from APS, CP, Cox; proprietary brands on sale to the public include Canesten® AF and Mycil Gold®
Solution, clotrimazole 1% in macrogol 400 (polyethylene glycol 400). Net price 20 mL = £2.32. For hairy areas
Additives: none as listed in section 13.1
Spray, clotrimazole 1%, in 30% isopropyl alcohol. Net price 40-mL atomiser = £4.99. Label: 15. For large or hairy areas
Additives: include propylene glycol
Dusting powder, clotrimazole 1%. Net price 30 g = £1.52
Additives: none as listed in section 13.1
Masnoderm® (Dominion)
Cream, clotrimazole 1%. Net price 20 g = £1.54
Additives: include benzyl alcohol, polysorbates

ECONAZOLE NITRATE
Indications; Side-effects: see under Clotrimazole
Administration: apply 2–3 times daily continuing
for 14 days after lesions have healed

Ecostatin® (Squibb)
Cream, econazole nitrate 1%. Net price 15 g =
£1.49; 30 g = £2.75
Additives: include butylated hydroxyanisole, fragrance
Pevaryl® (Janssen-Cilag)
Cream, econazole nitrate 1%. Net price 30 g =
£2.65
Additives: include butylated hydroxyanisole, fragrance
Lotion, econazole nitrate 1%. Net price 30 mL =
£3.33
Additives: include butylated hydroxyanisole, fragrance

KETOCONAZOLE
Indications; Side-effects: see under Clotrimazole

PoM **Nizoral®** (Janssen-Cilag)
NHS*Cream,* ketoconazole 2%. Net price 30 g =
£3.81
Additives: include polysorbates, propylene glycol
Apply 1–2 times daily, continuing for a few days after
lesions have healed
* except for seborrhoeic dermatitis and pityriasis versicolor and endorsed 'SLS'

MICONAZOLE NITRATE
Indications; Side-effects: see under Clotrimazole
Administration: apply twice daily continuing for
10 days after lesions have healed; nail infections,
apply daily under occlusive dressing

Daktarin® (Janssen-Cilag)
Cream, miconazole nitrate 2%. Net price 30 g =
£2.07
Additives: include butylated hydroxyanisole
Note. A generic version of miconazole nitrate 2% cream
is available from APS, Hillcross
NHS *Dusting powder,* miconazole nitrate 2%. Net
price 20 g = £1.81
Additives: none as listed in section 13.1
Spray powder, miconazole nitrate 0.16%, in an
aerosol basis. Net price 100 g = £2.27
Additives: none as listed in section 13.1

NYSTATIN
Indications: skin infections due to *Candida* spp.
Administration: apply 2–4 times daily, continuing
for 7 days after lesions have healed

PoM **Nystaform®** (Bayer)
Cream, nystatin 100 000 units/g, chlorhexidine
hydrochloride 1%. Net price 30 g = £2.62
Additives: include benzyl alcohol, polysorbate 60
PoM **Nystan®** (Squibb)
Cream, nystatin 100 000 units/g. Net price 30 g =
£2.18
Additives: include benzyl alcohol, propylene glycol, fragrance
Gel, nystatin 100000 units/g. Net price 30 g =
£2.66
Additives: include chlorocresol, fragrance
Ointment, nystatin 100 000 units/g, in *Plasti-
base®.* Net price 30 g = £1.75
Additives: none as listed in section 13.1

PoM **Tinaderm-M®** (Schering-Plough)
Cream, nystatin 100 000 units/g, tolnaftate 1%.
Net price 20 g = £1.83. For *Candida* infections
and tinea
Additives: include butylated hydroxytoluene, hydroxybenzoates
(parabens), fragrance

SALICYLIC ACID
Indications: fungal skin infections, particularly
tinea
Side-effects: hypersensitivity reactions

Phytex® (Pharmax)
Paint, salicylic acid 1.46% (total combined), tannic acid
4.89% and boric acid 3.12% (as borotannic complex), in
a vehicle containing alcohol and ethyl acetate. Net price
25 mL (with brush) = £1.29. For fungal nail infections
(onychomycosis)
Additives: none as listed in section 13.1
Apply twice daily
Caution: flammable; avoid in pregnancy and children
under 5 years

SULCONAZOLE NITRATE
Indications; Side-effects: see under Clotrimazole
Cautions: avoid contact with eyes (lens changes in
animals after high oral doses)

PoM **Exelderm®** (Zeneca)
Cream, sulconazole nitrate 1%. Net price 30 g =
£3.00
Apply 1–2 times daily continuing for 2–3 weeks after
lesions have healed
Additives: include polysorbates, propylene glycol

TERBINAFINE
Indications: fungal skin infections
Cautions: pregnancy, breast-feeding; avoid con-
tact with eyes
Side-effects: redness, itching, or stinging; rarely
allergic reactions (discontinue)

PoM **Lamisil®** (Novartis)
Cream, terbinafine hydrochloride 1%. Net price
15 g = £4.86; 30 g = £8.76
Apply thinly 1–2 times daily for up to 1 week in tinea
pedis, 1–2 weeks in tinea corporis and tinea cruris, 2
weeks in cutaneous candidiasis and pityriasis versicolor;
review after 2 weeks; CHILD not recommended
Additives: include benzyl alcohol, polysorbate 60
Tablets, see section 5.2

TIOCONAZOLE
Indications: see under preparation
Side-effects: local irritation, usually during first
week of treatment; discontinue if sensitivity reaction develops

Trosyl® (Pfizer)
PoM *Nail solution,* tioconazole 28%. Net price
12 mL (with applicator brush) = £27.38
Additives: none as listed in section 13.1
Administration: fungal nail infections, apply to nails and
surrounding skin twice daily for up to 6 months (may be
extended to 12 months)

UNDECENOATES

Indications: skin infections, particularly tinea pedis

Monphytol® (LAB)

Paint, methyl undecenoate 5%, propyl undecenoate 0.7%, salicylic acid 3%, methyl salicylate 25%, propyl salicylate 5%, chlorbutol 3%. Net price 18 mL (with brush) = £1.47. For fungal (particularly nail) infections

Additives: none as listed in section 13.1

Apply twice daily

Mycota® (Seton)

Cream, zinc undecenoate 20%, undecenoic acid 5%. Net price 25 g = £1.02

Additives: include fragrance

Dusting powder, zinc undecenoate 20%, undecenoic acid 2%. Net price 70 g = £1.50

Additives: include fragrance

Spray application, undecenoic acid 2.5%, dichlorophen 0.25% (pressurised aerosol pack). Net price 100 mL = £1.62

Additives: include fragrance

Apply 1–2 times daily

13.10.3   Antiviral preparations

Aciclovir cream is indicated for the treatment of initial and recurrent labial and genital *herpes simplex infections*; treatment should begin as early as possible. Systemic treatment is necessary for buccal or vaginal infections; *herpes zoster (shingles)* also requires systemic treatment (for details of systemic use see section 5.3). **Penciclovir** cream has been introduced recently; it is indicated for the treatment of labial *herpes simplex infection.*

Idoxuridine solution (5% in dimethyl sulphoxide) is of little value.

ACICLOVIR

(Acyclovir)

Indications: see notes above

Cautions: avoid contact with eyes and mucous membranes

Side-effects: transient stinging or burning; occasionally erythema or drying of the skin

PoM **Zovirax®** (GlaxoWellcome)

Cream, aciclovir 5%. Net price 2 g = £5.29; 10 g = £15.94

Administration: apply to lesions every 4 hours (5 times daily) for 5 days, started at first sign of attack

Additives: include propylene glycol

Note. A 2-g tube and a pump pack are on sale to the public for the treatment of cold sores (*Zovirax® Cold Sore Cream*); other brands on sale to the public include *Boots Avert®, Herpetad®* and *Soothelip®*

Eye ointment, see section 11.3.3

Tablets, see section 5.3

PENCICLOVIR

Indications: see notes above

Cautions: avoid contact with eyes and mucous membranes

Side-effects: transient stinging, burning, numbness

▼ PoM **Vectavir®** (SmithKline Beecham)

Cream, penciclovir 1%. Net price 2 g = £4.20

Administration: Herpes labialis, apply to lesions every 2 hours during waking hours for 4 days, starting at first sign of attack; CHILD under 16 years, not recommended

Additives: include propylene glycol

IDOXURIDINE IN DIMETHYL SULPHOXIDE

Indications: of little value, see notes above

Cautions: avoid contact with the eyes, mucous membranes, and textiles; breast-feeding (may taste unpleasant)

Contra-indications: pregnancy (toxicity in *animal* studies); **not** to be used in children

Side-effects: stinging on application, changes in taste; overuse may cause maceration

PoM **Herpid®** (Yamanouchi)

Application, idoxuridine 5% in dimethyl sulphoxide. Net price 5 mL (with applicator) = £6.25

Administration: herpes simplex or herpes zoster, apply to lesions 4 times daily for 4 days, starting at first sign of attack; CHILD under 12 years, not recommended

---

13.10.4   Parasiticidal preparations

Suitable quantities of parasiticidal preparations to be prescribed for specific areas of the body in adults are:

	Skin creams	Lotions	Cream rinses
Scalp (headlice)	—	50 mL	50–100 mL
Body (scabies)	30–60 g	100 mL	—
Body (crab lice)	30–60 g	100 mL	—

These amounts are usually suitable for an adult for single application.

SCABIES

Malathion and **permethrin** are indicated for *scabies (Sarcoptes scabiei).*

Aqueous preparations are preferable to alcoholic lotions, which are not recommended owing to irritation of excoriated skin and the genitalia.

Older preparations include benzyl benzoate, which is an irritant and should be avoided in children. Lindane and monosulfiram have been discontinued.

APPLICATION. Although acaricides have traditionally been applied after a hot bath, this is **not** necessary and there is even evidence that a hot bath may increase absorption into the bloodstream, removing them from their site of action on the skin.

All members of the affected household should be treated. Treatment should be applied to the whole body paying particular attention to the webs of the fingers and toes and brushing lotion under the ends of the nails. In the case of infants and young children (up to the age of about 2 years), the elderly, the immunocompromised, and those who have experienced treatment failure, application should be extended to the scalp, neck, face, and ears. Providing the application is done properly malathion and permethrin need only be applied once; in the case of benzyl benzoate up to three applications on consec-

---

    Prices are **net**, see p. 1

utive days may be needed. It is important to warn users **not** to wash their hands since this would require re-application. Patients with hyperkeratotic (crusted or 'Norwegian') scabies may require two or three applications of acaricide on consecutive days to ensure that enough penetrates the skin crusts to kill all the mites. **Ivermectin** (*Mectizan®*, MSD, not on UK market) in a single dose of 200 micrograms/kg has been used, in combination with topical drugs, for treatment of hyperkeratotic scabies that does not respond to topical treatment alone.

ITCHING. The *itch of scabies* persists for some weeks after the infestation has been eliminated and antipruritic treatment may be required. Application of **crotamiton** can be used to control itching after treatment with more effective acaricides, but caution is necessary if the skin is excoriated—**calamine** is probably more suitable. Oral administration of a **sedating antihistamine** (see section 3.4.1) at night may also be useful.

HEAD LICE

Malathion, **carbaryl** and the **pyrethroids** (permethrin and phenothrin) are effective against *head lice* (*Pediculus capitis*) but lice in some districts have developed resistance. Lotion, liquid or cream rinse formulations should be used. Shampoos are diluted too much in use to be effective. Aqueous formulations are preferred for asthmatic patients and small children, to avoid alcoholic fumes. A contact time of 12 hours or overnight treatment is recommended for lotions and liquids. A 2-hour treatment is no longer regarded as sufficient to ensure death of eggs.

In general, a course of treatment for head lice should be 2 applications of product 7 days apart to prevent lice emerging from any eggs that survive the first application.

The policy of rotating insecticides on a district-wide basis is now considered outmoded. The development of resistance requires a mosaic strategy whereby, if a course of treatment fails to cure, a different insecticide is used for the next treatment.

There is no published evidence that wet combing as a method of treatment can be successful in the community, although it may work for individuals. For successful treatment **30 minutes** combing, using a plastic detection comb, must be performed at 4-day intervals for a minimum of 2 weeks.

A **head lice repellant** containing piperonal 2% (*Rappell®*) is on sale to the public.

CRAB LICE

Malathion and **carbaryl** are effective for *crab lice* (*Pthirus pubis*). Aqueous lotions should be applied to **all** parts of the body (not merely the groins and axillae) for 12 hours or overnight; a second treatment is preferable after 7 days to kill lice emerging from surviving eggs. Alcoholic lotions are not recommended (owing to irritation of excoriated skin and the genitalia).

Aqueous **malathion** lotion is effective for *crab lice of the eye lashes* (but does not have a product licence for this indication).

BENZYL BENZOATE

Benzyl benzoate is effective for *scabies* but is not a first-choice for *scabies* (see notes above).

BENZYL BENZOATE
Indications: scabies (but see notes above)
Cautions: children (not recommended, see also under Administration, below), avoid contact with eyes and mucous membranes; do not use on broken or secondarily infected skin; pregnancy and breast-feeding
Side-effects: skin irritation, burning sensation especially on genitalia and excoriations, occasionally rashes
Administration: apply over the whole body; repeat without bathing on the following day and wash off 24 hours later; a third application may be required in some cases
Note. Not recommended for children—dilution to reduce irritant effect also reduces efficacy. Some manufacturers recommend application to the body but to exclude the head and neck, but in the elderly, the immunocompromised and those who have experienced treatment failure, application may need to be extended to the scalp, neck, face, and ears

Benzyl Benzoate Application, BP (Non-proprietary)
Application, benzyl benzoate 25% in an emulsion basis. Net price 500 mL = £2.43
Available from CP, Norton, Rhône-Poulenc Rorer (Ascabiol®)

CARBARYL

Carbaryl is recommended for *head lice* and *crab lice* (see notes above). In the light of conclusions (based on experimental data in *animals*) it would be prudent to consider carbaryl as a potential human carcinogen, it has recently been restricted to prescription only use. The Department of Health has emphasised that the risk is a theoretical one and that any risk from the intermittent use of head lice preparations is likely to be exceedingly small.

CARBARYL
(Carbaril)
Indications: see notes above and under preparations
Cautions: avoid contact with eyes; do not use on broken or secondarily infected skin; alcoholic lotions **not** recommended for pediculosis in asthmatics or small children, or for crab lice (see notes above); do not use lotion more than once a week for 3 weeks at a time; children under 6 months, medical supervision required
Side-effects: skin irritation
Administration: lotion—apply to dry hair and rub into the hair and scalp or affected areas, allow to dry naturally, comb, and remove by washing 12 hours later (see also notes above); shampoo—shampoo in, leave on hair for 5 minutes, rinse, repeat, rinse, allow to dry, comb, repeat twice at intervals of 3 days

---

PoM **Carylderm®** (Seton)

Lotion, carbaryl 0.5%, in an alcoholic basis. Net price 55 mL = £2.22; 160 mL = £4.90. Label: 15. For crab lice and head lice (alcoholic, see notes above)

NHS *Shampoo*, carbaryl 1%. Net price 100 mL = £3.25. For crab lice and head lice

PoM **Derbac® C** (Seton)

Liquid (= lotion), carbaryl 1% in an aqueous basis. Net price 50 mL = £2.22; 200 mL = £5.47. For head lice

PoM **Suleo-C®** (Seton)

Lotion, carbaryl 0.5%, in an alcoholic basis. Net price 50 mL = £2.22; 200 mL = £5.47. Label: 15. For head lice (alcoholic, see notes above)

MALATHION

Malathion is recommended for *scabies*, *head lice* and *crab lice* (for details see notes above).

MALATHION

Indications: see notes above and under preparations

Cautions: avoid contact with eyes; do not use on broken or secondarily infected skin; alcoholic lotions **not** recommended for pediculosis in asthmatics or small children, or for scabies or crab lice (see notes above); do not use lotion more than once a week for 3 weeks at a time; children under 6 months, medical supervision required

Side-effects: skin irritation

Administration: pediculosis—rub 0.5% lotion into dry hair, scalp, and affected area, comb, allow to dry naturally, remove by washing after 12 hours (see also notes above); apply 1% shampoo to hair for 5 minutes, rinse, repeat, rinse again, comb, repeat twice at intervals of 3 days

Scabies—apply 0.5% preparation over whole body, and wash off after 24 hours, see also notes above

Note. Manufacturer recommends application to the body but excludes the head and neck. In the case of young children, however, application may need to be extended to the scalp, neck, face, and ears. This extended application may also be necessary for the elderly, for the immunocompromised and for those who have experienced treatment failure

Derbac-M® (Seton)

Liquid, malathion 0.5% in an aqueous basis. Net price 50 mL = £2.05; 200 mL = £4.96. For crab lice, head lice and scabies

Prioderm® (Seton)

Lotion, malathion 0.5%, in an alcoholic basis. Net price 55 mL = £2.05; 160 mL = £4.39. Label: 15. For crab lice, head lice and scabies (alcoholic, see notes above)

NHS *Cream shampoo*, malathion 1%. Net price 40 g = £2.28. For crab lice and head lice

Quellada M® (Stafford-Miller)

Liquid, malathion 0.5% in an aqueous basis. Net price 50 mL = £1.94; 200 mL = £4.84. For crab lice, head lice and scabies

Cream shampoo, malathion 1%. Net price 40 g = £2.14. For crab lice and head lice

Suleo-M® (Seton)

Lotion, malathion 0.5%, in an alcoholic basis. Net price 50 mL = £2.05; 200 mL = £4.96. Label: 15. For head lice (alcoholic, see notes above)

PERMETHRIN

Permethrin is effective for *scabies* and *head lice* (for details see notes above).

PERMETHRIN

Indications: see notes above and under preparations

Cautions: avoid contact with eyes; do not use on broken or secondarily infected skin; pregnancy and breast-feeding; children under 6 months, medical supervision required for cream rinse (head lice); children aged 2 months—2 years, medical supervision required for dermal cream (scabies)

Side-effects: pruritus, erythema, and stinging; rarely rashes and oedema

Lyclear® (Warner Lambert)

Cream rinse, permethrin 1% in basis containing isopropyl alcohol 20%. Net price 59 mL = £2.14

Administration: head lice, apply to clean damp hair, leave on for 10 minutes, rinse and dry; not affected by chlorine in swimming pools

Dermal cream, permethrin 5%. Net price 30 g = £5.50. Label: 10 patient information leaflet

Administration: scabies, apply over whole body and wash off after 8–12 hours; CHILD apply over whole body including face, neck, scalp and ears. If hands are washed with soap and water within 8 hours of application, cream should be reapplied

Note. Manufacturer recommends application to the body but excludes the head and neck. In the case of young children, however, application may need to be extended to the scalp, neck, face, and ears. This extended application may also be necessary for the elderly, for the immunocompromised and for those who have experienced treatment failure.

Larger patients may require more than one 30-g pack for adequate treatment.

PHENOTHRIN

Phenothrin is recommended for *head lice* and *crab lice* (for details see notes above).

PHENOTHRIN

Indications: see notes above and under preparations

Cautions: avoid contact with eyes; do not use on broken or secondarily infected skin; children under 6 months, medical supervision required; may cause wheezing in asthmatics

Side-effects: skin irritation

Full Marks® (Seton)

Lotion, phenothrin 0.2% in basis containing iso-propyl alcohol 69.3%. Net price 55 mL = £2.07; 160 mL = £4.39. Label: 15

Administration: crab lice and head lice (alcoholic, see above), apply to dry hair, allow to dry naturally; sham-poo after 2 hours, comb while still wet

13.10.5 Preparations for minor cuts and abrasions

Some of the preparations listed are used in minor burns, and abrasions. They are applied as necessary. Preparations containing camphor, hydrargaphen, and sulphonamides should be **avoided**. Prepara-tions such as magnesium sulphate paste are also listed are now rarely used to treat carbuncles and boils as these are best treated with antibiotics (see section 5.1.1.2).

Cetrimide Cream, BP, cetrimide 0.5% in a suitable water-miscible basis such as cetostearyl alcohol 5%, liquid paraffin 50% in freshly boiled and cooled puri-fied water. Net price 50 g = 68p

Chlorhexidine Cream, BP 1988, chlorhexidine gluconate solution usually 5% (≡ chlorhexidine gluconate 1%), cetomacrogol emulsifying wax 25%, liquid paraffin 10%, in purified water, freshly boiled and cooled

Proflavine Cream, BPC, proflavine hemisulphate 0.1%, yellow beeswax 2.5%, chlorocresol 0.1%, liquid paraffin 67.3%, freshly boiled and cooled purified water 25%, wool fat 5%. Net price 100 mL = 86p

Caution: stains clothing

NHS **Anaflex®** (Geistlich)

Cream, polynoxylin 10%, in a water-miscible basis. Net price 50 g = £2.71

Betadine® (Seton)

Ointment, povidone-iodine 10%, in a water-misci-ble basis. Net price 20 g = £1.45; 80 g = £2.92. Avoid in children under 2 years

Additives: none as listed in section 13.1

Brulidine® (Rhône-Poulenc Rorer)

Cream, dibromopropamidine isethionate 0.15%, in a water-miscible basis. Net price 25 g = 95p

Additives: include hydroxybenzoates (parabens), fragrance

Cetavlex® (Zeneca)

Cream, cetrimide 0.5%, in a water-miscible basis. Net price 50 g = 54p

Additives: include hydroxybenzoates (parabens)

Crystacide® (Evans)

Cream, hydrogen peroxide 1% in a lipid-stabilised basis, net price 10 g = £2.85, 25 g = £4.78.

Additives: include disodium edetate, propylene glycol, salicylic acid

NHS **Dermalex®** (Sanofi Winthrop)

Skin lotion, allantoin 0.2%, hexachlorophane 0.5%, squalane 3% in an emulsion basis. Net price 250 mL = £5.22.

For prevention of pressure sores and prevention and treatment of urinary rash. Avoid in children under 2 years, except under medical supervision

Additives: include butylated hydroxyanisole, edetic acid, hydroxybenzoates (parabens), wool fat, fragrance

Vesagex® (Rybar)

Cream, cetrimide 1%. Net price 500 g = £6.23

Additives: include chlorocresol, fragrance

Preparations for boils

Magnesium Sulphate Paste, BP, dried magnesium sulphate 45 g, glycerol 55 g, phenol 500 mg. Net price 25 g = 51p; 50 g = 56p. Should be stirred before use

Apply under dressing

COLLODION

Flexible collodion may be used to seal minor cuts and wounds that have partially healed.

Collodion, Flexible, BP, castor oil 2.5%, colo-phony 2.5% in a collodion basis, prepared by dis-solving pyroxylin (10%) in a mixture of 3 volumes of ether and 1 volume of alcohol (90%). Net price 10 mL = 19p. Label: 15 (**important:** very highly inflammable)

SURGICAL TISSUE ADHESIVE

Enbucrilate is used as a tissue adhesive for closure of minor skin wounds and sealing sutured skin wounds. Within 20 seconds of contact with tissue moisture it polymerises with an exothermic reaction into a firm adhesive bond. It must therefore be applied very thinly (to avoid heat damage) and with proper technique (poor alignment cannot be cor-rected). Contact with eyes, internal organs, blood vessels, and nervous tissue should be **avoided**.

Hiotoooryl® (Sherwood Davis & Geck)

Tissue adhesive, sterile, enbucrilate with blue dye. Net price (single use) 500-mg vial = £10.20 (hosp. use only)

13.11 Disinfectants and cleansers

13.11.1 Alcohols and saline
13.11.2 Chlorhexidine salts
13.11.3 Cationic surfactants and soaps
13.11.4 Chlorine and iodine
13.11.5 Phenolics
13.11.6 Astringents, oxidisers, and dyes
13.11.7 Desloughing agents

The choice of *cleanser* is an important factor in treating skin conditions. For example, scaling disor-ders are best treated with **emulsifying ointment** (section 13.2.1) or other cleansers that do not irri-tate the skin.

Sodium chloride solution 0.9% is suitable for general cleansing of skin and wounds.

Useful *disinfectants* for skin cleansing include **cetrimide** (which has useful detergent properties), **chlorhexidine** and **potassium permanganate solution** 1 in 10 000. **Povidone-iodine** is preferred to chlorinated solutions (such as dilute sodium hypochlorite solution) which are too irritant and are no longer recommended. Topical preparations of **hexachlorophane** should be used with caution in neonates and should **not** be used on large raw sur-faces.

Astringent preparations, such as **potassium permanganate** solution are useful for oozing eczematous reactions (section 13.5.1). Silver nitrate lotion is now rarely used as it stains the skin black and may cause toxic effects if used for prolonged periods.

13.11.1   Alcohols and saline

ALCOHOL

Indications: skin preparation before injection

Cautions: flammable; avoid broken skin; patients have suffered severe burns when diathermy has been preceded by application of alcoholic skin disinfectants

Industrial Methylated Spirit, BP

Mixture of 19 volumes of ethanol (absolute alcohol) of an appropriate strength with 1 volume of approved wood naphtha and is Industrial Methylated Spirit of the quality known either as '66 OP' or as '74 OP'

Net price 100 mL = 18p. Label: 15

Surgical Spirit, BP, methyl salicylate 0.5 mL, diethyl phthalate 2%, castor oil 2.5%, in industrial methylated spirit. Net price 100 mL = 19p. Label: 15

SODIUM CHLORIDE

Indications: see notes above

Irriclens® (ConvaTec)

Solution in aerosol can, (sterile), sodium chloride 0.9%. Net price 240-mL can = £2.75

Normasol® (Seton)

Solution (sterile), sodium chloride 0.9%. Net price 25 × 25-mL sachet = £5.85; 6 × 100-mL sachet = £4.29

See also section 11.8.2

Sterac® Sodium Chloride (Galen)

Solution (sterile), sodium chloride 0.9%. Net price 150 mL = 83p

Sterijet® Sodium Chloride (Seton)

Solution (sterile), sodium chloride 0.9%. Net price 20 × 25-mL flexible ampoule = £6.20

Steripod® Sodium Chloride (Seton)

Steripod® sodium chloride 0.9% solution (sterile), sodium chloride 0.9%. Net price 25 × 20-mL sachet = £6.83

13.11.2   Chlorhexidine salts

CHLORHEXIDINE

Indications: see under preparations; bladder irrigation and catheter patency solutions (see section 7.4.4)

Cautions: avoid contact with eyes, brain, meninges and middle ear; not for use in body cavities; alcoholic solutions not suitable before diathermy

Side-effects: occasional sensitivity

Chlorhexidine 0.05% (Baxter)

2000 Solution (sterile), pink, chlorhexidine acetate 0.05%. Net price 1000 mL = 77p

For cleansing and disinfecting wounds and burns

CX Antiseptic Dusting Powder® (Adams)

Dusting powder, sterile, chlorhexidine acetate 1%. Net price 15 g = £2.25

For skin disinfection and antisepsis

Hibiscrub® (Zeneca)

Cleansing solution, red, chlorhexidine gluconate solution 20% (≡ 4% chlorhexidine gluconate), perfumed, in a surfactant solution. Net price 250 mL = £1.10; 500 mL = £1.61

Use instead of soap for pre-operative hand and skin preparation and for general hand and skin antisepsis

Hibisol® (Zeneca)

Solution, chlorhexidine gluconate solution 2.5% (≡ 0.5% chlorhexidine gluconate), in isopropyl alcohol 70% with emollients. Net price 500 mL = £1.68

To be used undiluted for hand and skin disinfection

Hibitane Obstetric® (Zeneca)

Cream, chlorhexidine gluconate solution 5% (≡ 1% chlorhexidine gluconate), in a pourable water-miscible basis. Net price 250 mL = 98p.

For use in obstetrics and gynaecology as an antiseptic and lubricant (for application to skin around vulva and perineum and to hands of midwife or doctor)

NHS **pHiso-Med®** (Sanofi Winthrop)

Solution, chlorhexidine gluconate 4% in an emulsion basis. Net price 150 mL = £4.64.

For use as a soap substitute in acne and seborrhoeic conditions; for bathing babies in maternity units (as 1 in 10 dilution) to prevent cross-infection and for pre-operative hand and skin preparation

Sterexidine® (Galen)

Solution (sterile), chlorhexidine gluconate 0.02%. Net price 150 mL = 83p

For disinfection and wound cleansing

Steripod® Chlorhexidine (Seton)

Steripod® Chlorhexidine solution, chlorhexidine gluconate solution 0.25% (≡ chlorhexidine gluconate 0.05%). Net price 25 × 20-mL vials = £6.83

For swabbing wounds and burns

Unisept® (Seton)

Solution (sterile), pink, chlorhexidine gluconate 0.05%. Net price 25 × 25-mL sachet = £5.85; 6 × 100-mL sachet = £4.29

For cleansing and disinfecting wounds and burns and swabbing in obstetrics

With cetrimide

Steripod® Chlorhexidine/Cetrimide (Seton)

Steripod® Chlorhexidine/Cetrimide solution, chlorhexidine gluconate solution 0.075% (≡ chlorhexidine gluconate 0.015%), cetrimide 0.15%. Net price 25 × 20-mL vials = £6.83

For cleansing and disinfecting wounds and burns

Tisept® (Seton)

Solution (sterile), yellow, chlorhexidine gluconate 0.015%, cetrimide 0.15%. Net price 25 × 25-mL sachet = £5.85; 6 × 100-mL sachet = £4.29

To be used undiluted for general skin disinfection and wound cleansing

Travasept 100® (Baxter)
Solution (sterile), yellow, chlorhexidine acetate 0.015%, cetrimide 0.15%. Net price 500 mL = 72p; 1000 mL = 77p
To be used undiluted in skin disinfection such as wound cleansing and obstetrics

CONCENTRATES

Hibitane 5% Concentrate® (Zeneca)
Solution, red, chlorhexidine gluconate solution 25% (≡ 5% chlorhexidine gluconate), in a perfumed aqueous solution. Net price 5 litres = £11.46
To be used diluted 1 in 10 (0.5%) with alcohol 70% for pre-operative skin preparation, or 1 in 100 (0.05%) with water for general skin disinfection
Note. Alcoholic solutions not suitable before diathermy (see Alcohol, above)

With cetrimide
Hibicet Hospital Concentrate® (Zeneca)
Solution, orange, chlorhexidine gluconate solution 7.5% (≡ chlorhexidine gluconate 1.5%), cetrimide 15%. Net price 5 litres = £8.54
To be used diluted 1 in 100 (1%) to 1 in 30 with water for skin disinfection and wound cleansing, and diluted 1 in 30 in alcohol 70% for pre-operative skin preparation
Note. Alcoholic solutions not suitable before diathermy (see Alcohol, above)

13.11.3   Cationic surfactants and soaps

BENZALKONIUM CHLORIDE
Indications: skin disinfection such as pre-operative skin preparation
Cautions: avoid contact with eyes and mucous membranes

Roccal® (Schein Rexodent)
Solution, blue, benzalkonium chloride 1%. Net price 2.25 litres = £12.85
To be used diluted 1 in 10 to 1 in 200
Additives: include fragrance
Roccal Concentrate 10X® (Schein Rexodent)
Concentrate, blue, benzalkonium chloride 10%. Net price 2.25 litres = £52.65
For preparation of Roccal Solution with freshly boiled and cooled purified water
Additives: include fragrance

CETRIMIDE
Indications: skin disinfection
Cautions: avoid contact with eyes; avoid use in body cavities
Side-effects: skin irritation and occasionally sensitisation

Preparations
Ingredient of Hibicet Hospital Concentrate®, Steripod®, Tisept®, and Travasept®100, see above

SOFT SOAP
Indications: removal of adherent crusts

Soap Spirit, BP, soft soap 65% in alcohol (90%). Net price 100 mL = 39p

13.11.4   Chlorine and iodine

CHLORINATED SOLUTIONS
Cautions: bleaches fabric; irritant (protect surrounding tissues with soft paraffin)

Chlorinated Soda Solution, Surgical, BPC,
(Dakin's Solution), boric acid, chlorinated lime, sodium carbonate, sufficient of each to provide a solution containing 0.5% of available chlorine in purified water, freshly boiled and cooled. Net price 500 mL = 75p. Has been used undiluted for cleansing wounds and ulcers but no longer recommended (too irritant)
NHS **Chlorasol®** (Seton)
Solution (sterile), sodium hypochlorite, containing 0.3–0.4% available chlorine. Net price 25 × 25-mL sachets = £8.89
Irritant therefore no longer recommended

IODINE COMPOUNDS
Indications: skin disinfection
Cautions: pregnancy, breast-feeding; broken skin (see below); renal impairment (see Appendix 3)
LARGE OPEN WOUNDS. The application of povidone-iodine to large wounds or severe burns may produce systemic adverse effects such as metabolic acidosis, hypernatraemia and impairment of renal function.
Contra-indications: avoid regular use in patients with thyroid disorders or those receiving lithium therapy
Side-effects: rarely sensitivity; may interfere with thyroid function tests

Betadine® (Seton)
Antiseptic paint, povidone-iodine 10% in an alcoholic solution. Net price 8 mL (with applicator brush) = £1.06
Apply undiluted to minor wounds and infections, twice daily
Alcoholic solution, povidone-iodine 10%. Net price 500 mL = £2.00
To be applied undiluted in pre- and post-operative skin disinfection; CHILD not recommended for regular use in neonates (and contra-indicated in very low birthweight infants)
Note. Flammable—caution in procedures involving hot wire cautery and diathermy
Antiseptic solution, povidone-iodine 10% in aqueous solution. Net price 500 mL = £1.83
To be applied undiluted in pre- and post-operative skin disinfection; CHILD not recommended for regular use in neonates (and contra-indicated in very low birthweight infants)
Note. Not for body cavity irrigation
Dry powder spray, povidone-iodine 2.5% in a pressurised aerosol unit. Net price 150-g unit = £2.92
For skin disinfection, particularly minor wounds and infections; CHILD under 2 years not recommended
Note. Not for use in serous cavities

Scalp and skin cleanser solution, povidone-iodine 7.5%, in a surfactant basis. Net price 250 mL = £2.43

Use for seborrhoeic conditions of scalp and acne vulgaris of face and neck 1–2 times daily; CHILD under 2 years not recommended

Skin cleanser solution, povidone-iodine 4%, in a surfactant basis. Net price 250 mL = £2.24

For infective conditions of the skin. Retain on skin for 3–5 minutes before rinsing; repeat twice daily; CHILD under 2 years not recommended

Surgical scrub, povidone-iodine 7.5%, in a non-ionic surfactant basis. Net price 500 mL = £1.65

To be used as a pre-operative scrub for hands and skin; CHILD not recommended for regular use in neonates (and contra-indicated in very low birthweight infants)

Savlon® Dry Powder (Novartis Consumer Health)

Savlon® Dry powder spray, povidone-iodine 1.14% in a pressurised aerosol unit. Net price 50-mL unit = £1.91; 150-mL = £2.71

For minor wounds

13.11.5   Phenolics

HEXACHLOROPHANE

(Hexachlorophene)

Indications: see under preparations (below)

Contra-indications: avoid use on badly burned or excoriated skin; pregnancy; children under 2 years except on medical advice

Side-effects: sensitivity; rarely photosensitivity

PoM **Ster-Zac DC Skin Cleanser®** (Seton)

Cream, hexachlorophane 3%. Net price 150 mL = £3.85

Use 3–5 mL instead of soap as pre-operative scrub for hands

Additives: include chlorocresol, edetic acid (EDTA), propylene glycol, wool fat, fragrance

Ster-Zac Powder® (Seton)

Dusting-powder, hexachlorophane 0.33%, zinc oxide 3%, talc 88.67%, starch 8% (sterile). Net price 30 g = 79p

Additives: include fragrance

Prevention of neonatal staphylococcal sepsis, after ligature of cord sprinkle on perineum, groin, front of abdomen, and axillas; after cutting cord and spraying with plastic dressing, powder stump and adjacent skin; after every napkin change powder stump, adjacent skin, perineum, groin, axillas, buttocks, and front of abdomen; continue until stump drops away and wound healed

Adjunct for treatment of recurrent furunculosis, powder daily area of skin normally subject to furunculosis

TRICLOSAN

Indications: skin disinfection

Cautions: avoid contact with eyes

Aquasept® (Seton)

Skin cleanser, blue, triclosan 2%. Net price 28.5 mL = 34p; 100 mL = 90p; 250 mL = £1.10; 500 mL = £1.68

For disinfection and pre-operative hand preparation
Additives: include chlorocresol, edetic acid (EDTA), propylene glycol, fragrance

Manusept® (Seton)

Antibacterial hand rub, triclosan 0.5%, isopropyl alcohol 70%. Net price 100 mL = 59p; 250 mL = £1.07; 500 mL = £1.56

For disinfection and pre-operative hand preparation
Additives: none as listed in section 13.1
Caution: flammable

Ster-Zac Bath Concentrate® (Seton)

Solution, triclosan 2%. Net price 28.5 mL = 40p; 500 mL = £4.46

For staphylococcal skin infections; prevention of cross-infection use 1 sachet/bath
Additives: include edetic acid (EDTA)

13.11.6   Astringents, oxidisers, and dyes

ALUMINIUM ACETATE

Indications: exudative eczematous reactions and wounds

Aluminium Acetate Lotion, aluminium acetate solution 5 mL, purified water, freshly boiled and cooled, to 100 mL. It should be freshly prepared. To be used undiluted as a wet dressing

Note. Aluminium acetate solution (13%) for the preparation of aluminium acetate lotion (0.65%) is available from Martindale (special order)

CRYSTAL VIOLET

(Methylrosanilinium Chloride; Gentian violet)

Indications: see below

Cautions: stains clothes and skin

Side-effects: mucosal ulcerations

Crystal Violet Paint, BP1980, crystal violet 0.5%, in purified water, freshly boiled and cooled. To be used undiluted

Note. Licensed for topical application on unbroken skin only; no longer recommended for application to mucous membranes or open wounds; restrictions do not apply to use for skin marking prior to surgery

HYDROGEN PEROXIDE

Indications: skin disinfection, particularly cleansing and deodorising wounds and ulcers

Cautions: large or deep wounds; avoid normal skin; bleaches fabric

Hydrogen Peroxide Solution, BP

Solution 6% (20 vols). Net price 100 mL = 14p

Solution 3% (10 vols). Net price 100 mL = 24p

Note. The BP directs that when hydrogen peroxide is prescribed, hydrogen peroxide solution 6% (20 vols) should be dispensed.

IMPORTANT. Strong solutions of hydrogen peroxide which contain 27% (90 vols) and 30% (100 vols) are only for the preparation of weaker solutions

Crystacide® see section 13.10.5

Hioxyl® see section 13.11.7

POTASSIUM PERMANGANATE

Indications: cleansing and deodorising suppurating eczematous reactions and wounds

Cautions: irritant to mucous membranes; stains skin and clothing

Administration: wet dressings or baths, approx. 0.01% solution

Potassium Permanganate Solution, potassium permanganate 0.1% (1 in 1000) in water

To be diluted 1 in 10 to provide a 0.01% (1 in 10 000) solution

Permitabs® (Bioglan)

Solution tablets, for preparation of topical solution, potassium permanganate 400 mg. Net price 30-tab pack = £3.67

1 tablet dissolved in 4 litres of water provides a 0.01% (1 in 10 000) solution

13.11.7   Desloughing agents

Desloughing agents for ulcers are second-line treatment and the underlying causes should be treated. The main beneficial effect is removal of slough and clot and the ablation of local infection. Preparations which absorb or help promote the removal of exudate may also help (Appendix 9). It should be noted that substances applied to an open area are easily absorbed and perilesional skin is easily sensitised. Gravitational dermatitis may be complicated by superimposed contact sensitivity to substances such as neomycin or lanolin. Enzyme preparations such as streptokinase-streptodornase or alternatively dextranomer (Appendix 9) are designed for sloughing ulcers and may help.

Aserbine® (Forley)

Cream, benzoic acid 0.025%, malic acid 0.375%, propylene glycol 1.75%, salicylic acid 0.006%. Net price 100 g = £2.00

Apply liberally to wound surface (best results with twice daily wound dressing but more frequent changes may be needed)

Additives: include hydroxybenzoates (parabens)

Solution, benzoic acid 0.15%, malic acid 2.25%, propylene glycol 40%, salicylic acid 0.0375%. Net price 500 mL = £3.00

Use as wash before each application of cream (or use as wet dressing)

Additives: include fragrance

Hioxyl® (Quinoderm Ltd)

Cream, hydrogen peroxide (stabilised) 1.5%. Net price 25 g = £1.99; 100 g = £6.23

For leg ulcers and pressure sores

Additives: none as listed in section 13.1

Apply when necessary and if necessary cover with a dressing

PoM **Varidase Topical®** (Lederle)

Powder, streptokinase 100 000 units, streptodornase 25 000 units. For preparing solutions for topical use. Net price per vial = £7.80; with sterile physiological saline 20 mL (combi-pack) = £8.20

Additives: none as listed in section 13.1

Reconstitute with 20 mL sterile physiological saline (or water for injections) and apply as wet dressing 1–2 times daily; cover with semi-occlusive dressing; irrigate lesion thoroughly with physiological saline and remove loosened material before next application; also used to dis-solve clots in the bladder or urinary catheters; *contra-indicated:* active haemorrhage; *side-effects:* infrequent allergic reactions (reduced by careful and frequent removal of exudate and thorough irrigation with physiological saline); transient burning reported

13.12   Antiperspirants

Aluminium chloride is a potent antiperspirant used in the treatment of severe hyperhidrosis.

ALUMINIUM CHLORIDE

Indications: hyperhidrosis affecting axillae, hands or feet

Cautions: avoid contact with eyes or mouth; do not shave axilla or use depilatories within 12 hours of use

Side-effects: skin irritation

Administration: apply at night to dry skin, wash off on following morning, initially daily then reduce frequency as condition improves—do not apply within 1 hour of taking a bath

Anhydrol Forte® (Dermal)

Solution (= application), aluminium chloride hexahydrate 20% in an alcoholic basis. Net price 60-mL bottle with roll-on applicator = £2.82. Label: 15

Driclor® (Stiefel)

Application, aluminium chloride hexahydrate 20% in an alcoholic basis. Net price 60-mL bottle with roll-on applicator = £2.82. Label: 15

Note. A 30-mL pack is on sale to the public (Driclor® Solution)

13.13   Wound management products and Elastic Hosiery

Preparations

See Appendix 9

13.14   Topical circulatory preparations

These preparations are used to improve circulation in conditions such as bruising, superficial thrombophlebitis, chilblains and varicose veins but are of little value. Chilblains are best managed by avoidance of exposure to cold; neither systemic nor topical vasodilator therapy is established as being effective. Sclerotherapy of varicose veins is described in section 2.13.

Rubefacients are described in section 10.3.2.

Hirudoid® (Sankyo)

Cream, heparinoid 0.3% in a vanishing-cream basis. Net price 50 g = £1.35

Additives: include hydroxybenzoates (parabens)

Gel, heparinoid 0.3%. Net price 50 g = £1.35

Additives: include propylene glycol, fragrance

Apply up to 4 times daily in superficial soft-tissue injuries and superficial thrombophlebitis

Lasonil® (Bayer)

Ointment, heparinoid 50 units, hyaluronidase 150 units/g. Net price 40 g = £1.08

Additives: include wool fat derivative

Apply 2–3 times daily in superficial soft-tissue injuries

14: Immunological products and
VACCINES

In this chapter, immunisation is discussed under the following headings:

14.1 Active immunity

Vaccines may consist of:

1. a *live attenuated* form of a virus (e.g. rubella or measles vaccine) or bacteria (e.g. BCG vaccine)
2. *inactivated* preparations of the virus (e.g. influenza vaccine) or bacteria, or
3. *extracts of* or *detoxified exotoxins* produced by a micro-organism (e.g. tetanus vaccine).

They stimulate production of antibodies and other components of the immune mechanism.

For **live attenuated** vaccines, immunisation is generally achieved with a single dose (but 3 doses are required with oral poliomyelitis and oral typhoid vaccines). Live attenuated vaccines usually produce a durable immunity but not always as long as that of the natural infection. When two live virus vaccines are required (and are not available as a combined preparation) they should be given either simultaneously at different sites or with an interval of at least 3 weeks.

Inactivated vaccines may require a primary series of injections of vaccine to produce adequate antibody response and in most cases booster (reinforcing) injections are required; the duration of immunity varies from months to many years.

Extracts of or **detoxified exotoxins** are more immunogenic if adsorbed onto an adjuvant (such as aluminium hydroxide). They require a primary series of injections followed by booster doses.

> Guidelines in this chapter reflect those in the handbook *Immunisation against Infectious Disease*, which in turn reflects the advice of the Joint Committee on Vaccination and Immunisation (JCVI). Copies can be obtained from:
>
> The Stationery Office
> The Publications Centre
> PO Box 276, London SW8 5DT
>
> Telephone orders, 0171-873 9090.

SIDE-EFFECTS. Some vaccines (e.g. poliomyelitis) produce very few reactions, while others (e.g. measles and rubella) may produce a very mild form of the disease. Some vaccines may produce discomfort at the site of injection and mild fever and malaise. Occasionally there are more serious untoward reactions and these should always be reported to the CSM. Anaphylactic reactions are very rare but can be fatal (see section 3.4.3 for management). For full details of side-effects, the product literature should always be consulted.

CONTRA-INDICATIONS. Most vaccines have some basic contra-indication to their use, and the product literature should always be consulted. In general, vaccination should be postponed if the subject is suffering from an *acute illness*. Minor infections without fever or systemic upset are not contra-indications. A definite severe reaction to a preceding dose is a contra-indication to further doses.

Some viral vaccines contain small quantities of antibiotics such as neomycin or polymyxin (or both); such vaccines may need to be withheld from individuals who are *sensitive to the antibiotic*. *Hypersensitivity to egg* contra-indicates influenza vaccine (residual egg protein present) and, if evidence of previous anaphylactic reaction, also yellow fever vaccine.

Live vaccines should not be routinely administered to *pregnant women* because of possible harm to the fetus but where there is a significant risk of exposure (e.g. to poliomyelitis or yellow fever), the need for vaccination outweighs any possible risk to the fetus. Live vaccines should not be given to individuals with *impaired immune response*, whether caused by disease (for special reference to *AIDS*, see below) or as a result of radiotherapy or treatment with high doses of corticosteroids or other immunosuppressive drugs[1,2]. They should not be given to those suffering from *malignant conditions* such as leukaemia and tumours of the reticulo-endothelial system[2].

The intramuscular route should not be used in patients with bleeding disorders such as haemophilia or thrombocytopenia.

VACCINES AND AIDS. The Department of Health has advised that HIV-positive subjects with or without symptoms can receive the following live vaccines:

measles[2] (or MMR), mumps, poliomyelitis[3], rubella;

and the following inactivated vaccines:

cholera, diphtheria, haemophilus influenzae type b, hepatitis A, hepatitis B, influenza, meningococcal, pertussis, pneumococcal, poliomyelitis[3], rabies, tetanus, typhoid (injection).

HIV-positive subjects should **not** receive:

BCG, yellow fever[4], typhoid (oral)

Note. The above advice differs from that for other immunocompromised patients.

1. Live vaccines should be postponed until at least 3 months after stopping corticosteroids and 6 months after stopping chemotherapy.
2. Consideration should be given to use of normal immunoglobulin after exposure to measles (see p. 531) and to varicella-zoster immunoglobulin after exposure to chickenpox or herpes zoster (see p. 532).
3. Virus may be excreted for longer periods than in normal subjects; contacts should be warned of this and of need for washing hands after changing a vaccinated infant's nappies; HIV-positive contacts are at greater risk than normal contacts. For HIV-positive symptomatic subjects inactivated poliomyelitis vaccine may be used at discretion of clinician.
4. Because insufficient evidence of safety.

Immunisation schedule

Vaccines for the childhood immunisation schedule should be obtained **via local Health Authorities** or (in England only) **direct from Farillon**—not for prescribing on FP10 (GP10 in Scotland) since not available to pharmacies.

During first year of life
Adsorbed Diphtheria, Tetanus and Pertussis Vaccine (triple vaccine)

3 doses at intervals of 4 weeks; first dose at 2 months of age

If pertussis component omitted from earlier immunisations 3 doses of Pertussis Vaccine can be given at monthly intervals to provide protection. If basic course against diphtheria and tetanus incomplete, triple vaccine (DTPer/Vac/Ads) may be used to begin or to complete course against pertussis to avoid more injections than necessary

plus

Haemophilus Influenzae type b Vaccine (Hib)

3 doses at intervals of 4 weeks; first dose at 2 months of age

also

Poliomyelitis Vaccine, Live (Oral)

3 doses at intervals of 4 weeks; first dose at 2 months of age

BCG Vaccine (for neonates at risk only)

See section 14.4, BCG Vaccines

During second year of life
Measles, Mumps and Rubella Vaccine, Live (MMR)

Single dose at 12–15 months of age

Haemophilus Influenzae type b Vaccine (Hib) (if not previously immunised)

Single dose at 13 months–4 years of age (over 4 years, see section 14.4, Haemophilus Influenzae type b Vaccine)

On entry into school or nursery school
Adsorbed Diphtheria and Tetanus Vaccine

Single booster dose

Preferably allow interval of at least 3 years after completing basic course; give at same session as MMR Vaccine but use separate syringe and needle, and give after MMR (MMR less painful) in different limb

also

Poliomyelitis Vaccine, Live (Oral)

Single booster dose

Preferably allow interval of at least 3 years after completing basic course

also

Measles, Mumps and Rubella Vaccine, Live (MMR)

Single booster dose

Give at same session as Adsorbed Diphtheria and Tetanus Vaccine but use separate syringe and needle; give MMR first (less painful) and use different limb—alternatively, second appointment can be made

Between 10–14 years of age
BCG Vaccine (for tuberculin-negative children)

Single dose

May be given simultaneously with another live vaccine; otherwise an interval of at least 3 weeks should be allowed between the two

On leaving school or before employment or further education
Adsorbed Diphtheria and Tetanus Vaccine for Adults and Adolescents

Single booster dose

Adsorbed Diphtheria and Tetanus Vaccine used at school entry **not** to be used for children aged over 10 years and adults

also

Poliomyelitis Vaccine, Live (Oral)

Single booster dose

During adult life
Poliomyelitis Vaccine, Live (Oral) (if not previously immunised)

3 doses at intervals of 4 weeks

No adult should remain unimmunised; health care workers in possible contact with poliomyelitis, and travellers to areas other than Australia, New Zealand, Northern and Western Europe and North America require booster dose if they have not received immunisation within last 10 years

Rubella Vaccine, Live (for susceptible women of child-bearing age)

Single dose

Women of child-bearing age should be tested for rubella antibodies and offered rubella immunisation if sero-negative—exclude pregnancy before immunisation, but see also section 14.4, Rubella Vaccine

Adsorbed Tetanus Vaccine (if not previously immunised)

3 doses at intervals of 4 weeks

Booster dose 10 years after primary course and again 10 years later maintains satisfactory level of protection—if diphtheria cover also needed give Adsorbed Diphtheria and Tetanus Vaccine for Adults and Adolescents

Adsorbed Diphtheria Vaccine for Adults and Adolescents (if not previously immunised)

3 doses at intervals of 4 weeks

Booster dose 10 years after primary course. If tetanus cover also needed give Adsorbed Diphtheria and Tetanus Vaccine for Adults and Adolescents

High-risk groups
For information on high-risk groups, see section 14.4 under individual vaccines

Hepatitis A Vaccine

Hepatitis B Vaccine

Influenza Vaccine

Pneumococcal Vaccine

Post-immunisation pyrexia—Joint Committee on
Vaccination and Immunisation recommendation.
The doctor should advise the parent that if pyrexia
develops after immunisation with triple vaccine the
child can be given a dose of paracetamol followed, if
necessary, by a second dose 4 to 6 hours later. The
dose of paracetamol for post-immunisation pyrexia
in an infant aged 2–3 months is 60 mg; an oral
syringe can be obtained from any pharmacy to give
the small dose-volume required. The doctor should
warn the parent that if the pyrexia persists after the
second dose medical advice should be sought.

For recommendation relating to advice after MMR
vaccine, see p. 525

For full range of paracetamol doses, see p. 196

14.2   Passive immunity

Immunity with immediate protection against certain
infective organisms can be obtained by injecting
preparations made from the plasma of immune individuals with adequate levels of antibody to the disease for which protection is sought (see under
Immunoglobulins, section 14.5). This passive
immunity lasts only a few weeks; where necessary
passive immunisation can be repeated.

Antibodies of human origin are usually termed
immunoglobulins. The term *antiserum* is applied to
material prepared in animals. Because of serum
sickness and other allergic-type reactions that may
follow injections of antisera, this therapy has been
replaced wherever possible by the use of immunoglobulins. Reactions are theoretically possible
after injection of human immunoglobulins but
reports of such reactions are very rare.

14.3   Storage and use

Care must be taken to store all vaccines and other
immunological products under the conditions recommended in the product literature, otherwise the
preparation may become denatured and totally ineffective. **Refrigerated storage** is usually necessary;
many vaccines need to be stored at 2–8°C and not
allowed to freeze. Vaccines should be protected
from light. Opened multidose vials which have not
been fully used should be disposed of *within one
hour* if no preservative is present (most live virus
vaccines) or *within 3 hours* or at the end of a session (when vaccines containing a preservative are
used but also including oral poliomyelitis vaccine).
Unused vaccines should be disposed of by incinera-
tion at a registered disposal contractor.

Particular attention must be paid to instructions
on the use of diluents. Vaccines which are liquid
suspensions or are reconstituted before use should
be adequately shaken to ensure uniformity of the
material to be injected.

Note. The Department of Health has advised *against the
use of jet guns* for vaccination owing to the risk of trans-
mitting blood-borne infections, such as HIV.

14.4   Vaccines and antisera

AVAILABILITY. Anthrax, rabies, and yellow fever
vaccines, botulism antitoxin, and snake and spider
venom antitoxins are available from local designated holding centres. Details of names, addresses,
and telephone numbers of holding centres are given
in:

The Health Service Supply Purchasing Guide, section D
pp. 1101–1199

For antivenom, see Emergency Treatment of
Poisoning, p. 26

Enquiries for vaccines not available commercially
can also be made to

Department of Health
Room 716
133–155 Waterloo Road
London SE1 8UG
Tel 0171-972 4476/7

In Scotland information about availability of vaccines can
be obtained from the Chief Administrative Pharmaceutical
Officer of the local Health Board. In Wales enquiries
should be directed to the Welsh Office, Cathays Park, Car-
diff CF1 3NQ (Tel 01222 825111, extn 4658) and in
Northern Ireland to the Department of Health and Social
Services, Castle Buildings, Stormont, Belfast BT4 3PP
(Tel 01232 520000).

For further details of availability, see under individual
vaccines.

ANTHRAX VACCINE

Anthrax immunisation is indicated for individuals
who handle infected animals, for those exposed to
imported infected animal products, and for laboratory staff who work with *Bacillus anthracis*. The
vaccine is the alum precipitate of an antigen from
Bacillus anthracis and, following the primary
course of injections, booster doses should be given
at about yearly intervals.

PoM **Anthrax Vaccine**
   Dose: initial course 3 doses of 0.5 mL by intramuscular
   injection at intervals of 3 weeks followed by a 4th dose
   after an interval of 6 months
   Booster doses: 0.5 mL annually
   Available from Public Health Laboratory Service

BCG VACCINES

BCG (Bacillus Calmette-Guérin) is a live attenuated strain derived from *Mycobacterium bovis*
which stimulates the development of hypersensitivity to *M. tuberculosis*. BCG vaccine should be
given intradermally by operators skilled in the technique (see below).

Within 2–6 weeks a small swelling appears at the
injection site which progresses to a papule or to a
benign ulcer about 10 mm in diameter and heals in
6–12 weeks. A dry dressing may be used if the
ulcer discharges, but air should **not** be excluded.

The CSM has reported that serious reactions with
BCG are uncommon and most often consist of prolonged ulceration or subcutaneous abscess formation
due to faulty injection technique.

BCG is recommended for the following groups if BCG immunisation, as evidenced by a characteristic scar, has not previously been carried out and they are negative for tuberculoprotein hypersensitivity:

contacts of those with active respiratory tuberculosis;

immigrants (including infants and children) from countries with a high incidence of tuberculosis should be immunised without delay. Their infants born in the UK should also be immunised within a few days of birth, or at two months of age at the same time as the first dose of routine childhood vaccines;

health service staff (including medical students, hospital medical staff, nurses, physiotherapists, radiographers, technical staff in pathology departments and any others considered to be at special risk because of the likelihood of contact with infective patients or their sputum; particularly important to test staff in contact with the immuno-compromised, e.g. in transplant, oncology and HIV units, and staff in maternity and paediatric departments);

children between 10 and 14 years of age (see schedule, section 14.1);

veterinary and other staff who handle animal species known to be susceptible to tuberculosis;

staff working in prisons, in residential homes and in hostels for refugees and the homeless;

those intending to stay for more than 1 month in countries with a high incidence of tuberculosis (section 14.6)

newly-born infants, children or adults where the parents or the adults request immunisation;

Apart from infants of up to 3 months, any person being considered for BCG immunisation must first be given a skin test for hypersensitivity to tuberculoprotein (see under Diagnostic agents, below).

BCG vaccine may be given simultaneously with another live vaccine (see also section 14.1), but if they are not given at the same time, an interval of at least 3 weeks should normally be allowed between them. However, when BCG is given to infants, there is no need to delay the primary immunisations, including poliomyelitis.

See section 14.1 for general contra-indications. BCG is also contra-indicated in subjects with generalised septic skin conditions (in the case of eczema, a vaccination site free from lesions should be chosen).

Intradermal
PoM **Bacillus Calmette-Guérin Vaccine.**
BCG Vaccine, Dried Tub/Vac/BCG. A freeze-dried preparation of live bacteria of a strain derived from the bacillus of Calmette and Guérin.
Dose: 0.1 mL (INFANT under 3 months 0.05 mL) by intradermal injection
Available from Health Authorities or (in England only) direct from Farillon
INTRADERMAL INJECTION TECHNIQUE. After swabbing with spirit and allowing to dry, skin is stretched between thumb and forefinger and needle (size 25G or 26G) inserted (bevel upwards) for about 2 mm into superficial layers of dermis (almost parallel with surface). Needle should be short with short bevel (can usually be seen through epidermis during insertion). Raised blanched bleb showing tips of hair follicles is sign of correct injection; 7 mm bleb ≡ 0.1 mL injection; if considerable resistance not felt, needle is removed and reinserted before giving more vaccine.

Injection site is at insertion of deltoid muscle onto humerus (sites higher on arm more likely to lead to keloid formation); tip of shoulder should be **avoided**; for cosmetic reasons, upper and lateral surface of thigh may be preferred and this is an acceptable alternative.
PoM **Bacillus Calmette-Guérin Vaccine, Isoniazid-Resistant.** A freeze-dried preparation of live bacteria of an isoniazid-resistant strain derived from the bacillus of Calmette and Guérin.
Dose: 0.1 mL (INFANT under 3 months 0.05 mL) by intradermal injection; for active immunisation of tuberculosis contacts receiving prophylactic treatment with isoniazid—but **no longer recommended**.
Available from Evans (special order)

Percutaneous
The percutaneous multiple puncture technique is an acceptable alternative **only** for young infants in whom the technique of intradermal injection may be difficult (18–20 puncture points are required)
PoM **Bacillus Calmette-Guérin Vaccine, Percutaneous** Tub/Vac/BCG(Perc). A preparation of live bacteria of a strain derived from the bacillus of Calmette and Guérin (**important:** this preparation must **not** be confused with the intradermal preparation)
Dose: about 0.03 mL by percutaneous administration but only recommended as an alternative for infants, see notes above
Available from Health Authorities or (in England only) direct from Farillon

DIAGNOSTIC AGENTS. In the *Mantoux test,* the diagnostic dose is by intradermal injection of Tuberculin Purified Protein Derivative (PPD):
Routine
    10 units PPD i.e. 0.1 mL of 100 units/mL (1 in 1000)
Special (hypersensitive or TB suspected)
    1 unit PPD i.e. 0.1 mL of 10 units/mL (1 in 10 000)
Special (low sensitivity)
    100 units PPD i.e. 0.1 mL of 1000 units/mL (1 in 100)

In the *Heaf test* (multiple puncture) a solution containing Tuberculin Purified Protein Derivative 100 000 units/mL is used; 1 mL is sufficient for up to about 20 tests.
Note. Tuberculin testing should not be carried out within 4 weeks of receiving a live viral vaccine since response to tuberculin may be inhibited.

PoM **Tuberculin PPD.** Prepared from the heat treated products of growth and lysis of the appropriate species of mycobacterium, and containing 100 000 units/mL. Net price 1-mL amp = £5.89. Also available diluted 1 in 100 (1000 units/mL), 1 in 1000 (100 units/mL), and 1 in 10 000 (10 units/mL). Net price 1 mL (all) = £2.22
Available from Health Authorities or (in England only) direct from Farillon

BOTULISM ANTITOXIN
A trivalent botulism antitoxin is available for the post-exposure prophylaxis of botulism and for the treatment of persons thought to be suffering from botulism. It specifically neutralises the toxins produced by *Clostridium botulinum* types A, B, and E. It is not effective against infantile botulism as the toxin (type A) is seldom, if ever, found in the blood in this type of infection.

Hypersensitivity reactions are a problem. It is essential to read the contra-indications, warnings, and details of sensitivity tests on the package insert. Prior to treatment checks should be made regarding previous administration of any antitoxin and history of any allergic condition, e.g. asthma, hay fever, etc. All patients should be tested for sensitivity (diluting the antitoxin if history of allergy).

PoM **Botulism Antitoxin.** A preparation containing the specific antitoxic globulins that have the power of neutralising the toxins formed by types A, B, and E of *Clostridium botulinum*.

Note. The BP title Botulinum Antitoxin is not used because the preparation currently available has a higher phenol content (0.45% against 0.25%).

Dose: prophylaxis, 20 mL by intramuscular injection as soon as possible after exposure; treatment, 20 mL (diluted to 100 mL with sodium chloride 0.9%) by slow intravenous infusion followed by 10 mL 2–4 hours later if necessary, and further doses at intervals of 12–24 hours.

Available from local designated centres. For supplies outside working hours apply to other designated centres and, as a last resort, to Department of Health Duty Officer (Tel 0171-210 5371).

CHOLERA VACCINE

Cholera vaccine contains heat-killed Inaba and Ogawa sub-types of *Vibrio cholerae*, Serovar O1. Cholera vaccine provides little protection and cannot control the spread of the disease. Laboratory staff who have direct contact with the cholera organism should be advised of the possible risk, and the need for vaccination determined. Cholera vaccine is no longer required for international travel. The Department of Health has advised:

the conventional vaccine provides poor protection and should no longer be given for international travel. In the rare circumstance where an unofficial demand may be anticipated, confirmation of non-requirement of cholera vaccine may be given on official notepaper signed and stamped by the medical practitioner.

Travellers to a country where cholera exists should be warned that scrupulous attention to food and water and personal hygiene is **essential**.

DIPHTHERIA VACCINES

Protection against diphtheria is essentially due to antitoxin, the production of which is stimulated by vaccines prepared from the toxin of *Corynebacterium diphtheriae*. These are more effective and cause fewer reactions if adsorbed onto a mineral carrier. Adsorbed diphtheria vaccines are recommended for the routine immunisation of babies and are usually given in the form of a triple vaccine, **adsorbed diphtheria, tetanus, and pertussis vaccine** (see schedule, section 14.1). Adsorbed diphtheria and tetanus vaccine is used in place of the triple vaccine when immunisation against pertussis is contra-indicated.

A booster dose of **adsorbed diphtheria and tetanus vaccine** is recommended at school entry (4–5 years of age). This should preferably be given after an interval of at least 3 years from the last dose of the basic course. A further booster dose is now recommended at school leaving; for this purpose **adsorbed diphtheria and tetanus vaccine for adults and adolescents** (a special low-dose version combined in a single injection with tetanus vaccine) is available. For details on booster doses of diphtheria vaccine in a child over 13 years who requires treatment of a tetanus-prone wound, see under Tetanus Vaccines (p. 529). If there is documented history of a fifth dose of tetanus vaccine having been given when the school-leaving booster dose of adsorbed diphtheria and tetanus vaccine for adults and adolescents is due, then a booster dose of single antigen adsorbed diphtheria vaccine for adults and adolescents should be given instead.

Other booster doses of adsorbed diphtheria vaccine are not recommended as a routine except for staff in contact with diphtheria patients, or handling clinical specimens which may be pathogenic, or working directly with *Corynebacterium diphtheriae;* they should be considered for a booster or for primary immunisation following a risk assessment. A low-dose vaccine, **adsorbed diphtheria vaccine for adults and adolescents**, is available for this purpose.

Unimmunised contacts of a diphtheria case require a primary course of 3 doses of adsorbed diphtheria vaccine at monthly intervals. *Immunised* contacts require a single booster dose (**important:** adults and children *over 10 years* must be given a **low-dose** vaccine); those also requiring tetanus cover can be given the appropriate strength of adsorbed diphtheria vaccine combined with tetanus vaccine.

Previously immunised travellers to countries where diphtheria is endemic or epidemic require a booster dose if their primary immunisation was more than 10 years ago. *Unimmunised travellers* require a full course of 3 doses at monthly intervals (**important:** adults and children *over 10 years* requiring either a primary course or a booster should be given a **low-dose** vaccine—those also requiring tetanus cover can be given the special low-dose version combined with tetanus vaccine).

See section 14.1 for general contra-indications.

Diphtheria vaccines for children

IMPORTANT. Not recommended for persons *aged 10 years or over* (use diphtheria vaccines for adults and adolescents instead)

With tetanus and pertussis (triple vaccine)

PoM **Adsorbed Diphtheria, Tetanus, and Pertussis Vaccine** DTPer/Vac/Ads. Prepared from diphtheria formol toxoid, tetanus formol toxoid, and pertussis vaccine adsorbed on a mineral carrier.

Dose: primary immunisation of children, 0.5 mL by intramuscular or deep subcutaneous injection at 2 months followed by second dose after 4 weeks and third dose after another 4 weeks (see schedule, section 14.1)

Available from Health Authorities or (in England only) direct from Farillon as Pasteur Mérieux brand or Evans (Trivax-AD®) brand

Important. Although some product literature (including patient information leaflets) may contra-indicate use of pertussis-containing vaccines in those with a personal or family history of epilepsy, it is recommended that the advice given under Pertussis Vaccine (Children with problem histories) is followed

Note. Adsorbed diphtheria, tetanus and pertussis vaccine is available in combination with Haemophilus influenzae type b vaccine, see under Haemophilus Influenzae type b Vaccine

With tetanus
PoM **Adsorbed Diphtheria and Tetanus Vaccine** DT/Vac/Ads(Child). Prepared from diphtheria formol toxoid and tetanus formol toxoid adsorbed on a mineral carrier.

Dose: primary immunisation of children omitting pertussis component, 0.5 mL by intramuscular or deep subcutaneous injection at 2 months followed by second dose after 4 weeks and third dose after another 4 weeks (see schedule, section 14.1); booster at school entry, 0.5 mL (see schedule, section 14.1)

Available from Health Authorities or (in England only) direct from Farillon as Evans brand or Pasteur Mérieux brand

Single antigen
PoM **Adsorbed Diphtheria Vaccine** Dip/Vac/Ads(Child). Prepared from diphtheria formol toxoid adsorbed on a mineral carrier. Net price 0.5-mL amp = £1.12

Note. Used only for contacts of a diphtheria case or carrier; *immunised children under 10 years* are given one dose of 0.5 mL by intramuscular or by deep subcutaneous injection, *unimmunised children under 10 years* are given three doses of 0.5 mL with an interval of 4 weeks between first and second doses and another 4 weeks between second and third; *adults and children over 10 years* must be given adsorbed diphtheria vaccine for adults and adolescents (see below).

Available from Health Authorities or (in England only) direct from Farillon

Diphtheria vaccines for adults and adolescents

IMPORTANT. Also for use in children aged *10 years or over*

The small quantity of diphtheria toxoid present in the preparations below is sufficient to recall immunity in individuals previously immunised against diphtheria but whose immunity may have diminished with time; it is insufficient to cause the serious reactions that may occur when diphtheria vaccine of conventional formulation is used in an individual who is already immune. The low dose vaccine must be used when immunising adults and children *over 10 years*; for school leavers a low-dose version combined in a single injection with tetanus vaccine is available (see notes above).

With tetanus
PoM **Adsorbed Diphtheria and Tetanus Vaccine for Adults and Adolescents** DT/Vac/Ads(Adult). Prepared from diphtheria formol toxoid and tetanus formol toxoid adsorbed on a mineral carrier.

Dose: primary immunisation in *patients over 10 years*, three doses each of 0.5 mL by intramuscular or deep subcutaneous injection separated by intervals of 4 weeks; booster, 0.5 mL after 10 years

Available from Health Authorities or (in England only) direct from Farillon as Pasteur Mérieux brand

Single antigen
PoM **Adsorbed Diphtheria Vaccine for Adults and Adolescents** Dip/Vac/Ads(Adult). Prepared from diphtheria formol toxoid adsorbed on a mineral carrier.

Dose: primary immunisation in *patients over 10 years*, three doses each of 0.5 mL by intramuscular or deep subcutaneous injection separated by intervals of 1 month; booster, 0.5 mL

Note. Unimmunised adults and children *over 10 years* who are contacts of a diphtheria case or carrier are given the primary immunisation course; immunised adults and children *over 10 years* are given the booster dose.

Available from Health Authorities or (in England only) direct from Farillon

DIPHTHERIA ANTITOXIN

Diphtheria antitoxin is used for passive immunisation; it is prepared in horses therefore reactions are common after administration.

It is now only used in suspected cases of diphtheria (without waiting for bacteriological confirmation); tests for hypersensitivity should be first carried out.

It is no longer used for prophylaxis because of the risk of hypersensitivity; unimmunised contacts should be promptly investigated and given erythromycin prophylaxis (see section 5.1, table 2) and vaccine (see notes above).

PoM **Diphtheria Antitoxin** Dip/Ser.

Dose: prophylactic 500 to 2000 units by intramuscular injection (but **not** used, see notes above); therapeutic 10 000 to 30 000 units increased to 40 000 to 100 000 units in severe cases; doses of up to 30 000 units should be given intramuscularly but for those over 40 000 units a portion is given intramuscularly followed by the bulk of the dose intravenously after an interval of ½–2 hours

Note. Children require the same dose as adults depending on the severity of the case.

Available from Communicable Disease Surveillance Centre (Tel 0181 200 6868) or in Northern Ireland from Public Health Laboratory, Belfast City Hospital (Tel 01232 329241).

HAEMOPHILUS INFLUENZAE TYPE B VACCINE

Children under the age of 13 months are at high risk of *Haemophilus influenzae* type b infection. **Haemophilus influenzae type b vaccine** (Hib) is a component of the primary course of childhood immunisation (see schedule, section 14.1). The course consists of 3 doses of Haemophilus influenzae type b vaccine with an interval of 1 month between each dose. If primary immunisations against diphtheria, tetanus, pertussis and poliomyelitis have already been commenced or completed, children under the age of 13 months should still receive 3 doses of Haemophilus influenzae type b vaccine at monthly intervals. Children over the age of 13 months are at a lower risk of infection and, if not previously immunised, need receive only 1 dose of the vaccine. The risk of infection falls sharply after the age of 4 years therefore the vaccine is not normally required for children over 4 years. However, it may be given to those over 4 years who are considered to be at increased risk of invasive *Haemophilus influenzae* type b disease (such as those with sickle cell disease and those receiving treatment for malignancy). Also, asplenic children and adults, irrespective of age or the interval from splenectomy, should receive a single dose of Haemophilus influenzae type b vaccine; those under one year should be given three doses. For elective splenectomy, the vaccine should ideally be given at least 2 weeks before the operation. Side-effects reported include fever, headache, malaise, irritability, prolonged crying, loss of appetite, vomiting, diarrhoea, and rash (including urticaria); convulsions, erythema multiforme, and transient cyanosis of the lower limbs have been reported.

See section 14.1 for general contra-indications

Single component
Each single component product may be used to complete a course started with any other single component product listed below

PoM **HibTITER®** (Wyeth)
Injection, capsular polysaccharide of *Haemophilus influenzae* type b (conjugated to a protein carrier). Net price 0.5-mL vial = £10.20
Dose: by intramuscular injection, 0.5 mL; for primary immunisation, 3 doses are required at intervals of 1 month (see schedule, section 14.1)
Note. If required, haemophilus influenzae type b vaccine is available in combination with adsorbed diphtheria, tetanus and pertussis vaccine (see below); alternatively, *HibTITER®* may be combined with *Trivax-AD®* brand of adsorbed diphtheria, tetanus and pertussis vaccine in the same syringe (final combined volume = 1 mL)
Available, as part of childhood immunisation schedule, from Health Authorities or (in England only) Farillon

PoM **ACT-HIB®** (Pasteur Mérieux)
Injection, powder for reconstitution, capsular polysaccharide of *Haemophilus influenzae* type b (conjugated to a protein carrier). Net price per vial with diluent = £9.25
Dose: by intramuscular or deep subcutaneous injection, 0.5 mL; for primary immunisation, 3 doses are required at intervals of 1 month (see schedule, section 14.1)
Note. If required, haemophilus influenzae type b vaccine is available in combination with adsorbed diphtheria, tetanus and pertussis vaccine (see below); alternatively, *ACT-HIB®* may be reconstituted with 0.5 mL of Pasteur Merieux brand of adsorbed diphtheria, tetanus and pertussis vaccine
Available, as part of childhood immunisation schedule, from Health Authorities or (in England only) Farillon

With diphtheria, tetanus and pertussis vaccines
Each combined product may be used to complete a course started with any other combined product listed below; **important** see also under Adsorbed Diphtheria, Tetanus and Pertussis Vaccine (p. 520)

▼ PoM **ACT-HIB®DTP dc** (Pasteur Mérieux)
Injection, powder for reconstitution, capsular polysaccharide of *Haemophilus influenzae* type b (conjugated to a protein carrier) with diluent containing diphtheria toxoid, tetanus toxoid and *Bordetella pertussis* cells. Net price per dual-chamber prefilled syringe = £10.90
Dose: CHILD under 4 years, by intramuscular or deep subcutaneous injection, 0.5 mL; for primary immunisation, 3 doses are required at intervals of 1 month (see schedule, section 14.1)
Available, as part of childhood immunisation schedule, from Health Authorities or (in England only) Farillon

▼ PoM **Trivax-HIB®** (SmithKline Beecham)
Injection, powder for reconstitution, capsular polysaccharide of *Haemophilus influenzae* type b (conjugated to a protein carrier) with diluent containing diphtheria toxoid, tetanus toxoid and *Bordetella pertussis* cells.
Dose: CHILD under 10 years, by intramuscular injection, 0.5 mL; for primary immunisation, 3 doses are required at intervals of 1 month (see schedule, section 14.1)
Available, as part of childhood immunisation schedule, from Health Authorities or (in England only) Farillon

HEPATITIS A VACCINE
Hepatitis A vaccine is prepared from formaldehyde-inactivated hepatitis A virus grown in human diploid cells.
Immunisation is recommended for:
laboratory staff who work directly with the virus;
haemophiliacs treated with Factor VIII or Factor IX concentrates or who have liver disease or who have been infected with hepatitis B or hepatitis C;
travellers to high-risk areas (see p. 533);
individuals who are at risk due to their sexual behaviour.
Immunisation should be considered for :
patients with chronic liver disease;
staff and residents of homes for those with severe learning difficulties;
workers at risk of exposure to untreated sewage.
Haemophiliacs and patients with chronic liver disease should be checked for previous exposure before immunisation.

Normal immunoglobulin (section 14.5) provides short-term protection against hepatitis A, but antibody titres after a primary course of hepatitis A vaccine are well in excess of those found after the administration of normal immunoglobulin.

Travellers to high-risk areas who require immunisation less than 10 days before departure may be given the single-dose vaccine plus normal immunoglobulin at a different injection site. Administration of normal immunoglobulin at the same time as the vaccine, at different injection sites, does not affect rate of seroconversion but the level of antibody may be reduced.

Side-effects of hepatitis A vaccine, usually mild, include transient soreness, erythema, and induration at the injection site. Less common effects include fever, malaise, fatigue, headache, nausea, and loss of appetite; generalised rashes are occasionally reported.

See section 14.1 for general contra-indications

Single component
▼ PoM **Avaxim®** (Pasteur Mérieux)
A suspension of formaldehyde-inactivated hepatitis A virus (GBM grown in human diploid cells) 320 antigen units/mL adsorbed onto aluminium hydroxide. Net price 0.5-mL prefilled syringe = £21.60
Dose: by intramuscular injection (see note below), 0.5 mL as a single dose; booster dose 0.5 mL 6 months following the initial dose; further booster doses, 0.5 mL every 10 years; CHILD under 16 years, not recommended
Note. The deltoid region is the preferred site of injection. The subcutaneous route may be used for patients with haemophilia

---

PoM **Havrix Monodose®** (SmithKline Beecham)

A suspension of formaldehyde-inactivated hepatitis A virus (HM 175 grown in human diploid cells) 1440 ELISA units/mL adsorbed onto aluminium hydroxide. Net price 1-mL (1440 ELISA units) prefilled syringe = £22.68; 0.5-mL (720 ELISA units) prefilled syringe (*Havrix Junior Monodose®*) = £18.03

Dose: by intramuscular injection (see note below), 1 mL as a single dose; booster dose, 1 mL 6–12 months following the initial dose; CHILD 1–15 years 0.5 mL

Note. The deltoid region is the preferred site of injection in adults. The subcutaneous route may be used for patients with haemophilia

▼ PoM **Vaqta® Paediatric and Adolescent** (Pasteur Mérieux)

A suspension of formaldehyde-inactivated hepatitis A virus (grown in human diploid cells) 50 antigen units/mL adsorbed onto aluminium hydroxide, net price 0.5-mL prefilled syringe = £16.39

Dose: by intramuscular injection (see note below) CHILD 2–17 years, 0.5 mL as a single dose; booster dose 0.5 mL 6–18 months following the initial dose; under 2 years of age, not recommended

Note. The deltoid region is the preferred site of injection

With hepatitis B vaccine
PoM **Twinrix® Adult**
See Hepatitis B Vaccine

HEPATITIS B VACCINE

Hepatitis B vaccine contains inactivated hepatitis B virus surface antigen (HBsAg) adsorbed on aluminium hydroxide adjuvant. It is made biosynthetically using recombinant DNA technology. The vaccine is used in individuals at high risk of contracting hepatitis B.

In the UK, high-risk groups include:
parenteral drug abusers;
individuals who change sexual partners frequently;
close family contacts of a case or carrier;
infants born to mothers who *either* have had hepatitis B during pregnancy, *or* are positive for both hepatitis B surface antigen and hepatitis B e-antigen *or* are surface antigen positive without e markers (or where they have not been determined); active immunisation of the infant is started immediately after delivery and *hepatitis B immunoglobulin* (see p. 532) is given at the same time as the vaccine. Infants born to mothers who are positive for hepatitis B surface antigen and for e-antigen antibody should receive the vaccine but not the immunoglobulin;
haemophiliacs, those receiving regular blood transfusions or blood products, and carers responsible for the administration of such products;
patients with chronic renal failure including those on haemodialysis. Haemodialysis patients should be monitored for antibodies annually and re-immunised if necessary;
health care personnel who have direct contact with blood or blood-stained body fluids or with patients' tissues;
trainee health care workers;
other occupational risk groups such as morticians and embalmers;
staff and patients of day-care or residential accommodation for those with severe learning difficulties;
inmates of custodial institutions;

those travelling to areas of high prevalence who intend to seek employment as health care workers or who plan to remain there for lengthy periods and who may therefore be at increased risk of acquiring infection as the result of medical or dental procedures carried out in those countries;
families adopting children from countries with a high prevalence of hepatitis B.

Short-term tourists or business travellers are not generally at increased risk of infection but may place themselves at risk by their sexual behaviour when abroad.

It should be borne in mind that immunisation takes up to 6 months to confer adequate protection; the duration of immunity is not known precisely, but a single booster 5 years after the primary course may be sufficient to maintain immunity for those who continue to be at risk.

More detailed guidance is given in the memorandum *Immunisation against Infectious Disease* . Immunisation does not eliminate the need for commonsense precautions for avoiding the risk of infection from known carriers by the routes of infection which have been clearly established, consult *Guidance for Clinical Health Care Workers: Protection against Infection with HIV and Hepatitis Viruses* and *Protecting Health Care Workers and Patients from Hepatitis B*. Accidental inoculation of hepatitis B virus-infected blood into a wound, incision, needle-prick, or abrasion may lead to infection, whereas it is unlikely that indirect exposure to a carrier will do so.

Specific **hepatitis B immunoglobulin** ('HBIG') is available for use with the vaccine in those accidentally infected and in infants (section 14.5).

See section 14.1 for general contra-indications.

Single component
PoM **Engerix B®** (SmithKline Beecham)

A suspension of hepatitis B surface antigen (rby, prepared from yeast cells by recombinant DNA technique) 20 micrograms/mL adsorbed onto aluminium hydroxide. Net price 0.5 mL (paediatric) vial = £9.85; 1-mL vial = £13.27; 1-mL prefilled syringe = £13.97

Dose: by intramuscular injection (see note below), 3 doses of 1 mL (20 micrograms), the second 1 month and the third 6 months after the first dose; more rapid (e.g. for travellers), third dose 2 months after first dose with booster at 12 months; CHILD birth to 12 years 3 doses of 0.5 mL (10 micrograms); INFANTS born to HBsAg-positive mothers (see also above), 3 doses of 0.5 mL (10 micrograms), first dose at birth with hepatitis B immunoglobulin injection (separate site)

Note. Deltoid muscle is preferred site of injection in adults; anterolateral thigh is preferred site in infants and children; not to be injected into the buttock (vaccine efficacy reduced); subcutaneous route used for patients with haemophilia.

PoM **HB-Vax® II** (Pasteur Mérieux)

A suspension of hepatitis B surface antigen (prepared from yeast cells by recombinant DNA technique) 10 micrograms/mL adsorbed onto aluminium hydroxide. Net price 1-mL prefilled syringe = £12.70; 1-mL vial = £11.95

Dose: by intramuscular injection (see note below) 3 doses of 1 mL (10 micrograms), the second 1 month and the third 6 months after the first dose; more rapid (e.g. for travellers), third dose 2 months after first dose with booster at 12 months; CHILD birth to 15 years 3 doses of 0.5 mL (5 micrograms); INFANTS born to HBsAg-positive mothers (see also above), 3 doses of 0.5 mL (5 micrograms), first dose at birth with hepatitis B immunoglobulin injection (separate site)

Note. Deltoid muscle is preferred site of injection in adults; anterolateral thigh is preferred site in infants and children; not to be injected into the buttock (vaccine efficacy reduced); subcutaneous route used for patients with haemophilia.

With hepatitis A vaccine

▼ PoM **Twinrix®** (SmithKline Beecham)

Inactivated hepatitis A virus 720 ELISA units and recombinant (DNA) hepatitis B surface antigen 20 micrograms/mL adsorbed onto aluminium hydroxide and aluminium phosphate. Net price 1-mL prefilled syringe (Adult) = £29.09; 0.5-mL prefilled syringe (Paediatric) = £22.36

Dose: by intramuscular injection into deltoid muscle (see note below); primary course of 3 doses of 1 mL, the second 1 month and the third 6 months after the first dose; 1 mL booster dose 5 years after the start of primary course for those at continued risk; CHILD 1–15 years 0.5 mL

Note. Primary course should be completed with *Twinrix®* (single component vaccines given at appropriate intervals may be used for booster dose); not to be injected into the buttock (vaccine efficacy reduced); subcutaneous route used for patients with haemophilia (but immune response may be reduced).

IMPORTANT. *Twinrix®* **not** recommended for post-exposure prophylaxis following percutaneous (needle-stick), ocular or mucous membrane exposure to hepatitis B virus.

INFLUENZA VACCINES

While most viruses are antigenically stable, the influenza viruses A and B (especially A) are constantly altering their antigenic structure as indicated by changes in the haemagglutinins (H) and neuraminidases (N) on the surface of the viruses. It is essential that influenza vaccines in use contain the H and N components of the prevalent strain or strains. Every year the World Health Organization recommends which strains should be included.

The recommended strains are grown in the allantoic cavity of chick embryos (therefore **contraindicated** in those hypersensitive to eggs).

Since **influenza vaccines** will not control epidemics they are recommended *only for persons at high risk*. Annual immunisation is strongly recommended for those of all ages, especially the elderly, with any of the following conditions:

chronic respiratory disease, including asthma;
chronic heart disease;
chronic renal failure;
diabetes mellitus;
immunosuppression due to disease or treatment, including asplenia or splenic dysfunction.

Influenza immunisation is also recommended for residents of nursing homes, residential homes for the elderly, and other long-stay facilities.

In non-pandemic years routine immunisation of Health Service Staff is not recommended, except for those at high risk (owing to medical disorders).

Interactions: Appendix 1 (influenza vaccine).

See section 14.1 for general contra-indications.

PoM **Inactivated Influenza Vaccine (Split Virion)** (Pasteur Mérieux)

Inactivated influenza vaccine (split virion) Flu/Vac/Split. Net price 0.5-mL disposable syringe = £5.10

Dose: 0.5 mL by deep subcutaneous or by intramuscular injection; CHILD 6–47 months, 0.25 mL repeated once after 4–6 weeks; 4–12 years, 0.5 mL repeated once after 4–6 weeks; single doses are appropriate for children who have already been immunised

PoM **Begrivac®** (Wyeth)

Inactivated influenza vaccine (split virion) Flu/Vac/Split. Net price 0.5-mL vial = £5.20

Dose: 0.5 mL by deep subcutaneous or by intramuscular injection; CHILD 9–12 years, 0.5 mL repeated once after 4–6 weeks; single doses are appropriate for children who have already been immunised.

PoM **Fluarix®** (SmithKline Beecham)

Inactivated influenza vaccine (split virion) Flu/Vac/Split. Net price 0.5-mL disposable syringe = £5.70

Dose: 0.5 mL by deep subcutaneous or by intramuscular injection; CHILD 6 months to 6 years, 0.25 mL repeated once after 4–6 weeks; single doses are appropriate for children who have already been immunised

PoM **Fluvirin®** (Evans)

Inactivated influenza vaccine (surface antigen) Flu/Vac/SA. Net price 0.5-mL disposable syringe = £5.09

Dose: 0.5 mL by deep subcutaneous or by intramuscular injection; CHILD 4–13 years, 0.5 mL repeated once after 4–6 weeks; single doses are appropriate for children who have already been immunised

PoM **Fluzone®** (Pasteur Mérieux)

Inactivated influenza vaccine (split virion) Flu/Vac/Split. Net price 0.5-mL disposable syringe = £5.18

Dose: 0.5 mL by deep subcutaneous or by intramuscular injection; CHILD 6–47 months, 0.25 mL repeated once after 4–6 weeks; 4–12 years, 0.5 mL repeated once after 4–6 weeks; single doses are appropriate for children who have already been immunised

PoM **Influvac Sub-unit®** (Solvay)

Inactivated influenza vaccine (surface antigen) Flu/Vac/SA. Net price 0.5-mL disposable syringe = £5.08

Dose: 0.5 mL by deep subcutaneous or by intramuscular injection; CHILD 6 months–4 years, 0.25 mL repeated once after 4–6 weeks; 4–13 years, 0.5 mL repeated once after 4–6 weeks; single doses are appropriate for children who have already been immunised

MEASLES VACCINE

Measles vaccine has been replaced by a combined measles/mumps/rubella vaccine (MMR vaccine) for all eligible children.

Administration of a measles-containing vaccine to children may be associated with a mild measles-like syndrome with a measles-like rash and pyrexia about a week after injection. Much less commonly, convulsions and, very rarely, encephalitis have been reported. Convulsions in infants are much less frequently associated with measles vaccines than with other conditions leading to febrile episodes.

MMR vaccine may be used in the control of outbreaks of measles (see under MMR Vaccine).

Single antigen vaccine

Available from Evans and Pasteur Mérieux on a named-patient basis

Combined vaccines, see under MMR vaccine

MMR VACCINE

A combined **measles/mumps/rubella vaccine** (MMR vaccine) has been introduced with the aim of eliminating rubella (and congenital rubella syndrome), measles, and mumps. Every child should receive two doses of MMR vaccine by entry to primary school, unless there is a valid contra-indication (see below) or parental refusal.

MMR vaccine has replaced measles vaccine for children of both sexes and should be given irrespective of previous measles, mumps or rubella infection.

The first dose of MMR vaccine is given to children aged 12–15 months. Since October 1996 a second (booster) dose has been given when starting school at 3–5 years of age (see schedule, section 14.1). Children presenting for their pre-school booster who have not received their first dose of MMR vaccine should be given a dose of MMR vaccine followed three months later by a second dose. At school-leaving age or at entry into further education, individuals of both sexes who have not received either MR or MMR vaccines should be offered MMR immunisation.

MMR vaccine may also be used in the control of outbreaks of measles and should be offered to susceptible children within 3 days of exposure to infection (**important:** MMR vaccine is not suitable for prophylaxis following exposure to mumps or rubella since the antibody response to the mumps and rubella components is too slow for effective prophylaxis).

Children with partially or totally impaired immune responsiveness should not receive live vaccines (for advice on AIDS see section 14.1). If they have been exposed to measles infection they should be given normal immunoglobulin (section 14.5).

Malaise, fever or a rash may occur following the first dose of MMR vaccine, most commonly about a week after immunisation and lasting about 2 to 3 days. Leaflets are available to provide parents with advice for reducing fever (including the use of paracetamol). Parotid swelling occasionally occurs, usually in the third week. After a second dose of MMR vaccine, adverse reactions are considerably less common than after the first dose. Post-vaccination meningoencephalitis was reported (rarely and with complete recovery) following immunisation with MMR vaccine containing Urabe mumps vaccine, which has now been discontinued; no cases have been confirmed in association with the currently-used Jeryl Lynn mumps vaccine. Children with post-vaccination symptoms are not infectious.

Contra-indications to MMR include:

children with untreated malignant disease or altered immunity, and those receiving immunosuppressive drugs or radiotherapy, or high-dose corticosteroids;

children who have received another live vaccine by injection within 3 weeks;

children with allergies to neomycin or kanamycin;

children with acute febrile illness (vaccination should be deferred);

if given to women, pregnancy should be avoided for 1 month (as for rubella vaccine);

should not be given within 3 months of an immuno-globulin injection.

It should be noted that:

children with a personal or close family history of convulsions should be given MMR vaccine, provided the parents understand that there may be a febrile response; immunoglobulin must not be given with MMR vaccine since the immune response to rubella and mumps may be inhibited; doctors should seek specialist paediatric advice rather than withold vaccination;

there is increasing evidence that MMR vaccine can be given safely even when the child has had an anaphylactic reaction to food containing egg (dislike of egg or refusal to eat is not a contra-indication).

PoM **MMR Vaccine**

Live measles, mumps, and rubella vaccine

Dose: 0.5 mL by deep subcutaneous or by intramuscular injection

Available from Health Authorities or (in England only) direct from Farillon as MMR II® (Pasteur Mérieux)

MENINGOCOCCAL POLYSACCHARIDE VACCINE

Meningococcal polysaccharide vaccine is indicated for visits of longer than 1 month to areas of the world where the risk of acquiring meningococcal infection is much higher than in the UK, particularly for travellers proposing to travel 'rough' or to live or work with local people. Travellers with asplenia (or severe dysfunction of the spleen) also particularly require protection.

These areas include Delhi, Nepal, Bhutan, Pakistan, Mecca (see below), and the meningitis belt of Africa, which encompasses southern sub-Saharan parts of Senegal, Mali, Niger, Chad, and Sudan; all of Gambia, Guinea, Togo, and Benin; South-west Ethiopia; northern parts of Sierra Leone, Liberia, Ivory Coast, Nigeria, Cameroon, Central African Republic, Uganda, and Kenya.

Saudi Arabia requires vaccination of pilgrims to Mecca during the Haj annual pilgrimage; this may apply to others visiting Saudi Arabia in the months leading up to August.

For advice on the immunisation of *close contacts* of disease cases of Group A and Group C meningococcal meningitis in the UK and on the role of the vaccine in the control of *local outbreaks*, consult the memorandum *Immunisation against Infectious Disease*.

The need for immunisation of laboratory staff who work directly with *Neisseria meningitidis* should be determined by assessing the risk.

See section 14.1 for general contra-indications.

PoM **AC Vax**® (SmithKline Beecham)
Meningococcal polysaccharide vaccine, Neimen/
Vac. Prepared from *Neisseria meningitidis*
(meningococcus) groups A and C. Net price single-dose vial (with diluent) = £6.86
Dose: ADULT and CHILD aged 2 months and over,
0.5 mL by deep subcutaneous or intramuscular injection

PoM **Mengivac (A+C)**® (Pasteur Mérieux)
Meningococcal polysaccharide vaccine, Neimen/
Vac. Prepared from *Neisseria meningitidis*
(meningococcus) groups A and C. Net price single-dose vial (with syringe containing diluent) =
£6.69
Dose: ADULT and CHILD aged over 18 months, 0.5 mL
by deep subcutaneous or intramuscular injection
Note. The lower age range for AC Vax® and Mengivac
(A+C)® differ; in the case of Mengivac (A+C)® the
product literature states that young children and infants
respond less well to the vaccine than older children and
adults, with little response to the Group C polysaccharide under 18 months of age and a poor response to
Group A polysaccharide under 3 months of age. Additionally, protection in infants under 18 months of age is
of shorter duration

MUMPS VACCINE

Mumps vaccine consists of a live attenuated strain
of virus grown in chick-embryo tissue culture.

See under MMR vaccine and section 14.1 for
contra-indications.

PoM **Mumpsvax**® (Pasteur Mérieux)
Mumps vaccine (Jeryl Lynn strain). Net price single-dose vial (with diluent) = £4.00
Dose: ADULT and CHILD over 1 year, 0.5 mL by subcutaneous injection

Combined vaccines
With measles and rubella
See MMR Vaccine

PERTUSSIS VACCINE

(Whooping-cough vaccine)
Pertussis vaccine is usually given combined with
diphtheria and tetanus vaccine (in triple vaccine)
starting at 2 months of age (see section 14.1).

With some vaccines available in the early 1960s
persistent screaming and collapse were reported
but these reactions are rarely observed with the vaccines now available. *Convulsions and encephalopathy* have been reported as rare complications, but
such conditions may arise from other causes and be
falsely attributed to the vaccine. Neurological complications *after whooping cough itself* are considerably more common than after the vaccine.

As with any other elective immunisation procedure it is advisable to postpone vaccination if the
child is suffering from any acute illness, until fully
recovered. Minor infections without fever or systemic upset are not reasons to delay immunisation.
Immunisation should not be carried out in children
who have a history of severe general reaction to a
preceding dose; in these children immunisation
should be completed with adsorbed diphtheria and
tetanus vaccine. Where there has been a severe

local reaction or pyrexia, acellular pertussis vaccine
may be used. The following reactions should be
regarded as severe:

Local—an extensive area of redness and swelling which
becomes indurated and involves most of the antero-lat-
eral surface of the thigh or a major part of the circumfer-
ence of the upper arm.

General—temperature of 39.5°C or more within 48
hours of vaccine, anaphylaxis, bronchospasm, laryngeal
oedema, generalised collapse, prolonged unresponsive-
ness, prolonged inconsolable screaming, and convulsions occurring within 72 hours.

A personal or family history of allergy is **not** a contra-indication to immunisation against whooping
cough; nor are stable neurological conditions such
as cerebral palsy or spina bifida.

Children with problem histories. When there is
a personal or family history of *febrile* convulsions,
there is an increased risk of these occurring after
pertussis immunisation. In such children, immunisation is *recommended* but advice on the *prevention
of fever* (see p. 518) should be given at the time of
immunisation.

In a British study, children with a family history
of epilepsy were immunised with pertussis vaccine
without any significant adverse events. These children's developmental progress has been normal. In
children with a close family history (first degree relatives) of *idiopathic epilepsy*, there may be a risk of
developing a similar condition, irrespective of
vaccine. Immunisation is *recommended* for these
children.

Where there is a *still evolving neurological problem*, immunisation should be *deferred* until the condition is stable. Children whose epilepsy is well
controlled may receive pertussis vaccine. When
there has been a documented history of *cerebral
damage in the neonatal period*, immunisation
should be *carried out unless there is evidence of an
evolving neurological abnormality*. If immunisation
is to be deferred, this should be stated on the neonatal discharge summary. Where there is doubt,
appropriate advice should be sought from a consultant paediatrician, district immunisation co-ordina-
tor or consultant in communicable disease control
rather than withholding vaccine.

Older children. There is no contra-indication to
administration of pertussis vaccine to unimmunised
older children in order to protect infants and sib-
lings. Since a course of 3 injections is required to
protect against pertussis, vaccine cannot be used to
control an outbreak.

▼ PoM **Acellular Pertussis Vaccine, APV**
(Lederle)
Unlicensed single-antigen acellular pertussis vaccine
(APV) has been made available by the Department of
Health under Crown Immunity only for completion
of immunisation against pertussis in those children
whose course of pertussis vaccine was not given (or
not completed) as part of their triple vaccine course
Dose: 0.5 mL by intramuscular or deep subcutaneous
injection, 3 doses at intervals of 1 month
Available from Farillon on a named-patient basis
Note. Should be ordered only when required for use

Combined vaccine (*pertussis, tetanus*, and *diphtheria*), see under Diphtheria vaccines

---

PNEUMOCOCCAL VACCINE

A polyvalent **pneumococcal polysaccharide vaccine** is recommended for the immunisation of persons over the age of 2 years with any of the following conditions:

Homozygous sickle cell disease;
Asplenia or severe dysfunction of the spleen;
Chronic renal disease or nephrotic syndrome;
Coeliac syndrome;
Immunodeficiency or immunosuppression due to disease or treatment, including HIV infection;
Chronic heart disease;
Chronic lung disease;
Chronic liver disease including cirrhosis;
Diabetes mellitus.

Where possible, the vaccine should be given at least 2 weeks before splenectomy and before chemotherapy; patients should be given advice about increased risk of pneumococcal infection (a patient card and information leaflet for patients with asplenia are available from the Department of Health). Prophylactic antibiotic therapy against pneumococcal infection should not be stopped after immunisation. The vaccine is effective in a single dose if the types of pneumonia in the community are reflected in the polysaccharides contained in the vaccine. It should not be given in pregnancy, or when breast-feeding, or when there is infection. Hypersensitivity reactions may occur.

REVACCINATION. Revaccination with the previously available 12- or 14-valent vaccines produced severe reactions in some subjects, especially if undertaken less than 3 years after the first injection; the same is likely to apply to revaccination with the currently available 23-valent vaccines. Revaccination is therefore not recommended except, after 5–10 years, in individuals in whom the antibody concentration is likely to decline more rapidly (e.g. asplenia, splenic dysfunction and nephrotic syndrome). If there is doubt about the need for revaccination, this should be discussed with a haematologist and measurement of antibody concentration considered.

IMPORTANT. Not for intradermal injection which may cause severe local reactions

See section 14.1 for general contra-indications.

PoM **Pneumovax® II** (Pasteur Mérieux)

Polysaccharide from each of 23 capsular types of pneumococcus. Net price 0.5-mL vial = £9.94

Dose: 0.5 mL by subcutaneous or intramuscular injection; CHILD under 2 years, not recommended (suboptimal response and also safety and efficacy not established)

PoM **Pnu-Imune®** (Wyeth)

Polysaccharide from each of 23 capsular types of pneumococcus. Net price 0.5-mL vial = £9.94

Dose: 0.5 mL by subcutaneous or intramuscular injection; CHILD under 2 years, not recommended

POLIOMYELITIS VACCINES

There are two types of poliomyelitis vaccine, poliomyelitis vaccine, live (oral) (Sabin) and poliomyelitis vaccine, inactivated (Salk). The oral vaccine, consisting of a mixture of attenuated strains of virus types 1, 2, and 3 is at present generally used in the UK.

A course of primary immunisation consists of 3 doses of **poliomyelitis vaccine, live (oral)**, starting at two months of age with an interval of 1 month between each dose (see schedule, section 14.1). The initial course of 3 doses should also be given to all unimmunised adults; no adult should remain unimmunised against poliomyelitis.

Two booster doses of poliomyelitis vaccine, live (oral), are recommended, the first at school entry and the second at school leaving (see schedule, section 14.1). Booster doses for adults are not necessary except for those at special risk such as travellers to endemic areas, or laboratory staff likely to be exposed to the viruses, or health care workers in possible contact with cases; booster doses should be given to such individuals every 10 years.

Vaccine-associated poliomyelitis and poliomyelitis in contacts of vaccinees are rare. In England and Wales there is an annual average of 1 recipient and 1 contact case for over 2 million doses of oral vaccine. The need for strict personal hygiene must be stressed; the contacts of a recently vaccinated baby should be advised particularly of the need to wash their hands after changing the baby's napkins.

Contra-indications to the use of oral poliomyelitis vaccine include vomiting and diarrhoea, and immunodeficiency disorders (or household contacts of patients with immunodeficiency disorders). See section 14.1 for further contra-indications.

Poliomyelitis vaccine (inactivated) may be used for those in whom poliomyelitis vaccine (oral) is contra-indicated because of immunosuppressive disorders (for advice on AIDS see section 14.1).

Either live (oral) vaccine or inactivated vaccine may be used to complete a course started with the other, except that live (oral) vaccine must **not** be used for immunosuppressed individuals or their household contacts (see also contra-indications).

TRAVELLERS. Travellers to areas other than Australia, New Zealand, Northern and Western Europe, and North America should be given a full course of oral poliomyelitis vaccine if they have not been immunised in the past. Those who have not received immunisation within the last 10 years should be given a booster dose of oral poliomyelitis vaccine.

Live (oral) (Sabin)

PoM **Poliomyelitis Vaccine, Live (Oral)** Pol/Vac (Oral)[1]. A suspension of suitable live attenuated strains of poliomyelitis virus, types 1, 2, and 3. Available in single-dose and 10-dose containers

Dose: 3 drops from a multidose container or the total contents of a single-dose container; for primary immunisation 3 doses are required (see schedule, section 14.1). May be given on a lump of sugar; not to be given with foods which contain preservatives

Available from Health Authorities or (in England and Scotland only) direct from Farillon

1. BP permits code OPV for vaccine in single doses provided it also appears on pack.

Note. Poliomyelitis vaccine loses potency once the container has been opened, therefore any vaccine remaining at the end of an immunisation session should be discarded; whenever possible sessions should be arranged to avoid undue wastage.

Inactivated (Salk)

PoM **Poliomyelitis Vaccine, Inactivated** Pol/ Vac (Inact). An inactivated suspension of suitable strains of poliomyelitis virus, types 1, 2, and 3.

Dose: 0.5 mL or as stated on the label by subcutaneous injection; for primary immunisation 3 doses are required at intervals of 4 weeks

Available direct from Farillon.

Note. Should be ordered one dose at a time (on a named-patient basis) and only when required for use

RABIES VACCINE

Pre-exposure, prophylactic immunisation with human diploid cell **rabies vaccine** should be offered to those at high risk—laboratory staff who handle the rabies virus, those working in quarantine stations, animal handlers, veterinary surgeons and field workers who are likely to be exposed to bites of possibly infected wild animals, certain port officials, licensed bat handlers and health workers who are likely to come into close contact with patients with rabies. Pre-exposure immunisation is also recommended for those living or travelling in enzootic areas who may be exposed to unusual risk.

The Department of Health has advised that for *prophylactic use* the vaccine produces a good anti-body response when given in a 3-dose schedule on days 0, 7, and 28, with a booster dose every 2–3 years to those at continued risk. For travellers to enzootic areas who are not animal handlers, 2 doses given 4 weeks apart may be acceptable *provided that post-exposure treatment is readily available;* for those who remain at continued risk a booster dose should be given 6–12 months later followed by a booster every 2–3 years.

Post-exposure treatment depends on the level of risk in the country concerned and the individual's immune status. For *post-exposure treatment of fully immunised patients:* countries with no risk, generally no treatment required; countries with low risk and high risk, two booster doses are needed (one on day 0 and one on day 3–7). For *post-exposure treatment of previously unimmunised patients* (or those whose prophylaxis is possibly inadequate): countries with no risk, generally no treatment required; countries with low risk, a course of injections should be started as soon as possible after exposure (days 0, 3, 7, 14 and 30); countries with high risk, as for countries with low risk, **plus** rabies immunoglobulin on day 0 (section 14.5). The course may be discontinued if it is proved that the patient was not at risk.

Staff in attendance on a patient who is highly suspected of, or known to be suffering from, rabies should be offered immunisation. Four intradermal doses of 0.1 mL of human diploid cell vaccine (Pasteur Mérieux) given on the same day at different sites (ensuring correct intradermal technique) has been suggested for this purpose [unlicensed route].

Advice on up-to-date country-by-country information and on post-exposure immunisation and treatment of rabies is available from the Virus Reference Division, Central Public Health Laboratory, Colindale, London NW9 5HT (Tel 0181-200 4400) or in Scotland from the Scottish Centre for Infection and Environmental Health (Tel 0141-946 7120).

There are no specific contra-indications to this diploid cell vaccine and its use should be considered whenever a patient has been attacked by an animal in a country where rabies is endemic, even if there is no direct evidence of rabies in the attacking animal.

PoM **Rabies Vaccine BP Pasteur Mérieux** (Pasteur Mérieux)

Freeze-dried inactivated Wistar rabies virus strain PM/WI 38 1503-3M cultivated in human diploid cells. Single-dose vial with syringe containing diluent

IMPORTANT. Studies have shown that when this vaccine is injected into the gluteal region there is a poor response. Concomitant administration of chloroquine may also affect the antibody response. Because of the potential consequences of inadequately treated rabies exposure and because there is no indication that fetal abnormalities have been associated with rabies vaccination, pregnancy is **not** considered a contra-indication to post-exposure prophylaxis. If there is substantial risk of exposure to rabies, pre-exposure prophylaxis may also be indicated during pregnancy

Dose: prophylactic, 1 mL by deep subcutaneous or intra-muscular injection in the deltoid region, on days 0, 7, and 28; also booster doses every 2–3 years to those at continued risk; see above for 2-dose schedule

Post-exposure, 1 mL by deep subcutaneous or intramuscular injection in the deltoid region, see notes above

Staff in attendance, see notes above

Also available from local designated centres (special workers and post-exposure treatment)

RUBELLA VACCINE

The selective policy of protecting women of child-bearing age from the risks of rubella (German measles) in pregnancy has been replaced by a policy of eliminating rubella in children; the single-antigen rubella immunisation programme for 10–14 year old girls has been discontinued. All children should be immunised with rubella-containing vaccine (measles, mumps and rubella) at 12–15 months and at 3–5 years (see MMR vaccine, p. 525). Immigrants who enter the UK after the age of school immunisation are particularly likely to require immunisation.

Every effort must be made to identify and immunise with rubella vaccine all *seronegative women of child-bearing age* (see schedule, section 14.1) as well as those who might put pregnant women at risk of infection (e.g. nurses and doctors in obstetric units).

Rubella vaccine may conveniently be offered to previously *unimmunised and seronegative post-partum women.* Immunising susceptible post-partum women a few days after delivery is important as far as the overall reduction of congenital abnormalities in the UK is concerned, for about 60% of these abnormalities occur in the babies of multiparous women.

PREGNANCY. Rubella immunisation should be avoided in early pregnancy, and women of child-bearing age should be advised not to become pregnant within 1 month of immunisation. However, despite active surveillance in the

UK, the USA, and Germany, no case of congenital rubella syndrome has been reported following inadvertent immunisation shortly before or during pregnancy. There is thus no evidence that the vaccine is teratogenic, and routine termination of pregnancy following inadvertent immunisation should **not** be recommended; potential parents should be given this information before making a decision about termination.

See section 14.1 for general contra-indications.

PoM **Rubella Vaccine, Live** Rub/Vac (Live).
Prepared from Wistar RA 27/3 strain propagated in human diploid cells
  Dose: 0.5 mL by deep subcutaneous or by intramuscular injection (see schedule, section 14.1 and notes above)
  Available from Health Authorities or (in England only) direct from Farillon as SmithKline Beecham brand (*Ervevax*®)

Combined vaccines, see under MMR vaccine

SMALLPOX VACCINE
Smallpox immunisation is no longer required routinely because global eradication has been achieved. Advice on the need for immunisation of workers in laboratories where pox viruses (such as vaccinia) are handled and of others whose work involves an identifiable risk of exposure to pox virus can be obtained from the Virus Reference Laboratory, Central Public Health Laboratory, Colindale (Tel 0181-200 4400) who will also supply the vaccine.

TETANUS VACCINES
(Tetanus toxoids)
Tetanus vaccines stimulate the production of the protective antitoxin. In general, adsorption on aluminium hydroxide, aluminium phosphate, or calcium phosphate improves antigenicity. Adsorbed tetanus vaccine is offered routinely to babies in combination with adsorbed diphtheria vaccine (DT/Vac/Ads(Child)) and more usually also combined with killed *Bordetella pertussis* organisms as a triple vaccine, adsorbed diphtheria, tetanus, and pertussis vaccine (DTPer/Vac/Ads), see schedule, section 14.1.

In children, the triple vaccine not only gives protection against tetanus in childhood but also gives the basic immunity for subsequent booster doses of adsorbed tetanus vaccine at school entry and at school leaving (combined with low-dose adsorbed diphtheria vaccine) and also when a potentially tetanus-contaminated injury has been received. Normally, booster doses of adsorbed tetanus vaccine should not be given unless more than 10 years have elapsed since the last booster dose because of the possibility that hypersensitivity reactions may develop. If a child over the age of 13 years requires a tetanus booster for a tetanus-prone wound then, provided more than 10 years have elapsed since the school-entry booster, adsorbed tetanus vaccine combined with low-dose adsorbed diphtheria vaccine can be given; the routine booster at school-leaving age is omitted.

Active immunisation is important for persons in older age groups who may never have had a routine or complete course of immunisation when younger. In these persons a course of adsorbed tetanus vaccine may be given. Very rarely, tetanus has developed after abdominal surgery; patients awaiting elective surgery should be asked about tetanus immunisation and immunised if necessary. All laboratory staff should be offered a primary course if unimmunised.

Any adult who has received 5 doses is likely to have life-long immunity; booster doses on injury should only be required if more than 10 years have elapsed since the last dose.

Wounds are considered to be tetanus-prone if they are sustained *either* more than 6 hours before surgical treatment *or* at any interval after injury and are puncture-type or show much devitalised tissue or are septic or are contaminated with soil or manure. All wounds should receive thorough surgical toilet. For *clean wounds,* a booster dose of adsorbed tetanus vaccine is given if the primary course (or booster dose) was given more than 10 years previously; non-immunised individuals (or whose immunisation status is not known) should be given a full course of the vaccine. For *tetanus-prone wounds,* treatment is as for clean wounds with the addition of a dose of tetanus immunoglobulin (section 14.5); in an immunised individual who has received a dose of adsorbed tetanus vaccine within the previous 10 years, the immunoglobulin may only be needed if the risk of infection is considered to be especially high (e.g. contamination with manure). Antibiotic treatment (with benzylpenicillin or co-amoxiclav) may also be required for tetanus-prone wounds.

See section 14.1 for general contra-indications

Single antigen vaccines
The BP directs that when Tetanus Vaccine is prescribed or demanded and the form is not stated, Adsorbed Tetanus Vaccine may be dispensed or supplied.
PoM **Adsorbed Tetanus Vaccine** Tet/Vac/Ads.
Prepared from tetanus formol toxoid with a mineral carrier (aluminium hydroxide).
  Dose: 0.5 mL or as stated on the label, by intramuscular or deep subcutaneous injection followed after 4 weeks by a second dose and after a further 4 weeks by a third
  Available from Evans (net price 0.5-mL amp = 71p, and as **Clostet**®, net price 0.5-mL single-dose syringe = £1.40) and from Pasteur Mérieux (net price 0.5-mL amp = 55p; 0.5-mL single-dose syringe = £1.20; 5-mL vial = £2.80)
Combined vaccines, see Diphtheria Vaccines

TYPHOID VACCINES
Typhoid immunisation is advised for travellers to countries where sanitation standards may be poor, although it is not a substitute for scrupulous personal hygiene (see section 14.6). Immunisation is also advised for laboratory workers handling specimens from suspected cases.

The original **whole cell typhoid vaccine** (no longer available) was normally given in 2 doses at intervals of 4–6 weeks for primary immunisation, with booster doses about every 3 years on continued exposure.

Capsular **polysaccharide typhoid vaccine** is given by *intramuscular or deep subcutaneous injection* with a booster dose every 3 years on continued exposure. Local reactions, including pain, swelling or erythema, may appear 48–72 hours after administration.

An **oral typhoid vaccine** is also available. It is a **live attenuated** vaccine contained in an enteric-coated capsule. It is taken *by mouth* as three doses of one capsule on alternate days, providing protection 7–10 days after the last dose. Protection may persist for up to 3 years in those constantly (or repeatedly) exposed to *Salmonella typhi*, but occasional travellers require a repeat course at intervals of 1 year. Oral typhoid vaccine is **contra-indicated** in individuals who are immunosuppressed (whether due to disease or its treatment) and is inactivated by concomitant administration of *antibiotics* or *sulphonamides*. Oral typhoid vaccine and oral poliomyelitis vaccine should be given at least 3 weeks apart on theoretical grounds. Administration of a dose of oral typhoid vaccine should be coordinated so that *mefloquine* is not taken for at least 12 hours before or after a dose (vaccination with oral typhoid vaccine should preferably be completed at least 3 days before the first dose of mefloquine). Side-effects to oral typhoid vaccine include nausea, vomiting, abdominal cramps, diarrhoea, headache, fever and hypersensitivity reactions including, rarely, anaphylaxis.

For general contra-indications to vaccines, see section 14.1.

Whole cell vaccine for injection

PoM **Typhoid Vaccine** Typhoid/Vac. A suspension of killed *Salmonella typhi* organisms.
Note. No longer available.

Polysaccharide vaccine for injection

PoM **Typhim Vi®** (Pasteur Mérieux)
Vi capsular polysaccharide typhoid vaccine, 50 micrograms/mL virulence polysaccharide antigen of *Salmonella typhi*. Net price 0.5-mL single-dose prefilled syringe = £10.68
Dose: 0.5 mL by deep subcutaneous or intramuscular injection; CHILD under 18 months, may show suboptimal response

Live oral vaccine

PoM **Vivotif®** (Evans)
Capsules, e/c, live attenuated *Salmonella typhi* (Ty 21a). Net price 3-cap pack = £14.85. Label: 23, 25, C, administration
Dose: ADULT and CHILD over 6 years, 1 capsule on days 1, 3, and 5; under 6 years, not recommended
COUNSELLING. Swallow as soon as possible after placing in mouth with a cold or lukewarm drink; it is important to store in refrigerator

YELLOW FEVER VACCINE

Yellow fever vaccine consists of a live attenuated yellow fever virus (17D strain) grown in developing chick embryos. Immunisation is indicated for those travelling or living in areas where infection is endemic (see p. 533) and for laboratory staff who handle the virus or who handle clinical material from suspected cases. Infants under 9 months of age should only be vaccinated if the risk of yellow fever is unavoidable since there is a small risk of encephalitis. The vaccine should not be given to those with impaired immune responsiveness, or who have had an anaphylactic reaction to egg; it should not be given during pregnancy (but where there is a significant risk of exposure the need for immunisation outweighs any risk to the fetus). See section 14.1 for further contra-indications. Reactions are few. The immunity which probably lasts for life is officially accepted for 10 years starting from 10 days after primary immunisation and for a further 10 years immediately after revaccination.

PoM **Yellow Fever Vaccine, Live** Yel/Vac.
A suspension of chick embryo proteins containing attenuated 17D strain virus
Dose: 0.5 mL by subcutaneous injection
Available (only to designated Yellow Fever Vaccination centres) as Arilvax® (Evans)

14.5   Immunoglobulins

Human immunoglobulins have replaced immunoglobulins of animal origin (antisera) which were frequently associated with hypersensitivity. Injection of immunoglobulins produces immediate protection lasting for several weeks.

The two types of human immunoglobulin preparation are **normal immunoglobulin** and **specific immunoglobulins**.

Further information about immunoglobulins is included in *Immunisation against Infectious Disease* (see section 14.1).

AVAILABILITY. **Normal immunoglobulin** is now only available from the *Public Health Laboratory Service* laboratories for contacts and the control of outbreaks. It is available commercially for other purposes.

Specific immunoglobulins are available from the *Public Health Laboratory Service* laboratories and *Regional Blood Transfusion Centres* in England and Wales with the exception of **tetanus immunoglobulin** which is distributed through *Regional Blood Transfusion Centres* to hospital pharmacies or blood transfusion departments and is also available to general medical practitioners. **Rabies immunoglobulin** is available from the *Central Public Health Laboratory, London.* The large amounts of **hepatitis B immunoglobulin** required by transplant centres should be obtained commercially.

In Scotland all immunoglobulins are available from the *Blood Transfusion Service.* **Tetanus immunoglobulin** is distributed by the *Blood Transfusion Service* to hospitals and general medical practitioners on demand.

NORMAL IMMUNOGLOBULIN
(Gamma Globulin)
Human **normal immunoglobulin** ('HNIG') is prepared from pools of at least 1000 donations of human plasma; it contains antibody to measles, mumps, varicella, hepatitis A, and other viruses that are currently prevalent in the general population.

CAUTIONS and SIDE-EFFECTS. Side-effects of immunoglobulins include malaise, chills, fever, and rarely anaphylaxis. Normal immunoglobulin is **contra-indicated** in patients with known class specific antibody to immunoglobulin A (IgA).

Normal immunoglobulin may **interfere with the immune response to live virus vaccines** which should therefore only be given **at least 3 weeks before or 3 months after** an injection of normal immunoglobulin (this does not apply to yellow fever vaccine since normal immunoglobulin does not contain antibody to this virus). For travellers, if there is insufficient time, the recommended interval may have to be ignored.

INTRAMUSCULAR

Normal immunoglobulin is administered by intramuscular injection for the protection of susceptible contacts against **hepatitis A** virus (infectious hepatitis), **measles** and, to a lesser extent, **rubella**.

HEPATITIS A. Control of hepatitis A depends on good hygiene and many studies have also shown the value of normal immunoglobulin in the prevention and control of outbreaks of this disease. It is recommended for controlling infection in contacts in closed institutions and also, under certain conditions, in school and home contacts, and for occasional or short-term travellers going to areas where the disease is highly endemic (all countries excluding Northern and Western Europe, North America, Australia, and New Zealand). **Hepatitis A vaccine** (see p. 522) is preferred for those visiting such countries frequently or who stay for longer than 3 months.

MEASLES. Normal immunoglobulin may be given for prophylaxis in children with compromised immunity (and in adults with compromised immunity who have no measles antibodies); it should be given as soon as possible after contact with measles. It should also be given to children under 12 months with recent severe illness for whom measles should be avoided; MMR vaccine should then be given (after an interval of **at least** 3 months) at around the usual age.

RUBELLA. Immunoglobulin after exposure does **not** prevent infection in non-immune contacts and is **not** recommended for protection of pregnant women exposed to rubella. It may however reduce the likelihood of a clinical attack which may possibly reduce the risk to the fetus. It should only be used when termination of pregnancy would be unacceptable when it should be given as soon as possible after exposure. Serological follow-up of recipients is essential. For routine prophylaxis, see **Rubella Vaccine** (p. 528).

REPLACEMENT THERAPY. Normal immunoglobulin may also be given intramuscularly for replacement therapy, but intravenous formulations (see below under Intravenous) are normally preferred.

For intramuscular use
PoM **Normal Immunoglobulin** Normal immunoglobulin injection. 250-mg vial; 750-mg vial
Dose: by deep intramuscular injection, Hepatitis A travel prophylaxis (2 months or less abroad), 250 mg; CHILD under 10 years 125 mg; longer travel prophylaxis

(3–5 months abroad, but see notes above) and to control outbreaks, 500 mg; CHILD under 10 years 250 mg
Measles prophylaxis, CHILD under 1 year 250 mg, 1–2 years 500 mg, 3 years and over 750 mg; to allow attenuated attack, CHILD under 1 year 100 mg, 1 year and over 250 mg
Rubella in pregnancy, prevention of clinical attack, 750 mg
Available from BPL and SNBTS and from Public Health Laboratory Service (for contacts and control of outbreaks only, see above)

PoM **Gammabulin®** (Immuno)
Normal immunoglobulin injection. Net price 2-mL vial = £3.12; 5-mL vial = £6.35; 10-mL vial = £10.70
Dose: see below

PoM **Kabiglobulin®** (Pharmacia & Upjohn)
Normal immunoglobulin injection 16%. Net price 2-mL amp = £2.78; 5-mL amp = £6.00
Dose: see below

Note. Doses for Gammabulin® and Kabiglobulin® are expressed in terms of volume:
Dose: by intramuscular injection,
Hepatitis A prophylaxis, ADULT and CHILD 0.02–0.04 mL/kg; greater exposure risk, 0.06–0.12 mL/kg
Measles prophylaxis, 0.2 mL/kg; to allow attenuated attack, 0.04 mL/kg
Rubella in pregnancy, prevention of clinical attack, 20 mL
Antibody deficiency syndromes, consult product literature

INTRAVENOUS

Special formulations for intravenous administration are available for replacement therapy for patients with congenital agammaglobulinaemia and hypogammaglobulinaemia, for the treatment of idiopathic thrombocytopenic purpura and Kawasaki syndrome, and for the prophylaxis of infection following bone marrow transplantation.

For intravenous use
PoM **Normal Immunoglobulin for Intravenous Use**
Available as: *Alphaglobin®* (2.5 g, 5 g, 10 g Alpha); *Gamimune-N®* (500 mg, 2.5 g, 5 g—Cutter); Human Immunoglobulin (3 g, 5 g, 10 g—SNBTS); *Octagam®* (2.5 g, 5 g, 10 g—Octapharma); *Sandoglobulin®* (1 g, 3 g, 6 g—Sandoz); *Vigam®S* (2.5 g, 5 g—BPL); *Vigam®Liquid* (5 g—BPL)

SPECIFIC IMMUNOGLOBULINS
Specific immunoglobulins are prepared by pooling the plasma of selected donors with high levels of the specific antibody required.

Although a hepatitis B vaccine is now available for those at high risk of infection, specific **hepatitis B immunoglobulin** ('HBIG') is available for use in association with the vaccine for the prevention of infection in laboratory and other personnel who have been accidentally inoculated with hepatitis B virus, and in infants born to mothers who have become infected with this virus in pregnancy or who are high-risk carriers.

Following exposure of an unimmunised individual to an animal in or from a high-risk country, specific **rabies immunoglobulin** of human origin should be injected at the site of the bite and also given intramuscularly. Rabies vaccine should also be given (for details see Rabies Vaccine, p. 528).

For tetanus-prone wounds, **tetanus immuno-globulin** of human origin ('HTIG') should be used in addition to wound toilet, antibiotic treatment and, where appropriate, adsorbed tetanus vaccine (see p. 529).

Varicella-zoster immunoglobulin (VZIG) is recommended for individuals who are at increased risk of severe varicella *and* who have no antibodies to varicella-zoster virus *and* who have significant exposure to chickenpox or herpes zoster. Those at increased risk include neonates of women who develop chickenpox 7 days before or 28 days after delivery, women exposed at any stage of pregnancy, and the immunosuppressed including those who have received corticosteroids in the previous 3 months at the following dose equivalents of prednisolone: *children* 2 mg/kg daily for at least 1 week or 1 mg/kg daily for 1 month; *adults* about 40 mg daily for more than 1 week. (**Important:** for full details consult *Immunisation against Infectious Disease*). **Varicella vaccine** is available on a named-patient basis from SmithKline Beecham or Pasteur Mérieux.

Cytomegalovirus immunoglobulin (available on a named-patient basis from Alpha as *Alphaglobin CMV®*) is indicated for prophylaxis in patients receiving immunosuppressive treatment

Hepatitis B

PoM **Hepatitis B Immunoglobulin** See notes above
Dose: by intramuscular injection (as soon as possible after exposure), ADULT 500 units; CHILD under 4 years 200 units, 5–9 years 300 units; NEONATE 200 units as soon as possible after birth; for full details consult *Immunisation against Infectious Disease*
Available from Public Health Laboratory Service (except for Transplant Centres, see p. 530), also available from BPL and SNBTS

Rabies

PoM **Rabies Immunoglobulin** (Antirabies Immunoglobulin Injection). See notes above
Dose: 20 units/kg, half by intramuscular injection and half by infiltration around wound
Available from Public Health Laboratory Service (also from BPL and SNBTS)

Tetanus

PoM **Tetanus Immunoglobulin** (Antitetanus Immunoglobulin Injection). See notes above
Dose: by intramuscular injection, prophylactic 250 units, increased to 500 units if more than 24 hours have elapsed or there is risk of heavy contamination
Therapeutic, 150 units/kg (multiple sites)
Available from BPL and SNBTS

PoM **Tetabulin®** (Immuno)
Tetanus immunoglobulin. Net price 250 unit prefilled syringe = £15.50
Dose: by intramuscular injection, prophylactic, 250 units, increased to 500 units if wound older than 12 hours or if risk of heavy contamination or if patient weighs more than 90 kg; second dose of 250 units given after 3–4 weeks if patient immunosuppressed or if active immunisation with tetanus vaccine contra-indicated
Therapeutic, 30–300 units/kg

PoM **Tetanus Immunoglobulin for Intravenous Use.** Used for proven or suspected clinical tetanus
Dose: by intravenous infusion, 5000–10 000 units
Available from SNBTS (2500-unit vial) on a named patient basis

Varicella–Zoster

PoM **Varicella-Zoster Immunoglobulin** (Antivaricella-zoster Immunoglobulin) See notes above
Dose: by deep intramuscular injection, prophylaxis (as soon as possible—not later than 10 days after exposure), CHILD up to 5 years 250 mg, 6–10 years 500 mg, 11–14 years 750 mg, over 15 years 1 g; second dose required if further exposure occurs after 3 weeks
Note. No evidence that effective in treatment of severe disease. An *intravenous* preparation of **normal immunoglobulin** (see Intravenous Therapy, p. 531) may be used to provide an immediate source of antibody.
Available from Public Health Laboratory Service (also from BPL and SNBTS)

ANTI-D (Rh$_0$) IMMUNOGLOBULIN

Anti-D (Rh$_0$) immunoglobulin is available to prevent a rhesus-negative mother from forming antibodies to fetal rhesus-positive cells which may pass into the maternal circulation during childbirth or abortion. It should be injected within 72 hours of the birth or abortion but even if a longer period has elapsed it may still give protection and should be administered. The objective is to protect any subsequent child from the hazard of haemolytic disease of the newborn.

Note. Rubella vaccine may be administered in the postpartum period simultaneously with anti-D (Rh$_0$) immunoglobulin injection providing separate syringes are used and the products are administered into contralateral limbs. If blood is transfused, the antibody response to the vaccine may be inhibited and a test for antibodies should be performed after 8 weeks and the subject revaccinated if necessary.

MMR vaccine should not be given within 3 months of an injection of anti-D (Rh$_0$) immunoglobulin injection.

PoM **Anti-D (Rh$_0$) Immunoglobulin**

Available from Regional Blood Transfusion Centres and from BPL and SNBTS
Dose: by deep intramuscular injection, to rhesus-negative woman for prevention of Rh$_0$(D) sensitisation:

Following abortion or birth of rhesus-positive infant, 500 units immediately or within 72 hours; for transplacental bleed in excess of 4–5 mL fetal red cells, extra 100–125 units per mL fetal red cells

Following any potentially sensitising episode (e.g. stillbirth, amniocentesis) up to 20 weeks' gestation 250 units per episode (after 20 weeks, 500 units) immediately or within 72 hours

Following Rh$_0$(D) incompatible blood transfusion, 125 units per mL transfused rhesus-positive red cells

Antenatal prophylaxis, 500 units may be given at weeks 28 and 34 of pregnancy; a further dose is still needed immediately or within 72 hours of delivery

PoM **Partobulin®** (Immuno)

Anti-D (Rh$_0$) immunoglobulin 1250 units/mL, net price 1-mL prefilled syringe = £16.48

Dose: by intramuscular injection, to rhesus-negative woman for prevention of Rh$_0$(D) sensitisation:

Following abortion, miscarriage or birth of rhesus-positive infant, 1250 units immediately or within 72 hours; for transplacental bleed in excess of 25 mL fetal blood (1% of fetal erythrocytes), 5000 units (*or* 50 units per mL fetal blood)

Following any potentially sensitising episode (e.g. amniocentesis) 1250 units immediately or within 72 hours

Following Rh$_0$(D) incompatible blood transfusion, at least 50–100 units per mL transfused rhesus-positive blood

Antenatal prophylaxis, 1250 units may be given at weeks 28 and 34 of pregnancy; a further dose is still needed immediately or within 72 hours of delivery

Note. Some UK authorities recommend lower doses for antenatal prophylaxis (see under Anti-D (Rh$_0$) Immunoglobulin, above)

INTERFERONS

Interferon gamma-1b is indicated for chronic granulomatous disease to reduce the frequency of serious infection.

INTERFERON GAMMA-1b

(Immune interferon)

Indications: adjunct to antibiotics to reduce frequency of serious infection in patients with chronic granulomatous disease

Cautions: severe hepatic or renal impairment; seizure disorders or compromised central nervous system function; pre-existing cardiac disease (including ischaemia, congestive heart failure, and arrhythmias); monitor before and during treatment: haematological tests (including full blood count, differential white cell count, and platelet count), blood chemistry tests (including renal and liver function tests) and urinalysis

DRIVING. May impair ability to drive or operate machinery; effects may be enhanced by alcohol

Side-effects: fever, headache, chills, myalgia, fatigue; nausea, vomiting, arthralgia, rashes and injection-site reactions reported

▼ PoM **Immukin®** (Boehringer Ingelheim)

Injection, recombinant human interferon gamma-1b 200 micrograms/mL. Net price 0.5-mL vial = £88.00

Dose: by subcutaneous injection, 50 micrograms/m^2 3 times a week; patients with body surface area of 0.5 m^2 or less, 1.5 micrograms/kg 3 times a week; not yet recommended for children under 6 months

14.6   International travel

Note. For advice on **malaria chemoprophylaxis**, see section 5.4.1.

No particular immunisation is required for travellers to the United States, Europe, Australia, or New Zealand although all travellers should have immu-

nity to tetanus and poliomyelitis (and childhood immunisations should be up to date). In Non-European areas surrounding the Mediterranean, in Africa, the Middle East, Asia, and South America, certain special precautions are required.

Long-term travellers to areas that have a high incidence of **poliomyelitis** or **tuberculosis** should be immunised with the appropriate vaccine; in the case of poliomyelitis previously immunised adults may be given a booster dose of oral poliomyelitis vaccine. BCG immunisation is recommended for travellers proposing to stay for longer than one month (or in close contact with the local population) in Asia, Africa, or Central and South America; it should preferably be given three months or more before departure.

Yellow fever immunisation is recommended for travel to much of Africa and South America. Many countries require an International Certificate of Vaccination from individuals arriving from, or who have been travelling through, endemic areas, whilst other countries require a certificate from all entering travellers (consult the Department of Health Handbook, *Health Information for Overseas Travel*).

Immunisation against **meningococcal meningitis** is recommended for a number of areas of the world (for details, see p. 525).

Protection against **hepatitis A** is recommended for travellers to high-risk areas outside Northern and Western Europe, North America, Australia and New Zealand. Hepatitis A vaccine (see p. 522) is preferred, particularly for frequent travellers or for stays longer than 3 months. Normal immunoglobulin (see p. 531) can be used as an alternative for short or infrequent travel (but may interfere with immune response to live viral vaccines, see section 14.5 under Normal Immunoglobulin).

Prophylactic immunisation against **rabies** (see p. 528) is recommended for travellers to enzootic areas on long journeys to remote areas out of reach of immediate medical attention.

Typhoid vaccine is indicated for travellers to those countries where typhoid is endemic but the vaccine is no substitute for personal precautions. Food should be freshly prepared and hot, and uncooked vegetables (including green salads) should be avoided; only fruits which can be peeled should be eaten. Only suitable bottled water, or tap water that has been boiled, or treated with sterilising tablets should be used for drinking. This advice also applies to cholera and other diarrhoeal diseases (including travellers' diarrhoea).

Cholera vaccine has little value in preventing infections and should **not** be given for international travel (see under Cholera Vaccine). It is no longer available.

Advice on **diphtheria,** on **Japanese encephalitis** (vaccine available on named-patient basis from Pasteur Mérieux) and on **tick-borne encephalitis** (vaccine available on named-patient basis from Immuno) is included in *Health Information for Overseas Travel*, see below.

Information on health advice for travellers

The Department of Health booklet, *Health Advice For Travellers* (code: T5) includes information on immunisation requirements (or recommendations) around the world. The booklet can be obtained from travel agents, post-offices or by telephoning 0800 555 777 (24-hour service).

The Department of Health handbook, *Health Information for Overseas Travel,* which draws together essential information *for doctors* regarding health advice for travellers, can be obtained from

The Stationery Office,
The Publications Centre,
PO Box 276, London SW8 5DT
Telephone orders, 0171 873 9090

Immunisation requirements change from time to time, and information on the current requirements for any particular country may be obtained from:

Communicable Disease Surveillance Centre Travel Unit, 61 Colindale Avenue, London NW9 5EQ (Tel 0181-200 6868), (for health care professionals only)

Communicable Diseases (Scotland) Unit, Ruchill Hospital, Bilslend Drive, Glasgow G20 9NB (Tel 0141-946 7120)

Scottish Office Department of Health, Public Health Policy Unit, St. Andrew's House, Edinburgh EH1 3DG (Tel 0131-556 8400)

Welsh Office, Cathays Park, Cardiff CF1 3NQ (Tel 01222 825111)

Department of Health and Social Services, Castle Buildings, Stormont, Belfast BT4 3PP (Tel 01232 520000)

or from the embassy or legation of the appropriate country.

     Prices are **net**, see p. 1

15: Drugs used in
ANAESTHESIA

This chapter describes briefly drugs used in anaesthesia; the reader is referred to other sources for more detailed information. The chapter is divided into two sections:
15.1 General anaesthesia
15.2 Local anaesthesia

15.1   General anaesthesia

15.1.1 Intravenous anaesthetics
15.1.2 Inhalational anaesthetics
15.1.3 Antimuscarinic drugs
15.1.4 Sedative and analgesic peri-operative drugs
15.1.5 Muscle relaxants
15.1.6 Anticholinesterases used in anaesthesia
15.1.7 Antagonists for central and respiratory depression
15.1.8 Drugs for malignant hyperthermia

Note. The drugs in section 15.1 should be used only by experienced personnel and where adequate resuscitative equipment is available.

ANAESTHESIA AND DRIVING. Patients given sedatives and analgesics during minor outpatient procedures should be very carefully warned about the risk of driving afterwards. For intravenous benzodiazepines and for a short general anaesthetic the risk extends to **at least 24 hours** after administration. Responsible persons should be available to take patients home. The dangers of taking **alcohol** should also be emphasised.

MODERN ANAESTHETIC TECHNIQUE. It is now common practice to administer several drugs with different actions to produce a state of surgical anaesthesia with minimal risk of toxic effects. An intravenous anaesthetic is usually used for induction, followed by maintenance with inhalational anaesthetics, perhaps supplemented by other drugs administered intravenously. Specific drugs are often used to produce muscular relaxation. These drugs interfere with spontaneous respiration so intermittent positive pressure ventilation by manual or mechanical means is commonly employed.

For certain procedures controlled hypotension may be required. Labetalol (see section 2.4), sodium nitroprusside (see section 2.5.1), and glyceryl trinitrate (see section 2.6.1) are used.

Beta-blockers (see section 2.4), adenosine, amiodarone (see section 2.3.2) or verapamil (see section 2.6.2) may be used to control arrhythmias during anaesthesia. Esmolol has a very short duration of action and is particularly suited to the peri- and intra-operative management of arrhythmias, including tachycardia, and hypertension (see section 2.4).

Glyceryl trinitrate (see section 2.6.1) is also used to control hypertension, particularly postoperatively.

SURGERY AND LONG-TERM MEDICATION. The risk of stopping long-term medication before surgery is often greater than the risk of continuing it during surgery; however, surgery itself may alter the need for continued drug therapy of certain conditions.

Patients with adrenal atrophy due to long-term corticosteroid use (section 6.3.2) may experience a precipitous fall in blood pressure unless corticosteroid cover is provided during anaesthesia and in the immediate postoperative period. Anaesthetists must therefore know whether a patient is, or has been, taking corticosteroids.

Other drugs that should not normally be stopped before surgery include analgesics, antiepileptics, bronchodilators, cardiovascular drugs, glaucoma drugs, and thyroid or antithyroid drugs. For general advice on surgery in diabetic patients see section 6.1.1.

Although it is possible to operate on patients taking oral anticoagulants when the INR is close to 2.0, many surgeons and anaesthetists prefer to stop oral anticoagulants. Individual circumstances will dictate whether it is appropriate to continue prophylaxis in the peri-operative period with either heparin or low molecular weight heparin until oral anticoagulation can be re-established; the haematologist should be consulted for further advice.

Drugs that should be stopped before surgery include combined oral contraceptives (discontinue 4 weeks before major elective surgery with adequate alternative contraceptive arrangements—see Surgery, section 7.3.1 for details); for advice on hormone replacement therapy, see section 6.4.1.1. In view of their hazardous interactions MAOIs should normally be stopped 2 weeks before surgery. Tricyclic antidepressants need not be stopped, but there may be an increased risk of arrhythmias and hypotension (and dangerous interaction with vasopressor drugs), therefore the anaesthetist should be informed if they are not. Lithium should be stopped 2 days before major surgery but the normal dose can be continued for minor surgery (with careful monitoring of fluids and electrolytes). To avoid withdrawal symptoms antidepressants need to be withdrawn gradually (see section 4.3).

It is vital that the anaesthetist should know of **all** drugs that a patient is (or has been) taking.

PROPHYLAXIS OF ACID ASPIRATION. Regurgitation and aspiration of gastric contents (Mendelson's syndrome) is an important complication of general anaesthesia, particularly in obstetrics and emergency surgery. The damage to the lung is influenced by both the pH and the volume of the gastric contents aspirated.

H₂-receptor antagonists (section 1.3.1) or **omeprazole** (section 1.3.5) may be used before surgery to increase the pH and reduce the volume of gastric fluid. They do not affect the pH of fluid already in the stomach and this limits their value in emergency procedures; oral H_2-receptor antagonists can be given 1–2 hours before the procedure but omeprazole must be given at least 12 hours earlier. Antacids are frequently used to neutralise the acidity of the fluid already in the stomach; 'clear' (nonparticulate) antacids such as sodium citrate are preferred.

GAS CYLINDERS

Each gas cylinder bears a label with the name of the gas contained in the cylinder. The name or chemical symbol of the gas appears on the shoulder of the cylinder and is also clearly and indelibly stamped on the cylinder valve.

The colours on the valve end of the cylinder extend down to the shoulder; in the case of mixed gases the colours for the individual gases are applied in four segments, two for each colour.

Gas cylinders should be stored in a cool well-ventilated room, free from flammable materials.

No lubricant of any description should be used on the cylinder valves.

15.1.1   Intravenous anaesthetics

Intravenous anaesthetics may be used alone to produce anaesthesia for short surgical procedures but are more commonly used for induction only. Intravenous anaesthetics nearly all produce their effect in one arm-brain circulation time and can cause apnoea and hypotension, and so adequate resuscitative facilities **must** be available. They are **contraindicated** if the anaesthetist is not confident of being able to maintain the airway (e.g. in the presence of a tumour in the pharynx or larynx). Extreme care is required in surgery of the mouth, pharynx, or larynx and in patients with acute cardiovascular failure (shock) or fixed cardiac output.

Individual requirements vary considerably and the recommended dosage is only a guide. Smaller dosage is indicated in ill, shocked, or debilitated patients, while robust individuals may require more. To facilitate tracheal intubation, induction is followed by a neuromuscular blocking drug (section 15.1.5).

TOTAL INTRAVENOUS ANAESTHESIA. This is a technique in which major surgery is carried out with all anaesthetic drugs given intravenously. Respiration is controlled, the lungs being inflated with oxygen-enriched air. Muscle relaxants are used to provide relaxation and prevent reflex muscle movements. The main problem to be overcome is the assessment of depth of anaesthesia.

ANAESTHESIA AND DRIVING. See previous page.

BARBITURATES

Thiopentone sodium (thiopental sodium) is a widely used intravenous anaesthetic, but has no analgesic properties. Induction is generally smooth and rapid, but owing to its narrow therapeutic mar-

gin, overdosage with cardiorespiratory depression may occur. The solution is highly alkaline and therefore irritant on misplaced injection outside the vein; arterial injection is particularly dangerous.

Awakening from a moderate dose of thiopentone is rapid due to redistribution of the drug in the whole body tissues. Metabolism is, however, slow and some sedative effects may persist for 24 hours. Repeated doses have a cumulative effect.

Methohexitone sodium (methohexital sodium) is less irritant to tissues than thiopentone. Recovery is marginally more rapid than in the case of thiopentone, but induction is less smooth with an incidence of hiccup, tremor, involuntary movements, and pain on injection.

Both thiopentone and methohexitone are **contraindicated** in porphyria (see section 9.8.2).

METHOHEXITONE SODIUM
(Methohexital Sodium)

Indications: induction and maintenance of anaesthesia for short procedures; with other anaesthetics for more prolonged anaesthesia

Cautions; Contra-indications; Side-effects: avoid or reduce dose in liver disease; see also under Thiopentone Sodium and notes above

Dose: *by intravenous injection,* usually as a 1% solution, 50–120 mg according to response at rate of 10 mg in 5 seconds; maintenance, 20–40 mg (2–4 mL of 1% solution) every 4–7 minutes; CHILD induction 1–1.5 mg/kg according to response

PoM **Brietal Sodium**® (Lilly)

Injection, powder for reconstitution, methohexitone sodium, net price 500 mg in 50-mL vial = £2.95

THIOPENTONE SODIUM
(Thiopental Sodium)

Indications: induction of general anaesthesia; anaesthesia of short duration

Cautions; Contra-indications; Side-effects: see notes above; reduce induction dose in severe liver disease; avoid in porphyria (see section 9.8.2); **interactions:** Appendix 1 (anaesthetics, general)

Dose: *by intravenous injection* as a 2.5% solution, in fit premedicated adults, initially 100–150 mg (reduced in elderly or debilitated) over 10–15 seconds (longer in elderly or debilitated), followed by further quantity if necessary according to response after 30–60 seconds; *or* up to 4 mg/kg; CHILD induction 2–7 mg/kg

PoM **Intraval Sodium**® (Rhône-Poulenc Rorer)

Injection 2.5%, powder for reconstitution, thiopentone sodium. Net price 500-mg amp = £1.35 (with water for injections £1.83); 2.5-g vial = £5.03 (with water for injections £5.90)

OTHER INTRAVENOUS ANAESTHETICS

Etomidate is an induction agent associated with rapid recovery without hangover effect. It causes less hypotension than other drugs used for induction. There is a high incidence of extraneous muscle movement and of pain on injection; these effects can be minimised by premedication with an opioid analgesic and the use of larger veins. There is evidence that repeated doses of etomidate have an undesirable suppressant effect on adrenocortical function.

Propofol is associated with rapid recovery without hangover effect and is very widely used. There is sometimes pain on intravenous injection, but significant extraneous muscle movements do not occur. The CSM have received reports of convulsions, anaphylaxis, and delayed recovery from anaesthesia after propofol administration; since some of the convulsions are delayed the CSM has advised special caution after day surgery. Propofol has been associated with bradycardia, occasionally profound; intravenous administration of an antimuscarinic may be necessary to prevent this.

Ketamine can be given by the intravenous or the intramuscular route, and has good analgesic properties when used in sub-anaesthetic dosage. The maximum effect occurs after more than one arm-brain circulation time. Muscle tone is increased. There is cardiovascular stimulation and arterial pressure may rise with tachycardia. The main disadvantage is the high incidence of hallucinations and other transient psychotic sequelae, though it is believed that these are much less significant in children. The incidence can be reduced when drugs such as diazepam are also used. Ketamine is **contra-indicated** in patients with hypertension and is best avoided in those prone to hallucinations. It is used mainly for paediatric anaesthesia, particularly when repeated administrations are required. Recovery is relatively slow.

ETOMIDATE

Indications: induction of anaesthesia

Cautions; Contra-indications; Side-effects: see notes above; porphyria (see section 9.8.2); **interactions:** Appendix 1 (anaesthetics, general)

Dose: by slow intravenous injection, 300 micrograms/kg; high-risk patients, 100 micrograms/kg/minute until anaesthetised (about 3 minutes)

PoM **Hypnomidate®** (Janssen-Cilag)

Injection, etomidate 2 mg/mL in propylene glycol 35%. Net price 10-mL amp = £1.58

KETAMINE

Indications: induction and maintenance of anaesthesia

Cautions; Contra-indications; Side-effects: see notes above; **interactions:** Appendix 1 (anaesthetics, general)

Dose: by intramuscular injection, short procedures, initially 6.5–13 mg/kg (10 mg/kg usually produces 12–25 minutes of surgical anaesthesia) Diagnostic manoeuvres and procedures not involving intense pain, initially 4 mg/kg

By intravenous injection over at least 60 seconds, short procedures, initially 1–4.5 mg/kg (2 mg/kg usually produces 5–10 minutes of surgical anaesthesia)

By intravenous infusion of a solution containing 1 mg/mL, longer procedures, induction, total dose of 0.5–2 mg/kg; maintenance (using microdrip infusion), 10–45 micrograms/kg/minute, rate adjusted according to response

PoM **Ketalar®** (P-D)

Injection, ketamine (as hydrochloride) 10 mg/mL, net price 20-mL vial = £3.52; 50 mg/mL, 10-mL vial = £7.31; 100 mg/mL, 10-mL vial = £13.42

PROPOFOL

Indications: see under Dose

Cautions; Contra-indications; Side-effects: see notes above; monitor blood lipid concentrations in patients at risk of fat overload; contra-indicated if history of propofol allergy (see CSM warning above); bacterial contamination (see below); **interactions:** Appendix 1 (anaesthetics, general)

BACTERIAL CONTAMINATION. In order to eliminate the **risk of infection** from bacterial contamination **strict aseptic technique** must be used when drawing-up propofol emulsion

Dose: induction of anaesthesia, *by intravenous injection,* 1.5–2.5 mg/kg (less in those over 55 years) at a rate of 20–40 mg every 10 seconds (lower end of range in those over 55 years); CHILD over 3 years 2.5 mg/kg adjusted as necessary

Maintenance of anaesthesia, *by intravenous infusion,* 4–12 mg/kg/hour *or by intravenous injection,* 25–50 mg repeated according to response; CHILD over 3 years 9–15 mg/kg/hour

Sedation during intensive care (with assisted ventilation), *by intravenous infusion,* 0.3–4 mg/kg/hour for up to 3 days; CHILD not recommended

Sedation for surgical and diagnostic procedures, initially *by intravenous injection,* 0.5–1 mg/kg over 1–5 minutes; maintenance, *by intravenous infusion,* 1.5–4.5 mg/kg/hour (in addition, if rapid increase in depth of sedation required, *by intravenous injection,* 10–20 mg); those over 55 years may require lower dose; CHILD not recommended

PoM **Diprivan®** (Zeneca)

Injection (emulsion), propofol 10 mg/mL, net price 20-mL amp = £3.88, 50-mL vial = £9.70, 50-mL prefilled syringe (for use with Diprifusor® TCI system) = £10.67, 100-mL vial = £19.40

Note. Diprifusor® TCI system is for use **only** for induction and maintenance of general anaesthesia in adults

15.1.2   Inhalational anaesthetics

Inhalational anaesthetics may be gases or volatile liquids. They can be used both for induction and maintenance of anaesthesia and may also be used following induction with an intravenous anaesthetic (section 15.1.1).

Gaseous anaesthetics require suitable equipment for storage and administration. They may be supplied via hospital pipelines or from metal cylinders. *Volatile liquid anaesthetics* are administered using calibrated vaporisers, using air, oxygen, or nitrous oxide–oxygen mixtures as the carrier gas. It should be noted that they can all trigger malignant hyperthermia (section 15.1.8).

To prevent hypoxia inhalational anaesthetics must be given with concentrations of oxygen greater than in air.

ANAESTHESIA AND DRIVING. See section 15.1.

VOLATILE LIQUID ANAESTHETICS

Halothane is a volatile liquid anaesthetic. Its advantages are that it is potent, induction is smooth, the vapour is non-irritant, pleasant to inhale, and seldom induces coughing or breath-holding. Despite these advantages, however, halothane is much less widely used than previously owing to its association with *severe hepatotoxicity* (**important:** see CSM advice, below).

Halothane causes cardiorespiratory depression. Respiratory depression results in elevation of arterial carbon dioxide tension and perhaps ventricular arrhythmias. Halothane also depresses the cardiac muscle fibres and may cause bradycardia. The result is diminished cardiac output and fall of arterial pressure. Adrenaline infiltrations should be avoided in patients anaesthetised with halothane as ventricular arrhythmias may result.

Halothane produces moderate muscle relaxation, but this may be inadequate for major abdominal surgery and specific muscle relaxants are then used.

CSM advice (halothane hepatotoxicity). In a publication on findings confirming that *severe hepatotoxicity* can follow halothane anaesthesia the CSM has reported that this occurs more frequently after repeated exposures to halothane and has a high mortality. The risk of severe hepatotoxicity appears to be increased by repeated exposures within a short time interval, but even after a long interval (sometimes of several years) susceptible patients have been reported to develop jaundice. Since there is no reliable way of identifying susceptible patients the CSM recommends the following precautions prior to use of halothane:

1. a careful anaesthetic history should be taken to determine previous exposure and previous reactions to halothane;
2. repeated exposure to halothane within a period of **at least** 3 months should be **avoided** unless there are **overriding** clinical circumstances;
3. a history of unexplained jaundice or pyrexia in a patient following exposure to halothane is an absolute **contra-indication** to its future use in that patient.

Enflurane is a volatile anaesthetic similar to halothane, but less potent, about twice the concentration being necessary for induction and maintenance.

Enflurane is a powerful cardiorespiratory depressant. Shallow respiration is likely to result in a rise of arterial carbon dioxide tension, but ventricular arrhythmias are uncommon and it is probably safe to use adrenaline infiltrations. Myocardial depression may result in a fall in cardiac output and in arterial hypotension. It may cause EEG changes and should be avoided in those liable to epileptic seizures. Enflurane may cause hepatotoxicity in those sensitised to halogenated anaesthetics but the risk is smaller than with halothane.

Enflurane is usually given to supplement nitrous oxide–oxygen mixtures.

Isoflurane is an isomer of enflurane. It has a potency intermediate between that of halothane and enflurane, and even less of an inhaled dose is metabolised than with enflurane. Heart rhythm is generally stable during isoflurane anaesthesia, but heart-rate may rise, particularly in younger patients. Systemic arterial pressure may fall, due to a decrease in systemic vascular resistance and with less decrease in cardiac output than occurs with halothane. Respiration is depressed. Muscle relaxation is produced and muscle relaxant drugs potentiated. Isoflurane may also cause hepatotoxicity in those sensitised to halogenated anaesthetics but the risk is appreciably smaller than with halothane.

Desflurane is reported to have about one-fifth the potency of isoflurane. Owing to limited experience it is not recommended in neurosurgical patients; owing to frequent occurrence of cough, breath-holding, apnoea, laryngospasm and increased secretions it is not recommended for induction in children. The risk of hepatotoxicity with desflurane in those sensitised to halogenated anaesthetics appears to be remote.

Sevoflurane is a newly introduced rapid acting volatile liquid anaesthetic. Patients may require early postoperative pain relief as emergence and recovery are particularly rapid.

VOLATILE ANAESTHETICS AND CARBOXYHAEMOGLOB-INAEMIA. Carboxyhaemoglobinaemia has been reported during anaesthesia with desflurane, enflurane, or isoflurane used in conjunction with carbon dioxide absorbents in breathing systems in the USA. This phenomenon was very rare and occurred when these absorbents became excessively dried out.

The use of barium hydroxide lime produces significantly more carbon monoxide than soda lime particularly at low water content.

Barium hydroxide lime is not available in the UK. The CSM has advised that no cases of carboxyhaemoglobinaemia have been reported in the UK and it seems unlikely that this problem will arise with the anaesthetic equipment currently in use in the UK.

DESFLURANE

Indications; Cautions; Contra-indications; Side-effects: see notes above; **interactions:** Appendix 1 (anaesthetics, general)

Dose: using a specifically designed calibrated vaporiser, *induction*, 4–11%; CHILD not recommended for induction

Maintenance, 2–6% in nitrous oxide; 2.5–8.5% in oxygen or oxygen-enriched air; max. 17%

PoM **Suprane®** (Pharmacia & Upjohn)
Desflurane. Net price 240 mL = £46.50

ENFLURANE

Indications; Cautions; Side-effects: see notes above; porphyria (section 9.8.2); caution is needed in epilepsy; **interactions:** Appendix 1 (anaesthetics, general)

Dose: using a specifically calibrated vaporiser, *induction*, increased gradually from 0.4% to max. of 4.5% in air, oxygen, or nitrous oxide–oxygen, according to response

Maintenance, 0.5–3% in nitrous oxide–oxygen

Enflurane (Abbott)
Enflurane. Net price 250 mL = £34.00

HALOTHANE

Indications; Cautions; Contra-indications; Side-effects: see notes above (**important:** CSM advice see also notes above); porphyria (section 9.8.2); **interactions:** Appendix 1 (anaesthetics, general)

Dose: using a specifically calibrated vaporiser, *induction*, increased gradually to 2–4% in oxygen or nitrous oxide–oxygen; CHILD 1.5–2%

Maintenance, 0.5–2%

Halothane (Concord)
Halothane. Net price 250 mL = £16.00
Fluothane® (Zeneca)
Halothane. Net price 250 mL = £16.36

ISOFLURANE

Indications; Cautions; Side-effects: see notes above; **interactions:** Appendix 1 (anaesthetics, general)

Dose: using a specifically calibrated vaporiser, *induction*, increased gradually from 0.5% to 3%, in oxygen or nitrous oxide–oxygen

Maintenance, 1–2.5% in nitrous oxide–oxygen; an additional 0.5–1% may be required when given with oxygen alone; caesarean section, 0.5–0.75% in nitrous oxide–oxygen

Isoflurane (Abbott)
Isoflurane. Net price 250 mL = £97.50

SEVOFLURANE

Indications; Cautions; Contra-indications; Side-effects: see notes above; agitation occurs frequently in children; **interactions:** Appendix 1 (anaesthetics, general)

IMPORTANT. In low-flow anaesthesia systems with soda lime, sevoflurane forms a vinyl ether ('Compound A') of unknown toxicity. Until further information becomes available, it would be wise to avoid the use of flow rates of less than 2 litres/minute with soda lime in patients with renal disease.

Dose: using a specifically calibrated vaporiser, *induction*, up to 5% in oxygen or nitrous oxide–oxygen; CHILD up to 7%

Maintenance, 0.5–3%

▼ PoM **Sevoflurane** (Abbott)
Sevoflurane. Net price 100 mL = £49.20

NITROUS OXIDE

Nitrous oxide is used for maintenance of anaesthesia and, in sub-anaesthetic concentrations, for analgesia. For *anaesthesia* it is commonly used in a concentration of 50 to 70% in oxygen as part of a balanced technique in association with other inhalational or intravenous agents. Nitrous oxide is unsatisfactory as a sole anaesthetic owing to lack of potency, but is useful as part of a sequence of drugs since it allows a significant reduction in dosage.

A mixture of nitrous oxide and oxygen containing 50% of each gas (*Entonox*®) is used to produce *analgesia without loss of consciousness*. Self-administration using a demand valve is popular and is used in obstetric practice, for changing painful dressings, as an aid to postoperative physiotherapy, and in emergency ambulances.

Nitrous oxide may have a deleterious effect if used in patients with an air-containing closed space since nitrous oxide diffuses into such a space with a resulting increase in pressure. This effect may be dangerous in the presence of a pneumothorax which may enlarge to compromise respiration.

Exposure of patients to nitrous oxide for prolonged periods, either by continuous or by intermittent administration, may result in megaloblastic anaemia due to interference with the action of vitamin B_{12}. For the same reason, exposure of theatre staff to nitrous oxide should be minimised. Depression of white cell formation may also occur.

NITROUS OXIDE

Indications; Cautions; Side-effects: see notes above; **interactions:** Appendix 1 (anaesthetics, general)

Dose: using a suitable anaesthetic apparatus, a mixture with 25–30% oxygen for *maintenance* of light anaesthesia

Analgesic, as a mixture with 50% oxygen, according to the patient's needs

15.1.3 Antimuscarinic drugs

Antimuscarinic premedication drugs are used (less commonly nowadays) to dry bronchial and salivary secretions which are increased by intubation and some inhalational anaesthetics. They are also used before or with neostigmine (section 15.1.6) to prevent bradycardia, excessive salivation, and other muscarinic actions of neostigmine. They are also used to prevent bradycardia and hypotension associated with agents such as halothane, propofol, and suxamethonium.

Atropine is now rarely used for premedication but still has an emergency role in the treatment of vagotonic side-effects. For its role in acute arrhythmias after myocardial infarction, see section 2.3.1; see also cardiopulmonary resuscitation algorithm, section 2.7.3.

Hyoscine effectively reduces secretions and also provides a degree of amnesia, sedation and anti-emesis. Unlike atropine it may produce bradycardia rather than tachycardia. In some patients, especially the elderly, hyoscine may cause the central anticholinergic syndrome (excitement, ataxia, hallucinations, behavioural abnormalities, and drowsiness).

Glycopyrronium produces good drying of salivary secretions. When given intravenously it produces less tachycardia than atropine. It is widely used with neostigmine for reversal of non-depolarising muscle relaxants (section 15.1.5).

Phenothiazines have too little drying activity to be effective when used alone.

ATROPINE SULPHATE

Indications: drying secretions, reversal of excessive bradycardia; with neostigmine for reversal of competitive neuromuscular block; other indications, see sections 1.2, 2.3.1, 11.5

Cautions: cardiovascular disease; see also section 1.2; **interactions:** Appendix 1 (antimuscarinics)

Side-effects: tachycardia; see also section 1.2

Dose: premedication, *by intravenous injection,* 300–600 micrograms immediately before induction of anaesthesia, and in incremental doses of 100 micrograms for the treatment of bradycardia

By intramuscular injection, 300–600 micrograms 30–60 minutes before induction; CHILD 20 micrograms/kg

For control of muscarinic side-effects of neostigmine in reversal of competitive neuromuscular block, *by intravenous injection,* 0.6–1.2 mg

Arrhythmias after myocardial infarction, see section 2.3.1; see also cardiopulmonary resuscitation algorithm, section 2.7.3

PoM **Atropine** (Non-proprietary)
Injection, atropine sulphate 600 micrograms/mL. Net price 1-mL amp = 32p
Note. Other strengths also available

PoM **Min-I-Jet® Atropine Sulphate** (IMS)
Injection, atropine sulphate 100 micrograms/mL, net price 5-mL disposable syringe = £3.78, 10-mL disposable syringe = £4.24, 30-mL disposable syringe = £7.75
Note. A 10-mL prefilled syringe containing atropine sulphate 300 micrograms/mL is also available from Aurum; net price 10-mL disposable syringe = £4.32

CD **Morphine and Atropine Injection,** see under Morphine Salts (section 15.1.4.3)

GLYCOPYRRONIUM BROMIDE

Indications; Cautions; Side-effects: see under Atropine Sulphate

Dose: premedication, *by intramuscular or intravenous injection,* 200–400 micrograms, *or* 4–5 micrograms/kg to a max. of 400 micrograms; CHILD, *by intramuscular or intravenous injection,* 4–8 micrograms/kg to a max. of 200 micrograms

Intra-operative use, *by intravenous injection,* as for premedication, repeated if necessary

Control of muscarinic side-effects of neostigmine in reversal of competitive neuromuscular block, *by intravenous injection,* 10–15 micrograms/kg with neostigmine 50 micrograms/kg; CHILD, 10 micrograms/kg with neostigmine 50 micrograms/kg

PoM **Robinul®** (Anpharm)
Injection, glycopyrronium bromide 200 micrograms/mL. Net price 1-mL amp = 63p; 3-mL amp = £1.06
Available as a generic from Antigen

PoM **Robinul-Neostigmine®,** see under Neostigmine Methylsulphate (section 15.1.6)

HYOSCINE HYDROBROMIDE
(Scopolamine Hydrobromide)

Indications: drying secretions, amnesia; other indications, see section 4.6

Cautions; Side-effects: see under Atropine Sulphate; may slow heart; avoid in the elderly (see notes above); porphyria (see section 9.8.2)

Dose: premedication, *by subcutaneous or intramuscular injection,* 200–600 micrograms 30–60 minutes before induction of anaesthesia, usually with papaveretum

PoM **Hyoscine** (Non-proprietary)
Injection, hyoscine hydrobromide 400 micrograms/mL, net price 1-mL amp = £2.67; 600 micrograms/mL, 1-mL amp = £2.69

CD **Papaveretum and Hyoscine Injection,** see under Papaveretum (section 15.1.4.3)

15.1.4   Sedative and analgesic perioperative drugs

15.1.4.1 Anxiolytics and neuroleptics
15.1.4.2 Non-opioid analgesics
15.1.4.3 Opioid analgesics

These drugs are given to allay the apprehension of the patient in the pre-operative period (including the night before operation), to relieve pain and discomfort when present, and to augment the action of subsequent anaesthetic agents. A number of the drugs used also provide some degree of pre-operative amnesia. The choice will vary with the individual patient, the nature of the operative procedure, the anaesthetic to be used and other prevailing circumstances such as outpatients, obstetrics, recovery facilities etc. The choice would also vary in elective and emergency operations.

PREMEDICATION IN CHILDREN. Oral administration is preferred to injections where possible but is not altogether satisfactory. Oral trimeprazine is still used but when given alone it may cause postoperative restlessness when pain is present.

Atropine or hyoscine is often given orally to children, but may be given intravenously immediately before induction.

ANAESTHESIA AND DRIVING. See section 15.1.

15.1.4.1 ANXIOLYTICS AND NEUROLEPTICS

Anxiolytic benzodiazepines are widely used whereas neuroleptics (e.g. chlorpromazine) are now rarely used.

BENZODIAZEPINES

Oral premedication with benzodiazepines is increasing in popularity, a short-acting oral benzodiazepine now being the most common premedicant.

Benzodiazepines are also of particular value for the production of light sedation during unpleasant procedures or during operations under local anaesthesia (including dentistry). The resultant amnesia is such that the patient is unlikely to have any unpleasant memories of the procedure (however, benzodiazepines, particularly when used for deep sedation, can sometimes induce sexual fantasies).

Benzodiazepines are also of particular value for sedation of patients in intensive care units, particularly those having assisted ventilation. Since they have no analgesic action they are often given in conjunction with opioid analgesics.

Benzodiazepines may on occasion cause marked respiratory depression and facilities for treatment of this are essential.

Diazepam is used to produce light sedation with amnesia. The 'sleep' dose shows too great an individual variation to recommend it for induction of anaesthesia. It is a long-acting drug with active metabolites, and a second period of drowsiness can occur 4–6 hours after its administration. Peri-operative use of diazepam in children is not generally recommended; its effect and timing of response are unreliable and paradoxical effects may occur.

Diazepam is relatively insoluble in water and preparations formulated in organic solvents are painful on intravenous injection and followed by a high incidence of venous thrombosis (which may not be noticed until a week after the injection); they are also painful on intramuscular injection, and absorption from the injection site is erratic. An emulsion preparation for intravenous injection is less irritant and is followed by a negligible incidence of venous thrombosis; it is not suitable for intramuscular injection. Diazepam is also available as a rectal solution.

Temazepam is given by mouth and has a shorter action and a relatively more rapid onset than diazepam by mouth. Used as a premedicant, anxiolytic and sedative effects are produced which continue for one and a half hours. After this period patients are usually fully alert but there may be residual drowsiness. It has proved useful as a premedicant in inpatient and day-case surgery.

Lorazepam produces more prolonged sedation than temazepam. In addition amnesia is commonplace. It is used as a premedicant the night before major surgery. A further, smaller, dose may be required the following morning if any delay in starting surgery is anticipated. Alternatively the first dose may be given in the early morning of the day of operation.

Midazolam is a water-soluble benzodiazepine which is often used in preference to diazepam. Recovery is faster than with diazepam. The incidence of side-effects is low but the CSM has received reports of respiratory depression (sometimes associated with severe hypotension) following intravenous administration. It is also associated with some major interactions (see below).

DIAZEPAM

Indications: premedication; sedation with amnesia, and in conjunction with local anaesthesia; other indications, see sections 4.1.2, 4.8.2, 10.2.2

Cautions; Contra-indications; Side-effects: see notes above and sections 4.1.2, 4.8.2

Dose: by mouth, 5 mg on night before minor or dental surgery then 5 mg 2 hours before procedure

By intravenous injection, into a large vein 10–20 mg over 2–4 minutes as sedative cover for minor surgical and medical procedures; premedication 100–200 micrograms/kg

By rectum in solution, 10 mg; ELDERLY 5 mg; CHILD not recommended (see notes above)

Note. Diazepam rectal solution doses in the BNF may differ from those in the product literature

Preparations
Section 4.1.2

LORAZEPAM

Indications: sedation with amnesia; as premedication; other indications, see sections 4.1.2, 4.8.2

Cautions; Contra-indications; Side-effects: see under Diazepam

Dose: by mouth, 2–3 mg the night before operation; 2–4 mg 1–2 hours before operation

By slow intravenous injection, preferably diluted with an equal volume of sodium chloride intravenous infusion 0.9% or water for injections, 50 micrograms/kg 30–45 minutes before operation

By intramuscular injection, diluted as above, 50 micrograms/kg 1–1½ hours before operation

Preparations
Section 4.1.2

MIDAZOLAM

Indications: sedation with amnesia, and in conjunction with local anaesthesia; premedication, induction

Cautions; Contra-indications; Side-effects: see under Diazepam; see notes above for CSM warning; **important:** profound sedation with erythromycin and possibly other drugs, see **interactions:** Appendix 1 (anxiolytics and hypnotics)

Dose: sedation, by intravenous injection over 30 seconds, 2 mg (elderly 1–1.5 mg) followed after 2 minutes by increments of 0.5–1 mg if sedation not adequate; usual range 2.5–7.5 mg (about 70 micrograms/kg), elderly 1–2 mg

Premedication, by intramuscular injection, 70–100 micrograms/kg 30–60 minutes before surgery; usual dose 5 mg (2.5 mg in elderly)

Induction, by slow intravenous injection, 200–300 micrograms/kg (elderly 100–200 micrograms/kg); CHILD over 7 years, 150 micrograms/kg

Sedation of patients receiving intensive care, by intravenous infusion, initially 30–300 micrograms/kg given over 5 minutes, then

30–200 micrograms/kg/hour; reduce dose (or omit initial dose) in hypovolaemia, vasoconstriction, or hypothermia; low doses may be adequate if opioid analgesic also used; avoid abrupt withdrawal after prolonged administration (safety after more than 14 days not established)

PoM **Hypnovel**® (Roche)
Injection, midazolam (as hydrochloride) 2 mg/mL, net price 5-mL amp = £1.01; 5 mg/mL, 2-mL amp = 85p

TEMAZEPAM
Indications: premedication before minor surgery; anxiety before investigatory procedures; hypnotic, (section 4.1.1)
Cautions; Contra-indications; Side-effects: see under Diazepam
Dose: by mouth, premedication, 20–40 mg (elderly, 10–20 mg) 1 hour before operation; CHILD 1 mg/kg (max. 30 mg)

Preparations
Section 4.1.1

CHLORMETHIAZOLE

Chlormethiazole (clomethiazole) is licensed for use as an intravenous infusion to maintain sleep during surgery carried out under regional anaesthesia, but is no longer in current use for this purpose.

CHLORMETHIAZOLE
(Clomethiazole)
Indications: sedative during regional anaesthesia (but see also notes above); other indications, see sections 4.1.1, 4.8.2, 4.10
Cautions; Contra-indications; Side-effects: see section 4.10
Dose: by intravenous infusion, as a 0.8% solution of chlormethiazole edisylate, induction 25 mL (200 mg)/minute for 1–2 minutes; maintenance 1–4 mL (8–32 mg)/minute
IMPORTANT. See special cautions for intravenous infusion, section 4.10

Preparations
See section 4.10

PHENOTHIAZINES AND RELATED DRUGS

Neuroleptics such as **chlorpromazine** and **droperidol** (section 4.2.1) are rarely used in the UK for premedication; although chlorpromazine is licensed to prevent shivering in induction of hypothermia, it is no longer in current use for this purpose. **Trimeprazine** is used as a premedicant for children.

PROMETHAZINE HYDROCHLORIDE
Indications: pre-operative sedative and antimuscarinic; anti-emetic, see section 4.6; other indications, see sections 3.4.1, 3.4.3
Cautions; Contra-indications; Side-effects: see section 4.6
Dose: premedication, *by mouth,* CHILD under 2 years not recommended, 2–5 years 15–20 mg, 5–10 years 20–25 mg
By deep intramuscular injection, 25–50 mg 1 hour before operation; CHILD 5–10 years, 6.25–12.5 mg

Preparations
Section 3.4.1 and section 15.1.4.3 (with pethidine)

TRIMEPRAZINE TARTRATE
(Alimemazine Tartrate)
Indications: pre-operative sedation, anti-emetic; other indications (section 3.4.1)
Cautions; Contra-indications; Side-effects: see notes above and section 3.4.1
Dose: by mouth, premedication, CHILD 2–7 years up to 2 mg/kg 1–2 hours before operation

Preparations
Section 3.4.1

15.1.4.2 NON-OPIOID ANALGESICS

Since non-steroidal anti-inflammatory drugs (NSAIDs) do not depress respiration, do not impair gastro-intestinal motility, and do not cause dependence, they may be useful alternatives (or adjuncts) to the use of opioids for the relief of postoperative pain. NSAIDs may be inadequate for the relief of severe pain.

Diclofenac, flurbiprofen, ketoprofen (section 10.1.1), and **ketorolac** are licensed for postoperative use. Diclofenac, ketoprofen and ketorolac can be given by injection as well as by mouth. Intramuscular injections of diclofenac and ketoprofen are given deep into the gluteal muscle to minimise pain and tissue damage; diclofenac can also be given by intravenous infusion for the treatment or prevention of postoperative pain. Ketorolac is less irritant on intramuscular injection but pain has been reported; it can also be given by intravenous injection.

Suppositories of diclofenac and ketoprofen may be effective alternatives to the parenteral use of these drugs. Flurbiprofen is also available as suppositories.

KETOROLAC TROMETAMOL
Indications: short-term management of moderate to severe acute postoperative pain
Cautions: reduce dose in elderly and in those weighing less than 50 kg; reduce dose and monitor in mild renal impairment (avoid if moderate or severe); heart failure, hepatic impairment and other conditions leading to reduction in blood volume or in renal blood flow (including those taking diuretics); cardiac decompensation, hypertension or similar conditions (fluid retention and oedema reported); **interactions:** Appendix 1 (NSAIDs)
GASTRO-INTESTINAL EFFECTS. Elderly and debilitated more prone to risk of gastro-intestinal effects (risk increases with increased dose and duration); see also under Contra-indications and Side-effects below

Contra-indications: history of hypersensitivity to aspirin or any other NSAID (severe anaphylactic reactions reported), history of asthma, complete or partial syndrome of nasal polyps, angioedema or bronchospasm; history of peptic ulceration or gastro-intestinal bleeding; haemorrhagic diatheses (including coagulation disorders) and operations with high risk of haemorrhage or incomplete haemostasis; confirmed or suspected cerebrovascular bleeding; moderate or severe renal impairment; hypovolaemia or dehydration; pregnancy (including labour and delivery) and breast-feeding

Side-effects: side-effects reported include anaphylaxis (with rash, bronchospasm, laryngeal oedema and hypotension), fluid retention (see Cautions), nausea, dyspepsia, abdominal discomfort, bowel changes, peptic ulceration, gastro-intestinal bleeding (elderly at greater risk, see also above), pancreatitis, drowsiness, dizziness, headache, sweating, dry mouth, excessive thirst, mental and sensory changes, convulsions, myalgia, aseptic meningitis, hyponatraemia, hyperkalaemia, raised blood urea and creatinine, urinary symptoms and acute renal failure, flushing or pallor, bradycardia, hypertension, purpura, thrombocytopenia, prolonged bleeding time, dyspnoea and pulmonary oedema, skin reactions (some severe, including Stevens-Johnson and Lyell's syndromes), postoperative wound haemorrhage, haematoma, epistaxis, oedema, liver function changes (discontinue if clinical symptoms); pain at injection site; for general side-effects of NSAIDs, see section 10.1.1

Dose: by mouth, PATIENT over 16 years, 10 mg every 4–6 hours (ELDERLY every 6–8 hours); max. 40 mg daily; max. duration of treatment 7 days; CHILD under 16 years, not recommended

By intramuscular injection or by intravenous injection over not less than 15 seconds, PATIENT over 16 years, initially 10 mg, then 10–30 mg every 4–6 hours when required (every 2 hours in initial postoperative period); max. 90 mg daily (ELDERLY and patients weighing less than 50 kg max. 60 mg daily); max. duration of treatment 2 days by either route; CHILD under 16 years, not recommended

Note. Pain relief may not occur upwards of 30 minutes after intravenous or intramuscular injection. When converting from parenteral to oral administration, total combined dose on the day of converting should not exceed 90 mg (60 mg in the elderly and patients weighing less than 50 kg) of which the oral component should not exceed 40 mg; patients should be converted to oral route as soon as possible

PoM **Toradol**® (Roche)
Tablets, ivory, f/c, ketorolac trometamol 10 mg, net price 20-tab pack = £6.52. Label: 17, 21
Injection, ketorolac trometamol 10 mg/mL, net price 1-mL amp = £1.06; 30 mg/mL, 1-mL amp = £1.28

15.1.4.3 OPIOID ANALGESICS

Opioid analgesics were formerly commonly used as premedicants given intramuscularly about an hour before operation, usually combined with an antisialogogue. Sometimes they were combined with a phenothiazine or droperidol. The main side-effects of opioid analgesics are respiratory depression, cardiovascular depression, and nausea and vomiting. The principal advantages were that opioid analgesics provided analgesia persisting into the operative period giving a reduced chance of awareness during anaesthesia with full doses of muscle relaxants. Nowadays anaesthetists are more likely to give potent opioids by the intravenous route at induction. For **patient controlled analgesia** (PCA) for the relief of postoperative pain consult **hospital protocols.**

INTRA-OPERATIVE ANALGESIA. Many of the conventional opioid analgesics are used to supplement general anaesthesia, usually in combination with nitrous oxide–oxygen and a muscle relaxant. Pethidine was the first to be used for this purpose but other drugs now available include alfentanil, fentanyl, nalbuphine, remifentanil, and tramadol (section 4.7.2).

Small doses of opioids given immediately before or with induction will reduce the induction dose and this is a popular technique in poor-risk patients. **Alfentanil** and **remifentanil** are particularly useful in this respect because they have an onset of action within 1–2 minutes. Alfentanil and **fentanyl** are suitable for use intra-operatively given as incremental boluses; alfentanil can also be used as an infusion, but accumulates with more prolonged use. Remifentanil should not be given as a bolus intra-operatively, but is very suitable for continuous infusion. The short duration of remifentanil enables it to be given for a prolonged period at high dosage, without accumulation, and with little risk of residual postoperative respiratory depression; supplemental analgesia will often be required after remifentanil.

Repeated intra-operative doses of fentanyl or alfentanil should be given with care, since not only may the respiratory depression persist into the postoperative period but it may become apparent for the first time postoperatively when the patient is away from immediate nursing attention. The specific opioid antagonist, naloxone (section 15.1.7), will immediately reverse this respiratory depression but the dose may have to be repeated. It is important to bear in mind that in clinical doses it will also reverse most of the analgesia—*careful titration* is necessary to *avoid* this. An alternative approach is to use the specific respiratory stimulant, doxapram (section 15.1.7), which can be given in an infusion and which will not affect the opioid analgesia. The use of intra-operative opioids should be borne in mind when prescribing postoperative analgesics. In many instances they will delay the need for the first dose but caution is necessary since there may be some residual respiratory depression potentiated by the postoperative analgesic.

Fentanyl may produce severe respiratory depression, especially in patients with decreased respiratory function or when other respiratory depressant drugs have been given. Respiratory depression may be treated by artificial ventilation or be reversed by naloxone or doxapram (see above). Alfentanil may also cause severe respiratory depression, especially when other respiratory depressant drugs have already been given; this may be reversed with naloxone.

Meptazinol can be used for analgesia during or after operation. It is associated with nausea and vomiting, but is claimed to have a reduced incidence of respiratory depression.

For general notes on analgesics, see section 4.7.

ALFENTANIL

Indications: analgesia especially during short operative procedure and outpatient surgery; enhancement of anaesthesia; analgesia and suppression of respiratory activity in patients receiving intensive care with assisted ventilation, for up to 4 days

Cautions; Contra-indications; Side-effects: see section 4.7.2 and notes above

Dose: by intravenous injection, spontaneous respiration, ADULT, initially up to 500 micrograms over 30 seconds; supplemental, 250 micrograms

With assisted ventilation, ADULT and CHILD, initially   30–50 micrograms/kg;   supplemental, 15 micrograms/kg

By intravenous infusion, with assisted ventilation, ADULT and CHILD, initially 50–100 micrograms/kg over 10 minutes *or* as a bolus, followed by maintenance of 0.5–1 micrograms/kg/minute

Analgesia and suppression of respiratory activity during intensive care, with assisted ventilation, *by intravenous infusion,* initially 2 mg/hour (approx. 30 micrograms/kg/hour) subsequently adjusted according to response (usual range 0.5–10 mg/hour); more rapid initial control may be obtained with an intravenous dose of 5 mg given in divided portions over 10 minutes (slowing if hypotension or bradycardia occur); additional doses of 0.5–1 mg may be given by intravenous injection during short painful procedures

CD Rapifen® (Janssen-Cilag)
Injection, alfentanil (as hydrochloride) 500 micrograms/mL. Net price 2-mL amp = 72p; 10-mL amp = £3.31
Intensive care injection, alfentanil (as hydrochloride) 5 mg/mL. To be diluted before use. Net price 1-mL amp = £2.65

BUPRENORPHINE

Indications: peri-operative analgesia; premedication; analgesia in other situations, see section 4.7.2

Cautions; Contra-indications; Side-effects: see section 4.7.2; effects only partially reversed by naloxone

Dose: pain, *by slow intravenous injection,* 300–450 micrograms
Premedication, *by sublingual administration,* 400 micrograms
By intramuscular injection, 300 micrograms

Preparations
Section 4.7.2

FENTANYL

Indications: analgesia during operation, enhancement of anaesthesia; respiratory depressant in assisted respiration

Cautions; Contra-indications; Side-effects: see section 4.7.2 and notes above

Dose: by intravenous injection, with spontaneous respiration,   50–200 micrograms,   then 50 micrograms   as   required;   CHILD   3–5 micrograms/kg,   then   1 microgram/kg   as required

With assisted ventilation, 0.3–3.5 mg, then 100–200 micrograms   as   required;   CHILD 15 micrograms/kg, then 1–3 micrograms/kg as required

▼ **CD Durogesic®**: see section 4.7.2
CD Sublimaze® (Janssen-Cilag)
Injection, fentanyl (as citrate) 50 micrograms /mL. Net price 2-mL amp = 24p; 10-mL amp = £1.17
Available as a generic from Antigen, Faulding DBL

MORPHINE SULPHATE

Indications: analgesia during and after operation; enhancement of anaesthesia; pre-operative sedation; analgesia in other situations, see section 4.7.2

Cautions; Contra-indications; Side-effects: see section 4.7.2 and notes above

Dose: by subcutaneous or intramuscular injection, up to 10 mg 1–1½ hours before operation; CHILD, *by intramuscular injection,* 150 micrograms/kg

Postoperative pain, *by subcutaneous or intramuscular injection,* 10 mg every 2–4 hours if necessary (15 mg for heavier well-muscled patients); CHILD up to 1 month 150 micrograms/kg, 1–12 months 200 micrograms/kg, 1–5 years 2.5–5 mg, 6–12 years 5–10 mg

Note. In the postoperative period, the patient should be closely monitored for pain relief as well as for side-effects especially respiratory depression

See also section 4.7.2 for analgesia

CD Morphine Sulphate Injection, morphine sulphate, 10 mg/mL. Net price 1-mL amp = 64p; other strengths see section 4.7.2

CD Morphine and Atropine Injection, morphine   sulphate   10 mg,   atropine   sulphate 600 micrograms/mL. Net price 1-mL amp = £1.96
Dose: premedication, by subcutaneous injection, 0.5–1 mL

NALBUPHINE HYDROCHLORIDE

Indications: peri-operative analgesia; premedication; analgesia in other situations, see section 4.7.2

Cautions; Contra-indications; Side-effects: see section 4.7.2 and notes above; also caution in ambulant patients (impairment of mental and physical ability)

Dose: acute pain, *by subcutaneous, intramuscular, or intravenous injection,* 10–20 mg, adjusted according   to   response;   CHILD   up   to 300 micrograms/kg repeated once or twice as necessary. See also section 4.7.2. for analgesia

Premedication, *by subcutaneous, intramuscular, or intravenous injection,* 100–200 micrograms/kg

Induction, *by intravenous injection,* 0.3–1 mg/kg over 10–15 minutes

Intra-operative analgesia, *by intravenous injection,* 250–500 micrograms /kg at 30-minute intervals

---

PoM **Nubain®** (Du Pont)

Injection, nalbuphine hydrochloride 10 mg/mL. Net price 1-mL amp = 73p; 2-mL amp = £1.13

PAPAVERETUM

IMPORTANT. Do **not** confuse with papaverine (see section 7.4.5)

A mixture of 253 parts of morphine hydrochloride, 23 parts of papaverine hydrochloride and 20 parts of codeine hydrochloride

REFORMULATION. *BP 1993, Addendum 1994,* includes the following explanation concerning the reformulation of papaveretum: *papaveretum injection* contains the three alkaloids *morphine, papaverine* and *codeine;* in reformulating the injection to remove *noscapine,* the amounts of the other three alkaloids have been maintained; thus the total amount of material per mL has decreased. Before reformulation the *lower strength injection* (which provides *the equivalent of 5 mg of the major component, morphine*) contained 10 mg per mL of the four-component material; it now contains *7.7 mg of papaveretum per mL.* Likewise, before reformulation the *higher strength injection* (which provides *the equivalent of 10 mg of morphine*) contained 20 mg per mL of the four-component material; it now contains *15.4 mg of papaveretum per mL.*

The **CSM** has advised that to avoid confusion the figures of 7.7 mg/mL or 15.4 mg/mL should be used for prescribing purposes.

Indications: postoperative analgesia; premedication

Cautions; Contra-indications; Side-effects: see section 4.7.2 and notes above

Dose: by subcutaneous, intramuscular, or intravenous injection, 7.7–15.4 mg repeated every 4 hours if necessary (ELDERLY initially 7.7 mg); CHILD up to 1 month 115.5 micrograms/kg, 1–12 months 115.5–154 micrograms/kg, 1–12 years 154–231 micrograms/kg

INTRAVENOUS DOSE. In general the intravenous dose should be quarter to half corresponding subcutaneous or intramuscular dose.

CD Papaveretum (Non-proprietary)

Injection, papaveretum 7.7 mg/mL (providing the equivalent of 5 mg of anhydrous morphine/mL), net price 1-mL amp = 71p; 15.4 mg/mL (providing the equivalent of 10 mg of anhydrous morphine/mL), 1-mL amp = 81p

Available from Martindale

Note. The name Omnopon® was formerly used for papaveretum preparations.

With hyoscine
CD Papaveretum and Hyoscine Injection,

papaveretum 15.4 mg (providing the equivalent of 10 mg of anhydrous morphine), hyoscine hydrobromide 400 micrograms/mL. Net price 1-mL amp = 83p

Dose: premedication, by subcutaneous or intramuscular injection, 0.5–1 mL

Available from Martindale

PETHIDINE HYDROCHLORIDE

Indications: peri-operative analgesia; premedication; analgesia in other situations, see section 4.7.2

Cautions; Contra-indications; Side-effects: convulsions may occur with excessive doses; see section 4.7.2 and notes above

Dose: premedication, *by intramuscular injection,* 25–100 mg 1 hour before operation; CHILD 0.5–2 mg/kg

Adjunct to nitrous oxide–oxygen, *by slow intravenous injection,* 10–25 mg repeated when required

Postoperative pain, *by subcutaneous or intramuscular injection,* 25–100 mg, every 2–3 hours if necessary; CHILD, *by intramuscular injection,* 0.5–2 mg/kg

Note. In the postoperative period, the patient should be closely monitored for pain relief as well as for side-effects especially respiratory depression

See also section 4.7.2 for analgesia

CD Pethidine (Non-proprietary)

Injection, pethidine hydrochloride 50 mg/mL, net price 1-mL amp = 39p; 2-mL amp = 39p; 10 mg/mL, 5-mL amp = 97p; 10-mL amp = £1.02

Various strengths available from Martindale, Roche

Tablets, see section 4.7.2

With promethazine
CD Pamergan P100® (Martindale)

Injection, pethidine hydrochloride 50 mg, promethazine hydrochloride 25 mg/mL. Net price 2-mL amp = 69p

Dose: premedication, 2 mL by intramuscular injection 1–1½ hours before operation; CHILD, by intramuscular injection, 8–12 years 0.75 mL, 13–16 years 1 mL

REMIFENTANIL

Indications: supplementation of general anaesthesia during induction and analgesia during maintenance of anaesthesia

Cautions; Contra-indications; Side-effects: see section 4.7.2 and notes above

Dose: induction, *by intravenous infusion,* 0.5–1 microgram/kg/minute, *with or without* an initial bolus *by intravenous injection* (of a solution containing 20–250 micrograms/mL) over not less than 30 seconds, 1 microgram/kg

Note. If patient is to be intubated more than 8 minutes after start of intravenous infusion, intial intravenous injection dose is unnecessary

Maintenance in ventilated patients, *by intravenous infusion,* 0.05–2 micrograms/kg/minute according to anaesthetic technique and adjusted according to response; supplemental doses in light anaesthesia, *by intravenous injection* every 2–5 minutes

Maintenance in spontaneous respiration anaesthesia, *by intravenous infusion,* initially 40 nanograms/kg/minute adjusted according to response, usual range 25–100 nanograms/kg/minute

CHILD 2–12 years, limited experience (see product literature)

▼ PoM **Ultiva®** (GlaxoWellcome)

Injection, powder for reconstitution, remifentanil (as hydrochloride), net price 1-mg vial = £5.50; 2-mg vial = £11.00; 5-mg vial = £27.50

15.1.5   Muscle relaxants

Muscle relaxants used in anaesthesia are also known as **neuromuscular blocking drugs**. By specific blockade of the neuromuscular junction they enable light levels of anaesthesia to be employed with adequate relaxation of the muscles of the abdomen and diaphragm. They also relax the vocal cords and allow the passage of a tracheal tube. Their action differs from the muscle relaxants acting on the spinal cord or brain which are used in musculoskeletal disorders (section 10.2.2).

Patients who have received a muscle relaxant should **always** have their respiration assisted or controlled until the drug has been inactivated or antagonised (section 15.1.6).

NON-DEPOLARISING MUSCLE RELAXANTS

Non-depolarising muscle relaxants (also known as competitive muscle relaxants) compete with acetylcholine for receptor sites at the neuromuscular junction and their action may be reversed with anticholinesterases such as neostigmine (section 15.1.6). Non-depolarising muscle relaxants may be divided into the aminosteroid group which includes **pancuronium**, **rocuronium** and **vecuronium**, and the benzylisoquinolinium group which includes **atracurium**, **cisatracurium**, **gallamine** and **mivacurium**.

Non-depolarising muscle relaxants have a slower onset of action than suxamethonium. These drugs can be classified by their duration of action as short-acting (15–30 minutes), intermediate-acting (30–40 minutes) and long-acting (60–120 minutes), although duration of action is dose-dependent. Drugs with a shorter or intermediate duration of action, such as atracurium and vecuronium, are more widely employed than those with a longer duration of action such as pancuronium.

Non-depolarising muscle relaxants have no sedative or analgesic effects and are not considered to be a triggering factor for malignant hyperthermia.

CAUTIONS. Allergic cross-reactivity between neuromuscular blocking agents has been reported; caution is advised in cases of hypersensitivity to these drugs. Their activity is prolonged in patients with myasthenia gravis and in hypothermia, therefore lower doses are required. Resistance may develop in patients with burns who may require increased doses; low plasma cholinesterase activity in these patients requires dose titration for mivacurium. **Interactions:** Appendix 1 (muscle relaxants)

SIDE-EFFECTS. Benzylisoquinolinium non-depolarising muscle relaxants (except cisatracurium) are associated with histamine release which can cause skin flushing, hypotension, tachycardia, bronchospasm and rarely, anaphylactoid reactions. Aminosteroid muscle relaxants are not associated with histamine release. Drugs possessing vagolytic activity can counteract any bradycardia that occurs during surgery.

Atracurium is a mixture of 10 isomers and is a benzylisoquinolinium muscle relaxant with an intermediate duration of action. It undergoes non-enzymatic metabolism which is independent of liver and kidney function, thus allowing its use in patients with hepatic or renal impairment. Cardiovascular effects are associated with significant histamine release.

Cisatracurium is a single isomer of atracurium. It is more potent and has a slightly longer duration of action than atracurium and provides greater cardiovascular stability because cisatracurium lacks histamine-releasing effects.

Mivacurium, a benzylisoquinolinium muscle relaxant, has a short duration of action. It is metabolised by plasma cholinesterase and muscle paralysis is prolonged in individuals deficient in this enzyme. It is not associated with vagolytic activity or ganglionic blockade although histamine release may occur, particularly with rapid injection.

Pancuronium, an aminosteroid muscle relaxant, has a long duration of action and is often used in patients receiving long-term mechanical ventilation in intensive care units. It lacks a histamine-releasing effect, but vagolytic and sympathomimetic effects can cause tachycardia and hypertension.

Rocuronium exerts an effect within 2 minutes and has the most rapid onset of any of the competitive muscle relaxants. It is an aminosteroid muscle relaxant with an intermediate duration of action. It is reported to have minimal histamine-releasing and cardiovascular effects; high doses produce mild vagolytic activity.

Vecuronium, an aminosteroid muscle relaxant, has an intermediate duration of action. It does not generally produce histamine release and lacks cardiovascular effects.

Gallamine has vagolytic and sympathomimetic properties and frequently increases pulse rate and blood pressure. It is rarely used since the other neuromuscular blocking drugs have a more predictable response and it should be avoided in patients with renal impairment.

ATRACURIUM BESYLATE
(Atracurium Besilate)

Indications: non-depolarising muscle relaxant of short to intermediate duration

Cautions: see notes above

Side-effects: see notes above

Dose: by intravenous injection, ADULT and CHILD over 1 month initially 300–600 micrograms/kg, then 100–200 micrograms/kg as required

By intravenous infusion, 5–10 micrograms/kg/minute (300–600 micrograms/kg/hour)

PoM **Tracrium**® (GlaxoWellcome)
Injection, atracurium besylate 10 mg/mL. Net price 2.5-mL amp = £1.86; 5-mL amp = £3.38; 25-mL amp = £14.53

CISATRACURIUM

Indications: non-depolarising muscle relaxant of intermediate duration

Cautions: see notes above

Side-effects: see notes above

Dose: by intravenous injection, intubation, 150 micrograms/kg; maintenance, 30 micrograms/kg approx. every 20 minutes

CHILD over 2 years, initially, 100 micrograms/kg; maintenance, 20 micrograms/kg approx. every 9 minutes

By intravenous infusion, ADULT and CHILD over 2 years, initially, 3 micrograms/kg/minute, *then after stabilisation,* 1–2 micrograms/kg/minute; dose reduced by up to 40% if used with enflurane or isoflurane

CHILD under 2 years not recommended

▼ PoM **Nimbex**® (GlaxoWellcome)

Injection, cisatracurium (as besylate) 2 mg/mL, net price 2.5-mL amp = £2.30, 10-mL amp = £8.50

Forte injection, cisatracurium (as besylate) 5 mg/mL, net price 30-mL vial = £35.00

GALLAMINE TRIETHIODIDE

Indications: non-depolarising muscle relaxant of intermediate duration

Cautions: see notes above

Contra-indications: renal impairment

Side-effects: see notes above

Dose: by intravenous injection, 80–120 mg, then 20–40 mg as required; NEONATE, 600 micrograms/kg; CHILD, 1.5 mg/kg

PoM **Flaxedil**® (Rhône-Poulenc Rorer)

Injection, gallamine triethiodide 40 mg/ml. Net price 2 mL amp = 72p

MIVACURIUM CHLORIDE

Indications: non-depolarising muscle relaxant of short duration

Cautions: see notes above; low plasma cholinesterase activity

Side-effects: see notes above

Dose: by intravenous injection, 70–250 micrograms/kg; maintenance 100 micrograms/kg every 15 minutes; CHILD 2–6 months initially 150 micrograms/kg, 7 months–12 years initially 200 micrograms/kg; maintenance (CHILD 2 months–12 years) 100 micrograms/kg every 6–9 minutes

Note. Doses up to 150 micrograms/kg may be given over 5–15 seconds, higher doses should be given over 30 seconds. In patients with asthma, cardiovascular disease or those who are sensitive to falls in arterial blood pressure give over 60 seconds

By intravenous infusion, maintenance of block, 8–10 micrograms/kg/minute, adjusted if necessary every 3 minutes by 1 microgram/kg/minute to usual dose of 6–7 micrograms/kg/minute; CHILD 2 months–12 years, usual dose 11–14 micrograms/kg/minute

PoM **Mivacron**® (GlaxoWellcome)

Injection, mivacurium (as chloride) 2 mg/mL , net price 5-mL amp = £2.86; 10-mL amp = £4.62

PANCURONIUM BROMIDE

Indications: non-depolarising muscle relaxant of long duration

Cautions: see notes above; hepatic impairment; reduce dose in renal impairment

Side-effects: see notes above

Dose: by intravenous injection, initially for intubation 50–100 micrograms/kg then 10–20 micrograms/kg as required; CHILD initially 60–100 micrograms/kg, then 10–20 micrograms/kg, NEONATE 30–40 micrograms/kg initially then 10–20 micrograms/kg

Intensive care, *by intravenous injection,* 60 micrograms/kg every 1–1½ hours

PoM **Pavulon**® (Organon-Teknika)

Injection, pancuronium bromide 2 mg/mL. Net price 2-mL amp = 72p

Available as a generic from Faulding DBL

ROCURONIUM BROMIDE

Indications: non-depolarising muscle relaxant of intermediate duration

Cautions: see notes above; hepatic and renal impairment

Side-effects: see notes above

Dose: by intravenous injection, intubation, 600 micrograms/kg; maintenance, 150 micrograms/kg

By intravenous infusion, 300–600 micrograms/kg/hour (after initial intravenous injection of 600 micrograms/kg)

CHILD similar sensitivity to adults; NEONATE not recommended

PoM **Esmeron**® (Organon-Teknika)

Injection, rocuronium bromide 10 mg/mL, net price 5-mL vial = £4.23, 10-mL vial = £8.46

VECURONIUM BROMIDE

Indications: non-depolarising muscle relaxant of intermediate duration

Cautions: see notes above; reduce dose in renal impairment

Side-effects: see notes above

Dose: by intravenous injection, intubation, 80–100 micrograms/kg; maintenance 20–30 micrograms/kg according to response; NEONATE and INFANT up to 4 months, initially 10–20 micrograms/kg then incremental doses to achieve response; CHILD over 5 months, as adult dose (up to 1 year onset more rapid and high intubation dose may not be required)

By intravenous infusion, 0.8–1.4 micrograms/kg/minute (after initial intravenous injection of 40–100 micrograms/kg)

PoM **Norcuron**® (Organon-Teknika)

Injection, powder for reconstitution, vecuronium bromide. Net price 10-mg vial = £4.44 (with water for injections)

Cautionary label wordings, see inside back cover

Prices are **net**, see p.1

DEPOLARISING MUSCLE RELAXANTS

Suxamethonium has the most rapid onset of action of any of the muscle relaxants and is ideal if fast onset and brief duration of action are required e.g. with tracheal intubation. Its duration of action is about 2 to 6 minutes following intravenous doses of about 1 mg/kg; repeated doses can be used for longer procedures.

Suxamethonium acts by mimicking acetylcholine at the neuromuscular junction but hydrolysis is much slower than for acetylcholine; depolarisation is therefore prolonged resulting in neuromuscular blockade. Unlike the non-depolarising muscle relaxants, its action cannot be reversed and recovery is spontaneous; anticholinesterases such as neostigmine potentiate the neuromuscular block.

Suxamethonium should be given after anaesthetic induction because paralysis is usually preceded by painful muscle fasciculations. Bradycardia may occur with repeated doses in adults and with the first dose in children. Premedication with atropine reduces bradycardia as well as the excessive salivation associated with suxamethonium use.

Prolonged paralysis may occur in **dual block**, which occurs with high or repeated doses of suxamethonium and is caused by the development of a non-depolarising block following the initial depolarising block. Individuals with myasthenia gravis are resistant to suxamethonium but can develop dual block resulting in delayed recovery. Prolonged paralysis may also occur in those with low or atypical plasma cholinesterase. Assisted ventilation should be continued until muscle function is restored.

SUXAMETHONIUM CHLORIDE

Indications: depolarising muscle relaxant of short duration

Cautions: see notes above; pregnancy (Appendix 4); patients with cardiac, respiratory or neuromuscular disease; raised intra-ocular pressure (avoid in penetrating eye injury); **interactions:** Appendix 1 (muscle relaxants)

Contra-indications: family history of malignant hyperthermia, low plasma cholinesterase activity, hyperkalaemia

Side-effects: see notes above; postoperative muscle pain, myoglobinaemia; tachycardia, arrhythmias, hypertension, hypotension, bronchospasm, apnoea, prolonged respiratory depression; hyperkalaemia; hyperthermia

Dose: by intravenous injection, ADULT 1 mg/kg (range 0.3–1.1 mg/kg); usual range 20–100 mg; max. 500 mg/hour; INFANT under 1 year, 2 mg/kg; CHILD 1–12 years, 1–2 mg/kg

By *intravenous infusion* as a 0.1–0.2% solution, 2–5 mg/minute; max. 500 mg/hour

By *intramuscular injection*, INFANT up to 4–5 mg/kg; CHILD up to 4 mg/kg; max. 150 mg

PoM **Suxamethonium Chloride** (Non-proprietary)
Injection, suxamethonium chloride 50 mg/mL, net price 2-mL amp = 24p
Available from Antigen
PoM **Anectine**® (GlaxoWellcome)
Injection, suxamethonium chloride 50 mg/mL, net price 2-mL amp = 73p

15.1.6   Anticholinesterases used in anaesthesia

Anticholinesterases reverse the effects of the non-depolarising (competitive) muscle relaxant drugs such as pancuronium but they prolong the action of the depolarising muscle relaxant drug suxamethonium.

Edrophonium has a transient action.

Neostigmine has a longer duration of action than edrophonium. It is the specific drug for reversal of non-depolarising (competitive) blockade. It acts within one minute of intravenous injection and lasts for 20 to 30 minutes; a second dose may then be necessary. Atropine or glycopyrronium (section 15.1.3) should be given before or with neostigmine in order to prevent bradycardia, excessive salivation, and other muscarinic actions of neostigmine.

EDROPHONIUM CHLORIDE

Indications: see under Dose

Cautions; Contra-indications; Side-effects: see section 10.2.1 and notes above. Atropine should also be given

Dose: brief reversal of non-depolarising neuromuscular blockade, *by intravenous injection* over several minutes, 500–700 micrograms/kg (after or with atropine sulphate 600 micrograms)
Diagnosis of myasthenia gravis, section 10.2.1

PoM **Edrophonium** (Non-proprietary)
Injection, edrophonium chloride 10 mg/mL. Net price 1-mL amp = £3.31
Available from Cambridge

NEOSTIGMINE METHYLSULPHATE

Indications: see under Dose

Cautions; Contra-indications; Side-effects: see section 10.2.1 and notes above. Atropine should also be given

Dose: reversal of non-depolarising neuromuscular blockade, *by intravenous injection* over 1 minute, 50–70 micrograms/kg (max. 5 mg) after or with atropine sulphate 0.6–1.2 mg
Myasthenia gravis, see section 10.2.1

PoM **Neostigmine** (Non-proprietary)
Injection, neostigmine methylsulphate 2.5 mg/mL. Net price 1-mL amp = 28p

With glycopyrronium
PoM **Robinul-Neostigmine**® (Anpharm)
Injection, neostigmine methylsulphate 2.5 mg, glycopyrronium bromide 500 micrograms/mL. Net price 1-mL amp = £1.06
Dose: by intravenous injection over 10–30 seconds, 1–2 mL *or* 0.02 mL/kg; CHILD 0.02 mL/kg (*or* 0.2 mL/kg of a 1 in 10 dilution using water for injections or sodium chloride injection 0.9%)

15.1.7   Antagonists for central and respiratory depression

The opioid antagonist **naloxone** can be used to reverse respiratory depression caused by opioid analgesics (**important:** unless the dosage is adjusted with considerable care, analgesia may also be reversed). **Doxapram** is a respiratory stimulant which does not reverse the other effects of opioid analgesics.

Flumazenil is a benzodiazepine antagonist for the reversal of the central sedative effects of benzodiazepines after anaesthetic and similar procedures. Flumazenil has a shorter half-life than that of diazepam and midazolam (and there is a risk that patients may become resedated).

DOXAPRAM HYDROCHLORIDE
Indications: see under Dose
Cautions: give with oxygen in severe irreversible airways obstruction or severely decreased lung compliance (because of increased work load of breathing); give with beta$_2$-adrenoceptor stimulant in bronchoconstriction; hypertension (avoid if severe), impaired cardiac reserve; hepatic impairment, pregnancy (compelling reasons only); **interactions:** Appendix 1 (doxapram)
Contra-indications: severe hypertension, status asthmaticus, coronary artery disease, thyrotoxicosis, epilepsy, physical obstruction of respiratory tract
Side-effects: moderate increase in blood pressure and heart rate; dizziness, perineal warmth; side-effects reported in postoperative period (causal effect not established) include muscle fasiculation, hyperactivity, sweating, confusion, hallucinations, cough, dyspnoea, laryngospasm, bronchospasm, sinus tachycardia, bradycardia, extrasystoles, nausea, vomiting and salivation
Dose: postoperative respiratory depression, *by intravenous injection* over at least 30 seconds, 1–1.5 mg/kg repeated if necessary after intervals of 1 hour *or* alternatively *by intravenous infusion*, 2–3 mg/minute adjusted according to response; CHILD not recommended
Acute respiratory failure, *by intravenous infusion*, 1.5–4 mg/minute adjusted according to response (given concurrently with oxygen and whenever possible monitor with frequent measurement of blood gas tensions); CHILD not recommended

PoM **Dopram**® (Anpharm)
Injection, doxapram hydrochloride 20 mg/mL. Net price 5-mL amp = £2.14
Intravenous infusion, doxapram hydrochloride 2 mg/mL in glucose 5%. Net price 500-mL bottle = £22.34

FLUMAZENIL
Indications: reversal of sedative effects of benzodiazepines in anaesthetic, intensive care, and diagnostic procedures

Cautions: short-acting (repeat doses may be necessary—benzodiazepine effects may persist for at least 24 hours); benzodiazepine dependence (may precipitate withdrawal symptoms); ensure neuromuscular blockade cleared before giving; avoid rapid injection in high-risk or anxious patients and following major surgery; hepatic impairment; severe head injury (rapid reversal of benzodiazepine sedation may increase risk of raised intracranial pressure); elderly, children, pregnancy and breast-feeding
Contra-indications: epileptics who have received prolonged benzodiazepine therapy
Side-effects: nausea, vomiting, and flushing; if wakening too rapid, agitation, anxiety, and fear; transient increase in blood pressure and heart-rate in intensive care patients; very rarely convulsions (particularly in epileptics)
Dose: by intravenous injection, 200 micrograms over 15 seconds, then 100 micrograms at 60-second intervals if required; usual dose range, 300–600 micrograms; max. total dose 1 mg (2 mg in intensive care); question aetiology if no response to repeated doses
By intravenous infusion, if drowsiness recurs after injection, 100–400 micrograms/hour, adjusted according to level of arousal

PoM **Anexate**® (Roche)
Injection, flumazenil 100 micrograms/mL. Net price 5-mL amp = £16.32

NALOXONE HYDROCHLORIDE
Indications: reversal of opioid-induced respiratory depression
Cautions: cardiovascular disease or those receiving cardiotoxic drugs (serious adverse cardiovascular effects reported); physical dependence on opioids (precipitates withdrawal); pain (see also under Titration of Dose, below); has short duration of action (repeated doses or infusion may be necessary to reverse effects of opioids with longer duration of action)
TITRATION OF DOSE. When used postoperatively, the dose should be titrated for each patient in order to obtain optimum respiratory response while maintaining **adequate** analgesia
Side-effects: nausea and vomiting reported; tachycardia and fibrillation also reported
Dose: by intravenous injection, 100–200 micrograms (1.5–3 micrograms/kg); if response inadequate, increments of 100 micrograms every 2 minutes; further doses *by intramuscular injection* after 1–2 hours if required
CHILD, *by intravenous injection*, 10 micrograms/kg; subsequent dose of 100 micrograms/kg if no response; if intravenous route not possible, may be given in divided doses *by intramuscular or subcutaneous injection*
NEONATE, *by subcutaneous, intramuscular, or intravenous injection*, 10 micrograms/kg, repeated every 2 to 3 minutes *or* 200 micrograms (60 micrograms/kg) *by intramuscular injection* as a single dose at birth (onset of action slower)

PoM **Naloxone** (Non-proprietary)
Injection, naloxone hydrochloride 20 micrograms/ mL. Net price 2-mL amp = £3.48
Injection, naloxone hydrochloride 400 micrograms/mL—see under Emergency Treatment of Poisoning p. 22
PoM **Narcan**® —see under Emergency Treatment of Poisoning p. 22
PoM **Narcan Neonatal**® (Du Pont)
Injection, naloxone hydrochloride 20 micrograms/ mL. Net price 2-mL amp = £3.48

15.1.8   Drugs for malignant hyperthermia

Dantrolene is used in the treatment of malignant hyperthermia which is a rare but potentially lethal complication of anaesthesia. It is characterised by a rapid rise in temperature, increasing muscle rigidity, tachycardia, and acidosis and can be triggered off by volatile anaesthetics, and suxamethonium. Dantrolene acts on skeletal muscle by interfering with calcium efflux in the muscle cell and stopping the contractile process. Known trigger agents should be avoided during anaesthesia.

DANTROLENE SODIUM
Indications: malignant hyperthermia
Cautions: avoid extravasation; **interactions:** Appendix 1 (muscle relaxants)
Dose: by rapid intravenous injection, 1 mg/kg, repeated as required to a cumulative max. of 10 mg/kg

PoM **Dantrium Intravenous**® (Procter & Gamble Pharm.)
Injection, powder for reconstitution, dantrolene sodium. Net price 20-mg vial = £22.52 (hosp. only)

15.2   Local anaesthesia

The use of local anaesthetics by injection or by application to mucous membranes to produce local analgesia is discussed in this section.

See also section 1.7 (colon and rectum), section 11.7 (eye), section 12.3 (oropharynx), and section 13.3 (skin).

USE OF LOCAL ANAESTHETICS. Local anaesthetic drugs act by causing a reversible block to conduction along nerve fibres. The drugs used vary widely in their potency, toxicity, duration of action, stability, solubility in water, and ability to penetrate mucous membranes. These variations determine their suitability for use by various routes, e.g. topical (surface), infiltration, plexus, epidural (extradural) or spinal block.

ADMINISTRATION. In estimating the safe dosage of these drugs it is important to take account of the rate at which they are absorbed and excreted as well as their potency. The patient's age, weight, physique, and clinical condition, the degree of vascularity of the area to which the drug is to be applied, and the duration of administration are other factors which must be taken into account.

Local anaesthetics do not rely on the circulation to transport them to their sites of action, but uptake into the general circulation is important in terminating their action. Following most regional anaesthetic procedures, maximum arterial plasma concentrations of anaesthetic develop within about 10 to 25 minutes, so **careful surveillance** for toxic effects is necessary during the first 30 minutes after injection. Great care must be taken to avoid accidental intravascular injection.

Epidural anaesthesia is commonly used during surgery, often combined with general anaesthesia, because of its protective effect against the stress response of surgery. It is often used when good postoperative pain relief is essential (e.g. aortic aneurysm surgery or major gut surgery).

TOXICITY. Toxic effects associated with the local anaesthetics are usually a result of excessively high plasma concentrations, and systemic effects whether associated with acute or cumulative overdose or with accidental intravascular injection. Effects initially include a feeling of inebriation and lightheadedness followed by sedation, circumoral paraesthesia and twitching; convulsions can occur in severe reactions. On intravenous injection convulsions and cardiovascular collapse may occur very rapidly. Hypersensitivity reactions occur mainly with the ester-type local anaesthetics such as amethocaine, benzocaine, cocaine, and procaine; reactions are less frequent with the amide types such as lignocaine, bupivacaine, prilocaine, and ropivacaine.

Toxicity may occur with repeated dosages due to accumulation of the drug, and reducing doses should therefore be given. Toxic effects may also occur if the injection is too rapid. Local anaesthetics should **not** be injected into inflamed or infected tissues nor should they be applied to the traumatised urethra. Under these conditions the drug may be so rapidly absorbed that a systemic rather than a local reaction is produced.

USE OF VASOCONSTRICTORS. Most local anaesthetics, with the exception of cocaine, cause dilation of blood vessels. The addition of a vasoconstrictor such as **adrenaline** (epinephrine) diminishes local blood flow, slows the rate of absorption of the local anaesthetic, and prolongs its local effect. Care is necessary when using adrenaline for this purpose because, in excess, it may produce ischaemic necrosis.

Adrenaline should **not** be added to injections used in digits and appendages. When adrenaline is included the final concentration should be 1 in 200 000 (5 micrograms/mL). In dental surgery, up to 1 in 80 000 (12.5 micrograms/mL) of adrenaline is used with local anaesthetics. There is no justification for using higher concentrations.

The total dose of adrenaline should **not** exceed 500 micrograms and it is essential not to exceed a concentration of 1 in 200 000 (5 micrograms/mL) if more than 50 mL of the mixture is to be injected. For general cautions associated with the use of adrenaline, see section 2.7.3. For drug interactions, see Appendix 1 (sympathomimetics).

LIGNOCAINE

Lignocaine (lidocaine) is effectively absorbed from mucous membranes and is a useful surface anaesthetic in concentrations of 2 to 4%. Except for surface anaesthesia, solutions should not usually exceed 1% in strength. The duration of the block (with adrenaline) is about 1½ hours.

LIGNOCAINE HYDROCHLORIDE
(Lidocaine Hydrochloride)

Indications: see under Dose; also dental anaesthesia (see next page); ventricular arrhythmias (section 2.3.2)

Cautions: epilepsy, hepatic or respiratory impairment, impaired cardiac conduction, bradycardia; porphyria (section 9.8.2); reduce dose in elderly or debilitated; resuscitative equipment should be available; see section 2.3.2 for effects on heart; **interactions:** Appendix 1 (lignocaine)

Contra-indications: hypovolaemia, complete heart block; do not use solutions containing adrenaline for anaesthesia in appendages

Side-effects: CNS effects include confusion, respiratory depression and convulsions; hypotension and bradycardia (may lead to cardiac arrest), hypersensitivity reported; see also notes above

Dose: infiltration anaesthesia, *by injection,* according to patient's weight and nature of procedure, max. 200 mg (or 500 mg if given in solutions containing adrenaline)—see also Administration on p. 550 and see also **important** warning below
Intravenous regional anaesthesia and nerve blocks, seek expert advice
Surface anaesthesia, usual strengths 2–4%, see preparations below

Important: the licensed doses stated above may not be appropriate in some settings and expert advice should be sought

Lignocaine hydrochloride injections
PoM **Lignocaine** (Non-proprietary)
Injection 0.5%, lignocaine hydrochloride 5 mg/mL, net price 10-mL amp = 25p
Injection 1%, lignocaine hydrochloride 10 mg/mL, net price 2-mL amp = 19p; 5-mL amp = 19p; 10-mL amp = 32p; 20-mL amp = 45p
Injection 2%, lignocaine hydrochloride 20 mg/mL, net price 2-mL amp = 24p; 5-mL amp = 21p

PoM **Min-I-Jet**® **Lignocaine Hydrochloride with Adrenaline** (IMS)
Injection 0.5% with adrenaline 1 in 200 000, lignocaine hydrochloride 5 mg/mL, adrenaline 1 in 200 000 (5 micrograms/mL). Net price 5-mL disposable syringe = £3.88

PoM **Xylocaine**® (Astra)
Injection 0.5%, anhydrous lignocaine hydrochloride 5 mg/mL. Net price 20-mL vial = 65p
Injection 0.5% with adrenaline 1 in 200 000, anhydrous lignocaine hydrochloride 5 mg/mL, adrena-

line 1 in 200 000 (5 micrograms/mL). Net price 20-mL vial = 67p
Injection 1%, anhydrous lignocaine hydrochloride 10 mg/mL. Net price 20-mL vial = 67p
Injection 1% with adrenaline 1 in 200 000, anhydrous lignocaine hydrochloride 10 mg/mL, adrenaline 1 in 200 000 (5 micrograms/mL). Net price 20-mL vial = 69p
Injection 2%, anhydrous lignocaine hydrochloride 20 mg/mL. Net price 20-mL vial = 71p
Injection 2% with adrenaline 1 in 200 000, anhydrous lignocaine hydrochloride 20 mg/mL, adrenaline 1 in 200 000 (5 micrograms/mL). Net price 20-mL vial = 73p

Lignocaine injections for dental use
Note. Consult expert dental sources for specific advice in relation to dose of lignocaine for dental anaesthesia
A large variety of lignocaine injections, plain or with adrenaline or noradrenaline, is also available in dental cartridges under the names **Lignospan**®, **Lignostab A**®, **Rexocaine**®, **Xylocaine**®, and **Xylotox**®.

Lignocaine for surface anaesthesia
Important. Rapid and extensive absorption may result in systemic side-effects
PoM **Emla**® (Astra)
Drug Tariff cream, lignocaine 2.5%, prilocaine 2.5%. Net price 5-g tube = £1.73
Surgical pack cream, lignocaine 2.5%, prilocaine 2.5%. Net price 30-g tube = £10.25
Premedication pack cream, lignocaine 2.5%, prilocaine 2.5%. Net price 10 × 5-g tube with 25 occlusive dressings = £19.50
Anaesthesia before e.g. venepuncture (not for infants), apply a thick layer under an occlusive dressing 1–5 hours before procedure; split skin grafting, apply a thick layer under an occlusive dressing 2–5 hours before procedure; genital warts (not for children), apply up to 10 g 5–10 minutes before removal
Cautions: not for wounds, mucous membranes (except genital warts in adults) or atopic dermatitis; avoid use near eyes or middle ear; although systemic absorption is low, caution in anaemia, or congenital or acquired methaemoglobinaemia (see also Prilocaine, p. 552); *side-effects* include transient paleness, redness, and oedema; **contra-indicated** in infants under 1 year

Instillagel® (CliniFlex)
Gel, lignocaine hydrochloride 2%, chlorhexidine gluconate solution 0.25%, in a sterile lubricant basis in disposable syringe. Net price 6-mL syringe = £1.51; 11-mL syringe = £1.69
Dose: 6–11 mL into urethra

PoM **Laryng-O-Jet** ® (IMS)
Jet spray 4% (disposable kit for laryngotracheal anaesthesia), lignocaine hydrochloride 40 mg/mL. Net price per unit (4-mL vial and disposable sterile cannula with cover and vial injector) = £4.55
Dose: usually 160 mg (4 mL) as a single dose instilled as jet spray into lumen of larynx and trachea (reduce dose according to size, age and condition of patient); max. 200 mg (5 mL)
Caution: may be rapidly and almost completely absorbed from respiratory tract and systemic side-effects may occur; extreme caution if mucosa has been traumatised or if sepsis present

---

Cautionary label wordings, see inside back cover

Xylocaine® (Astra)

Antiseptic gel, anhydrous lignocaine hydrochloride 2%, chlorhexidine gluconate solution 0.25% in a sterile lubricant basis. Net price 20 g = £1.06; 20-g single-use syringe (*Accordion®*) = 98p

Dose: into urethra, men 10 mL followed by 3–5 mL; women 5–10 mL

Gel, anhydrous lignocaine hydrochloride 2%, in a sterile lubricant water-miscible basis. Net price 20 g = 76p; 20-g single-use syringe (*Accordion®*) = 98p

Additives: include hydroxybenzoates (parabens)

Dose:
Into urethra, men 10 mL, followed by further 10 mL (total of up to 40 mL for cystoscopy); women 5–10 mL
Endoscopy, 10–20 mL
Endotracheal intubation, 5 mL applied to surface of tube (avoid introducing gel into lumen)

Ointment, lignocaine 5% in a water-miscible basis. Net price 15 g = 80p

Additives: include propylene glycol

Dose: max. 35 g in 24 hours

Spray (= pump spray), lignocaine 10% (100 mg/g) supplying 10 mg lignocaine/dose; 500 spray doses per container. Net price 50-mL bottle = £3.13

Dose: dental practice, 1–5 doses; maxillary sinus puncture, 3 doses; during delivery in obstetrics, up to 20 doses; procedures in pharynx, larynx, and trachea, up to 20 doses

Topical 4%, anhydrous lignocaine hydrochloride 40 mg/mL. Net price 30-mL bottle = £1.21

Additives: include hydroxybenzoates (parabens)

Dose: bronchoscopy, 2–3 mL with suitable spray; biopsy in mouth, 3–4 mL with suitable spray *or* swab (with adrenaline if necessary); max. 7.5 mL

BUPIVACAINE

The great advantage of bupivacaine over other local anaesthetics is its longer duration of action. It has a slow onset of action, taking up to 30 minutes for full effect. It is often used in lumbar epidural blockade and is particularly suitable for continuous epidural analgesia in labour. It is **contra-indicated** in intravenous regional anaesthesia (Bier's block). It is the principal drug for spinal anaesthesia in the UK.

BUPIVACAINE HYDROCHLORIDE

Indications: see under Dose

Cautions; Contra-indications; Side-effects: see under Lignocaine Hydrochloride and notes above; avoid accidental intravascular injection; myocardial depression may be more severe and more resistant to treatment; contra-indicated in intravenous regional anaesthesia (Bier's block); **interactions:** Appendix 1 (bupivacaine)

Dose: adjusted according to patient's weight and nature of procedure—**important**: see also under Administration, above

Local infiltration, 0.25% (up to 60 mL)

Peripheral nerve block, 0.25% (max. 60 mL), 0.375% (max. 40 mL), 0.5% (max. 30 mL)

Epidural block,
Surgery, *lumbar*, 0.5–0.75% (max. 20 mL of either)
   caudal, 0.5% (max. 30 mL)
Labour, *lumbar*, 0.25–0.5% (max. 12 mL of either)
   caudal, but rarely used, 0.25% (max. 20 mL), 0.375% (max. 20 mL), 0.5% (max. 20 mL)

Note. 0.75% **contra-indicated** for epidural use in obstetrics. **Important:** the licensed doses stated above may not be appropriate in some settings and expert advice should be sought

PoM **Marcain Heavy®** (Astra)

Injection, anhydrous bupivacaine hydrochloride 5 mg, glucose 80 mg/mL. Net price 4-mL amp = 98p

Dose: spinal anaesthesia, 2–4 mL

PoM **Marcain®** (Astra)

Injection, anhydrous bupivacaine hydrochloride 2.5 mg/mL (*Marcain®* 0.25%), net price 10-mL *Polyamp®* = £1.11; 3.75 mg/mL (*Marcain®* 0.375%), 10-mL *Polyamp®* = £1.22; 5 mg/mL (*Marcain®* 0.5%), 10-mL *Polyamp®* = £1.27; 7.5 mg/mL (*Marcain®* 0.75%), 10-mL *Polyamp®* = £1.90.

Note. Bupivacaine hydrochloride injection 0.25% and 0.5% also available from Antigen, Faulding DBL

PoM **Marcain with Adrenaline®** (Astra)

Injection 0.25%, bupivacaine hydrochloride 2.5 mg/mL, adrenaline 1 in 200 000 (5 micrograms/mL). Net price 10-mL amp = £1.40

Injection 0.5%, bupivacaine hydrochloride 5 mg/ mL, adrenaline 1 in 200 000 (5 micrograms/mL). Net price 10-mL amp = £1.23

PRILOCAINE

Prilocaine is a local anaesthetic of low toxicity which is similar to lignocaine. If used in high doses, methaemoglobinaemia may occur which can be treated with intravenous injection of methylene blue 1% using a dose of 1 mg/kg.

PRILOCAINE HYDROCHLORIDE

Indications: infiltration, intravenous regional anaesthesia, nerve block; also dental anaesthesia

Cautions; Contra-indications; Side-effects: see under Lignocaine Hydrochloride and notes above; caution in renal impairment; avoid in anaemia or congenital or acquired methaemoglobinaemia

Dose: adjusted according to site of operation and response of patient, to max. 400 mg used alone, or 600 mg if used with felypressin

PoM **Citanest®** (Astra)

Injection 0.5%, prilocaine hydrochloride 5 mg/mL. Net price 20-mL multidose vial = 71p; 50-mL multidose vial = 99p; 50-mL single dose vial = £1.27

Injection 1%, prilocaine hydrochloride 10 mg/mL. Net price 20-mL multidose vial = 73p; 50-mL multidose vial = £1.03

Injection 2%, prilocaine hydrochloride 20 mg/mL. Net price 10-mL single dose vial = 73p

Injection 4%, prilocaine hydrochloride 40 mg/mL. Net price 2-mL cartridge = 18p

---

PoM Citanest with Octapressin® (Astra)

Injection 3%, prilocaine hydrochloride 30 mg/mL, felypressin 0.03 unit/mL. For dental use. Net price 2-mL cartridge and self-aspirating cartridge (both) = 18p

PROCAINE

Procaine is now seldom used. It is as potent as lignocaine but has a shorter duration of action. It provides less intense analgesia because of reduced spread through the tissues. It is of no value as a surface anaesthetic.

PROCAINE HYDROCHLORIDE

Indications: local anaesthesia by infiltration and regional routes (but see notes above)

Cautions; Side-effects: see notes above

Dose: adjusted according to site of operation and patient's response

By injection, up to 1 g (200 mL of 0.5% solution or 100 mL of 1%) with adrenaline 1 in 200 000

PoM Procaine (Non-proprietary)

Injection, procaine hydrochloride 2% (20 mg/mL) in sodium chloride intravenous infusion. Net price 2-mL amp = £1.19; 5-mL amp = £3.49
Available from Martindale

AMETHOCAINE

Amethocaine (tetracaine) is an effective local anaesthetic for topical application; a 4% gel is indicated for anaesthesia prior to venepuncture or venous cannulation. It is rapidly absorbed from mucous membranes and should **never** be applied to inflamed, traumatised, or highly vascular surfaces. It should **never** be used to provide anaesthesia for bronchoscopy or cystoscopy, as lignocaine is a safer alternative. It is used in ophthalmology (section 11.7) and in skin preparations (section 13.3). Hypersensitivity to amethocaine has been reported.

AMETHOCAINE
(Tetracaine)

Indications: see under preparation below

Cautions; Contra-indications; Side effects: see notes above; side-effects include erythema, oedema and pruritus

Important. Rapid and extensive absorption may result in systemic side-effects (see also notes above)

Ametop® (S&N Hlth.)

Gel, amethocaine 4%. Net price 1.5-g tube = £1.20
Dose: apply contents of tube to site of venepuncture or venous cannulation and cover with occlusive dressing; remove gel and dressing after 30 minutes for venepuncture and after 45 minutes for venous cannulation; PREMATURE INFANT and INFANT under 1 month not recommended

ROPIVACAINE

Ropivacaine is a recently introduced amide type local anaesthetic agent.

ROPIVACAINE HYDROCHLORIDE

Indications: see under Dose

Cautions; Contra-indications; Side-effects: see under Lignocaine Hydrochloride and notes above

Dose: adjust according to patient's physical status and nature of procedure—see also under Administration on on p. 550

Surgical anaesthesia,
lumbar epidural, 15–20 mL of 10 mg/mL solution *or* 15–25 mL of 7.5 mg/mL solution; caesarean section, 15–20 mL of 7.5 mg/mL solution

thoracic epidural (to establish block for postoperative pain), 5–15 mL of 7.5 mg/mL solution

field block, up to 30 mL of 7.5 mg/mL solution

Acute pain,
lumbar epidural, 10–20 mL of 2 mg/mL solution followed by 10–15 mL of 2 mg/mL solution at intervals of at least 30 minutes *or* 6–10 mL/hour of 2 mg/mL solution as a continuous epidural infusion

thoracic epidural, 4–8 mL/hour of 2 mg/mL solution as a continuous infusion

field block, up to 100 mL of 2 mg/mL solution

▼ **PoM Naropin®** (Astra)

Injection, ropivacaine hydrochloride 2 mg/mL, net price 10-mL Polyamp® = £1.43; 7.5 mg/mL, 10-mL Polyamp® = £2.77; 10 mg/mL, 10-mL Polyamp® = £3.36

Epidural infusion, ropivacaine hydrochloride 2 mg/mL, net price 100-mL Polybag® = £8.62, 200-mL Polybag® = £15.13

OTHER LOCAL ANAESTHETICS

Benzocaine is a local anaesthetic of low potency and toxicity. It is an ingredient of some proprietary throat lozenges (section 12.3.3).

Mepivacaine is a local anaesthetic used in dentistry. It is available in dental cartridges with or without adrenaline as *Scandonest®*.

Cocaine readily penetrates mucous membranes and is an effective surface anaesthetic with an intense vasoconstrictor action. However, apart from its use in otolaryngology (see below), it has now been replaced by less toxic alternatives. It has marked sympathomimetic activity and should **never** be given by injection because of its toxicity. As a result of its intense stimulant effect it is a drug of addiction. In otolaryngology cocaine is applied to the nasal mucosa in concentrations of 4 to 10% (40–100 mg/mL). The maximum total dose recommended for application to the nasal mucosa in fit adults is a total of 1.5 mg/kg, which is equivalent to a total topical dose of approximately 100 mg for an adult male. It should be used only by those skilled in the precautions needed to *minimise absorption* and the *consequent risk of arrhythmias*. Although cocaine interacts with other drugs liable to induce arrhythmias, including adrenaline, some otolaryngologists consider that combined use of topical cocaine with topical adrenaline (in the form of a paste or a solution) improves the operative field and may possibly reduce absorption. Cocaine is a mydriatic as well as a local anaesthetic but owing to corneal toxicity it is now little used in ophthalmology. Cocaine should be avoided in porphyria (section 9.8.2).

Appendix 1: Interactions

Two or more drugs given at the same time may exert their effects independently or may interact. The interaction may be potentiation or antagonism of one drug by another, or occasionally some other effect. Adverse drug interactions should be reported to the CSM as for other adverse drug reactions.

Drug interactions may be **pharmacodynamic** or **pharmacokinetic**.

PHARMACODYNAMIC INTERACTIONS

These are interactions between drugs which have similar or antagonistic pharmacological effects or side-effects. They may be due to competition at receptor sites, or occur between drugs acting on the same physiological system. They are usually predictable from a knowledge of the pharmacology of the interacting drugs; in general, those demonstrated with one drug are likely to occur with related drugs. They occur to a greater or lesser extent in most patients who receive the interacting drugs.

PHARMACOKINETIC INTERACTIONS

These occur when one drug alters the absorption, distribution, metabolism, or excretion of another, thus increasing or reducing the amount of drug available to produce its pharmacological effects. They are not easily predicted and many of them affect only a small proportion of patients taking the combination of drugs. Pharmacokinetic interactions occurring with one drug cannot be assumed to occur with related drugs unless their pharmacokinetic properties are known to be similar.

Pharmacokinetic interactions are of several types:

AFFECTING ABSORPTION. The rate of absorption or the total amount absorbed can both be altered by drug interactions. Delayed absorption is rarely of clinical importance unless high peak plasma concentrations are required (e.g. when giving an analgesic). Reduction in the total amount absorbed, however, may result in ineffective therapy.

DUE TO CHANGES IN PROTEIN BINDING. To a variable extent most drugs are loosely bound to plasma proteins. Protein-binding sites are non-specific and one drug can displace another thereby increasing its proportion free to diffuse from plasma to its site of action. This only produces a detectable increase in effect if it is an extensively bound drug (more than 90%) that is not widely distributed throughout the body. Even so displacement rarely produces more than transient potentiation because this increased concentration of free drug results in an increased rate of elimination.

Displacement from protein binding plays a part in the potentiation of warfarin by phenylbutazone, sulphonamides, and tolbutamide but the importance of these interactions is due mainly to the fact that warfarin metabolism is also inhibited.

AFFECTING METABOLISM. Many drugs are metabolised in the liver. Induction of the hepatic microsomal enzyme system by one drug can gradually increase the rate of metabolism of another, resulting in lower plasma concentrations and a reduced effect. On withdrawal of the inducer plasma concentrations increase and toxicity may occur. Barbiturates, griseofulvin, most antiepileptics, and rifampicin are the most important enzyme inducers in man. Drugs affected include warfarin and the oral contraceptives.

Conversely when one drug inhibits the metabolism of another higher plasma concentrations are produced, rapidly resulting in an increased effect with risk of toxicity. Some drugs which potentiate warfarin and phenytoin do so by this mechanism.

AFFECTING RENAL EXCRETION. Drugs are eliminated through the kidney both by glomerular filtration and by active tubular secretion. Competition occurs between those which share active transport mechanisms in the proximal tubule. Thus probenecid delays the excretion of many drugs including penicillins, some cephalosporins, indomethacin, and dapsone; aspirin may increase the toxicity of methotrexate by a similar mechanism.

RELATIVE IMPORTANCE OF INTERACTIONS

Many drug interactions are harmless and many of those which are potentially harmful only occur in a small proportion of patients; moreover, the severity of an interaction varies from one patient to another. Drugs with a small therapeutic ratio (e.g. phenytoin) and those which require careful control of dosage (e.g. anticoagulants, antihypertensives, and antidiabetics) are most often involved.

Patients at increased risk from drug interactions include the elderly and those with impaired renal or liver function.

HAZARDOUS INTERACTIONS. The symbol • has been placed against interactions that are **potentially hazardous** and where combined administration of the drugs involved should be **avoided** (or only undertaken with caution and appropriate monitoring).

Interactions that have no symbol do not usually have serious consequences.

List of drug interactions

The following is an alphabetical list of drugs and their interactions; to avoid excessive cross-referencing each drug or group is listed twice: in the alphabetical list and also against the drug or group with which it interacts; changes in the interactions lists since BNF No. 34 (September 1997) are underlined.

For explanation of symbol • see previous page

Acarbose *see* Antidiabetics

ACE Inhibitors
Alcohol: enhanced hypotensive effect
Aldesleukin: enhanced hypotensive effect
Allopurinol: increased risk of toxicity with *captopril*, especially in renal impairment
Alprostadil: enhanced hypotensive effect
• Anaesthetics: enhanced hypotensive effect
• Analgesics: antagonism of hypotensive effect and increased risk of renal damage with *NSAIDs*; hyperkalaemia with *indomethacin, ketorolac and possibly other NSAIDs*
Antacids: absorption of *enalapril, fosinopril* and *possibly other ACE inhibitors* reduced
Anti-arrhythmics: *procainamide* increases risk of toxicity with *captopril*, especially in renal impairment
Antibacterials: absorption of *tetracyclines* reduced by *quinapril* (tablets contain magnesium carbonate excipient)
Antidepressants: enhanced hypotensive effect
Antidiabetics: hypoglycaemic effect possibly enhanced
other Antihypertensives: enhanced hypotensive effect; previous treatment with *clonidine* possibly delays antihypertensive effect of *captopril*
Antipsychotics: severe postural hypotension with *chlorpromazine and possibly other phenothiazines*
Anxiolytics and Hypnotics: enhanced hypotensive effect
Beta-blockers: enhanced hypotensive effect
Calcium-channel Blockers: enhanced hypotensive effect
Cardiac Glycosides: plasma concentration of *digoxin* possibly increased by *captopril*
Corticosteroids: antagonism of hypotensive effect
• Cyclosporin: increased risk of hyperkalaemia
• Diuretics: enhanced hypotensive effect (can be extreme); hyperkalaemia with *potassium-sparing diuretics*
Dopaminergics: *levodopa* enhances hypotensive effect
Epoetin: antagonism of hypotensive effect: increased risk of hyperkalaemia
• Lithium: *ACE inhibitors* reduce excretion of *lithium* (increased plasma-lithium concentration)
Muscle Relaxants: *baclofen* and *tizanidine* enhance hypotensive effect
Nitrates: enhance hypotensive effect
Oestrogens and Progestogens: *oestrogens* and *combined oral contraceptives* antagonise hypotensive effect
• Potassium Salts: increased risk of hyperkalaemia
Thymoxamine: enhanced hypotensive effect
Ulcer-healing Drugs: *carbenoxolone* antagonises hypotensive effect
Uricosurics: *probenecid* reduces excretion of *captopril*

Acebutolol *see* Beta-blockers
Aceclofenac *see* NSAIDs
Acemetacin *see* NSAIDs
Acetazolamide *see* Diuretics (carbonic anhydrase inhibitor)

Aciclovir and Famciclovir
Note. Interactions do not apply to topical preparations
other Antivirals: extreme lethargy reported on administration of *zidovudine* with *intravenous aciclovir*

Aciclovir and Famciclovir *(continued)*
Mycophenolate Mofetil: higher plasma concentrations of *aciclovir* and of *mycophenolate mofetil* on concomitant administration
Uricosurics: *probenecid* reduces *aciclovir* and possibly *famciclovir* excretion (increased plasma concentrations and risk of toxicity)

Acitretin *see* Retinoids
Acrivastine *see* Antihistamines
Adenosine
Note. Possibility of interaction with drugs tending to impair cardiac conduction
• Antiplatelet Drugs: effect enhanced and extended by *dipyridamole* (**important** risk of toxicity)
Theophylline: antagonism of anti-arrhythmic effect

Adrenaline *see* Sympathomimetics
Adrenergic Neurone Blockers
Alcohol: enhanced hypotensive effect
Alprostadil: enhanced hypotensive effect
• Anaesthetics: enhanced hypotensive effect
Analgesics: *NSAIDs* antagonise hypotensive effect
Anti-arrhythmics: increased risk of myocardial depression with *bretylium*
Antidepressants: *tricyclics* antagonise hypotensive effect
other Antihypertensives: enhanced hypotensive effect
Antipsychotics: *phenothiazines* enhance hypotensive effect (antagonism of hypotensive effect with higher doses of *chlorpromazine*)
Anxiolytics and Hypnotics: enhanced hypotensive effect
Beta-blockers: enhanced hypotensive effect
Calcium-channel Blockers: enhanced hypotensive effect
Corticosteroids: antagonism of hypotensive effect
Diuretics: enhanced hypotensive effect
Dopaminergics: *levodopa* enhances hypotensive effect
Muscle Relaxants: enhanced hypotensive effect with *tizanidine*
Nitrates: enhance hypotensive effect
Oestrogens and Progestogens: *oestrogens* and *combined oral contraceptives* antagonise hypotensive effect
Pizotifen: antagonism of hypotensive effect
• Sympathomimetics: *some anorectics, some cough and cold remedies (e.g. ephedrine)*, and *methylphenidate* antagonise hypotensive effect
Thymoxamine: enhanced hypotensive effect
Ulcer-healing Drugs: *carbenoxolone* antagonises hypotensive effect

Alcohol
ACE Inhibitors: enhanced hypotensive effect
Analgesics: sedative and hypotensive effect of *opioid analgesics* enhanced
• Antibacterials: disulfiram-like reaction with *cephamandole, metronidazole*, and *tinidazole*; increased risk of seizures with *cycloserine*
• Anticoagulants: *see* Warfarin
• Antidepressants: sedative effect of *tricyclics (and related)* enhanced; *tyramine* (contained in some alcoholic and dealcoholised beverages) interacts with *MAOIs* (hypertensive crisis)—but if no tyramine, enhanced hypotensive effect; effects of alcohol possibly enhanced by *SSRIs*

Alcohol *(continued)*
Antidiabetics: enhanced hypoglycaemic effect; flushing with *chlorpropamide* (in susceptible subjects); increased risk of lactic acidosis with *metformin*
Antiepileptics: CNS side-effects of *carbamazepine* possibly enhanced
Antihistamines: enhanced sedative effect
Antihypertensives: enhanced hypotensive effect; sedative effect of *indoramin* enhanced
Antimuscarinics: sedative effect of *hyoscine* enhanced
Antipsychotics: enhanced sedative effect
Anxiolytics and Hypnotics: enhanced sedative effect
Barbiturates and Primidone: enhanced sedative effect
Beta-blockers: enhanced hypotensive effect
Calcium-channel Blockers: plasma-alcohol concentration possibly increased by *verapamil*
Cytotoxics: disulfiram-like reaction with *procarbazine*
Dopaminergics: reduced tolerance to *bromocriptine*
Lofexidine: enhanced sedative effect
Muscle Relaxants: *baclofen* and *tizanidine* enhance sedative effect
Nabilone: enhanced sedative effect
Nitrates: enhanced hypotensive effect
Retinoids: *etretinate* formed from *acitretin* in presence of *alcohol*

Aldesleukin
Antihypertensives: enhanced hypotensive effect

Alendronic Acid *see* Bisphosphonates
Alfentanil *see* Opioid Analgesics
Alfuzosin *see* Alpha-blockers (post-synaptic)

Allopurinol
ACE Inhibitors: increased risk of toxicity with *captopril*, especially in renal impairment
Anticoagulants: effects of *nicoumalone* and *warfarin* possibly enhanced
Cyclosporin: plasma-cyclosporin concentration possibly increased (risk of nephrotoxicity)
• Cytotoxics: effects of *azathioprine* (*see also* p. 379) and *mercaptopurine* enhanced with increased toxicity

Alpha$_2$-adrenoceptor Stimulants
Antidepressants: manufacturers of *apraclonidine* and *brimonidine* advise avoid concomitant use with *tricyclics or related antidepressants* or *MAOIs*
Sympathomimetics: possible risk of hypertension with *adrenaline* and *noradrenaline*

Alpha-blockers
ACE Inhibitors: enhanced hypotensive effect
Alcohol: enhanced hypotensive effect; sedative effect of *indoramin* enhanced
Aldesleukin: enhanced hypotensive effect
Alprostadil: enhanced hypotensive effect
• Anaesthetics: enhanced hypotensive effect
Analgesics: *NSAIDs* antagonise hypotensive effect
• Antidepressants: enhanced hypotensive effect; manufacturer of *indoramin* advises avoid *MAOIs*
other Antihypertensives: additive hypotensive effect
Antipsychotics: enhanced hypotensive effect
Anxiolytics and Hypnotics: enhanced hypotensive and sedative effect
• Beta-blockers: enhanced hypotensive effect; increased risk of first-dose hypotensive effect of *post-synaptic alpha-blockers such as prazosin*
• Calcium-channel Blockers: enhanced hypotensive effect; increased risk of first-dose hypotensive effect of *post-synaptic alpha-blockers such as prazosin*
Corticosteroids : antagonism of hypotensive effect
• Diuretics: enhanced hypotensive effect; increased risk of first-dose hypotensive effect of *post-synaptic alpha-blockers such as prazosin*
Dopaminergics: *levodopa* enhances hypotensive effect

Alpha-blockers *(continued)*
Muscle Relaxants: *baclofen* and *tizanidine* enhance hypotensive effect
Nitrates: enhanced hypotensive effect
Oestrogens and Progestogens: *oestrogens and combined oral contraceptives* antagonise hypotensive effect
• Thymoxamine: possible severe postural hypotension
Ulcer-healing Drugs: *carbenoxolone* antagonises hypotensive effect

Alprazolam *see* Anxiolytics and Hypnotics

Alprostadil
Antihypertensives: enhanced hypotensive effect

Altretamine
• Antidepressants: risk of severe postural hypotension with *MAOIs* and *tricyclics*
• Pyridoxine: reduced response to altretamine

Aluminium Hydroxide *see* Antacids and Adsorbents

Amantadine
Antihypertensives: *methyldopa* and *metirosine* have extrapyramidal side-effects
Antimuscarinics: increased antimuscarinic side-effects
Antipsychotics: all have extrapyramidal side-effects
Metoclopramide and Domperidone: have extrapyramidal side-effects
Tetrabenazine: has extrapyramidal side-effects

Amifostine
Note. Limited information available—rapid clearance from plasma minimises risk of interactions; possibility of interactions with antihypertensives and other drugs which potentiate hypotension

Amikacin *see* Aminoglycosides
Amiloride *see* Diuretics (potassium-sparing)

Aminoglutethimide
• Anticoagulants: metabolism of *nicoumalone and warfarin* accelerated (reduced anticoagulant effect)
Antidiabetics: manufacturer advises metabolism of *oral antidiabetics* possibly accelerated
Cardiac Glycosides: metabolism of *digitoxin only* accelerated (reduced effect)
Corticosteroids: metabolism of *corticosteroids* accelerated (reduced effect)
Diuretics: increased risk of hyponatraemia
other Hormone Antagonists: plasma concentration of *tamoxifen* reduced
Oestrogens and Progestogens: *aminoglutethimide* reduces plasma concentration of *medroxy-progesterone*
Theophylline: metabolism of *theophylline* accelerated (reduced effect)

Aminoglycosides
other Antibacterials: increased risk of nephrotoxicity with *colistin*; increased risk of ototoxicity and nephrotoxicity with *capreomycin* and *vancomycin*
• Anticoagulants: *see* Phenindione and Warfarin
Antidiabetics: *neomycin* possibly enhances hypoglycaemic effect of *acarbose* and increases severity of gastro-intestinal effects
Antifungals: increased risk of nephrotoxicity with *amphotericin*
Bisphosphonates: increased risk of hypocalcaemia
• Botulinum Toxin: neuromuscular block enhanced (risk of toxicity)
• Cyclosporin: increased risk of nephrotoxicity
• Cytotoxics: increased risk of nephrotoxicity and possibly of ototoxicity with *cisplatin*
• Diuretics: increased risk of ototoxicity with *loop diuretics* (*see also* p. 252)
• Muscle Relaxants: effect of *non-depolarising muscle relaxants* enhanced
• Parasympathomimetics: antagonism of effect of *neostigmine and pyridostigmine*

Aminophylline *see* Theophylline

Amiodarone

Note. Amiodarone has a long half-life; there is a potential for drug interactions to occur for several weeks (or even months) after treatment with it has been stopped

• *other* Anti-arrhythmics: additive effect with *disopyramide, flecainide, procainamide, and quinidine* (increased risk of ventricular arrhythmias—avoid concomitant use); increased plasma concentrations of *flecainide, procainamide* and *quinidine*; increased myocardial depression with any anti-arrhythmic

• Antibacterials: increased risk of ventricular arrhythmias with *erythromycin* (parenteral) and *co-trimoxazole* (avoid concomitant use)

• Anticoagulants: metabolism of *nicoumalone and warfarin* inhibited (enhanced anticoagulant effect)

• Antidepressants: increased risk of ventricular arrhythmias with *tricyclics* (avoid concomitant use)

• Antiepileptics: metabolism of *phenytoin* inhibited (increased plasma concentration)

• Antihistamines: increased risk of ventricular arrhythmias with *astemizole* and *terfenadine* (avoid concomitant use)

• Antimalarials: increased risk of ventricular arrhythmias with *chloroquine, halofantrine, mefloquine* and *quinine* (avoid concomitant use)

• Antipsychotics: increased risk of ventricular arrhythmias with *phenothiazines, haloperidol, pimozide* and *sertindole* (avoid concomitant use)

• Antivirals: see Ritonavir, p. 581

• Beta-blockers: increased risk of bradycardia, AV block, and myocardial depression; increased risk of ventricular arrhythmias associated with *sotalol* (avoid concomitant use)

• Calcium-channel Blockers: *diltiazem and verapamil* increase risk of bradycardia, AV block, and myocardial depression

• Cardiac Glycosides: increased plasma concentration of *digoxin* (halve digoxin maintenance dose)

Cyclosporin: plasma concentration of *cyclosporin* possibly increased

Diuretics: toxicity increased if hypokalaemia occurs with *acetazolamide, loop diuretics, and thiazides*

Lithium: increased risk of hypothyroidism

• Pentamidine Isethionate: increased risk of ventricular arrhythmias with *amiodarone* (avoid concomitant use)

Thyroxine: for concomitant use see p. 69

Ulcer-healing Drugs: *cimetidine* increases plasma concentrations of *amiodarone*

Amisulpride *see* Antipsychotics
Amitriptyline *see* Antidepressants, Tricyclic
Amlodipine *see* Calcium-channel Blockers
Amoxapine *see* Antidepressants, Tricyclic
Amoxycillin *see* Penicillins
Amphetamines *see* Sympathomimetics

Amphotericin

Note. Close monitoring required with concomitant administration of nephrotoxic drugs or cytotoxics

Antibacterials: increased risk of nephrotoxicity with *aminoglycosides*

other Antifungals: *imidazoles* and *triazoles* possibly antagonise effect of amphotericin

• Cardiac Glycosides: increased toxicity if hypokalaemia occurs

• Corticosteroids: increased risk of hypokalaemia (avoid concomitant use unless corticosteroids needed to control reactions)

• Cyclosporin: increased risk of nephrotoxicity

Diuretics: increased risk of hypokalaemia with *loop diuretics* and *thiazides*

• Tacrolimus: increased risk of nephrotoxicity

Ampicillin *see* Penicillins
Amylobarbitone *see* Barbiturates and Primidone

Anabolic Steroids

• Anticoagulants: anticoagulant effect of *nicoumalone, phenindione, and warfarin* enhanced

Antidiabetics: hypoglycaemic effect possibly enhanced

Anaesthetics, General (*see also* Surgery and Long-term Medication, section 15.1)

• ACE Inhibitors: enhanced hypotensive effect

Antibacterials: possible potentiation of *isoniazid* hepatotoxicity; effect of *thiopentone* enhanced by *sulphonamides*; hypersensitivity-like reactions can occur with concomitant intravenous *vancomycin*

Antidepressants: risk of arrhythmias and hypotension increased with *tricyclics; MAOIs, see* section 15.1

• Antihypertensives: enhanced hypotensive effect

• Antipsychotics: enhanced hypotensive effect

Anxiolytics and Hypnotics: enhanced sedative effect

• Beta-blockers: enhanced hypotensive effect

• Calcium-channel Blockers: enhanced hypotensive effect and AV delay with *verapamil*; hypotensive effect of *dihydropyridines* enhanced by *isoflurane*

• Dopaminergics: risk of arrhythmias if *volatile liquid anaesthetics such as halothane* given with *levodopa*

Oxytocic: oxytocic effect possibly reduced by *volatile anaesthetics* (also enhanced hypotensive effect and risk of arrhythmias)

• Sympathomimetics: risk of arrhythmias if *adrenaline or isoprenaline* given with *volatile liquid anaesthetics such as halothane*

Theophylline: increased risk of arrhythmias with *halothane*

Anaesthetics, Local *see* Bupivacaine, Lignocaine
Analgesics *see* Aspirin, Nefopam, NSAIDs, Opioid Analgesics, and Paracetamol
Anion-exchange Resins *see* Cholestyramine and Colestipol

Antacids and Adsorbents

ACE Inhibitors: *antacids* reduce absorption of *enalapril, fosinopril* and *possibly other ACE inhibitors*

Analgesics: excretion of *aspirin* increased in alkaline urine; *antacids* reduce absorption of *diflunisal*

Anti-arrhythmics: excretion of *quinidine* reduced in alkaline urine (may occasionally increase plasma concentrations)

Antibacterials: *antacids* reduce absorption of *azithromycin, cefpodoxime, ciprofloxacin, isoniazid, nitrofurantoin, norfloxacin, ofloxacin, pivampicillin, rifampicin, and most tetracyclines*

Antiepileptics: *antacids* reduce absorption of *gabapentin* and *phenytoin*

Antifungals: *antacids* reduce absorption of *itraconazole* and *ketoconazole*

Antihistamines: *antacids* reduce absorption of *fexofenadine*

Antiplatelet Drugs: *dipyridamole* patient information leaflet advises avoidance of *antacids*

Antimalarials: *antacids* reduce absorption of *chloroquine and hydroxychloroquine*

Antipsychotics: *antacids* reduce absorption of *phenothiazines*

Bile Acids: *antacids* may reduce absorption of *chenodeoxycholic acid* and *ursodeoxycholic acid*

Bisphosphonates: *antacids* reduce absorption

Iron: *magnesium trisilicate* reduces absorption of *oral iron*

Lithium: *sodium bicarbonate* increases excretion (reduced plasma-lithium concentration)

Mycophenolate Mofetil: *antacids* reduce absorption of *mycophenolate mofetil*

Penicillamine: *antacids* reduce absorption

Antazoline *see* Antihistamines

Anti-arrhythmics *see* Adenosine; Amiodarone; Disopyramide; Flecainide; Lignocaine; Mexiletine; Moracizine; Procainamide; Propafenone; Quinidine

Anticholinergics *see* Antimuscarinics
Anticholinesterases *see* Parasympathomimetics
Anticoagulants *see* Heparin, Phenindione, and Warfarin
Antidepressants *see* Antidepressants, SSRI; Antidepressants, Tricyclic; MAOIs; Mianserin; Moclobemide; Nefazodone; Reboxetine; Trazodone; Tryptophan; Venlafaxine; Viloxazine

Antidepressants, SSRI

Alcohol: effects possibly enhanced

Anti-arrhythmics: plasma-flecainide concentration increased by *fluoxetine*

* Anticoagulants: effect of *nicoumalone and warfarin* possibly enhanced
* *other* Antidepressants: CNS effects of *SSRIs* increased by *MAOIs* (risk of serious toxicity); *SSRI* should not be started until 2 weeks after stopping *MAOI*; conversely, *MAOI* should not be started until at least 1 week after *citalopram* or *fluvoxamine* have been stopped, at least 5 weeks for *fluoxetine*, at least 2 weeks for *paroxetine* and *sertraline*; *moclobemide see* p. 182; plasma concentrations of some *tricyclics* increased; agitation and nausea with *tryptophan*
* Antiepileptics: antagonism (convulsive threshold lowered); plasma concentration of *carbamazepine* increased by *fluoxetine* and *fluvoxamine*; plasma concentration of *phenytoin* increased by *fluoxetine* and *fluvoxamine*; *phenytoin and possibly other antiepileptics* reduce plasma concentration of *paroxetine*
* Antihistamines: *fluvoxamine* increases risk of arrhythmias with *terfenadine*—avoid concomitant use
* Antipsychotics: plasma concentration of *clozapine* possibly increased by *fluoxetine* and *fluvoxamine*; plasma concentration of *haloperidol* increased by *fluoxetine*; plasma concentration of *sertindole* increased by *fluoxetine* and *paroxetine*
* Antivirals: see Ritonavir, p. 581
Anxiolytics and Hypnotics: plasma concentration of some *benzodiazepines* increased by *fluvoxamine*
* Barbiturates and Primidone: *see under* Antiepileptics, above
Beta-blockers: plasma concentration of *propranolol* increased by *fluvoxamine*
* Dopaminergics: hypertension and CNS excitation with *fluoxetine* and *selegiline*
* 5HT$_1$ Agonists: risk of CNS toxicity increased by *sumatriptan* (avoid concomitant use)
* Lithium: increased CNS effects (lithium toxicity reported)
Opioid Analgesics: *tramadol* possibly increases risk of convulsions
* Theophylline: plasma-theophylline concentration increased by *fluvoxamine* (concomitant use should usually be avoided, but where not possible halve theophylline dose and monitor plasma-theophylline concentration)

Antidepressants, Tricyclic

* Alcohol: enhanced sedative effect
Alpha$_2$-adrenoceptor Stimulants: manufacturers of *apraclonidine* and *brimonidine* advise avoid concomitant use
* Altretamine: risk of severe postural hypotension
Anaesthetics: risk of arrhythmias and hypotension increased
Analgesics: possibly increased side-effects with *nefopam*
* Anti-arrhythmics: increased risk of ventricular arrhythmias with drugs which prolong QT interval, including *amiodarone* (avoid concomitant use), *disopyramide*, *procainamide* and *quinidine*
Antibacterials: plasma concentrations of some *tricyclics* reduced by *rifampicin* (reduced antidepressant effect)

Antidepressants, Tricyclic *(continued)*

* *other* Antidepressants: CNS excitation and hypertension with *MAOIs; tricyclic or related antidepressant* should not be started until 2 weeks after stopping *MAOI*; conversely, *MAOI* should not be started until at least 1 week after *tricyclic or related antidepressant* has been stopped; *moclobemide see* p. 182; plasma concentrations of some *tricyclics* increased by *SSRIs*
* Antiepileptics: antagonism (convulsive threshold lowered); plasma concentrations of some *tricyclics* reduced (reduced antidepressant effect)
* Antihistamines: increased antimuscarinic and sedative effects; increased risk of ventricular arrhythmias with *astemizole* and *terfenadine*
* Antihypertensives: in general, hypotensive effect enhanced, but antagonism of effect of *adrenergic neurone blockers* and of *clonidine* (and increased risk of hypertension on clonidine withdrawal)
* Antimalarials: increased risk of ventricular arrhythmias with *halofantrine*
Antimuscarinics: increased antimuscarinic side-effects
Antipsychotics: increased plasma concentrations of *tricyclic antidepressants* and increased antimuscarinic side-effects with *phenothiazines*
* Antivirals: see Ritonavir, p. 581
Anxiolytics and Hypnotics: enhanced sedative effect
* Barbiturates and Primidone: *see under* Antiepileptics, above
* Beta-blockers: risk of ventricular arrhythmias associated with *sotalol* increased
Calcium-channel Blockers: *diltiazem* and *verapamil* and possibly *mibefradil* increase plasma concentration of *imipramine* and possibly *other tricyclics*
Disulfiram: inhibition of metabolism of *tricyclics* (increased plasma concentrations and increased disulfiram reaction reported with *alcohol with amitriptyline*)
Diuretics: increased risk of postural hypotension
Muscle Relaxants: enhanced muscle relaxant effect of *baclofen*
Nitrates: reduced effect of *sublingual nitrates* (owing to dry mouth)
Oestrogens and Progestogens: *oral contraceptives* antagonise antidepressant effect (but side-effects may be increased due to increased plasma concentrations of *tricyclics*)
Opioid Analgesics: *tramadol* possibly increases risk of convulsions
* Sympathomimetics: hypertension and arrhythmias with *adrenaline* (but local anaesthetics with adrenaline appear to be safe); hypertension with *noradrenaline*; *methylphenidate* may inhibit metabolism of *tricyclics*
Thyroxine: manufacturer of *lofepramine* advises avoid *thyroxine*
Ulcer-healing Drugs: plasma concentrations of *amitriptyline, doxepin, imipramine, nortriptyline, and probably other tricyclics* increased by *cimetidine* (inhibition of metabolism)

Antidiabetics

Note. Includes Acarbose; Insulin; Metformin; Sulphonylureas

ACE Inhibitors: possibly enhance hypoglycaemic effect

Alcohol: enhanced hypoglycaemic effect; flushing with *chlorpropamide* (in susceptible subjects); risk of lactic acidosis with *metformin*

Anabolic Steroids: possibly enhance hypoglycaemic effect

* Analgesics: *azapropazone, phenylbutazone* and possibly *other NSAIDs* enhance effect of *sulphonylureas*
Anion-exchange Resins: *cholestyramine* enhances hypoglycaemic effect of *acarbose*

Antidiabetics *(continued)*

- Antibacterials: *chloramphenicol, co-trimoxazole,* and *sulphonamides* enhance effect of *sulphonylureas; ciprofloxacin* possibly enhances effect of *glibenclamide; neomycin* possibly enhances hypoglycaemic effect of *acarbose* and increases severity of gastro-intestinal effects; *rifamycins* reduce effect of *sulphonylureas* (accelerate metabolism)

Anticoagulants: possibly enhanced hypoglycaemic effects of *sulphonylureas* and changes to anticoagulant effects of *warfarin and other coumarins*

Antidepressants: *MAOIs* enhance hypoglycaemic effect

Antiepileptics: *plasma-phenytoin* concentration transiently increased by *tolbutamide* (possibility of toxicity)

- Antifungals: *fluconazole* and *miconazole* increase plasma concentrations of *sulphonylureas*

Antihistamines: depressed thrombocyte count with concomitant use of *biguanides* and *ketotifen*

Antihypertensives: hypoglycaemic effect antagonised by *diazoxide*

Antipsychotics: *phenothiazines* possibly antagonise hypoglycaemic effect of *sulphonylureas*

Beta-blockers: enhanced hypoglycaemic effect (and masking of warning signs such as tremor)

Calcium-channel Blockers: *nifedipine* may occasionally impair glucose tolerance

Clofibrate Group: may improve glucose tolerance and have an additive effect

Corticosteroids: antagonism of hypoglycaemic effect

Diuretics: hypoglycaemic effect antagonised by *loop and thiazide diuretics; chlorpropamide increases risk of hyponatraemia with thiazides in combination with potassium-sparing diuretics*

Hormone Antagonists: manufacturer advises metabolism of *oral antidiabetics* possibly accelerated by *aminoglutethimide; octreotide* possibly reduces *insulin* and antidiabetic drug requirements in diabetes mellitus

Lithium: may occasionally impair glucose tolerance

Oestrogens and Progestogens: *oral contraceptives* antagonise hypoglycaemic effect

Pancreatin: hypoglycaemic effect of *acarbose* reduced by *pancreatin*

Testosterone: hypoglycaemic effect possibly enhanced

Ulcer-healing Drugs: *cimetidine* inhibits renal excretion of *metformin* (increased plasma-metformin concentrations); *cimetidine* and *ranitidine* enhance hypoglycaemic effect of *sulphonylureas*

- Uricosurics: *sulphinpyrazone* enhances effect of *sulphonylureas*

Antiepileptics *see* Carbamazepine; Chlormethiazole; Clonazepam; Ethosuximide; Gabapentin; Lamotrigine; Phenytoin; Topiramate; Valproate; Vigabatrin and p. 210

Antifungals *see* Amphotericin; Antifungals, Imidazole and Triazole; Griseofulvin; Terbinafine

Antifungals, Imidazole and Triazole

Note. Imidazole antifungals include clotrimazole, ketoconazole and miconazole; triazoles include fluconazole and itraconazole

In general, interactions relate to multiple-dose treatment

Analgesics: metabolism of *alfentanil* inhibited by *ketoconazole* (risk of prolonged or delayed respiratory depression)

Antacids and Adsorbents: *antacids* reduce absorption of *itraconazole* and *ketoconazole*

Antifungals, Imidazole and Triazole *(continued)*

- Antibacterials: *rifampicin* accelerates metabolism of *fluconazole, itraconazole* and *ketoconazole* (reduced plasma concentrations); plasma concentration of *rifampicin* may be reduced by *ketoconazole*; plasma concentration of *rifabutin* increased by *fluconazole* and *other triazoles* (risk of uveitis—possibly reduce rifabutin dose); plasma concentration of *ketoconazole* may be reduced by *isoniazid*

- Anticoagulants: effect of *nicoumalone* and *warfarin* enhanced by *fluconazole, itraconazole, ketoconazole,* and *miconazole* (note: oral gel absorbed)

- Antidiabetics: plasma concentrations of *sulphonylureas* increased by *fluconazole* and *miconazole*

- Antiepileptics: effect of *phenytoin* enhanced by *fluconazole* and *miconazole*; plasma concentrations of *itraconazole* and *ketoconazole* reduced by *phenytoin*

  other Antifungals: imidazoles and *triazoles* possibly antagonise effect of *amphotericin*

- Antihistamines: *fluconazole, itraconazole, ketoconazole* and possibly *other imidazoles* and *triazoles* inhibit *astemizole* and *terfenadine* metabolism (avoid concomitant use—cardiac toxicity reported); manufacturer advises possibility of increased plasma-loratadine concentration with *ketoconazole*

  Antimuscarinics: reduced absorption of *ketoconazole*

- Antipsychotics: *itraconazole* and *ketoconazole* inhibit metabolism of *sertindole* (increased toxicity)

- Antivirals: *ketoconazole* inhibits metabolism of *indinavir* (reduce dose of indinavir); on theoretical grounds, plasma-indinavir concentration significantly increased by *itraconazole* (avoid concomitant use); plasma concentration of *zidovudine* increased by *fluconazole* (increased risk of toxicity); see also Ritonavir, p. 581

- Anxiolytics and Hypnotics: plasma concentration of *midazolam* increased by *itraconazole, ketoconazole,* and possibly *fluconazole* (prolonged sedative effect)

  Calcium-channel Blockers: *itraconazole* inhibits metabolism of *felodipine* (increased plasma concentration)

- Cardiac Glycosides: plasma concentration of *digoxin* increased by *itraconazole*

- Cisapride: *fluconazole, itraconazole, ketoconazole* and *miconazole* inhibit metabolism (ventricular arrhythmias reported—avoid concomitant use)

- Cyclosporin: metabolism inhibited by *itraconazole, ketoconazole* and possibly *fluconazole* and *miconazole* (increased plasma-cyclosporin concentration)

  Cytotoxics: *ketoconazole* possibly inhibits metabolism of *paclitaxel; see also* Docetaxel; *itraconazole* may inhibit metabolism of *vincristine* (increased risk of neurotoxicity)

  Diuretics: plasma concentration of *fluconazole* increased by *hydrochlorothiazide*

- Lipid-regulating Drugs: *itraconazole* increases risk of myopathy with *simvastatin* (avoid concomitant use)

  Oestrogens and Progestogens: anecdotal reports of contraceptive failure with *fluconazole, itraconazole, ketoconazole* and possibly others

- Tacrolimus: *clotrimazole, fluconazole, ketoconazole* and possibly *other imidazoles* increase plasma-tacrolimus concentration

- Theophylline: plasma-theophylline concentration possibly increased by *fluconazole*

  Ulcer-healing Drugs: *histamine H₂- antagonists* reduce absorption of *itraconazole* and *ketoconazole; omeprazole* reduces absorption of *ketoconazole* and possibly *itraconazole; sucralfate* reduces absorption of *ketoconazole*

Antihistamines

Note. Sedative interactions apply to a lesser extent to the non-sedating antihistamines, and they do not appear to potentiate the effects of alcohol.

Interactions do not generally apply to antihistamines used for topical action (including inhalation)

Grapefruit juice increases plasma concentration of terfenadine

Alcohol: enhanced sedative effect

Antacids: reduced absorption of *fexofenadine*

- Anti-arrhythmics: increased risk of ventricular arrhythmias with *astemizole* and *terfenadine* (avoid concomitant use with *amiodarone, disopyramide, procainamide* and *quinidine*)

- Antibacterials: metabolism of *astemizole* and *terfenadine* inhibited by *clarithromycin* and *erythromycin* (avoid concomitant use—risk of hazardous arrhythmias); manufacturer advises possibility of increased plasma-loratadine concentration with *erythromycin*

- Antidepressants: *MAOIs* and *tricyclics* increase antimuscarinic and sedative effects; *tricyclics* increase risk of ventricular arrhythmias with *astemizole* and *terfenadine*; *fluvoxamine* and *nefazodone* increase risk of arrhythmias with terfenadine—avoid concomitant use

Antidiabetics: depressed thrombocyte count with concomitant use of *biguanides* and *ketotifen*

- Antifungals: *fluconazole, itraconazole, ketoconazole* and possibly *other imidazoles* and *triazoles* inhibit *astemizole* and *terfenadine* metabolism (avoid concomitant use—cardiac toxicity reported) ; manufacturer advises possibility of increased plasma-loratadine concentration with *ketoconazole*

- *other* Antihistamines: concomitant use of *astemizole* and *terfenadine* **not** recommended (risk of hazardous arrhythmias)

- Antimalarials: *halofantrine* and *quinine* increase risk of ventricular arrhythmias with *astemizole* and *terfenadine*

Antimuscarinics: increased antimuscarinic side-effects

- Antipsychotics: increased risk of ventricular arrhythmias with *astemizole* and *terfenadine*

- Antivirals: *indinavir, ritonavir,* and *saquinavir* increase risk of arrhythmias with *terfenadine*—avoid concomitant use

Anxiolytics and Hypnotics: enhanced sedative effect

- Beta-blockers: *sotalol* increases risk of ventricular arrhythmias with *astemizole* and *terfenadine*

Betahistine: antagonism (theoretical)

- Calcium-channel Blockers: *mibefradil* increases risk of arrhythmias with *astemizole* and *terfenadine*—avoid concomitant use

- Cisapride: increased risk of arrhythmias with *terfenadine*—avoid concomitant use

Cytotoxics: *see* Docetaxel

- Diuretics: hypokalaemia increases risk of ventricular arrhythmias with *astemizole* and *terfenadine*

Ulcer-healing Drugs: manufacturer advises possibility of increased plasma-loratadine concentration with *cimetidine*

Antihypertensives *see* individual drugs or groups

Antimalarials *see* individual drugs

Antimuscarinics

Note. Many drugs have antimuscarinic effects; concomitant use of two or three such drugs can increase side-effects such as dry mouth, urine retention, and constipation; concomitant use can also lead to confusion in the elderly; interactions do not generally apply to antimuscarinics used by inhalation

Alcohol: sedative effect of *hyoscine* enhanced

Analgesics: increased antimuscarinic effects with *nefopam*

Anti-arrhythmics: increased antimuscarinic effects with *disopyramide; atropine* delays absorption of *mexiletine*

Antimuscarinics *(continued)*

Antidepressants: increased antimuscarinic side-effects with *tricyclics and MAOIs*

Antifungals: reduced absorption of *ketoconazole*

Antihistamines: increased antimuscarinic side-effects

Antipsychotics: increased antimuscarinic side-effects of *phenothiazines* (but reduced plasma concentrations)

Cisapride: antagonism of gastro-intestinal effect

Dopaminergics: increased antimuscarinic side-effects with *amantadine*

Metoclopramide and Domperidone: *antimuscarinics such as propantheline* antagonise gastro-intestinal effects

Nitrates: reduced effect of *sublingual nitrates* (failure to dissolve under tongue owing to dry mouth)

Parasympathomimetics: antagonism of effect

Antiplatelet Drugs *see* Aspirin and Dipyridamole

Antipsychotics

Note. Increased risk of arrhythmias when antipsychotics given with other drugs which prolong QT interval—avoid concomitant use of pimozide, sertindole and thioridazine with anti-arrhythmics (particularly amiodarone, disopyramide, procainamide and quinidine), antihistamines such as astemizole and terfenadine, tricyclic antidepressants

Increased risk of toxicity with myelosuppressive drugs—clozapine in particular should not be used concurrently with drugs associated with a substantial potential for causing agranulocytosis, such as carbamazepine, co-trimoxazole, chloramphenicol, sulphonamides, pyrazolone analgesics such as azapropazone, penicillamine, or cytotoxics; also avoid clozapine with long-acting depot antipsychotics (have myelosuppressive potential)

ACE Inhibitors: severe postural hypotension with *chlorpromazine* and possibly *other phenothiazines*

Alcohol: enhanced sedative effect

- Anaesthetics: enhanced hypotensive effect

Analgesics: enhanced sedative and hypotensive effect with *opioid analgesics*; severe drowsiness possible if *indomethacin* given with *haloperidol*

Antacids: reduced absorption of *phenothiazines*

- Anti-arrhythmics: increased risk of ventricular arrhythmias with drugs which prolong QT interval (avoid concomitant use with amiodarone)

- Antibacterials: risk of arrhythmias if *clarithromycin* and possibly *erythromycin* given with *pimozide* (avoid concomitant use); *erythromycin* possibly increases plasma concentration of *clozapine* (possible increased risk of convulsions) and *sertindole*; *rifampicin* accelerates metabolism of *haloperidol* (reduced plasma-haloperidol concentration)

- Antidepressants: increased plasma concentrations and increased antimuscarinic effects notably on administration of *tricyclics* with *phenothiazines; fluoxetine* and *fluvoxamine* possibly increase plasma concentration of *clozapine; fluoxetine* increases plasma concentration of *haloperidol; fluoxetine* and *paroxetine* increase plasma concentration of *sertindole; oxypertine* causes CNS excitation and hypertension with *MAOIs; clozapine* possibly enhances central effects of *MAOIs*

Antidiabetics: hypoglycaemic effect of *sulphonylureas* possibly antagonised

- Antiepileptics: antagonism (convulsive threshold lowered); *carbamazepine* accelerates metabolism of *haloperidol, olanzapine,* and *risperidone* (reduced plasma concentrations); *carbamazepine* and *phenytoin* accelerate metabolism of *sertindole* (reduced plasma concentration); *phenytoin* accelerates metabolism of *clozapine* and *quetiapine*

- Antifungals: *itraconazole* and *ketoconazole* inhibit metabolism of *sertindole* (increased toxicity)

- Antihistamines: increased risk of ventricular arrhythmias with *astemizole* and *terfenadine*

Antipsychotics (*continued*)

Antihypertensives: enhanced hypotensive effect; higher doses of *chlorpromazine* antagonise hypotensive effect of *adrenergic neurone blockers*; increased risk of extrapyramidal effects on administration of *methyldopa* and *metirosine*

- Antimalarials: increased risk of ventricular arrhythmias with *halofantrine;* avoid concomitant use of *pimozide* with *mefloquine* and *quinine*

Antimuscarinics: antimuscarinic side-effects of *phenothiazines* increased (but reduced plasma concentrations)

- Antivirals: see Ritonavir, p. 581

Anxiolytics and Hypnotics: enhanced sedative effect

- Beta-blockers: *phenothiazines* increase risk of ventricular arrhythmias with *sotalol*; *propranolol* increases plasma concentration of *chlorpromazine*

Calcium-channel Blockers: enhanced hypotensive effect

Desferrioxamine: manufacturer advises avoid *prochlorperazine* (also *methotrimeprazine* on theoretical grounds)

Diuretics: hypokalaemia increases risk of ventricular arrhythmias with *pimozide*

Dopaminergics: antagonism of hypoprolactinaemic and antiparkinsonian effects of *bromocriptine* and *cabergoline*; antagonism of effect of *apomorphine, levodopa, lysuride,* and *pergolide*

Lithium: increased risk of extrapyramidal effects and possibility of neurotoxicity with *clozapine, haloperidol and phenothiazines*

Metoclopramide and Domperidone: increased risk of extrapyramidal effects with *metoclopramide*

Sympathomimetics: antagonise pressor action

Tetrabenazine: increased risk of extrapyramidal effects

Ulcer-healing Drugs: *cimetidine* may enhance effects of *chlorpromazine, clozapine,* and possibly *other antipsychotics*

Antivirals *see* Aciclovir and Famciclovir; Didanosine; Ganciclovir; Indinavir; Ritonavir; Saquinavir; Stavudine; Valaciclovir; Zalcitabine; Zidovudine

Anxiolytics and Hypnotics

Alcohol: enhanced sedative effect

Anaesthetics: enhanced sedative effect

Analgesics: *opioid analgesics* enhance sedative effect

- Antibacterials: *erythromycin* inhibits metabolism of *midazolam* (increased plasma-midazolam concentration, with profound sedation) and *zopiclone*; *isoniazid* inhibits metabolism of *diazepam*; *rifampicin* increases metabolism of *diazepam* and possibly *other benzodiazepines*

Anticoagulants: *chloral hydrate* and *triclofos* may transiently enhance anticoagulant effect of *nicoumalone and warfarin*

Antidepressants: enhanced sedative effect; manufacturer contra-indicates *buspirone* with *MAOIs*; plasma concentrations of some *benzodiazepines* increased by *fluvoxamine*

Antiepileptics: metabolism of *clonazepam* accelerated (reduced effect); plasma-phenytoin concentrations increased or decreased by *diazepam* and possibly *other benzodiazepines*

- Antifungals: *itraconazole, ketoconazole,* and possibly *fluconazole* increase plasma concentration of *midazolam* (prolonged sedative effect)

Antihistamines: enhanced sedative effect

Antihypertensives: enhanced hypotensive effect; enhanced sedative effect with *alpha-blockers* and possibly *moxonidine*

Antipsychotics: enhanced sedative effect

- Antivirals: see Ritonavir, p. 581

Calcium-channel Blockers: *diltiazem* and *verapamil* inhibit metabolism of *midazolam* (increased plasma-midazolam concentration, with increased sedation)

Anxiolytics and Hypnotics (*continued*)

Disulfiram: metabolism of *benzodiazepines* inhibited, with enhanced sedative effect (*temazepam* toxicity reported)

Dopaminergics: *benzodiazepines* occasionally antagonise effect of *levodopa*

Lofexidine: enhanced sedative effect

Muscle Relaxants: *baclofen* and *tizanidine* enhance sedative effect

Nabilone: enhanced sedative effect

Ulcer-healing Drugs: *cimetidine* inhibits metabolism of *benzodiazepines and chlormethiazole* (increased plasma concentrations); *omeprazole* inhibits metabolism of *diazepam* (increased plasma concentration)

Apomorphine

Antipsychotics: antagonism of effects

Appetite Suppressants *see* Sympathomimetics

Apraclonidine *see* Alpha$_2$-adrenoceptor Stimulants

Aspirin

other Analgesics: avoid concomitant administration of other *NSAIDs* (increased side-effects)

Antacids and Adsorbents: excretion of *aspirin* increased in alkaline urine

- Anticoagulants: increased risk of bleeding due to antiplatelet effect

Antiepileptics: enhancement of effect of *phenytoin* and *valproate*

Corticosteroids: increased risk of gastro-intestinal bleeding and ulceration

- Cytotoxics: reduced excretion of *methotrexate* (increased toxicity)

Diuretics: antagonism of diuretic effect of *spironolactone;* reduced excretion of *acetazolamide* (risk of toxicity)

Metoclopramide and Domperidone: *metoclopramide* enhances effect of *aspirin* (increased rate of absorption)

Mifepristone: manufacturer recommends avoid *aspirin* until 8–12 days after *mifepristone*

Uricosurics: effect of *probenecid* and *sulphinpyrazone* reduced

Astemizole *see* Antihistamines

Atenolol *see* Beta-blockers

Atorvastatin *see* Statins

Atovaquone

- Antibacterials: plasma atovaquone concentration reduced by *rifampicin* and by *tetracycline* (possible therapeutic failure of *atovaquone*)

Metoclopramide and Domperidone: plasma-atovaquone concentration reduced by *metoclopramide*

Atracurium *see* Muscle Relaxants (non-depolarising)

Atropine *see* Antimuscarinics

Auranofin *see* Gold

Azapropazone *see* NSAIDs

Azatadine *see* Antihistamines

Azathioprine

- Allopurinol: enhancement of effect with increased toxicity (*see also* p. 379)
- Antibacterials: manufacturer reports interaction with *rifampicin* (transplants possibly rejected)

Azelastine *see* Antihistamines

Azithromycin *see* Erythromycin and other Macrolides

Azlocillin *see* Penicillins

Aztreonam

- Anticoagulants: anticoagulant effect of *nicoumalone and warfarin* possibly enhanced

Baclofen *see* Muscle Relaxants

Bambuterol *see* Sympathomimetics, Beta$_2$

Barbiturates and Primidone

Alcohol: enhanced sedative effect

Anti-arrhythmics: metabolism of *disopyramide and quinidine* increased (reduced plasma concentrations)

Barbiturates and Primidone *(continued)*

Antibacterials: metabolism of *chloramphenicol, doxycycline, and metronidazole* accelerated (reduced effect); *sulphonamides* enhance effect of *thiopentone*

• Anticoagulants: metabolism of *nicoumalone and warfarin* accelerated (reduced anticoagulant effect)

• Antidepressants: antagonism of anticonvulsant effect (convulsive threshold lowered); metabolism of *mianserin* and *tricyclics* accelerated (reduced plasma concentrations)

• Antiepileptics: concomitant administration of *phenobarbitone or primidone* with other antiepileptics may enhance toxicity without a corresponding increase in antiepileptic effect; moreover interactions can complicate monitoring of treatment; interactions include enhanced effects, increased sedation, and reductions in plasma concentrations; for further details see p. 210

Antifungals: *phenobarbitone* reduces absorption of *griseofulvin* (reduced effect)

• Antipsychotics: antagonism of anticonvulsant effect (convulsive threshold lowered)

Antivirals: plasma concentration of *indinavir* possibly reduced

• Calcium-channel Blockers: effect of *felodipine, isradipine* and probably *nicardipine, nifedipine* and *other dihydropyridines, diltiazem,* and *verapamil* reduced

Cardiac Glycosides: metabolism of *digitoxin only* accelerated (reduced effect)

• Corticosteroids: metabolism of *corticosteroids* accelerated (reduced effect)

• Cyclosporin: metabolism of *cyclosporin* accelerated (reduced effect)

Hormone Antagonists: metabolism of *toremifene* possibly accelerated

• Oestrogens and Progestogens: metabolism of *gestrinone, tibolone,* and *oral contraceptives* accelerated (reduced contraceptive effect, **important:** see p. 351)

Theophylline: metabolism of *theophylline* accelerated (reduced effect)

Thyroxine: metabolism of thyroxine accelerated (may increase thyroxine requirements in hypothyroidism)

Vitamins: *vitamin D* requirements possibly increased

Beclomethasone see Corticosteroids

Belladonna Alkaloids see Antimuscarinics

Bendrofluazide see Diuretics (thiazide)

Benorylate see Aspirin *and* Paracetamol

Benperidol see Antipsychotics

Benzhexol see Antimuscarinics

Benzodiazepines see Anxiolytics and Hypnotics

Benzthiazide see Diuretics (thiazide)

Benztropine see Antimuscarinics

Benzylpenicillin see Penicillins

Beta-blockers

Note. Since systemic absorption may follow topical application of beta-blockers to the eye the possibility of interactions, in particular, with drugs such as verapamil should be borne in mind

ACE Inhibitors: enhanced hypotensive effect

Alcohol: enhanced hypotensive effect

Aldesleukin: enhanced hypotensive effect

Alprostadil: enhanced hypotensive effect

• Anaesthetics: enhanced hypotensive effect; increased risk of *bupivacaine* toxicity with *propranolol*

Analgesics: *NSAIDs* antagonise hypotensive effect

Beta-blockers *(continued)*

• Anti-arrhythmics: increased risk of myocardial depression and bradycardia; with *amiodarone* increased risk of bradycardia and AV block; increased risk of *lignocaine* toxicity with *propranolol*; *propafenone* increases plasma concentration of *metoprolol* and *propranolol*; risk of ventricular arrhythmias associated with *sotalol* increased by *amiodarone, disopyramide, procainamide,* and *quinidine* (avoid concomitant use)

Antibacterials: *rifampicin* accelerates metabolism of *bisoprolol* and *propranolol* (reduced plasma concentration)

• Antidepressants: *fluvoxamine* increases plasma concentration of *propranolol*; risk of ventricular arrhythmias associated with *sotalol* increased by *tricyclics*

Antidiabetics: enhanced hypoglycaemic effect (and masking of warning signs such as tremor)

• Antihistamines: risk of ventricular arrhythmias associated with *sotalol* increased by *astemizole* and *terfenadine*

• Antihypertensives: enhanced hypotensive effect; increased risk of withdrawal hypertension with *clonidine*; increased risk of first-dose hypotensive effect with *post-synaptic alpha-blockers such as prazosin*

• Antimalarials: risk of ventricular arrhythmias associated with *sotalol* increased by *halofantrine*; increased risk of bradycardia with *mefloquine*

• Antipsychotics: risk of ventricular arrhythmias associated with *sotalol* increased by *phenothiazines*; plasma concentration of *chlorpromazine* increased by *propranolol*

Anxiolytics and Hypnotics: enhanced hypotensive effect

• Calcium-channel Blockers: increased risk of bradycardia and AV block with *diltiazem*; severe hypotension and heart failure occasionally with *nifedipine*; asystole, severe hypotension, and heart failure with *verapamil* (see p. 101); increased risk of bradycardia with *mibefradil*

Cardiac Glycosides: increased AV block and bradycardia

Corticosteroids: antagonism of hypotensive effect

Diuretics: enhanced hypotensive effect; risk of ventricular arrhythmias associated with *sotalol* increased by hypokalaemia

Ergotamine: increased peripheral vasoconstriction

Muscle Relaxants: *propranolol* enhances effect; possible enhanced hypotensive effect and bradycardia with *tizanidine*

Oestrogens and Progestogens: *oestrogens* and *combined oral contraceptives* antagonise hypotensive effect

Parasympathomimetics: risk of arrhythmias possibly increased by *pilocarpine*; *propranolol* antagonises effect of *neostigmine* and *pyridostigmine*

• Sympathomimetics: severe hypertension with *adrenaline* and *noradrenaline* and possibly with *dobutamine* (especially with *non-selective beta-blockers*); severe hypertension also possible with *sympathomimetics in anorectics* and *cough and cold remedies*

Theophylline: *beta-blockers* should be avoided on pharmacological grounds (bronchospasm)

• Thymoxamine: possible severe postural hypotension

Thyroxine: metabolism of *propranolol* accelerated (reduced effect)

Ulcer-healing Drugs: plasma concentrations of *labetalol* and *propranolol* increased by *cimetidine*; hypotensive effect antagonised by *carbenoxolone*

Xamoterol: antagonism of effect of *xamoterol* and reduction in beta-blockade

Betahistine
Antihistamines: antagonism (theoretical)
Betamethasone *see* Corticosteroids
Betaxolol *see* Beta-blockers
Bethanechol *see* Parasympathomimetics
Bethanidine *see* Adrenergic Neurone Blockers
Bezafibrate *see* Clofibrate Group
Bicalutamide
Anticoagulants: effect of *warfarin* possibly enhanced
Bile Acids
Antacids: may reduce absorption of bile acids
Cholestyramine and Colestipol: may reduce absorption of bile acids
• Clofibrate group: *clofibrate* increases elimination of cholesterol in bile
• Oestrogens and Progestogens: *oestrogens* increase elimination of cholesterol in bile
Biperiden *see* Antimuscarinics
Bismuth Chelate *see* Tripotassium Dicitratobismuthate
Bisoprolol *see* Beta-blockers
Bisphosphonates
Analgesics: bioavailability of *tiludronic acid* increased by *indomethacin*; *alendronic acid* possibly increases gastro-intestinal side-effects of *NSAIDs*
Antacids: reduced absorption
Antibacterials: increased risk of hypocalcaemia with *aminoglycosides*
Calcium Salts: reduced absorption
Iron: reduced absorption
Botulinum Toxin
• Antibacterials: effects enhanced by *aminoglycosides* and *spectinomycin* (risk of toxicity)
• Muscle Relaxants: effects enhanced by *non-depolarising muscle relaxants*
Bretylium *see* Adrenergic Neurone Blockers
Brimonidine see Alpha₂-adrenoceptor Stimulants
Bromazepam *see* Anxiolytics and Hypnotics
Bromocriptine and Cabergoline
Alcohol: reduced tolerance to *bromocriptine*
Antibacterials: *erythromycin* and possibly *other macrolides* increase plasma concentration (increased risk of toxicity)
Antipsychotics: antagonism of hypoprolactinaemic and antiparkinsonian effects
Metoclopramide and Domperidone: antagonise hypoprolactinaemic effect
• Sympathomimetics: increased risk of toxicity with *bromocriptine* and *isometheptene* or *phenylpropanolamine*
Brompheniramine *see* Antihistamines
Buclizine *see* Antihistamines
Budesonide *see* Corticosteroids
Bumetanide *see* Diuretics (loop)
Bupivacaine
Anti-arrhythmics: increased myocardial depression
Beta-blockers: increased risk of *bupivacaine* toxicity with *propranolol*
Buprenorphine *see* Opioid Analgesics
Buspirone *see* Anxiolytics and Hypnotics
Butobarbitone *see* Barbiturates and Primidone
Cabergoline *see* Bromocriptine and Cabergoline
Calcium Salts
Antibacterials: reduced absorption of *tetracyclines*
Bisphosphonates: reduced absorption
Cardiac Glycosides: large intravenous doses of *calcium* can precipitate arrhythmias
Diuretics: increased risk of hypercalcaemia with *thiazides*
Calcium-channel Blockers
Note. Grapefruit juice increases plasma concentration of dihydropyridine calcium-channel blockers (except amlodipine) and verapamil
Dihydropyridine calcium-channel blockers include amlodipine, felodipine, isradipine, lacidipine, nicardipine, nifedipine, nimodipine and nisoldipine

Calcium-channel Blockers *(continued)*
ACE Inhibitors: enhanced hypotensive effect
Alcohol: plasma-alcohol concentration possibly increased by *verapamil*
Aldesleukin: enhanced hypotensive effect
Alprostadil: enhanced hypotensive effect
• Anaesthetics: *verapamil* increases hypotensive effect of *general anaesthetics* and risk of AV delay; *isoflurane* enhances hypotensive effect of *dihydropyridines*
• Anti-arrhythmics: *amiodarone-induced* risk of bradycardia, AV block, and myocardial depression increased by *diltiazem* and *verapamil*; plasma-concentration of *quinidine* reduced by *nifedipine*; increased risk of myocardial depression and asystole if *verapamil* given with *disopyramide* and *flecainide*; with *verapamil* raised plasma concentration of *quinidine* (extreme hypotension may occur)
• Antibacterials: *erythromycin* possibly inhibits metabolism of *felodipine* (increased plasma concentration); *rifampicin* increases metabolism of *diltiazem, nifedipine, verapamil* and possibly *isradipine, nicardipine* and *nisoldipine* (plasma concentrations significantly reduced)
Antidepressants: *diltiazem, verapamil* and possibly *mibefradil* increase plasma concentration of *imipramine* and possibly other *tricyclics*
Antidiabetics: *nifedipine* may occasionally impair glucose tolerance
• Antiepileptics: effect of *carbamazepine* enhanced by *diltiazem* and *verapamil*; *diltiazem* and *nifedipine* increase plasma concentration of *phenytoin*; effect of *felodipine* and *isradipine* and probably *nicardipine, nifedipine* and *other dihydropyridines* reduced by *carbamazepine, phenobarbitone, phenytoin, and primidone*; effect of *diltiazem* and *verapamil* reduced by *phenobarbitone* and *phenytoin*
• Antifungals: *itraconazole* inhibits metabolism of *felodipine* (increased plasma concentration)
• Antihistamines: *mibefradil* increases risk of arrhythmias with *astemizole* and *terfenadine—* avoid concomitant use
• Antihypertensives: enhanced hypotensive effect; increased risk of first-dose hypotensive effect of *post-synaptic alpha-blockers such as prazosin*
Antimalarials: possible increased risk of bradycardia with some *calcium-channel blockers* and *mefloquine*
Antipsychotics: enhanced hypotensive effect
• Antivirals: see Ritonavir, p. 581
Anxiolytics and Hypnotics: *diltiazem* and *verapamil* inhibit metabolism of *midazolam* (increased plasma-midazolam concentration, with increased sedation)
• Barbiturates and Primidone: *see under* Antiepileptics, above
• Beta-blockers: increased risk of bradycardia and AV block with *diltiazem;* occasionally severe hypotension and heart failure with *nifedipine;* asystole, severe hypotension, and heart failure with *verapamil* (see p. 101); increased risk of bradycardia with *mibefradil*
other Calcium-channel Blockers: clearance of *nifedipine* reduced by *diltiazem* (increased plasma-nifedipine concentration)
• Cardiac Glycosides: plasma concentration of *digoxin* increased by *diltiazem, nifedipine, verapamil* and possibly *nifedipine*; increased AV block and bradycardia with *verapamil*
• Cisapride: risk of arrhythmias with mibefradil—avoid concomitant use

Calcium-channel Blockers *(continued)*
* Cyclosporin: plasma-cyclosporin concentrations increased by *diltiazem, mibefradil, nicardipine, and verapamil;* possibly increases plasma concentration of *nifedipine*
  Diuretics: enhanced hypotensive effect
* Lipid-regulating Drugs: *mibefradil* increases bioavailability of *simvastatin* and possibly *atorvastatin* and *cerivastatin* (increased risk of rhabdomyolysis—avoid concomitant use)
  Lithium: neurotoxicity may occur without increased plasma-lithium concentrations in patients given *diltiazem* and *verapamil*
  Muscle Relaxants: *nifedipine* and *verapamil* enhance effect of *non-depolarising muscle relaxants;* hypotension, myocardial depression, and hyperkalaemia with *verapamil* and intravenous *dantrolene;* risk of arrhythmias with *diltiazem* and intravenous *dantrolene;* enhanced hypotensive effect with *tizanidine*
* Theophylline: *diltiazem, verapamil* and possibly *other calcium-channel blockers* (increased plasma-theophylline concentration)
  Thymoxamine: enhanced hypotensive effect
  Ulcer-healing Drugs: *cimetidine* inhibits metabolism of *some calcium-channel blockers* (increased plasma concentrations)
Candesartan as for ACE Inhibitors
Canrenoate *see* Diuretics *(as for* spironolactone)
Capreomycin
  other Antibacterials: increased risk of nephrotoxicity with *colistin;* increased risk of nephrotoxicity and ototoxicity with *aminoglycosides and vancomycin*
  Cytotoxics: increased risk of nephrotoxicity and ototoxicity with *cisplatin*
Captopril *see* ACE Inhibitors
Carbachol *see* Parasympathomimetics
Carbamazepine
  Alcohol: CNS side-effects of *carbamazepine* possibly enhanced
* Analgesics: *dextropropoxyphene* enhances effect of *carbamazepine;* effect of *tramadol* decreased by *carbamazepine*
* Antibacterials: metabolism of *doxycycline* accelerated (reduced effect); plasma-carbamazepine concentration increased by *clarithromycin, erythromycin* and *isoniazid* (also isoniazid hepatotoxicity possibly increased); plasma-carbamazepine concentration reduced by *rifabutin*
* Anticoagulants: metabolism of *nicoumalone* and *warfarin* accelerated (reduced anticoagulant effect)
* Antidepressants: antagonism of anticonvulsant effect (convulsive threshold lowered); plasma concentration of *carbamazepine* increased by *fluoxetine, fluvoxamine,* and *viloxazine;* metabolism of *mianserin* and *tricyclics* accelerated (reduced plasma concentrations); manufacturer advises avoid with *MAOIs* or within 2 weeks of *MAOIs*
* *other* Antiepileptics: concomitant administration of *two or more antiepileptics* may enhance toxicity without a corresponding increase in antiepileptic effect; moreover interactions between individual antiepileptics can complicate monitoring of treatment; interactions include enhanced effects, increased sedation, and reductions in plasma concentrations; for further details, see p. 210
* Antimalarials: *chloroquine* and *mefloquine* antagonise anticonvulsant effect
* Antipsychotics: antagonism of anticonvulsant effect (convulsive threshold lowered); metabolism of *haloperidol, olanzapine, risperidone,* and *sertindole* accelerated (reduced plasma concentrations)
* Antivirals: plasma-concentration of *indinavir* possibly reduced; see also Ritonavir, p. 581

Carbamazepine *(continued)*
* Calcium-channel Blockers: *diltiazem and verapamil* enhance effect of *carbamazepine;* effect of *felodipine, isradipine* and probably *nicardipine, nifedipine* and *other dihydropyridines* reduced
  Cardiac Glycosides: metabolism of *digitoxin only* accelerated (reduced effect)
* Corticosteroids: metabolism accelerated (reduced effect)
* Cyclosporin: metabolism accelerated (reduced plasma-cyclosporin concentration)
  Diuretics: increased risk of hyponatraemia
* Hormone Antagonists: *danazol* inhibits metabolism of *carbamazepine* (enhanced effect); metabolism of *toremifene* possibly accelerated
  Lithium: neurotoxicity may occur without increased plasma-lithium concentration
  Muscle Relaxants: effect of *non-depolarising muscle relaxants* antagonised (recovery from neuromuscular blockade accelerated)
* Oestrogens and Progestogens: *carbamazepine* accelerates metabolism of *oral contraceptives* (reduced contraceptive effect, **important:** see p. 351) and of *gestrinone and tibolone*
  Retinoids: plasma concentration possibly reduced by *isotretinoin*
  Theophylline: metabolism of *theophylline* accelerated (reduced effect)
  Thyroxine: metabolism accelerated (may increase thyroxine requirements in hypothyroidism)
* Ulcer-healing Drugs: metabolism inhibited by *cimetidine* (increased plasma-carbamazepine concentration)
  Vitamins: *carbamazepine* possibly increases *vitamin D* requirements
Carbenoxolone
  Note. Interactions do not apply to small amounts used topically on oral mucosa
  Antihypertensives: antagonism of hypotensive effect
  Cardiac Glycosides: toxicity increased if hypokalaemia occurs
  Corticosteroids: increased risk of hypokalaemia
  Diuretics: antagonism of diuretic effect; increased risk of hypokalaemia with *acetazolamide, thiazides,* and *loop diuretics;* inhibition of ulcer healing with *amiloride* and *spironolactone*
Carbonic Anhydrase Inhibitors *see* Diuretics
Cardiac Glycosides
  ACE Inhibitors: *captopril* possibly increases plasma concentration of *digoxin*
  Analgesics: *NSAIDs* may exacerbate heart failure, reduce GFR and increase plasma-cardiac glycoside concentrations
  Anion-exchange Resins: absorption possibly reduced by *cholestyramine* and *colestipol*
* Anti-arrhythmics: plasma concentration of *digoxin* increased by *amiodarone, propafenone, and quinidine* (halve maintenance dose of digoxin)
  Antibacterials: *erythromycin* and possibly *other macrolides* enhance effect of *digoxin; rifamycins* accelerate metabolism of *digitoxin only* (reduced effect)
  Antiepileptics: metabolism of *digitoxin only* accelerated (reduced effect)
* Antifungals: increased toxicity if hypokalaemia occurs with *amphotericin;* plasma concentration of *digoxin* increased by *itraconazole*
* Antimalarials: *quinine* (includes use of quinine for cramp) *hydroxychloroquine* and *possibly chloroquine* raise plasma concentration of *digoxin;* possible increased risk of bradycardia with *mefloquine*
  Barbiturates and Primidone: *see under* Antiepileptics, above
  Beta-blockers: increased AV block and bradycardia
  Calcium Salts: large intravenous doses of *calcium* can precipitate arrhythmias

Cardiac Glycosides *(continued)*
- Calcium-channel Blockers: plasma concentration of *digoxin* increased by *diltiazem, nicardipine, verapamil* and possibly *nifedipine*; increased AV block and bradycardia with *verapamil*

  Corticosteroids: increased risk of hypokalaemia
- Diuretics: increased toxicity if hypokalaemia occurs with *acetazolamide, loop diuretics, and thiazides*; effects of *digoxin* enhanced by *spironolactone*

  Hormone Antagonists: *aminoglutethimide* accelerates metabolism of *digitoxin only* (reduced effect)

  Lipid-regulating Drugs: plasma concentration of *digoxin* possibly increased by *atorvastatin*

  Muscle Relaxants: arrhythmias with *suxamethonium*; possible bradycardia with *tizanidine*

  Sulphasalazine: absorption of *digoxin* possibly reduced

  Ulcer-healing Drugs: increased toxicity if hypokalaemia occurs with *carbenoxolone*; plasma concentration of *digoxin* possibly increased by *proton pump inhibitors*; absorption possibly reduced by *sucralfate*

Carisoprodol *see* Anxiolytics and Hypnotics
Carteolol *see* Beta-blockers
Carvedilol *see* Beta-blockers
Cefaclor *see* Cephalosporins
Cefadroxil *see* Cephalosporins
Cefixime *see* Cephalosporins
Cefodizime *see* Cephalosporins
Cefotaxime *see* Cephalosporins
Cefoxitin *see* Cephalosporins
Cefpirome *see* Cephalosporins
Cefpodoxime *see* Cephalosporins
Ceftazidime *see* Cephalosporins
Ceftibuten *see* Cephalosporins
Ceftriaxone *see* Cephalosporins
Cefuroxime *see* Cephalosporins
Celiprolol *see* Beta-blockers
Cephalexin *see* Cephalosporins
Cephalosporins
  Alcohol: disulfiram-like reaction with *cephamandole*
  Antacids and Adsorbents: *antacids* reduce absorption of *cefpodoxime*
- Anticoagulants: anticoagulant effect of *warfarin and nicoumalone* enhanced by *cephamandole* and possibly others

  Ulcer-healing Drugs: *histamine H_2-antagonists* reduce absorption of *cefpodoxime*

  Uricosurics: excretion of *cephalosporins* reduced by *probenecid* (increased plasma concentrations)

Cephamandole *see* Cephalosporins
Cephazolin *see* Cephalosporins
Cephradine *see* Cephalosporins
Cerivastatin *see* Statins
Certoparin *see* Heparin
Cetirizine *see* Antihistamines
Chenodeoxycholic Acid *see* Bile Acids
Chloral *see* Anxiolytics and Hypnotics
Chloramphenicol
  other Antibacterials: *rifampicin* accelerates metabolism (reduced chloramphenicol-plasma concentration)
- Anticoagulants: anticoagulant effect of *nicoumalone and warfarin* enhanced
- Antidiabetics: effect of *sulphonylureas* enhanced
- Antiepileptics: metabolism accelerated by *phenobarbitone* (reduced chloramphenicol-plasma concentration); increased plasma concentration of *phenytoin* (risk of toxicity)
- Barbiturates and Primidone: *see under* Antiepileptics, above

Chlordiazepoxide *see* Anxiolytics and Hypnotics
Chlormethiazole *see* Anxiolytics and Hypnotics

Chloroquine and Hydroxychloroquine
  Antacids: reduced absorption
- Anti-arrhythmics: *chloroquine* increases risk of ventricular arrhythmias with *amiodarone* (avoid concomitant use)
  Antiepileptics: antagonism of anticonvulsant effect
  other Antimalarials: increased risk of convulsions with *mefloquine;* increased risk of arrhythmias with *halofantrine* (**important:** see also CSM advice under Halofantrine, p. 287)
- Cardiac Glycosides: *hydroxychloroquine* and possibly *chloroquine* increase plasma concentration of *digoxin*
- Cyclosporin: *chloroquine* increases plasma-cyclosporin concentration (increased risk of toxicity)
  Parasympathomimetics: *chloroquine* and *hydroxychloroquine* have potential to increase symptoms of myasthenia gravis and thus diminish effect of *neostigmine* and *pyridostigmine*
  Ulcer-healing Drugs: *cimetidine* inhibits metabolism of *chloroquine* (increased plasma concentration)
  Vaccines: *see* Rabies Vaccine p. 528
Chlorothiazide *see* Diuretics (thiazide)
Chlorpheniramine *see* Antihistamines
Chlorpromazine *see* Antipsychotics
Chlorpropamide *see* Antidiabetics (sulphonylurea)
Chlortetracycline *see* Tetracyclines
Chlorthalidone *see* Diuretics (thiazide-related)
Cholestyramine and Colestipol
  Note. Other drugs should be taken at least 1 hour before or 4–6 hours after cholestyramine or colestipol to reduce possible interference with absorption
  Analgesics: absorption of *paracetamol* and *phenylbutazone* reduced by *cholestyramine*
  Antibacterials: *cholestyramine* antagonises effect of oral *vancomycin*
- Anticoagulants: anticoagulant effect of *nicoumalone, phenindione,* and *warfarin* enhanced or reduced
  Antidiabetics: hypoglycaemic effect of *acarbose* enhanced by *cholestyramine*
  Antiepileptics: absorption of *valproate* possibly reduced
  Bile Acids: absorption of chenodeoxycholic acid and ursodeoxycholic acid possibly reduced
  Cardiac Glycosides: possibly reduced absorption
  Diuretics: reduced absorption of *thiazides* (give at least 2 hours apart)
  Mycophenolate Mofetil: absorption of *mycophenolate mofetil* reduced
  Thyroxine: reduced absorption
Cholinergics *see* Parasympathomimetics
Cilastatin [ingredient] *see* Primaxin®
Cilazapril *see* ACE Inhibitors
Cimetidine *see* Histamine H_2-antagonists
Cinnarizine *see* Antihistamines
Cinoxacin *see* 4-Quinolones
Ciprofibrate *see* Clofibrate Group
Ciprofloxacin *see* 4-Quinolones
Cisapride
  Analgesics: *opioid analgesics* possibly antagonise effect on gastro-intestinal motility
- Antibacterials: *clarithromycin* and *erythromycin* possibly inhibit metabolism of *cisapride* (risk of ventricular arrhythmias—avoid concomitant use)
  Anticoagulants: effect of *oral anticoagulants* possibly enhanced
- Antifungals: *fluconazole, itraconazole, ketoconazole* and *miconazole* inhibit metabolism of *cisapride* (ventricular arrhythmias reported—avoid concomitant use)
- Antihistamines: increased risk of arrhythmias with *terfenadine*—avoid concomitant use
  Antimuscarinics: antagonism of effect on gastro-intestinal motility
  Antivirals: see Ritonavir, p. 581
- Calcium-channel Blockers: risk of arrhythmias with *mibefradil*—avoid concomitant use

Cisatracurium *see* Muscle Relaxants (non-depolarising)
Cisplatin
* Antibacterials: *aminoglycosides* and *capreomycin* increase risk of nephrotoxicity and possibly of ototoxicity
  Diuretics: increased risk of nephrotoxicity and ototoxicity
Citalopram *see* Antidepressants, SSRI
Cladribine
  Note. Increased risk of myelosuppression with other myelosuppressive drugs
Clarithromycin *see* Erythromycin and other Macrolides
Clemastine *see* Antihistamines
Clindamycin
  Muscle Relaxants: enhancement of effect of *non-depolarising muscle relaxants*
  Parasympathomimetics: antagonism of effect of *neostigmine* and *pyridostigmine*
Clobazam *see* Anxiolytics and Hypnotics
Clodronate Sodium *see* Bisphosphonates
Clofibrate Group
* Anticoagulants: enhancement of effect of *nicoumalone, phenindione,* and *warfarin*
  Antidiabetics: may improve glucose tolerance and have additive effect
* Bile Acids: *clofibrate* increases elimination of cholesterol in bile
  other Lipid-regulating Drugs: increased risk of myopathy with *statins*
Clomipramine *see* Antidepressants, Tricyclic
Clonazepam (general sedative interactions *as for* Anxiolytics and Hypnotics)
Clonidine (for general hypotensive interactions *see also* Hydralazine)
  ACE Inhibitors: previous treatment with *clonidine* possibly delays antihypertensive effect of *captopril*
* Antidepressants: *tricyclics* antagonise hypotensive effect and also increase risk of rebound hypertension on *clonidine* withdrawal
* Beta-blockers: increased risk of hypertension on *clonidine* withdrawal
Clopamide *see* Diuretics (thiazide)
Clorazepate *see* Anxiolytics and Hypnotics
Clotrimazole *see* Antifungals, Imidazole and Triazole
Clozapine *see* Antipsychotics
Co-amoxiclav *see* Penicillins
Co-beneldopa *see* Levodopa
Co-careldopa *see* Levodopa
Codeine *see* Opioid Analgesics
Co-fluampicil *see* Penicillins
Colchicine
* Cyclosporin: possibly increases risk of nephrotoxicity and myotoxicity (increased plasma-cyclosporin concentration)
Cold and Cough Remedies *see* Antihistamines and Sympathomimetics
Colestipol *see* Cholestyramine and Colestipol
Colistin (other interactions *as for* Aminoglycosides)
  Muscle Relaxants: enhanced muscle relaxant effect
Contraceptives, Oral
  Note. Also covers oestrogens taken alone; in case of hormone replacement therapy low dose unlikely to induce interactions
  ACE Inhibitors: *oestrogens* and *combined oral contraceptives* antagonise hypotensive effect
* Antibacterials: *rifamycins* accelerate metabolism of both *combined* and *progestogen-only oral contraceptives* (reduced contraceptive effect, **important:** see p. 351); when *broad-spectrum antibiotics such as ampicillin and tetracycline* given with *combined oral contraceptives* possibility of reduced contraceptive effect (risk probably small, but see p. 351)
* Anticoagulants: antagonism of anticoagulant effect of *nicoumalone, phenindione,* and *warfarin*

Contraceptives, Oral *(continued)*
  Antidepressants: antagonism of antidepressant effect has been reported, but side-effects of *tricyclics* may be increased due to higher plasma concentrations
  Antidiabetics: antagonism of hypoglycaemic effect
* Antiepileptics: *carbamazepine, phenobarbitone, phenytoin, primidone* and *topiramate* accelerate metabolism (reduced effect of both combined and progestogen-only contraceptives, **important:** see p. 351)
* Antifungals: *griseofulvin* accelerates metabolism (reduced contraceptive effect, **important:** see p. 351); anecdotal reports of contraceptive failure with *fluconazole, itraconazole, ketoconazole* and possibly others
  Antihypertensives: *combined oral contraceptives* antagonise hypotensive effect
* Antivirals: *ritonavir* accelerates metabolism of *combined oral contraceptives* (reduced contraceptive effect)
* Barbiturates and Primidone: *see under* Antiepileptics, above
  Beta-blockers: *oestrogens* and *combined oral contraceptives* antagonise hypotensive effect
* Bile Acids: *oestrogens* increase elimination of cholesterol in bile
* Cyclosporin: increased plasma-cyclosporin concentration
  Diuretics: *combined oral contraceptives* antagonise diuretic effect
* Retinoids: oral *tretinoin* reduces efficacy of *progesterone-only* and possibly *combined oral contraceptives*
  Tacrolimus: efficacy of *oral contraceptives* possibly decreased
  Theophylline: *combined oral contraceptives* delay excretion (increased plasma-theophylline concentration)
  Ulcer-healing drugs: manufacturer advises *lansoprazole* possibly accelerates metabolism
Corticosteroids
  Note. Do not generally apply to corticosteroids used for topical action (including inhalation)
  Analgesics: increased risk of gastro-intestinal bleeding and ulceration with *aspirin* and *NSAIDs*
* Antibacterials: *rifamycins* accelerate metabolism of *corticosteroids* (reduced effect)
  Antidiabetics: antagonism of hypoglycaemic effect
* Antiepileptics: *carbamazepine, phenobarbitone, phenytoin, and primidone* accelerate metabolism of *corticosteroids* (reduced effect)
* Antifungals: increased risk of hypokalaemia with *amphotericin* (avoid concomitant use unless corticosteroids required to control reactions)
  Antihypertensives: antagonism of hypotensive effect
  Antivirals: plasma concentration of *indinavir* possibly reduced by *dexamethasone*
* Barbiturates and Primidone: *see under* Antiepileptics, above
  Cardiac Glycosides: increased toxicity if hypokalaemia occurs with *corticosteroids*
* Cyclosporin: plasma-cyclosporin concentration increased by high-dose *methylprednisolone*; *cyclosporin* increases plasma concentration of *prednisolone*
  Diuretics: antagonism of diuretic effect; *acetazolamide, loop diuretics, and thiazides* increase risk of hypokalaemia
  Hormone Antagonists: *aminoglutethimide* accelerates metabolism of *corticosteroids* (reduced effect)
  Sympathomimetics: increased risk of hypokalaemia if high doses of *corticosteroids* given with high doses of *bambuterol, eformoterol, fenoterol, reproterol, ritodrine, salbutamol, salmeterol, terbutaline* and *tulobuterol; see also* CSM advice, p. 126; *ephedrine* accelerates metabolism of *dexamethasone*

Corticosteroids *(continued)*
 Ulcer-healing Drugs: *carbenoxolone* increases risk of
 hypokalaemia
 Vaccines: see p. 516

Co-trimoxazole and Sulphonamides
 Anaesthetics: effect of *thiopentone* enhanced
- Anti-arrhythmics: co-trimoxazole increases risk of
 ventricular arrhythmias with *amiodarone* (avoid
 concomitant use)
- Anticoagulants: effect of *nicoumalone* and *warfarin*
 enhanced
- Antidiabetics: effect of *sulphonylureas* enhanced
- Antiepileptics: antifolate effect and plasma
 concentration of *phenytoin* increased by *co-
 trimoxazole* and possibly *other sulphonamides*
- Antimalarials: increased risk of antifolate effect with
 pyrimethamine (includes *Fansidar®* and
 Maloprim®)
- Cyclosporin: increased risk of nephrotoxicity;
 plasma-cyclosporin concentration possibly reduced
 by *sulphadiazine*
 Cytotoxics: antifolate effect of *methotrexate*
 increased by *co-trimoxazole*
 Potassium Aminobenzoate: inhibits effect of
 sulphonamides

Cyclizine *see* Antihistamines
Cyclobarbitone *see* Barbiturates
Cyclopenthiazide *see* Diuretics (thiazide)
Cyclopentolate *see* Antimuscarinics
Cyclophosphamide and Ifosfamide
- Anticoagulants: *ifosfamide* possibly enhances effect
 of *warfarin*
 Muscle Relaxants: *cyclophosphamide* enhances
 effect of *suxamethonium*

Cycloserine
- Alcohol: increased risk of seizures
 other Antibacterials: increased CNS toxicity with
 isoniazid
- Antiepileptics: increased plasma concentration of
 phenytoin (risk of toxicity)

Cyclosporin
 Note. Grapefruit juice increases plasma-cyclosporin con-
 centration (risk of toxicity)
- ACE Inhibitors: increased risk of hyperkalaemia
 Allopurinol: possibly increases plasma-cyclosporin
 concentration (risk of toxicity)
- Analgesics: increased risk of nephrotoxicity with
 NSAIDs; *cyclosporin* increases plasma
 concentration of *diclofenac* (halve diclofenac dose)
 Anti-arrhythmics: *amiodarone* and *propafenone*
 possibly increase plasma-cyclosporin
 concentration
- Antibacterials: *aminoglycosides, co-trimoxazole* (and
 trimethoprim alone), and *4-quinolones* increase
 risk of nephrotoxicity; *doxycycline* possibly
 increases plasma-cyclosporin concentration;
 erythromycin and possibly *other macrolides*
 increase plasma-cyclosporin concentration;
 *rifampicin, intravenous sulphadimidine,
 intravenous trimethoprim* (and possibly
 sulphadiazine) reduce plasma-cyclosporin
 concentration
- Antiepileptics: *carbamazepine, phenobarbitone,
 phenytoin, and primidone* accelerate metabolism
 (reduced plasma-cyclosporin concentration)
- Antifungals: *amphotericin* increases risk of
 nephrotoxicity; *griseofulvin* possibly reduces
 plasma-cyclosporin concentration; *itraconazole,
 ketoconazole,* and possibly *fluconazole* and
 miconazole inhibit metabolism (increased plasma-
 cyclosporin concentration)
- Antimalarials: *chloroquine* increases plasma-
 cyclosporin concentration (risk of toxicity)
- Barbiturates and Primidone: *see under* Antiepileptics,
 above

Cyclosporin *(continued)*
- Calcium-channel Blockers: *diltiazem, mibefradil,
 nicardipine,* and *verapamil* increase plasma-
 cyclosporin concentration; *cyclosporin* possibly
 increases plasma concentration of *nifedipine*
- Colchicine: possibly increases risk of nephrotoxicity
 and myotoxicity (increased plasma-cyclosporin
 concentration)
- Corticosteroids: *high-dose methylprednisolone*
 increases plasma-cyclosporin concentration;
 cyclosporin increases plasma concentration of
 prednisolone
- Cytotoxics: increased risk of neurotoxicity with
 doxorubicin; increased risk of nephrotoxicity with
 melphalan; increased toxicity with *methotrexate;
 see also* Docetaxel
- Diuretics: *potassium-sparing diuretics* increase risk
 of hyperkalaemia
- Hormone Antagonists: *danazol* inhibits metabolism
 (increased plasma-cyclosporin concentration);
 octreotide reduces absorption (reduced plasma-
 cyclosporin concentration)
- Lipid-regulating Drugs: increased risk of myopathy
 with *statins*
- Oestrogens and Progestogens: *progestogens* inhibit
 metabolism (increased plasma-cyclosporin
 concentration)
- Potassium Salts: increased risk of hyperkalaemia
- Tacrolimus: plasma-cyclosporin half-life prolonged
 (increased risk of toxicity)
- Ulcer-healing Drugs: *cimetidine* possibly increases
 plasma-cyclosporin concentration
 Vaccines: *see* p. 516

Cyproheptadine *see* Antihistamines
Cytarabine
 Flucytosine: plasma flucytosine concentration
 possibly reduced
Cytotoxics *see under* individual drugs
Dalteparin *see* Heparin
Danazol
- Anticoagulants: effect of *nicoumalone and warfarin*
 enhanced (inhibits metabolism)
- Antiepileptics: inhibits metabolism of *carbamazepine*
 (increased plasma-carbamazepine concentration)
- Cyclosporin: inhibits metabolism (increased plasma-
 cyclosporin concentration)
 Tacrolimus: plasma-tacrolimus concentration
 possibly increased

Dantrolene *see* Muscle Relaxants
Dapsone
 Antibacterials: plasma concentration reduced by
 rifamycins
 Probenecid: *dapsone* excretion reduced (increased
 risk of side-effects)

Debrisoquine *see* Adrenergic Neurone Blockers
Deflazacort *see* Corticosteroids
Demecarium *see* Parasympathomimetics
Demeclocycline *see* Tetracyclines
Desferrioxamine
 Antipsychotics: manufacturer advises avoid
 prochlorperazine (also *methotrimeprazine* on
 theoretical grounds)
Desflurane *see* Anaesthetics, General (volatile liquid)
Desmopressin
 Analgesics: effect of *desmopressin* potentiated by
 indomethacin
Desogestrel *see* Progestogens
Dexamethasone *see* Corticosteroids
Dexamphetamine *see* Sympathomimetics
Dextromoramide *see* Opioid Analgesics
Dextropropoxyphene *see* Opioid Analgesics
Diamorphine *see* Opioid Analgesics
Diazepam *see* Anxiolytics and Hypnotics
Diazoxide (general hypotensive interactions *as for*
 Hydralazine)
 Antidiabetics: antagonism of hypoglycaemic effect
Diclofenac *see* NSAIDs

Dicyclomine see Antimuscarinics
Didanosine
   Note. Antacids in formulation affect absorption of other drugs, see also Antacids and Adsorbents, p. 557
      other Antivirals: plasma-didanosine concentration possibly increased by *ganciclovir*
Diflunisal see NSAIDs
Digitoxin see Cardiac Glycosides
Digoxin see Cardiac Glycosides
Dihydrocodeine see Opioid Analgesics
Diltiazem see Calcium-channel Blockers
Dimenhydrinate see Antihistamines
Diphenhydramine see Antihistamines
Diphenylpyraline see Antihistamines
Diphenoxylate see Opioid Analgesics
Dipipanone see Opioid Analgesics
Dipivefrine see Sympathomimetics (*as for* adrenaline)
Dipyridamole
   Antacids: patient information leaflet advises avoidance of *antacids*
 • Anti-arrhythmics: effect of *adenosine* enhanced and extended (**important** risk of toxicity)
 • Anticoagulants: enhanced effect due to antiplatelet action of *dipyridamole*
   Cytotoxics: efficacy of *fludarabine* possibly reduced
Disodium Etidronate see Bisphosphonates
Disodium Pamidronate see Bisphosphonates
Disopyramide
 • *other* Anti-arrhythmics: *amiodarone* increases risk of ventricular arrhythmias (avoid concomitant use); increased myocardial depression with any *anti-arrhythmic*
 • Antibacterials: plasma concentration of *disopyramide* reduced by *rifampicin* but increased by *erythromycin* and possibly *clarithromycin* (risk of toxicity)
 • Antidepressants: increased risk of ventricular arrhythmias with *tricyclics*
   Antiepileptics: plasma concentration of *disopyramide* reduced by *phenobarbitone, phenytoin, and primidone*
 • Antihistamines: increased risk of ventricular arrhythmias with *astemizole* and *terfenadine*
 • Antimalarials: increased risk of ventricular arrhythmias with *halofantrine*
   Antimuscarinics: increased antimuscarinic side-effects
 • Antipsychotics: increased risk of ventricular arrhythmias with *phenothiazines*
   Barbiturates and Primidone: *see under* Antiepileptics, above
 • Beta-blockers: increased myocardial depression; increased risk of ventricular arrhythmias associated with *sotalol* (avoid concomitant use)
 • Calcium-channel blockers: increased myocardial depression with *verapamil*
 • Diuretics: cardiac toxicity of *disopyramide* increased if hypokalaemia occurs with *acetazolamide, loop diuretics, and thiazides*
   Nitrates: reduced effect of *sublingual nitrates* (failure to dissolve under tongue owing to dry mouth)
Distigmine see Parasympathomimetics
Disulfiram
   Alcohol: disulfiram reaction (*see* section 4.10)
   Antibacterials: psychotic reaction with *metronidazole* reported
 • Anticoagulants: effect of *nicoumalone and warfarin* enhanced
   Antidepressants: inhibition of metabolism of *tricyclic antidepressants* (increased plasma concentrations); increased disulfiram reaction with *alcohol* reported if *amitriptyline* also taken
 • Antiepileptics: inhibition of metabolism of *phenytoin* (increased risk of toxicity)
   Anxiolytics and Hypnotics: inhibition of metabolism of *benzodiazepines*, with enhanced sedative effect (*temazepam* toxicity reported)
   Theophylline: inhibition of metabolism (increased risk of toxicity)

Diuretics
 • ACE Inhibitors: enhanced hypotensive effect (can be extreme); risk of hyperkalaemia with *potassium-sparing diuretics*
   Alprostadil: enhanced hypotensive effect
   Analgesics: *diuretics* increase risk of nephrotoxicity of *NSAIDs*; *NSAIDs notably indomethacin* and *ketorolac* antagonise diuretic effect; *indomethacin* and *possibly other NSAIDs* increase risk of hyperkalaemia with *potassium-sparing diuretics*; occasional reports of decreased renal function when *indomethacin* given with *triamterene*; diuretic effect of *spironolactone* antagonised by *aspirin*; *aspirin* reduces excretion of *acetazolamide* (risk of toxicity)
   Anion-exchange Resins: *cholestyramine and colestipol* reduce absorption of *thiazides* (give at least 2 hours apart)
 • Anti-arrhythmics: cardiac toxicity of *amiodarone, disopyramide, flecainide, and quinidine* increased if hypokalaemia occurs; action of *lignocaine* and *mexiletine* antagonised by hypokalaemia; *acetazolamide* reduces excretion of *quinidine* (increased plasma concentration)
 • Antibacterials: *loop diuretics* increase ototoxicity of *aminoglycosides* (*see also* section 5.1.4), *colistin, and vancomycin*
   Antidepressants: increased risk of postural hypotension with *tricyclics*
   Antidiabetics: hypoglycaemic effect antagonised by *loop and thiazide diuretics*; *chlorpropamide* increases risk of hyponatraemia associated with *thiazides* in combination with *potassium-sparing diuretics*
   Antiepileptics: increased risk of hyponatraemia with *carbamazepine*; *carbonic anhydrase inhibitors* possibly increase risk of osteomalacia with *antiepileptics* such as *phenytoin*
   Antifungals: increased risk of hypokalaemia if *loop diuretics* and *thiazides* given with *amphotericin*; *hydrochlorothiazide* increases plasma concentration of *fluconazole*
 • Antihistamines: hypokalaemia increases risk of ventricular arrhythmias with *astemizole* and *terfenadine*
 • Antihypertensives: enhanced hypotensive effect; increased risk of first-dose hypotensive effect of post-synaptic *alpha-blockers such as prazosin*; increased risk of hypokalaemia with *indapamide*
 • Antimalarials: electrolyte disturbances increase risk of ventricular arrhythmias with *halofantrine*
   Antipsychotics: in hypokalaemia increased risk of ventricular arrhythmias with *pimozide*
   Beta-blockers: enhanced hypotensive effect; in hypokalaemia increased risk of ventricular arrhythmias with *sotalol*
   Calcium Salts: risk of hypercalcaemia with *thiazides*
   Calcium-channel Blockers: enhanced hypotensive effect
 • Cardiac Glycosides: increased toxicity if hypokalaemia occurs with *acetazolamide, loop diuretics, and thiazides;* effect enhanced by *spironolactone*
   Corticosteroids: increased risk of hypokalaemia with *acetazolamide, loop diuretics, and thiazides;* antagonism of diuretic effect
 • Cyclosporin: increased risk of hyperkalaemia with *potassium-sparing diuretics*
   Cytotoxics: increased risk of nephrotoxicity and ototoxicity with *cisplatin*
   other Diuretics: increased risk of hypokalaemia if *acetazolamide, loop diuretics or thiazides* given together; profound diuresis possible if *metolazone* given with *frusemide*

Diuretics *(continued)*

   Hormone Antagonists: increased risk of hyponatraemia with *aminoglutethimide*; *thiazides* increase risk of hypercalcaemia with *toremifene*; *trilostane* increases risk of hyperkalaemia with *potassium-sparing diuretics*

• Lithium: *lithium* excretion reduced by *loop diuretics, potassium-sparing diuretics and thiazides* (increased plasma-lithium concentration and risk of toxicity—*loop diuretics* safer than *thiazides*); *lithium* excretion increased by *acetazolamide*

   Muscle Relaxants: enhanced hypotensive effect with *baclofen* and *tizanidine*

   Oestrogens and Progestogens: *oestrogens and combined oral contraceptives* antagonise diuretic effect

• Potassium Salts: hyperkalaemia with *potassium-sparing diuretics*

   Sympathomimetics: increased risk of hypokalaemia if *acetazolamide, loop diuretics,* and *thiazides* given with high doses of *bambuterol, eformoterol, fenoterol, reproterol, ritodrine, salbutamol, salmeterol, terbutaline,* and *tulobuterol*; see also CSM advice, p. 126

   Thymoxamine: enhanced hypotensive effect

   Ulcer-healing Drugs: increased risk of hypokalaemia if *acetazolamide, loop diuretics,* and *thiazides* given with *carbenoxolone; carbenoxolone* antagonises diuretic effect; *amiloride and spironolactone* antagonise ulcer-healing effect of *carbenoxolone*

   Vitamins: increased risk of hypercalcaemia if *thiazides* given with *vitamin D*

Dobutamine *see* Sympathomimetics

Docetaxel

   Note. No formal clinical studies but *in-vitro* studies suggest possible interaction with cyclosporin, erythromycin, ketoconazole, terfenadine—consult product literature

Domperidone

   Analgesics: *opioid analgesics* antagonise effect on gastro-intestinal activity

   Antimuscarinics: antagonism of effect on gastro-intestinal activity

   Dopaminergics: antagonism of hypoprolactinaemic effect of *bromocriptine*

Donepezil *see* Parasympathomimetics

Dopamine *see* Sympathomimetics

Dopaminergics *see* Amantadine, Bromocriptine and Cabergoline, Levodopa, Lysuride, Quinagolide and Ropinirole

Dopexamine *see* Sympathomimetics

Dorzolamide *see* Diuretics (carbonic anhydrase inhibitor)

   Note. Since systemic absorption may follow topical application of dorzolamide to the eye, the possibility of interactions should be borne in mind

Dothiepin *see* Antidepressants, Tricyclic

Doxapram

   Sympathomimetics: risk of hypertension

   Theophylline: increased CNS stimulation

Doxazosin *see* Alpha-blockers (post-synaptic)

Doxepin *see* Antidepressants, Tricyclic

Doxorubicin

• Cyclosporin: increased risk of neurotoxicity

   Stavudine: may inhibit effect of *stavudine*

Doxycycline *see* Tetracyclines

Doxylamine *see* Antihistamines

Droperidol *see* Antipsychotics

Dydrogesterone *see* Progestogens

Ecothiopate *see* Parasympathomimetics

Edrophonium *see* Parasympathomimetics

Eformoterol *see* Sympathomimetics, Beta$_2$

Enalapril *see* ACE Inhibitors

Enflurane *see* Anaesthetics, General (volatile liquid)

Enoxaparin *see* Heparin

Ephedrine *see* Sympathomimetics

Epoetin

   ACE Inhibitors: antagonism of hypotensive effect; increased risk of hyperkalaemia

Ergotamine

• Antibacterials: ergotism with *erythromycin* and possibly *azithromycin*

   Antidepressants: possibly increased blood pressure with *reboxetine*

   Beta-blockers: increased peripheral vasoconstriction

• 5HT$_1$ Agonists: increased risk of vasospasm (avoid ergotamine for 6 hours after both sumatriptan and zolmitriptan; avoid sumatriptan for 24 hours and zolmitriptan for 6 hours after ergotamine)

Erythromycin and other Macrolides

   Note. Interactions do not apply to small amounts used topically

   Analgesics: plasma concentration of *alfentanil* increased by *erythromycin*

   Antacids and Adsorbents: *antacids* reduce absorption of *azithromycin*

• Anti-arrhythmics: plasma concentration of *disopyramide* increased by *erythromycin* and possibly *clarithromycin* (risk of toxicity); erythromycin (parenteral) increases risk of ventricular arrhythmias with *amiodarone* (avoid concomitant use)

• *other* Antibacterials: *clarithromycin* and possibly *other macrolides* increase plasma concentration of *rifabutin* (risk of uveitis—reduce rifabutin dose)

• Anticoagulants: effect of *nicoumalone and warfarin* enhanced by *erythromycin* and possibly enhanced by *clarithromycin* and some *other macrolides*

• Antiepileptics: *clarithromycin* and *erythromycin* inhibit metabolism of *carbamazepine* (increased plasma-carbamazepine concentration)

• Antihistamines: *clarithromycin* and *erythromycin* inhibit metabolism of *astemizole* and *terfenadine* (avoid concomitant use—risk of hazardous arrhythmias, see pp. 142 and 143); manufacturer advises possibility of increased plasma-loratadine concentration with *erythromycin*

• Antipsychotics: risk of arrhythmias if *clarithromycin* and possibly *erythromycin* given with *pimozide* (avoid concomitant use); *erythromycin* possibly increases plasma concentration of *clozapine* (possible increased risk of convulsions) and *sertindole*

• Antivirals: *clarithromycin tablets* reduce absorption of *zidovudine*; see also Ritonavir, p. 581

• Anxiolytics and Hypnotics: *erythromycin* inhibits metabolism of *midazolam* (increased plasma-midazolam concentration, with profound sedation) and *zopiclone*

   Calcium-channel Blockers: *erythromycin* possibly inhibits metabolism of *felodipine* (increased plasma concentration)

   Cardiac Glycosides: effect of *digoxin* enhanced by *erythromycin* and possibly enhanced by *other macrolides*

• Cisapride: *clarithromycin* and *erythromycin* possibly inhibit metabolism of *cisapride* (risk of ventricular arrhythmias—avoid concomitant use)

• Cyclosporin: *erythromycin* and possibly *other macrolides* inhibit metabolism (increased plasma-cyclosporin concentration)

   Cytotoxics: *see* Docetaxel

   Dopaminergics: plasma concentration of *bromocriptine* and *cabergoline* increased by *erythromycin*

• Ergotamine: ergotism reported

• Tacrolimus: *clarithromycin* and *erythromycin* increase plasma-tacrolimus concentration

• Theophylline: *clarithromycin* and *erythromycin* inhibit metabolism (increased plasma-theophylline concentration) (if erythromycin given by mouth, also decreased plasma-erythromycin concentration)

   Ulcer-healing Drugs: *cimetidine* increases plasma-erythromycin concentration (increased risk of toxicity, including deafness)

Erythropoietin *see* Epoetin
Esmolol *see* Beta-blockers
Estropipate *see* Contraceptives, Oral
Ethacrynic Acid *see* Diuretics (loop)
Ethinyloestradiol *see* Contraceptives, Oral
Ethosuximide
- Antibacterials: *isoniazid* increases plasma concentrations (increased risk of toxicity)
- Antidepressants: antagonism (convulsive threshold lowered)
- *other* Antiepileptics: concomitant administration of two or more antiepileptics may enhance toxicity without a corresponding increase in antiepileptic effect; moreover interactions between individual antiepileptics can complicate monitoring of treatment; interactions include enhanced effects, increased sedation, and reductions in plasma concentrations; for further details, see p. 210
- Antipsychotics: antagonism (convulsive threshold lowered)

Ethynodiol *see* Progestogens
Etidronate Disodium *see* Bisphosphonates
Etodolac *see* NSAIDs
Etomidate *see* Anaesthetics, General
Famciclovir *see* Aciclovir and Famciclovir
Famotidine *see* Histamine H$_2$-antagonists
Fansidar® *contains* Sulfadoxine and Pyrimethamine
Felodipine *see* Calcium-channel Blockers
Fenbufen *see* NSAIDs
Fenofibrate *see* Clofibrate Group
Fenoprofen *see* NSAIDs
Fenoterol *see* Sympathomimetics, Beta$_2$
Fentanyl *see* Opioid Analgesics
Ferrous Salts *see* Iron
Fexofenadine *see* Antihistamines
Filgrastim
  Note. Use not recommended in period from 24 hours before to 24 hours after chemotherapy—for further details consult product literature
  Cytotoxics: possible exacerbation of neutropenia with *fluorouracil*
Finasteride
  Note. No clinically important interactions reported
Flavoxate *see* Antimuscarinics
Flecainide
- *other* Anti-arrhythmics: *amiodarone* increases plasma-flecainide concentration (and increases risk of ventricular arrhythmias—avoid concomitant use); increased myocardial depression with any *anti-arrhythmic*
- Antidepressants: *fluoxetine* increases plasma-flecainide concentration; increased risk of arrhythmias with *tricyclics*
- Antihistamines: increased risk of ventricular arrhythmias with *astemizole* and *terfenadine*
- Antimalarials: *quinine* increases plasma concentration of *flecainide*; increased risk of arrhythmias with *halofantrine* (**important:** see p. 287)
- Antivirals: see Ritonavir, p. 581
- Beta-blockers: increased myocardial depression and bradycardia
- Calcium-channel Blockers: increased myocardial depression and asystole with *verapamil*
- Diuretics: cardiac toxicity increased if hypokalaemia occurs
  Ulcer-healing Drugs: *cimetidine* inhibits metabolism of *flecainide* (increased plasma-flecainide concentration)
Flucloxacillin *see* Penicillins
Fluconazole *see* Antifungals, Imidazole and Triazole
Flucytosine
  Cytotoxics: *cytarabine* possibly reduces plasma-flucytosine concentrations

Fludarabine
  Antiplatelet Drugs: efficacy possibly reduced by *dipyridamole*
- *other* Cytotoxics: increased pulmonary toxicity with *pentostatin* (unacceptably high incidence of fatalities)
Fludrocortisone *see* Corticosteroids
Flunisolide *see* Corticosteroids
Flunitrazepam *see* Anxiolytics and Hypnotics
Fluorouracil
  Antibacterials: *metronidazole* inhibits metabolism (increased toxicity)
  Filgrastim: possible exacerbation of neutropenia
  Ulcer-healing Drugs: *cimetidine* inhibits metabolism (increased plasma-fluorouracil concentration)
Fluoxetine *see* Antidepressants, SSRI
Flupenthixol *see* Antipsychotics
Fluphenazine *see* Antipsychotics
Flurazepam *see* Anxiolytics and Hypnotics
Flurbiprofen *see* NSAIDs
Flutamide
- Anticoagulants: effect of *warfarin* enhanced
Fluticasone *see* Corticosteroids
Fluvastatin *see* Statins
Fluvoxamine *see* Antidepressants, SSRI
Folic Acid *see* Vitamins
Fosinopril *see* ACE Inhibitors
Framycetin *see* Aminoglycosides
Frusemide *see* Diuretics (loop)
Gabapentin
  Antacids and Adsorbents: *antacids* reduce absorption
  other Antiepileptics: none demonstrated with *carbamazepine, phenobarbitone, phenytoin,* or *valproate*
Gallamine *see* Muscle Relaxants (non-depolarising)
Ganciclovir
  Note: Increased risk of myelosuppression with other myelosuppressive drugs—consult product literature
- Antibacterials: increased toxicity with *Primaxin®* (convulsions reported)
- *other* Antivirals: plasma concentration of *didanosine* possibly increased; profound myelosuppression with *zidovudine* (see also p. 280)
  Uricosurics: *probenecid* reduces renal excretion (increased plasma half-life)
Gemfibrozil *see* Clofibrate Group
Gentamicin *see* Aminoglycosides
Gestodene *see* Progestogens
Gestrinone
  Antibacterials: *rifampicin* accelerates metabolism (reduced plasma concentration)
  Antiepileptics: *carbamazepine, phenobarbitone, phenytoin, and primidone* accelerate metabolism (reduced plasma concentration)
  Barbiturates and Primidone: *see under* Antiepileptics, above
Gestronol *see* Progestogens
Glibenclamide *see* Antidiabetics (sulphonylurea)
Gliclazide *see* Antidiabetics (sulphonylurea)
Glipizide *see* Antidiabetics (sulphonylurea)
Gliquidone *see* Antidiabetics (sulphonylurea)
Glyceryl Trinitrate (general hypotensive interactions *as for* Hydralazine)
  Anti-arrhythmics: *disopyramide* may reduce effect of *sublingual nitrates* (owing to dry mouth)
- Anticoagulants: excretion of *heparin* increased by *glyceryl trinitrate infusion* (reduced anticoagulant effect)
  Antidepressants: *tricyclics* may reduce effect of *sublingual nitrates* (owing to dry mouth)
  Antimuscarinics: *antimuscarinics such as atropine and propantheline* may reduce effect of *sublingual nitrates* (owing to dry mouth)
Gold
  Note. Increased risk of toxicity with other nephrotoxic and myelosuppressive drugs

Griseofulvin
- Anticoagulants: metabolism of *nicoumalone and warfarin* accelerated (reduced anticoagulant effect)

  Antiepileptics: absorption reduced by *phenobarbitone* (reduced effect)

  Barbiturates and Primidone: *see under* Antiepileptics, above

  Cyclosporin: plasma-cyclosporin concentration possibly reduced
- Oestrogens and Progestogens: metabolism of *oral contraceptives* accelerated (reduced contraceptive effect, **important:** see p. 351)

Guanethidine *see* Adrenergic Neurone Blockers

Guar Gum

  Antibacterials: absorption of *phenoxymethylpenicillin* reduced

Halofantrine
- Anti-arrhythmics: increased risk of ventricular arrhythmias with drugs which prolong QT interval (including amiodarone, disopyramide, flecainide, procainamide and quinidine)
- Antidepressants: increased risk of ventricular arrhythmias with *tricyclics*
- Antihistamines: increased risk of ventricular arrhythmias with *astemizole* and *terfenadine*
- *other* Antimalarials: increased risk of arrhythmias with *chloroquine*, *mefloquine* and *quinine* (**important:** see also CSM advice under Halofantrine, p. 287)
- Antipsychotics: increased risk of ventricular arrhythmias with *phenothiazines*
- Beta-blockers: increased risk of ventricular arrhythmias with *sotalol*
- Diuretics: increased risk of ventricular arrhythmias if electrolyte disturbances occur

Haloperidol *see* Antipsychotics

Halothane *see* Anaesthetics, General (volatile liquid)

Heparin
- Analgesics: *aspirin* enhances anticoagulant effect; increased risk of haemorrhage with *parenteral diclofenac* and *ketorolac* (avoid concomitant use, including low-dose heparin)

  Antiplatelet Drugs: *aspirin and dipyridamole* enhance anticoagulant effect
- Nitrates: *glyceryl trinitrate infusion* increases excretion (reduced anticoagulant effect)

Hexamine

  Potassium Citrate: urine should be acid

Histamine H₁-antagonists *see* Antihistamines

Histamine H₂-antagonists

  Analgesics: *cimetidine* inhibits metabolism of *opioid analgesics notably pethidine* (increased plasma concentrations); *cimetidine* possibly increases plasma concentration of *azapropazone*

  Anthelmintics: *cimetidine* possibly inhibits metabolism of *mebendazole* (increased plasma concentration)
- Anti-arrhythmics: *cimetidine* increases plasma concentrations of *amiodarone, flecainide, lignocaine, procainamide, propafenone, quinidine,* and possibly *moracizine*

  Antibacterials: absorption of *cefpodoxime* reduced; *cimetidine* increases plasma-erythromycin concentration (increased risk of toxicity, including deafness); *rifampicin* accelerates metabolism of *cimetidine* (reduced plasma-cimetidine concentration); *cimetidine* inhibits metabolism of *metronidazole* (increased plasma-metronidazole concentration)
- Anticoagulants: *cimetidine* enhances anticoagulant effect of *nicoumalone and warfarin* (inhibits metabolism)

  Antidepressants: *cimetidine* inhibits metabolism of *amitriptyline, doxepin, imipramine, moclobemide, and nortriptyline* (increased plasma concentrations)

Histamine H₂-antagonists *(continued)*

  Antidiabetics: *cimetidine* inhibits renal excretion of *metformin* (increased plasma concentration); *cimetidine* and *ranitidine* enhance hypoglycaemic effect of *sulphonylureas*
- Antiepileptics: *cimetidine* inhibits metabolism of *carbamazepine, phenytoin, and valproate* (increased plasma concentrations)

  Antifungals: absorption of *itraconazole and ketoconazole* reduced; plasma concentration of *terbinafine* increased by *cimetidine*

  Antihistamines: manufacturer advises possibility of increased plasma-loratadine concentration with *cimetidine*

  Antimalarials: *cimetidine* inhibits metabolism of *chloroquine* and *quinine* (increased plasma concentrations)

  Antipsychotics: *cimetidine* possibly enhances effect of *chlorpromazine, clozapine, and possibly other antipsychotics*

  Anxiolytics and Hypnotics: *cimetidine* inhibits metabolism of *benzodiazepines* and *chlormethiazole* (increased plasma concentrations)

  Beta-blockers: *cimetidine* inhibits metabolism of *beta-blockers* such as *labetalol* and *propranolol* (increased plasma concentrations)

  Calcium-channel Blockers: *cimetidine* inhibits metabolism of *some calcium-channel blockers* (increased plasma concentrations)
- Cyclosporin: *cimetidine* possibly increases plasma-cyclosporin concentration

  Cytotoxics: *cimetidine* increases plasma concentration of *fluorouracil*

  Hormone Antagonists: *octreotide* possibly delays absorption of *cimetidine*
- Theophylline: *cimetidine* inhibits metabolism (increased plasma-theophylline concentration)

Homatropine *see* Antimuscarinics

Hormone Antagonists *see* Aminoglutethimide; Bicalutamide; Danazol; Finasteride; Flutamide; Gestrinone; Octeotide; Tamoxifen; Toremifene; Trilostane

5HT₁ Agonists

  Note. There are currently no recognised drug interactions with naratriptan
- Antidepressants: risk of CNS toxicity with MAOIs including *moclobemide* (avoid sumatriptan for 2 weeks after MAOI, reduce dose of zolmitriptan when given with moclobemide); *sumatriptan* increases risk of CNS toxicity with *SSRIs* (avoid concomitant use)
- Ergotamine: increased risk of vasospasm (avoid ergotamine for 6 hours after both sumatriptan and zolmitriptan; avoid sumatriptan for 24 hours and zolmitriptan for 6 hours after ergotamine)
- Lithium: *sumatriptan* increases risk of CNS toxicity (avoid concomitant use)

Hydralazine

  ACE Inhibitors: enhanced hypotensive effect

  Alcohol: enhanced hypotensive effect

  Aldesleukin: enhanced hypotensive effect

  Alprostadil: enhanced hypotensive effect
- Anaesthetics: enhanced hypotensive effect

  Analgesics: *NSAIDs* antagonise hypotensive effect

  Antidepressants: enhanced hypotensive effect

  other Antihypertensives: additive hypotensive effect

  Antipsychotics: enhanced hypotensive effect

  Anxiolytics and Hypnotics: enhanced hypotensive effect

  Beta-blockers: enhanced hypotensive effect

  Calcium-channel Blockers: enhanced hypotensive effect

  Corticosteroids: antagonism of hypotensive effect

  Diuretics: enhanced hypotensive effect

  Dopaminergics: *levodopa* enhances hypotensive effect

Hydralazine *(continued)*
Muscle Relaxants: *baclofen* and *tizanidine* enhance hypotensive effect
Nitrates: enhanced hypotensive effect
Oestrogens and Progestogens: *oestrogens* and *combined oral contraceptives* antagonise hypotensive effect
Thymoxamine: enhanced hypotensive effect
Ulcer-healing Drugs: *carbenoxolone* antagonises hypotensive effect
Hydrochlorothiazide *see* Diuretics (thiazide)
Hydrocortisone *see* Corticosteroids
Hydroflumethiazide *see* Diuretics (thiazide)
Hydroxychloroquine *see* Chloroquine and Hydroxychloroquine
Hydroxyprogesterone *see* Progestogens
Hydroxyzine *see* Antihistamines
Hyoscine *see* Antimuscarinics (for general sedative interactions *see also* Antihistamines)
Hypnotics *see* Anxiolytics and Hypnotics
Ibesartan as for ACE Inhibitors
Ibuprofen *see* NSAIDs
Ifosfamide *see* Cyclophosphamide and Ifosfamide
Imipenem *see* Primaxin®
Immunoglobulins
Note. For advice on immunoglobulins and live virus vaccines, see under Normal Immunoglobulin section 14.5
Imipramine *see* Antidepressants, Tricyclic
Indapamide *see* Diuretics (thiazide-related)
Indinavir
• Antibacterials: concomitant administration of *indinavir* and *rifabutin* increases plasma-rifabutin concentration and decreases plasma-indinavir concentration (reduce dose of rifabutin and increase dose of indinavir); metabolism enhanced by *rifampicin* (plasma-indinavir concentration significantly reduced—avoid concomitant use)
Anti-epileptics: plasma-indinavir concentration possibly reduced by *carbamazepine, phenobarbitone* and *phenytoin*
• Antifungals: metabolism inhibited by *ketoconazole* (reduce dose of indinavir); on theoretical grounds, plasma-indinavir concentration significantly increased by *itraconazole* (avoid concomitant use)
• Antihistamines: increased risk of arrhythmias with *terfenadine*—avoid concomitant use
Barbiturates and Primidone: *see under* Antiepileptics, above
Corticosteroids: plasma-indinavir concentration possibly reduced by *dexamethasone*
Indomethacin *see* NSAIDs
Indoramin *see* Alpha-blockers
Influenza Vaccine
Anticoagulants: effect of *warfarin* occasionally enhanced
Antiepileptics: effect of *phenytoin* enhanced
Theophylline: effect occasionally enhanced
Insulin *see* Antidiabetics
Interferons
Note. Consult product literature for interactions of interferon beta and gamma
Theophylline: *interferon alfa* inhibits metabolism of *theophylline* (enhanced effect)
Ipratropium *see* Antimuscarinics
Iron
Antacids: *magnesium trisilicate* reduces absorption of *oral iron*
Antibacterials: *tetracyclines* reduce absorption of *oral iron* (and *vice versa*); absorption of *ciprofloxacin, norfloxacin,* and *ofloxacin* reduced by *oral iron*
Bisphosphonates: reduced absorption
Dopaminergics: absorption of *levodopa* may be reduced
Penicillamine: reduced absorption of *penicillamine*
Trientine: reduced absorption of *oral iron*
Zinc: reduced absorption of *oral iron* (and *vice versa*)

Isocarboxazid *see* MAOIs
Isoflurane *see* Anaesthetics, General (volatile liquid)
Isometheptene *see* Sympathomimetics
Isoniazid
Anaesthetics: hepatotoxicity possibly potentiated by *isoflurane*
Antacids and Adsorbents: *antacids* reduce absorption
other Antibacterials: increased CNS toxicity with *cycloserine*
• Antiepileptics: metabolism of *carbamazepine, ethosuximide, and phenytoin* inhibited (enhanced effect); also, with *carbamazepine,* isoniazid hepatotoxicity possibly increased
Antifungals: plasma concentration of *ketoconazole* may be reduced
Anxiolytics and Hypnotics: metabolism of *diazepam* inhibited
Theophylline: *isoniazid* possibly increases plasma *theophylline* concentration
Isoprenaline *see* Sympathomimetics
Isosorbide Dinitrate *see* Glyceryl Trinitrate
Isosorbide Mononitrate *see* Glyceryl Trinitrate
Isotretinoin *see* Retinoids
Isradipine *see* Calcium-channel Blockers
Itraconazole *see* Antifungals, Imidazole and Triazole
Kanamycin *see* Aminoglycosides
Kaolin *see* Antacids and Adsorbents
Ketamine *see* Anaesthetics, General
Ketoconazole *see* Antifungals, Imidazole and Triazole
Ketoprofen *see* NSAIDs
Ketorolac *see* NSAIDs
Ketotifen *see* Antihistamines
Labetalol *see* Beta-blockers
Lacidipine *see* Calcium-channel Blockers
Lamivudine
Antibacterials: *trimethoprim* increases plasma concentration
Lamotrigine
• *other* Antiepileptics: concomitant administration of *two or more antiepileptics* may enhance toxicity without a corresponding increase in antiepileptic effect; moreover interactions between individual antiepileptics can complicate monitoring of treatment; interactions include enhanced effects, increased sedation, and reductions in plasma concentrations; for further details, see p. 210
Lansoprazole *see* Proton Pump Inhibitors
Lenograstim
Note. Use not recommended from 1 day before until 24 hours after chemotherapy—for further details consult product literature
Levobunolol *see* Beta-blockers
Levocabastine *see* Antihistamines
Levodopa
• Anaesthetics: risk of arrhythmias with *volatile liquid anaesthetics such as halothane*
• Antidepressants: hypertensive crisis with *MAOIs* (including *moclobemide*)—avoid for at least 2 weeks after stopping MAOI
Antihypertensives: enhanced hypotensive effect
Antipsychotics: antagonism of effect
Anxiolytics and Hypnotics: occasional antagonism of effect by *chlordiazepoxide, diazepam, lorazepam* and possibly *other benzodiazepines*
Iron: absorption of *levodopa* may be reduced
Metoclopramide and Domperidone: levodopa-plasma concentrations increased by *metoclopramide*
Vitamins: effect of *levodopa* antagonised by *pyridoxine* unless a *dopa decarboxylase inhibitor* also given
Levonorgestrel *see* Progestogens

Lignocaine
  other Anti-arrhythmics: increased myocardial depression
  Beta-blockers: increased risk of myocardial depression; increased risk of *lignocaine* toxicity with *propranolol*
  Diuretics: effect of *lignocaine* antagonised by hypokalaemia with *acetazolamide, loop diuretics, and thiazides*
  Ulcer-healing Drugs: *cimetidine* inhibits metabolism of *lignocaine* (increased risk of toxicity)
Lipid-regulating Drugs *see* Cholestyramine and Colestipol; Clofibrate Group; Nicotinic Acid; Statins
Lisinopril *see* ACE Inhibitors
Lithium
• ACE Inhibitors: *lithium* excretion reduced (increased plasma-lithium concentration)
• Analgesics: excretion of *lithium* reduced by *azapropazone, diclofenac, ibuprofen, indomethacin, ketorolac* (avoid concomitant use), *mefenamic acid, naproxen, phenylbutazone, piroxicam,* and probably *other NSAIDs* (risk of toxicity)
  Antacids and Adsorbents: *sodium bicarbonate* increases excretion of *lithium* (reduced plasma-lithium concentrations)
  Anti-arrhythmics: increased risk of hypothyroidism with *amiodarone*
  Antibacterials: *lithium* toxicity reported with *metronidazole* and *spectinomycin*
• Antidepressants: *SSRIs* increase risk of CNS effects (lithium toxicity reported)
  Antidiabetics: *lithium* may occasionally impair glucose tolerance
  Antiepileptics: neurotoxicity may occur with *carbamazepine* and *phenytoin* without increased plasma-lithium concentration
• Antihypertensives: neurotoxicity may occur with *methyldopa* without increased plasma-lithium concentration
  Antipsychotics: increased risk of extrapyramidal effects and possibility of neurotoxicity (notably with *haloperidol*)
  Calcium-channel Blockers: neurotoxicity may occur with *diltiazem and verapamil* without increased plasma-lithium concentration
• Diuretics: *lithium* excretion reduced by *loop diuretics, potassium-sparing diuretics, and thiazides* (increased plasma-lithium concentration and risk of toxicity—*loop diuretics* safer than *thiazides); lithium* excretion increased by *acetazolamide*
• 5HT$_1$ Agonists: *sumatriptan* increases risk of CNS toxicity
  Metoclopramide and Domperidone: increased risk of extrapyramidal effects and possibility of neurotoxicity with *metoclopramide*
  Muscle Relaxants: muscle relaxant effect enhanced; *baclofen* possibly aggravates hyperkinesis
  Parasympathomimetics: *lithium* antagonises effect of *neostigmine* and *pyridostigmine*
  Theophylline: *lithium* excretion increased (reduced plasma-lithium concentration)
Lofepramine *see* Antidepressants, Tricyclic
Lofexidine
  Alcohol: enhanced sedative effect
  Anxiolytics and Hypnotics: enhanced sedative effect
Loprazolam *see* Anxiolytics and Hypnotics
Loratadine *see* Antihistamines
Lorazepam *see* Anxiolytics and Hypnotics
Lormetazepam *see* Anxiolytics and Hypnotics
Losartan as for ACE Inhibitors
Loxapine *see* Antipsychotics
Lymecycline *see* Tetracyclines
Lysuride
  Antipsychotics: antagonism of effect
Macrolides *see* Erythromycin and other Macrolides

Magnesium Salts (*see also* Antacids and Adsorbents)
  Muscle Relaxants: effect of *non-depolarising muscle relaxants* enhanced by *parenteral magnesium salts*
Magnesium Trisilicate *see* Antacids and Adsorbents
Maloprim® *contains* Dapsone and Pyrimethamine
MAOIs
  Note. For interactions of reversible MAO-A inhibitors (RIMAs) see Moclobemide, and for interactions of MAO-B inhibitors see Selegiline
• Alcohol: some *alcoholic* and *dealcoholised beverages* contain *tyramine* which interacts with *MAOIs* (hypertensive crisis)—but if no tyramine, enhanced hypotensive effect; foods, *see* section 4.3.2
  Alpha$_2$-adrenoceptor Stimulants: manufacturers of *apraclonidine* and *brimonidine* advise avoid concomitant use
• Altretamine: risk of severe postural hypotension
• Analgesics: CNS excitation or depression (hypertension or hypotension) with *pethidine* and possibly *other opioid analgesics*—avoid concomitant use and for 2 weeks after MAOI discontinued; manufacturer advises avoid *nefopam*
  Anaesthetics: *see* section 15.1
• Anorectics: *see* Sympathomimetics, below
• *other* Antidepressants: enhancement of CNS effects and toxicity with *other MAOIs* (avoid for at least a week after stopping *previous MAOIs* then start with reduced dose); increased risk of toxicity with *nefazodone* (**important:** if MAOIs discontinued shortly before, initiate nefazodone cautiously with gradual dose increase); CNS effects of *SSRIs* increased by *MAOIs* (risk of serious toxicity); SSRI should not be started until 2 weeks after stopping *MAOI*; conversely, *MAOI* should not be started until at least 1 week after *citalopram* or *fluvoxamine* have been stopped, at least 5 weeks for *fluoxetine*, at least 2 weeks for *paroxetine* and *sertraline*; CNS excitation and hypertension with most *tricyclics and related antidepressants* (avoid for at least 2 wweeks after stopping MAOI, and avoid MAOI for at least 1 week after stopping tricyclic); CNS excitation and confusion with *tryptophan* (reduce tryptophan dose); enhancement of CNS effects and toxicity possible with *reboxetine* and *venlafaxine* (avoid for at least 2 weeks after stopping MAOI, and avoid MAOI for at least 1 week after stopping reboxetine or venlafaxine)
  Antidiabetics: effect of *insulin, metformin, and sulphonylureas* enhanced
• Antiepileptics: antagonism of anticonvulsant effect (convulsive threshold lowered); manufacturer advises avoid *carbamazepine* with or within 2 weeks of *MAOIs*
• Antihypertensives: hypotensive effect enhanced; manufacturer advises avoidance of *indoramin*
  Antihistamines: increased antimuscarinic and sedative effects
  Antimuscarinics: increased side-effects
• Antipsychotics: CNS excitation and hypertension with *oxypertine*; *clozapine* possibly enhances central effects
  Anxiolytics and Hypnotics: manufacturer advises avoidance of *buspirone*
• Barbiturates and Primidone: *see under* Antiepileptics, above
• Dopaminergics: hypertensive crisis with *levodopa* (avoid for at least 2 weeks after stopping MAOI); hypotension with *selegiline*
• 5HT$_1$ Agonists: risk of CNS toxicity (avoid sumatriptan for 2 weeks after MAOI)
• Sympathomimetics: hypertensive crisis with *sympathomimetics* such as *dexamphetamine and other amphetamines, dopamine, dopexamine, ephedrine, isometheptene, methylphenidate, phentermine, phenylephrine, phenylpropanolamine,* and *pseudoephedrine*

MAOIs *(continued)*
- Tetrabenazine: CNS excitation and hypertension
  <u>Tolcapone</u>: manufacturer advises avoid concomitant use

Maprotiline *see* Antidepressants, Tricyclic

Mebendazole
   Ulcer-healing Drugs: metabolism possibly inhibited by *cimetidine* (increased plasma-mebendazole concentration)

Medroxyprogesterone *see* Progestogens

Mefenamic Acid *see* NSAIDs

Mefloquine
- <u>Anti-arrhythmics</u>: increased risk of ventricular arrhythmias with *amiodarone* (avoid concomitant use) and *quinidine*
- Antiepileptics: antagonism of anticonvulsant effect *other* Antimalarials: increased risk of convulsions with *chloroquine* and *quinine*, but should not prevent use of intravenous quinine in severe cases; for full precautions see footnote on p. 282 (also applies to *quinidine*); increased risk of ventricular arrhythmias with *halofantrine* (**important:** see also CSM advice under Halofantrine, p. 287)
- <u>Antipsychotics</u>: increased risk of ventricular arrhythmias—avoid concomitant use with *pimozide*
  Beta-blockers: possible increased risk of bradycardia
  Calcium-channel Blockers: possible increased risk of bradycardia with some *calcium-channel blockers*
  Cardiac Glycosides: possible increased risk of bradycardia with *digoxin*
  Vaccines: *see* Typhoid Vaccine, p. 529

Mefruside *see* Diuretics (thiazide)

Megestrol *see* Progestogens

Meloxicam *see* NSAIDs

Melphalan
   Antibacterials: increased toxicity with *nalidixic acid*
- Cyclosporin: increased risk of nephrotoxicity

Mepacrine
   Antimalarials: increased plasma concentration of *primaquine* (risk of toxicity)

Meprobamate *see* Anxiolytics and Hypnotics

Meptazinol *see* Opioid Analgesics

Mequitazine *see* Antihistamines

Mercaptopurine
- Allopurinol: enhancement of effect (increased toxicity)

Mestranol *see* Contraceptives, Oral

Metaraminol *see* Sympathomimetics (*as* noradrenaline)

Metformin *see* Antidiabetics

Methadone *see* Opioid Analgesics

Methocarbamol *see* Muscle Relaxants

Methohexitone *see* Anaesthetics, General

Methotrexate
- Analgesics: excretion reduced by *aspirin, azapropazone* (avoid concomitant use), *diclofenac, indomethacin, ketoprofen, naproxen, phenylbutazone, and probably other NSAIDs* (increased risk of toxicity)
   Antibacterials: antifolate effect increased by *co-trimoxazole and trimethoprim*; excretion reduced by *penicillins* (increased risk of toxicity)
   Antiepileptics: *phenytoin* increases antifolate effect
   Antimalarials: antifolate effect increased by *pyrimethamine* (ingredient of *Fansidar®* and *Maloprim®*)
- Cyclosporin: increased toxicity
- Retinoids: plasma concentration of *methotrexate* increased by *acitretin* (also increased risk of hepatotoxicity)
- Uricosurics: excretion reduced by *probenecid* (increased risk of toxicity)

Methotrimeprazine *see* Antipsychotics

Methoxamine *see* Sympathomimetics (*as* noradrenaline)

Methyldopa
   Alcohol: enhanced hypotensive effect
   <u>Alprostadil</u>: enhanced hypotensive effect
- Anaesthetics: enhanced hypotensive effect
   Analgesics: *NSAIDs* antagonise hypotensive effect
   Antidepressants: enhanced hypotensive effect
   other Antihypertensives: enhanced hypotensive effect
   Antipsychotics: increased risk of extrapyramidal effects; enhanced hypotensive effect
   Anxiolytics and Hypnotics: enhanced hypotensive effect
   Beta-blockers: enhanced hypotensive effect
   Calcium-channel Blockers: enhanced hypotensive effect
   Corticosteroids: antagonism of hypotensive effect
   Diuretics: enhanced hypotensive effect
   Dopaminergics: antagonism of antiparkinsonian effect; *levodopa* enhances hypotensive effect
- Lithium: neurotoxicity may occur without increased plasma-lithium concentration
- Muscle Relaxants: enhanced hypotensive effect with *baclofen* and *tizanidine*
   Nitrates: enhance hypotensive effect
   Oestrogens and Progestogens: *oestrogens and combined oral contraceptives* antagonise hypotensive effect
   Sympathomimetics: *see* Sympathomimetics (main list)
   <u>Thymoxamine</u>: enhanced hypotensive effect
   Ulcer-healing Drugs: *carbenoxolone* antagonises hypotensive effect

Methylphenidate *see* Sympathomimetics

Methylphenobarbitone *see* Barbiturates

Methylprednisolone *see* Corticosteroids

Metipranolol *see* Beta-blockers

Metirosine
   Antipsychotics: increased risk of extrapyramidal effects
   Dopaminergics: antagonism

Metoclopramide
   Analgesics: increased absorption of *aspirin and paracetamol* (enhanced effect); *opioid analgesics* antagonise effect on gastro-intestinal activity
   Antimuscarinics: antagonism of effect on gastro-intestinal activity
   Antipsychotics: increased risk of extrapyramidal effects
   Atovaquone: plasma concentration reduced by *metoclopramide*
   Dopaminergics: antagonism of hypoprolactinaemic effect of *bromocriptine*; increased plasma concentration of *levodopa*; antagonism of antiparkinsonian effects of *pergolide*
   Lithium: increased risk of extrapyramidal effects and possibility of neurotoxicity
   Tetrabenazine: increased risk of extrapyramidal effects

Metolazone *see* Diuretics (thiazide-related)

Metoprolol *see* Beta-blockers

Metronidazole
   Alcohol: disulfiram-like reaction
- Anticoagulants: effect of *nicoumalone and warfarin* enhanced
- Antiepileptics: *metronidazole* inhibits metabolism of *phenytoin* (increased plasma-phenytoin concentration); *phenobarbitone* accelerates metabolism of *metronidazole* (reduced plasma-metronidazole concentration)
- Barbiturates and Primidone: *see under* Antiepileptics, above
   Cytotoxics: *metronidazole* inhibits metabolism of *fluorouracil* (increased toxicity)
   Disulfiram: psychotic reactions reported
   Lithium: increased toxicity reported
   Ulcer-healing Drugs: *cimetidine* inhibits metabolism (increased plasma-metronidazole concentration)

Mexiletine

Analgesics: *opioid analgesics* delay absorption
• *other* Anti-arrhythmics: increased myocardial depression with any combination of *anti-arrhythmics*

Antibacterials: *rifampicin* accelerates metabolism (reduced plasma-mexiletine concentration)

Antiepileptics: *phenytoin* accelerates metabolism (reduced plasma-mexiletine concentration)

Antimuscarinics: *atropine* delays absorption

Diuretics: action of *mexiletine* antagonised by hypokalaemia due to *acetazolamide, loop diuretics, and thiazides*

Theophylline: plasma-theophylline concentration increased

Mianserin

Alcohol: enhanced effect

other Antidepressants: as for Antidepressants, Tricyclic
• Antiepileptics: antagonism (convulsive threshold lowered); metabolism accelerated by *carbamazepine, phenobarbitone,* and *phenytoin* (reduced plasma-mianserin concentration)

Anxiolytics and Hypnotics: enhanced effect
• Barbiturates and Primidone: *see under* Antiepileptics, above

Miconazole *see* Antifungals, Imidazole and Triazole

Midazolam *see* Anxiolytics and Hypnotics

Mifepristone

Analgesics: manufacturer recommends avoid *aspirin* and *NSAIDs* until 8–12 days after *mifepristone* administration

Minocycline *see* Tetracyclines

Minoxidil *see* Hydralazine for general hypotensive interactions

Mirtazapine

Alcohol: enhanced sedative effect
• *other* Antidepressants: as for Antidepressants, tricyclic

Anxiolytics and Hypnotics: enhanced sedative effect

Misoprostol

Analgesics: increased risk of CNS toxicity with *phenylbutazone*

Mivacurium *see* Muscle Relaxants (non-depolarising)

Moclobemide

Note. Moclobemide is a reversible MAO-A inhibitor (RIMA), see also p. 182
• Analgesics: CNS excitation or depression (hypertension or hypotension) with *codeine , pethidine,* and possibly *fentanyl , morphine,* and *other opioid analgesics*; effects of *ibuprofen* and possibly *other NSAIDs* enhanced
• Anorectics: as for MAOIs (see main list)
• *other* Antidepressants: see p. 182
• Dopaminergics: hypertensive crisis with *levodopa*
• 5HT₁ Agonists: risk of CNS toxicity (reduce dose of zolmitriptan)
• Sympathomimetics: as for MAOIs (see main list)

Ulcer-healing Drugs: *cimetidine* inhibits metabolism (increased plasma-moclobemide concentration)

Moexipril *see* ACE Inhibitors

Monoamine-oxidase Inhibitors *see* MAOIs, Moclobemide, and Selegiline

Moracizine

other Anti-arrhythmics: increased myocardial depression with any *anti-arrhythmic*

Theophylline: metabolism of *theophylline* accelerated (reduced effect)

Ulcer-healing Drugs: *cimetidine* possibly increases plasma-moracizine concentration

Morphine *see* Opioid Analgesics

Moxonidine

Alprostadil: enhanced hypotensive effect

other Antihypertensives: enhanced hypotensive effect

Anxiolytics and Hypnotics: sedative effect of *benzodiazepines* possibly enhanced

Moxonidine *(continued)*

Muscle Relaxants: enhanced hypotensive effect with *baclofen* and *tizanidine*

Thymoxamine: enhanced hypotensive effect

Muscle Relaxants

ACE Inhibitors: enhanced hypotensive effect with *baclofen* and *tizanidine*

Alcohol: enhanced sedative effect with *baclofen* and *tizanidine*

Analgesics: *ibuprofen* and *possibly other NSAIDs* reduce excretion of *baclofen* (increased risk of toxicity)
• Anti-arrhythmics: *procainamide* and *quinidine* enhance muscle relaxant effect
• Antibacterials: effect of *non-depolarising muscle relaxants* enhanced by *aminoglycosides, azlocillin, clindamycin, colistin* and *piperacillin*

Antidepressants: *tricyclics* enhance muscle relaxant effect of *baclofen*

Antiepileptics: effect of *non-depolarising muscle relaxants* antagonised by *carbamazepine* and *phenytoin* (recovery from neuromuscular blockade accelerated)

Antihypertensives: enhanced hypotensive effect with *baclofen* and *tizanidine*

Anxiolytics and Hypnotics: enhanced sedative effect with *baclofen* and *tizanidine*

Beta-blockers: *propranolol* enhances muscle relaxant effect; possible enhanced hypotensive effect and bradycardia with *tizanidine*
• Botulinum Toxin: neuromuscular block enhanced by *non-depolarising muscle relaxants* (risk of toxicity)

Calcium-channel Blockers: *nifedipine* and *verapamil* enhance effect of *non-depolarising muscle relaxants*; hypotension, myocardial depression, and hyperkalaemia reported with intravenous *dantrolene* and *verapamil*; risk of arrhythmias with *diltiazem* and intravenous *dantrolene*

Cardiac Glycosides: arrhythmias if *suxamethonium* given with *digoxin*; possible bradycardia if *tizanidine* given with *digoxin*

Cytotoxics: *cyclophosphamide* and *thiotepa* enhance effect of *suxamethonium*

Diuretics: enhanced hypotensive effect with *baclofen* and *tizanidine*

Lithium: *lithium* enhances muscle relaxant effect; *baclofen* possibly aggravates hyperkinesis

Magnesium Salts: *parenteral magnesium* enhances effect of *non-depolarising muscle relaxants*

Parasympathomimetics: *demecarium* and *ecothiopate* eye-drops, *neostigmine* and *pyridostigmine,* and possibly *donepezil* enhance effect of *suxamethonium* but antagonise effect of *non-depolarising muscle relaxants*

Sympathomimetics: *bambuterol* enhances effect of *suxamethonium*

Mycophenolate Mofetil

Anion-exchange Resins: *cholestyramine* reduces absorption

Antacids and Adsorbents: *antacids* reduce absorption

Antivirals: higher plasma concentrations of *mycophenolate mofetil* and of *aciclovir* on concomitant administration

Nabilone

Alcohol: sedative effect of *nabilone* enhanced

Anxiolytics and Hypnotics: enhanced sedative effect

Nabumetone *see* NSAIDs

Nadolol *see* Beta-blockers

Nalbuphine *see* Opioid Analgesics

Nalidixic Acid *see* 4-Quinolones

Nandrolone *see* Anabolic Steroids

Naproxen *see* NSAIDs

Naratriptan *see* 5HT₁ Agonists

Nefazodone

Note. Although interactions with alcohol, antipsychotics, and lithium have not been reported, caution should be observed on concomitant use with nefazodone

Antidepressants: increased risk of toxicity with *MAOIs* (**important:** if MAOIs discontinued shortly before, initiate cautiously with gradual dosage increase)

* Antihistamines: increased risk of arrhythmias with *terfenadine*—avoid concomitant use

Antihypertensives: hypotensive effect possibly enhanced

Anxiolytics and Hypnotics: possibly enhanced sedative effect with *benzodiazepines*

Nefopam

* Antidepressants: manufacturer recommends avoid *MAOIs;* possibly increased side-effects with *tricyclics*

Antimuscarinics: increased side-effects

Neomycin *see* Aminoglycosides

Neostigmine *see* Parasympathomimetics

Netilmicin *see* Aminoglycosides

Nicardipine *see* Calcium-channel Blockers

Nicorandil

Note. Interactions not observed with beta-blockers, digoxin, rifampicin, cimetidine, nicoumalone, calcium-channel blockers, or frusemide; possibility of hypotensive interaction with vasodilators, tricyclics, or alcohol

Nicotine and Tobacco

Theophylline: *tobacco smoking* increases metabolism (reduced plasma-theophylline concentration)

Nicotinic Acid

Note. Interactions apply to lipid-regulating doses of nicotinic acid

* *other* Lipid-regulating Drugs: increased risk of myopathy with *statins*

Nicoumalone *see* Warfarin and other Coumarins

Nifedipine *see* Calcium-channel Blockers

Nimodipine *see* Calcium-channel Blockers

Nisoldipine *see* Calcium-channel Blockers

Nitrates *see* Glyceryl Trinitrate

Nitrazepam *see* Anxiolytics and Hypnotics

Nitrofurantoin

Antacids and Adsorbents: *magnesium trisilicate* reduces absorption

Uricosurics: *probenecid* reduces excretion of *nitrofurantoin* (risk of toxicity)

Nitroprusside *as for* Hydralazine

Nitrous Oxide *see* Anaesthetics, General

Nizatidine *see* Histamine H_2-antagonists

Noradrenaline *see* Sympathomimetics

Norethisterone *see* Progestogens

Norfloxacin *see* 4-Quinolones

Norgestimate *see* Progestogens

Norgestrel *see* Progestogens

Nortriptyline *see* Antidepressants, Tricyclic

NSAIDs (*see also* Aspirin)

Note. Interactions do not generally apply to topical NSAIDS

* ACE Inhibitors: antagonism of hypotensive effect; increased risk of renal damage and increased risk of hyperkalaemia on administration with *indomethacin, ketorolac* and possibly *other NSAIDs*

* *other* Analgesics: avoid concomitant administration of two or more *NSAIDs*, including *aspirin* (increased side-effects)

Anion-exchange Resins: *cholestyramine* reduces absorption of *phenylbutazone*

Antacids and Adsorbents: *antacids* reduce absorption of *diflunisal*

Antibacterials: *NSAIDs* possibly increase risk of convulsions with *4-quinolones*

NSAIDs *(continued)*

* Anticoagulants: anticoagulant effect of *nicoumalone* and *warfarin* seriously enhanced by *azapropazone* and *phenylbutazone* (avoid concomitant use), and possibly enhanced by *diclofenac, diflunisal, flurbiprofen, mefenamic acid, piroxicam, sulindac, and other NSAIDs*; increased risk of haemorrhage with *parenteral diclofenac* and *ketorolac* and all *anticoagulants,* including *low-dose heparin* (avoid concomitant use)

Antidepressants: *moclobemide* enhances effect of *ibuprofen* and possibly *other NSAIDs*

* Antidiabetics: effect of *sulphonylureas* enhanced by *azapropazone, phenylbutazone* and possibly *other NSAIDs*

* Antiepileptics: effect of *phenytoin* enhanced by *azapropazone* (avoid concomitant use), *phenylbutazone* and possibly *other NSAIDs*

Antihypertensives: antagonism of hypotensive effect

Antipsychotics: severe drowsiness possible if *indomethacin* given with *haloperidol*

* Antivirals: see Ritonavir, p. 581

Beta-blockers: antagonism of hypotensive effect

Bisphosphonates: bioavailability of *tiludronic acid* increased by *indomethacin; alendronic acid* possibly increases gastro-intestinal side-effects of *NSAIDs*

Cardiac Glycosides: *NSAIDs* may exacerbate heart failure, reduce GFR, and increase plasma-cardiac glycoside concentration

Corticosteroids: increased risk of gastro-intestinal bleeding and ulceration

* Cyclosporin: increased risk of nephrotoxicity; *cyclosporin* increases plasma concentration of *diclofenac* (halve diclofenac dose)

* Cytotoxics: excretion of *methotrexate* reduced by *aspirin, azapropazone* (avoid concomitant use), *diclofenac, indomethacin, ketoprofen, naproxen, phenylbutazone and probably other NSAIDs* (increased risk of toxicity)

Desmopressin: effect potentiated by *indomethacin*

Diuretics: risk of nephrotoxicity of *NSAIDs* increased; *NSAIDs* notably *indomethacin* and *ketorolac* antagonise diuretic effect; *indomethacin* and possibly *other NSAIDs* increase risk of hyperkalaemia with *potassium-sparing diuretics*; occasional reports of decreased renal function when *indomethacin* given with *triamterene*

* Lithium: excretion of *lithium* reduced by *azapropazone, diclofenac, ibuprofen, indomethacin, ketorolac* (avoid concomitant use), *mefenamic acid, naproxen, phenylbutazone, piroxicam,* and probably *other NSAIDs* (risk of toxicity)

Mifepristone: manufacturer recommends avoid *aspirin* and *NSAIDs* until 8-12 days after *mifepristone* administration

Muscle Relaxants: *ibuprofen* and possibly *other NSAIDs* reduce excretion of *baclofen* (increased risk of toxicity)

* Tacrolimus: *ibuprofen* increases risk of nephrotoxicity

Thyroxine: false low total plasma-thyroxine concentration with *phenylbutazone*

Ulcer-healing Drugs: plasma concentration of *azapropazone* possibly increased by *cimetidine;* risk of CNS toxicity with *phenylbutazone* increased by *misoprostol*

* Uricosurics: *probenecid* delays excretion of *indomethacin, ketoprofen, ketorolac* (avoid concomitant use), and *naproxen* and increases plasma-NSAID concentration

* Vasodilators: risk of ketorolac-associated bleeding increased by *oxpentifylline* (avoid concomitant use)

Octreotide

Antidiabetics: possibly reduces *insulin* and *antidiabetic drug* requirements in diabetes mellitus

Cyclosporin: absorption of *cyclosporin* reduced (reduced plasma concentration)

Ulcer-healing Drugs: absorption of *cimetidine* possibly delayed

Oestrogens *see* Contraceptives, Oral

Ofloxacin *see* 4-Quinolones

Olanzapine *see* Antipsychotics

Omeprazole *see* Proton Pump Inhibitors

Opioid Analgesics

Alcohol: enhanced sedative and hypotensive effect

Anti-arrhythmics: delayed absorption of *mexiletine*

Antibacterials: *rifampicin* accelerates metabolism of *methadone* (reduced effect); *erythromycin* increases plasma concentration of *alfentanil;* manufacturer of *ciprofloxacin* advises avoid premedication with *opioid analgesics* (reduced plasma-ciprofloxacin concentration)

• Anticoagulants: *dextropropoxyphene* may enhance effect of *nicoumalone* and *warfarin*

• Antidepressants: CNS excitation or depression (hypertension or hypotension) if *pethidine* and possibly *other opioid analgesics* given to patients receiving *MAOIs* (including *moclobemide*)—avoid concomitant use and for 2 weeks after *MAOI* discontinued; *tramadol* possibly increases risk of convulsions with *SSRIs* and *tricyclics*

• Antiepileptics: *dextropropoxyphene* enhances effect of *carbamazepine*; effect of *tramadol* decreased by *carbamazepine*; *phenytoin* accelerates *methadone* metabolism (reduced effect and risk of withdrawal effects)

Antifungals: metabolism of *alfentanil* inhibited by *ketoconazole* (risk of prolonged or delayed respiratory depression)

Antipsychotics: enhanced sedative and hypotensive effect

• Antivirals: *methadone* possibly increases plasma concentration of *zidovudine*; see also Ritonavir, p. 581

Anxiolytics and Hypnotics: enhanced sedative effect

Cisapride: possible antagonism of gastro-intestinal effect

• Dopaminergics: hyperpyrexia and CNS toxicity reported with *selegiline*

Metoclopramide and Domperidone: antagonism of gastro-intestinal effects

Ulcer-healing Drugs: *cimetidine* inhibits metabolism of opioid analgesics notably *pethidine* (increased plasma concentration)

Orciprenaline *see* Sympathomimetics

Orphenadrine *see* Antimuscarinics

Oxazepam *see* Anxiolytics and Hypnotics

Oxitropium *see* Antimuscarinics

Oxpentifylline

• Analgesics: increased risk of bleeding with *ketorolac* (avoid concomitant use)

Oxprenolol *see* Beta-blockers

Oxybutynin *see* Antimuscarinics

Oxymetazoline *see* Sympathomimetics

Oxypertine *see* Antipsychotics

Oxytetracycline *see* Tetracyclines

Oxytocin

Anaesthetics: *inhalational anaesthetics* possibly reduce oxytocic effect (also enhanced hypotensive effect and risk of arrhythmias)

Prostaglandins: uterotonic effect potentiated

Sympathomimetics: enhancement of vasopressor effect of *vasoconstrictor sympathomimetics*

Paclitaxel

Antifungals: *ketoconazole* possibly inhibits metabolism of *paclitaxel*

Pamidronate Sodium *see* Bisphosphonates

Pancreatin

Antidiabetics: hypoglycaemic effect of *acarbose* reduced

Pancuronium *see* Muscle Relaxants (non-depolarising)

Pantoprazole *see* Proton Pump Inhibitors

Papaveretum *see* Opioid Analgesics

Paracetamol

Anion-exchange Resins: *cholestyramine* reduces absorption of *paracetamol*

Anticoagulants: prolonged regular use of *paracetamol* possibly enhances *warfarin*

Metoclopramide and Domperidone: *metoclopramide* accelerates absorption of *paracetamol* (enhanced effect)

Parasympathomimetics

Anti-arrhythmics: *procainamide, quinidine* and possibly *propafenone* antagonise effect of *neostigmine* and *pyridostigmine*

• Antibacterials: *aminoglycosides, clindamycin* and *colistin* antagonise effect of *neostigmine* and *pyridostigmine*

Antimalarials; *chloroquine* and *hydroxychloroquine* have potential to increase symptoms of myasthenia gravis and thus diminish effect of *neostigmine* and *pyridostigmine*

Antimuscarinics: antagonism of effect

Beta-blockers: risk of arrhythmias possibly increased by *pilocarpine*; *propranolol* antagonises effect of *neostigmine* and *pyridostigmine*

Lithium: antagonism of effect of *neostigmine* and *pyridostigmine*

Muscle Relaxants: *demecarium* and *ecothiopate* eye-drops, *neostigmine* and *pyridostigmine,* and possibly *donepezil* enhance effect of *suxamethonium,* but antagonise effect of *non-depolarising muscle relaxants*

Paroxetine *see* Antidepressants, SSRI

Penicillamine

Antacids: reduced absorption of *penicillamine*

Iron: reduced absorption of *penicillamine*

Zinc: reduced absorption of *penicillamine*

Penicillins

Antacids: reduced absorption of *pivampicillin*

Anticoagulants: *see* Phenindione and Warfarin

Cytotoxics: reduced excretion of *methotrexate* (increased risk of toxicity)

Guar Gum: reduced absorption of *phenoxymethylpenicillin*

Muscle Relaxants: effects of *non-depolarising muscle relaxants* enhanced by *azlocillin* and *piperacillin*

Oestrogens and Progestogens: *see* Contraceptives, Oral

Uricosurics: excretion of *penicillins* reduced by *probenecid*

Pentaerythritol Tetranitrate *see* Glyceryl Trinitrate

Pentamidine Isethionate

• Anti-arrhythmics: increased risk of ventricular arrhythmias with *amiodarone* (avoid concomitant use)

Pentazocine *see* Opioid Analgesics

Pentostatin

• *other* Cytotoxics: increases pulmonary toxicity of *fludarabine* (unacceptably high incidence of fatalities)

Pergolide

Antipsychotics: antagonism of effect

Metoclopramide and Domperidone: *metoclopramide* antagonises effect

Pericyazine *see* Antipsychotics

Perindopril *see* ACE Inhibitors

Perphenazine *see* Antipsychotics

Pethidine *see* Opioid Analgesics

Phenazocine *see* Opioid Analgesics

Phenelzine *see* MAOIs

Phenindamine *see* Antihistamines

Phenindione

Note. Change in patient's clinical condition, particularly associated with liver disease, intercurrent illness, or drug administration, necessitates more frequent testing. Major changes in diet (especially involving salads and vegetables) and in alcohol consumption may also affect anticoagulant control

- Anabolic Steroids: anticoagulant effect enhanced by *oxymetholone, stanozolol and others*
- Analgesics: anticoagulant effect enhanced by *aspirin*; increased risk of haemorrhage with *parenteral diclofenac* and *ketorolac* (avoid concomitant use)

  Anion-exchange Resins: anticoagulant effect enhanced or reduced by *cholestyramine*

  Antibacterials: although studies have failed to demonstrate interaction, common experience in anticoagulant clinics is that INR can be altered by course of *oral broad-spectrum antibiotics* such as *ampicillin* (may also apply to antibiotics given for local action on gut such as *neomycin*)

- Antiplatelet Drugs: anticoagulant effect enhanced by *aspirin* and *dipyridamole*
- Clofibrate Group: enhanced anticoagulant effect
- Oestrogens and Progestogens: anticoagulant effect antagonised by *oral contraceptives*
- Testosterone: anticoagulant effect enhanced
- Thyroxine: enhanced anticoagulant effect
- Vitamins: anticoagulant effect antagonised by *vitamin K* (present in some enteral feeds)

Pheniramine *see* Antihistamines

Phenobarbitone *see* Barbiturates

Phenoperidine *see* Opioid Analgesics

Phenothiazines *see* Antipsychotics

Phenoxymethylpenicillin *see* Penicillins

Phentermine *see* Sympathomimetics

Phentolamine *see* Alpha-blockers

Phenylbutazone *see* NSAIDs

Phenylephrine *see* Sympathomimetics

Phenylpropanolamine *see* Sympathomimetics

Phenytoin

- Analgesics: plasma-phenytoin concentration increased by *aspirin, azapropazone* (avoid concomitant use), *phenylbutazone* and possibly *other NSAIDs*; metabolism of *methadone* accelerated (reduced effect and risk of withdrawal effects)

  Antacids: reduced *phenytoin* absorption

- Anti-arrhythmics: *amiodarone* increases plasma-phenytoin concentration; *phenytoin* reduces plasma concentrations of *disopyramide, mexiletine*, and *quinidine*

- Antibacterials: plasma-phenytoin concentration increased by *chloramphenicol, cycloserine, isoniazid*, and *metronidazole*; plasma-phenytoin concentration and antifolate effect increased by *co-trimoxazole* and *trimethoprim* and possibly by *other sulphonamides*; plasma-phenytoin concentration reduced by *rifamycins*; plasma concentration of *doxycycline* reduced by *phenytoin*

- Anticoagulants: metabolism of *nicoumalone* and *warfarin* accelerated (possibility of reduced anticoagulant effect, but enhancement also reported)

- Antidepressants: antagonism of anticonvulsant effect (convulsive threshold lowered); *fluoxetine, fluvoxamine*, and *viloxazine* increase plasma-phenytoin concentration; *phenytoin* reduces plasma concentrations of *mianserin, paroxetine*, and *tricyclics*

  Antidiabetics: plasma-phenytoin concentration transiently increased by *tolbutamide* (possibility of toxicity)

Phenytoin *(continued)*

- *other* Antiepileptics: concomitant administration of *two or more antiepileptics* may enhance toxicity without a corresponding increase in antiepileptic effect; moreover interactions between individual antiepileptics can complicate monitoring of treatment; interactions include enhanced effects, increased sedation, and reductions in plasma concentrations; for further details see p. 210

- Antifungals: plasma-phenytoin concentration increased by *fluconazole* and *miconazole*; plasma concentration of *itraconazole* and *ketoconazole* reduced

- Antimalarials: antagonism of anticonvulsant effect; increased risk of antifolate effect with *pyrimethamine* (includes *Fansidar®* and *Maloprim®*)

  Antiplatelet Drugs: plasma-phenytoin concentration increased by *aspirin*

- Antipsychotics: antagonism of anticonvulsant effect (convulsive threshold lowered); *phenytoin* accelerates metabolism of *clozapine, quetiapine* and *sertindole* (reduced plasma concentrations)

  Antivirals: plasma concentration of *indinavir* possibly reduced; plasma-phenytoin concentrations increased or decreased by *zidovudine*

  Anxiolytics and Hypnotics: *diazepam* and possibly *other benzodiazepines* increase or decrease plasma-phenytoin concentration

- Calcium-channel Blockers: *diltiazem* and *nifedipine* increase plasma concentration of *phenytoin*; effect of *felodipine, isradipine* and probably *nicardipine, nifedipine* and *other dihydropyridines, diltiazem*, and *verapamil* reduced

  Cardiac Glycosides: metabolism of *digitoxin only* accelerated (reduced effect)

- Corticosteroids: metabolism of *corticosteroids* accelerated (reduced effect)

- Cyclosporin: metabolism of *cyclosporin* accelerated (reduced plasma concentration)

  Cytotoxics: reduced absorption of *phenytoin*; increased antifolate effect with *methotrexate*

- Disulfiram: plasma-phenytoin concentration increased

  Diuretics: increased risk of osteomalacia with *carbonic anhydrase inhibitors*

  Food: some *enteral foods* may interfere with absorption of *phenytoin*

  Hormone Antagonists: metabolism of *toremifene* possibly accelerated

  Lithium: neurotoxicity may occur without increased plasma-lithium concentration

  Muscle Relaxants: effect of *non-depolarising muscle relaxants* antagonised (recovery from neuromuscular blockade accelerated)

- Oestrogens and Progestogens: metabolism of *gestrinone, tibolone*, and *oral contraceptives* accelerated (reduced contraceptive effect, **important:** see p. 351)

  Sympathomimetics: plasma-phenytoin concentration increased by *methylphenidate*

  Theophylline: metabolism of *theophylline* accelerated (reduced plasma-theophylline concentration)

  Thyroxine: metabolism of *thyroxine* accelerated (may increase thyroxine requirements in hypothyroidism)

- Ulcer-healing Drugs: *cimetidine* inhibits metabolism (increased plasma-phenytoin concentration); *sucralfate* reduces absorption; *omeprazole* enhances effect of *phenytoin* (interaction with *lansoprazole* possibly differs)

- Uricosurics: plasma-phenytoin concentration increased by *sulphinpyrazone*

  Vaccines: effect enhanced by *influenza vaccine*

  Vitamins: plasma-phenytoin concentration occasionally reduced by *folic acid*; vitamin D requirements possibly increased

Physostigmine *see* Parasympathomimetics
Phytomenadione *see* Vitamins (Vitamin K)
Pilocarpine *see* Parasympathomimetics
Pimozide *see* Antipsychotics
Pindolol *see* Beta-blockers
Piperacillin *see* Penicillins
Pipothiazine *see* Antipsychotics
Piroxicam *see* NSAIDs
Pivampicillin *see* Penicillins
Pizotifen
  Antihypertensives: hypotensive effect of *adrenergic neurone blockers* antagonised
Polymyxins *see* Colistin
Polythiazide *see* Diuretics (thiazides)
Potassium Aminobenzoate
  Antibacterials: effect of *sulphonamides* inhibited
Potassium Salts (includes Salt Substitutes)
* ACE Inhibitors: increased risk of hyperkalaemia
* Cyclosporin: increased risk of hyperkalaemia
* Diuretics: hyperkalaemia with *potassium-sparing diuretics*
Pravastatin *see* Statins
Prazosin *see* Alpha-blockers (post-synaptic)
Prednisolone *see* Corticosteroids
Prednisone *see* Corticosteroids
Primaquine
  Mepacrine: increased plasma concentration of *primaquine* (risk of toxicity)
Primaxin®
* Antivirals: increased toxicity with *ganciclovir* (convulsions reported)
Primidone *see* Barbiturates and Primidone
Probenecid
  ACE Inhibitors: reduced excretion of *captopril*
* Analgesics: *aspirin* antagonises effect; excretion of *indomethacin, ketoprofen, ketorolac* (avoid concomitant use), and *naproxen* delayed and increased plasma-NSAID concentrations
  Antibacterials: reduced excretion of *cephalosporins, cinoxacin, ciprofloxacin, dapsone, nalidixic acid, nitrofurantoin, norfloxacin,* and *penicillins* (increased plasma-concentrations); antagonism by *pyrazinamide*
  Antivirals: reduced excretion of *aciclovir, ganciclovir, zidovudine,* and possibly *famciclovir* (increased plasma concentrations and risk of toxicity)
* Cytotoxics: reduced excretion of *methotrexate* (increased risk of toxicity)
Procainamide
  ACE Inhibitors: increased risk of toxicity with *captopril*, especially in renal impairment
* *other* Anti-arrhythmics: *amiodarone* increases procainamide-plasma concentrations (increased risk of ventricular arrhythmias—avoid concomitant use); increased myocardial depression with *any anti-arrhythmic*
  Antibacterials: *trimethoprim* increases plasma concentration of *procainamide*
* Antidepressants: increased risk of ventricular arrhythmias with *tricyclics*
* Antihistamines: increased risk of ventricular arrhythmias with *astemizole* and *terfenadine*
* Antimalarials: increased risk of ventricular arrhythmias with *halofantrine*
* Antipsychotics: increased risk of ventricular arrhythmias with *phenothiazines*
* Beta-blockers: increased risk of ventricular arrhythmias associated with *sotalol* (avoid concomitant use)
* Muscle Relaxants: muscle relaxant effect enhanced
  Parasympathomimetics: antagonism of effect of *neostigmine* and *pyridostigmine*
* Ulcer-healing Drugs: *cimetidine* inhibits excretion (increased plasma-procainamide concentration)
Procarbazine
  Alcohol: disulfiram-like reaction
Prochlorperazine *see* Antipsychotics

Procyclidine *see* Antimuscarinics
Progestogens (*see also* Contraceptives, Oral)
  Antibacterials: metabolism accelerated by *rifamycins* (reduced effect)
* Cyclosporin: increased plasma-cyclosporin concentration (inhibition of metabolism)
  Hormone Antagonists: *aminoglutethimide* reduces plasma concentration of *medroxyprogesterone*
Proguanil
* Anticoagulants: effect of *warfarin* possibly enhanced
Promazine *see* Antipsychotics
Promethazine *see* Antihistamines
Propafenone
  other Anti-arrhythmics: *quinidine* increases plasma concentration of *propafenone*; increased myocardial depression with any *anti-arrhythmic*
* Antibacterials: *rifampicin* reduces plasma concentration of *propafenone* (reduced effect)
* Anticoagulants: increased plasma concentration of *warfarin* and *nicoumalone* (enhanced effect)
* Antidepressants: increased risk of arrhythmias with *tricyclics*
* Antihistamines: increased risk of ventricular arrhythmias with *astemizole* and *terfenadine*
* Antivirals: see Ritonavir, p. 581
  Beta-blockers: increased plasma concentration of *metoprolol* and *propranolol*
* Cardiac Glycosides: increased plasma concentrations of *digoxin* (halve maintenance dose of digoxin)
  Cyclosporin: plasma-cyclosporin concentration possibly increased
  Parasympathomimetics: possible antagonism of effect of *neostigmine* and *pyridostigmine*
  Theophylline: increased plasma-theophylline concentration
* Ulcer-healing Drugs: *cimetidine* increases plasma-propafenone concentration
Propantheline *see* Antimuscarinics
Propofol *see* Anaesthetics, General
Propranolol *see* Beta-blockers
Prostaglandins
  Oxytocin: uterotonic effect enhanced
Proton Pump Inhibitors
  Note. There are currently no recognised drug interactions with pantoprazole
* Anticoagulants: effects of *warfarin* enhanced by *omeprazole*; interaction with *lansoprazole* possibly differs
* Antiepileptics: effects of *phenytoin* enhanced by *omeprazole*; interaction with *lansoprazole* possibly differs
  Antifungals: absorption of *ketoconazole* and possibly *itraconazole* reduced
  Anxiolytics and Hypnotics: metabolism of *diazepam* inhibited by *omeprazole* (increased effect possible)
  Cardiac Glycosides: plasma concentration of *digoxin* possibly increased
  Oestrogens and Progestogens: manufacturer advises that *lansoprazole* possibly accelerates metabolism of *oral contraceptives*
  Tacrolimus: *omeprazole* possibly increases plasma-tacrolimus concentration
Protriptyline *see* Antidepressants, Tricyclic
Pseudoephedrine *see* Sympathomimetics
Pyrazinamide
  Uricosurics: antagonism of effect of *probenecid and sulphinpyrazone*
Pyridostigmine *see* Parasympathomimetics
Pyridoxine *see* Vitamins
Pyrimethamine
* Antibacterials: increased antifolate effect with *co-trimoxazole* and *trimethoprim*
  Antiepileptics: increased antifolate effect with *phenytoin*
  Cytotoxics: increased antifolate effect with *methotrexate*

Quetiapine *see* Antipsychotics
Quinagolide
  Note. No interactions reported; theoretical possibility of reduced effect with dopamine antagonists (eg phenothiazines)
Quinalbarbitone *see* Barbiturates and Primidone
Quinapril *see* ACE Inhibitors
Quinidine
  Antacids: reduced excretion in alkaline urine (plasma-quinidine concentration occasionally increased)
• *other* Anti-arrhythmics: *amiodarone* increases plasma-quinidine concentrations (and increases risk of ventricular arrhythmias—avoid concomitant use); plasma concentration of *propafenone* increased; increased myocardial depression with *any anti-arrhythmic*
  Antibacterials: *rifamycins* accelerate metabolism (reduced plasma-quinidine concentration)
  Anticoagulants: effect of *nicoumalone* and *warfarin* may be enhanced
• Antidepressants: increased risk of ventricular arrhythmias with *tricyclics*
  Antiepileptics: *phenobarbitone, phenytoin,* and *primidone* accelerate metabolism (reduced plasma-quinidine concentration)
• Antihistamines: increased risk of ventricular arrhythmias with *astemizole* and *terfenadine*
• Antimalarials: increased risk of ventricular arrhythmias with *halofantrine* and *mefloquine*
• Antipsychotics: increased risk of ventricular arrhythmias with *phenothiazines*
  Antivirals: see Ritonavir, p. 581
  Barbiturates and Primidone: *see under* Antiepileptics, above
• Beta-blockers: increased risk of ventricular arrhythmias associated with *sotalol* (avoid concomitant use)
• Calcium-channel Blockers: *nifedipine* reduces plasma-quinidine concentration; *verapamil* increases plasma-quinidine concentration (possibility of extreme hypotension)
• Cardiac Glycosides: plasma concentration of *digoxin* increased (halve digoxin maintenance dose)
• Diuretics: *acetazolamide* reduces excretion (plasma-quinidine concentration occasionally increased); quinidine toxicity increased if hypokalaemia occurs with *acetazolamide, loop diuretics,* and *thiazides*
• Muscle Relaxants: muscle relaxant effect enhanced
  Parasympathomimetics: antagonism of effect of *neostigmine and pyridostigmine*
• Ulcer-healing Drugs: *cimetidine* inhibits metabolism (increased plasma-quinidine concentration)
Quinine
• Anti-arrhythmics: plasma concentration of *flecainide* increased; increased risk of ventricular arrhythmias with *amiodarone* (avoid concomitant use)
• Antihistamines: increased risk of ventricular arrhythmias with *astemizole* and *terfenadine*
• Antipsychotics: increased risk of ventricular arrhythmias—avoid concomitant use with *pimozide*
• *other* Antimalarials: *see* Halofantrine, Mefloquine
• Cardiac Glycosides: plasma concentration of *digoxin* increased (halve digoxin maintenance dose); includes use of *quinine* for cramps
  Ulcer-healing Drugs: *cimetidine* inhibits metabolism (increased plasma-quinine concentration)
4-Quinolones
  Analgesics: possible increased risk of convulsions with *NSAIDs*; manufacturer of *ciprofloxacin* advises avoid premedication with *opioid analgesics* (reduced plasma-ciprofloxacin concentration)
  Antacids and Adsorbents: *antacids* reduce absorption of *ciprofloxacin, norfloxacin* and *ofloxacin*
• Anticoagulants: anticoagulant effect of *nicoumalone* and *warfarin* enhanced by *ciprofloxacin, nalidixic acid, norfloxacin* and *ofloxacin*

4-Quinolones *(continued)*
  Antidiabetics: effect of *glibenclamide* possibly enhanced by *ciprofloxacin*
• Cyclosporin: increased risk of nephrotoxicity
  Cytotoxics: toxicity of *melphalan* increased by *nalidixic acid*
  Iron: absorption of *ciprofloxacin, norfloxacin,* and *ofloxacin* reduced by *oral iron*
• Theophylline: *ciprofloxacin* and *norfloxacin* increase plasma-theophylline concentration
  Ulcer-healing Drugs: *sucralfate* reduces absorption of *ciprofloxacin, norfloxacin,* and *ofloxacin*
  Uricosurics: *probenecid* reduces excretion of *cinoxacin, ciprofloxacin, nalidixic acid* and *norfloxacin*
  Zinc Salts: *zinc* reduces absorption of *ciprofloxacin* and *norfloxacin*
Rabies Vaccine *see* p. 528
Ramipril *see* ACE Inhibitors
Ranitidine *see* Histamine H$_2$-antagonists
Ranitidine Bismuth Citrate *see* Histamine H$_2$-antagonists
Reboxetine
  Note. Limited clinical data available, but manufacturers advise avoid concomitant administration with anti-arrhythmics, antipsychotics, cyclosporin, imidazole and triazole antifungals, fluvoxamine, macrolide antibiotics and tricyclic antidepressants
• *other* Antidepressants: risk of increased toxicity with *MAOIs* (reboxetine should not be started until 2 weeks after stopping MAOI, and conversely MAOI should not be started until at least 1 week after stopping reboxetine)
  Ergotamine: possibly increased blood pressure
Remifentanil *see* Opioid Analgesics
Reproterol *see* Sympathomimetics, Beta$_2$
Retinoids
  Alcohol: etretinate formed from *acitretin* in presence of *alcohol*
  Antibacterials: possible increased risk of benign intracranial hypertension with *tetracyclines* and *acitretin, isotretinoin* and *tretinoin*
• Anticoagulants: *acitretin* possibly reduces anticoagulant effect of *warfarin*
  Antiepileptics: plasma concentration of *carbamazepine* possibly reduced by *isotretinoin*
• Cytotoxics: *acitretin* increases plasma concentration of *methotrexate* (also increased risk of hepatotoxicity)
• Oestrogens and Progestogens: *tretinoin* reduces efficacy of *progesterone-only* and possibly *combined oral contraceptives*
  Vitamins: risk of hypervitaminosis A with *vitamin A* and *acitretin, isotretinoin* and *tretinoin*
Rifabutin *see* Rifamycins
Rifampicin *see* Rifamycins
Rifamycins
  Analgesics: metabolism of *methadone* accelerated (reduced effect)
  Antacids: reduced absorption of *rifampicin*
• Anti-arrhythmics: metabolism accelerated—reduced plasma concentrations of *disopyramide, mexiletine, propafenone, and quinidine*
• *other* Antibacterials: metabolism of *chloramphenicol* accelerated by *rifampicin* (reduced plasma concentration); plasma concentration of *dapsone* reduced; plasma concentration of *rifabutin* increased by *clarithromycin* and possibly *other macrolides* (risk of uveitis—reduce rifabutin dose)
• Anticoagulants: metabolism of *nicoumalone and warfarin* accelerated (reduced anticoagulant effect)
  Antidepressants: metabolism of some *tricyclics* accelerated by *rifampicin* (reduced plasma concentration)
• Antidiabetics: metabolism of *chlorpropamide, tolbutamide and possibly other sulphonylureas* accelerated (reduced effect)

Rifamycins *(continued)*

- Antiepileptics: metabolism of *carbamazepine* and *phenytoin* accelerated (reduced plasma concentration)
- Antifungals: metabolism of *fluconazole, itraconazole* and *ketoconazole* accelerated by *rifampicin* (reduced plasma concentrations); plasma concentration of *rifampicin* may be reduced by *ketoconazole*; plasma concentration of *terbinafine* reduced by *rifampicin*; plasma concentration of *rifabutin* increased by *fluconazole* and possibly *other triazoles* (risk of uveitis—reduce rifabutin dose)

  Antipsychotics: metabolism of *haloperidol* accelerated by *rifampicin* (reduced plasma concentration)

- Antivirals: concomitant administration of *indinavir* and *rifabutin* increases plasma-rifabutin concentration and decreases plasma-indinavir concentration (reduce dose of rifabutin and increase dose of indinavir); metabolism of *indinavir* enhanced by *rifampicin* (plasma-indinavir concentration significantly reduced—avoid concomitant use); plasma concentration of *rifabutin* increased by *ritonavir* (risk of uveitis—avoid concomitant use); plasma concentration of *saquinavir* reduced

  Anxiolytics and Hypnotics: metabolism of *diazepam* and possibly *other benzodiazepines* accelerated (reduced plasma concentration)

- Atovaquone: plasma concentration reduced by *rifampicin* (possible therapeutic failure of atovaquone)

  Beta-blockers: metabolism of *bisoprolol* and *propranolol* accelerated by *rifampicin* (plasma concentrations significantly reduced)

- Calcium-channel Blockers: metabolism of *diltiazem, nifedipine,* and *verapamil* and possibly *isradipine, nicardipine* and *nisoldipine* accelerated by *rifampicin* (plasma concentrations significantly reduced)

- Cardiac Glycosides: metabolism of *digitoxin only* accelerated (reduced effect)

- Corticosteroids: metabolism of *corticosteroids* accelerated (reduced effect)

- Cyclosporin: metabolism accelerated (reduced plasma-cyclosporin concentration)

- Cytotoxics: manufacturer reports interaction with *azathioprine* (transplants possibly rejected)

  Lipid-regulating Drugs: metabolism of *fluvastatin* accelerated (reduced effect)

- Oestrogens and Progestogens: metabolism accelerated (contraceptive effect of *both combined and progestogen-only oral contraceptives* reduced, **important:** see p. 351)

- Tacrolimus: *rifampicin* decreases plasma-tacrolimus concentration

  Theophylline: metabolism accelerated by *rifampicin* (reduced plasma-theophylline concentration)

  Thyroxine: metabolism of *thyroxine* accelerated by *rifampicin* (may increase requirements in hypothyroidism)

  Ulcer-healing Drugs: metabolism of *cimetidine* accelerated by *rifampicin* (reduced plasma concentration)

Riluzole

  Note. No clinical data available but since riluzole extensively metabolised by the liver, possibility of interactions with a number of drugs—consult product literature for details

Risperidone *see* Antipsychotics

Ritodrine *see* Sympathomimetics, Sympathomimetics, Beta$_2$, and p. 346

Ritonavir

- *Note.* Ritonavir is a potent inhibitor of several hepatic microsomal systems, therefore possibility of interactions with a number of drugs; manufacturer advises that concomitant use of some analgesics, anti-arrhythmics, anticoagulants, antidepressants, antiepileptics, antifungals, antihistamines, antipsychotics, anxiolytics and hypnotics, calcium-channel blockers, cisapride, and macrolide antibacterials requires monitoring or should be avoided—consult product literature for details

- Antibacterials: plasma concentration of *rifabutin* increased by *ritonavir* (risk of uveitis—avoid concomitant use)

- Antihistamines: increased risk of arrhythmias with *terfenadine*—avoid concomitant use

- Oestrogens and Progestogens: metabolism accelerated by *ritonavir* (contraceptive effect of combined oral contraceptives reduced)

- Theophylline: metabolism accelerated by *ritonavir* (reduced plasma-theophylline concentration)

Rocuronium *see* Muscle Relaxants (non-depolarising)

Ropinirole

  Note. Limited clinical data available, but possibility of interactions—consult product literature for details

Rowachol®

  Anticoagulants: effect of *nicoumalone and warfarin* possibly reduced

Salbutamol *see* Sympathomimetics, Beta$_2$

Salmeterol *see* Sympathomimetics, Beta$_2$

Salt Substitutes *see* Potassium Salts

Saquinavir

  Note. Limited clinical data available, but possibility of interactions with a number of drugs—consult product literature for details

- Antibacterials: metabolism accelerated by *rifamycins* (reduced plasma concentration)

- Antihistamines: increased risk of arrhythmias with *terfenadine*—avoid concomitant use

Selegiline

  Note. Selegiline is an MAO-B inhibitor

- Analgesics: hyperpyrexia and CNS toxicity with *pethidine*

- Antidepressants: hypertension and CNS excitation with *fluoxetine*; hypotension with *MAOIs*

Sermorelin

  Note. Avoid preparations which affect release of growth hormone, see p. 331

Sertindole *see* Antipsychotics

Sertraline *see* Antidepressants, SSRI

Sevoflurane *see* Anaesthetics, General (volatile liquid)

Simvastatin *see* Statins

Sodium Aurothiomalate *see* Gold

Sodium Bicarbonate *see* Antacids and Adsorbents

Sodium Clodronate *see* Bisphosphonates

Sodium Valproate *see* Valproate

Sotalol *see* Beta-blockers

Spectinomycin

- Botulinum Toxin: neuromuscular block enhanced (risk of toxicity)

  Lithium: increased toxicity reported

Spironolactone *see* Diuretics (potassium-sparing)

Stanozolol *see* Anabolic Steroids

Statins

  Antibacterials: metabolism of *fluvastatin* accelerated by *rifampicin* (reduced effect)

- Anticoagulants: effect of *nicoumalone* and *warfarin* enhanced by *simvastatin*

- Antifungals: *itraconazole* increases risk of myopathy with *simvastatin* (avoid concomitant use)

  Cardiac Glycosides: plasma-digoxin concentration possibly increased by *atorvastatin*

- Calcium-channel Blockers: *mibefradil* increases bioavailability of *simvastatin* and possibly *atorvastatin* and *cerivastatin* (increased risk of rhabdomyolysis—avoid concomitant use)

- Cyclosporin: increased risk of myopathy

Statins *(continued)*
- *other* Lipid-regulating Drugs: increased risk of myopathy with *clofibrate group* and *nicotinic acid*

Stavudine
Cytotoxics: *doxorubicin* may inhibit effect of *stavudine*

Streptomycin *see* Aminoglycosides

Sucralfate
Antibacterials: reduced absorption of *ciprofloxacin, norfloxacin, ofloxacin,* and *tetracycline*
- Anticoagulants: absorption of *warfarin* possibly reduced
- Antiepileptics: reduced absorption of *phenytoin*
Antifungals: reduced absorption of *ketoconazole*
Cardiac Glycosides: absorption of *cardiac glycosides* possibly reduced
Thyroxine: reduced absorption of *thyroxine*

Sulfadoxine *see* Co-trimoxazole and Sulphonamides

Sulfametopyrazine *see* Co-trimoxazole and Sulphonamides

Sulindac *see* NSAIDs

Sulphadiazine *see* Co-trimoxazole and Sulphonamides

Sulphadimidine *see* Co-trimoxazole and Sulphonamides

Sulphasalazine
Cardiac Glycosides: absorption of *digoxin* possibly reduced

Sulphinpyrazone
Analgesics: *aspirin* antagonises uricosuric effect
Antibacterials: *pyrazinamide* antagonises effect
- Anticoagulants: anticoagulant effect of *nicoumalone* and *warfarin* enhanced
- Antidiabetics: effect of *sulphonylureas* enhanced
- Antiepileptics: plasma concentration of *phenytoin* increased
Theophylline: plasma-theophylline concentration reduced

Sulphonamides *see* Co-trimoxazole and Sulphonamides

Sulphonylureas *see* Antidiabetics

Sulpiride *see* Antipsychotics

Sumatriptan *see* 5HT$_1$ Agonists

Suxamethonium *see* Muscle Relaxants

Sympathomimetics *(see below* for Beta$_2$-Sympathomimetics)
Alpha$_2$-adrenoceptor Stimulants: possible risk of hypertension with *adrenaline* and *noradrenaline*
- Anaesthetics: risk of arrhythmias if *adrenaline and isoprenaline* given with *volatile liquid anaesthetics* such as *halothane*
- Antidepressants: with *tricyclics* administration of *adrenaline* and *noradrenaline* may cause hypertension and arrhythmias (but local anaesthetics with adrenaline appear to be safe); *methylphenidate* may inhibit metabolism of *tricyclics*; with *MAOIs* administration of inotropics such as *dopamine* and *dopexamine* may cause hypertensive crisis; also with *MAOIs* administration of *dexamphetamine and other amphetamines, ephedrine, isometheptene, methylphenidate, phentermine, phenylephrine, phenylpropanolamine,* and *pseudoephedrine* may cause hypertensive crisis (these drugs are contained in anorectics or cold and cough remedies)
Antiepileptics: *methylphenidate* increases plasma concentration of *phenytoin* and possibly of *phenobarbitone* and *primidone*
- Antihypertensives: sympathomimetics in *anorectics* and *cold and cough remedies (see* above) and *methylphenidate* antagonise hypotensive effect of *adrenergic neurone blockers*
Barbiturates and Primidone: *see under* Antiepileptics, above

Sympathomimetics *(continued)*
- Beta-blockers: severe hypertension with *adrenaline* and *noradrenaline* and possibly with *dobutamine* (especially with non-selective beta-blockers); severe hypertension also possible with sympathomimetics in *anorectics and cold and cough remedies, see* above
Corticosteroids: *ephedrine* accelerates metabolism of *dexamethasone*
- Dopaminergics: increased risk of toxicity when *isometheptene* or *phenylpropanolamine* given with *bromocriptine*
Doxapram: risk of hypertension
Oxytocin: hypertension with *vasoconstrictor sympathomimetics*
- *other* Sympathomimetics: *dopexamine* possibly potentiates effect of *adrenaline* and *noradrenaline*

Sympathomimetics, Beta$_2$
Corticosteroids: increased risk of hypokalaemia if high doses of *corticosteroids* given with high doses of *bambuterol, eformoterol, fenoterol, reproterol, ritodrine, salbutamol, salmeterol, terbutaline* and *tulobuterol; see also* CSM advice, p. 126
Diuretics: increased risk of hypokalaemia if *acetazolamide, loop diuretics,* and *thiazides* given with high doses of *bambuterol, eformoterol, fenoterol, reproterol, ritodrine, salbutamol, salmeterol, terbutaline,* and *tulobuterol; see also* CSM advice, p. 126
Muscle Relaxants: effect of *suxamethonium* enhanced by *bambuterol*
Theophylline: increased risk of hypokalaemia if given with high doses of *bambuterol, eformoterol, fenoterol, reproterol, ritodrine, salbutamol, salmeterol, terbutaline,* and *tulobuterol; see also* CSM advice. p. 126

Tacrolimus
- Analgesics: *ibuprofen* increases risk of nephrotoxicity
- Antibacterials: *clarithromycin* and *erythromycin* increase plasma-tacrolimus concentration; *rifampicin* decreases plasma-tacrolimus concentration
- Antifungals: *amphotericin* increases risk of nephrotoxicity; *clotrimazole, fluconazole, ketoconazole* and possibly *other imidazoles* increase plasma-tacrolimus concentration
- Cyclosporin: plasma-cyclosporin half-life prolonged (increased risk of toxicity)
Hormone Antagonists: *danazol* possibly increases plasma-tacrolimus concentration
Oestrogens and Progestogens: efficacy of *oral contraceptives* possibly decreased
Ulcer-healing Drugs: *omeprazole* possibly increases plasma-tacrolimus concentration

Tamoxifen
- Anticoagulants: anticoagulant effect of *nicoumalone and warfarin* enhanced
other Hormone Antagonists: *aminoglutethimide* reduces plasma-tamoxifen concentration

Tamsulosin *see* Alpha-blockers (post-synaptic)

Temazepam *see* Anxiolytics and Hypnotics

Temocillin *see* Penicillins

Tenoxicam *see* NSAIDs

Terazosin *see* Alpha-blockers (post-synaptic)

Terbinafine
Antibacterials: plasma concentration reduced by *rifampicin*
Ulcer-healing Drugs: plasma concentration increased by *cimetidine*

Terbutaline *see* Sympathomimetics, Beta$_2$

Terfenadine *see* Antihistamines

Testosterone
- Anticoagulants: anticoagulant effect of *warfarin, nicoumalone* and *phenindione* enhanced
Antidiabetics: hypoglycaemic effect possibly enhanced

Tetrabenazine (general extrapyramidal interactions *as for* Antipsychotics)
* Antidepressants: CNS excitation and hypertension with *MAOIs*

Tetracyclines
ACE Inhibitors: *quinapril* reduces absorption (tablets contain magnesium carbonate excipient)
Antacids: reduced absorption
Anticoagulants: *see* Phenindione and Warfarin
Antiepileptics: *carbamazepine, phenobarbitone, phenytoin,* and *primidone* increase metabolism of *doxycycline* (reduced plasma concentration)
Atovaquone: plasma-atovaquone concentration reduced
Barbiturates and Primidone: *see under* Antiepileptics, above
Calcium Salts: reduced absorption of *tetracyclines*
* Cyclosporin: *doxycycline* possibly increases plasma-cyclosporin concentration
Dairy products: reduced absorption (except *doxycycline* and *minocycline*)
Iron: absorption of *oral iron* reduced by *tetracyclines* and *vice versa*
Oestrogens and Progestogens: *see* Contraceptives, Oral (main list)
Retinoids: possible increased risk of benign intracranial hypertension with *tetracyclines* and *acitretin, isotretinoin* and *tretinoin*
Ulcer-healing Drugs: *tripotassium dicitrato-bismuthate* and *sucralfate* reduce absorption
Zinc Salts: reduced absorption (and *vice versa*)

Theophylline
Anaesthetics: increased risk of arrhythmias with *halothane*
Anthelmintics: *thiabendazole* may increase plasma-theophylline concentration
Anti-arrhythmics: antagonism of anti-arrhythmic effect of *adenosine*; plasma-theophylline concentration increased by *mexiletine* and *propafenone*; plasma-theophylline concentration reduced by *moracizine*
* Antibacterials: plasma-theophylline concentration increased by *ciprofloxacin, clarithromycin, erythromycin* (if erythromycin given by mouth, also decreased plasma-erythromycin concentration), and *norfloxacin* and possibly increased by *isoniazid*; plasma-theophylline concentration reduced by *rifampicin*
* Antidepressants: plasma-theophylline concentration increased by *fluvoxamine* (concomitant use should usually be avoided, but where not possible halve theophylline dose and monitor plasma-theophylline concentration) and *viloxazine*
Antiepileptics: plasma-theophylline concentration reduced by *carbamazepine, phenobarbitone, phenytoin,* and *primidone*
* Antifungals: plasma-theophylline concentration possibly increased by *fluconazole*
* Antivirals: plasma-theophylline concentration reduced by *ritonavir*
Barbiturates and Primidone: *see under* Antiepileptics, above
Beta-blockers: should be avoided on pharmacological grounds (bronchospasm)
* Calcium-channel Blockers: plasma-theophylline concentration increased by *diltiazem, verapamil,* and possibly *other calcium-channel blockers*
Disulfiram: increases plasma-theophylline concentration
Doxapram: increased CNS stimulation
Hormone Antagonists: plasma-theophylline concentration reduced by *aminoglutethimide*
Interferons: plasma-theophylline concentration increased by *interferon alfa*
Lithium: *lithium* excretion accelerated (reduced plasma-lithium concentration)

Theophylline *(continued)*
Nicotine and Tobacco: plasma-theophylline concentration reduced by *tobacco smoking*
Oestrogens and Progestogens: plasma-theophylline concentration increased by *combined oral contraceptives*
Sympathomimetics: increased risk of hypokalaemia if *theophylline* given with high doses of *bambuterol, eformoterol, fenoterol, reproterol, ritodrine, salbutamol, salmeterol, terbutaline,* and *tulobuterol; see also* CSM advice, p. 126
* Ulcer-healing Drugs: plasma-theophylline concentration increased by *cimetidine*
Uricosurics: plasma-theophylline concentration reduced by *sulphinpyrazone*
Vaccines: plasma-theophylline concentration occasionally increased by *influenza vaccine*

Thiabendazole
Theophylline: plasma concentration may be increased

Thiopentone *see* Anaesthetics, General
Thioridazine *see* Antipsychotics
Thiotepa
Muscle Relaxants: effect of *suxamethonium* enhanced

Thymoxamine
* Alpha-blockers: possible severe postural hypotension
other Antihypertensives: enhanced hypotensive effect
* Beta-blockers: possible severe postural hypotension

Thyroxine
Analgesics: false low total plasma-thyroxine concentration with *phenylbutazone*
Anion exchange Resins: *cholestyramine* reduces absorption of *thyroxine*
Anti-arrhythmics: for use with *amiodarone*, see p. 69
Antibacterials: *rifampicin* accelerates metabolism of thyroxine (may increase requirements in hypothyroidism)
* Anticoagulants: effect of *nicoumalone, phenindione,* and *warfarin* enhanced
Antidepressants: manufacturer of *lofepramine* advises avoid *thyroxine*
Antiepileptics: *carbamazepine, phenobarbitone, phenytoin,* and *primidone* accelerate metabolism of *thyroxine* (may increase requirements in hypothyroidism)
Barbiturates and Primidone: *see under* Antiepileptics, above
Beta-blockers: metabolism of *propranolol* accelerated (reduced effect)
Ulcer-healing Drugs: *sucralfate* reduces absorption of *thyroxine*

Tiaprofenic Acid *see* NSAIDs
Tibolone
Antibacterials: *rifampicin* accelerates metabolism (reduced plasma concentration)
Antiepileptics: *carbamazepine, phenobarbitone, phenytoin,* and *primidone* accelerate metabolism (reduced plasma concentration)
Barbiturates and Primidone: *see* Antiepileptics, above

Tiludronic Acid *see* Bisphosphonates
Timentin® *see* Penicillins
Timolol *see* Beta-blockers
Tinidazole
Alcohol: disulfiram-like reaction

Tinzaparin *see* Heparin
Tobramycin *see* Aminoglycosides
Tolazamide *see* Antidiabetics (sulphonylurea)
Tolbutamide *see* Antidiabetics (sulphonylurea)
Tolcapone
Antidepressants: manufacturer advises avoid concomitant use with *MAOIs*

Tolfenamic Acid *see* NSAIDs

Topiramate
- *other* Antiepileptics: concomitant administration of *two or more antiepileptics* may enhance toxicity without a corresponding increase in antiepileptic effect; moreover, interactions between individual antiepileptics can complicate monitoring of treatment; interactions include enhanced effects, increased sedation, and reductions in plasma concentrations; for further details, see p. 210

Oestrogens and Progestogens: metabolism of *oral contraceptives* accelerated (reduced contraceptive effect, **important:** see p. 351)

Torasemide *see* Diuretics (loop)

Toremifene
- Anticoagulants: anticoagulant effect of *nicoumalone* and *warfarin* possibly enhanced

Antiepileptics: metabolism possibly accelerated by *carbamazepine, phenobarbitone* and *phenytoin* (reduced plasma-toremifene concentration)

Diuretics: increased risk of hypercalcaemia with *thiazides*

Tramadol *see* Opioid Analgesics

Trandolapril *see* ACE Inhibitors

Tranylcypromine *see* MAOIs

Trazodone
Alcohol: enhanced sedative effect
- other Antidepressants: as for Antidepressants, Tricyclic
- Antiepileptics: antagonism of anticonvulsant effect

Anxiolytics and Hypnotics: enhanced sedative effect

Triamcinolone *see* Corticosteroids

Triamterene *see* Diuretics (potassium-sparing)

Triclofos *see* Anxiolytics and Hypnotics

Trientine
Iron: absorption of *oral iron* reduced

Trifluoperazine *see* Antipsychotics

Trilostane
Diuretics: increased risk of hyperkalaemia with *potassium-sparing diuretics*

Trimeprazine *see* Antihistamines

Trimethoprim
Anti-arrhythmics: plasma concentration of *procainamide* increased

Anticoagulants: effect of *nicoumalone* and *warfarin* possibly enhanced

Antiepileptics: plasma concentration and antifolate effect of *phenytoin* increased
- Antimalarials: increased risk of antifolate effect with *pyrimethamine* (in *Fansidar®* and *Maloprim®*)

Antivirals: plasma concentration of *lamivudine* increased
- Cyclosporin: increased risk of nephrotoxicity; plasma-cyclosporin concentration possibly reduced by *intravenous trimethoprim*

Cytotoxics: antifolate effect of *methotrexate* increased

Trimetrexate
Note. Limited clinical data, but potential for serious interactions—consult product literature for details

Trimipramine *see* Antidepressants, Tricyclic

Tripotassium Dicitratobismuthate
Antibacterials: reduced absorption of *tetracyclines*

Triprolidine *see* Antihistamines

Tropicamide *see* Antimuscarinics

Tryptophan
- *other* Antidepressants: CNS excitation and confusion with *MAOIs* (reduce tryptophan dose); agitation and nausea with *fluoxetine, fluvoxamine, paroxetine, and sertraline*

Tulobuterol *see* Sympathomimetics, Beta$_2$

Typhoid Vaccine *see* p. 529

Ulcer-healing Drugs *see* individual drugs

Uricosurics *see* individual drugs

Ursodeoxycholic Acid *see* Bile Acids

Vaccines *see* Influenza Vaccine (p. 572), Rabies Vaccine (p. 528), Typhoid Vaccine (p. 529)
Note. For a general warning on *live vaccines* and *high doses of corticosteroids* or *other immunosuppressive drugs,* see section 14.1; for advice on *live vaccines* and *immunoglobulins,* see under Normal Immunoglobulin, section 14.5

Valaciclovir *see* Aciclovir and Famciclovir
Note. Interactions as for aciclovir

Valproate
Analgesics: *aspirin* enhances effect

Anion-exchange Resins: *cholestyramine* possibly reduces absorption

Anticoagulants: anticoagulant effect of *nicoumalone* and *warfarin* possibly increased
- Antidepressants: antagonism of anticonvulsant effect (convulsive threshold lowered)
- *other* Antiepileptics: concomitant administration of *two or more antiepileptics* may enhance antiepileptic effect; moreover, interactions between individual antiepileptics can complicate monitoring of treatment; interactions include enhanced effects, increased sedation, and reductions in plasma concentrations; for further details, see p. 210
- Antimalarials: *chloroquine* and *mefloquine* antagonise anticonvulsant effect
- Antipsychotics: antagonism of anticonvulsant effect (convulsive threshold lowered)

Ulcer-healing Drugs: *cimetidine* inhibits metabolism (increased plasma-valproate concentration)

Valsartan as for ACE Inhibitors

Vancomycin
Anaesthetics: hypersensitivity-like reactions can occur with concomitant vancomycin infusion

Anion-exchange Resins: antagonism of *oral vancomycin* by *cholestyramine*
other Antibacterials: increased risk of ototoxicity and nephrotoxicity with *aminoglycosides and capreomycin*

Diuretics: increased risk of ototoxicity with *loop diuretics*

Vecuronium *see* Muscle Relaxants (non-depolarising)

Venlafaxine
- *other* Antidepressants: CNS effects of *MAOIs* increased (risk of toxicity); *venlafaxine* should not be started until 2 weeks after stopping *MAOI;* conversely, *MAOI* should not be started until at least 1 week after stopping *venlafaxine*

Verapamil *see* Calcium-channel Blockers

Vigabatrin
- *other* Antiepileptics: concomitant administration of *two or more antiepileptics* may enhance toxicity without a corresponding increase in antiepileptic effect; moreover, interactions between individual antiepileptics can complicate monitoring of treatment; interactions include enhanced effects, increased sedation, and reductions in plasma concentrations; for further details, see p. 210

Viloxazine
- *other* Antidepressants: as for Antidepressants, Tricyclic
- Antiepileptics: increased plasma concentrations of *carbamazepine* and *phenytoin*

Theophylline: increased plasma-theophylline concentration

Vincristine
Antifungals: *itraconazole* may inhibit metabolism (increased risk of neurotoxicity)

Vitamins
- Altretamine: *pyridoxine* reduces response to *altretamine*
- Anticoagulants: anticoagulant effect of *nicoumalone, phenindione, and warfarin* antagonised by *vitamin K* (present in some enteral feeds)

Vitamins *(continued)*

Antiepileptics: *folic acid* occasionally reduces plasma-phenytoin concentration; *vitamin D* requirements possibly increased by *carbamazepine, phenobarbitone, phenytoin,* and *primidone*

Barbiturates and Primidone: *see* Antiepileptics, above

Diuretics: increased risk of hypercalcaemia if *thiazides* given with *vitamin D*

Dopaminergics: effect of *levodopa* antagonised by *pyridoxine* (unless a dopa decarboxylase inhibitor also given)

<u>Retinoids</u>: risk of hypervitaminosis A with *vitamin A* and *acitretin, isotretinoin* and *tretinoin*

Warfarin and other Coumarins

Note. Change in patient's clinical condition, particularly associated with liver disease, intercurrent illness, or drug administration, necessitates more frequent testing. Major changes in diet (especially involving salads and vegetables) and in alcohol consumption may also affect warfarin control

- Alcohol: enhanced anticoagulant effect with large amounts (see also above)

Allopurinol: anticoagulant effect possibly enhanced

- Anabolic Steroids: *oxymetholone, stanozolol and others* enhance anticoagulant effect
- Analgesics: *aspirin* increases risk of bleeding due to antiplatelet effect; anticoagulant effect seriously enhanced by *azapropazone* and *phenylbutazone* (avoid concomitant use), and possibly enhanced by *diclofenac, diflunisal, flurbiprofen, mefenamic acid, piroxicam, sulindac, and other NSAIDs*; anticoagulant effect possibly also enhanced by *dextropropoxyphene* and by prolonged regular use of *paracetamol*; increased risk of haemorrhage with *parenteral diclofenac* and *ketorolac* (avoid concomitant use)
- Anion-exchange Resins: *cholestyramine* may enhance or reduce anticoagulant effect
- Anti-arrhythmics: *amiodarone and propafenone* enhance anticoagulant effect; *quinidine* may enhance anticoagulant effect
- Antibacterials: anticoagulant effect reduced by *rifamycins*; anticoagulant effect enhanced by *cephamandole, chloramphenicol, ciprofloxacin, co-trimoxazole, erythromycin, metronidazole, ofloxacin,* and *sulphonamides*; anticoagulant effect possibly also enhanced by *aztreonam, clarithromycin* and some *other macrolides, nalidixic acid, neomycin, norfloxacin, tetracyclines,* and *trimethoprim*; although studies have failed to demonstrate interaction, common experience in anticoagulant clinics is that INR can be altered following course of oral *broad-spectrum antibiotic, such as ampicillin* (may also apply to antibiotics given for local action on gut such as *neomycin*)
- Antidepressants: *SSRIs* possibly enhance anticoagulant effect

<u>Antidiabetics</u>: possibly enhanced hypoglycaemic effects of *sulphonylureas* and changes to anticoagulant effect

- Antiepileptics: reduced anticoagulant effect with *carbamazepine, phenobarbitone, and primidone*; anticoagulant effect possibly increased by *valproate*; both reduced and enhanced effects reported with *phenytoin*
- Antifungals: anticoagulant effect reduced by *griseofulvin;* anticoagulant effect enhanced by *fluconazole, itraconazole, ketoconazole, and miconazole* (note: oral gel absorbed)
- Antimalarials: anticoagulant effect possibly enhanced by *proguanil*
- Antiplatelet Drugs: *aspirin and dipyridamole* increase risk of bleeding due to antiplatelet effect
- Antivirals: see Ritonavir, p. 581

Warfarin and other Coumarins *(continued)*

Anxiolytics and Hypnotics: *chloral* and *triclofos* may transiently enhance anticoagulant effect

- Barbiturates and Primidone: anticoagulant effect reduced

Cisapride: effect of *oral anticoagulants* possibly enhanced

- Cytotoxics: anticoagulant effect possibly enhanced by *ifosfamide*
- Disulfiram: enhanced anticoagulant effect
- Hormone Antagonists: *aminoglutethimide* reduces anticoagulant effect; *danazol, flutamide, tamoxifen* and possibly *bicalutamide* and *toremifene* enhance anticoagulant effect
- Lipid-regulating Drugs: *clofibrate group* and *simvastatin* enhance anticoagulant effect
- Oestrogens and Progestogens: *oral contraceptives* reduce anticoagulant effect
- Retinoids: *acitretin* possibly reduces anticoagulant effect

Rowachol®: possibly reduced anticoagulant effect

- Testosterone: anticoagulant effect of *warfarin* and *nicoumalone* enhanced
- Thyroxine: enhanced anticoagulant effect
- Ulcer-healing Drugs: *sucralfate* possibly reduces anticoagulant effect (reduced absorption); *cimetidine and omeprazole* enhance anticoagulant effect
- Uricosurics: *sulphinpyrazone* enhances anticoagulant effect

Vaccines: *influenza vaccine* occasionally enhances anticoagulant effect

- Vitamins: *vitamin K* reduces anticoagulant effect; major changes in diet (especially involving vegetables) may affect control; *vitamin K* also present in some enteral feeds

Xamoterol

Beta-blockers: antagonism of effect of *xamoterol* and reduction in beta-blockade

Xipamide *see* Diuretics (thiazide-related)

Xylometazoline *see* Sympathomimetics

Zalcitabine

Note. Clinical data limited. Avoid use with other drugs which have potential to cause peripheral neuropathy—for further details consult product literature

Zidovudine

Note. Increased risk of toxicity with nephrotoxic and myelosuppressive drugs—for further details consult product literature

Analgesics: *methadone* possibly increases plasma-zidovudine concentration

Antibacterials: *clarithromycin tablets* reduce absorption of *zidovudine*

Antiepileptics: plasma-phenytoin concentrations increased or decreased

Antifungals: plasma concentration of *zidovudine* increased by *fluconazole* (increased risk of toxicity)

- *other* Antivirals: extreme lethargy reported on administration of *intravenous aciclovir*; profound myelosuppression with *ganciclovir* (see also p. 280)

Uricosurics: *probenecid* increases plasma-zidovudine concentration and risk of toxicity

Zinc

Antibacterials: reduced absorption of *ciprofloxacin* and *norfloxacin; tetracyclines* reduce absorption of *zinc* (and *vice versa*)

Iron: reduced absorption of *oral iron* (and *vice versa*)

Penicillamine: reduced absorption of *penicillamine*

Zolmitriptan *see* 5HT$_1$ Agonists

Zolpidem *see* Anxiolytics and Hypnotics

Zopiclone *see* Anxiolytics and Hypnotics

Zuclopenthixol *see* Antipsychotics

Appendix 2: Liver Disease

Liver disease may alter the response to drugs in several ways as indicated below, and drug prescribing should be kept to a minimum in all patients with severe liver disease. The main problems occur in patients with jaundice, ascites, or evidence of encephalopathy.

IMPAIRED DRUG METABOLISM. Metabolism by the liver is the main route of elimination for many drugs, but the hepatic reserve appears to be large and liver disease has to be severe before important changes in drug metabolism occur. Routine liver-function tests are a poor guide to the capacity of the liver to metabolise drugs, and in the individual patient it is not possible to predict the extent to which the metabolism of a particular drug may be impaired.

A few drugs, e.g. rifampicin and fusidic acid, are excreted in the bile unchanged and may accumulate in patients with intrahepatic or extrahepatic obstructive jaundice.

HYPOPROTEINAEMIA. The hypoalbuminaemia in severe liver disease is associated with reduced protein binding and increased toxicity of some highly protein-bound drugs such as phenytoin and prednisolone.

REDUCED CLOTTING. Reduced hepatic synthesis of blood-clotting factors, indicated by a prolonged prothrombin time, increases the sensitivity to oral anticoagulants such as warfarin and phenindione.

HEPATIC ENCEPHALOPATHY. In severe liver disease many drugs can further impair cerebral function and may precipitate hepatic encephalopathy. These include all sedative drugs, opioid analgesics, those diuretics that produce hypokalaemia, and drugs that cause constipation.

FLUID OVERLOAD. Oedema and ascites in chronic liver disease may be exacerbated by drugs that give rise to fluid retention, e.g. NSAIDs, corticosteroids, and carbenoxolone.

HEPATOTOXIC DRUGS. Hepatotoxicity is either dose-related or unpredictable (idiosyncratic). Drugs causing dose-related toxicity may do so at lower doses than in patients with normal liver function, and some drugs producing reactions of the idiosyncratic kind do so more frequently in patients with liver disease. These drugs should be avoided.

Table of drugs to be avoided or used with caution in liver disease

The list of drugs given below is not comprehensive and is based on current information concerning the use of these drugs in therapeutic dosage. Products introduced or amended since publication of BNF No. 34 (September 1997) are underlined.

Drug	Comment	Drug	Comment
Acamprosate	Avoid in severe liver disease	Anastrozole	Avoid in moderate to severe liver disease
Acarbose	Avoid	Androgens	Preferably avoid— dose-related toxicity with some, and produce fluid retention
ACE Inhibitors	Use of prodrugs such as cilazapril, enalapril, fosinopril, moexipril, perindopril, quinapril, ramipril, and trandolapril requires close monitoring in patients with impaired liver function		
		Antacids	In patients with fluid retention, avoid those containing large amounts of sodium, e.g. magnesium trisilicate mixture, Gaviscon®
Aceclofenac see NSAIDs			
Acemetacin see NSAIDs			Avoid those causing constipation—can precipitate coma
Acitretin	Avoid—further impairment of liver function may occur		
Acrivastine see Antihistamines		Anticoagulants, Oral	Avoid, especially if prothrombin time is already prolonged
Alfentanil see Opioid Analgesics			
Alfuzosin	Reduce dose in mild to moderate liver disease; avoid if severe	Antidepressants, MAOI see MAOIs	
		Antidepressants, SSRI	Reduce dose or avoid in severe liver disease
Alprazolam see Anxiolytics and Hypnotics		Antidepressants, Tricyclic (and related)	Tricyclics preferable to MAOIs but sedative effects increased (avoid in severe liver disease)
Altretamine	Rare reports of hepatotoxicity		
Amifostine	Manufacturer advises avoid		
Aminophylline see Theophylline			
Amitriptyline see Antidepressants, Tricyclic			
Amlodipine	Half-life prolonged—may need dose reduction	Antihistamines	Avoid—may precipitate coma; astemizole and terfenadine, see also pp. 142 and 143
Amoxapine see Antidepressants, Tricyclic			
Anabolic Steroids	Preferably avoid—dose-related toxicity		
Analgesics see Aspirin, NSAIDs, Opioid Analgesics and Paracetamol			

Table of drugs to be avoided or used with caution in liver disease (*continued*)

Drug	Comment	Drug	Comment
Antipsychotics	All can precipitate coma; phenothiazines are hepatotoxic; see also Clozapine, Olanzapine, Quetiapine, Risperidone and Sertindole	Chlorpromazine *see* Antipsychotics	
		Chlorpropamide *see* Sulphonylureas	
		Chlortetracycline *see* Tetracyclines	
		Chlorthalidone *see* Thiazides	
Anxiolytics and Hypnotics	All can precipitate coma; small dose of oxazepam or temazepam probably safest; reduce oral dose of chlormethiazole; reduce dose of zopiclone (avoid if severe)	Cholestyramine	Interferes with absorption of fat-soluble vitamins and may aggravate malabsorption in primary biliary cirrhosis; likely to be ineffective in complete biliary obstruction
Aspirin	Avoid—increased risk of gastro-intestinal bleeding	Cidofovir	No information—manufacturer advises caution
Astemizole *see* Antihistamines		Cilazapril *see* ACE Inhibitors	
Atorvastatin *see* Statins		Cimetidine	Increased risk of confusion; reduce dose
Atovaquone	Manufacturer advises caution—monitor more closely	Cinnarizine *see* Antihistamines	
Auranofin *see* Gold		Cinoxacin *see* 4-Quinolones	
Aurothiomalate *see* Gold		Ciprofibrate	Avoid in severe liver disease
Azapropazone *see* NSAIDs		Ciprofloxacin *see* 4-Quinolones	
Azatadine *see* Antihistamines		Cisapride	Halve dose initially
Azathioprine	May need dose reduction	Citalopram	Use doses at lower end of range
Azithromycin	Avoid; jaundice reported	Clarithromycin	Hepatic dysfunction including jaundice reported
Bambuterol	Avoid in severe liver disease	Clavulanic Acid [ingredient] *see* Co-amoxiclav and *Timentin*®	
Bendrofluazide *see* Thiazides			
Benorylate [aspirin-paracetamol ester] *see* Aspirin		Clemastine *see* Antihistamines	
Benperidol *see* Antipsychotics		Clindamycin	Reduce dose
Bezafibrate	Avoid in severe liver disease	Clobazam *see* Anxiolytics and Hypnotics	
Bicalutamide	Increased accumulation possible in moderate to severe impairment	Clofibrate	Avoid in severe liver disease
		Clomiphene	Avoid in severe liver disease
Bromazepam *see* Anxiolytics and Hypnotics		Clomipramine *see* Antidepressants, Tricyclic	
Brompheniramine *see* Antihistamines		Clopamide *see* Thiazides	
Buclizine *see* Antihistamines		Clorazepate *see* Anxiolytics and Hypnotics	
Bumetanide *see* Loop Diuretics		Clozapine	Initial dose 12.5 mg daily increased slowly with regular monitoring of liver function; avoid in symptomatic or progressive liver disease or liver failure
Bupivacaine *see* Lignocaine			
Buprenorphine *see* Opioid Analgesics			
Cabergoline	Reduce dose or avoid in liver disease		
Candesartan	Halve initial dose in mild or moderate disease; avoid if severe	Co-amoxiclav	Monitor liver function in liver disease. Cholestatic jaundice, see p. 241
		Codeine *see* Opioid Analgesics	
Carbamazepine	Metabolism impaired in advanced liver disease. For advice on counselling for all patients, see p. 211	Contraceptives, Oral	Avoid in active liver disease and if history of pruritus or cholestasis during pregnancy
		Cyclizine *see* Antihistamines	
Carbenoxolone	Produces sodium and water retention and hypokalaemia	Cyclofenil	Avoid in severe liver disease
		Cyclopenthiazide *see* Thiazides	
Carvedilol	Avoid	Cyclosporin	May need dose adjustment
Ceftriaxone	Reduce dose and monitor plasma concentration if both hepatic and severe renal impairment	Cyproheptadine *see* Antihistamines	
		Cyproterone Acetate	Dose-related toxicity; *see also* CSM advice on p. 388
Cerivastatin *see* Statins		Dalteparin *see* Heparin	
Certoparin *see* Heparin		Danaparoid *see* Heparin	
Cetirizine *see* Antihistamines		Dantrolene	Avoid—may cause severe liver damage
Chenodeoxycholic Acid	Avoid in chronic liver disease; patients with non-functioning gall-bladder do not respond	Debrisoquine	May need dose reduction
		Demeclocycline *see* Tetracyclines	
Chloral Hydrate *see* Anxiolytics and Hypnotics		Desflurane	Reduce dose
Chloramphenicol	Avoid—increased risk of bone-marrow depression	Desogestrel *see* Progestogens	
		Dexfenfluramine	Manufacturer advises avoid
Chlordiazepoxide *see* Anxiolytics and Hypnotics		Dextromethorphan *see* Opioid Analgesics	
Chlormethiazole *see* Anxiolytics and Hypnotics		Dextromoramide *see* Opioid Analgesics	
Chlorothiazide *see* Thiazides		Dextropropoxyphene *see* Opioid Analgesics	
Chlorpheniramine *see* Antihistamines		Diamorphine *see* Opioid Analgesics	

Table of drugs to be avoided or used with caution in liver disease (*continued*)

Drug	Comment	Drug	Comment
Diazepam *see* Anxiolytics and Hypnotics		Fosinopril *see* ACE Inhibitors	
Diclofenac *see* NSAIDs		Frusemide *see* Loop Diuretics	
Didanosine	Reduce initial dose	Fusidic Acid	Impaired biliary excretion; may be increased risk of hepato-toxicity; avoid or reduce dose
Diflunisal *see* NSAIDs			
Dihydrocodeine *see* Opioid Analgesics			
Diltiazem	Reduce dose	Gemcitabine	Monitor liver function
Dimenhydrinate *see* Antihistamines		Gemfibrozil	Avoid in liver disease
Diphenoxylate *see* Opioid Analgesics		Gestodene *see* Progestogens	
Diphenylpyraline *see* Antihistamines		Gestrinone	Avoid in severe liver disease
Dipipanone *see* Opioid Analgesics		Gestronol *see* Progestogens	
Disopyramide	Half-life prolonged—may need dose reduction	Glibenclamide *see* Sulphonylureas	
		Gliclazide *see* Sulphonylureas	
Docetaxel	Monitor liver function—reduce dose according to liver enzymes	Glimepiride	Manufacturer advises avoid in severe liver impairment
		Glipizide *see* Sulphonylureas	
Dothiepin *see* Antidepressants, Tricyclic		Gliquidone *see* Sulphonylureas	
Doxazosin	No information—manufacturer advises caution	Gold (auranofin, aurothiomalate)	Avoid in severe liver disease—hepatotoxicity may occur
Doxepin *see* Antidepressants, Tricyclic		Haloperidol *see* Antipsychotics	
Doxorubicin	Reduce dose according to bilirubin concentration	Halothane *see* p. 538	
		Heparin	Reduce dose in severe disease
Doxycycline *see* Tetracyclines		Hydrochlorothiazide *see* Thiazides	
Doxylamine *see* Antihistamines		Hydroflumethiazide *see* Thiazides	
Droperidol *see* Antipsychotics		Hydromorphone *see* Opioid Analgesics	
Dydrogesterone *see* Progestogens		Hydroxyprogesterone Hexanoate *see* Progestogens	
Eformoterol	Metabolism possibly reduced in severe cirrhosis	Hydroxyzine *see* Antihistamines	
		Hypnotics *see* Anxiolytics and Hypnotics	
Enalapril *see* ACE Inhibitors		Ibuprofen *see* NSAIDs	
Enoxaparin *see* Heparin		Idarubicin	Reduce dose according to bilirubin concentration
Epirubicin	Reduce dose according to bilirubin concentration		
		Imipramine *see* Antidepressants, Tricyclic	
Epoetin	Manufacurers advise caution in chronic liver failure	Indapamide *see* Thiazides	
		Indinavir	Reduce dose to 600 mg every 8 hours in mild to moderate impairment; not studied in severe impairment
Ergometrine	Avoid in severe liver disease		
Ergotamine	Avoid in severe liver disease—risk of toxicity increased		
		Indomethacin *see* NSAIDs	
Erythromycin	May cause idiosyncratic hepatotoxicity	Interferon alfa	Close monitoring in mild to moderate impairment; avoid if severe
Estropipate *see* Oestrogens			
Ethacrynic Acid *see* Loop Diuretics		Interferon beta	Avoid in decompensated liver disease
Ethinyloestradiol *see* Oestrogens			
Ethynodiol Diacetate *see* Progestogens		Irinotecan	Monitor closely or avoid according to bilirubin concentration
Etodolac *see* NSAIDs			
Famciclovir	Usual dose in well compensated liver disease (information not available on decompensated)	Isocarboxazid *see* MAOIs	
		Isoniazid	Avoid if possible—idiosyncratic hepatotoxicity more common; *see also* p. 263
Felodipine	Reduce dose	Isotretinoin	Avoid—further impairment of liver function may occur
Fenbufen *see* NSAIDs			
Fenofibrate *see* Clofibrate		Isradipine	Reduce dose
Fenoprofen *see* NSAIDs		Itraconazole	Half-life prolonged—plasma concentration monitoring advised
Fentanyl *see* Opioid Analgesics			
Fexofenadine *see* Antihistamines			
Flecainide	Avoid (or reduce dose) in severe liver disease	Ketoconazole	Induces hepatitis-like reaction; may accumulate in severe liver disease; contra-indicated unless no alternative; *see also* p. 270
Flucloxacillin	Cholestatic jaundice, see p. 239		
Fluconazole	Toxicity with related drugs		
Flunitrazepam *see* Anxiolytics and Hypnotics			
Fluoxetine *see* Antidepressants, SSRI		Ketoprofen *see* NSAIDs	
Flupenthixol *see* Antipsychotics		Ketorolac *see* NSAIDs	
Fluphenazine *see* Antipsychotics		Ketotifen *see* Antihistamines	
Flurazepam *see* Anxiolytics and Hypnotics		Labetalol	Avoid—severe hepatocellular injury reported
Flurbiprofen *see* NSAIDs			
Fluvastatin *see* Statins			
Fluvoxamine *see* Antidepressants, SSRI			
Fosfestrol *see* Oestrogens			

Table of drugs to be avoided or used with caution in liver disease (*continued*)

Drug	Comment	Drug	Comment
Lacidipine	Antihypertensive effect possibly increased	Mivacurium	Reduce dose
Lamotrigine	Manufacturer advises avoid	Moclobemide	Reduce dose in severe liver disease
Lansoprazole	In severe liver disease dose should not exceed 30 mg daily	Moexipril *see* ACE Inhibitors	
Levonorgestrel *see* Progestogens		Monoamine-oxidase Inhibitors *see* MAOIs	
Lignocaine	Avoid (or reduce dose) in severe liver disease	Morphine *see* Opioid Analgesics	
		Moxonidine	Avoid in severe liver disease
Lofepramine *see* Antidepressants, Tricyclic		Nabumetone *see* NSAIDs	
Loop Diuretics	Hypokalaemia may precipitate coma (use potassium-sparing diuretic to prevent this); increased risk of hypomagnesaemia in alcoholic cirrhosis	Nalbuphine *see* Opioid Analgesics	
		Nalidixic Acid *see* 4-Quinolones	
		Nandrolone *see* Anabolic Steroids	
		Naproxen *see* NSAIDs	
		Naratriptan	Max. 2.5 mg in 24 hours in moderate hepatic impairment; avoid if severe
Loprazolam *see* Anxiolytics and Hypnotics			
Lorazepam *see* Anxiolytics and Hypnotics		Nefazodone	Reduce dose
Lormetazepam *see* Anxiolytics and Hypnotics		Neomycin	Absorbed from gastro-intestinal tract in liver disease—increased risk of ototoxicity
Losartan	Consider lower dose		
Loxapine *see* Antipsychotics			
Lymecycline *see* Tetracyclines			
Magnesium Salts	Avoid in hepatic coma if risk of renal failure	Nicardipine	Reduce dose
		Nifedipine	Reduce dose
MAOIs	May cause idiosyncratic hepatotoxicity	Nisoldipine *see* p. 101	
		Nitrazepam *see* Anxiolytics and Hypnotics	
Maprotiline *see* Antidepressants, Tricyclic (and related)		Nitrofurantoin	Cholestatic jaundice and chronic active hepatitis reported
Medroxyprogesterone Acetate *see* Progestogens			
Mefenamic Acid *see* NSAIDs		Nitroprusside	Avoid in severe liver disease
Mefloquine	Avoid for prophylaxis in severe liver disease	Norethisterone *see* Progestogens	
		Norfloxacin *see* 4-Quinolones	
Mefruside *see* Thiazides		Norgestimate *see* Progestogens	
Megestrol Acetate *see* Progestogens		Norgestrel *see* Progestogens	
Meloxicam *see* NSAIDs		Nortriptyline *see* Antidepressants, Tricyclic	
Meprobamate *see* Anxiolytics and Hypnotics		NSAIDs	Increased risk of gastro-intestinal bleeding and can cause fluid retention; avoid in severe liver disease
Meptazinol *see* Opioid Analgesics			
Mequitazine *see* Antihistamines			
Meropenem	Monitor transaminase and bilirubin concentrations		
		Oestradiol *see* Oestrogens	
Mesterolone *see* Androgens		Oestriol *see* Oestrogens	
Mestranol *see* Oestrogens		Oestrogens	Avoid; *see also* Contraceptives, Oral
Metformin	Avoid—increased risk of lactic acidosis		
		Ofloxacin *see* 4-Quinolones	
Methadone *see* Opioid Analgesics		Olanzapine	Consider initial dose of 5 mg daily
Methohexitone	Avoid or reduce dose		
Methotrexate	Dose-related toxicity—avoid in non-malignant conditions (e.g. psoriasis)	Omeprazole	In liver disease not more than 20 mg daily should be needed
		Ondansetron	Reduce dose; not more than 8 mg daily in severe liver disease
Methotrimeprazine *see* Antipsychotics			
Methoxsalen	Avoid or reduce dose		
Methyldopa	Avoid—increased risk of hepatotoxicity	Opioid Analgesics	Avoid or reduce dose—may precipitate coma
		Oral Contraceptives *see* Contraceptives, Oral	
Metoclopramide	Reduce dose	Oxazepam *see* Anxiolytics and Hypnotics	
Metolazone *see* Thiazides		Oxprenolol	Reduce dose
Metoprolol	Reduce oral dose	Oxypertine *see* Antipsychotics	
Metronidazole	Reduce dose in severe liver disease	Oxytetracycline *see* Tetracyclines	
		Paclitaxel	Avoid in severe liver disease
Mexiletine	Avoid (or reduce dose) in severe liver disease	Pantoprazole	In cirrhosis, administer on alternate days
Mianserin *see* Antidepressants, Tricyclic (and related)		Papaveretum *see* Opioid Analgesics	
		Paracetamol	Dose-related toxicity—avoid large doses
Mibefradil	Monitor response in mild or moderate liver disease. Manufacturer advises avoid in severe liver disease	Paroxetine *see* Antidepressants, SSRI	
		Pentazocine *see* Opioid Analgesics	
		Pericyazine *see* Antipsychotics	
Miconazole	Avoid	Perindopril *see* ACE Inhibitors	
Minocycline *see* Tetracyclines			

Table of drugs to be avoided or used with caution in liver disease (*continued*)

Drug	Comment	Drug	Comment
Perphenazine *see* Antipsychotics		Rifampicin	Impaired elimination; may be increased risk of hepato-toxicity; avoid or do not exceed 8mg/kg daily; *see also* p. 264
Pethidine *see* Opioid Analgesics			
Phenazocine *see* Opioid Analgesics			
Phenelzine *see* MAOIs		Riluzole	Avoid
Phenindamine *see* Antihistamines		Risperidone	Manufacturer advises initial dose of 500 micrograms twice daily increased in steps of 500 micrograms twice daily to 1–2 mg twice daily
Pheniramine *see* Antihistamines			
Phenobarbitone	May precipitate coma		
Phenoperidine *see* Opioid Analgesics			
Phenothiazines *see* Antipsychotics			
Phenylbutazone *see* NSAIDs		Ritonavir	Avoid in severe hepatic impairment
Phenytoin	Reduce dose to avoid toxicity		
Pholcodine *see* Opioid Analgesics		Rocuronium	Reduce dose
Pilocarpine	Reduce oral dose	Ropinirole	Avoid in severe hepatic impairment
Pimozide *see* Antipsychotics			
Piperazine	Manufacturer advises avoid	Saquinavir	Plasma concentration possibly increased in severe hepatic impairment
Pipothiazine *see* Antipsychotics			
Piracetam	Avoid		
Piroxicam *see* NSAIDs		Sertindole	Slower titration and lower maintenance dose in mild to moderate impairment; avoid if severe
Polyestradiol *see* Oestrogens			
Polythiazide *see* Thiazides			
Pravastatin *see* Statins			
Prazosin	Initially 500 micrograms daily; increased with caution		
		Sertraline *see* Antidepressants, SSRI	
Prednisolone	Side-effects more common	Simvastatin *see* Statins	
Prednisone	Prednisolone is preferable (prednisone needs conversion to prednisolone by liver before active)	Sodium Aurothiomalate *see* Gold	
		Sodium Bicarbonate *see* Antacids	
		Sodium Fusidate *see* Fusidic Acid	
		Sodium Nitroprusside *see* Nitroprusside	
Primidone	Reduce dose; may precipitate coma	Sodium Valproate *see* Valproate	
		Stanozolol *see* Anabolic Steroids	
Procainamide	Avoid or reduce dose	Statins	Avoid in active liver disease or unexplained persistent elevations in serum transaminases
Prochlorperazine *see* Antipsychotics			
Progesterone *see* Progestogens			
Progestogens	Avoid; *see also* Contraceptives, Oral		
		Stilboestrol *see* Oestrogens	
Promazine *see* Antipsychotics		Sulindac *see* NSAIDs	
Promethazine *see* Antihistamines		Sulphonylureas	Increased risk of hypoglycaemia in severe liver disease; avoid or use small dose; can produce jaundice
Propafenone	Reduce dose		
Propranolol	Reduce oral dose		
Propylthiouracil			
Protriptyline *see* Antidepressants, Tricyclic		Sulpiride *see* Antipsychotics	
Pyrazinamide	Avoid—idiosyncratic hepatotoxicity more common; *see also* p. 263	Sumatriptan	Use half oral dose
		Suxamethonium	Prolonged apnoea may occur in severe liver disease due to reduced hepatic synthesis of pseudocholinesterase
Quetiapine	Manufacturer advises initial dose of 25 mg daily, increased daily in steps of 25–50 mg		
		Tacrolimus	Reduce dose
Quinapril *see* ACE Inhibitors		Temazepam *see* Anxiolytics and Hypnotics	
4-Quinolones	See section 5.1.12; hepatitis with necrosis reported with *ciprofloxacin*; hepatitis also reported for *norfloxacin; nalidixic acid* partially conjugated in liver; reduce dose of *ofloxacin* in severe liver disease	Tenoxicam *see* NSAIDs	
		Terbinafine	Reduce dose
		Terfenadine *see* Antihistamines	
		Testosterone *see* Androgens	
		Tetracyclines	Avoid (or use with caution)—dose-related toxicity by i/v route; SLE syndrome and hepatic damage reported with minocycline
Ramipril *see* ACE Inhibitors			
Ranitidine	Increased risk of confusion; reduce dose		
Reboxetine	Initial dose 2 mg twice daily, increased according to tolerance	Theophylline	Reduce dose
		Thiazides	Avoid in severe liver disease; hypokalaemia may precipitate coma (potassium-sparing diuretic can prevent); increased risk of hypo-magnesaemia in alcoholic cirrhosis
Remifentanil *see* Opioid Analgesics			
Rifabutin	Reduce dose in severe hepatic impairment		

Table of drugs to be avoided or used with caution in liver disease (*continued*)

Drug	Comment	Drug	Comment
Thiopentone	Reduce dose for induction in severe liver disease	Trimipramine *see* Antidepressants, Tricyclic	
Thioridazine *see* Antipsychotics		Triprolidine *see* Antihistamines	
Tiaprofenic acid *see* NSAIDs		Tulobuterol	Avoid
Tibolone	Avoid in severe liver disease	Valproate	Avoid if possible—hepato-toxicity and liver failure may occasionally occur (usually in first 6 months); *see also* p. 215
Timentin®	Cholestatic jaundice, see p. 244		
Tinzaparin *see* Heparin			
Tizanidine	Avoid in severe liver disease	Valsartan	Halve dose in mild to moderate hepatic impairment; avoid if severe
Tolazamide *see* Sulphonylureas			
Tolbutamide *see* Sulphonylureas			
Tolcapone	May accumulate in moderate cirrhotic liver disease; dose should remain below 200 mg 3 times daily	Venlafaxine	Halve dose in moderate hepatic impairment; avoid if severe
		Verapamil	Reduce oral dose
Tolfenamic Acid *see* NSAIDs		Vinblastine	Dose reduction may be necessary
Topotecan	Avoid in severe hepatic impairment	Vincristine	Dose reduction may be necessary
Torasemide *see* Loop Diuretics		Vindesine	Dose reduction may be necessary
Toremifene	Elimination decreased in hepatic impairment—avoid if severe	Vinorelbine	Dose reduction may be necessary
Tramadol *see* Opioid Analgesics		Xipamide *see* Thiazides	
Trandolapril *see* ACE Inhibitors		Zalcitabine	Further impairment of liver function may occur
Tranylcypromine *see* MAOIs			
Trazodone *see* Antidepressants, Tricyclic (and related)		Zidovudine	Accumulation may occur
Tretinoin (oral)	Reduce dose	Zolpidem *see* Anxiolytics and Hypnotics	
Triclofos *see* Anxiolytics and Hypnotics		Zopiclone *see* Anxiolytics and Hypnotics	
Trifluoperazine *see* Antipsychotics		Zuclopenthixol *see* Antipsychotics	
Trimeprazine *see* Antihistamines			

Appendix 3: Renal Impairment

The use of drugs in patients with reduced renal function can give rise to problems for several reasons:

failure to excrete a drug or its metabolites may produce toxicity;

sensitivity to some drugs is increased even if elimination is unimpaired;

many side-effects are tolerated poorly by patients in renal failure;

some drugs cease to be effective when renal function is reduced.

Many of these problems can be avoided by reducing the dose or by using alternative drugs.

Principles of dose adjustment in renal impairment

The level of renal function below which the dose of a drug must be reduced depends on whether the drug is eliminated entirely by renal excretion or is partly metabolised, and on how toxic it is.

For many drugs with only minor or no dose-related side-effects very precise modification of the dose regimen is unnecessary and a simple scheme for dose reduction is sufficient.

For more toxic drugs with a small safety margin dose regimens based on glomerular filtration rate should be used. For those where both efficacy and toxicity are closely related to plasma concentrations recommended regimens should be seen only as a guide to initial treatment; subsequent treatment must be adjusted according to clinical response and plasma concentration.

The total daily maintenance dose of a drug can be reduced either by reducing the size of the individual doses or by increasing the interval between doses. For some drugs, if the size of the maintenance dose is reduced it will be important to give a loading dose if an immediate effect is required. This is because when a patient is given a regular dose of any drug it takes more than five times the half-life to achieve steady-state plasma concentrations. As the plasma half-life of drugs excreted by the kidney is prolonged in renal failure it may take many days for the reduced dosage to achieve a therapeutic plasma concentration. The loading dose should usually be the same size as the initial dose for a patient with normal renal function.

Nephrotoxic drugs should, if possible, be avoided in patients with renal disease because the consequences of nephrotoxicity are likely to be more serious when the renal reserve is already reduced.

Use of dosage table

Dose recommendations are based on the severity of renal impairment. This is expressed in terms of glomerular filtration rate (GFR), usually measured by the **creatinine clearance**. The serum-creatinine concentration can usually be used instead as a measure of renal function but is only a rough guide unless corrected for age, weight, and sex. Nomograms are available for making the correction and should be used where accuracy is important.

For prescribing purposes renal impairment is arbitrarily divided into 3 grades:

Grade	GFR	Serum creatinine (approx.)
Mild	20–50 mL/minute	150–300 µmol/litre
Moderate	10–20 mL/minute	300–700 µmol/litre
Severe	<10 mL/minute	> 700 µmol/litre

Note. Conversion factors are:
Litres/24 hours = mL/minute × 1.44
mL/minute = Litres/24 hours × 0.69

DIALYSIS. For prescribing in patients on continuous ambulatory peritoneal dialysis (CAPD) or haemodialysis, consult specialist literature.

Renal function declines with age; many elderly patients have a glomerular filtration rate below 50 mL/minute which, because of reduced muscle mass, may not be indicated by a raised serum creatinine. It is wise to assume at least mild impairment of renal function when prescribing for the elderly.

The following table may be used as a guide to drugs which are known to require a reduction in dose in renal impairment, and to those which are potentially harmful or are ineffective. Drug prescribing should be kept to the minimum in all patients with severe renal disease.

If even mild renal impairment is considered likely on clinical grounds, renal function should be checked before prescribing **any** drug which requires dose modification.

Table of drugs to be avoided or used with caution in renal impairment

Products introduced or amended since publication of BNF No. 34 (September 1997) are <u>underlined</u>.

Drug and Degree of impairment	Comment	Drug and Degree of impairment	Comment
Acamprosate		**Aminoglycosides**	
Mild	Avoid; excreted in urine	Mild	Reduce dose; monitor plasma concentrations; ototoxic; nephrotoxic; *see also* p. 252
Acarbose			
Moderate to severe	Manufacturer advises avoid —no information available	**Amisulpride**	
ACE Inhibitors		Mild	Manufacturer advises reduce dose by half
Mild to moderate	Use with caution and monitor response (see also p. 87). Hyperkalaemia and other side-effects more common. Initial doses: captopril 12.5 mg twice daily, cilazapril 500 micrograms once daily, enalapril 2.5 mg once daily, moexipril 3.75 mg once daily, perindopril 2 mg once daily (2 mg once daily on alternate days in moderate impairment), quinapril 2.5 mg once daily, ramipril 1.25 mg once daily, trandolapril 500 micrograms once daily	Moderate	Manufacturer advises reduce dose by two-thirds
		Severe	Manufacturer advises dose reduction and intermittent treatment
		Amoxycillin	
		Severe	Reduce dose; rashes more common
		Amphotericin	
		Mild	Use only if no alternative; nephrotoxicity may be reduced with use of complexes (*see also* p. 270)
		Ampicillin	
		Severe	Reduce dose; rashes more common
Acebutolol *see* Beta-blockers		**Amylobarbitone**	
Aceclofenac *see* NSAIDs		Severe	Reduce dose; active metabolite accumulates
Acemetacin *see* NSAIDs		**Analgesics** *see* Opioid Analgesics and NSAIDs	
Acetazolamide		**Anastrozole**	
Mild	Avoid; metabolic acidosis	Moderate to severe	Avoid—no information available
Aciclovir		**Antipsychotics**	
Moderate to severe	Reduce dose; possible transient increase in plasma urea	Severe	Start with small doses; increased cerebral sensitivity; *see also* Amisulpride, Clozapine, Olanzapine, Quetiapine, Risperidone, Sertindole and Sulpiride
Acipimox			
Mild	Reduce dose		
Acitretin			
Mild	Avoid; increased risk of toxicity	**Anxiolytics and Hypnotics**	
Acrivastine		Severe	Start with small doses; increased cerebral sensitivity
Moderate	Avoid; excreted by kidney	**Aspirin**	
Adrenergic Neurone Blockers		Severe	Avoid; sodium and water retention; deterioration in renal function; increased risk of gastro-intestinal bleeding
Moderate to severe	Avoid; increased postural hypotension; decrease in renal blood flow		
Alendronic Acid		**Atenolol** *see* Beta-blockers	
Moderate to severe	Avoid	**Atovaquone**	Manufacturer advises caution—monitor more closely
Alfentanil *see* Opioid Analgesics			
Alfuzosin		**Auranofin** *see* Gold	
Moderate	Reduce dose	**Aurothiomalate** *see* Gold	
Allopurinol		**Azapropazone** *see* NSAIDs (excreted by kidney)	
Moderate	100mg daily; increased toxicity; rashes	**Azathioprine**	
Severe	100mg on alternate days	Severe	Reduce dose
Alprazolam *see* Anxiolytics and Hypnotics		**Azithromycin**	
Alteplase		Moderate to severe	No information available
Moderate	Risk of hyperkalaemia	**Azlocillin**	
Altretamine		Moderate	Reduce dose
Mild	Nephrotoxic; if renal function deteriorates reduce dose or discontinue	**Aztreonam**	
		Moderate	Reduce dose
Aluminium Salts		**Baclofen**	
Severe	Aluminium is absorbed and may accumulate	Mild	Use smaller doses (e.g. 5 mg daily); excreted by kidney
Note. Absorption of aluminium from aluminium salts is increased by citrates, which are contained in many effervescent preparations (such as effervescent analgesics)		**Bambuterol**	
		Mild	Reduce dose
Amantadine		**Bendrofluazide** *see* Thiazides	
Mild to moderate	Reduce dose; excreted by kidney	**Benorylate** [aspirin-paracetamol ester] *see* Aspirin	
Severe	Avoid	**Benperidol** *see* Antipsychotics	
Amifostine	Manufacturer advises avoid	**Benzodiazepines** *see* Anxiolytics and Hypnotics	
Amikacin *see* Aminoglycosides			
Amiloride *see* Diuretics, Potassium-sparing			

Table of drugs to be avoided or used with caution in renal impairment (*continued*)

Drug and Degree of impairment	Comment	Drug and Degree of impairment	Comment
Benzylpenicillin		Cefuroxime	
Severe	Max. 6 g daily; neurotoxicity—high doses may cause convulsions	Moderate to severe	Reduce parenteral dose
		Celiprolol *see* Beta-blockers	
Beta-blockers		Cephalexin	
Moderate	Start with small dose of acebutolol (active metabolite accumulates); reduce dose of atenolol, nadolol, pindolol, sotalol (all excreted unchanged)	Severe	Max. 500 mg daily
		Cephamandole	
		Mild	Reduce dose
		Cephazolin	
		Mild	Reduce dose
		Cephradine	
Severe	Start with small dose; higher plasma concentrations after oral administration; may reduce renal blood flow and adversely affect renal function in severe impairment; manufacturer advises avoid celiprolol and sotalol	Mild	Reduce dose
		Certoparin *see* Heparin	
		Cetirizine	
		Moderate	Use half dose
		Cerivastatin	
		Moderate to severe	Max. 200 micrograms daily
		Chloral Hydrate *see* Anxiolytics and Hypnotics	
		Chloramphenicol	
Betaxolol *see* Beta-blockers		Severe	Avoid unless no alternative; dose-related depression of haematopoiesis
Bethanidine *see* Adrenergic Neurone Blockers			
Bezafibrate		Chlordiazepoxide *see* Anxiolytics and Hypnotics	
Mild to moderate	Reduce dose; further deterioration in renal function	Chlormethiazole *see* Anxiolytics and Hypnotics	
		Chloroquine	
Severe	Avoid	Mild to moderate	Reduce dose (but for malaria prophylaxis see section 5.4.1)
Bicarbonate *see* Sodium Bicarbonate			
Bismuth Chelate *see* Tripotassium Dicitratobismuthate		Severe	Avoid (but for malaria prophylaxis see section 5.4.1)
Bisoprolol *see* Beta-blockers			
Bleomycin		Chlorothiazide *see* Thiazides	
Moderate	Reduce dose	Chlorpromazine *see* Antipsychotics	
Bromazepam *see* Anxiolytics and Hypnotics		Chlorpropamide	
Bumetanide		Mild	Avoid; tolbutamide and gliquidone suitable alternatives
Moderate	May need high doses		
Buprenorphine *see* Opioid Analgesics			
Calcitonin		Chlortetracycline *see* Tetracyclines	
Moderate	Reduce dose	Chlorthalidone *see* Thiazides	
Candesartan		Cidofovir	
Moderate	Halve initial dose	Mild	Avoid; nephrotoxic
Severe	Avoid	Cilastatin [ingredient] *see* Primaxin®	
Capreomycin		Cilazapril *see* ACE Inhibitors	
Mild	Reduce dose; nephrotoxic; ototoxic	Cimetidine	
		Mild to moderate	600–800 mg daily; occasional risk of confusion
Captopril *see* ACE Inhibitors			
Carbamazepine	Manufacturer advises caution	Severe	400 mg daily
Carbenoxolone		Cinoxacin	
Moderate	Avoid; fluid retention	Moderate	Avoid; nausea, rashes
Carboplatin *see* Cisplatin		Ciprofibrate	
Cefadroxil		Moderate	100 mg on alternate days
Moderate	Reduce dose	Severe	Avoid
Cefixime		Ciprofloxacin	
Moderate	Reduce dose	Moderate	Use half dose
Cefodizime		Cisapride	
Moderate	Reduce dose	Moderate	Start with half dose
Cefotaxime		Cisplatin	
Severe	Use half dose	Mild	Avoid if possible; nephrotoxic and neurotoxic
Cefoxitin			
Mild	Reduce dose	Citalopram	
Cefpirome		Moderate to severe	No information available
Mild	Usual initial dose, then use half dose	Citrates	Absorption of aluminium from aluminium salts is increased by citrates, which are contained in many effervescent preparations (such as effervescent analgesics)
Moderate to severe	Usual initial dose, then one-quarter dose		
Cefpodoxime			
Moderate	Reduce dose		
Ceftazidime		Clarithromycin	
Mild	Reduce dose	Moderate to severe	Use half dose
Ceftibuten		Clavulanic acid [ingredient] *see* Co-amoxiclav, Timentin®	
Mild	Reduce dose		
Ceftriaxone		Clobazam *see* Anxiolytics and Hypnotics	
Severe	Reduce dose; also monitor plasma concentration if both severe renal and hepatic impairment	Clodronate sodium	
		Mild to moderate	Use half dose and monitor serum creatinine
		Severe	Avoid

Table of drugs to be avoided or used with caution in renal impairment (*continued*)

Drug and Degree of impairment	Comment
Clofibrate	
Mild to moderate	Reduce dose; further deterioration in renal function; myopathy
Severe	Avoid
Clopamide *see* Thiazides	
Clorazepate *see* Anxiolytics and Hypnotics	
Clozapine	
Mild to moderate	Initial dose 12.5 mg daily increased slowly
Severe	Avoid
Co-amoxiclav	
Moderate to severe	Reduce dose
Codeine *see* Opioid Analgesics	
Colchicine	
Severe	Avoid or reduce dose if no alternative
Colistin	
Mild	Reduce dose; nephrotoxic, neurotoxic
Co-trimoxazole	
Moderate	Reduce dose; rashes and blood disorders; may cause further deterioration in renal function
Cyclopenthiazide *see* Thiazides	
Cyclophosphamide	
Moderate	Reduce dose
Cycloserine	
Mild to moderate	Reduce dose
Severe	Avoid
Cyclosporin *see* p. 381 (*see also* p. 493 if used in atopic dermatitis or psoriasis and p. 440 if used in rheumatoid arthritis)	
Dalteparin *see* Heparin	
Danaparoid *see* Heparin	
Debrisoquine *see* Adrenergic Neurone Blockers	
Demeclocycline *see* Tetracyclines	
De-Nol®, De-Noltab®	
Severe	Avoid
Desflurane	
Moderate	Reduce dose
Desmopressin	Antidiuretic effect may be reduced; **important:** *see also* p. 332
Dextromethorphan *see* Opioid Analgesics	
Dextromoramide *see* Opioid Analgesics	
Dextropropoxyphene *see* Opioid Analgesics	
Diamorphine *see* Opioid Analgesics	
Diazepam *see* Anxiolytics and Hypnotics	
Diazoxide	
Severe	75–150 mg i/v; increased sensitivity to hypotensive effect
Diclofenac *see* NSAIDs	
Didanosine	
Mild to moderate	Reduce dose; excreted by kidney
Diflunisal *see* NSAIDs (excreted by kidney)	
Digitoxin	
Severe	Max. 100 micrograms daily; *see also* Digoxin
Digoxin	
Mild	Reduce dose; toxicity increased by electrolyte disturbances; *see also* p. 59
Dihydrocodeine *see* Opioid Analgesics	
Diltiazem	Start with smaller dose
Dimenhydrinate	
Severe	Manufacturer advises may accumulate
Diphenoxylate *see* Opioid Analgesics	
Dipipanone *see* Opioid Analgesics	
Disodium Etidronate *see* Etidronate Disodium	
Disodium Pamidronate *see* Pamidronate Disodium	

Drug and Degree of impairment	Comment
Disopyramide	
Mild	100 mg every 8 hours *or* 150 mg every 12 hours
Moderate	100 mg every 12 hours
Severe	150 mg every 24 hours
Note. Sustained release preparations may be unsuitable; monitor plasma-disopyramide concentrations	
Diuretics, Potassium-sparing	
Mild	Monitor plasma K+; high risk of hyperkalaemia in renal impairment; amiloride excreted by kidney unchanged
Moderate	Avoid
Domperidone	
Severe	Reduce dose by 30–50%
Doxycycline *see* Tetracyclines	
Droperidol *see* Antipsychotics	
Enalapril *see* ACE Inhibitors	
Enflurane	
Severe	Avoid
Enoxaparin *see* Heparin	
Ephedrine	
Severe	Avoid; increased CNS toxicity
Ergometrine	
Severe	Manufacturer advises avoid
Ergotamine	
Moderate	Avoid; nausea and vomiting; risk of renal vasoconstriction
Erythromycin	
Severe	Max. 1.5 g daily (ototoxicity)
Esmolol *see* Beta-blockers	
Ethacrynic Acid	
Severe	Avoid; ototoxic
Ethambutol	
Mild	Reduce dose; optic nerve damage
Etidronate Disodium	
Mild	Max. 5 mg/kg daily; excreted by kidney
Moderate	Avoid
Etodolac *see* NSAIDs	
Etoposide	
Mild	Reduce dose
Famciclovir	
Mild to moderate	Reduce dose
Famotidine	
Severe	Reduce dose
Fenbufen *see* NSAIDs	
Fenofibrate	
Mild	67 mg twice daily
Moderate	67 mg daily
Severe	Avoid
Fenoprofen *see* NSAIDs	
Fentanyl *see* Opioid Analgesics	
Flecainide	
Mild	Max. initial dose 100 mg daily
Flucloxacillin	
Severe	Reduce dose
Fluconazole	
Mild	Reduce dose or increase interval for multiple dose therapy
Flucytosine	
Mild	Reduce dose
Fludarabine	
Mild	Reduce dose and monitor response
Moderate	Avoid
Flunitrazepam *see* Anxiolytics and Hypnotics	
Fluoxetine	
Mild to moderate	Reduce dose (give on alternate days)
Severe	Avoid
Flupenthixol *see* Antipsychotics	
Fluphenazine *see* Antipsychotics	

Table of drugs to be avoided or used with caution in renal impairment (*continued*)

Drug and Degree of impairment	Comment	Drug and Degree of impairment	Comment
Flurazepam *see* Anxiolytics and Hypnotics		Ifosfamide	
Flurbiprofen *see* NSAIDs		Moderate	Reduce dose
Fluvastatin		Imipenem *see Primaxin*®	
Severe	Avoid	Indapamide *see* Thiazides	
Fluvoxamine		Indomethacin *see* NSAIDs	
Moderate	Start with smaller dose	Inosine Pranobex	
Foscarnet		Mild	Avoid; metabolised to uric acid
Mild	Reduce dose; consult product literature	Insulin	
Fosinopril *see* ACE Inhibitors		Severe	May need dose reduction; insulin requirements fall; compensatory response to hypoglycaemia is impaired
Frusemide			
Moderate	May need high doses; deafness may follow rapid i/v injection		
Fybogel Mebeverine®		Interferon alfa	
Severe	Avoid; contains 7 mmol potassium per sachet	Mild to moderate	Close monitoring required
		Severe	Avoid
Gabapentin		Interferon beta	No information available—monitoring advised
Mild	Reduce dose; consult product literature		
Gallamine		Irinotecan	No information available
Moderate	Avoid; prolonged paralysis	Isoniazid	
Ganciclovir		Severe	Max. 200 mg daily; peripheral neuropathy
Mild	Reduce dose; consult product literature		
Gaviscon®		Isotretinoin	
Severe	Avoid; high sodium content	Mild	Avoid; increased risk of toxicity
Gemcitabine		Itraconazole	Bioavailability possibly reduced—plasma concentration monitoring advised
Mild	Monitor renal function		
Gemfibrozil			
Severe	Start with 900 mg daily	Kanamycin *see* Aminoglycosides	
Gentamicin *see* Aminoglycosides		Ketoprofen *see* NSAIDs	
Gestrinone		Ketorolac *see* NSAIDs	
Severe	Avoid	Lamotrigine	
Glibenclamide		Moderate to severe	Metabolite may accumulate
Severe	Avoid; increased risk of prolonged hypoglycaemia	Lamivudine	
		Mild	Reduce dose
Gliclazide		Levocabastine	
Severe	Start with small dose; increased risk of hypoglycaemia	Severe	Manufacturer advises avoid
		Lisinopril *see* ACE Inhibitors	
Glimepiride		Lithium	
Severe	Manufacturer advises avoid	Mild	Avoid if possible or reduce dose and monitor plasma concentration carefully
Glipizide			
Severe	Start with small dose; increased risk of hypoglycaemia	Moderate	Avoid
		Loprazolam *see* Anxiolytics and Hypnotics	
Gliquidone		Lorazepam *see* Anxiolytics and Hypnotics	
Severe	May need dose reduction; increased risk of hypoglycaemia	Lormetazepam *see* Anxiolytics and Hypnotics	
		Losartan	
Gold (auranofin, aurothiomalate)		Moderate to severe	Start with 25 mg once daily
Mild	Avoid; nephrotoxic	Loxapine *see* Antipsychotics	
Guanethidine *see* Adrenergic Neurone Blockers		Lymecycline *see* Tetracyclines	
Haloperidol *see* Antipsychotics		Magnesium Salts	
Heparin		Moderate	Avoid or reduce dose; increased risk of toxicity; magnesium carbonate mixture and magnesium trisilicate mixture also have high sodium content
Severe	Risk of bleeding increased		
Hetastarch			
Severe	Avoid; excreted by kidney		
Hexamine			
Mild	Avoid; ineffective	*Malarone*®	
Hydralazine		Severe	Manufacturer advises caution in acute renal failure
Moderate	Start with small dose; increased hypotensive effect		
Hydrochlorothiazide *see* Thiazides		Mefenamic Acid *see* NSAIDs	
Hydroflumethiazide *see* Thiazides		Mefruside *see* Thiazides	
Hydromorphone *see* Opioid Analgesics		Meloxicam *see* NSAIDs	
Hydroxychloroquine		Melphalan	
Mild to moderate	Reduce dose; only on prolonged use	Moderate	Reduce dose
		Severe	Avoid high intravenous doses
Severe	Avoid	Meprobamate *see* Anxiolytics and Hypnotics	
Hypnotics *see* Anxiolytics and Hypnotics		Meptazinol *see* Opioid Analgesics	
Ibuprofen *see* NSAIDs		Mercaptopurine	
Idarubicin		Moderate	Reduce dose
Mild	Reduce dose		

Table of drugs to be avoided or used with caution in renal impairment (*continued*)

Drug and Degree of impairment	Comment	Drug and Degree of impairment	Comment
Meropenem		**Nifedipine**	
Mild	Increase dose interval to every 12 hours	Moderate	Start with small dose; reversible deterioration in renal function has been reported
Moderate	Half dose every 12 hours		
Severe	Half dose every 24 hours		
Mesalazine		**Nitrazepam** *see* Anxiolytics and Hypnotics	
Mild	Avoid; nephrotoxic	**Nitrofurantoin**	
Metformin		Mild	Avoid; peripheral neuropathy; ineffective because of inadequate urine concentrations
Mild	Avoid; increased risk of lactic acidosis		
Methadone *see* Opioid Analgesics			
Methocarbamol		**Nitroprusside**	
Mild	Avoid; increased plasma urea and acidosis due to solvent in injection	Moderate	Avoid prolonged use
		Nizatidine	
		Mild	Use half dose
Methotrexate		Moderate	Use one-quarter dose
Mild	Reduce dose; accumulates; nephrotoxic	**Norfloxacin**	
		Severe	Use half dose
Moderate	Avoid	**NSAIDs**	
Methotrimeprazine *see* Antipsychotics		Mild	Use lowest effective dose and monitor renal function; sodium and water retention; deterioration in renal function possibly leading to renal failure; deterioration also reported after topical use
Methyldopa			
Moderate	Start with small dose; increased sensitivity to hypotensive and sedative effect		
Metoclopramide			
Severe	Avoid or use small dose; increased risk of extrapyramidal reactions	Moderate to severe	Avoid if possible
		Ofloxacin	
Metolazone *see* Thiazides		Mild	Usual initial dose, then use half dose
Metoprolol *see* Beta-blockers			
Midazolam *see* Anxiolytics and Hypnotics		Moderate	Usual initial dose, then 100 mg every 24 hours
Milrinone			
Mild	Reduce dose and monitor response	Olanzapine	Consider initial dose of 5 mg daily
Minocycline *see* Tetracyclines			
Mivacurium		**Olsalazine**	
Severe	Reduce dose; prolonged paralysis	Mild	Manufacturer advises avoid if significant renal impairment
Moexipril *see* ACE Inhibitors		**Opioid Analgesics**	
Morphine *see* Opioid Analgesics		Moderate to severe	Reduce doses or avoid; increased and prolonged effect; increased cerebral sensitivity
Moxonidine			
Mild	Max. single dose 200 micrograms and max. daily dose 400 micrograms		
		Oxazepam *see* Anxiolytics and Hypnotics	
Moderate to severe	Avoid	Oxpentifylline	
Nabumetone *see* NSAIDs		Mild	Reduce dose by 30–50% if creatinine clearance less than 30 mL/minute
Nadolol *see* Beta-blockers			
Nalbuphine *see* Opioid Analgesics			
Nalidixic Acid		**Oxprenolol** *see* Beta-blockers	
Moderate	Avoid; increased risk of nausea, vomiting, rashes, photosensitivity; ineffective because of inadequate urine concentration	**Oxypertine** *see* Antipsychotics	
		Oxytetracycline *see* Tetracyclines	
		Pamidronate Disodium	
		Moderate to severe	Max. infusion rate 20 mg/hour
Naproxen *see* NSAIDs		**Pancuronium**	
Naratriptan		Severe	Prolonged duration of block
Moderate	Max. 2.5 mg in 24 hours	**Papaveretum** *see* Opioid Analgesics	
Severe	Avoid	**Paroxetine**	
Narcotic Analgesics *see* Opioid Analgesics		Moderate	Usual initial dose; small increments if necessary
Nefazodone			
Severe	Reduce dose	**Penicillamine**	
Neomycin		Mild	Avoid if possible or reduce dose; nephrotoxic
Mild	Avoid; ototoxic; nephrotoxic		
Neostigmine		**Pentamidine**	
Moderate	May need dose reduction	Mild	Reduce dose; consult product literature
Netilmicin *see* Aminoglycosides			
Nicardipine		**Pentazocine** *see* Opioid Analgesics	
Moderate	Start with small dose	**Pericyazine** *see* Antipsychotics	
Nicotine		**Perindopril** *see* ACE Inhibitors	
Severe	May affect clearance of nicotine or its metabolites	**Perphenazine** *see* Antipsychotics	
		Pethidine *see* Opioid Analgesics	
		Phenazocine *see* Opioid Analgesics	
		Phenobarbitone	
		Severe	Avoid large doses
		Phenoperidine *see* Opioid Analgesics	
		Phenothiazines *see* Antipsychotics	

Table of drugs to be avoided or used with caution in renal impairment (*continued*)

Drug and Degree of impairment	Comment	Drug and Degree of impairment	Comment
Phenylbutazone *see* NSAIDs		Ranitidine	
Pholcodine *see* Opioid Analgesics		Severe	Use half normal dose; occasional risk of confusion
Pimozide *see* Antipsychotics		Ranitidine Bismuth Citrate	
Pindolol *see* Beta-blockers		Severe	Avoid
Piperacillin		Reboxetine	Initial dose 2 mg twice daily, increased according to tolerance
Adult:			
Mild	Max. daily dose 16 g		
Moderate	Max. daily dose 12 g		
Severe	Max. daily dose 8 g	*Regulan*®	
Child 1 month–12 years:		Severe	Avoid; contains 6.4 mmol potassium per sachet
Moderate to severe	Reduce dose; consult product literature	Rifabutin	
		Moderate	Use half dose
Piperazine		Riluzole	No information available—manufacturer advises avoid
Severe	Reduce dose; neurotoxic		
Pipothiazine *see* Antipsychotics		Risperidone	Manufacturer advises initial dose of 500 micrograms twice daily increased in steps of 500 micrograms twice daily to 1–2 mg twice daily
Piracetam			
Mild	Use half dose		
Moderate	Use one-quarter dose		
Severe	Avoid		
Piroxicam *see* NSAIDs		Rocuronium	
Pivampicillin		Moderate	Reduce dose; prolonged paralysis
Severe	Reduce dose; rashes more common	Ropinirole	
Polythiazide *see* Thiazides		Severe	Avoid
Potassium Salts		Salcatonin *see* Calcitonin	
Moderate	Avoid routine use; high risk of hyperkalaemia	Salicylates *see* Aspirin	
		Salt Substitutes	
Povidone-iodine		Moderate	Avoid routine use; high risk of hyperkalaemia (*see* section 9.2.1.1)
Severe	Avoid regular application to inflamed or broken mucosa		
Pravastatin		Saquinavir	
Moderate to severe	Start at lower end of dosage range	Severe	Dose adjustment possibly required
		Sertraline	Manufacturer advises caution
Prazosin		Simvastatin	
Moderate to severe	Initially 500 micrograms daily; increased with caution	Moderate to severe	Doses above 10 mg daily should be used with caution
		Sodium Aurothiomalate *see* Gold	
Primaxin®		Sodium Bicarbonate	
Mild	Reduce dose	Severe	Avoid; specialised role in some forms of renal disease
Primidone			
Severe	Avoid large doses	Sodium Cellulose Phosphate	
Probenecid		Mild to moderate	Reduce dose
Moderate	Avoid; ineffective and toxicity increased	Severe	Avoid
		Sodium Clodronate *see* Clodronate Sodium	
Procainamide		Sodium Nitroprusside *see* Nitroprusside	
Mild	Avoid or reduce dose	Sodium Salts	
Procarbazine		Severe	Avoid
Moderate	Reduce dose	*Solpadeine*®	
Prochlorperazine *see* Antipsychotics		Severe	Avoid; contains 18.5 mmol sodium per tablet
Proguanil			
Mild	100 mg once daily	*Solpadol*®	
Moderate	50 mg on alternate days	Severe	Avoid; contains 18.6 mmol sodium per tablet
Severe	50 mg once weekly; increased risk of haematological toxicity	Sotalol *see* Beta-blockers	
		Spironolactone *see* Diuretics, Potassium-sparing	
Promazine *see* Antipsychotics		Stavudine	
Propranolol *see* Beta-blockers		Mild	20 mg twice daily (15 mg if <60 kg)
Propylthiouracil			
Mild to moderate	Reduce dose by 25%	Moderate	20 mg once daily (15 mg if <60 kg)
Severe	Reduce dose by 50%		
Pseudoephedrine		Severe	Information not available
Severe	Avoid; increased CNS toxicity	Streptomycin *see* Aminoglycosides	
Pyridostigmine		Sucralfate	
Moderate	Reduce dose; excreted by kidney	Severe	Avoid; aluminium is absorbed and may accumulate
Quetiapine	Manufacturer advises initial dose of 25 mg daily; increased daily in steps of 25–50 mg	Sulfametopyrazine *see* Sulphonamides	
		Sulindac *see* NSAIDs	
Quinapril *see* ACE Inhibitors		Sulphadiazine	
Raltitrexed		Severe	Avoid; high risk of crystalluria
Mild	Reduce dose	Sulphadimidine *see* Sulphonamides	
Moderate to severe	Avoid		
Ramipril *see* ACE Inhibitors			

Table of drugs to be avoided or used with caution in renal impairment (*continued*)

Drug and Degree of impairment	Comment	Drug and Degree of impairment	Comment
Sulphasalazine		Tolbutamide	
Severe	Ensure high fluid intake; rashes and blood disorders; crystalluria a risk	Severe	May need dose reduction; increased risk of hypoglycaemia
Sulphinpyrazone		Tolfenamic Acid *see* NSAIDs	
Moderate	Avoid; ineffective as uricosuric	Topiramate	
		Moderate to severe	Longer time to steady-state plasma concentrations
Sulphonamides		Topotecan	
Moderate	Ensure high fluid intake; rashes and blood disorders; crystalluria a risk	Moderate	Reduce dose
		Severe	Avoid
Sulphonylureas *see under* individual drugs		Torasemide	
Sulpiride		Moderate	May need high doses
Moderate	Avoid if possible, or reduce dose	Tramadol *see* Opioid Analgesics	
		Trandolapril *see* ACE Inhibitors	
Tazobactam [ingredient] *see* Tazocin®		Tretinoin (oral)	
Tazocin®		Mild	Reduce dose
Mild	Reduce dose	Triamterene *see* Diuretics, Potassium-sparing	
Teicoplanin		Triclofos *see* Anxiolytics and Hypnotics	
Mild	Reduce dose after 4 days; consult product literature	Trifluoperazine *see* Antipsychotics	
		Trimeprazine	
Temazepam *see* Anxiolytics and Hypnotics		Severe	Avoid
Temocillin		Trimethoprim	
Moderate	Reduce dose	Moderate	Reduce dose
Tenoxicam *see* NSAIDs		Tripotassium	
Terbinafine		Dicitratobismuthate	
Mild	Use half normal dose	Severe	Avoid
Tetracyclines (except doxycycline and minocycline)		Tulobuterol	
Mild	Avoid—use doxycycline or minocycline if necessary; anti-anabolic effect, increased plasma urea, further deterioration in renal function	Mild	May need dose reduction; excreted by kidney
		Moderate to severe	Avoid
		Tylex®	
		Moderate to severe	Avoid effervescent tablets; contain 13.6 mmol sodium per tablet
Thiazides and Related Diuretics		Valaciclovir as for Aciclovir	
Moderate	Avoid; ineffective (metolazone remains effective but risk of excessive diuresis)	Valsartan	
		Moderate to severe	Start with 40 mg once daily
Thioguanine		Vancomycin	
Moderate	Reduce dose	Mild	Avoid parenteral use if possible; ototoxic; nephrotoxic
Thioridazine *see* Antipsychotics		Vecuronium	
Tiaprofenic Acid *see* NSAIDs		Severe	Reduce dose; duration of block possibly prolonged
Ticarcillin [ingredient] *see* Timentin®		Venlafaxine	
Tiludronic Acid		Moderate	Use half dose
Moderate to severe	Avoid	Severe	Avoid
Timentin®		Vigabatrin	
Moderate to severe	Reduce dose	Mild	Excreted by kidney—lower maintenance dose may be required
Timolol *see* Beta-blockers		Xamoterol	
Tinzaparin		Moderate	Reduce dose; excreted by kidney
Severe	May need dose reduction	Xipamide *see* Thiazides	
Tizanidine		Zidovudine	
Mild	Initially 2 mg once daily; increase once-daily dose gradually before increasing frequency	Mild	Excreted by kidney; increased risk of toxicity
Tobramycin *see* Aminoglycosides		Zopiclone *see* Anxiolytics and Hypnotics	
Tolazamide		Zuclopenthixol *see* Antipsychotics	
Severe	May need dose reduction; increased risk of hypoglycaemia		

Appendix 4: Pregnancy

Drugs can have harmful effects on the fetus at any time during pregnancy. It is important to bear this in mind when prescribing for a woman of *childbearing age*.

During the *first trimester* drugs may produce congenital malformations (teratogenesis), and the period of greatest risk is from the third to the eleventh week of pregnancy.

During the *second* and *third trimesters* drugs may affect the growth and functional development of the fetus or have toxic effects on fetal tissues; and drugs given shortly before term or during labour may have adverse effects on labour or on the neonate after delivery.

The following list includes drugs which may have harmful effects in pregnancy and indicates the trimester of risk. It is based on human data but information on *animal* studies has been included for some newer drugs when its omission might be misleading.

Drugs should be prescribed in pregnancy only if the expected benefit to the mother is thought to be greater than the risk to the fetus, and all drugs should be avoided if possible during the first trimester. Drugs which have been extensively used in pregnancy and appear to be usually safe should be prescribed in preference to new or untried drugs; and the smallest effective dose should be used.

Few drugs have been shown conclusively to be teratogenic in man but no drug is safe beyond all doubt in early pregnancy. Screening procedures are available where there is a known risk of certain defects.

Absence of a drug from the list does not imply safety. It should be noted that the BNF provides independent advice and may not always agree with the product literature.

Information on drugs and pregnancy is also available from the National Teratology Information Service (telephone: 0191-232 1525).

Table of drugs to be avoided or used with caution in pregnancy

Products introduced or amended since publication of BNF No. 34 (September 1997) are underlined.

Drug (Trimester of risk)	Comment	Drug (Trimester of risk)	Comment
Acamprosate	Manufacturer advises avoid	Alcohol	
Acarbose	Manufacturer advises avoid	(1, 2)	Regular daily drinking is teratogenic (fetal alcohol syndrome) and may cause growth retardation; occasional single drinks are probably safe
ACE Inhibitors (1, 2, 3)	Avoid; may adversely affect fetal and neonatal blood pressure control and renal function; also possible skull defects and oligohydramnios; toxicity in *animal* studies		
		(3)	Withdrawal syndrome may occur in babies of alcoholic mothers
Acebutolol *see* Beta-blockers		Alendronic Acid *see* Bisphosphonates	
Aceclofenac *see* NSAIDs		Alfentanil *see* Opioid Analgesics	
Acemetacin *see* NSAIDs		Alglucerase	Information not available
Acetazolamide *see* Diuretics		Allopurinol	Toxicity not reported; manufacturer advises avoid; use only if no safer alternative and disease carries risk for mother or child
Aciclovir	Experience limited— manufacturers advise use only when potential benefits outweigh possibility of unknown risks; limited absorption from topical preparations		
		Alpha-blockers (post-synaptic)	No evidence of teratogenicity; manufacturers advise use only when potential benefit outweighs potential risk
Acitretin (1, 2, 3)	Teratogenic; effective contraception must be used for at least 1 month before treatment, during treatment, and for at least 2 years after stopping	Alprazolam *see* Anxiolytics and Hypnotics	
		Alprostadil (urethral application only)	Manufacturer advises barrier contraception if partner pregnant
Acrivastine *see* Antihistamines		Alteplase *see* Streptokinase	
Adapalene	Manufacturer advises teratogenicity in *animal* studies and recommends effective contraception during treatment	Altretamine *see* Cytotoxic Drugs	
		Amantadine	Avoid; toxicity in *animal* studies
Albendazole	Manufacturer advises teratogenic in *animal* studies	Amifostine	No information available— manufacturer advises avoid
Alclometasone *see* Corticosteroids		Amikacin *see* Aminoglycosides	
		Amiloride *see* Diuretics	
		Aminoglutethimide	Avoid; toxicity in *animal* studies and may affect fetal sexual development

Table of drugs to be avoided or used with caution in pregnancy (*continued*)

Drug (Trimester of risk)	Comment	Drug (Trimester of risk)	Comment
Aminoglycosides (2, 3)	Auditory or vestibular nerve damage; risk greatest with streptomycin; probably very small with gentamicin and tobramycin, but avoid unless essential (if given, monitor plasma concentration)	Antiepileptics	Benefit of treatment outweighs risk to fetus; risk of teratogenicity greater if more than one drug used; **important**: *see also* carbamazepine, ethosuximide, phenobarbitone, phenytoin, valproate, vigabatrin, and p. 210
Aminophylline *see* Theophylline			
Amiodarone (2, 3)	Possible risk of neonatal goitre; use only if no alternative	Antihistamines	No evidence of teratogenicity; some packs of antihistamines sold to the public carry warning to avoid in pregnancy; manufacturer of astemizole advises avoid (see p. 142)
Amisulpride	Manufacturer advises avoid		
Amitriptyline *see* Antidepressants, Tricyclic			
Amlodipine *see* Calcium-channel Blockers			
Amorolfine	No information available; systemic absorption very low, but manufacturer advises avoid	Antimalarials (1, 3)	Benefit of prophylaxis and treatment in malaria outweighs risk; **important**: *see also* individual drugs and pp. 283 and 284
Amoxapine *see* Antidepressants, Tricyclic			
Amphotericin	Not known to be harmful but manufacturers advise avoid unless expected benefit outweighs potential risk	Antipsychotics	*See also* amisulpride, clozapine, olanzapine, quetiapine, risperidone, sertindole
Amylobarbitone *see* Barbiturates			
Anabolic Steroids (1, 2, 3)	Masculinisation of female fetus	(3)	Extrapyramidal effects in neonate occasionally reported
Anaesthetics, General (3)	Depress neonatal respiration	Anxiolytics and Hypnotics (1)	Avoid if possible; manufacturer of buspirone advises toxicity in *animal studies*
Anaesthetics, Local (3)	With large doses, neonatal respiratory depression, hypotonia, and bradycardia after paracervical or epidural block; neonatal methaemoglobinaemia with prilocaine and procaine	(3)	Depress neonatal respiration. Benzodiazepines cause neonatal drowsiness, hypotonia, and withdrawal symptoms; avoid large doses and regular use; short-acting benzodiazepines preferable to long-acting
Analgesics *see* Opioid Analgesics, Nefopam, NSAIDs and Paracetamol		Apomorphine	Avoid
Androgens (1, 2, 3)	Masculinisation of female fetus	Aspirin (3)	Impaired platelet function and risk of haemorrhage; delayed onset and increased duration of labour with increased blood loss; avoid analgesic doses if possible in last few weeks (low doses probably not harmful); with high doses, closure of fetal ductus arteriosus *in utero* and possibly persistent pulmonary hypertension of newborn; kernicterus in jaundiced neonates
Anistreplase *see* Streptokinase			
Anticoagulants			
Heparin (1, 2, 3)	Osteoporosis has been reported after prolonged use		
Oral Anticoagulants (1, 2, 3)	Congenital malformations; fetal and neonatal haemorrhage *See also* section 2.8		
Antidepressants *see* individual drugs (and groups)		Astemizole *see* Antihistamines	
Antidepressants, SSRI (1, 2, 3)	Manufacturers advise use only if potential benefit outweighs possible risk (no evidence of teratogenicity); adverse effects with sertraline in *animals* (manufacturer recommends avoid)	Atenolol *see* Beta-blockers	
		Atorvastatin *see* Statins	
		Atovaquone	Information not available
		Auranofin *see* Gold	
		Aurothiomalate *see* Gold	
		Azapropazone *see* NSAIDs	
Antidepressants, Tricyclic (and related) (3)	Tachycardia, irritability, and muscle spasms in neonate reported with imipramine	Azatadine *see* Antihistamines	
		Azathioprine *see* p. 368	
		Azelastine *see* Antihistamines	
		Azithromycin	Not known to be harmful but manufacturer advises use only if adequate alternatives not available

Table of drugs to be avoided or used with caution in pregnancy (*continued*)

Drug (Trimester of risk)	Comment	Drug (Trimester of risk)	Comment
Aztreonam	Manufacturer advises avoid (but no evidence of teratogenicity)	Carbamazepine (1)	Risk of teratogenesis including increased risk of neural tube defects (counselling and screening and adequate folate supplements advised, e.g. 5 mg daily); *see also* Antiepileptics and p. 210
Baclofen	Manufacturer advises toxicity in *animal* studies		
Bambuterol *see* section 3.1.1 [text]			
Barbiturates (3)	Withdrawal effects in neonate; *see also* Phenobarbitone	(3)	Because of neonatal bleeding tendency associated with some antiepileptics, manufacturer advises prophylactic vitamin K₁ for mother before delivery (as well as for neonate)
Beclomethasone *see* Corticosteroids			
Bendrofluazide *see* Diuretics			
Benorylate [aspirin-paracetamol ester] *see* Aspirin		Carbenoxolone (3)	Avoid; causes sodium retention with oedema
Benperidol *see* Antipsychotics		Carbimazole (2, 3)	Neonatal goitre and hypo-thyroidism; has been associated with aplasia cutis of the neonate
Benserazide [ingredient] *see* Madopar®			
Benzodiazepines *see* Anxiolytics and Hypnotics			
Beta-blockers	May cause intra-uterine growth retardation, neonatal hypoglycaemia, and bradycardia; risk greater in severe hypertension *See also* section 2.5	Carvedilol *see* Beta-blockers	
		Celiprolol *see* Beta-blockers	
		Cephalosporins	Not known to be harmful
		Cerivastatin *see* Statins	
Betamethasone *see* Corticosteroids		Certoparin *see* Anticoagulants (Heparin)	
Betaxolol *see* Beta-blockers		Cetirizine *see* Antihistamines	
Bethanidine *see* Guanethidine		Chenodeoxycholic Acid (1, 2, 3)	Theoretical risk of effects on fetal metabolism
Bezafibrate *see* Clofibrate			
Bismuth Chelate	Manufacturer advises avoid on theoretical grounds	Chloral *see* Anxiolytics and Hypnotics	
Bisoprolol *see* Beta-blockers		Chloramphenicol (3)	Neonatal 'grey syndrome'
Bisphosphonates	Manufacturers advise avoid	Chlordiazepoxide *see* Anxiolytics and Hypnotics	
Botulinum Toxin	Manufacturers advise avoid	Chlormethiazole *see* Anxiolytics and Hypnotics	
Bromazepam *see* Anxiolytics and Hypnotics		Chloroquine *see* Antimalarials	
Brompheniramine *see* Antihistamines		Chlorothiazide *see* Diuretics	
Buclizine *see* Antihistamines		Chlorpheniramine *see* Antihistamines	
Budesonide *see* Corticosteroids		Chlorpromazine *see* Antipsychotics	
Bumetanide *see* Diuretics		Chlorpropamide *see* Sulphonylureas	
Bupivacaine *see* Anaesthetics, Local		Chlortetracycline *see* Tetracyclines	
Buprenorphine *see* Opioid Analgesics		Chlorthalidone *see* Diuretics	
Buserelin	Avoid	Cidofovir	Avoid (toxicity in animal studies); effective contraception required during and after treatment; also men should avoid fathering a child during and for 3 months after treatment
Buspirone *see* Anxiolytics and Hypnotics			
Cabergoline	Once regular ovulatory cycles have been achieved manufacturer advises discontinuation for one month before intended conception (although no evidence of teratogenicity)		
		Cilastatin [ingredient] *see* Primaxin®	
		Cilazapril *see* ACE Inhibitors	
Calcipotriol	Manufacturer advises avoid if possible	Cinnarizine *see* Antihistamines	
		Ciprofibrate *see* Clofibrate	
Calcitonin	Information not available	Ciprofloxacin *see* 4-Quinolones	
Calcium-channel Blockers	May inhibit labour and manufacturers advise that diltiazem, mibefradil and some dihydro-pyridines are teratogenic in *animals*, but risk to fetus should be balanced against risk of uncontrolled maternal hypertension	Cisapride	Manufacturer advises avoid
		Cisatracurium	Information not available
		Citalopram	Information not available; *see also* Antidepressants, SSRI
		Cladribine *see* Cytotoxic Drugs	
Candesartan	As for ACE Inhibitors	Clarithromycin	Not known to be harmful but manufacturer advises avoid unless expected benefit outweighs potential risk
Capreomycin	Manufacturer advises teratogenic in *animal* studies		
Captopril *see* ACE Inhibitors			

Table of drugs to be avoided or used with caution in pregnancy *(continued)*

Drug (Trimester of risk)	Comment
Clemastine *see* Antihistamines	
Clindamycin	Not known to be harmful
Clobazam *see* Anxiolytics and Hypnotics	
Clobetasol *see* Corticosteroids	
Clobetasone *see* Corticosteroids	
Clodronate Sodium *see* Bisphosphonates	
Clofibrate (1, 2, 3)	Avoid—theoretical possibility of interference with embryonic growth and development due to anticholesterol effect
Clomiphene	Possible effects on fetal development
Clomipramine *see* Antidepressants, Tricyclic	
Clomocycline *see* Tetracyclines	
Clonazepam *see* Antiepileptics	
Clorazepate *see* Anxiolytics and Hypnotics	
<u>Clozapine</u>	Manufacturer advises avoid
Co-amoxiclav	No evidence of teratogenicity but manufacturer advises avoid unless essential
Codeine *see* Opioid Analgesics	
Colistin (2, 3)	Avoid—possible risk of fetal toxicity
Contraceptives, Oral	Epidemiological evidence suggests no harmful effects on fetus
Corticosteroids (2, 3)	Benefit of treatment, e.g. in asthma, outweighs risk; high systemic doses (>10 mg prednisolone daily) may produce fetal and neonatal adrenal suppression; corticosteroid cover required by mother during labour; monitor closely if fluid retention
Co-trimoxazole	
(1)	Theoretical teratogenic risk (trimethoprim a folate antagonist)
(3)	Neonatal haemolysis and methaemoglobinaemia; fear of increased risk of kernicterus in neonates appears to be unfounded
Cromoglycate	Not known to be harmful; *see also* section 3.1.1 [text]
Cyclizine *see* Antihistamines	
Cyclopenthiazide *see* Diuretics	
Cyclosporin *see* p. 368	
Cyproheptadine *see* Antihistamines	
Cyproterone [ingredient] *see Dianette*®	
Cytotoxic Drugs (1)	Most are teratogenic; *see* section 8.1
Dalteparin *see* Anticoagulants (Heparin)	
Danaparoid	Insufficient information available
Danazol (1, 2, 3)	Avoid; has weak androgenic effects and virilisation of female fetus reported

Drug (Trimester of risk)	Comment
Dapsone (3)	Neonatal haemolysis and methaemoglobinaemia; adequate folate supplements should be given to mother
Debrisoquine *see* Guanethidine	
Deflazacort *see* Corticosteroids	
Demeclocycline *see* Tetracyclines	
Desferrioxamine	Manufacturer advises toxicity in *animal* studies
Desflurane *see* Anaesthetics, General	
Desmopressin	Has low oxytocic effect
Desogestrel *see* Contraceptives, Oral	
Desonide *see* Corticosteroids	
Desoxymethasone *see* Corticosteroids	
Dexamethasone *see* Corticosteroids	
Dexamphetamine	Manufacturer advises avoid (retrospective evidence of uncertain significance suggesting possible embryotoxicity)
Dextromethorphan *see* Opioid Analgesics	
Dextromoramide *see* Opioid Analgesics	
Dextropropoxyphene *see* Opioid Analgesics	
Diamorphine *see* Opioid Analgesics	
Dianette® (1, 2, 3)	Feminisation of male fetus (due to cyproterone)
Diazepam *see* Anxiolytics and Hypnotics	
Diazoxide (2, 3)	Prolonged use may produce alopecia and impaired glucose tolerance in neonate, inhibits uterine activity during labour
Diclofenac *see* NSAIDs	
Didanosine	Information not available; manufacturer advises use only when potential benefit outweighs possible risk
Diflucortolone *see* Corticosteroids	
Diflunisal *see* NSAIDs	
Digoxin	May need dosage adjustment
Dihydrocodeine *see* Opioid Analgesics	
Dihydroergotamine *see* Ergotamine	
Diltiazem *see* Calcium-channel Blockers	
Dimenhydrinate *see* Antihistamines	
Diphenhydramine *see* Antihistamines	
Diphenoxylate *see* Opioid Analgesics	
Diphenylpyraline *see* Antihistamines	
Dipipanone *see* Opioid Analgesics	
Disodium Etidronate *see* Bisphosphonates	
Disodium Pamidronate *see* Bisphosphonates	
Disopyramide (3)	May induce labour
Distigmine	Manufacturer advises avoid (may stimulate uterine contractions)
Disulfiram (1)	High concentrations of acetaldehyde which occur in presence of alcohol may be teratogenic

Table of drugs to be avoided or used with caution in pregnancy (*continued*)

Drug (Trimester of risk)	Comment	Drug (Trimester of risk)	Comment
Diuretics	Not used to treat hypertension in pregnancy	Fenofibrate (1, 2, 3)	Manufacturer advises toxicity in *animal* studies; *see also* Clofibrate
(1)	Manufacturers advise avoid acetazolamide and torasemide (toxicity in *animal* studies)	Fenoprofen *see* NSAIDs	
(3)	Thiazides may cause neonatal thrombocytopenia	Fenoterol *see* section 3.1.1 [text]	
Docetaxel *see* Cytotoxic Drugs		Fentanyl *see* Opioid Analgesics	
Domperidone	Manufacturer advises avoid	Fenticonazole	Manufacturer advises avoid unless essential
Dornase alfa	No evidence of teratogenicity; manufacturer advises use only when benefit outweighs risk	Fexofenadine *see* Antihistamines	
Dothiepin *see* Antidepressants, Tricyclic		Filgrastim	Toxicity in *animal* studies; manufacturer advises use only if expected therapeutic benefit outweighs possible risk
Doxazosin *see* Alpha-blockers (post-synaptic)			
Doxepin *see* Antidepressants, Tricyclic		Finasteride (1, 2, 3)	Avoid unprotected intercourse (see section 6.4.2). May cause feminisation of male fetus
Doxycycline *see* Tetracyclines			
Doxylamine *see* Antihistamines		Flavoxate	Manufacturer advises avoid unless no safer alternative
Droperidol *see* Antipsychotics			
Dydrogesterone *see* Progestogens		Flecainide	Manufacturer advises toxicity in *animal* studies
Econazole	Not known to be harmful		
Eformoterol	Manufacturers advise use only when potential benefit outweighs risk; *see also* section 3.1.1.1 [text]	Fluclorolone *see* Corticosteroids	
		Fluconazole	Manufacturer advises avoid (toxicity at high doses in *animal* studies)
Enalapril *see* ACE Inhibitors			
Enflurane *see* Anaesthetics, General		Flucytosine (1)	Possible teratogenic risk
Enoxaparin *see* Anticoagulants (Heparin)			
Ephedrine	Not known to be harmful	Fludarabine *see* Cytotoxic Drugs	
Epoetin	Information not available— manufacturers advise avoid unless essential	Flunisolide *see* Corticosteroids	
		Flunitrazepam *see* Anxiolytics and Hypnotics	
Ergotamine (1, 2, 3)	Oxytocic effects on the pregnant uterus	Fluocinolone *see* Corticosteroids	
		Fluocinonide *see* Corticosteroids	
Erythromycin	Not known to be harmful	Fluocortolone *see* Corticosteroids	
Esmolol *see* Beta-blockers		Fluoxetine *see* Antidepressants, SSRI	
Ethacrynic acid *see* Diuretics		Flupenthixol *see* Antipsychotics	
Ether *see* Anaesthetics, General		Fluphenazine *see* Antipsychotics	
Ethinyloestradiol *see* Contraceptives, Oral		Flurandrenolone *see* Corticosteroids	
Ethionamide (1)	May be teratogenic	Flurazepam *see* Anxiolytics and Hypnotics	
		Flurbiprofen *see* NSAIDs	
Ethosuximide (1)	May possibly be teratogenic; *see* Antiepileptics	Fluticasone *see* Corticosteroids	
		Fluvastatin *see* Statins	
Ethynodiol *see* Contraceptives, Oral		Fluvoxamine *see* Antidepressants, SSRI	
Etidronate Disodium *see* Bisphosphonates		Foscarnet	Manufacturer advises avoid
Etodolac *see* NSAIDs		Fosinopril *see* ACE Inhibitors	
Etomidate *see* Anaesthetics, General		Framycetin *see* Aminoglycosides	
Etoposide *see* Cytotoxic Drugs		Frusemide *see* Diuretics	
Famciclovir *see* Aciclovir		Gabapentin *see* Antiepileptics	
Fansidar®		Gamolenic Acid	Manufacturer advises caution (but no teratogenic effects in *animals*)
(1)	Possible teratogenic risk (pyrimethamine a folate antagonist)		
		Ganciclovir	Avoid—teratogenic risk; *see also* p. 280
(3)	Neonatal haemolysis and methaemoglobinaemia; fear of increased risk of kernicterus in neonates appears to be unfounded *see also* Antimalarials	Gemcitabine *see* Cytotoxic Drugs	
		Gemfibrozil *see* Clofibrate	
		Gentamicin *see* Aminoglycosides	
		Gestodene *see* Contraceptives, Oral	
		Gestrinone (1, 2, 3)	Avoid
Felodipine *see* Calcium-channel Blockers		Glibenclamide *see* Sulphonylureas	
Fenbufen *see* NSAIDs		Gliclazide *see* Sulphonylureas	

Table of drugs to be avoided or used with caution in pregnancy (*continued*)

Drug (Trimester of risk)	Comment
Glimepiride *see* Sulphonylureas	
Glipizide *see* Sulphonylureas	
Gliquidone *see* Sulphonylureas	
Gold	
Auranofin	Manufacturer advises teratogenicity in *animal* studies; effective contraception should be used during and for at least 6 months after treatment
Aurothiomalate (1, 2, 3)	Manufacturer advises avoid
Goserelin	Avoid—manufacturer advises theoretical risk of toxicity
Granisetron	Information not available; manufacturer advises use only when compelling reasons
Griseofulvin	Avoid (fetotoxicity and teratogenicity in *animals*); effective contraception required during and for at least 1 month after treatment (**important:** effectiveness of oral contraceptives reduced, see p. 272); also men should avoid fathering a child during and for at least 6 months after treatment
Growth Hormone *see* Somatropin	
Guanethidine (3)	Postural hypotension and reduced uteroplacental perfusion, should not be used to treat hypertension in pregnancy
Halcinonide *see* Corticosteroids	
Halofantrine (1)	Manufacturer advises toxicity in *animal* studies
Haloperidol *see* Antipsychotics	
Halothane *see* Anaesthetics, General	
Heparin *see* Anticoagulants	
5HT₁ Agonists	Limited experience—manufacturers advise avoid unless expected benefit to mother outweighs any possible risk to fetus
Hydralazine (1)	Manufacturer advises toxicity in *animal* studies
Hydrochlorothiazide *see* Diuretics	
Hydrocortisone *see* Corticosteroids	
Hydroflumethiazide *see* Diuretics	
Hydromorphone *see* Opioid Analgesics	
Hydroxychloroquine	Avoid for rheumatic disease (but for malaria *see* Antimalarials)
Hydroxyprogesterone *see* Progestogens	
Hydroxyzine *see* Antihistamines	
Hypnotics *see* Anxiolytics and Hypnotics	
Ibuprofen *see* NSAIDs	
Idarubicin *see* Cytotoxic Drugs	
Idoxuridine	Manufacturers advise toxicity in *animal* studies

Drug (Trimester of risk)	Comment
Imipenem [ingredient] *see* Primaxin®	
Imipramine *see* Antidepressants, Tricyclic	
Immunosuppressants *see* section 8.1	
Indapamide *see* Diuretics	
Indinavir	Information not available; manufacturer advises use only if potential benefit justifies potential risk
Indomethacin *see* NSAIDs	
Insulin (1, 2, 3)	Insulin requirements should be assessed frequently by an experienced diabetic physician
Interferons	Manufacturers recommend avoid unless compelling reasons
Iodine and Iodides (2, 3)	Neonatal goitre and hypothyroidism
Radioactive iodine (1, 2, 3)	Permanent hypothyroidism—avoid
Iodoform *see* Povidone-iodine	
Irbesartan	As for ACE Inhibitors
Irinotecan *see* Cytotoxic Drugs	
Isocarboxazid *see* MAOIs	
Isoflurane *see* Anaesthetics, General	
Isotretinoin (1, 2, 3)	Teratogenic; effective contraception must be used for at least 1 month before oral treatment, during treatment and for at least 1 month after stopping; also avoid topical treatment
Isradipine *see* Calcium-channel Blockers	
Itraconazole	Manufacturer advises use only in life-threatening situations (toxicity at high doses in *animal* studies)
Kanamycin *see* Aminoglycosides	
Ketamine *see* Anaesthetics, General	
Ketoconazole	Manufacturer advises teratogenicity in *animal* studies; packs carry a warning to avoid in pregnancy
Ketoprofen *see* NSAIDs	
Ketorolac *see* NSAIDs	
Ketotifen *see* Antihistamines	
Labetalol *see* Beta-blockers	
Lacidipine *see* Calcium-channel Blockers	
Lamivudine	Information not available; manufacturer advises avoid during first trimester
Lamotrigine *see* Antiepileptics	
Lansoprazole	Manufacturer advises avoid
Latanoprost	Manufacturer advises avoid
Lenograstim	Toxicity in *animal* studies; manufacturer advises use only if expected therapeutic benefit outweighs possible risk
Levocabastine *see* Antihistamines	
Levodopa	Manufacturers advise toxicity in *animal* studies

Table of drugs to be avoided or used with caution in pregnancy (*continued*)

Drug (Trimester of risk)	Comment	Drug (Trimester of risk)	Comment
Levonorgestrel *see* Contraceptives, Oral		Metaraminol (1, 2, 3)	Avoid—may reduce placental perfusion
Lignocaine *see* Anaesthetics, Local		Metformin (1, 2, 3)	Avoid
Lisinopril *see* ACE Inhibitors			
Lithium (1, 2, 3)	Dose requirements increased; neonatal goitre reported; lithium toxicity (hypotonia and cyanosis) in neonate if maternal therapy poorly controlled	Methadone *see* Opioid Analgesics	
		Methohexitone *see* Anaesthetics, General	
		Methotrexate *see* Cytotoxic Drugs; for additional advice relating to women and men, *see also* p. 493	
		Methotrimeprazine *see* Antipsychotics	
Lofepramine *see* Antidepressants, Tricyclic		Methylphenidate	Limited experience; manufacturer advises avoid unless potential benefit outweighs risk
Loprazolam *see* Anxiolytics and Hypnotics			
Loratadine *see* Antihistamines			
Lorazepam *see* Anxiolytics and Hypnotics			
Lormetazepam *see* Anxiolytics and Hypnotics		Methylphenobarbitone *see* Antiepileptics	
Losartan	As for ACE Inhibitors	Methylprednisolone *see* Corticosteroids	
Lymecycline *see* Tetracyclines		Metoclopramide	Not known to be harmful but manufacturer advises use only when compelling reasons
Madopar® *see* Levodopa			
Malarone®	Manufacturer advises avoid unless essential		
		Metolazone *see* Diuretics	
Maloprim®		Metoprolol *see* Beta-blockers	
(1)	Possible teratogenic risk (pyrimethamine a folate antagonist)	Metronidazole	Manufacturer advises avoidance of high-dose regimens
(3)	Neonatal haemolysis and methaemoglobinaemia (due to dapsone); adequate folate supplements should be given to mother; *see also* Antimalarials	Metyrapone	Avoid (may impair biosynthesis of fetal-placental steroids)
		Mianserin *see* Antidepressants, Tricyclic (and related)	
		Mibefradil *see* Calcium-channel blockers	
MAOIs (including moclobemide) (1, 2, 3)	No evidence of harm but manufacturers advise avoid unless compelling reasons	Miconazole	Manufacturer advises avoid unless essential
		Mifepristone	Manufacturer advises that if treatment fails, essential that pregnancy be terminated by another method
Maprotiline *see* Antidepressants, Tricyclic (and related)			
Mebendazole	Manufacturer advises toxicity in *animal* studies		
		Minocycline *see* Tetracyclines	
Mefenamic Acid *see* NSAIDs		Minoxidil (3)	Neonatal hirsutism reported
Mefloquine (1)	Manufacturer advises teratogenicity in *animal* studies; avoid for prophylaxis, *see* p. 284		
		Misoprostol (1, 2, 3)	Avoid; increases uterine tone
		Mitomycin *see* Cytotoxic Drugs	
Mefruside *see* Diuretics		Moclobemide *see* MAOIs	
Meloxicam *see* NSAIDs		Moexipril *see* ACE Inhibitors	
Melphalan *see* Cytotoxic Drugs		Molgramostim	Manufacturer advises toxicity in *animal* studies
Menadiol (3)	Neonatal haemolytic anaemia, hyperbilirubinaemia and increased risk of kernicterus in jaundiced infants		
		Moracizine	Information not available
		Morphine *see* Opioid Analgesics	
		Moxonidine	Information not available
Meprobamate *see* Anxiolytics and Hypnotics		Mycophenolate Mofetil	Avoid; effective contraception required during and for 6 weeks after discontinuation of treatment
Meptazinol *see* Opioid Analgesics			
Meropenem	Information not available; manufacturer advises use only if potential benefit justifies potential risk		
		Nabumetone *see* NSAIDs	
		Nadolol *see* Beta-blockers	
Mesalazine	Negligible quantities cross placenta	Nafarelin	Avoid
		Nalbuphine *see* Opioid Analgesics	
Mesna	Not known to be harmful; *see also* section 8.1	Nalidixic acid *see* 4-Quinolones	
		Naloxone	Manufacturer advises use only if expected benefit outweighs potential risk
Mesterolone *see* Androgens			
Mestranol *see* Contraceptives, Oral			

Table of drugs to be avoided or used with caution in pregnancy (*continued*)

Drug (Trimester of risk)	Comment	Drug (Trimester of risk)	Comment
Nandrolone *see* Anabolic Steroids		Olanzapine	Manufacturer advises use only if potential benefit outweighs risk
Naproxen *see* NSAIDs			
Naratriptan *see* 5HT$_1$ Agonists			
Narcotic Analgesics *see* Opioid Analgesics		Omeprazole	Manufacturer advises toxicity in *animal* studies
Nedocromil *see* section 3.1.1 [text]			
Nefazodone	Information not available; manufacturer advises use only if clearly needed	Ondansetron	No information available; manufacturer advises avoid unless potential benefit outweighs possible risk
Nefopam	Information not available; manufacturer advises avoid unless no safer treatment	Opioid Analgesics (3)	Depress neonatal respiration; withdrawal effects in neonates of dependent mothers; gastric stasis and risk of inhalation pneumonia in mother during labour
Neomycin *see* Aminoglycosides			
Neostigmine (3)	Neonatal myasthenia with large doses		
Netilmicin *see* Aminoglycosides			
Nicardipine *see* Calcium-channel Blockers		Orphenadrine	Information not available
Nicorandil	Information not available	Oxazepam *see* Anxiolytics and Hypnotics	
Nicotine (1,2,3)	Avoid	Oxprenolol *see* Beta-blockers	
		Oxybutynin	Manufacturer advises toxicity at high doses in *animal* studies
Nifedipine *see* Calcium-channel Blockers			
Nimodipine *see* Calcium-channel Blockers		Oxypertine *see* Antipsychotics	
Nisoldipine *see* Calcium-channel Blockers		Oxytetracycline *see* Tetracyclines	
Nitrazepam *see* Anxiolytics and Hypnotics		Paclitaxel *see* Cytotoxic Drugs	
Nitrofurantoin (3)	May produce neonatal haemolysis if used at term	Pamidronate Disodium *see* Bisphosphonates	
		Pancreatin	Not known to be harmful
Nitrous oxide *see* Anaesthetics, General		Pantoprazole	Information not available; manufacturer advises avoid unless benefit exceeds potential risk
Nizatidine	Manufacturer advises toxicity at high doses in *animal* studies		
Noradrenaline (1, 2, 3)	Avoid—may reduce placental perfusion	Papaveretum *see* Opioid Analgesics	
		Paracetamol	Not known to be harmful
Norethisterone *see* Contraceptives, Oral		Paroxetine *see* Antidepressants, SSRI	
Norfloxacin *see* 4-Quinolones		Penicillamine (1, 2, 3)	Fetal abnormalities reported rarely; avoid if possible
Norgestimate *see* Contraceptives, Oral			
Nortriptyline *see* Antidepressants, Tricyclic		Penicillins	Not known to be harmful
NSAIDs	Most manufacturers advise avoid (or avoid unless expected benefit outweighs potential risk); ketorolac contra-indicated during pregnancy, labour and delivery	Pentamidine isethionate	Manufacturer advises avoid unless essential
		Pentazocine *see* Opioid Analgesics	
		Pericyazine *see* Antipsychotics	
		Perindopril *see* ACE Inhibitors	
(3)	With regular use closure of fetal ductus arteriosus *in utero* and possibly persistent pulmonary hypertension of the newborn. Delayed onset and increased duration of labour	Perphenazine *see* Antipsychotics	
		Pethidine *see* Opioid Analgesics	
		Phenelzine *see* MAOIs	
		Phenindamine *see* Antihistamines	
		Phenindione *see* Anticoagulants, Oral	
		Pheniramine *see* Antihistamines	
Nystatin	Information not available, but absorption from gastro-intestinal tract negligible	Phenobarbitone (1, 3)	Congenital malformations. Neonatal bleeding tendency—prophylactic vitamin K$_1$ for mother before delivery (as well as for neonate); *see also* Antiepileptics
Octreotide (1, 2, 3)	Avoid; possible effect on fetal growth		
Oestrogens *see* Contraceptives, Oral		Phenothiazines *see* Antipsychotics	
Ofloxacin *see* 4-Quinolones		Phentolamine	Information not available

Table of drugs to be avoided or used with caution in pregnancy (*continued*)

Drug (Trimester of risk)	Comment	Drug (Trimester of risk)	Comment
Phenytoin (1, 3)	Congenital malformations (screening advised); adequate folate supplements should be given to mother (e.g. folic acid 5 mg daily). Neonatal bleeding tendency—prophylactic vitamin K_1 for mother before delivery (as well as for neonate). Caution in interpreting plasma concentrations—bound may be reduced but free (i.e. effective) unchanged; *see also* Antiepileptics	Propofol *see* Anaesthetics, General	
		Propranolol *see* Beta-blockers	
		Propylthiouracil (2, 3)	Neonatal goitre and hypothyroidism
		Prothionamide (1)	May be teratogenic
		Protriptyline *see* Antidepressants, Tricyclic	
		Pseudoephedrine	Not known to be harmful
		Pyridostigmine (3)	Neonatal myasthenia with large doses
Pholcodine *see* Opioid Analgesics		Pyrimethamine (1)	Theoretical teratogenic risk (folate antagonist); adequate folate supplements should be given to mother; *see also* Antimalarials
Pilocarpine	Avoid—smooth muscle stimulant		
Pimozide *see* Antipsychotics			
Pindolol *see* Beta-blockers			
Piperazine	No clinical evidence of harm but packs sold to the general public carry a warning to avoid in pregnancy except on medical advice	Quetiapine	Manufacturer advises use only if potential benefit outweighs risk
		Quinagolide	Manufacturer advises discontinue when pregnancy confirmed unless medical reason for continuing
Piperacillin *see* Penicillins			
Pipothiazine *see* Antipsychotics			
Piracetam	Manufacturer advises avoid	Quinapril *see* ACE Inhibitors	
Piroxicam *see* NSAIDs		Quinine (1)	High doses are teratogenic; but in malaria benefit of treatment outweighs risk
Podophyllotoxin	Avoid		
Podophyllum resin (1, 2, 3)	Avoid—neonatal death and teratogenesis have been reported	4-Quinolones (1, 2, 3)	Arthropathy in *animal* studies
		Raltitrexed *see* Cytotoxic Drugs	
Polythiazide *see* Diuretics		Ramipril *see* ACE Inhibitors	
Povidone-iodine (2, 3)	Sufficient iodine may be absorbed to affect the fetal thyroid	Reboxetine	No information available— manufacturer advises avoid (and discontinue if pregnancy occurs)
Pravastatin *see* Statins			
Prazosin *see* Alpha-blockers (post-synaptic)		Remifentanil	Information not available; *see also* Opioid Analgesics
Prednisolone *see* Corticosteroids			
Prednisone *see* Corticosteroids		Reproterol *see* section 3.1.1 [text]	
Prilocaine (3)	Neonatal methaemoglobinaemia; *see also* Anaesthetics, Local	Reteplase *see* Streptokinase	
		Rifabutin	Information not available
Primaquine (3)	Neonatal haemolysis and methaemoglobinaemia; *see also* Antimalarials	Rifampicin (1)	Manufacturers advise very high doses teratogenic in *animal* studies; *see also* p. 261
Primaxin®	Manufacturer advises toxicity in *animal* studies	(3)	Risk of neonatal bleeding may be increased
Primidone *see* Phenobarbitone		Riluzole	No information available; manufacturer advises avoid
Procaine (3)	Neonatal methaemoglobinaemia; *see also* Anaesthetics, Local	Risperidone	Manufacturer advises use only if potential benefit outweighs risk
Prochlorperazine *see* Antipsychotics			
Progestogens (1)	High doses may possibly be teratogenic	Ritodrine	For use in premature labour see section 7.1.3
Proguanil	Adequate folate supplements should be given to mother; *see also* Antimalarials	Ritonavir	No information available; manufacturer advises use only if potential benefit clearly outweighs potential risk
Promazine *see* Antipsychotics		Salbutamol	For use in asthma *see* section 3.1.1 [text]
Promethazine *see* Antihistamines		(3)	For use in premature labour *see* section 7.1.3
Propafenone	Information not available; manufacturer advises avoid	Salcatonin *see* Calcitonin	

Table of drugs to be avoided or used with caution in pregnancy (*continued*)

Drug (Trimester of risk)	Comment
Salicylates *see* Aspirin	
Salmeterol *see* section 3.1.1 [text]	
Saquinavir	No information available
Sertindole	Manufacturer advises avoid
Sertraline *see* Antidepressants, SSRI	
Sevoflurane *see* Anaesthetics, General	
Simvastatin *see* Statins	
Sodium Aurothiomalate *see* Gold	
Sodium Clodronate *see* Bisphosphonates	
Sodium Cromoglycate *see* Cromoglycate	
Sodium Valproate *see* Valproate	
Somatropin	Discontinue if pregnancy occurs—no information available but theoretical risk
Sotalol *see* Beta-blockers	
Spironolactone	Manufacturers advise toxicity in *animal* studies
Stanozolol *see* Anabolic Steroids	
Statins	Avoid—congenital anomalies reported; decreased synthesis of cholesterol possibly affects fetal development
Stavudine	No information available
Stilboestrol (1)	High doses associated with vaginal carcinoma, urogenital abnormalities, and reduced fertility in female offspring
Streptokinase (1, 2, 3)	Possibility of premature separation of placenta in first 18 weeks; theoretical possibility of fetal haemorrhage throughout pregnancy; avoid postpartum use—maternal haemorrhage
Streptomycin *see* Aminoglycosides	
Sulfadoxine *see* Sulphonamides	
Sulfametopyrazine *see* Sulphonamides	
Sulindac *see* NSAIDs	
Sulphadiazine *see* Sulphonamides	
Sulphadimidine *see* Sulphonamides	
Sulphasalazine (3)	Theoretical risk of neonatal haemolysis; adequate folate supplements should be given to mother
Sulphonamides (3)	Neonatal haemolysis and methaemoglobinaemia; fear of increased risk of kernicterus in neonates appears to be unfounded
Sulphonylureas (3)	Neonatal hypoglycaemia; insulin is normally substituted in all diabetics; if oral drugs are used therapy should be stopped at least 2 days before delivery
Sulpiride *see* Antipsychotics	
Sumatriptan *see* 5HT$_1$ Agonists	
Suxamethonium	Mildly prolonged maternal paralysis may occur
Tacrolimus	Avoid; manufacturer advises toxicity in *animal* studies
Tamoxifen	Avoid—possible effects on fetal development; effective contraception must be used during treatment and for 2 months after stopping
Tazarotene	Avoid; effective contraception required
Temazepam *see* Anxiolytics and Hypnotics	
Tenoxicam *see* NSAIDS	
Terazosin *see* Alpha-blockers (post-synaptic)	
Terbinafine	Information not available
Terbutaline	For use in asthma *see* section 3.1.1 [text]
(3)	For use in premature labour *see* section 7.1.3
Terfenadine *see* Antihistamines	
Testosterone *see* Androgens	
Tetracyclines (1)	Effects on skeletal development in *animal* studies
(2, 3)	Dental discoloration; maternal hepatotoxicity with large parenteral doses
Theophylline (3)	Neonatal irritability and apnoea have been reported
Thiabendazole (1)	Teratogenic in *animal* studies
Thiazides (3)	May cause neonatal thrombocytopenia; *see also* Diuretics
Thiopentone *see* Anaesthetics, General	
Thioridazine *see* Antipsychotics	
Thymoxamine	Manufacturer advises avoid
Thyroxine *see* section 6.2.1	
Tiaprofenic Acid *see* NSAIDs	
Tiludronic Acid *see* Bisphosphonates	
Timolol *see* Beta-blockers	
Tinidazole	Manufacturer advises avoid in first trimester
Tinzaparin	Manufacturer advises avoid unless no safer alternative
Tizanidine	Information not available; manufacturer advises use only when potential benefit outweighs risk
Tobramycin *see* Aminoglycosides	
Tocopheryl Acetate (1, 2, 3)	No evidence of safety of high doses
Tolbutamide *see* Sulphonylureas	
Tolcapone	Manufacturer advises avoid unless potential benefit outweighs risk
Tolfenamic Acid *see* NSAIDs	
Topiramate	Manufacturer advises avoid unless potential benefit outweighs potential risk; *see also* Antiepileptics
Topotecan *see* Cytotoxic Drugs	
Torasemide *see* Diuretics	

Table of drugs to be avoided or used with caution in pregnancy (*continued*)

Drug (Trimester of risk)	Comment	Drug (Trimester of risk)	Comment
Tramadol	Information not available; *see also* Opioid Analgesics	Vaccines (live) (1)	Theoretical risk of congenital malformations, but need for vaccination may outweigh possible risk to fetus (*see also* p. 516); avoid MMR and Rubella vaccines but see p.528
Trandolapril *see* ACE Inhibitors			
Tranylcypromine *see* MAOIs			
Trazodone *see* Antidepressants, Tricyclic (and related)		Valaciclovir	Information not available; *see also* Aciclovir
Tretinoin (1, 2, 3)	Teratogenic; effective contraception must be used for at least 1 month before oral treatment, during treatment and for at least 1 month after stopping; also avoid topical treatment	Valproate (1, 3)	Increased risk of neural tube defects (counselling and screening advised— **important**: see also p. 210); neonatal bleeding and neonatal hepatotoxicity also reported; *see also* Antiepileptics
Triamcinolone *see* Corticosteroids		Valsartan	As for ACE Inhibitors
Triamterene *see* Diuretics		Vancomycin	Little information available; manufacturer advises avoid unless expected benefit outweighs potential risk
Tribavirin	Avoid; manufacturer advises teratogenicity in *animal* studies		
Triclofos *see* Anxiolytics and Hypnotics		Venlafaxine	Information not available
Trifluoperazine *see* Antipsychotics		Verapamil *see* Calcium-channel Blockers	
Trilostane (1, 2, 3)	Interferes with placental sex hormone production	Vigabatrin	Congenital anomalies reported—manufacturer advises avoid; *see also* Antiepileptics
Trimeprazine *see* Antihistamines			
Trimetaphan (3)	Avoid; risk of paralytic ileus in newborn	Viloxazine *see* Antidepressants, Tricyclic (and related)	
Trimethoprim (1)	Theoretical teratogenic risk (folate antagonist)	Vinorelbine *see* Cytotoxic Drugs	
Trimetrexate	Avoid (fetotoxicity and teratogenicity in *animals*); avoid conception for at least 6 months after administration to woman or man	Vitamin A (1)	Excessive doses may be teratogenic; *see also* p. 417
		Warfarin *see* Anticoagulants, Oral	
Trimipramine *see* Antidepressants, Tricyclic		Xamoterol	Manufacturer advises toxicity in *animal* studies
Tripotassium Dicitratobismuthate *see* Bismuth Chelate		Xipamide *see* Diuretics	
Triprolidine *see* Antihistamines		Zalcitabine	Limited information available; use only if potential benefit to mother justifies potential risk to fetus
Tropisetron	Manufacturer advises toxicity in *animal* studies		
Tulobuterol *see* section 3.1.1 [text]		Zidovudine	Limited information available; manufacturer advises use only if clearly indicated; *see also* p. 278
Urokinase (1, 2, 3)	Avoid; possibility of premature separation of placenta in first 18 weeks; theoretical possibility of fetal haemorrhage throughout pregnancy; also avoid postpartum use—maternal haemorrhage		
		Zolmitriptan *see* 5HT$_1$ Agonists	
		Zolpidem *see* Anxiolytics and Hypnotics	
		Zopiclone *see* Anxiolytics and Hypnotics	
		Zuclopenthixol *see* Antipsychotics	

Appendix 5: Breast-feeding

Administration of some drugs (e.g. ergotamine) to nursing mothers may cause toxicity in the infant, whereas administration of others (e.g. digoxin), has little effect on the neonate. Some drugs inhibit lactation (e.g. bromocriptine).

Toxicity to the infant can occur if the drug enters the milk in pharmacologically significant quantities. Milk concentrations of some drugs (e.g. iodides), may exceed those in the maternal plasma so that therapeutic doses in the mother may cause toxicity to the infant. Some drugs inhibit the infant's sucking reflex (e.g. phenobarbitone). Drugs in breast milk may, at least theoretically, cause hypersensitivity in the infant even when concentrations are too low for a pharmacological effect.

The following table lists drugs:

which should be used with caution or which are contra-indicated in breast-feeding for the reasons given above;

which, on present evidence, may be given to the mother during breast-feeding, because they appear in milk in amounts which are too small to be harmful to the infant;

which are not known to be harmful to the infant although they are present in milk in significant amounts.

For many drugs there is insufficient evidence available to provide guidance and it is advisable only to administer essential drugs to a mother during breast-feeding. Because of the inadequacy of currently available information on drugs in breast milk the following table should be used only as a guide; absence from the table does not imply safety.

Table of drugs present in breast milk

Products introduced or amended since publication of BNF No. 34 (September 1997) are <u>underlined</u>.

Drug	Comment	Drug	Comment
Acamprosate	Manufacturer advises avoid	<u>Amisulpride</u>	No information available—manufacturer advises avoid
Acarbose	Manufacturer advises avoid		
Acebutolol *see* Beta-blockers		Amitriptyline *see* Antidepressants, Tricyclic	
Aceclofenac	No information available—manufacturer advises avoid	Amlodipine	No information available—manufacturer advises avoid
Acemetacin	Manufacturer advises avoid	Amorolfine	No information available—manufacturer advises avoid
Acetazolamide	Amount too small to be harmful		
Acetohexamide *see* Sulphonylureas		Amoxapine *see* Antidepressants, Tricyclic	
Aciclovir	Significant amount in milk after systemic administration	Amphetamines	Significant amount in milk. Avoid
Acitretin	Avoid	Amphotericin	No information available
Acrivastine *see* Antihistamines		Amylobarbitone *see* Barbiturates	
Adapalene	No information available—manufacturer advises avoid (if used, avoid application to chest)	Androgens	Avoid; may cause masculinisation in the female infant or precocious development in the male infant; high doses suppress lactation
Alcohol	Large amounts may affect infant and reduce milk consumption		
Alendronic Acid	No information available	Anthraquinones	Avoid; large doses may cause increased gastric motility and diarrhoea (particularly cascara and danthron)
Alfacalcidol *see* Vitamin D			
Alglucerase	No information available		
<u>Allopurinol</u>	Present in milk	Anticoagulants, Oral	Risk of haemorrhage; increased by vitamin-K deficiency; warfarin appears safe but phenindione should be avoided
Alprazolam *see* Benzodiazepines			
<u>Altretamine</u> *see* Cytotoxic Drugs			
Amantadine	Avoid; present in milk; toxicity in infant reported	Antidepressants, SSRI *see* individual entries	
Amethocaine	No information available	Antidepressants, Tricyclic (and related)	Amount of tricyclic antidepressants (including related drugs such as mianserin and trazodone) too small to be harmful but most manufacturers advise avoid; accumulation of doxepin metabolite may cause sedation and respiratory depression
Amifostine	No information available		
Amiloride	No information available—manufacturer advises avoid		
Aminoglutethimide	Avoid		
Aminophylline *see* Theophylline			
Amiodarone	Avoid; present in milk in significant amounts; theoretical risk from release of iodine; *see also* Iodine		

Table of drugs excreted in breast milk (*continued*)

Drug	Comment
Antihistamines	Significant amount of some antihistamines; although not known to be harmful some manufacturers advise avoid; drowsiness in infant reported with clemastine
Antipsychotics	Although amount excreted in milk probably too small to be harmful, *animal* studies indicate possible adverse effects of these drugs on developing nervous system therefore avoid unless absolutely necessary; *see also* amisulpride, chlorpromazine, clozapine, olanzapine, quetiapine, risperidone, sertindole, sulpiride
Apomorphine	No information available
Aspirin	Avoid—possible risk of Reye's syndrome; regular use of high doses could impair platelet function and produce hypoprothrombinaemia in infant if neonatal vitamin K stores low
Astemizole	Manufacturer advises avoid (*see also* section 3.4.1)
Atenolol *see* Beta-blockers	
Atorvastatin	No information available—manufacturer advises avoid
Atropine	May possibly have antimuscarinic effects in infants
Atovaquone	No information available
Auranofin *see* Gold	
Aurothiomalate *see* Gold	
Azapropazone	Avoid—small amounts in milk
Azatadine *see* Antihistamines	
Azithromycin	No information available
Baclofen	Amount too small to be harmful
Barbiturates	Avoid if possible (*see also* phenobarbitone); large doses may cause drowsiness
Beclomethasone *see* Corticosteroids	
Bendrofluazide *see* Thiazides	
Benperidol *see* Antipsychotics	
Benzodiazepines	Avoid repeated doses; lethargy and weight loss may occur in infant
Beta-blockers and Labetalol	Monitor infant; possible toxicity due to beta-blockade but amount of most beta-blockers excreted in milk too small to affect infant; acebutolol, atenolol, nadolol, and sotalol are present in greater amounts than other beta-blockers; manufacturer advises avoid celiprolol
Betamethasone *see* Corticosteroids	
Betaxolol *see* Beta-blockers	
Bezafibrate	Manufacturer advises avoid
Bisoprolol *see* Beta-blockers	
Botulinum Toxin	Manufacturers advise avoid
Bromazepam *see* Benzodiazepines	
Bromocriptine	Suppresses lactation
Brompheniramine *see* Antihistamines	
Buclizine *see* Antihistamines	

Drug	Comment
Bumetanide	No information available—manufacturer advises avoid if possible
Bupivacaine	Amount too small to be harmful
Buprenorphine	Amount too small to be harmful
Buserelin	Small amount present in milk—manufacturer advises avoid
Butobarbitone *see* Barbiturates	
Cabergoline	Suppresses lactation
Caffeine	Regular intake of large amounts can affect infant
Calciferol *see* Vitamin D	
Calcipotriol	No information available
Calcitonin	Avoid; inhibits lactation in *animals*
Calcitriol *see* Vitamin D	
Candesartan	Manufacturer advises avoid
Captopril	Excreted in milk—manufacturers advise avoid
Carbamazepine	Amount probably too small to be harmful but severe skin reaction reported in 1 infant
Carbimazole	Amounts in milk may be sufficient to affect neonatal thyroid function therefore lowest effective dose should be used (*see also* section 6.2.2)
Carisoprodol	Concentrated in milk; no adverse effects reported but best avoided
Carvedilol *see* Beta-blockers	
Cascara *see* Anthraquinones	
Celiprolol *see* Beta-blockers	
Cephalosporins	Excreted in low concentrations
Cerivastatin	Manufacturer advises avoid
Cetirizine *see* Antihistamines	
Chloral Hydrate	Sedation in infant
Chloramphenicol	Use another antibiotic; may cause bone-marrow toxicity in infant; concentration in milk usually insufficient to cause 'grey syndrome'
Chlordiazepoxide *see* Benzodiazepines	
Chlormethiazole	Amount too small to be harmful
Chloroquine	Amount probably too small to be harmful; inadequate for reliable protection against malaria, see section 5.4.1
Chlorothiazide *see* Thiazides	
Chlorpheniramine *see* Antihistamines	
Chlorpromazine	Drowsiness in infant reported; *see* Antipsychotics
Chlorpropamide *see* Sulphonylureas	
Chlortetracycline *see* Tetracyclines	
Chlorthalidone *see* Thiazides	
Cholecalciferol *see* Vitamin D	
Cidofovir	Manufacturer advises avoid
Cilastatin [ingredient] *see Primaxin*®	
Cilazapril	No information available—manufacturer advises avoid
Cimetidine	Significant amount—not known to be harmful but manufacturer advises avoid
Ciprofibrate	No information available

Table of drugs excreted in breast milk (*continued*)

Drug	Comment	Drug	Comment
Ciprofloxacin	Avoid—high concentrations in breast milk	Dapsone	Haemolytic anaemia; although significant amount in milk risk to infant very small
Cisapride	Although amount in milk small manufacturer advises avoid	Deflazacort *see* Corticosteroids	
Cisatracurium	No information available	Demeclocycline *see* Tetracyclines	
Citalopram	Present in milk—manufacturer advises caution	Desogestrel *see* Contraceptives, Oral	
Cladribine *see* Cytotoxic Drugs		Dexamethasone *see* Corticosteroids	
Clarithromycin	Excreted in milk	Dexamphetamine *see* Amphetamines	
Clavulanic acid (in co-amoxiclav, Timentin®)	Trace amounts in milk	Dextropropoxyphene	Amount too small to be harmful
Clemastine *see* Antihistamines		Diamorphine	Therapeutic doses unlikely to affect infant; withdrawal symptoms in infants of dependent mothers; breast-feeding no longer considered best method of treating dependence in offspring of dependent mothers and should be stopped
Clindamycin	Amount probably too small to be harmful but bloody diarrhoea reported in 1 infant		
Clobazam *see* Benzodiazepines			
Clodronate Sodium	No information available		
Clofibrate	Excreted in milk—manufacturer advises avoid	Diazepam *see* Benzodiazepines	
Clomipramine *see* Antidepressants, Tricyclic		Diclofenac	Amount too small to be harmful
Clomocycline *see* Tetracyclines		Didanosine	Breast-feeding not advised in HIV infection
Clorazepate *see* Benzodiazepines		Diflunisal	Manufacturer advises avoid
Clozapine	Manufacturer advises avoid	Digoxin	Amount too small to be harmful
Co-amoxiclav	Trace amounts in milk	Dihydrotachysterol *see* Vitamin D	
Codeine	Amount too small to be harmful	Diltiazem	Significant amount—manufacturers advise avoid
Colchicine	Caution because of its cytotoxicity	Diphenhydramine *see* Antihistamines	
Contraceptives, Oral	Avoid combined oral contraceptives until weaning or for 6 months after birth (adverse effects on lactation); progestogen-only contraceptives do not affect lactation (start 3 weeks after birth or later)	Diphenylpyraline *see* Antihistamines	
		Disodium Etidronate	No information available
		Disodium Pamidronate	Manufacturer advises avoid
		Disopyramide	Present in milk—use only if essential and monitor infant for antimuscarinic effects
Corticosteroids	Continuous therapy with high doses (>10 mg prednisolone daily) could possibly affect infant's adrenal function—monitor carefully	Docetaxel *see* Cytotoxic Drugs	
		Domperidone	Amount probably too small to be harmful
Cortisone Acetate *see* Corticosteroids		Dothiepin *see* Antidepressants, Tricyclic	
Co-trimoxazole	Small risk of kernicterus in jaundiced infants and of haemolysis in G6PD-deficient infants (due to sulphamethoxazole)	Doxazosin	Accumulates in milk—manufacturer advises avoid
		Doxepin *see* Antidepressants, Tricyclic	
		Doxycycline *see* Tetracyclines	
Cough mixtures containing iodides	Use alternative cough mixtures; *see* Iodine	Doxylamine *see* Antihistamines	
		Droperidol *see* Antipsychotics	
Cromoglycate	Unlikely to be excreted in milk	Eformoterol	Manufacturers advise avoid
Cyclopenthiazide *see* Thiazides		Enalapril	Amount probably too small to be harmful
Cycloserine	Amount too small to be harmful	Ephedrine	Irritability and disturbed sleep reported
Cyclosporin	Excreted in milk—manufacturer advises avoid	Epoetin	No information available—manufacturers advise avoid
Cyproheptadine *see* Antihistamines		Ergocalciferol *see* Vitamin D	
Cyproterone Acetate	Caution; possibility of anti-androgen effects in neonate	Ergotamine	Avoid; ergotism may occur in infant; repeated doses may inhibit lactation
Cytotoxic Drugs	Discontinue breast-feeding	Erythromycin	Only small amounts in milk
Danaparoid	No information available	Esmolol *see* Beta-blockers	
Danazol	No data available but avoid because of possible androgenic effects in infant	Ethambutol	Amount too small to be harmful
		Ethamsylate	Significant amount but not known to be harmful
Danthron *see* Anthraquinones			

Table of drugs excreted in breast milk (*continued*)

Drug	Comment
Ethinyloestradiol *see* Contraceptives, Oral	
Ethosuximide	Avoid—significant amount in milk; hyperexcitability and poor suckling reported
Ethynodiol *see* Contraceptives, Oral	
Etidronate Disodium	No information available
Etodolac	Manufacturer advises avoid
Etoposide *see* Cytotoxic Drugs	
Famciclovir	No information available
Famotidine	Amount too small to be harmful
Fansidar®	Small risk of kernicterus in jaundiced infants and of haemolysis in G6PD-deficient infants (due to sulfadoxine)
Felodipine	Appears in milk
Fenbufen	Amount too small to be harmful
Fenoprofen	Amount too small to be harmful
Fentanyl	Manufacturer advises avoid
Fenticonazole	No information available
Fexofenadine *see* Antihistamines	
Filgrastim	No information available—manufacturer advises avoid
Flavoxate	No information available
Flecainide	Significant amount but not known to be harmful
Fluconazole	Significant amount—manufacturer advises avoid
Flucytosine	Manufacturer advises avoid
Fludarabine *see* Cytotoxic Drugs	
Flunitrazepam *see* Benzodiazepines	
Fluoxetine	Significant amounts in milk reported—manufacturer advises avoid
Flupenthixol *see* Antipsychotics	
Fluphenazine *see* Antipsychotics	
Flurazepam *see* Benzodiazepines	
Flurbiprofen	Amount too small to be harmful
Fluticasone *see* Corticosteroids	
Fluvastatin	Manufacturer advises avoid
Fluvoxamine	Manufacturer advises avoid
Fosinopril	Excreted in milk—manufacturer advises avoid
Frusemide	Amount too small to be harmful
Gabapentin	No information available
Ganciclovir	Avoid; *see also* p. 280
Gemcitabine *see* Cytotoxic Drugs	
Gemfibrozil	No information available
Gestodene *see* Contraceptives, Oral	
Gestrinone	Manufacturer advises avoid
Glibenclamide *see* Sulphonylureas	
Gliclazide *see* Sulphonylureas	
Glimepiride *see* Sulphonylureas	
Glipizide *see* Sulphonylureas	
Gliquidone *see* Sulphonylureas	
Glymidine *see* Sulphonylureas	
Gold (auranofin, aurothiomalate)	Caution—excreted in milk; theoretical possibility of rashes and idiosyncratic reactions
Goserelin	Manufacturer advises avoid

Drug	Comment
Granisetron	No information available
Growth Hormone *see* Somatropin	
Halofantrine	Avoid
Haloperidol *see* Antipsychotics	
Halothane	Excreted in milk
Hepatitis A Vaccine	No information available
Hydrochlorothiazide *see* Thiazides	
Hydrocortisone *see* Corticosteroids	
Hydroflumethiazide *see* Thiazides	
Hydroxychloroquine	Avoid—risk of toxicity in infant
Hydroxyzine *see* Antihistamines	
Hyoscine	Amount too small to be harmful
Ibuprofen	Amount too small to be harmful but some manufacturers advise avoid (including topical use)
Idarubicin *see* Cytotoxic Drugs	
Idoxuridine	May possibly make milk taste unpleasant
Imipenem [ingredient] *see* *Primaxin*®	
Imipramine *see* Antidepressants, Tricyclic	
Indapamide	No information available—manufacturer advises avoid
Indinavir	Breast-feeding not advised in HIV infection
Indomethacin	Amount probably too small to be harmful but convulsions reported in one infant—manufacturers advise avoid
Insulin	Amount too small to be harmful
Interferons	No information available
Iodine	Stop breast-feeding; danger of neonatal hypothyroidism or goitre; appears to be concentrated in milk
Radioactive iodine	Breast-feeding contra-indicated after therapeutic doses. With diagnostic doses withhold breast-feeding for at least 24 hours
Irbesartan	Manufacturer advises avoid
Irinotecan *see* Cytotoxic Drugs	
Isoniazid	Monitor infant for possible toxicity; theoretical risk of convulsions and neuropathy; prophylactic pyridoxine advisable in mother and infant
Isotretinoin	Avoid
Itraconazole	Small amounts excreted in milk
Ketoprofen	Amount probably too small to be harmful but manufacturer advises avoid unless essential
Ketorolac	Avoid
Ketotifen *see* Antihistamines	
Labetalol *see* Beta-blockers	
Lacidipine	No information available
Lamivudine	Breast-feeding not advised in HIV infection
Lamotrigine	No information available
Lansoprazole	No information available
Latanoprost	May be present in milk—manufacturer advises avoid

Table of drugs excreted in breast milk (*continued*)

Drug	Comment	Drug	Comment
Lenograstim	No information available	Metronidazole	Significant amount in milk; manufacturer advises avoid large single doses
Levocabastine	Amount too small to be harmful		
Levodopa	No information available	Mexiletine	Amount too small to be harmful
Levonorgestrel *see* Contraceptives, Oral		Mianserin *see* Antidepressants, Tricyclic (and related)	
Lignocaine	Amount too small to be harmful		
Liothyronine	May interfere with neonatal screening for hypothyroidism	Mibefradil	Present in milk—manufacturer advises avoid
Lisinopril	No information available— manufacturer advises caution	Miconazole	No information available
		Mifepristone	No information available— manufacturer advises stop breast-feeding for 14 days after administration
Lithium salts	Present in milk and risk of toxicity in infant— manufacturers advise avoid		
Lofepramine *see* Antidepressants, Tricyclic		Minocycline *see* Tetracyclines	
Loprazolam *see* Benzodiazepines		Minoxidil	Significant amount but not known to be harmful
Loratadine	Excreted in milk—manufacturer advises avoid	Misoprostol	No information available— manufacturer advises avoid
Lorazepam *see* Benzodiazepines			
Lormetazepam *see* Benzodiazepines		Moclobemide	Amount too small to be harmful, but patient leaflet advises avoid
Losartan	Manufacturer advises avoid		
Lymecycline *see* Tetracyclines		Moexipril	No information available— manufacturer advises avoid
Lysuride	May suppress lactation		
Malarone®	Manufacturer advises avoid	Molgramostim	No information available— manufacturer advises avoid (potential for adverse effects in infant)
Maloprim®	Haemolytic anaemia (due to dapsone); risk to infant very small		
Maprotiline *see* Antidepressants, Tricyclic (and related)		Moracizine	Excreted in milk—manufacturer advises avoid
Mebendazole	No information available	Morphine	Therapeutic doses unlikely to affect infant; withdrawal symptoms in infants of dependent mothers; breast-feeding not best method of treating dependence in offspring and should be stopped
Mebeverine	Amount too small to be harmful		
Medroxyprogesterone Acetate *see* Progestogens			
Mefenamic Acid	Amount too small to be harmful, but manufacturer advises avoid		
Mefloquine	Avoid—excreted in milk		
Mefruside *see* Thiazides		Moxonidine	Excreted in milk— manufacturer advises avoid
Meloxicam	No information available— manufacturer advises avoid	Mycophenolate Mofetil	No information available— manufacturer advises avoid
Meprobamate	Avoid; concentration in milk may exceed maternal plasma concentrations fourfold and may cause drowsiness in infant	Nabumetone	No information available— manufacturer advises avoid
Mequitazine *see* Antihistamines		Nadolol *see* Beta-blockers	
Meropenem	Manufacturer advises avoid unless potential benefit justifies potential risk	Nafarelin	No information available
		Nalidixic Acid	Risk to infant very small but one case of haemolytic anaemia reported
Mesalazine	Diarrhoea reported but manufacturers advise negligible amounts detected in breast milk		
		Naloxone	No information available
Mestranol *see* Contraceptives, Oral		Naproxen	Amount too small to be harmful but manufacturers advise avoid
Methadone	Withdrawal symptoms in infant; breast-feeding permissible during maintenance but dose should be as low as possible and infant monitored to avoid sedation	Naratriptan	No information available— manufacturer advises caution
		Nefazodone	No information available
		Neostigmine	Amount probably too small to be harmful; monitor infant
Methotrimeprazine *see* Antipsychotics		Nicardipine	Manufacturer advises avoid
Methyldopa	Amount too small to be harmful	Nicorandil	No information available— manufacturer advises avoid
Methylphenidate	No information available— manufacturer advises avoid		
		Nicotine	Avoid—present in milk
Methylprednisolone *see* Corticosteroids		Nicoumalone *see* Anticoagulants, Oral	
Metoclopramide	Although amount in milk small, avoid unless essential	Nifedipine	Amount too small to be harmful but manufacturers advise avoid
Metolazone *see* Thiazides		Nisoldipine	Manufacturer advises avoid
Metoprolol *see* Beta-blockers		Nitrazepam *see* Benzodiazepines	

Table of drugs excreted in breast milk (*continued*)

Drug	Comment	Drug	Comment
Nitrofurantoin	Only small amounts in milk but could be enough to produce haemolysis in G6PD-deficient infants	Phenytoin	Small amount excreted in milk; manufacturer advises avoid—*but see* section 4.8.1
Nizatidine	Amount too small to be harmful	Pilocarpine	No information available—manufacturer advises avoid
Norethisterone *see* Contraceptives, Oral		Pimozide *see* Antipsychotics	
Norfloxacin	No information available—manufacturer advises avoid	Pindolol *see* Beta-blockers	
		Piperacillin *see* Penicillins	
Norgestimate *see* Contraceptives, Oral		Piracetam	Manufacturer advises avoid
Nortriptyline *see* Antidepressants, Tricyclic		Piroxicam	Amount too small to be harmful
NSAIDs *see* individual entries		Pizotifen	Amount probably too small to be harmful, but patient information leaflet advises avoid
Nystatin	No information available, but absorption from gastro-intestinal tract negligible		
		Polythiazide *see* Thiazides	
Octreotide	Avoid	Povidone-iodine	Avoid; iodine absorbed from vaginal preparations is concentrated in milk
Oestrogens	Avoid; adverse effects on lactation; *see also* Contraceptives, Oral		
		Pravastatin	Small amount excreted in milk—manufacturer advises avoid
Ofloxacin	Manufacturer advises avoid		
Olanzapine	No information available—manufacturer advises avoid	Prazosin	Amount probably too small to be harmful
Omeprazole	No information available	Prednisolone *see* Corticosteroids	
Ondansetron	No information available—manufacturer advises avoid	Prednisone *see* Corticosteroids	
		Primaxin®	No information available—manufacturer advises avoid
Opioid Analgesics *see* individual entries			
Orphenadrine	Excreted in milk—manufacturer advises avoid	Primidone *see* Phenobarbitone	
		Probenecid	No information available
Oxazepam *see* Benzodiazepines		Prochlorperazine *see* Antipsychotics	
Oxitropium	No information available	Procainamide	Excreted in milk—manufacturer advises avoid
Oxprenolol *see* Beta-blockers			
Oxybutynin	Present in milk—manufacturers advise avoid	Progestogens	High doses suppress lactation but *see also* Contraceptives, Oral
Oxypertine *see* Antipsychotics		Proguanil *see* Chloroquine	
Oxytetracycline *see* Tetracyclines		Promazine *see* Antipsychotics	
Pamidronate Disodium	Manufacturer advises avoid	Promethazine *see* Antihistamines	
		Propafenone	No information available—manufacturer advises avoid
Pantoprazole	No information available		
Papaveretum *see* Morphine		Propranolol *see* Beta-blockers	
Paracetamol	Amount too small to be harmful	Propylthiouracil	Monitor infant's thyroid status but amounts in milk probably too small to affect infant; high doses might affect neonatal thyroid function
Paroxetine	Manufacturer advises avoid unless potential benefit outweighs possible risk		
Penicillins	Trace amounts in milk		
Pentamidine isethionate	Manufacturer advises avoid unless essential	Protriptyline *see* Antidepressants, Tricyclic	
		Pseudoephedrine	Amount too small to be harmful
Pergolide	May suppress lactation	Pyrazinamide	Amount too small to be harmful
Pericyazine *see* Antipsychotics		Pyridostigmine	Amount probably too small to be harmful
Perindopril	No information available—manufacturer advises avoid		
		Pyrimethamine	Significant amount—avoid administration of other folate antagonists to infant
Perphenazine *see* Antipsychotics			
Phenindamine *see* Antihistamines			
Phenindione *see* Anticoagulants, Oral		Quetiapine	No information available—manufacturer advises avoid
Pheniramine *see* Antihistamines			
Phenobarbitone	Avoid when possible; drowsiness may occur but risk probably small; one report of methaemo-globinaemia with phenobarbitone and phenytoin	Quinagolide	Suppresses lactation
		Quinalbarbitone *see* Barbiturates	
		Quinapril	No information available—manufacturer advises caution
		Quinidine	Significant amount but not known to be harmful
Phenolphthalein	Avoid; increased gastric motility, diarrhoea, and possibly rash	Raltitrexed *see* Cytotoxic Drugs	
Phentolamine	No information available	Ramipril	Manufacturer advises avoid
Phenylbutazone	Avoid—small amounts in milk	Ranitidine	Significant amount but not known to be harmful

Table of drugs excreted in breast milk (*continued*)

Drug	Comment	Drug	Comment
Ranitidine Bismuth Citrate	No information available—manufacturer advises avoid	Terbutaline	Amount too small to be harmful
Reboxetine	No information available—manufacturer advises avoid	Terfenadine *see* Antihistamines	
Remifentanil	No information available	Tetracyclines	Avoid (although absorption and therefore discoloration of teeth in infant probably usually prevented by chelation with calcium in milk)
Rifabutin	No information available		
Rifampicin	Amount too small to be harmful		
Riluzole	No information available—manufacturer advises avoid		
Risperidone	No information available—manufacturer advises avoid	Theophylline	Irritability in infant reported; modified-release preparations probably safe
Ritonavir	Breast-feeding not advised in HIV infection	Thiamine	Severely thiamine-deficient mothers should avoid breast-feeding as toxic methyl-glyoxal excreted in milk
Saquinavir	Breast-feeding not advised in HIV infection		
Senna *see* Anthraquinones		Thiazides	Amount too small to be harmful; large doses may suppress lactation
Sertindole	No information available—manufacturer advises avoid	Thioridazine *see* Antipsychotics	
Sertraline	No information available	Thyroxine	May interfere with neonatal screening for hypothyroidism
Simvastatin	No information available—manufacturer advises avoid	Tiaprofenic Acid	Amount too small to be harmful
Sodium Clodronate	No information available	Tiludronic Acid	No information available
Sodium Cromoglycate *see* Cromoglycate		Timolol *see* Beta-blockers	
Sodium Valproate *see* Valproate		Tinzaparin	No information available—manufacturer advises avoid
Somatropin	No information available	Tizanidine	No information available—manufacturer advises use only if potential benefit outweighs risk
Sotalol *see* Beta-blockers			
Stavudine	Breast-feeding not advised in HIV infection	Tolazamide *see* Sulphonylureas	
Sulfametopyrazine *see* Sulphonamides		Tolbutamide *see* Sulphonylureas	
Sulindac	No information available	Tolcapone	Present in milk—manufacturer advises avoid
Sulphadiazine *see* Sulphonamides		Tolfenamic Acid	Amount too small to be harmful
Sulphadimidine *see* Sulphonamides		Topiramate	Manufacturer advises avoid
Sulphasalazine	Small amounts in milk (1 report of bloody diarrhoea and rashes); theoretical risk of neonatal haemolysis especially in G6PD-deficient infants	Topotecan *see* Cytotoxic Drugs	
		Torasemide	No information available
		Tramadol	Amount probably too small to be harmful, but manufacturer advises avoid
Sulphinpyrazone	No information available	Trandolapril	Manufacturers advise avoid
Sulphonamides	Small risk of kernicterus in jaundiced infants particularly with long-acting sulphonamides, and of haemolysis in G6PD-deficient infants	Trazodone as for Antidepressants, Tricyclic	
		Tretinoin	Avoid
		Triamcinolone *see* Corticosteroids	
Sulphonylureas	Caution; theoretical possibility of hypoglycaemia in infant	Trifluoperazine *see* Antipsychotics	
		Trimeprazine *see* Antihistamines	
Sulpiride	Best avoided; significant amounts in milk; *see also* Antipsychotics	Trimethoprim	Excreted in milk—short-term use not known to be harmful
Sumatriptan	Present in milk after subcutaneous injection—withhold breast-feeding for 24 hours	Trimetrexate	Manufacturer advises termination of breast-feeding; also breast-feeding not advised in HIV infection
Tacrolimus	Avoid—excreted in milk	Trimipramine *see* Antidepressants, Tricyclic	
Tamoxifen	No information available—manufacturer advises avoid	Triprolidine *see* Antihistamines	
		Tropisetron	No information available
Tazarotene	Manufacturer advises avoid	Tulobuterol	No information available
Teicoplanin	No information available	Valaciclovir	No information available; *see also* Aciclovir
Temazepam *see* Benzodiazepines			
Tenoxicam	No information available	Valproate	Amount too small to be harmful
Terazosin	No information available	Valsartan	Manufacturer advises avoid
Terbinafine	Excreted in milk— manufacturer advises avoid	Vancomycin	Excreted in milk—manufacturer advises avoid
		Venlafaxine	No information available

Table of drugs excreted in breast milk (*continued*)

Drug	Comment
Verapamil	Amount too small to be harmful
Vigabatrin	No information available—manufacturer advises avoid
Viloxazine *see* Antidepressants, Tricyclic (and related)	
Vinorelbine *see* Cytotoxic Drugs	
Vitamin A	Theoretical risk of toxicity in infants of mothers taking large doses
Vitamin D (and related compounds)	Caution with high doses; may cause hypercalcaemia in infant
Warfarin *see* Anticoagulants, Oral	
Xipamide	No information available
Zalcitabine	Breast-feeding not advised in HIV infection
Zidovudine	Breast-feeding not advised in HIV infection
Zolmitriptan	No information available—manufacturer advises caution
Zolpidem	Small amounts excreted in milk—manufacturer advises avoid
Zopiclone	Excreted in milk—manufacturer advises avoid
Zuclopenthixol *see* Antipsychotics	

Appendix 6: Intravenous Additives

INTRAVENOUS ADDITIVES POLICIES. A local policy on the addition of drugs to intravenous fluids should be drawn up by a multi-disciplinary team in each Health Authority and issued as a document to the members of staff concerned.

Centralised additive services are provided in a number of hospital pharmacy departments and should be used in preference to making additions on wards.

The information that follows should be read in conjunction with local policy documents.

Guidelines

1. Drugs should only be added to infusion containers when constant plasma concentrations are needed or when the administration of a more concentrated solution would be harmful.
2. In general, only one drug should be added to any infusion container and the components should be compatible. Ready-prepared solutions should be used whenever possible. Drugs should not normally be added to blood products, mannitol, or sodium bicarbonate. Only specially formulated additives should be used with fat emulsions or amino-acid solutions (see section 9.3).
3. Solutions should be thoroughly mixed by shaking and checked for absence of particulate matter before use.
4. Strict asepsis should be maintained throughout and in general the giving set should not be used for more than 24 hours.
5. The infusion container should be labelled with the patient's name, the name and quantity of additives, and the date and time of addition (and the new expiry date or time). Such additional labelling should not interfere with information on the manufacturer's label that is still valid. When possible, containers should be retained for a period after use in case they are needed for investigation.
6. It is good practice to examine intravenous infusions from time to time while they are running. If cloudiness, crystallisation, change of colour, or any other sign of interaction or contamination is observed the infusion should be discontinued.

Problems

MICROBIAL CONTAMINATION. The accidental entry and subsequent growth of micro-organisms converts the infusion fluid pathway into a potential vehicle for infection with micro-organisms, particularly species of Candida, Enterobacter, and Klebsiella. Ready-prepared infusions containing the additional drugs, or infusions prepared by an additive service (when available) should therefore be used in preference to making extemporaneous additions to infusion containers on wards etc. However, when this is necessary strict aseptic procedure should be followed.

INCOMPATIBILITY. Physical and chemical incompatibilities may occur with loss of potency, increase in toxicity, or other adverse effect. The solutions may become opalescent or precipitation may occur, but in many instances there is no visual indication of incompatibility. Interaction may take place at any point in the infusion fluid pathway, and the potential for incompatibility is increased when more than one substance is added to the infusion fluid.

Common incompatibilities. Precipitation reactions are numerous and varied and may occur as a result of pH, concentration changes, 'salting-out' effects, complexation or other chemical changes. Precipitation or other particle formation must be avoided since, apart from lack of control of dosage on administration, it may initiate or exacerbate adverse effects. This is particularly important in the case of drugs which have been implicated in either thrombophlebitis (e.g. diazepam) or in skin sloughing or necrosis caused by extravasation (e.g. sodium bicarbonate and certain cytotoxic drugs). It is also especially important to effect solution of colloidal drugs and to prevent their subsequent precipitation in order to avoid a pyrogenic reaction (e.g. amphotericin).

It is considered undesirable to mix beta-lactam antibiotics, such as semi-synthetic penicillins and cephalosporins, with proteinaceous materials on the grounds that immunogenic and allergenic conjugates could be formed.

A number of preparations undergo significant loss of potency when added singly or in combination to large volume infusions. Examples include ampicillin in infusions that contain glucose or lactates, mustine hydrochloride in isotonic saline and gentamicin/carbenicillin combinations. The breakdown products of dacarbazine have been implicated in adverse effects.

Blood. Because of the large number of incompatibilities, drugs should not normally be added to blood and blood products for infusion purposes. Examples of incompatibility with blood include hypertonic mannitol solutions (irreversible crenation of red cells), dextrans (rouleaux formation and interference with cross-matching), glucose (clumping of red cells), and oxytocin (inactivated).

If the giving set is not changed after the administration of blood, but used for other infusion fluids, a fibrin clot may form which, apart from blocking the set, increases the likelihood of microbial growth.

Intravenous fat emulsions may break down with coalescence of fat globules and separation of phases when additions such as antibiotics or electrolytes are made, thus increasing the possibility of embolism. Only specially formulated products such as Vitlipid N® (see section 9.3) may be added to appropriate intravenous fat emulsions.

Other infusions that frequently give rise to incompatibility include amino acids, mannitol, and sodium bicarbonate.

Bactericides such as chlorocresol 0.1% or phenylmercuric nitrate 0.001% are present in some injection solutions. The total volume of such solutions added to a container for infusion on one occasion should not exceed 15 mL.

Method

Ready-prepared infusions should be used whenever available. **Potassium chloride** is usually available in concentrations of 20, 27, and 40 mmol/litre in sodium chloride intravenous infusion (0.9%), glucose intravenous infusion (5%) or sodium chloride and glucose intravenous infusion. **Lignocaine hydrochloride** is usually available in concentrations of 0.1 or 0.2% in glucose intravenous infusion (5%).

When addition is required to be made extemporaneously, any product reconstitution instructions such as those relating to concentration, vehicle, mixing, and handling precautions should be strictly followed using an aseptic technique throughout. Once the product has been reconstituted, addition to the infusion fluid should be made immediately in order to minimise microbial contamination and, with certain products, to prevent degradation or other formulation change which may occur; e.g. reconstituted ampicillin injection degrades rapidly on standing, and also may form polymers which could cause sensitivity reactions.

It is also important in certain instances that an infusion fluid of specific pH be used (e.g. **frusemide** injection requires dilution in infusions of pH greater than 5.5).

When drug additions are made it is important to mix thoroughly; additions should not be made to an infusion container that has been connected to a giving set, as mixing is hampered. If the solutions are not thoroughly mixed a concentrated layer of the additive may form owing to differences in density. **Potassium chloride** is particularly prone to this 'layering' effect when added without adequate mixing to infusions packed in non-rigid infusion containers; if such a mixture is administered it may have a serious effect on the heart.

A time limit between addition and completion of administration must be imposed for certain admixtures to guarantee satisfactory drug potency and compatibility. For admixtures in which degradation occurs without the formation of toxic substances, an acceptable limit is the time taken for 10% decomposition of the drug. When toxic substances are produced stricter limits may be imposed. Because of the risk of microbial contamination a maximum time limit of 12 hours should be imposed for additions made elsewhere than in hospital pharmacies offering central additive service.

Certain injections must be protected from light during continuous infusion to minimise oxidation, e.g. amphotericin, dacarbazine, and sodium nitroprusside.

Dilution with a small volume of an appropriate vehicle and administration using a motorised infusion pump is advocated for preparations such as heparin where strict control over administration is required. In this case the appropriate dose may be dissolved in a convenient volume (e.g. 24 to 48 mL) of sodium chloride intravenous infusion (0.9%).

Use of table

The table lists preparations given by three methods:

continuous infusion,

intermittent infusion, and

addition via the drip tubing.

Drugs for **continuous infusion** must be diluted in a large volume infusion. Penicillins and cephalosporins are not usually given by continuous infusion because of stability problems and because adequate plasma and tissue concentrations are best obtained by intermittent infusion. Where it is necessary to administer them by continuous infusion, detailed literature should be consulted.

Drugs that are both compatible and clinically suitable may be given by **intermittent infusion** in a relatively small volume of infusion over a short period of time, e.g. 100 mL in 30 minutes. The method is used if the product is incompatible or unstable over the period necessary for continuous infusion; the limited stability of ampicillin or amoxycillin in large volume glucose or lactate infusions may be overcome in this way.

Intermittent infusion is also used if adequate plasma and tissue concentrations are not produced by continuous infusion as in the case of drugs such as carbenicillin, dacarbazine, gentamicin, and ticarcillin.

An in-line burette may be used for intermittent infusion techniques in order to achieve strict control over the time and rate of administration, especially for infants and children and in intensive care units. Intermittent infusion may also make use of the 'piggy-back' technique provided that no additions are made to the primary infusion. In this method the drug is added to a small secondary container connected to a Y-type injection site on the primary infusion giving set; the secondary solution is usually infused within 30 minutes.

Addition *via* the drip tubing is indicated for a number of cytotoxic drugs in order to minimise extravasation. The preparation is added aseptically *via* the rubber septum of the injection site of a fast-running infusion. In general, drug preparations intended for a bolus effect should be given directly into a separate vein where possible. Failing this, administration may be made *via* the drip tubing provided that the preparation is compatible with the infusion fluid when given in this manner.

Table of drugs given by intravenous infusion

Covers addition to *Glucose intravenous infusion* 5 and 10%, *Sodium chloride intravenous infusion* 0.9%, *Compound sodium chloride intravenous infusion* (Ringer's solution), and *Compound sodium lactate intravenous infusion* (Hartmann's solution). Compatibility with glucose 5% and with sodium chloride 0.9% indicates compatibility with *Sodium chloride and glucose intravenous infusion*. Infusion of a large volume of hypotonic solution should be avoided therefore care should be taken if water for injections is used. The information in the Table relates to the proprietary preparations indicated; for other preparations suitability should be checked with the manufacturer

Abciximab (*ReoPro®*)

Continuous *in* Glucose 5% *or* Sodium chloride 0.9%
Withdraw from vial (through a non-pyrogenic low protein-binding 0.2 or 0.22 micron filter), dilute in infusion fluid and give *via* infusion pump through a non-pyrogenic low protein-binding 0.2 or 0.22 micron filter

Acetylcysteine (*Parvolex®*)

Continuous *in* Glucose 5%
See Emergency Treatment of Poisoning

Aciclovir sodium (*Zovirax IV®*; *Aciclovir IV*, Faulding DBL; *Aciclovir Sodium*, Lennon)

Intermittent *in* Sodium chloride 0.9% *or* Sodium chloride and glucose *or* Compound sodium lactate
For *Zovirax IV®* and *Aciclovir Sodium* (Lennon) initially reconstitute to 25 mg/mL in water for injections or sodium chloride 0.9% then dilute to not more than 5 mg/mL with the infusion fluid; minimum volume 50 mL; to be given over 1 hour; alternatively, may be administered in a concentration of 25 mg/mL using a suitable infusion pump and given over 1 hour; for *Aciclovir IV* (Faulding DBL) dilute to not more than 5 mg/mL with infusion fluid; give over 1 hour

Aclarubicin hydrochloride (*Aclacin®*)

Intermittent *in* Glucose 5% *or* Sodium chloride 0.9%
Dissolve initially in 10 mL water for injections or sodium chloride 0.9% then dilute with 200–500 mL infusion fluid to a concentration of 200–500 micrograms/mL; give over 30–60 minutes and protect from light during administration; pH of glucose infusion should be between 5 and 6

Aldesleukin (*Proleukin®*)

Continuous *in* Glucose 5%
Reconstitute each vial with 1.2 mL water for injections (do not shake or allow to foam); dilute in up to 500 mL glucose 5% containing albumin 0.1% (albumin added and thoroughly mixed in glucose 5% solution before adding aldesleukin); polypropylene, PVC, polyolefin, or glass containers with polyethylene or PVC giving sets may be used; do not use in-line filter

Alfentanil hydrochloride (*Rapifen®* preparations)

Continuous *or* intermittent *in* Glucose 5% *or* Sodium chloride 0.9% *or* Compound sodium lactate

Alglucerase (*Ceredase®*)

Intermittent *in* Sodium chloride 0.9%
Dilute requisite dose of concentrate with infusion fluid to give a final volume of 100 mL; administer over 1–2 hours; use within 3 hours after dilution; use in-line filter

Alprostadil (*Prostin VR®*)

Continuous *in* Glucose 5% *or* Sodium chloride 0.9%
Add directly to the infusion solution avoiding contact with the walls of plastic containers

Alteplase (*Actilyse®*)

Continuous *or* intermittent *in* Sodium chloride 0.9%
Dissolve in water for injections to a concentration of 1 mg/mL and infuse intravenously; alternatively dilute the solution further in the infusion fluid to a concentration of not less than 200 micrograms/mL; not to be infused in glucose solution

Amifostine (*Ethyol®*)

Intermittent *in* Sodium chloride 0.9%
Give over 15 minutes

Amikacin sulphate (*Amikin®*)

Intermittent *in* Glucose 5% *or* Sodium chloride 0.9% *or* Compound sodium lactate
To be given over 30 minutes

Aminophylline

Continuous *in* Glucose 5% *or* Sodium chloride 0.9% *or* Compound sodium lactate

Amiodarone hydrochloride (*Cordarone X®*)

Continuous *or* intermittent *in* Glucose 5%
Suggested initial infusion volume 250 mL given over 20–120 minutes; for repeat infusions up to 1.2 g in max. 500 mL; infusion in extreme emergency see section 2.3.2; should not be diluted to less than 600 micrograms/mL; incompatible with sodium chloride infusion

Amoxycillin sodium (*Amoxil®*)

Intermittent *in* Glucose 5% *or* Sodium chloride 0.9%
Reconstituted solutions diluted and given without delay; suggested volume 100 mL given over 30–60 minutes
via drip tubing *in* Glucose 5% *or* Sodium chloride 0.9% *or* Ringer's solution *or* Compound sodium lactate
Continuous infusion not usually recommended

Amphotericin (colloidal) (*Amphocil®*)

Intermittent *in* Glucose 5%
Initially reconstitute with water for injections (50 mg in 10 mL, 100 mg in 20 mL), shaking gently to dissolve (fluid may be opalescent) then dilute to a concentration of 625 micrograms/mL (1 volume of reconstituted solution with 7 volumes of infusion fluid); give at a rate of 1–2 mg/kg/hour or slower if not tolerated (initial test dose 2 mg of a 100 microgram/mL solution over 10 minutes); incompatible with sodium chloride or other electrolyte solutions, flush existing intravenous line with glucose 5% or use separate line

Amphotericin (lipid complex) (*Abelcet®*)

Intermittent *in* Glucose 5%
Allow suspension to reach room temperature, shake gently to ensure no yellow settlement, withdraw requisite dose (using 17–19 gauge needle) into one or more 20-mL syringes; replace needle on syringe with a 5-micron filter needle provided (fresh needle for each syringe) and dilute to a concentration of 1 mg/mL; preferably give *via* an infusion pump at a rate of 2.5 mg/kg/hour (initial test dose of 1 mg given over 15 minutes); an in-line filter (pore size no less than 5 micron) may be used; do not use sodium chloride or other electrolyte solutions, flush existing intravenous line with glucose 5% or use separate line

Amphotericin (liposomal) (*AmBisome®*)

Intermittent *in* Glucose 5%
Reconstitute each vial with 12 mL water for injections and shake vigorously to produce a preparation containing 4 mg/mL; withdraw requisite dose from vial and introduce into infusion fluid through the 5 micron filter provided to produce a final concentration of 0.2–2 mg/mL; infuse over 30–60 minutes (initial test dose 1 mg over 10 minutes); incompatible with sodium chloride solutions, flush existing intravenous line with glucose 5% or use separate line

Amphotericin sodium deoxycholate complex (*Fungizone®*)

Intermittent *in* Glucose 5%

Reconstitute each vial with 10 mL water for injections and shake immediately to produce a 5 mg/mL colloidal solution; dilute further in infusion fluid to a concentration of 100 micrograms/mL; pH of the glucose must not be below 4.2 (check each container—see product literature for details of buffer); infuse over 2–4 hours, or longer if not tolerated (initial test dose 1 mg over 20–30 minutes); begin infusion immediately after dilution and protect from light; incompatible with sodium chloride solutions, flush existing intravenous line with glucose 5% or use separate line

Ampicillin sodium (*Penbritin®*)

Intermittent *in* Glucose 5% *or* Sodium chloride 0.9%
Reconstituted solutions diluted and given without delay; suggested volume 100 mL given over 30–60 minutes
via drip tubing *in* Glucose 5% *or* Sodium chloride 0.9% *or* Ringer's solution *or* Compound sodium lactate
Continuous infusion not usually recommended

Ampicillin/cloxacillin (sodium salts) (*Ampiclox®*)

Intermittent *in* Glucose 5% *or* Sodium chloride 0.9%
Reconstituted solutions diluted and given without delay; suggested volume 100 mL given over 30–60 minutes
via drip tubing *in* Glucose 5% *or* Sodium chloride 0.9% *or* Ringer's solution *or* Compound sodium lactate

Amsacrine (*Amsidine®*)

Intermittent in Glucose 5%
Reconstitute with diluent provided and dilute to suggested volume 500 mL; give over 60–90 minutes; use glass syringes; incompatible with sodium chloride infusion

Atenolol (*Tenormin®*)

Intermittent *in* Glucose 5% *or* Sodium chloride 0.9%
Suggested infusion time 20 minutes

Atracurium besylate (*Tracrium®*)

Continuous *in* Glucose 5% *or* Sodium chloride 0.9% *or* Compound sodium lactate
Stability varies with diluent

Azathioprine (sodium salt) (*Imuran®*)

via drip tubing *in* Glucose 5% *or* Sodium chloride 0.9%

Azlocillin sodium (*Securopen® 5 g*)

Intermittent *in* Glucose 5 and 10% *or* Sodium chloride 0.9% *or* Ringer's solution
Intermittent infusion suggested for doses over 2 g; to be given over 20–30 minutes

Aztreonam (*Azactam®*)

Intermittent *in* Glucose 5% *or* Sodium chloride 0.9% *or* Ringer's solution *or* Compound sodium lactate
Dissolve initially in water for injections (1 g per 3 mL) then dilute to a concentration of less than 20 mg/mL; to be given over 20–60 minutes

Benzylpenicillin sodium (*Crystapen®*)

Intermittent *in* Glucose 5% *or* Sodium chloride 0.9%
Suggested volume 100 mL given over 30–60 minutes
Continuous infusion not usually recommended

Betamethasone sodium phosphate (*Betnesol®*)

Continuous *or* intermittent *or via* drip tubing *in* Glucose 5% *or* Sodium chloride 0.9%

Bleomycin sulphate Intermittent *in* Sodium chloride 0.9%

To be given slowly; suggested volume 200 mL

Bumetanide (*Burinex®*)

Intermittent *in* Glucose 5% *or* Sodium chloride 0.9%
Suggested volume 500 mL given over 30–60 minutes

Calcium folinate (*Calcium Leucovorin®, Refolinon®*)

Continuous *in* Sodium chloride 0.9%
Calcium Leucovorin® can also be infused in Glucose 5 and 10% or Compound sodium lactate

Calcium gluconate

Continuous *in* Glucose 5% *or* Sodium chloride 0.9%
Avoid bicarbonates, phosphates, or sulphates

Carboplatin (*Paraplatin®*)

Intermittent *in* Glucose 5% *or* Sodium chloride 0.9%
Final concentration as low as 500 micrograms/mL; give over 15–60 minutes

Carmustine (*BiCNU®*)

Intermittent *in* Glucose 5% *or* Sodium chloride 0.9%
Reconstitute with diluent provided; give over 1–2 hours

Cefodizime sodium (*Timecef®*)

Intermittent *in* Glucose 5% *or* Sodium chloride 0.9% *or* Ringer's solution *or* Compound sodium lactate *or* Water for injections
Dissolve in 40 mL infusion fluid and give over up to 30 minutes

Cefotaxime sodium (*Claforan®*)

Intermittent *in* Glucose 5% *or* Sodium chloride 0.9% *or* Compound sodium lactate *or* Water for injections
Suggested volume 40–100 mL given over 20–60 minutes

Cefoxitin sodium (*Mefoxin®*)

Intermittent *or via* drip tubing in Glucose 5 and 10% *or* Sodium chloride 0.9%
Continuous infusion not usually recommended

Ceftazidime pentahydrate (*Fortum®*, *Kefadim®*)

Intermittent *or via* drip tubing *in* Glucose 5 and 10% *or* Sodium chloride 0.9% *or* Compound sodium lactate
Dissolve 2 g initially in 10 mL (3 g in 15 mL) infusion fluid; for *Fortum®* dilute further to a concentration of 40 mg/mL; for *Kefadim®* dilute further to a concentration of 20 mg/mL; give over up to 30 minutes

Ceftriaxone (sodium salt) (*Rocephin®*)

Intermittent *or via* drip tubing *in* Glucose 5 and 10% *or* Sodium chloride 0.9%
Reconstitute 2-g vial with 40 mL infusion fluid; give intermittent infusion over at least 30 minutes (60 minutes in neonates); not to be given with infusion fluids containing calcium

Cefuroxime sodium (*Zinacef®*)

Intermittent *or via* drip tubing *in* Glucose 5% *or* Sodium chloride 0.9% *or* Compound sodium lactate
Dissolve initially in water for injections (at least 2 mL for each 250 mg, 15 mL for 1.5 g); suggested volume 50–100 mL given over 30 minutes

Cephamandole nafate (*Kefadol®*)

Intermittent *or via* drip tubing *in* Glucose 5 and 10% *or* Sodium chloride 0.9%
Continuous infusion not usually recommended

Cephazolin sodium (*Kefzol*®)
Intermittent *or* via drip tubing *in* Glucose 5 and 10% *or* Sodium chloride 0.9% *or* Compound sodium lactate
Reconstitute initially with water for injections; dilute to 50–100 mL with infusion fluid

Cephradine (*Velosef*®)
Continuous *or* intermittent *in* Glucose 5 and 10% *or* Sodium chloride 0.9% *or* Ringer's solution *or* Compound sodium lactate

Chloramphenicol sodium succinate (*Kemicetine*®)
Intermittent *or* via drip tubing *in* Glucose 5% *or* Sodium chloride 0.9%

Chloroquine sulphate (*Nivaquine*®)
Continuous *in* Sodium chloride 0.9%
See also section 5.4.1

Cidofovir (*Vistide*®)
Intermittent *in* Sodium chloride 0.9%
Dilute requisite dose with 100 mL infusion fluid; infuse over 1 hour

Cimetidine (*Tagamet*®)
Continuous *or* intermittent *in* Glucose 5% *or* Sodium chloride 0.9%
For intermittent infusion suggested volume 100 mL given over 30–60 minutes

Cisatracurium (*Nimbex*®, *Nimbex Forte*®)
Continuous *in* Glucose 5% *or* Sodium chloride 0.9%
Solutions of 2 mg/mL and 5 mg/mL may be infused undiluted; alternatively dilute with infusion fluid to a concentration of 0.1–2 mg/mL

Cisplatin (*Cisplatin*, Lederle; *Cisplatin powder for injection*, Lederle)
Continuous *in* Sodium chloride 0.9% *or* Sodium chloride and glucose
Reconstitute cisplatin powder for injection with water for injections (10 mg in 10 mL, 50 mg in 50 mL); suggested volume 2 litres given over 6–8 hours

Cladribine (*Leustat*®)
Continuous *in* Sodium chloride 0.9%
Dilute with 100–500 mL and give over 24 hours; glucose solutions are unsuitable

Clarithromycin (*Klaricid*® I.V.)
Intermittent *in* Glucose 5% *or* Sodium chloride 0.9% *or* Ringer's solution *or* Compound sodium lactate
Dissolve initially in water for injections (500 mg in 10 mL) then dilute to a concentration of 2 mg/mL; give over 60 minutes

Clindamycin phosphate (*Dalacin*® C Phosphate)
Continuous *or* intermittent *in* Glucose 5% *or* Sodium chloride 0.9%
Give over at least 10–60 minutes (1.2 g over at least 60 minutes; higher doses by continuous infusion)

Clomipramine hydrochloride (*Anafranil*®)
Intermittent *in* Glucose 5% *or* Sodium chloride 0.9%
See product literature for details of initial dose to test tolerance; suggested volume 125–500mL given over 45–180 minutes

Clonazepam (*Rivotril*®)
Intermittent *in* Glucose 5 and 10% *or* Sodium chloride 0.9%
Suggested volume 250 mL

Co-amoxiclav (*Augmentin*®)
Intermittent *in* Sodium chloride 0.9% *or* Water for injections; see also package leaflet
Suggested volume 50–100 mL given over 30–40 minutes and completed within 4 hours of reconstitution
via drip tubing *in* Glucose 5% *or* Sodium chloride 0.9%

Co-fluampicil (sodium salts) (*Magnapen*®)
Intermittent *in* Glucose 5% *or* Sodium chloride 0.9%
Reconstituted solutions diluted and given without delay; suggested volume 100 mL given over 30–60 minutes
via drip tubing *in* Glucose 5% *or* Sodium chloride 0.9% *or* Ringer's solution *or* Compound sodium lactate

Colistin sulphomethate sodium (*Colomycin*®)
Continuous *or* intermittent *in* Glucose 5% *or* Sodium chloride 0.9% *or* Ringer's solution
Max. 6 hours between addition and completion of administration

Co-trimoxazole (*Septrin*® for infusion)
Intermittent *in* Glucose 5 and 10% *or* Sodium chloride 0.9% *or* Ringer's solution
Dilute contents of 1 ampoule (5 mL) to 125 mL, 2 ampoules (10 mL) to 250 mL or 3 ampoules (15 mL) to 500 mL; suggested duration of infusion 90 minutes (but may be adjusted according to fluid requirements); if fluid restriction necessary, 1 ampoule may be diluted with 75 mL glucose 5%

Cyclophosphamide (*Endoxana*®)
Intermittent *or* via drip tubing *in* Glucose 5% *or* Sodium chloride 0.9% *or* Water for injections
For intermittent infusion suggested volume 50–100 mL given over 5–15 minutes
via drip tubing in Glucose 5%

Cyclosporin (*Sandimmun*®)
Continuous *in* Glucose 5% *or* Sodium chloride 0.9%
Dilute to a concentration of 50 mg in 20–100 mL; give over 2–6 hours; not to be used with PVC equipment

Cytarabine (*Cytosar*®)
Continuous *or* intermittent *or* via drip tubing *in* Glucose 5% *or* Sodium chloride 0.9%
Reconstitute *Cytosar*® with water for injections or with infusion fluid; check container for haze or precipitate during administration

Dacarbazine (*DTIC-Dome*®)
Intermittent *in* Glucose 5% *or* Sodium chloride 0.9%
Reconstitute initially with water for injections then dilute in 125–250 mL infusion fluid; give over 15–30 minutes; protect infusion from light

Dactinomycin (*Cosmegen Lyovac*®)
Intermittent *or* via drip tubing *in* Glucose 5% *or* Sodium chloride 0.9%
Reconstitute with water for injections

Daunorubicin (as hydrochloride) (*Cerubidin*®)
via drip tubing *in* Sodium chloride 0.9%
Reconstitute vial with 4 mL water for injections to give 5 mg/mL solution; dilute requisite dose with infusion fluid to a concentration of 1 mg/mL; give over 20 minutes

Daunorubicin (liposomal) (*DaunoXome*®)
Intermittent *in* Glucose 5%
Dilute to a concentration of 0.2–1 mg/mL; give over 30–60 minutes; incompatible with sodium chloride solutions; in-line filter not recommended (if used, pore size should be no less than 5 micron)

Desferrioxamine mesylate (*Desferal*®)
Continuous *or* intermittent *in* Glucose 5% *or* Sodium chloride 0.9%
Dissolve initially in water for injections (500 mg in 5 mL) then dilute with infusion fluid

Desmopressin (*DDAVP*®)
Intermittent *in* Sodium chloride 0.9%
Dilute with 50 mL and give over 20 minutes

Dexamethasone sodium phosphate
(*Decadron*®; *Dexamethasone*, Organon)
Continuous *or* intermittent *or via* drip tubing *in* Glucose 5% *or* Sodium chloride 0.9%
Dexamethasone (Organon) can also be infused in Ringer's solution *or* Compound sodium lactate

Diamorphine hydrochloride (*Diamorphine Injection*, CP)
Continuous *in* Glucose 5% *or* Sodium chloride 0.9%
Glucose is preferred as infusion fluid

Diazepam (solution) (*Valium*®)
Continuous *in* Glucose 5% *or* Sodium chloride 0.9%
Dilute to a concentration of not more than 40 mg in 500 mL; max. 6 hours between addition and completion of administration; adsorbed to some extent by the plastics of the infusion set

Diazepam (emulsion) (*Diazemuls*®)
Continuous *in* Glucose 5 and 10%
May be diluted to a max. concentration of 200 mg in 500 mL; max. 6 hours between addition and completion of administration; adsorbed to some extent by the plastics of the infusion set
via drip tubing *in* Glucose 5 and 10% *or* Sodium chloride 0.9%
Adsorbed to some extent by the plastics of the infusion set

Diclofenac sodium (*Voltarol*®)
Continuous *or* intermittent *in* Glucose 5% *or* Sodium chloride 0.9%
Dilute 75 mg with 100–500 mL infusion fluid (previously buffered with 0.5 mL sodium bicarbonate 8.4% solution *or* with 1 mL sodium bicarbonate 4.2% solution); for intermittent infusion give over 30–120 minutes

Digoxin (*Lanoxin*®)
Continuous *in* Glucose 5% *or* Sodium chloride 0.9%
To be given slowly; see also section 2.1.1

Digoxin-specific antibody fragments
(*Digibind*®)
Intermittent *in* Sodium chloride 0.9%
Dissolve initially in water for injections (4 mL/vial) then dilute with the sodium chloride 0.9% and give through a 0.22 micron sterile, disposable filter over 30 minutes

Dinoprostone (*Prostin E2*®)
Continuous *or* intermittent *in* Glucose 5% *or* Sodium chloride 0.9%

Disodium etidronate (*Didronel IV*®)
Continuous *in* Sodium chloride 0.9%
Dilute in large-volume infusion, suggested minimum volume 250 mL; minimum period of infusion 2 hours

Disodium pamidronate (*Aredia*®)
Continuous *in* Sodium chloride 0.9%
Reconstitute initially with water for injections (15 mg in 5 mL, 30 mg or 90 mg in 10 mL); dilute with infusion fluid to a concentration of not more than 60 mg in 250 mL; give at a rate not exceeding 1 mg/minute; not to be given with infusion fluids containing calcium

Disopyramide phosphate (*Rythmodan*®)
Continuous *or* intermittent *in* Glucose 5% *or* Sodium chloride 0.9% *or* Ringer's solution *or* Compound sodium lactate
Max. rate by continuous infusion 20–30 mg/hour (or 400 micrograms/kg/hour)

Dobutamine hydrochloride (*Dobutrex*®, *Posiject*®)
Continuous *in* Glucose 5% *or* Sodium chloride 0.9%
Dilute to a concentration of 0.5–1 mg/mL and give *via* a controlled infusion device; give higher concentration (max. 5 mg/mL) with infusion pump; incompatible with bicarbonate

Docetaxel (*Taxotere*®)
Intermittent *in* Glucose 5% *or* Sodium chloride 0.9%
Stand docetaxel vials and solvent at room temperature for 5 minutes; add solvent to produce a concentrate containing 10 mg/mL; dilute the requisite dose with 250 mL infusion fluid to a final concentration of 300–900 micrograms/mL; infuse over 1 hour

Dopamine hydrochloride (*Intropin*®)
Continuous *in* Glucose 5% *or* Sodium chloride 0.9% *or* Compound sodium lactate
Dilute to a concentration of 1.6 mg/mL; incompatible with bicarbonate

Dopexamine hydrochloride (*Dopacard*®)
Continuous *in* Glucose 5% *or* Sodium chloride 0.9%
Dilute to a concentration of 400 or 800 micrograms/mL; max. concentration *via* large peripheral vein 1 mg/mL, concentrations up to 4 mg/mL may be infused *via* central vein; give *via* infusion pump or other device which provides accurate control of rate; contact with metal should be minimised; incompatible with bicarbonate

Doxorubicin hydrochloride (*Doxorubicin Rapid Dissolution*, *Doxorubicin Solution*) (both Pharmacia & Upjohn)
via drip tubing *in* Glucose 5% *or* Sodium chloride 0.9%
Reconstitute *Doxorubicin Rapid Dissolution* with water for injections or sodium chloride 0.9% (10 mg in 5 mL, 50 mg in 25 mL); give over 2–3 minutes

Doxorubicin hydrochloride (liposomal) (*Caelyx*®)
via drip tubing *in* Glucose 5%
Dilute requisite dose in 250 mL infusion fluid; give over 30 minutes

Electrolytes (*Addiphos*®)
Continuous *in* Glucose 5 and 10%
Suggested volume 500 mL

Enoximone (*Perfan*®)
Continuous *or* intermittent *in* Sodium chloride 0.9% *or* Water for injections
Dilute to a concentration of 2.5 mg/mL; incompatible with glucose solutions; use only plastic containers or syringes

Epirubicin hydrochloride (*Pharmorubicin*® *Rapid Dissolution*, *Pharmorubicin*® *Solution*)
via drip tubing *in* Sodium chloride 0.9%
Reconstitute *Pharmorubicin*® *Rapid Dissolution* with sodium chloride 0.9% or with water for injections (10 mg in 5 mL, 20 mg in 10 mL, 50 mg in 25 mL); give over 3–5 minutes

Epoetin beta (*Recormon*®)
Intermittent *in* Sodium chloride 0.9%
Reconstitute with water for injections provided and dilute in at least 100 mL infusion fluid; complete administration within 2 hours of preparation; avoid glass, use only plastic materials for infusion

Epoprostenol (*Flolan*®)
Continuous *in* Sodium chloride 0.9%
Reconstitute with the diluent provided (pH 10.5) to make a concentrate; use this concentrate within 12 hours and store at 2–8°C; dilute with not more than 6 times the volume of sodium chloride 0.9% before use

Erythromycin lactobionate
Continuous *or* intermittent *in* Glucose 5% (neutralised with sodium bicarbonate) *or* Sodium chloride 0.9%
Dissolve initially in water for injections (1 g in 20 mL) then dilute to a concentration of 1 mg/mL for continuous infusion and 1–5 mg/mL for intermittent infusion; give intermittent infusion over 20–60 minutes

Esmolol hydrochloride (*Brevibloc*®)
Continuous *or* intermittent *in* Glucose 5% *or* Sodium chloride 0.9%
Dilute to a concentration of 10 mg/mL; for continuous infusion use a suitable infusion control device; incompatible with bicarbonate

Ethacrynic acid (sodium salt) (*Edecrin*®)
via drip tubing *in* Glucose 5% *or* Sodium chloride 0.9%
pH of glucose infusion should be adjusted to above 5

Ethanol
Continuous *in* Glucose 5% *or* Sodium chloride 0.9% *or* Ringer's solution *or* Compound sodium lactate
Dilute to a concentration of 5–10%

Etoposide (*Vepesid*®; *Etoposide*, Du Pont)
Intermittent *in* Sodium chloride 0.9%
For *Vepesid*® dilute to a concentration of not more than 250 micrograms/mL and give over not less than 30 minutes; for *Etoposide* (Du Pont) dilute with either sodium chloride 0.9% or glucose 5% to a concentration of 200 micrograms/mL and give over 30–60 minutes; check container for haze or precipitate during infusion

Filgrastim (*Neupogen*®)
Continuous *or* intermittent *in* Glucose 5%
For a filgrastim concentration of less than 1 500 000 units/mL (15 micrograms/mL) albumin solution (human serum albumin) is added to produce a final albumin concentration of 2 mg/mL; should not be diluted to a filgrastim concentration of less than 200 000 units/mL (2 micrograms/mL) and should not be diluted with sodium chloride solution

Flecainide acetate (*Tambocor*®)
Continuous *or* intermittent *in* Glucose 5% *or* Sodium chloride 0.9% *or* Compound sodium lactate
Minimum volume in infusion fluids containing chlorides 500 mL

Flucloxacillin sodium (*Floxapen*®)
Intermittent *in* Glucose 5% *or* Sodium chloride 0.9%
Suggested volume 100 mL given over 30–60 minutes
via drip tubing *in* Glucose 5% *or* Sodium chloride 0.9% *or* Ringer's solution *or* Compound sodium lactate
Continuous infusion not usually recommended

Fludarabine phosphate (*Fludara*®)
Intermittent *in* Sodium chloride 0.9%
Reconstitute each 50 mg with 2 mL water for injections and dilute requisite dose in 100 mL; give over 30 minutes

Flumazenil (*Anexate*®)
Continuous *in* Glucose 5% *or* Sodium chloride 0.9%

Fluorouracil sodium
Continuous *or via* drip tubing *in* Glucose 5%
For continuous infusion suggested volume 500 mL given over 4 hours

Foscarnet sodium (*Foscavir*®)
Intermittent *in* Glucose 5% *or* Sodium chloride 0.9%
Dilute to a concentration of 12 mg/mL for infusion into peripheral vein (undiluted solution *via* central venous line only); infuse over at least 1 hour

Frusemide (sodium salt) (*Lasix*®)
Continuous *in* Sodium chloride 0.9% *or* Ringer's solution
Infusion pH must be above 5.5 and rate should not exceed 4 mg/minute; glucose solutions are unsuitable

Fusidic acid (sodium salt) (*Fucidin*®)
Continuous *in* Glucose 5% (but see below) *or* Sodium chloride 0.9%
Reconstitute with the buffer solution provided and dilute to 500 mL; give through central venous line over 2 hours (or over 6 hours if superficial vein used); incompatible in solution of pH less than 7.4

Ganciclovir (sodium salt) (*Cymevene*®)
Intermittent *in* Glucose 5% *or* Sodium chloride 0.9% *or* Ringer's solution *or* Compound sodium lactate
Reconstitute initially in water for injections (500 mg/10 mL) then dilute to not more than 10 mg/mL with infusion fluid (usually 100 mL); give over 1 hour

Gemcitabine (*Gemzar*®)
Intermittent *in* Sodium chloride 0.9%
Reconstitute initially with sodium chloride 0.9% (200 mg in at least 5 mL, 1 g in at least 25 mL); may be diluted further with infusion fluid; give over 30 minutes

Gentamicin sulphate (*Cidomycin*®)
Intermittent *or via* drip tubing *in* Glucose 5% *or* Sodium chloride 0.9%
Suggested volume for intermittent infusion 50–100 mL given over 20 minutes

Glyceryl trinitrate (*Nitrocine*®, *Nitronal*®, *Tridil*®)
Continuous *in* Glucose 5% *or* Sodium chloride 0.9%
For *Tridil*® dilute to a concentration of not more than 400 micrograms/mL; for *Nitrocine*® suggested infusion concentration 100 micrograms/mL; incompatible with polyvinyl chloride infusion containers such as *Viaflex*® or *Steriflex*®; use glass or polyethylene containers or give *via* a syringe pump

Granisetron hydrochloride (*Kytril*®)
Intermittent *in* Glucose 5% *or* Sodium chloride 0.9% *or* Compound sodium lactate
Dilute 3 mL in 20–50 mL infusion fluid (up to 3 mL in 10–30 mL for children); give over 5 minutes

Heparin sodium
Continuous *in* Glucose 5% *or* Sodium chloride 0.9%
Administration with a motorised pump advisable

Hydralazine hydrochloride (*Apresoline*®)
Continuous *in* Sodium chloride 0.9% *or* Ringer's solution
Suggested infusion volume 500 mL

Hydrocortisone sodium phosphate (*Efcortesol*®)
Continuous *or* intermittent *or via* drip tubing *in* Glucose 5% *or* Sodium chloride 0.9%

Hydrocortisone sodium succinate (*Efcortelan Soluble*®, *SoluCortef*®)
Continuous *or* intermittent *or via* drip tubing *in* Glucose 5% *or* Sodium chloride 0.9%

Idarubicin hydrochloride (*Zavedos®*)
via drip tubing *in* Sodium chloride 0.9%
  Reconstitute with water for injections; give over 5–10 minutes

Ifosfamide (*Mitoxana®*)
Continuous *or* intermittent *or via* drip tubing *in* Glucose 5% *or* Sodium chloride 0.9%
  For continuous infusion, suggested volume 3 litres given over 24 hours; for intermittent infusion, give over 30–120 minutes

Imipenem/cilastatin (sodium salt) (*Primaxin®*)
Intermittent *in* Glucose 5% *or* Sodium chloride 0.9%
  Dilute to a concentration of 5 mg (as imipenem)/mL; infuse 250–500 mg (as imipenem) over 20–30 minutes, 1 g over 40–60 minutes
Continuous infusion not usually recommended

Insulin (soluble)
Continuous *in* Sodium chloride 0.9% *or* Compound sodium lactate
  Adsorbed to some extent by plastics of infusion set; see also section 6.1.3; ensure insulin is not injected into 'dead space' of injection port of the infusion bag

Irinotecan hydrochloride (*Campto®*)
Intermittent *in* Glucose 5% *or* Sodium chloride 0.9%
  Dilute requisite dose in 250 mL infusion fluid; give over 30–90 minutes

Isoprenaline hydrochloride (*Saventrine IV®*)
Continuous *in* Glucose 5% *or* Sodium chloride and glucose
  Dilute in a large-volume infusion; suggested minimum volume 500 mL; pH of the infusion must be below 5

Isosorbide dinitrate (*Isoket 0.05%®*, *Isoket 0.1%®*)
Continuous *in* Glucose 5% *or* Sodium chloride 0.9%
  Adsorbed to some extent by polyvinyl chloride infusion containers; preferably use glass or polyethylene containers or give *via* a syringe pump; *Isoket 0.05%®* can alternatively be administered undiluted using a syringe pump with a glass or rigid plastic syringe

Kanamycin sulphate (*Kannasyn®*)
Intermittent *in* Glucose 5% *or* Sodium chloride 0.9%
  Dilute to 2.5 mg/mL and give at a rate of 3–4 mL/minute

Ketamine hydrochloride (*Ketalar®*)
Continuous *in* Glucose 5% *or* Sodium chloride 0.9%
  Dilute to 1 mg/mL; microdrip infusion for maintenance of anaesthesia

Labetalol hydrochloride (*Trandate®*)
Intermittent *in* Glucose 5% *or* Sodium chloride and glucose
  Dilute to a concentration of 1 mg/mL; suggested volume 200 mL; adjust rate with in-line burette

Lenograstim (*Granocyte®*)
Intermittent *in* Sodium chloride 0.9%
  Initially reconstitute with 1 mL water for injection provided (do not shake vigorously) then dilute with up to 50 mL infusion fluid for each vial of *Granocyte-13* or up to 100 mL infusion fluid for *Granocyte-34*; give over 30 minutes

Magnesium sulphate
Continuous *in* Glucose 5% *or* Sodium chloride 0.9%
  Suggested concentration up to 200 mg/mL

Melphalan (*Alkeran®*)
Intermittent *or via* drip tubing *in* Sodium chloride 0.9%
  Reconstitute with the solvent-diluent provided then dilute with infusion fluid; max. 90 minutes between addition and completion of administration; incompatible with glucose infusion

Meropenem (*Meronem®*)
Intermittent *in* Glucose 5 and 10% *or* Sodium chloride 0.9%
  Dilute in 50–200 mL infusion fluid and give over 15–30 minutes

Mesna (*Uromitexan®*)
Continuous *or via* drip tubing *in* Glucose 5% *or* Sodium chloride 0.9%

Metaraminol tartrate (*Aramine®*)
Continuous *or via* drip tubing *in* Glucose 5% *or* Sodium chloride 0.9% *or* Ringer's solution *or* Compound sodium lactate
Suggested infusion volume 500mL

Methocarbamol (*Robaxin®*)
Intermittent *in* Glucose 5% *or* Sodium chloride 0.9%
  Dilute to a concentration of not less than 1 g in 250 mL

Methotrexate sodium (*Methotrexate*) (Lederle)
Continuous *or via* drip tubing *in* Glucose 5% *or* Sodium chloride 0.9% *or* Compound sodium lactate *or* Ringer's solution
  Dilute in a large-volume infusion; max. 24 hours between addition and completion of administration

Methyldopate hydrochloride (*Aldomet®*)
Intermittent *in* Glucose 5%
  Suggested volume 100 mL given over 30–60 minutes

Methylprednisolone sodium succinate (*Solu-Medrone®*)
Continuous *or* intermittent *or via* drip tubing *in* Glucose 5% *or* Sodium chloride 0.9%
  Reconstitute initially with water for injections; doses up to 250 mg should be given over at least 5 minutes, high doses over at least 30 minutes

Metoclopramide hydrochloride (*Maxolon High Dose®*)
Continuous *or* intermittent *in* Glucose 5% *or* Sodium chloride 0.9% *or* Compound sodium lactate
  Continuous infusion recommended; loading dose, dilute with 50–100 mL and give over 15–20 minutes; maintenance dose, dilute with 500 mL and give over 8–12 hours; for intermittent infusion dilute with at least 50 mL and give over at least 15 minutes

Mexiletine hydrochloride (*Mexitil®*)
Continuous *in* Glucose 5% *or* Sodium chloride 0.9%

Milrinone (*Primacor®*)
Continuous *in* Glucose 5% *or* Sodium chloride 0.9%
  Dilute to a suggested concentration of 200 micrograms/mL

Mitozantrone hydrochloride (*Novantrone®*)
via drip tubing *in* Glucose 5% *or* Sodium chloride 0.9%
  Suggested volume at least 50 mL given over at least 3–5 minutes

Mivacurium chloride (*Mivacron®*)
Continuous *in* Glucose 5% *or* Sodium chloride 0.9%
  Dilute to a concentration of 500 micrograms/mL; may also be given undiluted

Molgramostim (Leucomax®)

Intermittent *in* Glucose 5% *or* Sodium chloride 0.9%

Reconstitute each vial with 1 mL water for injections; dilute with 25–100 mL infusion fluid to a concentration of not less than 80 000 units/mL; give over 4–6 hours; infusion through low protein binding 0.2 or 0.22 micron filter recommended; some infusion sets (e.g. *Port-A-Cath*®) adsorb molgramostim and should not be used

Mustine hydrochloride (Knoll)

via drip tubing *in* Glucose 5% *or* Sodium chloride 0.9%

Naloxone (Min-I-Jet® Naloxone Hydrochloride, Narcan®)

Continuous *in* Glucose 5% *or* Sodium chloride 0.9%

Dilute to a concentration of 4 micrograms/mL

Netilmicin sulphate (Netillin®)

Intermittent *or via* drip tubing *in* Glucose 5 and 10% *or* Sodium chloride 0.9%

For intermittent infusion suggested volume 50–200 mL given over 90–120 minutes

Nimodipine (Nimotop®)

via drip tubing *in* Glucose 5% *or* Sodium chloride 0.9% *or* Ringer's solution

Not to be added to infusion container; administer *via* an infusion pump through a Y-piece into a central catheter; incompatible with polyvinyl chloride giving sets or containers; protect infusion from light

Nizatidine (Axid®)

Continuous *or* intermittent *in* Glucose 5% *or* Sodium chloride 0.9% *or* Compound sodium lactate

For continuous infusion, dilute 300 mg in 150 mL and give at a rate of 10 mg/hour; for intermittent infusion, dilute 100 mg in 50 mL and give over 15 minutes

Noradrenaline acid tartrate (Levophed®)

Continuous *in* Glucose 5% *or* Sodium chloride and glucose

Give *via* controlled infusion device; for administration *via* syringe pump, dilute 4 mg noradrenaline acid tartrate (2 mL solution) with 48 mL; for administration *via* drip counter dilute 40 mg (20 mL solution) with 480 mL; give through a central venous catheter; incompatible with alkalis

Ondansetron hydrochloride (Zofran®)

Continuous *or* intermittent *in* Glucose 5% *or* Sodium chloride 0.9% *or* Ringer's solution

For intermittent infusion, dilute 32 mg in 50–100 mL and give over at least 15 minutes

Oxytocin (Syntocinon®)

Continuous *in* Glucose 5%

Preferably given *via* a variable-speed infusion pump in a concentration appropriate to the pump; if given by drip infusion for *induction or enhancement of labour*, dilute 5 units in 500 mL infusion fluid; for *postpartum uterine haemorrhage* dilute 5–20 units in 500 mL; if high doses given for prolonged period (e.g. for inevitable or missed abortion or for postpartum haemorrhage), use low volume of an electrolyte-containing infusion fluid (not Glucose 5%) given at higher concentration than for induction or enhancement of labour; close attention to patient's fluid and electrolyte status essential

Paclitaxel (Taxol®)

Continuous *in* Glucose 5% *or* Sodium chloride 0.9%

Begin infusion within 3 hours of dilution; dilute to a concentration of 0.3–1.2 mg/mL and give through a 0.22 micron in-line filter over 3 hours; not to be used with PVC equipment (short PVC inlet or outlet on filter may be acceptable)

Pentamidine isethionate (Pentacarinat®)

Intermittent *in* Glucose 5% *or* Sodium chloride 0.9%

Dissolve initially in water for injections (300 mg in 3–5 mL) then dilute in 50–250 mL; give over at least 60 minutes

Pentostatin (Nipent®)

Intermittent *in* Glucose 5% *or* Sodium chloride 0.9%

Dilute with 25–50 mL and give over 20–30 minutes

Phenoxybenzamine hydrochloride

Intermittent *in* Sodium chloride 0.9%

Dilute in 200–500 mL infusion; give over at least 2 hours; max. 4 hours between dilution and completion of administration

Phentolamine mesylate (Rogitine®)

Intermittent *in* Glucose 5% *or* Sodium chloride 0.9%

Phenylephrine hydrochloride

Intermittent *in* Glucose 5% *or* Sodium chloride 0.9%

Dilute 10 mg in 500 mL infusion fluid

Phenytoin sodium (Epanutin®)

Intermittent *in* Sodium chloride 0.9%

Flush intravenous line with Sodium chloride 0.9% before and after infusion; dilute in 50–100 mL infusion fluid (final concentration not to exceed 10 mg/mL) and give through an in-line filter (0.22–0.50 micron) at a rate not exceeding 50 mg/minute (neonates, give at a rate of 1–3 mg/kg/minute); complete administration within 1 hour of preparation

Phytomenadione (in mixed micelles vehicle) (Konakion® MM)

Intermittent *in* Glucose 5%

Dilute with 55 mL; may be injected into lower part of infusion apparatus

Piperacillin sodium (Pipril®)

Intermittent *in* Glucose 5% *or* Sodium chloride 0.9% *or* Compound sodium lactate *or* Water for injections

Minimum volume 50 mL given over 20–40 minutes

Piperacillin/tazobactam (sodium salts) (Tazocin®)

Intermittent *in* Glucose 5% *or* Sodium chloride 0.9% *or* Water for injections

Reconstitute initially with water for injections or sodium chloride infusion 0.9% (2.25 g in 10 mL, 4.5 g in 20 mL) then dilute to at least 50 mL with infusion fluid; give over 20–30 minutes

Potassium canrenoate (Spiroctan-M®)

Intermittent *in* Glucose 5% *or* Sodium chloride 0.9%

Suggested volume 250 mL

Potassium chloride

Continuous *in* Glucose 5% *or* Sodium chloride 0.9%

Dilute in a large-volume infusion; mix thoroughly to avoid 'layering', especially in non-rigid infusion containers; use ready-prepared solutions when possible

Procainamide hydrochloride (Pronestyl®)

Continuous *or* intermittent *in* Glucose 5%

For maintenance, dilute to a concentration of *either* 2 mg/mL and give at a rate of 1–3 mL/minute *or* 4 mg/mL and give at a rate of 0.5–1.5 mL/minute

Propofol (emulsion) (*Diprivan*®)

via drip tubing *in* Glucose 5% *or* Sodium chloride 0.9%

To be administered *via* a Y-piece close to injection site
Continuous *in* Glucose 5%

Dilute to a concentration not less than 2 mg/mL; administer using suitable device to control infusion rate; use glass or PVC containers (if PVC bag used it should be full—withdraw volume of infusion fluid equal to that of propofol to be added); give within 6 hours of preparation; propofol may alternatively be infused undiluted using a suitable infusion pump

Quinine dihydrochloride

Continuous *in* Sodium chloride 0.9%

To be given over 4 hours; see also section 5.4.1

Ranitidine hydrochloride (*Zantac*®)

Intermittent *in* Glucose 5% *or* Sodium chloride 0.9% *or* Compound sodium lactate

Remifentanil (*Ultiva*®)

Intermittent *or via* drip tubing *in* Glucose 5% *or* Sodium chloride 0.9% *or* Water for injections

Reconstitute with infusion fluid to a concentration of 1 mg/mL then dilute further to a concentration of 20–250 micrograms/mL (50 micrograms/mL recommended for general anaesthesia)

Rifampicin (*Rifadin*®, *Rimactane*®)

Intermittent *in* Glucose 5 and 10% *or* Sodium chloride 0.9% *or* Ringer's solution

Reconstitute with solvent provided then dilute with 250 mL (*Rimactane*®) or 500 mL (*Rifadin*®) infusion fluid; give over 2–3 hours

Ritodrine hydrochloride (*Yutopar*®)

Continuous *in* Glucose 5%

Give *via* controlled infusion device, preferably a syringe pump; if syringe pump available dilute to a concentration of 3 mg/mL or if syringe pump not available dilute to a concentration of 300 micrograms/mL; close attention to patient's fluid and electrolyte status essential

Rocuronium bromide (*Esmeron*®)

Continuous *or via* drip tubing *in* Glucose 5% *or* Sodium chloride 0.9%

Salbutamol sulphate (*Ventolin*® *For Intravenous Infusion*)

Continuous *in* Glucose 5%

For *bronchodilatation* dilute 5 mg with 500 mL glucose 5% or sodium chloride 0.9%; for *premature labour* dilute with glucose 5% to a concentration not exceeding 500 micrograms/mL (preferable to use low volume); give *via* controlled infusion device; close attention to patient's fluid and electrolyte status essential

Salcatonin (*Miacalcic*®)

Continuous *in* Sodium chloride 0.9%

Diluted solution given without delay; dilute in 500 mL and give over at least 6 hours; glass or hard plastic containers should not be used; approx. 20% loss of potency on dilution (take into account when calculating dose)

Sodium calciumedetate (*Ledclair*®)

Continuous *in* Glucose 5% *or* Sodium chloride 0.9%

Dilute to a concentration of not more than 3%; suggested volume 250–500 mL given over at least 1 hour

Sodium clodronate (*Bonefos*® *Concentrate*, *Loron*®)

Continuous *in* Sodium chloride 0.9%

Dilute 300 mg in 500 mL and give over at least 2 hours or 1.5 g in 500 mL and give over at least 4 hours; *Bonefos*® Concentrate can also be diluted in Glucose 5%

Sodium nitroprusside (*Faulding DBL*)

Continuous *in* Glucose 5%

Reconstitute 50 mg with 2–3 mL glucose 5% then dilute immediately with 250–1000 mL. infusion fluid; preferably infuse *via* infusion device to allow precise control; protect infusion from light

Sodium valproate (*Epilim*®)

Continuous *or* intermittent *in* Glucose 5% *or* Sodium chloride 0.9%

Reconstitute with solvent provided then dilute with infusion fluid

Sotalol hydrochloride (*Sotacor*®)

Continuous *or* intermittent *in* Glucose 5% *or* Sodium chloride 0.9%

Dilute to a concentration of between 0.01–2 mg/mL

Streptokinase (*Kabikinase*®, *Streptase*®)

Continuous *or* intermittent *in* Glucose 5% *or* Sodium chloride 0.9%

Reconstitute *Kabikinase*® with water for injections and *Streptase*® with sodium chloride 0.9% then dilute further with infusion fluid

Sulphadiazine sodium

Continuous *in* Sodium chloride 0.9%

Suggested volume 500 mL; ampoule solution has a pH of over 10

Suxamethonium chloride (*Anectine*®)

Continuous *in* Glucose 5% *or* Sodium chloride 0.9%

Tacrolimus (*Prograf*®)

Continuous *in* Glucose 5% *or* Sodium chloride 0.9%

Dilute concentrate in infusion fluid to a final concentration of 4–100 micrograms/mL; give over 24 hours; incompatible with PVC

Teicoplanin (*Targocid*®)

Intermittent *in* Glucose 5% *or* Sodium chloride 0.9% *or* Compound sodium lactate

Reconstitute initially with water for injections provided; infuse over 30 minutes

Continuous infusion not usually recommended

Temocillin sodium (*Temopen*®)

Intermittent *in* Glucose 5% *or* Sodium chloride 0.9% *or* Ringer's solution *or* Compound sodium lactate

Dissolve initially in water for injections (500 mg in 10 mL; 1–2 g in 20 mL) then dilute with infusion fluid and give over 30–40 minutes

Terbutaline sulphate (*Bricanyl*®)

Continuous *in* Glucose 5%

For *bronchodilatation* dilute 1.5–2.5 mg with 500 mL glucose 5% or sodium chloride 0.9% and give over 8–10 hours; for *premature labour* dilute in glucose 5% and give *via* controlled infusion device preferably a syringe pump; if syringe pump available dilute to a concentration of 100 micrograms/mL; if syringe pump not available dilute to a concentration of 10 micrograms/mL; close attention to patient's fluid and electrolyte status essential

Tetracycline hydrochloride (*Achromycin*® *Intravenous*)

Continuous *in* Glucose 5% *or* Sodium chloride 0.9% *or* Compound sodium lactate

Reconstitute initially with water for injections (250 mg in 5 mL, 500 mg in 10 mL) then dilute to at least 100 mL (max. 1 litre) and give at a rate not exceeding 100 mL in 5 minutes preferably through a 0.22 micron filter

Ticarcillin sodium/clavulanic acid (*Timentin*®)
Intermittent *in* Glucose 5% *or* Water for injections
  Suggested volume glucose 5%, 50–150 mL (depending on dose) or water for injections, 25–100 mL; given over 30–40 minutes

Tobramycin sulphate (*Nebcin*®)
Intermittent *or via* drip tubing *in* Glucose 5% *or* Sodium chloride 0.9%
  For adult intermittent infusion suggested volume 50–100 mL (children proportionately smaller volume) given over 20–60 minutes

Topotecan hydrochloride (*Hycamtin*®)
Intermittent *in* Glucose 5% *or* Sodium chloride 0.9%
  Reconstitute 4 mg with 4 mL water for injections then dilute to a final concentration of 25–50 micrograms/mL; give over 30 minutes

Tramadol hydrochloride (*Zydol*®)
Continuous *or* intermittent *in* Glucose 5% *or* Sodium chloride 0.9% *or* Ringer's solution *or* Compound sodium lactate

Tranexamic acid (*Cyklokapron*®)
Continuous *in* Glucose 5% *or* Sodium chloride 0.9% *or* Ringer's solution

Treosulfan (*Treosulfan*) (Medac)
Intermittent *in* Water for injections
  Infusion suggested for doses above 5 g; dilute to a concentration of 5 g in 100 mL

Trimetaphan camsylate (Cambridge)
Intermittent *in* Sodium chloride 0.9% *or* Sodium chloride and glucose
  Dilute to a concentration of 0.05–0.1% (0.25% if fluid restriction necessary)

Trimethoprim lactate (*Monotrim*®)
via drip tubing *in* Glucose 5% *or* Sodium chloride 0.9% *or* Compound sodium lactate *or* Ringer's solution

Trimetrexate (*Neutrexin*®)
Intermittent *in* Glucose 5%
  Reconstitute each 25 mg with 2 mL glucose 5% or water for injections; dilute further with infusion fluid to a concentration of 0.25–2 mg/mL; infuse over 60–90 minutes; incompatible with solutions containing sodium chloride or other electrolytes, flush intravenous line with glucose 5%

Trisodium edetate (*Limclair*®)
Continuous *in* Glucose 5% *or* Sodium chloride 0.9%
  Dilute to a concentration of 10 mg/mL; give over 2–3 hours

Tropisetron hydrochloride (*Navoban*®)
Intermittent *or via* drip tubing *in* Glucose 5% *or* Sodium chloride 0.9% *or* Ringer's solution
  Suggested concentration for infusion 50 micrograms/mL

Urokinase (*Urokinase*, Leo; *Ukidan*®)
Continuous *in* Sodium chloride 0.9%

Vancomycin hydrochloride (*Vancocin*®)
Intermittent *in* Glucose 5% *or* Sodium chloride 0.9%
  Reconstitute each 500 mg with 10 mL water for injections and dilute to 100–200 mL with infusion fluid; give over at least 60 minutes (rate not to exceed 10 mg/minute for doses over 500 mg); use continuous infusion only if intermittent not feasible

Vasopressin, synthetic (*Pitressin*®)
Intermittent *in* Glucose 5%
  Suggested concentration 20 units/100 mL given over 15 minutes

Vecuronium bromide (*Norcuron*®)
Continuous *in* Glucose 5% *or* Sodium chloride 0.9% *or* Ringer's solution
  Reconstitute with the solvent provided

Vinblastine sulphate (*Velbe*®)
via drip tubing *in* Sodium chloride 0.9%
  Reconstitute with the diluent provided; give within approx. 1 minute

Vincristine sulphate (*Oncovin*®)
via drip tubing *in* Glucose 5% *or* Sodium chloride 0.9%

Vindesine sulphate (*Eldisine*®)
via drip tubing *in* Glucose 5% *or* Sodium chloride 0.9%
  Reconstitute with the diluent provided; give over 1–3 minutes

Vitamins B & C (*Pabrinex*® *I/V High potency*)
Intermittent *or via* drip tubing *in* Glucose 5% *or* Sodium chloride 0.9%
  Ampoule contents should be mixed, diluted, and administered without delay; give over 10 minutes (see CSM advice, section 9.6.2)

Vitamins, multiple
(*Cernevit*®)
Intermittent *in* Glucose 5% *or* Sodium chloride 0.9%
  Dissolve initially in 5 mL water for injections (or infusion fluid)
(*Multibionta*®)
Intermittent *in* Glucose 5% *or* Sodium chloride 0.9%
  Dilute 10 mL in not less than 250 mL of infusion fluid (adults); see also section 9.3
(*Solivito N*®)
Intermittent *in* Glucose 5 and 10%
  Suggested volume 500–1000 mL given over 2–3 hours; see also section 9.3

Zidovudine (*Retrovir*®)
Intermittent *in* Glucose 5%
  Dilute to a concentration of 2 mg/mL or 4 mg/mL and give over 1 hour

Appendix 7: Borderline Substances

In certain conditions some foods (and toilet preparations) have characteristics of drugs and the Advisory Committee on Borderline Substances advises as to the circumstances in which such substances may be regarded as drugs. Prescriptions issued in accordance with the Committee's advice and endorsed 'ACBS' will normally not be investigated.

General Practitioners are reminded that the ACBS recommends products on the basis that they may be regarded as drugs for the management of specified conditions. Doctors should satisfy themselves that the products can safely be prescribed, that patients are adequately monitored and that, where necessary, expert hospital supervision is available.

FOODS WHICH MAY BE PRESCRIBED ON FP10

Note. This is a list of food products which the ACBS has approved. The clinical condition for which the product has approval follows each entry.

Advera® (Abbott)

Liquid, providing protein 14.2 g, carbohydrate 48.3 g, fat 5.4 g, energy 1262 kJ (299 kcal)/237 mL, with vitamins and minerals. Gluten-free. Orange and chocolate flavours. Net price 237-mL can = £2.67. For use as a necessary nutritional supplement prescribed on medical grounds for: short-bowel syndrome, intractable malabsorption, pre-operative preparation of patients who are undernourished, proven inflammatory bowel disease, following total gastrectomy, bowel fistulas, disease-related malnutrition. Not to be prescribed for any child under 5 years of age

Aglutella® (Ultrapharm)

Rice, low protein. Net price 500 g = £3.95. For inherited metabolic disorders, renal or liver failure requiring a low-protein diet

AL 110® (Nestlé)

Powder, protein 14 g, fat 25 g, carbohydrate 55.3 g, energy 2100 kJ (502 kcal)/100 g with vitamins and minerals. Net price 400 g = £7.27. For proven lactose intolerance in pre-school children, galactosaemia, and galactokinase deficiency

Alcoholic Beverages *see under* Rectified Spirit

Alembicol D® (Alembic Products)

Fractionated coconut oil. Net price 5 kg = £188.33. For steatorrhoea associated with cystic fibrosis of the pancreas, intestinal lymphangiectasia, surgery of the intestine, chronic liver disease, liver cirrhosis, other proven malabsorption syndromes; in a ketogenic diet in the management of epilepsy; type 1 hyperlipoproteinaemia

Alfare® (Nestlé)

Powder, protein 16.5 g, fat 24 g, carbohydrate 51.7 g, energy 2010 kJ (480 kcal)/100 g with vitamins and minerals. Net price 400 g = £5.49. For disaccharide and/or whole protein intolerance, or where amino acids or peptides are indicated in conjunction with medium chain triglycerides (MCT)

Aminex® (Gluten Free Foods Ltd)

Low-protein. Biscuits, net price 200 g = £3.75. Cookies, 150 g = £3.75. Rusks, 200 g = £3.75. For inherited metabolic disorders, renal or liver failure requiring a low-protein diet

Amino Acid Modules (SHS)

Leucine-Free Amino Acid Mix, powder, essential and non-essential amino acids 93%, except leucine. Net price 200 g = £49.59. For isovaleric acidaemia

Methionine-Free Amino Acid Mix, powder, essential and non-essential amino acids 93%, except methionine. Net price 200 g = £49.59. For homocystinuria or hypermethioninaemia

Methionine, Threonine, Valine-Free and Isoleucine-Low Amino Acid Mix, powder, essential and non-essential amino acids 93%, except methionine, threonine, and valine, with trace amounts of isoleucine. Net price 200 g = £49.59. For methylmalonic acidaemia or propionic acidaemia

Phenylalanine, Tyrosine, and Methionine-Free Amino Acid Mix, powder, essential and non-essential amino acids 93%, except methionine, phenylalanine, and tyrosine. Net price 200 g = £49.59. For tyrosinaemia type I where plasma concentrations are above normal

Tyrosine and Phenylalanine-Free Amino Acid Mix, powder, essential and non-essential amino acids 93%, except phenylalanine and tyrosine. Net price 200 g = £52.07. For tyrosinaemia where plasma methionine concentrations are normal

Aminogran® (UCB Pharma)

Food Supplement, powder, containing all essential amino acids except phenylalanine, for use with mineral mixture (see below). Net price 500 g = £42.77. For phenylketonuria

Mineral Mixture, powder, containing all appropriate minerals for use with the above food supplement and other synthetic diets. Net price 250 g = £7.24. For phenylketonuria and as a mineral supplement in synthetic diets

Analog® (SHS)

Note. Analog products are generally intended for use in children up to 1 year

MSUD Analog, powder, essential and non-essential amino acids 15.5% except isoleucine, leucine and valine, with carbohydrate, fat, vitamins, minerals, and trace elements. Net price 400 g = £24.00. For maple syrup urine disease

RVHB Analog, powder, essential and non-essential amino acids 15.5% except methionine, with carbohydrate, fat, vitamins, minerals, and trace elements. Net price 400 g = £24.00. For hypermethioninaemia; homocystinuria

XLeu Analog, powder, essential and non-essential amino acids 15.5% except leucine, with carbohydrate, fat, vitamins, minerals, and trace elements. Net price 400 g = £24.00. For isovaleric acidaemia

Ingredients: include arachis oil (peanut oil)

XLys Analog, powder, essential and non-essential amino acids 15.5% except lysine, with carbohydrate, fat, vitamins, minerals, and trace elements. Net price 400 g = £24.00. For hyperlysinaemia

XLys, Try Low Analog, powder, essential and non-essential amino acids 15.5% except lysine, and low tryptophan, with carbohydrate, fat, vitamins, minerals, and trace elements. Net price 400 g = £24.00. For type 1 glutaric aciduria

XMet, Thre, Val, Isoleu, Analog, powder, essential and non-essential amino acids 15.5% except methionine, threonine, valine and low isoleucine, with carbohydrate, fat, vitamins, minerals, and trace elements. Net price 400 g = £24.00. For methylmalonic acidaemia or propionic acidaemia

XP Analog, powder, essential and non-essential amino acids 15.5% except phenylalanine, with carbohydrate, fat, vitamins, minerals, and trace elements. Net price 400 g = £16.00. For phenylketonuria

XPhen, Tyr Analog, powder, essential and non-essential amino acids 15.5% except phenylalanine and tyrosine, with carbohydrate, fat, vitamins, minerals and trace elements. Net price 400 g = £24.00. For tyrosinaemia

XPhen, Tyr, Met Analog, powder, essential and non-essential amino acids 15.5% except phenylalanine, tyrosine and methionine, with carbohydrate, fat, vitamins, minerals and trace elements. Net price 400 g = £24.00. For tyrosinaemia

Aproten® (Ultrapharm)

Gluten-free. Flour. Net price 300 g = £1.84. For gluten-sensitive enteropathies including steatorrhoea due to gluten sensitivity, coeliac disease, and dermatitis herpetiformis

Low protein. Low Na+ and K+. Net prices: biscuits 180 g (36) = £2.80; bread mix 250 g = £2.00; cake mix 300 g = £2.10; crispbread 260 g = £3.95; pasta (anellini,ditalini, rigatini, spaghetti) 500 g = £3.95; tagliatelle 250 g = £2.10. For inherited metabolic disorders, renal or liver failure requiring a low-protein diet

L-Arginine (SHS)

Powder, net price 100 g = £7.44. For use as a supplement in urea cycle disorders other than arginase deficiency, such as hyperammonaemia types I and II, citrullaemia, arginosuccinic aciduria, and deficiency of N-acetyl glutamate synthetase

Arnott® (Ultrapharm)

Rice Cookies, gluten-free. Net price 200 g = £1.68. For gluten-sensitive enteropathies including steatorrhoea due to gluten sensitivity, coeliac disease, and dermatitis herpetiformis

Barkat® (Gluten Free Foods Ltd)

Bread mix, gluten-free. Net price 500 g = £4.12. For gluten-sensitive enteropathies including steatorrhoea due to gluten sensitivity, coeliac disease, and dermatitis herpetiformis

Bi-Aglut® (Ultrapharm)

Biscuits, gluten-free. Net price 180 g (36) = £2.60

Cracker toast, gluten-, lactose-, and milk-protein-free. Net price 240 g (40) – £3.60

Both for gluten-sensitive enteropathies including steatorrhoea due to gluten sensitivity, coeliac disease, dermatitis herpetiformis

Calogen® (SHS)

Emulsion, arachis oil (peanut oil) 50% in water. Net price 250 mL = £3.67; 1 litre = £13.66. For disease-related malnutrition, malabsorption states or other conditions requiring fortification with a high-fat supplement

Caloreen® (Nestlé Clinical)

Powder, water-soluble dextrins, with less than 1.8 mmol of Na+ and 0.3 mmol of K+/100 g. Net price 250 g = £1.51. For disease-related malnutrition, malabsorption states or other conditions requiring fortification with a high or readily available carbohydrate supplement

Calsip® (Fresenius)

Liquid, maltodextrin 50%. Flavours: apple, pineapple, neutral. Net price 200-mL carton = 89 p. For disease-related malnutrition, malabsorption states or other conditions requiring fortification with a high or readily available carbohydrate supplement

Caprilon® (Cow & Gate)

Powder, protein 11.8%, carbohydrate 55.1%, fat 28.3% (medium chain triglycerides 21.3%). Low in lactose, gluten- and sucrose-free. Used as a 12.7% solution. Net price 420 g = £10.10. For disorders in which a high intake of MCT is beneficial

Carobel, Instant® (Cow & Gate)

Powder, carob seed flour. Net price 45 g = £2.63. For thickening feeds in the treatment of vomiting

Casilan 90® (Heinz)

Powder, whole protein, containing all essential amino acids, 90% with less than 0.1% Na+. Net price 250 g = £4.82. For biochemically proven hypoproteinaemia

Clara's Kitchen® (Gluten Free Foods Ltd)

Gluten-free. Bread mix, net price 500 g = £3.53; hi-fibre bread mix, 500 g = £3.53. For gluten-sensitive enteropathies including steatorrhoea due to gluten-sensitivity, coeliac disease and dermatis herpetiformis

Clinifeed® (Nestlé Clinical)

Clinifeed 1.0, protein 3.8 g, carbohydrate 12.5 g, fat 3.9 g, energy 420 kJ (100 kcal)/100 mL, with vitamins, minerals and trace elements, neutral flavour. Gluten- and lactose-free. Net price 375-mL can = £1.80; 500-mL Dripac® = £2.60; 1-litre Dripac® = £5.14. For use as the sole source of nutrition or as a necessary nutritional supplement prescribed on medical grounds for: short-bowel syndrome, intractable malabsorption, pre-operative preparation of patients who are undernourished, proven inflammatory bowel disease, following total gastrectomy, dysphagia, bowel fistulas, disease-related malnutrition. Not to be prescribed for any child under one year; use with caution for young children up to 5 years of age

Clinifeed 1.5, protein 5.6 g, carbohydrate 18.8 g, fat 6.0 g, energy 640 kJ (150 kcal)/100 mL, with vitamins, minerals and trace elements, neutral flavour. Gluten- and lactose-free. Net price 500-mL Dripac® = £2.90; 1-litre Dripac® = £5.70. For indications see under *Clinifeed 1.0*

Clinifeed fibre, protein 3.8 g, carbohydrate 12.5 g, fat 3.9 g, fibre 1.5 g, energy 420 kJ (100 kcal)/100 mL with vitamins, minerals and trace elements, neutral flavour. Gluten- and lactose-free. Net price 500-mL Dripac® = £3.20; 1-litre Dripac®= £6.20. For indications see under *Clinifeed 1.0*

Clinifeed Iso, protein 10.5 g, carbohydrate 49.2 g, fat 15.4 g, energy 1575 kJ (375 kcal)/375 mL, with vitamins and minerals, vanilla flavour. Fructose- and sucrose-free, and low sodium. Net price 375-mL can = £1.80. For indications see under *Clinifeed 1.0*

Comminuted Chicken Meat (Cow & Gate)

Suspension (aqueous). Net price 150 g = £2.01. For carbohydrate intolerance in association with possible or proven intolerance of milk; glucose and galactose intolerance

Corn flour and corn starch For hypoglycaemia associated with glycogen-storage disease

Dextrose *see* Glucose

Dialamine® (SHS)

Powder, essential amino acids 30%, with carbohydrate 62%, energy 1500 kJ (360 kcal)/100 g, with ascorbic acid, minerals, and trace elements. Flavour: orange. Net price 200 g = £20.13. For oral feeding where essential amino acid supplements are required; e.g. chronic renal failure, hypoproteinaemia, wound fistula leakage with excessive protein loss, conditions requiring a controlled nitrogen intake, and haemodialysis

dp® (SHS)

Cookies, low-protein, butterscotch- or chocolate-flavoured chip cookies. Net price 170 g = £5.70. For inherited metabolic disorders, renal or liver failure requiring a low-protein diet

Duobar® (SHS)

Bar, protein-free (phenylalanine nil added), carbohydrate 56 g, fat 42 g, energy 2450 kJ (600 kcal)/100 g. Low sodium and potassium. Strawberry and vanilla flavours. Net price 45-g bar = 98 p. For disease-related malnutrition, malabsorption states or other conditions requiring fortification with fat/carbohydrate supplement

Duocal® (SHS)

Liquid, emulsion providing carbohydrate 23.4 g, fat 7.1 g, energy 628 kJ (150 kcal)/100 mL. Low-electrolyte, gluten-, lactose-, and protein-free. Net price 250 mL = £2.02; 1 litre = £7.20

MCT Powder, carbohydrate 74 g, fat 23.2 g (of which MCT 83%), energy 2116 kJ (505 kcal)/100 g. Low electrolyte, gluten-, protein- and lactose-free. Net price 400 g = £12.40

Cautionary label wordings, see inside back cover   Prices are **net**, see p.1

Super Soluble Powder, carbohydrate 72.7 g, fat 22.3 g, energy 1988 kJ (473 kcal)/100 g. Low electrolyte, gluten-, protein-, and lactose-free. Net price 400 g = £11.26

All for disease-related malnutrition, malabsorption states or other conditions requiring fortification with fat/carbohydrate supplement

Elemental 028® (SHS)

028 Powder, amino acids 12%, carbohydrate 70.5–72%, fat 6.64%, energy 1544–1568 kJ (364–370 kcal)/100 g with vitamins and minerals. For preparation with water before use. Net price 100-g box (orange flavoured or plain) = £3.82

028 Extra powder, amino acids 15%, carbohydrate 59%, fat 17.45%, energy 1860 kJ (443 kcal)/100 g, with vitamins, minerals, and trace elements. For preparation with water before use. Net price 100 g (plain) = £4.20; also available orange-flavoured (carbohydrate 55%, energy 1793 kJ (427 kcal)/100 g), 100 g = £4.20

028 Extra liquid, amino acids 7.5 g, carbohydrate 27.5 g, fat 8.7 g, energy 896 kJ (215 kcal)/250 mL, with vitamins, minerals, and trace elements. Flavours: grapefruit, orange and pineapple, summer fruits. Net price 250-mL carton = £2.37

All for use as the sole source of nutrition or as a necessary nutritional supplement prescribed on medical grounds for: short-bowel syndrome, intractable malabsorption, proven inflammatory bowel disease, bowel fistulas. Not to be prescribed for any child under one year; use with caution for young children up to 5 years of age

Emelis® (Nestlé Clinical)

Cream dessert, protein 11.82 g, carbohydrate 19.39 g, fat 3.25 g, energy 642 kJ (153 kcal)/125 g, with vitamins and minerals. Flavours: caramel, chocolate, peach, vanilla. Net price 125-g pot = £1.05. For use as a necessary nutritional supplement prescribed on medical grounds for: short-bowel syndrome, intractable malabsorption, pre-operative preparation of patients who are undernourished, proven inflammatory bowel disease, following total gastrectomy, dysphagia, bowel fistulas, disease-related malnutrition, continuous ambulatory peritoneal dialysis (CAPD), and haemodialysis. Not to be precribed for any child under one year; use with caution for young children up to 5 years of age

Emsogen® (SHS)

Powder, amino acids 15%, carbohydrate 60%, fat 16.4%, energy 1839 kJ (436 kcal)/100 g, with vitamins, minerals, and trace elements. For preparation with water before use. Net price 100 g = £4.20; also available orange-flavoured (carbohydrate 55%, energy 1754 kJ (418 kcal)/100 g), 100 g = £4.20. For use as the sole source of nutrition or as a necessary nutritional supplement prescribed on medical grounds for short-bowel syndrome, intractable malabsorption, proven inflammatory bowel disease, bowel fistulas. Not to be prescribed for any child under one year; use with caution for young children up to 5 years of age

Ener-G® (General Dietary)

Gluten-free. Rice bread (sliced), brown, net price 474 g = £3.75; white, 456 g = £3.75. Rice loaf, 612 g = £3.75. Brown rice and maize bread, 742 g = £3.75. Tapioca bread (sliced), 480 g = £3.75. Rice pasta (macaroni, shells, small shells, and lasagne), 454 g = £3.45; spaghetti, 447 g = £3.45; tagliatelle, 400 g = £3.45; vermicelli, 300 g = £3.45; cannelloni, 284 g = £3.45. Brown rice pasta: lasagne, 454 g = £3.45; macaroni, 454 g = £3.45; spaghetti, 447 g = £3.45. For gluten-sensitive enteropathies including steatorrhoea due to gluten sensitivity, coeliac disease, and dermatitis herpetiformis

Low protein egg replacer, carbohydrate 94 g, energy 1574 kJ (376 kcal)/100 g. Egg-, gluten- and lactose-free. Net price 454 g = £3.00. For phenylketonuria, similar amino acid abnormalities, renal failure, liver failure and liver cirrhosis.

Enlive® (Abbott)

Liquid, protein 9.6 g, carbohydrate 65.4 g, energy 1274 kJ (300 kcal)/240 mL, with vitamins and minerals; fat-free. Flavours: apple, fruit punch, grapefruit, lemon and lime, orange, peach, pineapple, strawberry. Net price 240-mL Tetrapak® = £1.56. For use as a necessary nutritional supplement prescribed on medical grounds: for short-bowel syndrome, intractable malabsorption, pre-operative preparation of patients who are undernourished, proven inflammatory bowel disease, following total gastrectomy, dysphagia, bowel fistulas, disease-related malnutrition. Not to be prescribed for any child under 1 year; use with caution for young children up to 5 years of age

Enrich® (Abbott)

Liquid with dietary fibre, providing protein 9.4 g, carbohydrate 34.9 g, fat 8.8 g, fibre 3.4 g, energy 1079 kJ (256 kcal)/250 mL with vitamins and minerals. Lactose- and gluten-free. Vanilla and chocolate flavours. Net price 250-mL can = £1.99. For use as the sole source of nutrition or as a necessary nutritional supplement prescribed on medical grounds for: short-bowel syndrome, intractable malabsorption, pre-operative preparation of patients who are undernourished, proven inflammatory bowel disease, following total gastrectomy, dysphagia, disease-related malnutrition. Not to be prescribed for any child under one year; use with caution for young children up to 5 years of age

Ensure® (Abbott)

Liquid, protein 10.0 g, fat 8.4 g, carbohydrate 33.9 g, energy 1057 kJ (251 kcal)/250 mL with minerals and vitamins, lactose- and gluten-free. Vanilla, chocolate, coffee, eggnog, nut, chicken, mushroom, and asparagus flavours. Net price 250-mL can = £1.69

Powder, same composition as Ensure liquid when reconstituted. Vanilla flavour. Net price 400 g = £11.06

Both for use as the sole source of nutrition or as a necessary nutritional supplement prescribed on medical grounds for: short-bowel syndrome, intractable malabsorption, pre-operative preparation of patients who are undernourished, proven inflammatory bowel disease, following total gastrectomy, dysphagia, bowel fistulas, disease-related malnutrition. Neither to be prescribed for any child under one year; use with caution for young children up to 5 years of age

Ensure Plus® (Abbott)

Liquid, protein 12.5 g, fat 10.0 g, carbohydrate 40.0 g, with vitamins and minerals, lactose- and gluten-free, energy 1260 kJ (300 kcal)/200 mL. Vanilla flavour. Net price 250-mL can = £1.94; 500-mL bottle = £3.72; 1-litre bottle = £7.44. Caramel, chocolate, strawberry, banana, fruit of the forest, raspberry, orange, coffee, black currant and vanilla flavours. Net price 200-mL Tetrapak = £1.49. As a necessary nutritional supplement prescribed on medical grounds for: short-bowel syndrome, intractable malabsorption, pre-operative preparation of patients who are undernourished, proven inflammatory bowel disease, following total gastrectomy, dysphagia, bowel fistulas, disease-related malnutrition, continuous ambulatory peritoneal dialysis (CAPD), and haemodialysis. Not to be prescribed for any child under one year; use with caution for young children up to 5 years of age

Entera® (Fresenius)

Liquid, protein 11.3 g, carbohydrate 37.6 g, fat 11.66 g, energy 1260 kJ (300 kcal)/200 mL, with vitamins and minerals. Net price 200-mL carton = £1.48 (flavours: vanilla, strawberry, butterscotch, black currant, banana, orange, pineapple, chocolate-mint, vegetable cream, and neutral); 500-mL bottle = £3.40 (flavour: neutral); 500-mL EasyBag® = £3.50. For use as sole source of nutrition or as a necessary nutritional supplement prescribed on medical grounds for: short-bowel syndrome, intractable malabsorption, pre-operative preparation of patients who are undernourished, proven inflammatory bowel disease, following total gastrectomy, dysphagia, bowel fistulas, disease-related malnutrition. Not to be prescribed for any child under one year; use with caution for young children up to 5 years of age

Farley's Soya Formula (Farley)

Powder, providing protein 2%, carbohydrate 7%, fat 3.8% with vitamins and minerals when reconstituted. Gluten-, sucrose-, and lactose-free. Net price 450 g = £3.53. For proven lactose and associated sucrose intolerance in pre-school children, galactokinase deficiency, galactos-aemia, and cow's milk protein intolerance

Formance® (Abbott)

Semi-solid, protein 6.8 g, carbohydrate 34.0 g, fat 9.7 g, energy 1052 kJ (250 kcal)/142 g with vitamins and minerals. Gluten-free. Vanilla, chocolate, and butterscotch flavours. Net price 142-g can = £1.76. As a necessary nutritional supplement prescribed on medical grounds for: short-bowel syndrome, intractable malabsorption, pre-operative preparation of patients who are undernourished, proven inflammatory bowel disease, following total gastrectomy, dysphagia, bowel fistulas, disease-related malnutrition, continuous ambulatory peritoneal dialysis (CAPD), and haemodialysis. Not to be prescribed for any child under one year; use with caution for young children up to 5 years of age

Fortijuce® (Nutricia Clinical)

Liquid, protein 8 g, carbohydrate 56.8 g, energy 1046 kJ (250 kcal)/200 mL, with vitamins, minerals and trace elements. Fat-free. Flavours: apricot, black currant, dandelion and burdock, lemon and lime, peach and orange, pineapple, summer fruit. Net price 200-mL carton = £1.50. As a necessary nutritional supplement prescribed on medical grounds for: short-bowel syndrome, intractable malabsorption, pre-operative preparation of patients who are undernourished, proven inflammatory bowel disease, following total gastrectomy, dysphagia, bowel fistulas, disease-related malnutrition. Not to be prescribed for any child under 1 year; use with caution for young children up to 5 years of age

Fortimel® (Nutricia Clinical)

Liquid, protein 19.4 g, carbohydrate 20.8 g, fat 4.2 g, energy 840 kJ (200 kcal)/200 mL with vitamins and minerals. Vanilla, strawberry, chocolate, coffee, apricot, and forest fruits flavours. Net price 200-mL carton = £1.16. As a necessary nutritional supplement prescribed on medical grounds for: short-bowel syndrome, intractable malabsorption, pre-operative preparation of patients who are undernourished, proven inflammatory bowel disease, following total gastrectomy, dysphagia, bowel fistulas, disease-related malnutrition. Not to be prescribed for any child under one year; use with caution for young children up to 5 years of age

Fortipudding® (Nutricia Clinical)

Semi-solid, protein 15.3 g, carbohydrate 24 g, fat 4.5 g, energy 840 kJ (198 kcal)/150 g with vitamins and minerals. Vanilla, chocolate, and coffee flavours. Net price 150-g tub = £1.31. As a necessary nutritional supplement prescribed on medical grounds for: short-bowel syndrome, intractable malabsorption, pre-operative preparation of patients who are undernourished, proven inflammatory bowel disease, following total gastrectomy, dysphagia, bowel fistulas, disease-related malnutrition, continuous ambulatory peritoneal dialysis (CAPD) and haemodialysis. Not to be prescribed for any child under one year; use with caution for young children up to 5 years of age

Fortisip® (Nutricia Clinical)

Liquid, protein 10 g, carbohydrate 35.8 g, fat 13 g, energy 1260 kJ (300 kcal)/200 mL, with vitamins, minerals and trace elements. Gluten-free and low lactose. Vanilla, banana, chocolate, orange, strawberry, tropical fruits, toffee, chicken, mushroom, and neutral flavours. Net price 200 mL = £1.46. As a necessary nutritional supplement prescribed on medical grounds for: short-bowel syndrome, intractable malabsorption, pre-operative

preparation of patients who are undernourished, proven inflammatory bowel disease, following total gastrectomy, dysphagia, bowel fistulas, disease-related malnutrition. Not to be prescribed for any child under one year; use with caution for young children up to 5 years of age

Frebini® (Fresenius)

Liquid, protein 5 g, carbohydrate 27 g, fat 8 g, energy 840 kJ (200 kcal)/200 mL, with vitamins, minerals and trace elements. Flavour: neutral. Net price 200-mL bottle = £1.68. For use as the sole source of nutrition or as a necessary nutritional supplement prescribed on medical grounds for short-bowel syndrome, intractable malabsorption, pre-operative preparation of patients who are undernourished, proven inflammatory bowel disease, following total gastrectomy, dysphagia, bowel fistulas, disease-related malnutrition and/or growth failure. Not to be prescribed for any child under one year of age

Fresenius OPD® *see* Survimed OPD®

Fresubin® (Fresenius)

Liquid, protein 7.6 g, carbohydrate 27.6 g, fat 6.8 g, energy 840 kJ (200 kcal)/200 mL with vitamins and minerals. Gluten-free, low lactose and cholesterol. Net price 200-mL carton (nut, peach, black currant, chocolate, mocha, and vanilla flavours) = £1.35; 500-mL bottle (nut, peach and neutral flavours) = £2.70; 500-mL EasyBag® = £2.80; 1-litre EasyBag® = £5.60. For use as the sole source of nutrition or as a necessary nutritional supplement prescribed on medical grounds for: short-bowel syndrome, intractable malabsorption, pre-operative preparation of patients who are undernourished, proven inflammatory bowel disease, following total gastrectomy, dysphagia, bowel fistulas, disease-related malnutrition, and Refsum's disease. Not to be prescribed for any child under one year; use with caution for young children up to 5 years of age

Fresubin 750 MCT® (Fresenius)

Liquid, protein 37.5 g, carbohydrate 85 g, fat 30 g, energy 3150 kJ (750 kcal)/500 mL with vitamins, minerals, and trace elements. Gluten-free and low lactose. Vanilla flavour. Net price 500-mL bottle = £3.10; 500-mL EasyBag® = £3.20. As a necessary nutritional supplement prescribed on medical grounds for: short-bowel syndrome, intractable malabsorption, pre-operative preparation of patients who are undernourished, proven inflammatory bowel disease, following total gastrectomy, dysphagia, bowel fistulas, disease-related malnutrition, continuous ambulatory peritoneal dialysis (CAPD), and haemodialysis. Not to be prescribed for any child under one year; use with caution for young children up to 5 years of age

Fresubin Isofibre® (Fresenius)

Liquid with dietary fibre, protein 19 g, carbohydrate 69 g, fat 17 g, energy 2100 kJ (500 kcal)/500 mL, with vitamins and minerals. Flavour: neutral. Net price 500-mL bottle = £3.20; 500-mL EasyBag® = £3.20; 1-litre EasyBag® = £6.40. For use as sole source of nutrition or as a necessary nutritional supplement prescribed on medical grounds for: short-bowel syndrome, intractable malabsorption, pre-operative preparation of patients who are undernourished, proven inflammatory bowel disease, following total gastrectomy, dysphagia, disease-related malnutrition. Not to be prescribed for any child under 2 years; use with caution for young children up to 5 years of age

Fructose (laevulose). For proven glucose/galactose intolerance

Galactomin® (Cow & Gate)

Formula 17, powder, protein 14.5 g, fat 25.9 g, carbohydrate 56.9 g, mineral salts 3.4 g/100 g. Used as a 13.1% solution with additional vitamins in place of milk. Net price 400 g = £9.30. For proven lactose intolerance in preschool children, galactosaemia and galactokinase deficiency

Formula 19, powder, protein 14.6 g, fat 30.8 g, carbohydrate 49.7 g (fructose as carbohydrate source), mineral salts 2.1 g/100 g, with vitamins. Used as a 12.9% solution in place of milk. Net price 400 g = £24.50. For glucose plus galactose intolerance

Generaid® (SHS)

Powder, whey protein and additional branched-chain amino acids (protein equivalent 81%). Net price 200 g (unflavoured) = £20.39. For patients with chronic liver disease and/or porto-hepatic encephalopathy

Plus Powder, whey protein and additional branched-chain amino acids (protein equivalent 11%) carbohydrate 62%, fat 19% with vitamins, minerals and trace elements. Net price 400 g = £14.16. For children over one year of age with hepatic disorders

Glucose (dextrose monohydrate). Net price 100 g = 16p. For glycogen storage disease and sucrose/isomaltose intolerance

Glutafin® (Nutricia Dietary)

Gluten-free. White loaf (sliced or unsliced), net price 400 g = £2.32; part-baked, 400 g = £2.59. Multigrain white loaf (sliced or unsliced), 400 g = £2.59. Fibre loaf (sliced or unsliced), 400 g = £2.32. Multigrain fibre loaf (sliced and unsliced), 400 g = £2.59. Bread with soya bran (dispensed in tin), 280 g = £1.57. White rolls, 400 g = £2.59. White rolls (part-baked), 4 = £2.59. Multigrain fibre rolls, 400 g = £2.59. Mixes (white, multigrain white, fibre and multigrain fibre), 500 g = £4.83. Biscuits, savoury or tea, 125 g = £1.43. Biscuits, digestive or sweet, 150 g = £1.44. Biscuits, 200 g = £3.21. Crackers, 200 g = £2.34. High fibre crackers, 200 g = £1.96. Pasta (penne, spirals, spaghetti), 500 g = £4.88; (lasagne, tagliatelle), 250 g = £2.56. Pizza bases, 2× 100 g = £3.30. For gluten-sensitive enteropathies including steatorrhoea due to gluten sensitivity, coeliac disease, and dermatitis herpetiformis

Glutano® (Gluten Free Foods Ltd)

Gluten-free. Biscuits, net price 125 g = £1.43. Crackers, 150 g = £1.47. Flour mix, 750 g = £4.12. Pasta (macaroni, spaghetti, spirals, tagliatelle), 250 g = £1.58. Wholemeal bread (sliced or par-baked), 500 g = £2.24. For gluten-sensitive enteropathies including steatorrhoea due to gluten sensitivity, coeliac disease, and dermatitis herpetiformis

Hycal® (SmithKline Beecham Healthcare)

Liquid, protein-free, low-electrolyte, glucose syrup solids 49.5%. Flavours: black currant, lemon, orange, and raspberry. Net price 171 mL = 73p. For disease-related malnutrition, malabsorption states or other conditions requiring fortification with high or readily available carbohydrate supplement

InfaSoy® (Cow & Gate)

Powder, carbohydrate 7.1%, fat 3.6%, and protein 1.8% with vitamins and minerals when used as a 12.7% solution. Net price 450 g = £3.61; 900 g = £6.92. For proven lactose and associated sucrose intolerance in preschool children, galactokinase deficiency, galactosaemia, and proven whole cow's milk sensitivity

Instant Carobel *see* **Carobel, Instant**®

Isomil® (Abbott)

Powder, protein 1.8%, carbohydrate 6.9%, fat 3.7% with vitamins and minerals when reconstituted. Lactose-free. Net price 400 g = £3.38. For proven lactose intolerance in preschool children, galactokinase deficiency, galactosaemia, and proven whole cow's milk sensitivity

Jevity® (Abbott)

Liquid, protein 4 g, fat 3.5 g, carbohydrate 13.1 g, dietary fibre 1.4 g, energy 421 kJ (100 kcal)/100 mL, with vitamins and minerals. Gluten-, lactose-, and sucrose-free. Net price 500-mL bottle = £3.23, 1-litre bottle = £6.46, 1.5-litre bottle = £9.69. For use as the sole source of nutrition or as a necessary nutritional supplement prescribed on medical grounds for: short-bowel syndrome, intractable malabsorption, pre-operative preparation of patients who are undernourished, proven inflammatory

bowel disease, following total gastrectomy, dysphagia, disease-related malnutrition. Not to be prescribed for any child under 1 year; use with caution for young children up to 5 years of age

Juvela® (SHS)

Gluten-free. Harvest mix, fibre mix, and flour mix, net price 500 g = £4.80. Bread (whole or sliced), 400-g loaf = £2.28. Fibre bread (sliced and unsliced), 400-g loaf = £2.28. Bread rolls, 3 × 5 = £9.18, fibre bread rolls, 3 × 5 = £9.18, part-baked rolls, 3 × 5 = £9.57. Crispbread, 210 g = £2.68. Digestive biscuits, 160 g = £1.69. Savoury biscuits, 110 g = £1.58. Tea biscuits, 160 g = £1.69. For gluten-sensitive enteropathies including steatorrhoea due to gluten sensitivity, coeliac disease, and dermatitis herpetiformis

Low Protein. Mix, net price 500 g = £4.85. Bread (whole or sliced), 400-g loaf = £2.28. Bread rolls, 3 × 5 rolls = £8.73. Biscuits, orange and cinnamon flavour, 150 g = £4.52; chocolate chip, 130 g = £4.52. For inherited metabolic disorders, renal or liver failure requiring a low-protein diet

Kindergen PROD® (SHS)

Powder, protein 7.6 g, carbohydrate 60.6 g, fat 26.1 g, energy 2060 kJ (492 kcal)/100 g with vitamins and minerals. Net price 400 g = £14.48. For complete nutritional support or supplementary feeding for infants and children with chronic renal failure who are receiving peritoneal rapid overnight dialysis

Leucine-Free Amino Acid Mix *see* Amino Acid Modules

Lifestyle® (Ultrapharm)

Gluten-free. Brown bread (sliced and unsliced), net price 400 g = £2.28. White bread (sliced and unsliced), 400 g = £2.28. High fibre bread (unsliced), 400 g = £2.38. Bread rolls, 400 g = £2.38. For gluten-sensitive enteropathies including steatorrhoea due to gluten sensitivity, coeliac disease, and dermatitis herpetiformis

Liga® (Jacobs)

Rusks, gluten-free, low sugar. Net price 6 = 88p. For gluten-sensitive enteropathies including steatorrhoea due to gluten sensitivity, coeliac disease, and dermatitis herpetiformis

Liquigen® (SHS)

Emulsion, medium chain triglycerides 52%. Net price 250 mL = £5.75; 1 litre = £21.22. For steatorrhoea associated with cystic fibrosis of the pancreas; intestinal lymphangiectasia, surgery of the intestine; chronic liver disease and liver cirrhosis; other proven malabsorption syndromes; ketogenic diet in the management of epilepsy; type I hyperlipoproteinaemia

Locasol® (Cow & Gate)

Powder, protein 14.6 g, carbohydrate 56.5 g, fat 26.1 g, mineral salts 1.9 g, not more than 55 mg of Ca²⁺/100 g and vitamins. Used as a 13.1% solution in place of milk. Net price 400 g = £12.93. For calcium intolerance

Lofenalac® (Bristol-Myers)

Powder, protein 15%, carbohydrate 60%, fat 18%, phenylalanine not more than 0.1% with vitamins and minerals. Gluten-, sucrose-, and lactose-free. Net price 450 g = £11.61. For phenylketonuria

Loprofin® (SHS)

Low protein. Sweet biscuits, net price 150 g = £1.44; chocolate cream-filled biscuits, 125 g = £1.44; cookies (chocolate chip or cinnamon), 100 g = £4.70; wafers (orange, vanilla, or chocolate), 100 g = £1.41. Egg replacer, 250 g = £4.05. Bread (sliced or whole), 400-g loaf = £2.32. Bread (white, with or without salt), 227 g = £1.58. Fibre bread (sliced and unsliced), 400 g = £2.32. Mix, 500 g = £4.88. Crackers, 150 g = £1.98. Pasta (macaroni, pasta spirals, spaghetti, vermicelli), 250 g = £2.56. For inherited metabolic disorders, renal or liver failure requiring a low-protein diet

PKU Drink, protein 1 g (phenylalanine 30 mg), lactose 9.4 g, fat 4 g, energy 300 kJ (72 kcal)/200 mL. Net price 200-mL bottle = 47p. For phenylketonuria

Low protein drink (Milupa)

Powder, protein 0.4%, carbohydrate 5.1%, fat 2% when reconstituted. Net price 400 g = £7.23. For inherited disorders of amino acid metabolism in childhood

Note. Termed Milupa lpd by manufacturer

Maxamaid® (SHS)

Note. Maxamaid products are generally intended for use in children aged 1 to 8 years

MSUD Maxamaid, powder, essential and non-essential amino acids 30% except isoleucine, leucine, and valine, with carbohydrate, fat less than 0.5%, vitamins, minerals, and trace elements. Net price 500 g = £52.76. For maple syrup urine disease

RVHB Maxamaid, powder, essential and non-essential amino acids 30% except methionine, with carbohydrate, fat less than 0.5%, vitamins, minerals, and trace elements. Net price 500 g = £52.76. For hypermethioninaemia, homocystinuria

XLeu Maxamaid, powder, essential and non-essential amino acids 28.6% except leucine, with carbohydrate, fat less than 0.5%, vitamins, minerals, and trace elements. Net price 454 g = £46.51. For isovaleric acidaemia

XLys Maxamaid, powder, essential and non-essential amino acids 30% except lysine, with carbohydrate, fat less than 0.5%, vitamins, minerals, and trace elements. Net price 500 g = £51.22. For hyperlysinaemia

XLys,Try, Maxamaid, powder, essential and non-essential amino acids 30% except lysine and tryptophan, with carbohydrate, fat less than 0.5%, vitamins, minerals, and trace elements. Net price 500 g = £52.76. For glutaric aciduria

XMet, Thre, Val, Isoleu Maxamaid, powder, essential and non-essential amino acids 30% except methionine, threonine, valine and low isoleucine, with carbohydrate, fat less than 0.5%, vitamins, minerals, and trace elements. Net price 500 g = £51.22. For methylmalonic acidaemia or propionic acidaemia

XP Maxamaid, essential and non-essential amino acids 30% except phenylalanine, with carbohydrate, vitamins, minerals, and trace elements. Net price 25-g bar = £1.35; powder (unflavoured), 500 g = £33.26; (orange-flavoured), 500 g = £33.26. For phenylketonuria. Not to be prescribed for children under 2 years of age

Ingredients: of 25-g bar include arachis oil (peanut oil)

XP Maxamaid Concentrate, powder, essential and non-essential amino acids 65% except phenylalanine, with carbohydrate, fat less than 0.5%, vitamins, minerals, and trace elements. Unflavoured. Net price 200 g = £39.66. For phenylketonuria. Not to be prescribed for children under 2 years of age

XPhen, Tyr Maxamaid, powder, essential and non-essential amino acids 30% except phenylalanine and tyrosine, with carbohydrate, fat less than 0.5%, vitamins, minerals, and trace elements. Net price 500 g = £51.22. For tyrosinaemia

Maxamum® (SHS)

Note. Maxamum products are generally intended for use in children aged over 8 years

MSUD Maxamum, powder, essential and non-essential amino acids 47% except isoleucine, leucine, and valine, with carbohydrate, fat less than 0.5%, vitamins, minerals, and trace elements. Orange-flavoured or unflavoured. Net price 500 g = £84.58. For maple syrup urine disease

RVHB Maxamum, powder, essential and non-essential amino acids 47% except methionine, with carbohydrate, fat less than 0.5%, vitamins, minerals, and trace elements. Unflavoured. Net price 500 g = £84.58. For hypermethioninaemia, homocystinuria

XMet, Thre, Val, Isoleu Maxamum, powder, essential and non-essential amino acids 47% except methionine, threonine, valine, and low isoleucine, with carbohydrate, fat less than 0.5%, vitamins, minerals, and trace elements.

Unflavoured. Net price 500 g = £82.12. For methylmalonic acidaemia or propionic acidaemia

XP Maxamum, powder, essential and non-essential amino acids 47% except phenylalanine, with carbohydrates, vitamins, minerals, and trace elements. Orange flavoured or unflavoured. Net price 500 g = £51.40. For phenylketonuria. Not to be prescribed for children under 8 years

Maxijul® (SHS)

Liquid, carbohydrate 50%, with potassium 0.004%, sodium 0.023%. Gluten-, lactose-, and fructose-free. Flavours: black currant, lemon and lime, orange, and natural. Net price 200 mL = 80p

LE Powder, modification of Maxijul® with lower concentrations of sodium and potassium. Net price 200 g = £2.93, 2 kg = £19.43

Super Soluble Powder, glucose polymer, potassium 0.004%, sodium 0.046%. Gluten-, lactose-, and fructose-free. Net price 4 × 132-g sachet pack = £2.98, 200 g = £1.52, 2.5 kg = £12.68

All for disease-related malnutrition; malabsorption states or other conditions requiring fortification with high or readily available carbohydrate supplement

Maxipro Super Soluble® (SHS)

Powder, whey protein and additional amino acids (protein equivalent 80%). Net price 200 g = £6.25; 1 kg = £25.01. For biochemically proven hypoproteinaemia. Not to be prescribed for any child under one year; unsuitable as a sole source of nutrition

Maxisorb® (SHS)

Powder, protein 12 g, carbohydrate 9 g, fat 6 g, energy 565 kJ (135 kcal)/30 g with minerals. Vanilla, strawberry and chocolate flavours. Net price 5 × 30-g sachets = £2.69. For biochemically proven hypoproteinaemia. Not to be prescribed for any child under one year; use with caution for young children up to 5 years of age

MCT Oil

Triglycerides from medium chain fatty acids. For steatorrhoea associated with cystic fibrosis of the pancreas; intestinal lymphangiectasia; surgery of the intestine; chronic liver disease and liver cirrhosis; other proven malabsorption syndromes; in a ketogenic diet in the management of epilepsy; in type I hyperlipoproteinaemia

Available from Bristol-Myers (net price 950 mL = £12.18); Cow & Gate (net price 500 mL = £7.27)

MCT Pepdite® (SHS)

Powder, essential and non-essential amino acids, peptides, medium chain triglycerides, monoglyceride of sunflower oil, with carbohydrate, fat, vitamins, minerals, and trace elements.

MCT Pepdite 0–2. Net price 400 g = £11.43

MCT Pepdite 2+. Net price 400 g = £11.43

Both for disorders in which a high intake of medium chain triglyceride is beneficial

Metabolic Mineral Mixture® (SHS)

Powder, essential mineral salts. Net price 100 g = £7.10. For mineral supplementation in synthetic diets

Methionine-Free Amino Acid Mix *see* Amino Acid Modules

Methionine, Threonine, Valine-Free and Isoleucine-Low Amino Acid Mix *see* Amino Acid Modules

Milupa® lpd *see under* Low Protein Drink

Milupa® PKU2 and PKU3 *see under* PKU2 and PKU3

Monogen® (SHS)

Powder, protein 11.4 g, carbohydrate 68 g, fat 11.4 g (of which MCT 93%), energy 1772 kJ (420 kcal)/100 g, with vitamins, minerals and trace elements. Net price 400 g = £11.30. For long-chain acyl-CoA dehydrogenase deficiency (LCAD), carnitine palmitoyl transferase deficiency (CPTD), primary and secondary lipoprotin lipase deficiency

MSUD Aid III® (SHS)

Powder, containing full range of amino acids except iso-leucine, leucine, and valine, with vitamins, minerals, and trace elements. Net price 200 g = £49.59. For maple syrup urine disease and related conditions where it is necessary to limit the intake of branched chain amino acids

Neocate® (SHS)

Powder, essential and non-essential amino acids, malto-dextrin, fat, vitamins, minerals, and trace elements. Net price 400 g = £18.28. For proven whole protein intoler-ance, short-bowel syndrome, intractable malabsorption, proven inflammatory bowel disease, and bowel fistulas

Nepro® (Abbott)

Liquid, protein 16.6 g, carbohydrate 51.1 g, fat 22.7 g, energy 1991 kJ (475 kcal)/237 mL with vitamins and minerals. Net price 237-mL can = £2.28. For patients with chronic renal failure who are on haemodialysis or continuous ambulatory peritoneal dialysis (CAPD), or patients with cirrhosis or other conditions requiring a high energy, low fluid, low electrolyte diet

Nestargel® (Nestlé)

Powder, carob seed flour 96.5%, calcium lactate 3.5%. Net price 125 g = £3.46. For thickening feeds in the treatment of vomiting

Nutramigen® (Bristol-Myers)

Powder, protein 13%, carbohydrate 62%, fat 18% with vitamins and minerals. Gluten-, sucrose-, and lactose-free. Net price 425 g = £7.44. For disaccharide and/or whole protein intolerance where additional medium chain triglyceride is not indicated

Nutrison® (Nutricia Clinical)

Energy Plus, liquid, protein 30 g, carbohydrate 92 g, fat 29 g, energy 3200 kJ (755 kcal)/500 mL. Net price 500 mL = £3.09; 1 litre (Steriflo®) = £6.40. As a neces-sary nutritional supplement prescribed on medical grounds for: short-bowel syndrome, intractable mal-absorption, pre-operative preparation of patients who are undernourished, proven inflammatory bowel disease, following total gastrectomy, dysphagia, bowel fistulas, disease-related malnutrition. Not to be prescribed for any child under one year; use with caution for young children up to 5 years of age

Fibre, liquid, protein 20 g, carbohydrate 61.5 g, fat 19.5 g, fibre 7.5 g, energy 2125 kJ (505 kcal)/500 mL. Net price 500-mL bottle = £2.99; 1 litre (Steriflo®) = £6.10. For use as the sole source of nutrition or as a necessary nutritional supplement prescribed on medical grounds for: short-bowel syndrome, intractable malabsorption, pre-operative preparation of patients who are undernour-ished, proven inflammatory bowel disease, following total gastrectomy, dysphagia, disease-related malnutri-tion. Not to be prescribed for any child under one year; use with caution for young children up to 5 years of age

Soya, liquid, protein 20 g, carbohydrate 61.5 g, fat 19.5 g, energy 2125 kJ (505 kcal)/500 mL, with vitamins and minerals. Gluten-free. Net price 500 mL = £2.87; 1 litre (Steriflo®) = £6.36. For indications see under Nutrison Standard

Standard, liquid, protein 20 g, carbohydrate 61.5 g, fat 19.5 g, energy 2125 kJ (505 kcal)/500 mL, with vitamins and minerals. Net price 500 mL = £2.73; 1 litre (Steri-flo®) = £5.46. For use as the sole source of nutrition or as a necessary nutritional supplement prescribed on medical grounds for: short-bowel syndrome, intractable malabsorption, pre-operative preparation of patients who are undernourished, proven inflammatory bowel disease, following total gastrectomy, dysphagia, bowel fistulas, disease-related malnutrition. Not to be pre-scribed for any child under one year; use with caution for young children up to 5 years of age

Nutrison MCT® (Nutricia Clinical)

Liquid, protein 25 g, carbohydrate 61.5 g, fat 16.5 g, energy 2095 kJ (500 kcal)/500 mL with vitamins and minerals. Gluten- and fructose-free, low lactose. Vanilla

flavour. Net price 500 mL = £2.80. As a necessary nutri-tional supplement prescribed on medical grounds for: short-bowel syndrome, intractable malabsorption, pre-operative preparation of patients who are undernour-ished, proven inflammatory bowel disease, following total gastrectomy, dysphagia, bowel fistulas, disease-related malnutrition. Not to be prescribed for any child under one year; use with caution for young children up to 5 years of age

Nutrison Paediatric® (Nutricia Clinical)

Energy Plus, liquid, protein 6.8 g, carbohydrate 37.6 g, fat 13.6 g, energy 1260 kJ (300 kcal)/200 mL. Net price 200-mL bottle = £2.19. For use as the sole source of nutrition or as a necessary nutritional supplement pre-scribed on medical grounds for: disease-related mal-nutrition and growth failure

Standard, liquid, protein 5.5 g, carbohydrate 24.4 g, fat 9 g, energy 840 kJ (200 kcal)/200 mL. Net price 200-mL bottle = £1.82. For use as the sole source of nutrition or as a necessary nutritional supplement prescribed on medical grounds for: short-bowel syndrome, intractable malabsorption, pre-operative preparation of patients who are undernourished, dysphagia, bowel fistulas, dis-ease-related malnutrition and/or growth failure. Not to be prescribed for any child under one year

Nutrison Pepti® (Nutricia Clinical)

Liquid, protein 20 g, fat 5 g, carbohydrate 94 g, energy 2100 kJ (500 kcal)/500 mL with vitamins and minerals. Gluten-free. Net price 500 mL = £3.87; 1 litre (Steri-flo®) = £8.20

Powder, same composition as Pepti-2000 LF® liquid when reconstituted. Net price 126-g sachet = £4.60

Both for use as the sole source of nutrition or as a neces-sary nutritional supplement prescribed on medical grounds for: short-bowel syndrome, intractable mal-absorption, proven inflammatory bowel disease, bowel fistulas. Not to be prescribed for any child under one year; use with caution for young children up to 5 years of age

Osmolite® (Abbott)

Liquid, protein 10.0 g, carbohydrate 33.9 g, fat 8.5 g, energy 1060 kJ (252 kcal)/250 mL with vitamins and minerals. Gluten- and lactose-free. Net price 250-mL can = £1.47; 500-mL bottle = £2.84, 1-litre bottle = £5.68, 1.5-litre bottle = £8.52. For use as the sole source of nutrition or as a necessary nutritional supplement pre-scribed on medical grounds for: short-bowel syndrome, intractable malabsorption, pre-operative preparation of patients who are undernourished, proven inflammatory bowel disease, following total gastrectomy, bowel fistu-las, disease-related malnutrition. Not to be prescribed for any child under one year; use with caution for young children up to 5 years of age

Paediasure® (Abbott)

Liquid, protein 7.5 g, fat 12.5 g, carbohydrate 27.4 g, with minerals and vitamins, gluten-free, energy 1054 kJ (252 kcal)/250 mL. Vanilla flavour. Net price 250-mL can = £2.26. For use as the sole source of nutrition or as a necessary nutritional supplement prescribed on medi-cal grounds for: short-bowel syndrome, intractable mal-absorption, pre-operative preparation of patients who are undernourished, dysphagia, bowel fistulas, and disease-related malnutrition and/or growth failure. Not to be pre-scribed for any child under one year

Paediatric Seravit® (SHS)

Powder, vitamins, minerals, low sodium and potassium, and trace elements. Net price 200 g (unflavoured) = £10.00; pineapple flavour, 200 g = £10.66. For vitamin and mineral supplementation in restrictive therapeutic diets in infants and children

Pepdite® (SHS)

Powder, essential and non-essential amino acids, peptides, with carbohydrate, fat, vitamins, minerals, and trace elements.

Pepdite 0–2. Providing 1925 kJ (460 kcal)/100 g. Net price 400 g = £10.70

Ingredients: include arachis oil (peanut oil)

Pepdite 2+. Providing 1787 kJ (425 kcal)/100 g. Net price 400 g = £10.70

Both for disaccharide and/or whole protein intolerance, or where amino acids or peptides are indicated in conjunction with medium chain triglycerides

Peptamen® (Nestlé Clinical)

Liquid, protein 4%, carbohydrate 12.7%, fat 3.9%, energy 420 kJ (100 kcal)/100 mL, with vitamins and minerals. Lactose- and gluten-free. Flavours: vanilla, unflavoured. Net price 250-mL can = £2.95. For use as the sole source of nutrition or as a necessary nutritional supplement prescribed on medical grounds for: short-bowel syndrome, intractable malabsorption, proven inflammatory bowel disease, bowel fistulas. Not to be prescribed for any child under one year; use with caution for young children up to 5 years of age

Flavour sachets, chocolate, strawberry and banana, cappucino flavours. Net price 24-sachet pack = £7.50

Pepti-Junior® (Cow & Gate)

Powder, protein 15.3 g, fat 28.3 g, carbohydrate 55.1 g, energy 2140 kJ (507 kcal)/100 g with vitamins and minerals. Used as a 13.1% solution in place of milk. Net price 450 g = £8.22. For disaccharide and/or whole protein intolerance or where amino acids and peptides are indicated in conjunction with medium chain triglycerides

Perative® (Abbott)

Liquid, providing protein 15.8 g, carbohydrate 42 g, fat 8.8 g, energy 1308 kJ (310 kcal)/237 mL, with vitamins and minerals. Gluten-free, unflavoured. Net price 237-mL can = £2.49, 1-litre bottle = £9.96. For use as a necessary nutritional supplement prescribed on medical grounds for: short-bowel syndrome, intractable malabsorption, pre-operative preparation of patients who are undernourished, proven inflammatory bowel disease, following total gastrectomy, bowel fistulas, disease-related malnutrition. Not to be prescribed for any child under 5 years of age

Phenylalanine, Tyrosine and Methionine-Free Amino Acid Mix *see* Amino Acid Modules

Phlexy-10® Exchange System (SHS)

Bar, essential and non-essential amino acids except phenylalanine 8.33 g, carbohydrate 20.5 g, fat 4.5 g/42-g bar. Citrus fruit flavour. Net price per bar = £3.61

Capsules, essential and non-essential amino acids except phenylalanine 416 mg/capsule. Net price 200-cap pack = £24.40

Drink Mix, powder, containing essential and non-essential amino acids except phenylalanine 10 g, carbohydrate 6.8 g/20-g sachet. Blackcurrant and apple flavour. Net price 20-g sachet = £2.44

All for phenylketonuria

PK Aid 4® (SHS)

Powder, containing essential and non-essential amino acids except phenylalanine. Net price 500 g = £81.84. For phenylketonuria

PKU 2® (Milupa)

Granules, containing essential and non-essential amino acids except phenylalanine; with vitamins, minerals, trace elements, 7.1% sucrose. Flavour: vanilla. Net price 500 g = £49.73. For phenylketonuria

PKU 3® (Milupa)

Granules, containing essential and non-essential amino acids except phenylalanine, vitamins, minerals, and trace elements, with 3.4% sucrose. Flavour: vanilla. Net price 500 g = £49.73. For phenylketonuria, not recommended for child under 8 years

Polial® (Ultrapharm)

Biscuits. Gluten- and lactose-free. Net price 200-g pack = £2.85. For gluten-sensitive enteropathies including steatorrhea due to gluten sensitivity, coeliac disease, and dermatitis herpetiformis

Polycal® (Nutricia Clinical)

Powder, glucose, maltose, and polysaccharides, providing 161 kJ (380 kcal)/100 g. Net price 400 g = £2.73

Liquid , glucose polymers providing carbohydrate 61.5 g/100 mL. Low-electrolyte, protein-free. Flavours: apple, black currant, lemon, orange, and neutral. Net price 200 mL = £1.07

Both for disease-related malnutrition; malabsorption states or other conditions requiring fortification with a high or readily available carbohydrate supplement

Polycose® (Abbott)

Powder, glucose polymers, providing carbohydrate 94 g, energy 1598 kJ (376 kcal)/100 g. Net price 350-g can = £3.22. For disease-related malnutrition; malabsorption states or other conditions requiring fortification with a high or readily available carbohydrate supplement

Pregestimil® (Bristol-Myers)

Powder, protein 12.8%, carbohydrate 61.6%, fat 18.3% with vitamins and minerals. Gluten-, sucrose-, and lactose-free. Net price 450 g = £8.49. For disaccharide and/or whole protein intolerance or where amino acids or peptides are indicated in conjunction with medium chain triglycerides

Prejomin® (Milupa)

Granules, protein 13.3 g, carbohydrate 57 g, fat 24.2 g, energy 2090 kJ (499 kcal)/100 g, with vitamins and minerals. Gluten-free. For preparation with water before use. Net price 400 g = £9.04. For disaccharide and/or whole protein intolerance where additional medium chain triglyceride is not indicated

ProMod® (Abbott)

Powder, protein 75 g, carbohydrate 7.5 g, fat 6.9 g/100 g. Gluten-free. Net price 275-g can = £8.60. For biochemically proven hypoproteinaemia

Prosobee® (Bristol Myers)

Liquid concentrate, protein 4.1%, carbohydrate 13.7%, fat 7.2% with vitamins and minerals. Gluten-, sucrose-, and lactose-free. Net price 385 mL = £1.28

Powder, protein 15.6%, carbohydrate 51.4%, fat 27.9% with vitamins and minerals. Gluten-, sucrose-, and lactose-free. Net price 400 g = £3.22

Both for proven lactose and associated sucrose intolerance in pre-school children, galactokinase deficiency, galactosaemia, and proven whole cow's milk sensitivity

Protein Forte® (Fresenius)

Liquid, protein 20 g, carbohydrate 19 g, fat 5.2 g, energy 840 kJ (200 kcal)/200 mL, with vitamins, minerals, and trace elements. Gluten-free. Vanilla, strawberry, and chocolate flavours. Net price 200-mL carton = £1.15. As a necessary nutritional supplement prescribed on medical grounds for: short-bowel syndrome, intractable malabsorption, pre-operative preparation of patients who are undernourished, proven inflammatory bowel disease, following total gastrectomy, dysphagia, bowel fistulas, disease-related malnutrition, continuous ambulatory peritoneal dialysis (CAPD) and haemodialysis. Not to be prescribed for any child under one year; use with caution for young children up to 5 years of age

Protifar® (Nutricia Clinical)

Powder, protein 88.5%. Low lactose, gluten- and sucrose-free. Net price 225 g = £5.46. For biochemically proven hypoproteinaemia

Provide® (Fresenius)

Liquid, protein 3.6 g, carbohydrate 11 g, fat less than 1 g, energy 250 kJ (60 kcal)/100 mL with vitamin C and minerals. Gluten- and lactose-free. Apple, black currant, lemon and lime, and tropical fruit flavour. Net price 250-mL carton = £1.20

Xtra Liquid, protein 3.75 g, carbohydrate 27.5 g, energy 525 kJ (125 kcal)/100 mL with vitamins, minerals and trace elements. Gluten-free. Apple, blackcurrant, cherry, citrus cola, lemon & lime, melon, orange & pineapple flavour. Net price 200-mL carton = £1.45.

Both for use as a necessary nutritional supplement prescribed on medical grounds for: short-bowel syndrome, intractable malabsorption, pre-operative preparation of patients who are undernourished, proven inflammatory bowel disease, following total gastrectomy, dysphagia, bowel fistulas, disease-related malnutrition. Not to be prescribed for any child under one year; use with caution for young children up to 5 years of age

Rectified Spirit. Where the therapeutic qualities of alcohol are required rectified spirit (suitably flavoured and diluted) should be prescribed

Renamil® (Kimal)

Powder, protein 4.7 g, carbohydrate 70.2 g, fat 18.7 g, 1984 kJ (468 kcal)/100 g, with vitamins and minerals. Net price 1 kg = £26.60. For chronic renal failure. Not suitable for infants and children under 1 year of age

Renapro® (Kimal)

Powder, whey protein providing protein 92 g, carbohydrate <300 mg, fat 500 mg, 1562 kJ (367 kcal)/100 g. Net price 100 g = £9.28. For dialysis and hypoproteinaemia. Not suitable for infants and children under 1 year of age

Rite-Diet® (SHS)

Gluten-free. White bread (sliced and unsliced), 400 g = £2.32. Fibre bread (sliced and unsliced), 400 g = £2.32. White rolls, 4 = £2.34. Fibre rolls, 4 = £2.34. For gluten-sensitive enteropathies including steatorrhoea due to gluten sensitivity, coeliac disease, and dermatitis herpetiformis

Low protein. Baking mix. Net price 500 g = £4.88. Flour mix. 400 g = £4.83. For inherited metabolic disorders, renal or liver failure requiring a low-protein diet

SHS Modjul® Flavour System (SHS)

Powder, black currant, orange, pineapple, and savoury tomato flavours. Net price 100 g = £6.50. For use with any unflavoured products based on peptides or amino acids

Scandishake® (SHS)

Powder, protein 4 g, carbohydrate 58 g, fat 21 g, energy 1831 kJ (437 kcal)/sachet. For reconstitution with milk. Flavours: chocolate, strawberry, vanilla. Net price 85 g sachet = £1.72. For disease-related malnutrition; malabsorption states or other conditions requiring fortification with a fat/carbohydrate supplement

Schar® (Schär)

Gluten-free. Bread. Net price 250 g = £1.41. Baguette (french bread), 400 g = £2.39. Wholemeal bread, 300 g = £1.72. Bread rolls, 150 g = £1.41. Lunch rolls, 150 g = £1.21. White bread buns, 200 g = £1.41. Bread mix, 1 kg = £5.00. Cake mix, 500 g = £3.95. Flour mix, 1 kg = £5.00. Wholemeal flour, 1 kg = £5.00. Cracker toast, 150 g = £1.72. Crackers, 200 g = £2.15. Crispbread, 250 g = £2.82. Pasta (bavette, fusilli, penne, rigati), 500 g = £3.30; lasagne, 250 g = £2.80; spaghetti, 500 g = £3.41. Pizza bases, 250 g (2 × 125 g) = £4.12. Savoy biscuits, 200 g = £2.15. For gluten-sensitive enteropathies including steatorrhoea due to gluten sensitivity, coeliac disease, and dermatitis herpetiformis

Sno-Pro® (SHS)

Drink, protein 220 mg (phenylalanine 12.5 mg), carbohydrate 8 g, fat 3.8 g, energy 272 kJ (65 kcal)/100 mL. Net price 200 mL = 59p. For phenylketonuria, chronic renal failure, and other inborn errors of metabolism

Sunnyvale® (Everfresh)

Mixed grain bread, gluten-free. Net price 400 g = £1.31. For gluten-sensitive enteropathies including steatorrhoea due to gluten sensitivity, coeliac disease and dermatitis herpetiformis

Suplena® (Abbott)

Liquid, protein 7.1 g, carbohydrate 60.7 g, fat 22.7 g, energy 1994 kJ (476 kcal)/237 mL. Flavour: vanilla. Net price 237-mL can = £2.28. For patients with chronic or

acute renal failure who are not undergoing dialysis; chronic or acute liver disease with fluid restriction; other conditions requiring a high-energy, low-protein, low-electrolyte, low-volume enteral feed

Survimed OPD® (Fresenius)

Liquid, protein 22.5 g, carbohydrate 75 g, fat 13 g, energy 2100 kJ (500 kcal)/500 mL, with vitamins, minerals, and trace elements. Gluten-free, and low lactose. Net price 500-mL bottle = £4.35; 500-mL EasyBag® = £4.45. As a necessary nutritional supplement prescribed on medical grounds for: short-bowel syndrome, intractable malabsorption, pre-operative preparation of patients who are undernourished, proven inflammatory bowel disease, following total gastrectomy, dysphagia, bowel fistulas, disease-related malnutrition. Not to be prescribed for any child under one year; use with caution for young children up to 5 years of age

Thick and Easy® (Fresenius)

Powder. Modified maize starch. Net price 225-g can = £3.75; 4.54 kg = £63.75. For thickening of foods in dysphagia. Not to be prescribed for children under one year except in cases of failure to thrive

Thixo-D® (Sutherland)

Powder, modified maize starch, gluten-free. Net price 375-g tub = £5.10. For thickening of foods in dysphagia. Not to be prescribed for children under one year except in cases of failure to thrive

Tinkyada® (General Dietary)

Gluten-free. Brown rice pasta (elbows, fettucini, fusilli, penne, shells, spaghetti, spirals). Net price 454 g = £3.00. For gluten-sensitive enteropathies due to gluten-sensitivity, coeliac disease and dermatitis herpetiformis

Tonexis® (Nestlé Clinical)

Tonexis, liquid, protein 15%, carbohydrate 55%, fat 30%, energy 840 kJ (200 kcal)/200 mL. Flavours: chocolate, coffee, strawberry-raspberry, vanilla. Net price 200-mL Tetrabrik® = £1.18

Tonexis 1.5, liquid, protein 15%, carbohydrate 55%, fat 30%, energy 1260 kJ (300 kcal)/200 mL. Flavours: apricot, banana, chocolate, red fruits, vanilla. Net price 200-mL Tetrabrik® = £1.40

Both for use as necessary nutritional supplements prescribed on medical grounds for: short-bowel syndrome, intractable malabsorption, pre-operative preparation of patients who are undernourished, proven inflammatory bowel disease, following total gastrectomy, dysphagia, bowel fistulas, disease-related malnutrition. Not to be prescribed for any child under one year; use with caution for young children up to 5 years of age

Tritamyl® (Gluten Free Foods Ltd)

Gluten-free. Flour, net price 1 kg = £5.60. Brown bread mix, 1 kg = £5.60. White bread mix, 1 kg = £5.60. For gluten-sensitive enteropathies including steatorrhoea due to gluten sensitivity, coeliac disease and dermatitis herpetiformis

Trufree® (Larkhall)

Gluten-free, wheat-free flours. For gluten-sensitive enteropathies including steatorrhoea due to gluten sensitivity, coeliac disease, and dermatitis herpetiformis

No. 1, net price 1 kg = £5.59. *No. 2 with rice bran*, 1 kg = £5.93. *No. 3 for Cantabread®*, 1 kg = £6.34. *No. 4 white*, 1 kg = £5.59. *No. 5 brown*, 1 kg = £5.59. *No. 6 plain*, 1 kg = £5.06. *No. 7 self-raising*, 1 kg = £5.44. *No. 8 special dietary*, 1 kg = £4.84

L-Tyrosine (SHS)

Powder, net price 100 g = £11.16. For use as a supplement in maternal phenylketonurics who have low plasma tyrosine concentrations

Tyrosine and Phenylalanine-Free Amino Acid Mix

see Amino Acid Modules

Ultra® (Ultrapharm)

Gluten-free. Baguette, net price 400 g = £2.39. Bread, net price 400 g = £2.39. High-fibre bread, 500 g = £3.26. Bread rolls, 400 g = £2.39. Crackerbread, 100 g = £1.72. Pizza base, net price 400 g = £2.58. For gluten-sensitive enteropathies including steatorrhoea due to gluten sensitivity, coeliac disease and dermatitis herpetiformis

Low protein. Brown bread (canned). Net price 500 g = £3.80. White bread (canned), 350 g = £2.75. PKU bread, 400 g = £2.10. PKU flour, 500 g = £2.98. PKU biscuits, 200 g = £2.15. PKU cookies, 250 g = £2.25. PKU pizza base, 400 g = £2.15. PKU savoy biscuits, 150 g = £2.00. For inherited metabolic disorders, renal or liver failure requiring a low-protein diet

Valpiform® (General Dietary)

Gluten-free. Bread mix. Net price 1 kg = £5.18. Pastry mix, 1 kg = £5.18. Petites baguettes, 2 x 300 g = £2.39. For gluten-sensitive enteropathies including steatorrhoea due to gluten sensitivity, coeliac disease, and dermatitis herpetiformis

Low protein. Shortbread biscuits. Net price 120 g = £3.38. For inherited metabolic disorders, renal or liver failure requiring a low-protein diet

Vitajoule® (Vitaflo)

Powder, glucose polymers, providing carbohydrate 96 g, energy 1610 kJ (380 kcal)/100 g. Net price 40 × 125 g = £32.80, 500 g = £2.32. For disease-related malnutrition; malabsorption states or other conditions requiring fortification with a high or readily available carbohydrate supplement

Vitamins and Minerals. Only for use in the management of actual or potential vitamin or mineral deficiency; not to be prescribed as dietary supplements or 'pick-me-ups'

Vitapro® (Vitaflo)

Powder, whole milk proteins, containing all essential amino acids, 75%. Net price 250 g = £4.60. For biochemically proven hypoproteinaemia

Vitaquick® (Vitaflo)

Powder. Modified maize starch. Net price 50 × 10-g sachet = £16.20, 100 g = £2.10, 250 g = £3.60; 1 kg = £11.33. For thickening of foods in dysphagia. Not to be prescribed for children under one year old except in cases of failure to thrive

Wysoy® (Wyeth)

Powder, carbohydrate 6.9%, fat 3.6%, and protein 2.1% with vitamins and minerals when reconstituted. Net price 430 g = £3.98; 860 g = £7.58. For proven lactose and associated sucrose intolerance in preschool children, galactokinase deficiency, galactosaemia and proven whole cow's milk sensitivity

CONDITIONS FOR WHICH FOODS MAY BE PRESCRIBED ON FP10

Note. This is a list of clinical conditions for which the ACBS has approved food products. It is essential to check the list of products (above) for availability.

Amino acid metabolic disorders and similar protein disorders: low protein drink (Milupa); see also histidinaemia; homocystinuria; maple syrup urine disease; phenylketonuria; low-protein products; synthetic diets; tyrosinaemia.

Bowel fistulas:

Complete foods: Clinifeed 1.0, 1.5, Fibre and Iso; Elemental 028 and 028 Extra; Emsogen; Enrich; Ensure; Ensure Powder; Entera; Frebini; Fresubin Liquid and Sip Feeds; Jevity; Nutrison Fibre, Paediatric, Pepti, Soya and Standard; Osmolite; Paediasure; Peptamen.

Nutritional supplements: Advera; Emelis; Enlive; Ensure Plus; Formance; Fortijuce; Fortimel; Fortipudding; Fortisip; Fresubin 750 MCT; Nutrison Energy Plus and

MCT; Perative; Protein Forte; Provide and Provide Xtra; Survimed OPD; Tonexis and 1.5.

Calcium intolerance: Locasol New Formula.

Carbohydrate malabsorption: Duobar. See also synthetic diets; malabsorption states.

(a) Disaccharide intolerance: Alfare; Caloreen; Calsip; Duocal Super Soluble and Duocal Liquid; Maxijul LE, Liquid, Super Soluble; Nutramigen; Pepdite; Pepti-Junior; Polycal; Polycal Liquid; Polycose powder; Pregestimil; Prejomin; Vitajoule. See also lactose intolerance; lactose with associated sucrose intolerance.

(b) Glucose and galactose intolerance: Comminuted Chicken Meat (Cow & Gate); Fructose; Galactomin Formula 19 (fructose formula).

(c) Isomaltose intolerance: Glucose (dextrose).

(d) Lactose intolerance: AL 110; Comminuted chicken meat (Cow & Gate); Farley's Soya Formula; Galactomin Formula 17; InfaSoy; Isomil Formula; Nutramigen; Pepdite; Pregestimil; Prejomin; Prosobee; Wysoy.

(e) Lactose with associated sucrose intolerance: Comminuted Chicken Meat (Cow & Gate); Farley's Soya Formula; Galactomin Formula 17; InfaSoy; Nutramigen; Pepti-Junior; Pregestimil; Prejomin; Prosobee; Wysoy.

(f) Sucrose intolerance: Glucose (dextrose) and see also synthetic diets; malabsorption states; lactose with associated sucrose intolerance.

Note. Lactose or sucrose intolerance is defined as a condition of intolerance to an intake of the relevant disaccharide confirmed by demonstrated clinical benefit of the effectiveness of the disaccharide-free diet, and presence of reducing substances and/or excessive acid in the stools, a low concentration of the corresponding disaccharidase enzyme on intestinal biopsy, or by breath tests or lactose tolerance tests

Carnitine palmitoyl transferase deficiency (CPTD): Monogen

Coeliac disease: see gluten-sensitive enteropathies.

Continuous Ambulatory Peritoneal Dialysis (CAPD): see dialysis.

Cystic fibrosis: see malabsorption states.

Dermatitis Herpetiformis: see gluten-sensitive enteropathies.

Dialysis (nutritional supplements for haemodialysis or continuous ambulatory peritoneal dialysis (CAPD) patients): Emelis; Ensure Plus; Formance; Fortipudding; Fresubin 750 MCT; Kindergen PROD; Nepro; Protein Forte; Renapro; Suplena.

Disaccharide intolerance: see carbohydrate malabsorption.

Dysphagia:

Complete foods: Clinifeed 1.0, 1.5, Fibre and Iso; Enrich; Ensure; Ensure Powder; Entera; Frebini; Fresubin Liquid and Sip Feeds, Isofibre; Jevity; Nutrison Fibre, Paediatric, Soya and Standard; Paediasure.

Nutritional supplements: Advera; Emelis; Enlive; Ensure Plus; Formance; Fortijuce; Fortimel; Fortipudding; Fortisip; Fresubin 750 MCT; Nutrison Energy Plus and MCT; Protein Forte; Provide and Provide Xtra; Survimed OPD; Tonexis and 1.5.

Thickeners: Thick & Easy; Thixo-D; Vitaquick.

Note. Dysphagia is defined as that associated with intrinsic disease of the oesophagus, e.g. oesophagitis; neuromuscular disorders, e.g. multiple sclerosis and motor neurone disease; major surgery and/or radiotherapy for cancer of the upper digestive tract; protracted severe inflammatory disease of the upper digestive tract, e.g. Stevens-Johnson syndrome and epidermolysis bullosa

Epilepsy (ketogenic diet in): Alembicol D; Liquigen; Medium-Chain Triglyceride Oil (MCT).

Flavouring (for use with any unflavoured product based on peptides or amino acids): SHS Flavour Modjul

Galactokinase deficiency and galactosaemia:

AL 110; Farley's Soya Formula; Galactomin Formula 17; InfaSoy; Isomil powder; Prosobee; Wysoy.

Gastrectomy (total):

Complete foods: Clinifeed 1.0, 1.5, Fibre and Iso; Enrich; Ensure; Ensure Powder; Entera; Frebini; Fresubin Liquid and Sip Feeds, Isofibre; Jevity; Nutrison Fibre, Soya and Standard; Osmolite.

Nutritional supplements: Advera; Emelis; Enlive; Ensure Plus; Formance; Fortijuce; Fortimel; Fortipudding; Fortisip; Fresubin 750 MCT; Nutrison Energy Plus and MCT; Perative; Protein Forte; Provide and Provide Xtra; Survimed OPD; Tonexis and 1.5.

Glucose/galactose intolerance: see carbohydrate malabsorption.

Glutaric aciduria: XLys, Try Maxamaid

Gluten-sensitive enteropathies: Aproten flour; Arnott gluten-free rice cookies; Barkat gluten-free bread mix; Bi-Aglut biscuits, and gluten-free cracker toast; Clara's Kitchen gluten-free bread mix and hi-fibre bread mix; Ener-G brown and white rice bread, brown rice and maize bread, gluten-free tapioca bread, rice loaf, gluten-free rice pasta (cannelloni, lasagna, macaroni, shells, small shells, spaghetti, tagliatelli, vermicelli); brown rice pasta (lasagna, macaroni, spaghetti); Glutafin bread, bread with soya bran (dispensed in tin), multigrain white loaf (sliced or unsliced), white rolls, fibre bread, mixes (white, multigrain white, fibre, multigrain fibre), biscuits (digestive, savoury, sweet (without chocolate or sultanas), tea), crackers, high fibre crackers and pasta (spirals, macaroni, spaghetti, vermicelli); Glutano gluten-free biscuits, crackers, flour mix, pastas (macaroni, spaghetti, spirals, tagliatelle), wholemeal bread (sliced or par-baked); Juvela gluten-free harvest mix, loaf and high-fibre loaf (sliced and unsliced), bread rolls, fibre bread rolls, part-baked rolls, crispbread, mix and fibre mix; digestive biscuits, savoury biscuits and tea biscuits; Lifestyle gluten-free bread rolls, brown and white bread; Liga gluten-free rusks (Jacobs); Polial gluten-free biscuits; Rite-Diet gluten-free fibre rolls, high-fibre bread (sliced and unsliced), white bread (sliced and unsliced), white rolls; Schar gluten-free bread, bread mix, bread rolls, cake mix, crackers, cracker toast, crispbread, flour mix, french bread (baguette), pasta (bavette, fusilli, lasagne, penne, rigati, spaghetti), pizza base, savoy biscuits, white bread buns, wholemeal bread, wholemeal flour mix; Sunnyvale gluten-free bread; Tinkyada gluten-free brown rice pasta (elbows, fettucini, fusilli, penne, shells, spaghetti, spirals); Tritamyl flour, brown bread mix and white bread mix; Trufree gluten-free flours No. 1, No. 2 with rice bran, No. 3 for Cantabread, No. 4 white, No. 5 brown, No. 6 plain, No. 7 self-raising, No. 8 special dietary; Ultra gluten-free baguette, high-fibre bread, crackerbread, pizza base; Valpiform bread mix, pastry mix, petites baguettes

Glycogen storage disease: Caloreen; Corn Flour or Corn Starch; Glucose (dextrose); Maxijul LE, Liquid (orange flavour), and Super Soluble; Polycal; Polycal Liquid; Polycose; Vitajoule.

Growth Failure (disease related): Frebini; Nutrison Paediatric and Energy Plus; Paediasure; Survimed OPD.

Haemodialysis: see dialysis.

Histidinaemia: see low-protein products; synthetic diets.

Homocystinuria: Analog RVHB; Methionine-Free Amino Acid Mix; RVHB Maxamaid; RVHB Maxamum, and see also low-protein products; synthetic diets.

Hyperlipoproteinaemia type 1: Alembicol D; Liquigen; Medium Chain Triglyceride Oil.

Hyperlysinaemia: Analog XLys; XLys Maxamaid

Hypermethioninaemia: Analog RVHB; Methionine-Free Amino Acid Mix; RVHB Maxamaid; RVHB Maxamum.

Hypoglycaemia: Corn Flour or Corn Starch; and see also glycogen storage disease.

Hypoproteinaemia: Casilan 90; Dialamine; Maxipro Super Soluble; Maxisorb; ProMod; Protifar; Renapro; Vitapro.

Inflammatory Bowel Disease:

Complete foods: Clinifeed 1.0, 1.5, Fibre and Iso; Elemental 028; Elemental 028 Extra; Emsogen; Enrich; Ensure; Ensure Powder; Entera; Frebini; Fresubin Liquid, Sip Feeds and Isofibre; Jevity; Nutrison Fibre, Pepti, Soya and Standard; Osmolite; Peptamen.

Nutritional supplements: Advera; Emelis; Enlive; Ensure Plus; Formance; Fortijuce; Fortimel; Fortipudding; Fortisip; Fresubin 750 MCT; Nutrison Energy Plus and MCT; Perative; Protein Forte; Provide and Provide Xtra; Survimed OPD; Tonexis and 1.5.

Intestinal lymphangiectasia: see malabsorption states.

Intestinal surgery: see malabsorption states

Isomaltose intolerance: see carbohydrate malabsorption.

Isovaleric acidaemia: Leucine-Free Amino Acid Mix; XLeu Analog; XLeu Maxamaid.

Lactose intolerance: see carbohydrate malabsorption.

Lipoprotein lipase deficiency (primary and secondary): Monogen

Liver failure: Aglutella low-protein rice; Alembicol D; Aminex low-protein biscuits, cookies and rusks; Aproten products (anellini, biscuits, bread mix; cake mix, crispbread, ditalini, rigatini, spaghetti, tagliatelle); dp Low-Protein butterscotch-flavoured or chocolate-flavoured chip cookies; Ener-G low protein egg replacer; Generaid; Generaid Plus; Juvela low-protein (chocolate chip, orange, and cinnamon flavour) cookies, loaf (sliced and unsliced), bread rolls, mix; Liquigen; Loprofin egg replacer; Loprofin low-protein bread (sliced and unsliced), bread (canned, with or without salt), fibre bread (sliced and unsliced), mix, pasta (macaroni, penne, spaghetti long, pasta spirals, vermicelli), sweet biscuits, chocolate cream-filled biscuits, crackers, cookies (chocolate chip, cinnamon), wafers (orange, chocolate, vanilla); Medium Chain Triglyceride Oil; Nepro; Rite-Diet low-protein baking mix, flour mix; Suplena; Ultra low-protein, canned bread (brown and white); Ultra PKU biscuits, bread, cookies, flour, pizza base and savoy biscuits; Valpiform shortbread biscuits

Long chain acyl-CoA dehydrogenase deficiency (LCAD): Monogen

Low-protein products: Aglutella low-protein rice; Aminex low-protein biscuits, cookies and rusks; Aproten products (anellini, biscuits, bread mix, cake mix, crispbread, ditalini, rigatini, spaghetti, tagliatelle); dp Low-Protein butterscotch-flavoured or chocolate-flavoured chip cookies; Ener-G low protein egg replacer; Juvela low-protein (chocolate chip, orange, and cinnamon flavour) cookies, loaf (sliced and unsliced), mix, bread rolls; Loprofin egg replacer; Loprofin low-protein bread (sliced and unsliced), bread (canned, with or without salt), fibre bread (sliced and unsliced), mix, pasta (macaroni, penne, spaghetti long, pasta spirals, vermicelli); sweet biscuits, chocolate cream-filled biscuits, crackers, cookies (chocolate chip, cinnamon), wafers (orange, chocolate, vanilla); Rite-Diet low-protein flour mix, baking mix; Ultra low-protein, canned bread (brown and white); Ultra PKU biscuits, bread, cookies, flour, pizza base and savoy biscuits; Valpiform shortbread biscuits.

Malabsorption states: (see also gluten-sensitive enteropathies; liver failure; carbohydrate malabsorption; intestinal lymphangiectasia; milk intolerance and synthetic diets).

(a) Protein sources: Caprilon Formula; Comminuted Chicken Meat (Cow & Gate); Duocal Super Soluble and Liquid; Maxipro Super Soluble; MCT Pepdite; Neocate; Pepdite.

(b) Fat sources: Alembicol D; Calogen; Caprilon Formula; Liquigen; MCT Pepdite; Medium Chain Triglyceride Oil.

(c) Carbohydrate: Caloreen; Calsip; Hycal; Maxijul LE, Liquid, and Super Soluble; Polycal; Polycal Liquid; Polycose; Vitajoule.

(d) Fat/carbohydrate sources: Duobar; Duocal Liquid and Super Soluble; Scandishake.

(e) Complete Feeds. For use as the sole source of nutrition or as a necessary nutritional supplement prescribed on medical grounds: Caprilon Formula; Clinifeed 1.0, 1.5, Fibre and Iso; Elemental 028; Elemental 028 Extra; Emsogen; Enrich; Ensure; Ensure Powder; Entera; Frebini; Fresubin Liquid, Sip Feeds and Isofibre; Jevity; MCT Pepdite; Nutrison Fibre, Paediatric, Pepti, Soya and Standard; Osmolite; Paediasure; Pepdite; Peptamen; Pepti-Junior; Pregestimil.

(f) Nutritional supplements. Necessary nutritional supplements prescribed on medical grounds: Advera; Emelis; Enlive; Ensure Plus; Formance; Fortijuce; Fortimel; Fortipudding; Fortisip; Fresubin 750 MCT; Nutrison Energy Plus and MCT; Perative; Protein Forte; Provide and Provide Xtra; Survimed OPD; Tonexis and 1.5.

(g) Minerals: Aminogran Mineral Mixture; Metabolic Mineral Mixture.

(h) Vitamins: As appropriate, and see synthetic diets.

(i) Vitamins and Minerals: Paediatric Seravit

Malnutrition (disease-related):
Complete foods: Calogen; Caloreen; Calsip; Clinifeed 1.0, 1.5, Fibre and Iso; Duobar; Duocal Liquid and Super Soluble; Enrich; Ensure; Ensure Powder; Entera; Frebini; Fresubin Liquid, Sip Feeds and Isofibre; Hycal; Jevity; Maxijul LE, Liquid and Super Soluble; Nutrison Fibre, Paediatric, Paediatric Energy Plus, Soya and Standard; Osmolite; Paediasure; Polycal Liquid and Powder; Polycose; Scandishake; Vitajoule.

Nutritional supplements: Advera; Clinifeed 400 and Protein Rich; Emelis; Enlive; Ensure Plus; Formance; Fortijuce; Fortimel; Fortipudding; Fortisip; Fresubin 750 MCT; Nutrison Energy Plus and MCT; Perative; Protein Forte; Provide and Provide Xtra; Survimed OPD; Tonexis and 1.5.

Maple syrup urine disease: Analog MSUD; MSUD Maxamaid; MSUD Maxamum; MSUD Aid III, and see also low-protein products; synthetic diets.

Methylmalonic acidaemia: Analog XMet, Thre, Val, Isoleu; XMet, Thre, Val, Isoleu Maxamaid; XMet, Thre, Val, Isoleu Maxamum; Methionine, Threonine, Valine-Free and Isoleucine-Low Amino Acid Mix.

Milk protein sensitivity: Comminuted Chicken Meat (Cow & Gate); Farley's Soya Formula; InfaSoy; Isomil powder; Nutramigen; Prosobee; Wysoy, and see also synthetic diets.

Nutritional support for adults
A. **Nutritionally complete feeds.** For use as the sole source of nutrition or as a necessary nutritional supplement prescribed on medical grounds:
(i) Gluten-Free: Clinifeed Iso; Entera; Fresubin Liquid and Sip Feeds; Nutrison Fibre and Standard.
(ii) Lactose- and Gluten-Free: Clinifeed 1.0 and 1.5; Enrich; Ensure, Ensure Powder; Fresubin Isofibre; Nutrison Soya; Osmolite.
(iii) Containing fibre: Clinifeed Fibre; Enrich; Fresubin Isofibre; Jevity; Nutrison Fibre.
(iv) Elemental Feeds: Elemental 028; Elemental 028 Extra; Emsogen; Nutrison Pepti; Peptamen.
B. **Nutritional source supplements:** see synthetic diets; malabsorption states.
(a) General supplements. Necessary nutritional supplements prescribed on medical grounds: Advera; Emelis; Enlive; Ensure; Ensure Plus; Formance; Fortijuce; Fortimel; Fortipudding; Fortisip; Fresubin 750 MCT; Maxisorb; Nutrison Energy Plus and MCT; Perative; Protein Forte; Provide and Provide Xtra; Survimed OPD; Tonexis and 1.5.
(b) Carbohydrates; lactose-free and gluten-free; Caloreen*; Calsip*; Hycal*; Maxijul LE*, Liquid, and Super Soluble; Polycal*; Polycal Liquid*; Polycose; Vitajoule.
*Have low electrolyte content.
(c) Fat: Alembicol D; Calogen; Liquigen; MCT Oil.

(d) Fat/carbohydrate sources: Duobar; Duocal Liquid, MCT Powder and Super Soluble (low-electrolyte content); Scandishake.

(e) Nitrogen sources: Casilan 90 (whole protein based, low-sodium); Maxipro Super Soluble (whey protein based, low-sodium); Pro-Mod (whey protein based, low-sodium).

(f) Minerals: Aminogran Mineral Mixture; Metabolic Mineral Mixture.

Phenylketonuria: Aglutella low-protein rice; Aminex low-protein biscuits, cookies and rusks; Aminogran Food Supplement and Mineral Mixture; Analog XP; Aproten products (annellini, biscuits, bread mix, cake mix, crispbread, ditalini, rigatini, spaghetti, tagliatelle); dp Low-Protein butterscotch-flavoured or chocolate-flavoured chip cookies; Ener-G low protein egg replacer; Juvela low-protein loaf (sliced and unsliced), bread rolls, cookies (chocolate chip, orange, and cinnamon flavour), mix; Lofenalac; Loprofin egg replacer; Loprofin low-protein bread (sliced and unsliced), bread (canned, with or without salt), fibre bread (sliced and unsliced), mix and pasta (macaroni, penne, spaghetti long, pasta spirals, vermicelli), sweet biscuits, chocolate cream-filled biscuits, crackers, cookies (chocolate chip, cinnamon), wafers (orange, chocolate, vanilla); Loprofin PKU drink; Metabolic Mineral Mixture; Milupa PKU2 and PKU3; Phlexy-10 exchange system; PK Aid 4; Rite-Diet low-protein baking mix, flour mix; Sno-Pro; L-Tyrosine supplement; Ultra low-protein, canned white bread; Ultra PKU biscuits, bread, cookies, flour, pizza base, savoy biscuits; Valpiform shortbread biscuits; XP Maxamaid; XP Bar Maxamaid; XP Concentrate Maxamaid; XP Maxamum; and see low-protein products and synthetic diets

Propionic acidaemia: Analog XMet, Thre, Val, Isoleu; XMet, Thre, Val, Isoleu Maxamaid; XMet Thre, Val, Isoleu Maxamum; Methionine, Threonine, Valine-Free and Isoleucine-Low Amino Acid Mix.

Protein intolerance: *see* amino acid metabolic disorders; low protein products; milk protein sensitivity; synthetic diets, and whole protein sensitivity.

Refsum's Disease: Fresubin Liquid and Sip Feeds.

Renal dialysis: *see* Dialysis.

Renal failure: Aglutella low-protein rice; Aminex low-protein biscuits, cookies and rusks; Aproten products (annellini, biscuits, bread mix, cake mix, crispbread, ditalini, rigatini, spaghetti, tagliatelle); Dialamine; dp Low-Protein butterscotch-flavoured or chocolate-flavoured chip cookies; Ener-G low protein egg replacer; Juvela low-protein (chocolate chip, orange, and cinnamon flavour) cookies, loaf (sliced and unsliced), bread rolls and flour mix; Kindergen PROD; Loprofin egg replacer; Loprofin low-protein bread (sliced and unsliced), bread (canned, with or without salt), fibre bread (sliced and unsliced), mix and pasta (macaroni, penne, spaghetti long, pasta spirals, vermicelli), sweet biscuits, chocolate cream-filled biscuits, crackers, cookies (chocolate chip, cinnamon), wafers (orange, chocolate, vanilla); Nepro; Renamil; Rite-Diet low-protein flour mix, baking mix, Sno-Pro Drink; Suplena; Ultra low-protein, canned bread (brown and white); Ultra PKU biscuits, cookies, flour, pizza base and savoy biscuits; Valpiform shortbread biscuits.

Short bowel syndrome: *see* Malabsorption states.

Sicca Syndrome: Glandosane; Luborant; Oralbalance; Saliva Orthana; Salivace; Saliveze; Salivix.

Sucrose intolerance: *see* Carbohydrate malabsorption.

Synthetic diets:
(a) Fat: Alembicol D; Calogen; Liquigen; Medium Chain Triglyceride Oil.
(b) Carbohydrate: Caloreen; Calsip; Hycal; Maxijul LE, Liquid, Super Soluble; Polycal; Polycal Liquid; Polycose powder; Vitajoule.

(c) Fat/carbohydrate sources: Duobar; Duocal Liquid, MCT Powder and Super Soluble (low-electrolyte content); Scandishake.

(d) Minerals: Aminogran Mineral Mixture; Metabolic Mineral Mixture.

(e) Protein sources: see malabsorption states, complete feeds.

(f) Vitamins: as appropriate and see malabsorption states, nutritional support for adults.

(g) Vitamins and Minerals: Paediatric Seravit.

Tyrosinaemia: Analog XPhen, Tyr; Analog XPhen, Tyr, Met; XPhen, Tyr Maxamaid; Phenylalanine, Tyrosine and Methionine-Free Amino Acid Mix; Tyrosine and Phenylalanine-Free Amino Acid Mix.

Urea cycle disorders: L-Arginine supplement

Vomiting in infancy: Instant Carobel, Nestargel.

Whole protein sensitivity: Alfare; Caprilon Formula; MCT Pepdite; Neocate; Nutramigen; Pepdite; Pepti-Junior; Pregestimil; Prejomin.

Note. Defined as intolerance to whole protein, proven by at least two withdrawal and challenge tests, as suggested by an accurate dietary history

Xerostomia: Glandosane; Luborant; Saliva Orthana; Salivace; Saliveze; Salivix.

CONDITIONS FOR WHICH TOILET PREPARATIONS MAY BE PRESCRIBED ON FP10

Note. This is a list of clinical conditions for which the ACBS has approved toilet preparations. For details of the preparations see Chapter 13.

Birthmarks: see disfiguring skin lesions.

Dermatitis: Aveeno Bath Oil; Aveeno Cream; Aveeno sachets (regular and oilated); E45 Emollient Bath Oil; E45 Emollient Wash Oil; Vaseline Dermacare Cream and Lotion.

Dermatitis herpetiformis: see gluten-sensitive enteropathies.

Disfiguring skin lesions (birthmarks, mutilating lesions, scars, vitiligo): Boots Covering Cream; Covermark classic foundation and finishing powder; Dermablend Cover Creme, Leg and Body Cover, and Setting Powder; Dermacolor Camouflage cream and fixing powder; Keromask masking cream and finishing powder; Veil Cover cream and Finishing Powder. (Cleansing Creams, Cleansing Milks, and Cleansing Lotions are excluded.)

Eczema: see dermatitis.

Photodermatoses (skin protection in): Ambre Solaire Total Screen for Sun-Sensitive skin SPF60; Coppertone Ultrashade 23; Piz Buin Sunblock Lotion 20; RoC Dermatological Minesol Total Sunblock SPF 44; RoC Total Sunblock Cream SPF 25 (Colourless and tinted); Spectraban 25; Spectraban Ultra 28; Sun E45 Lotion SPF 15, SPF 25, Sunblock SPF 50; Uvistat Babysun Cream 22; Uvistat Lipscreen 15; Uvistat Sun Block Cream 20; Uvistat Tinted Lotion 25; Uvistat Ultrablock Sun Cream 30.

Pruritus: see dermatitis.

Appendix 8: Urinary and Stoma Appliances

This Appendix includes incontinence appliances, urethral catheters, and stoma products.

Incontinence appliances and urethral catheters

Incontinence appliances are listed in Part IXB of *Drug Tariff* or Part 5 of *Scottish Drug Tariff*; urethral catheters are included in Part IXA of *Drug Tariff* or Part 3 of *Scottish Drug Tariff*

DRAINABLE DRIBBLING APPLIANCES

Re-usable for at least 1 month (with exception of Alexa®)

Bullen range
Bags (Bullen)
 Net price 10 Dribblet® bags = £21.78; 10 Dribblet® sheath bags = £48.88

DePuy range
Aquadry® (DePuy)
 Drip type urinal. Net price 1 = £50.54

Henleys range
Alexa® dribbler bag (Henleys)
 Plain disposable bag, with draw strings. Net price 100 bags = £4.22; 100 bags with non-reflux valve = £16.25

Jade-Euro-Med range
Bag (Jade-Euro-Med)
 Dribbling bag with loops and tapes. Net price 1 = £16.33
Urinal (Jade-Euro-Med)
 Drip male urinal with tap. Net price 1 = £43.87; 1 replacement belt = £10.82

Rüsch range
Peoplecare® (Rüsch)
 Male drip urinal. Net price 1 = £48.49

Ward range
Bags (Ward)
 Male dribbling bag with diaphragm and belt. Net price 1 = £27.24

INCONTINENCE BELTS

Average life 6 months

Jade-Euro-Med range
Waist belt for kipper bags (Jade-Euro-Med)
 Net price 1 = £5.40; 1 (with webbing band) = £5.40

Rüsch range
Peoplecare® (Rüsch)
 Waist and support strap for kipper bag. Net price 1 = £6.28

SIMS Portex range
Belts (SIMS Portex)
 Rubber belt. Net price 1 = £5.51
 Web belt (small, medium, or large) = £10.82

Ward range
Belts (Ward)
 Waist belt for black kipper bag. Net price 1 = £5.00
 Rubber belt for PP (pubic pressure) urinal. Net price 1 = £4.33

INCONTINENCE SHEATHS

Unless otherwise indicated the incontinence sheaths (also known as penile sheaths or external catheters) listed below are of the soft, flexible, latex type. Each sheath may be left in place for 1 to 3 days between changes

Bard range
Integrity® (Bard)
 Incontinence sheath, self-adhesive. Net price 30 sheaths (25, 30, or 35 mm) = £39.49
Reliasheath® (Bard)
 Incontinence sheath with adhesive strip. Net price 30 sheaths (20, 25, 30, 35, or 40 mm) = £36.21
Uriplan® (Bard)
 Incontinence sheath. Net price 30 sheaths (20, 25, 30, 35, or 40 mm) = £24.25
 Uro sheath® (washable; may be used many times). Net price 1 (25, 35, or 40 mm) = £5.06

Camp range
Posey® (Camp)
 Incontinence sheath. 'Fastflow' incontinence sheath Net price 10 sheaths (25, 30, or 35 mm) = £6.38

Cliniflex range
Medimates® (CliniFlex)
 Incontinence sheath with single-sided adhesive strip. Net price 30 sheaths (straight, 20, 25, 30, 35, or 40 mm; bulb, 25, 30, or 35 mm) = £29.35
 Incontinence sheath with double-sided adhesive strip. Net price 30 sheaths (straight, 20, 25, 30, 35, or 40 mm; bulb, 25, 30, or 35 mm) = £31.31

Coloplast range
Conveen® (Coloplast)
 Incontinence sheath, with anti-kink design and Uriliner® adhesive strip. Net price 30 sheaths (very small, small, medium, large, or extra-large) = £42.54; 30 Security® sheaths (small, medium, or large) = £42.54
Conveen self-sealing Urisheath® (Coloplast)
 Incontinence sheath. Net price 30 sheaths (small, medium, or large) = £42.09; 30 Security® sheaths (small, medium, or large) = £42.09

DePuy range
Aquadry® (DePuy)
 Incontinence sheath. Net price 10 sheaths (small, medium, large, or extra-large) = £10.04; 30 sheaths with bulbous end (small, medium, standard, large, or extra-large) = £30.12
Aquadry Freedom® (DePuy)
 Freedom® incontinence sheath, self-adhesive. Net price 30 sheaths (small, medium, standard, large, or extra-large) = £41.14
 Freedom Plus® incontinence sheath, self-adhesive. Net price 30 sheaths (small, medium, standard, large, or extra-large) = £41.14
Clear Advantage® (DePuy)
 Incontinence sheath, silicone, self-adhesive . Net price 30 sheaths (small, medium, large, extra-large) = £40.94

EMS Medical range
Sheaths (EMS)

Incontinence sheath. Net price 100 sheaths (25, 30, or 35 mm) = £44.29; 30 sheaths (with liner; 25, 30, or 35 mm) = £32.29

Hollister range
InCare® (Hollister)

Incontinence sheath, self-adhesive. Net price 30 sheaths (22–25 mm; 26–30 mm; 31–35 mm; 36–39 mm) = £40.38

Hospital Management and Supplies range
Macrodom® (Hospital Management & Supplies)

Incontinence sheath, including adhesive strip. Net price 30 sheaths (with 2-inch tube) = £22.30; 25 sheaths (with 5-inch tube) = £23.33

Macrodom Plus® (Hospital Management & Supplies)

Incontinence sheath, including adhesive strip. Net price 30 sheaths (small, medium, or large) = £23.00

North West Medical range
Uridrop® (North West)

Incontinence sheath. Net price 30 sheaths (paediatric = 42 or 55 mm; sizes 1, 2, 3, or 4 = 70, 80, 100, or 107 mm) = £12.70

Incontinence sheath, with Uristrip® adhesive strip. Net price 30 sheaths (paediatric = 42 or 55 mm; sizes 1, 2, 3, or 4 = 70, 80, 100, or 107 mm) = £25.40

Payne range
Incontiaid® (Payne)

Incontinence sheath. Net price 10 sheaths, with adhesive strip (sizes 20, 25, 30, 35 or 40 mm) = £13.05; 1 sheath, without adhesive strip (sizes 20, 25, 30, 35 or 40 mm) = 82p; 10 adhesive strips = £4.24

Rüsch range
Dryaid® (Rüsch)

Incontinence sheath. Net price 20 sheaths (with adhesive strip; small, medium, large, or extra-large) = £26.13; 20 sheaths (without adhesive strip; small, medium, large, or extra-large) = £15.14

Portasheath® (Rüsch)

Incontinence sheath. Net price 25 sheaths (25, 30, or 35 mm) = £21.25

Secure external catheter kit, with adhesive strip. Net price 10 sheaths (25, 30, or 35 mm) = £8.70

Salts range
Heritage Cohesive /Sheath Pack® (Salts)

Incontinence sheath, with adhesive. Net price 30 sheaths (17, 22, 25, 32, or 34 mm) = £33.59

Male continence sheath (Salts)

Incontinence sheath. Net price 10 sheaths (17, 22, 25, 32, or 34 mm) = £7.57

Seton range
Incontinence sheath (Seton)

Incontinence sheath. Net price 30 sheaths (small, medium, large, or extra-large) = £31.70; 30 sheaths with self-adhesive liner (small, medium, or extra-large) = £37.77

Sherwood range
Texas Catheter® (Sherwood)

Incontinence sheath, with adhesive strip. Net price 12 sheaths = £8.64

Uri Drain® (Sherwood)

Incontinence sheath, with double-sided adhesive strap (25, 30, or 35 mm). Net price 10 = £8.00

Simpla range
U-Sheath Plus® (Simpla)

Incontinence sheath, with external liner. Net price 30 sheaths (small, medium, large, or extra-large) = £28.19

Incontinence sheath, with Uriseal® liner. Net price 30 sheaths (small, medium, large, or extra-large) = £39.96

U-Sheath® (Simpla)

Incontinence sheath, with Uriseal® liner. Net price 30 sheaths (small, medium, large, or extra-large) = £36.54

SIMS Portex range
Continence sheath (SIMS Portex)

Incontinence sheath. Net price 1 sheath (small, medium, large, or extra-large) = £1.42

Uro Flo® (SIMS Portex)

Incontinence sheath, straight, including adhesive liner. Net price 30 sheaths (small, medium, or large) = £39.30

Uro Flo Mk2® (SIMS Portex)

Incontinence sheath, bulbous, with adhesive liner. Net price 30 sheaths (small, medium or large) = £39.30

Male incontinence sheath (SIMS Portex)

Incontinence sheath. Net price 100 sheaths = £65.11

FIXING STRIPS AND ADHESIVES

Bio Diagnostics®
Urifix® tape. Net price 5 m = £4.90

Camp®
Posey® sheath holder. Net price 12 (adult) = £13.25; 12 (paediatric) = £10.20

CliniFlex®
MediMates® adhesive strips. Net price 30 = £10.00

ConvaTec®
Urihesive® strips. Net price 15 = £6.27

DePuy
Aquadry® penile liners. Net price 20 = £8.22

EMS Medical
Urifix® tape. Net price 5 m = £6.12

North West Medical
Uristrip® adhesive strip. Net price 30 = £12.70

Payne
Incontiaid® sheath holder. Net price 1 = 96p

Rüsch
Dryaid® strip. Net price 20 strips = £10.99

Salts
Heritage® sheath collar pack. Net price 30 = £3.86

NHS Cohesive® strips for use with sheaths. Net price 10 = £4.97

LEG BAGS

Most plastic bags suitable for use for 5–7 days; rubber bags re-usable for 4–6 months

Bard range
Uriplan® (Bard)

Leg bag, plastic, shaped, with tap outlet and elastic Velcro straps. Net price 10 bags (350 mL, direct inlet) = £24.48; 10 bags (350 mL, 12 inch inlet tube) = £24.26; 10 bags (500 mL, direct inlet) = £24.66; 10 bags (500 mL, 4 or 12 inch inlet tube) = £24.75; 10 bags (750 mL, direct inlet, or 4, 12, or 15 inch inlet tube) = £24.84

Seton Urisac® (Bard)

Leg bag, plastic. Net price 10 bags (350 mL, short tube) = £12.48; 10 bags (350 mL, long tube) = £12.85; 10 bags (500 mL, short tube) = £13.59; 10 bags (500 mL, long tube) = £13.97; 10 bags (750 mL, short tube) = £14.33; 10 bags (750 mL, long tube) = £14.94

Coloplast range
Conveen® (Coloplast)

Security leg bag, plastic. Net price 10 bags (500 mL, 25 or 50 cm tube) = £20.19

Contour leg bag, plastic, shaped, sterile with sample port. Net price, with 1 set Velcro bands, 10 bags (600 mL, 5 or 30 cm tube; 800 mL, 45 cm tube) = £24.76; 10 non-sterile bags (600 mL, 45 cm adjustable tube) = £24.76

ConvaTec range
Accuseal® (ConvaTec)

Leg bag, plastic. Net price 10 bags (500 mL) = £18.18

DePuy range
Aquadry® (DePuy)

Catheter drainage bag, plastic. Net price 10 bags (small) = £22.61; 10 bags (large) = £23.21

Leg bag, plastic. Net price 10 bags (350, 500, or 750 mL, short or long tube) = £22.43

Leg bag, with Aquasleeve® support. Net price 10 bags (500 mL short or long tube, 750 mL long tube; small, medium or large support) – £21.89

EMS Medical range
Leg drainage bags (EMS)

Leg bag, plastic. Net price 10 bags (500 mL, short or long tube) = £15.94

Incare range
Urinary leg bag (Incare)

Leg bag, plastic. Net price 10 bags (540 mL, 37 cm tube) = £24.91; 10 bags (540 mL, direct in-let) = £24.31

Jade-Euro-Med range
Leg bags (Jade-Euro-Med)

Kipper bag, black, white, or clear. Net price 1 bag = £24.85

Leg drainage bag, plastic, with tap outlet. Net price 10 bags (350 or 500 mL) = £21.32; 10 bags (750 mL) = £22.24

Maersk range
Careline® (Maersk)

Leg bag, plastic, with tap outlet and overnight connection tube. Net price, with 1 pair Velcro straps, 10 bags (350 mL, short or long tube) = £21.87; 10 bags (500 mL, short or long tube) = £22.45; 10 bags (750 mL, short or long tube) = £22.92

Manfred Sauer range
Discreet® (Manfred Sauer)

Leg bag, female with overnight connection tube and fabric/velcro leg straps. Net price 10 bags (450 mL with inlet tube suitable for suprapubic catheter) = £21.25; 10 bags (400 mL with straight inlet tube) = £21.25

Sauer leg bag (Manfred Sauer)

Leg bag, plastic, with tap outlet and overnight connection tube and fabric/velcro leg straps. Net price 10 bags (700 or 1300 mL, short or long tube) = £19.31; 10 bags, sterile (700 or 1300 mL, short or long tube) = £22.30

Payne range
Incontiaid® (Payne)

Leg bag, plastic. Net price 1 bag (500 or 750 mL) = £2.44

Single-chambered GU Black Kipper Bags (Payne)

Leg bag, single-chambered. Net price 1 bag (rubber, with box outlet tap) = £38.62; 1 rubber bag (for night use) = £51.99; 1 bag (for female use) = £38.62; 1 bag (rubber, kipper-style) = £47.60; 1 bag (rubber, Ross type) = £44.08

Leg bags (formerly Willis range)

Rubber bag, for catheter drainage, short neck leg strap. Net price 1 bag = £26.47; 1 bag with web belt and support strap) = £30.98

Rubber bag, female, drainage bag, with conical mount. Net price 1 bag = £25.12; 1 bag (with web belt and support strap) = £29.62

Rüsch range
Leg bag (Rüsch)

Leg bag, plastic. Net price 10 bags (short tube, 350 or 500 mL) = £13.48; 10 bags (long tube, 350 or 500 mL) = £14.41; 10 bags (750 mL) = £9.64

Kipper bags (Rüsch)

Leg bag. Net price 1 bag (clear/white plastic or all black plastic or rubber, with strap and buckle) = £26.24; 1 bag (clear/white plastic, without strap and buckle) = £21.51

Salts range
Heritage® (Salts)

Leg bag, plastic. Net price 10 bags (500 mL, short tube) = £13.99; 10 bags (500 mL, long tube) = £14.24; 10 bags (750 mL, short tube) = £15.59; 10 bags (750 mL, long tube) = £15.96; 5 leg bag packs = £9.99

Sherwood range
Argyle® (Sherwood)

Leg bag, plastic. Net price (350, 500 or 750 mL, short or long tube) = £21.30

Simpla range
Trident® T1 (Simpla)

Leg bag, plastic. Net price 10 bags (350 mL, short tube) = £24.55; 10 bags (500 mL, short or long tube) = £24.75; 10 bags (750 mL, short, long, or adjustable long tube) = £24.86

Trident® T2 (Simpla)

Leg bag, plastic. Net price 10 bags (350 mL, short tube) = £24.79; 10 bags (500 mL, short tube or long tube) = £25.06; 10 bags (750 mL, short tube, long tube or adjustable long tube) = £25.18

SIMS Portex range
Leg bags (SIMS Portex)

Leg bag, with valve outlet, natural latex straps, and plastic tube. Net price 10 bags (350 mL, short tube) = £23.68; 10 bags (350 mL, long tube) = £24.11; 10 bags (500 mL, short tube) = £24.14; 10 bags (500 mL, long tube) = £24.77; 10 bags (750 mL, short tube) = £24.50; 10 bags (750 mL, long tube) = £24.64

Leg bag, with twist tap, elastic straps, and plastic tube. Net price 10 bags (750 mL, short tube) = £24.54; 10 bags (750 mL, long tube, 30 cm) = £24.68

Tri-form® leg bag, plastic. Net price 10 bags (500 mL, short tube) = £23.88; 10 bags (500 mL, medium tube) = £24.16; 10 bags (500 mL, long tube) = £24.37

NHS Meredith® (SIMS Portex)

Top outlet bag. Net price 25 bags (2 litres) = £47.28

PVC drainage bag (SIMS Portex)

Leg bag, plastic. Net price 1 bag (small or large) = £3.74

Rubber bags (SIMS Portex)

Leg bag, rubber, with leg strap. Net price = £36.00

Uro-Flo® (SIMS Portex)

Standard leg bag, plastic. Net price 10 bags (350, 500 or 750 mL, 5 or 30 cm tube) = £14.66

Universal range
Unicorn® (Universal)

Leg bag, plastic. Net price 10 bags (350 mL, short tube) = £17.60; 10 bags (500 mL, short or long tube) = £17.80; 10 bags (750 mL, short or long tube) = £18.00

Ward range
Kipper bag (Ward)

Leg bag, kipper type, rubber. Net price 1 bag (black, clear, or white) = £22.75

Leg drainage bag (Ward)

Leg bag, plastic. Net price 10 bags (350 mL) = £10.99; 10 bags (500 mL) = £11.33; 10 bags (750 mL) = £12.00

St Peters Pattern (Ward)

Leg bag. Net price 5 bags = £30.41

Comfort® (Ward)

Leg bag, plastic. Net price 10 bags (350 mL) = £11.03; 10 bags (500 mL) = £11.35; 10 bags (750 mL) = £11.93

NIGHT DRAINAGE BAGS

Suitable for night-time use for collection of urine from indwelling catheters or from incontinence sheaths; bag hangers normally supplied through community nursing service.

Drainage bags have life of 5–7 nights

Bard

Uriplan® drainage bag. Net price 10 bags = £11.10; Collection bag (non-drainable), 10 bags = £2.19

Coloplast

Conveen® 1.5 litre drainage bag with 90 cm tube. Net price 10 bags = £12.44

ConvaTec

Surgicare System® 2 litre drainage bag. Net price 5 bags (Accuseal®) = £7.39; 5 bags (night) = £7.39

Dansac

Dansac® 2 litre night drainage bag. Net price 10 bags = £10.55

DePuy

Aqua® range 2 litre urine drainage bag. Net price 10 bags (Aqua® 2, non-drainable) = £2.06; 10 bags (Aqua® 4) = £9.70

Jade-Euro-Med

2 litre drainage bag with tap outlet. Net price 1 bag = £1.44

Maersk

Careline® range, 2 litre urine drainage bag with 90 cm inlet tube. Net price 10 bags (Careline® E1, non- drainable) = £1.91; 10 bags (Careline® E2, non-drainable, with non-reflux valve) = £2.05; bags (Careline® E4, with non-reflux valve and tap outlet) = £5.01

Rand Rocket

Urine drainage bag (non-drainable, short or long tube). Net price 25 bags = £3.87

Rüsch

Drainage bags, 2 litre. Net price 10 bags (C) = £10.37; 10 bags with non-reflux valve and plug (CV) = £11.51; 10 bags with non-reflux valve and tap (CVT) = £11.93; 10 bags with non-reflux valve and wide bore tap (DVT) = £11.00

Salts

2 litre H2 urine drainage bag. Net price 10 bags with non-reflux valve and tap = £11.61

Sherwood

Argyle® 2 litre urinary drainage bag. Net price 10 bags = £9.60

Simpla

S5 (formerly S4 Plus®) overnight drainage bag. Net price 10 bags = £10.56

Urine drainage bag. Net price 10 bags (S1, non-drainable) = £2.25; 10 bags (S2, non-drainable with non-reflux valve) = £2.38; 10 bags (S4, short tube) = £11.37; 10 bags (S4, long tube) = £11.75

SIMS Portex

Inbeds 2 litre drainage bag with twist tap. Net price 10 bags = £13.13

Mirage® night drainage bag. Net price 10 bags = £10.30

Uro-flo® night drainage bag. Net price 10 bags (female or male) = £14.22

Ward

2 litre drainage bag with push/pull outlet. Net price 10 bags = £11.94

SUSPENSORY SYSTEMS

Drainage bag with support; bags may be used for 5–7 days

Bard

Urisac® Portabag® with belt. Net price 10 bags (plastic) = £11.63; 1 belt = £6.81

EMS Medical

Drainage bag with Shepheard Sporran belt. Net price 10 bags (plastic) = £15.94; 1 belt = £8.10

Rüsch

Portabag® with Portabelt®. Net price 10 bags (plastic) = £15.45; 1 belt = £8.63

SIMS Portex

Holster bag with leg bag holster. Net price 10 bags (400 mL, plastic) = £18.49; 1 holster (24–30, 30–36, or 36–44 inch) = £8.64

TUBING AND ACCESSORIES

Bard

Adaptor for Uro sheath® (penile sheath to leg bag) 8 inch. Net price 1 = £1.04

Uriplan® leg bag straps (washable). Net price 5 pairs = £12.12

Latex leg bag straps. Net price 10 pairs = £2.48

Seton range foam/Velcro leg bag straps. Net price 10 pairs = £4.72

Urisleeve® leg bag holder. Net price 4 (small: 24–39 cm; medium: 36–55 cm; large: 40–70 cm) = £6.90

Coloplast

Velcro bands (washable). Net price 10 pairs = £34.89

ConvaTec

Accuseal® leg bag extension tube. Net price 10 tubes = £6.71

DePuy

Leg bag connecting tube. Net price 10 = £6.95

Aquadry® leg straps. Net price 5 pairs = £9.25

Aquasleeve®. Net price 4 (small: 24–33 cm; standard: 34–39 cm; medium: 40–46 cm; large: 47–64 cm) = £6.90

EMS Medical

Velcro leg straps. Net price 10 = £5.58

Incare

Leg bag straps. Net price 1 pair (14 inch, calf or 23 inch, thigh) = £2.73

Jade-Euro-Med

Velcro leg straps. Net price 1 pair = £1.75

Leg bag connecting tube. Net price 1 = £1.36; 1 (with mount) = £2.33

Maersk

Careline® leg bag straps. Net price 10 = £12.18

Payne

Rubber extension tube, 6 inch. Net price = £3.27

Rubber leg strap. Net price 1 = £1.14

Velcro leg strap. Net price 1 = 90p

Portex

Paul (Penrose) tubing. Net price 10 (6, 13, 19, or 25 mm) = £13.12; 10 (32, 38, 44, or 51 mm) = £13.12 [G3]

Tapered adaptor (catheter to leg bag). Net price 1 = £6.12; 1(stepped) = £8.64

Rüsch

Connecting tubes, net price 1 tube for kipper bag = £2.61; 14-inch connecting tube for drip urinal = £2.60; 1 connecting tube for all urinals with female connector = £3.97

Salts

Heritage® leg bag extension tube. Net price 2 tubes = £2.00

Sherwood

Argyle® foam and Velcro strap, washable. Net price 1 (75 cm, leg) = £1.69; 1 (150 cm, abdomen) = £3.17

Argyle Suregrip® general purpose tube, internal diameter 7 mm, length 2.7 m. Net price 50 tubes = £36.00

Argyle Penrose® tubing, internal diameter 6, 8, 10, 13, 16, 19, or 25 mm and length 44 cm. Net price 50 = £30.75

Simpla

Leg bag straps. Net price 20 pairs (foam) = £12.84; 5 pairs (elasticated, washable) = £12.78

G-Strap. Net price 'adult' or 'short', 5 = £11.71 'abdomen', 5 = £12.91

SIMS Portex

Stopcock for Chiron plastic urinal bags (in place of screwcap). Net price 1 = £4.44

Rubber extension tube (with mounts). Net price = £4.59

Rubber tubing (length, 1.5 m). Net price 1 = £10.72

Plastic connector with tube. Net price 1 = £3.05

Female connector for Mitcham bag. Net price = £2.05

Night bag connector. Net price 1 = £1.24

Spare 'O' rings for pubic pressure urinal. Net price 5 = £1.17

Uro-Flo® elastic Velcro leg straps. Net price 5 pairs = £4.21

Leg bag extension tube. Net price 10 (30 cm) = £23.46; 10 (60 cm) = £26.32

Silgrip® leg straps. Net price 5 pairs (elasticated or Side-Fix thigh-fitting) = £12.18; 5 pairs (Side-Fix calf-fitting) = £11.58

URINAL SYSTEMS

Patients generally have two urinal systems (one to wash and one to wear). Each appliance should last for 6 months

Bard

Uriplan Maguire® urinal and adaptor. Net price (waist sizes 66–81 cm, 81–96 cm, or 96–112 cm) = £59.21

Mobile paraplegic day and night urinal. Net price 1 = £48.31

Uriplan Maguire® adaptor and tubing. Net price = £7.99

Bell and Croyden

Fridjohn male urinal. Net price 1 = £40.61

Male urinal, day and night use. Net price 1 (with long or short bag) = £37.35

Bullen

Male urinal. Net price 1 (with large-size long bag) = £72.01

DePuy

Aquadry® urinal. Net price 1 cross cut diaphragm and scrotal support; inner sheath and rubber understrap (1.125, 1.25, 1.375, 1.5, or 1.625 inch); pubic pressure: pressure ring, tapered inner sleeve trimmed to fit and rubber understrap; pressure ring, diaphragm and rubber understrap (1, 1.25, or 1.5 inch); pressure ring, diaphragm and scrotal support (1, 1.25, or 1.5 inch) = £54.27

Spares

Bag (for all standard urinals). Net price 5 (250 or 325 mL) = £11.51; rubber leg bag connecting tube with female attachment, net price 1 = £2.73

Flange (child: 0.5, 0.675, 0.75, 0.875, 1, 1.125, or 1.25 inch; adult: 1, 1.125, 1.25, 1.375, 1.5, 1.625, or 1.75 inch). Net price 1 = £25.95

Cones. Net price 1 (small, medium, or large; curved or straight) = £11.22

Rubber belt. Net price 1 (24, 28, 36, or 44 inch) = £3.13

Ellis

Hallam modular urinal. Net price 1 = £31.63; 1 spare bag = £1.68; 1 spare belt = £3.75

Jade-Euro-Med

Male day and night urinal with tap, covered bag, with band and suspensory, and leg strap with air vent. Net price 1 = £51.49

Male night urinal with tap, covered bag, with band and suspensory. Net price 1 = £62.66

Male day and night urinal with tap, long tube, covered bag, with band and suspensory with air vent. Net price 1 = £60.89

Male day and night urinal with tap, double bag, air vent, inflating rim, with band understraps. Net price 1 = £64.49

Male day and night urinal with tap, covered bag, diaphragm top, and air vent. Net price 1 = £55.72

Male day and night urinal with tap, improved pattern, inflating rim, short air vent, with band and understrap. Net price 1 = £61.16; 1 (with extension tube) = £64.55; 1 (with long bag) = £62.03

Male day and night urinal with tap, air vent, diaphragm top, with band and understrap. Net price 1 (with long bag) = £59.33; 1 (with short bag) = £54.98

Male day and night urinal with tap, air vent, with band and suspensory. Net price 1 (long bag) = £52.83

Male day urinal with tap, to contain penis and scrotum. Net price 1 (short bag, with band and understrap) = £49.82; 1 (with inner sheath and air vent) = £51.75

Male jockey appliance with tap. Net price 1 = £55.10

Spares

Replacement belt. Net price 1 = £10.82

Outer receiver. Net price 1 = £12.60

Inner sheath. Net price 5 = £12.60

Plastic bags. Net price 5 = £13.88

Rubber bag. Net price 1 = £23.14

Ring. Net price 1 = 92p

Stoke Mandeville male urinal with tap (specify sheath size). Net price 1 = £58.49; 1 (with double bag) = £70.23; 1 replacement sheath (specify size) = £5.78

Male pubic pressure urinal with tap (specify sheath size). Net price 1 (with rubber bag) = £62.55; 1 (with 5 plastic bags) = £58.87

Spares

Flange with sheaths. Net price 1 = £29.23

Cone. Net price (curved, small, medium, or large; straight, small, medium, large, or extra-large) = £11.59

Plastic bag. Net price 1 (small or large) = £13.88

Rubber bag. Net price 1 = £22.68

Rubber belt. Net price 1 = £4.16

Progress® long life plastic urinal. Net price 1 (inner sheath or scrotal) = £24.71

Fridjohn urinal. Net price 1 = £73.88

YB wet urinal. Net price 1 = £59.96

Essex appliance. Net price 1 = £50.05

One-piece belt. Net price 1 (rubber or plastic bag coverlet) = £50.10

LRC

Dry sheaths. Net price 144 = £14.42

Payne

Male incontinence appliance with rubber belt. Net price 1 (MK1 with combined rubber flange and understraps) = £60.42; 1 (MK2 with rubber flange and fabric facepiece) = £64.97; 1 (MK3 with combined rubber flange, understraps, and coned top) = £53.62; 1 (MK9, with rubber flange and fabric facepiece) = £67.70

Lightweight male incontinence appliance. Net price 1 (MK4 with fabric facepiece and separate long flanged plastic bag with foam pad) = £38.30; 1 (MK5, with fabric facepiece, with belt combined, separate flange, and long flanged plastic bag) = £53.80; 1 (MK6 with combined flange and understraps and long flanged plastic bag with rubber bag) = £47.18; 1 (MK10, with fabric facepiece, with belt combined, separate flange, and long flanged plastic bag) = £56.55

Spares

Rubber flange. Net price 1 (with feathered diaphragm, MK2, MK5, MK9, MK10) = £17.50; 1 (MK1, MK6) = £27.08; 1 (with feathered diaphragm and combined reinforced top, MK3) = £30.72

Material facepiece. Net price 1 facepiece with belt and loop (MK2, MK4, MK5) = £20.28; 1 facepiece with support belt, loop and scrotal = £23.01

Flange support with wide belt and scrotal support (MK9, MK10). Net price 1 = £23.01

Reinforced cone top (MK1, MK2, MK9). Net price 1 = £11.77

Bag (MK1, MK2, MK3, MK9). Net price 1 plastic bag = £2.96; 1 rubber bag = £17.80

Bag, long flange plastic. Net price 1 MK4 bag = £4.54; 1 MK5, MK6, MK10 bag = £4.00

Belt (MK1, MK3, MK6). Net price 1 (elastic) = £8.08; 1 (web) = £5.65; 1 (rubber) = £3.81

Night connector (MK1, MK2, MK3, MK9). Net price 1 = £3.81

Payne's urine director. Net price 1 = £21.62

Stoke Mandeville condom urinal complete. Net price 1 = £49.86

Spares

Kipper bag. Net price 1 = £28.05

Belt. Net price 1 (38, 46, or 60 inch) = £5.95

Rubber tube and connector. Net price 1 = £2.18; rubber tubing = £4.49 per metre; nylon connector (GU or SM) 1 = £1.27

Dry incontinence sheath. Net price 144 = £14.51

Pubic pressure urinal complete with bag. Net price 1 (rubber or plastic bag) = £60.42

Spares

Pubic pressure flange with sheath (1-inch flange with 0.5, 0.625, 0.75, or 0.875 inch sheath; 1.25-inch flange with 0.875 or 1 inch sheath; 1.5-inch flange with 1.125 or 1.25 inch sheath; 1.75-inch flange with 1.375, 1.5, or 1.625 inch sheath). Net price 1 = £27.08

Coned top. Net price 1 (straight or curved: small, medium, or large; straight: extra-large) = £11.77

Replacements

Rubber bag with vent tube (MK1, MK2, MK3, MK9). Net price 1 = £21.37

Reinforced cone top with vent tube (MK1, MK2, MK3, MK9). Net price 1 = £15.48

Latex tubing, 8 or 10 mm bore. Net price per metre = £4.49

GU Condom set. Net price 1 = £51.99; 1 (with 40 oz bag) = £64.50

Urinal replacement parts

Nylon stud (GU or SM). Net price 1 = £1.27; 1 (with latex tube) = £2.18

Waist belt for single-chambered bag. Net price 1 (38, 46, or 60 inch) = £5.95

(formerly Willis range)

Male urinal, day and night, air tube to bag, inner sheath and diaphragm to receiver, web belt and cotton suspensory bag. Net price 1 = £48.91; 1 (long narrow Coutil®-covered bag, web belt and cotton suspensory bag) = £50.91

Male urinal, receiver to contain penis and scrotum, web waist band, and tape understraps. Net price 1 (day, night, or small build) = £46.71

Male urinal, long rubber bag with 2 leg straps, loops and straps, flanged receiver, air tube, diaphragm and short conical inner sheath, web band and cotton suspensory bag. Net price 1 (day and night) = £48.32

Male urinal, short rubber bag, detachable bag and night tube, web belt and cotton suspensory bag. Net price 1 (day and night) = £38.94

Spares for above urinals

Suspension bag. Net price 1 (small, medium, or large) = £4.92

Rüsch

Thames urinal with bag and connecting tube. Net price 1 (standard or long bag) = £76.24

Severn urinal with bag and connecting tube. Net price 1 (standard, long, or 5 plastic bags) = £76.24; 5 Severn spare sheaths = £29.89

Mersey urinal with bag and connecting tube. Net price 1 (standard, long, or 5 plastic bags) = £76.24

Wye, male, MkII, light-weight urinal. Net price 1 (with separate connecting tube and on/off valve) = £24.64; 1 (with long night extension tube) = £28.72; 1 (with short or long bag) =£41.03

Arizona male urinal. Net price 1 = £76.24

'55' male urinal for paraplegic patients. Net price 1 = £75.09; 6 spare sheaths = £34.05

Stoke Mandeville pattern male urinal with double chamber rubber collection bag. Net price 1 (20, 24, 25, 28, 32, 35, 38, 42, 45, 48, 51, 54, 57, 60, or 63 mm sheath) =£76.24; 1 spare sheath = £7.03

Sahara one-piece top pubic pressure urinal with bag. Net price 1 paediatric (with small rubber collection bag or 5 small plastic collection bags) = £72.68; 1 standard or large (with standard or long rubber collection bag or 5 medium plastic collection bags, and connecting tube) = £72.68

Peoplecare® pubic pressure male urinal. Net price 1 paediatric (flange 25 mm and sheath 13, 16, 19, or 22 mm; or flange 29 mm and sheath 22 or 25 mm; or flange 32 mm and sheath 19, 22, or 25 mm) = £23.60; 1 adult (flange 38 mm and sheath 19, 22, 25, 29, or 32 mm; or flange 44 mm and sheath 35, 38, or 41 mm) = £23.60

Spares

Pubic pressure bag, standard. Net price 1 (medium) = £12.18; 1 (large) = £15.10; 1 (curved top, small, medium, or large) = £9.19; 1 (straight top, small, medium, large, or extra-large) = £9.19

Transverse rubber bag with tap. Net price 1 = £24.94

Pubic pressure flange for transverse rubber bag with tap. Net price 1 (double-based) = £23.60; 1 (adult, rubber) = £27.21

Kipper inco set with 1 black rubber kipper bag, 10 penile sheaths, waist and support strap, and connecting tube. Net price 1 = £40.84

Salts

Male pubic pressure urinal with rubber bag or 4 plastic bags. Net price 1 = £49.62

Spares

Pubic pressure flange with sheath (1-inch flange with 0.5, 0.625, 0.75, or 0.875 inch sheath; 1.25-inch flange with 0.75, 0.875, or 1 inch sheath; 1.5-inch flange with 0.75, 0.875, 1, or 1.125 inch sheath; 1.75-inch flange with 1.375, 1.5, or 1.625 inch sheath). Net price 1 = £23.59

Cone. Net price 1 (small, medium, or large: straight or curved; extra-large: straight) = £10.50

Pubic pressure flange belt. Net price 1 = £20.72

Bags. Net price 4 (plastic, child or adult) = £11.54; 1 (rubber, child, adult, or transverse) = £11.54

Belt. Net price = £3.51

SIMS Portex

Male pubic pressure urinal, child, with integral flange. Net price 1 (rubber bag, straight cone, medium) = £60.72; 1 (plastic bag, curved cone, small or medium) = £59.36

Spares

Pubic pressure flange with integral sheath for child. Net price 1 (25-mm flange with 13, 16, 19, or 22 mm sheath; 29-mm flange with 25 mm sheath; 32-mm flange with 25 mm sheath) = £33.42

Cone. Net price 1 (small, medium, or large, straight or curved; extra-large, straight) = £14.13

Pubic pressure flange, double-based. Net price 1 (child, 32 mm; adult, 38 or 44 mm) = £29.87

Chailey male urinal. Net price 1 (child, plastic bag) = £62.48; 1 (adolescent or adult, rubber bag) = £56.02; 1 (adolescent or adult, plastic bag) = £70.96

Spares

Curved top with integral sheath and straps. Net price 1 (child: 22-mm sheath; adult: 22, 25, 29, 32, 35, 38, or 44 mm sheath) = £37.38

Belt, rubber. Net price 1 (61 or 91 cm) = £5.51

Bags, plastic (also suitable for pubic pressure and Chiron® urinals). Net price 1 (wide neck, adult, or child) = £3.67

Bags, rubber (also suitable for pubic pressure and Chiron® urinals). Net price 1 child size = £17.78; 1 adult size = £24.36

Male pubic pressure urinal, adult, with integral flange. Net price 1 (rubber bag, various sizes) = £70.35; 1 (plastic bag, various sizes) = £65.55

Replacement pubic pressure flange. Net price 1 = £33.42

Male pubic pressure urinal, adult, with double-based flange. Net price 1 (rubber bag, various sizes) = £68.63; 1 (plastic bag, various sizes) = £65.55

Replacement sheath. Net price 10 = £1.28

Bag, rubber, for pubic pressure urinals. Net price 1 (adult, with vent tube) = £29.16; 1 (adult, double) = £31.23

Stoke Mandeville urinal. Net price 1 (sheath type) = £64.09; 1 (double rubber bag) = £83.29

Spares

Sheath. Net price 1 = £8.74; 10 (for sheath type) = £3.84

Chiron male rubber urinal with webbing belt. Net price 1 = £57.68

Male one-piece urinal. Net price = £54.91

Surrey model lightweight urinal. Net price (MKI or MKII) = £52.17

Spares

Foam pad. Net price 5 (76 mm/32 mm) = £6.47

Chiron urinal. Net price 1 (male, plastic, rubber sheaths) = £29.85; 1 (geriatric, film-type sheaths) = £43.34; 1 (rubber sheaths) = £43.34

Spares

Sheath. Net price 1 (rubber) = £5.51; 10 (non-allergenic film type) = £1.01

Net suspensory. Net price 1 = £12.96

Male urinal for bed use. Net price 1 = £48.69

Pubic flange, large opening. Net price 1 = £22.39

Transverse rubber bag and stopcock. Net price 1 (child) = £32.95

Ward

Jockey male urinal. Net price 1 = £71.36

Varsity male urinal. Net price 1 = £55.08

Male urinal. Net price 1 (day use, covered bag, complete with belt suspensory and thigh strap) = £45.57; 1 (day and night, covered bag, air vent, belt suspensory) = £47.16; 1 (day and night, short bag and belt) = £48.82; 1 (day and night, short covered bag and belt) = £52.92; 1 (day and night, double chamber bag) = £55.00; 1 (day and night, long bag and belt) = £48.82

Paraplegic male urinal. Net price 1 = £66.72

Stoke Mandeville Pattern. Net price 1 = £64.11; 1 (removable rubber sheath, double chamber rubber bag, thigh strap and belt) = £57.58

Spare sheath. Net price 1 = £5.94

Male pubic pressure urinal. Net price 1 (rubber bag) = £59.74; 1 (plastic bag) = £52.93

Spares

Pubic pressure flange. Net price 1 = £27.40

Pubic pressure cone. Net price 1 = £10.83

Bags. Net price 1 (rubber) = £14.84; 1 (plastic) = £2.97

Male urinal. Net price 1 (day, covered bag complete with belt) = £43.38; 1 (day and night or night, covered bag complete with belt, suspensory, and thigh strap) = £57.31; 1 (day and night, long tube, air vent, rubber bag, complete with belt and thigh strap) = £52.03

Male urinal. Net price 1 (night, covered bag complete with belt, suspensory, and thigh strap) = £57.31

Male dribbling bag and tapes. Net price 1 = £21.17

Male urinal. Net price 1 (day and night, short covered bag or short bag and belt) = £48.82

Male urinal. Net price 1 (sheath and disc type with long rubber belt or sheath and suspensory with short or long covered bag) = £53.24

Night urinal. Net price 1 (with long tube) = £25.73

Stoke Mandeville sheath-type urinal, with 30 rubber film sheaths, rubber bag, and thigh strap and belt. Net price 1 = £50.97

Webbing belt. Net price 1 = £9.01

Elastic leg strap. Net price 10 = £5.15

Net suspensory. Net price 1 = £11.85

Spare rubber bag with vent. Net price 1 = £25.75

Spare receiver. Net price 1 = £37.08

URETHRAL CATHETERS

Urethral catheter sizes are designated by the Charrière (Ch) gauge system; when the size is not stated by the prescriber the Drug Tariff recommends that size 14 or 16 be supplied. For the Foley catheter, if the balloon size is not stated, the 10 mL size should be supplied for adults, 5 mL for paediatric use (balloon sizes are defined as the amount of fluid required to fully inflate the volume of lumen).

Foley catheters for short-/medium-term use in adults
Bard
Uriplan®, teflon-coated latex, male or female. Net price, male (12–26 Ch: 10-mL balloon; 16–26 Ch: 30-mL balloon), 1 catheter = £2.23; female (Ch 12–22: 10-mL balloon), 1 catheter = £3.33; pre-filled with sterile water (Ch 12–22: 10-mL balloon), 1 catheter = £2.54

Rüsch
Soft Simplastic®, PVC, male or female. Net price, male (12–26 Ch: 10-mL balloon; 16–26 Ch: 30 mL balloon), 1 catheter = £4.52; female (12–22 Ch: 10-mL balloon; 16–22 Ch: 30-mL balloon), 1 catheter = £4.52

100 plus®, teflon-coated latex, male or female. Net price male (12–26 Ch: 10-mL balloon; 16–26 Ch: 30-mL balloon), 1 catheter = £1.95; female (12–22 Ch: 10-mL balloon; 16–32 Ch: 30-mL balloon), 1 catheter = £2.48

SIMS Portex
Eschmann Folatex®, latex, male or female. Net price, male (12–28 Ch: 10- or 30-mL balloon), 1 catheter = £2.04; female (12–28 Ch: 10- or 30-mL balloon), 1 catheter = £2.04

Foley catheters for short-/medium-term use in children
All 8–10 Ch: 5-mL balloon
Bard
Uriplan®, teflon-coated latex. Net price 1 catheter = £6.15

Rüsch
100 plus®, teflon-coated latex. Net price 1 catheter = £4.16

SIMS Portex
Eschmann Folatex®, latex. Net price 1 catheter = £3.69

Foley catheters for long-term use in adults
Bard
Biocath®, hydrogel-coated, male or female. Net price, male (12–26 Ch: 10- or 30-mL balloon), 1 catheter = £6.88; female (12–22 Ch: 10-mL balloon), 1 catheter = £6.97; pre-filled with sterile water, (12–22 Ch: 10-mL balloon), 1 male catheter = £7.14; 1 female catheter = £7.14

Silastic®, silicone-coated. Net price (12–24 Ch: 10-mL balloon; 16–28 Ch: 30-mL balloon), 1 catheter = £7.23

Bard®, silicone elastomer-coated latex, male or female. Net price, male (12–22 Ch: 10-mL balloon; 16–22 Ch: 30-mL balloon), 1 catheter = £7.56; female (16–22 Ch: 30-mL balloon), 1 catheter = £7.56; pre-filled with sterile water, male or female (12–22 Ch: 10-mL balloon), 1 catheter = £8.17

Bard®, all silicone. Net price male (12–22 Ch: 10-mL balloon; 16–22 Ch: 30-mL balloon), 1 catheter = £7.80; female (12–16 Ch: 10-mL balloon), 1 catheter = £7.48

Medasil
All silicone, male or female. Net price, male (12–26 Ch: 10-mL balloon; 16–26 Ch: 30-mL balloon), 1 catheter = £4.62; female (12–26 Ch: 10-mL balloon; 16–26 Ch: 30-mL balloon), 1 catheter = £4.62

Rüsch
Silikon 100®, male or female. Net price male (12–26 Ch: 10-mL balloon; 18–20 Ch: 20-mL balloon; 22–26 Ch: 30-mL balloon), 1 catheter = £6.50; female (12–22 Ch: 10-mL balloon; 18–20 Ch: 20-mL balloon; 22 Ch: 30-mL balloon), 1 catheter = £6.50

Ultrasil®, silicone elastomer-coated latex, male. Net price (12–26 Ch: 10-mL balloon; 16–26 Ch: 30-mL balloon), 1 catheter = £5.42

Sherwood

Argyle®, all silicone, male or female. Net price, male (12–24 Ch: 10-mL balloon; 16 Ch: 20-mL balloon; 18–26 Ch: 30-mL balloon), 1 catheter = £5.83; female (12–18 Ch: 10-mL balloon), 1 catheter = £5.83

Simpla

All silicone, male or female. Net price, male (12–26 Ch: 10-mL balloon; 16–18 Ch: 20-mL balloon; 20–26 Ch: 30-mL balloon), 1 catheter = £7.78; female (12–18 Ch: 10-mL balloon; 20–26 Ch: 30-mL balloon), 1 catheter = £7.73

Trident®, silicone elastomer-coated latex, male. Net price (12–22 Ch: 10-mL balloon; 16–24 Ch: 30-mL balloon), 1 catheter = £4.82

Foley catheters for long-term use in children
All 8–10 Ch: 5-mL balloon

Bard

Biocath®, hydrogel-coated. Net price 1 catheter = £6.97

Medasil

All silicone. Net price 1 catheter = £4.62

Rüsch

Silikon 100®. Net price 1 catheter = £6.50

Sherwood

Argyle®, all silicone. Net price 1 catheter = £6.29

Simpla

All silicone. Net price 1 catheter = £7.84

Nélaton catheters ('ordinary' cylindrical catheter)

Bard

Reliacath®, teflon-coated latex, 14 Ch. Net price 5-catheter pack = £6.65

Reliacath®, plastic, male, female, or paediatric. Net price, male or female (12–18 Ch), 5-catheter pack = £6.13; paediatric (8–10 Ch), 5-catheter pack = £6.13

DePuy

Aquadry® *Self-cath*, male, female or paediatric. Net price, male (8–18 Ch), 5-catheter pack = £5.00; female (10–14 Ch), 5-catheter pack = £5.00; paediatric (8–10 Ch), 5-catheter pack = £5.00

EMS

PVC, male, female or paediatric. Net price, male (10–18 Ch), 5-catheter pack = £4.91; female (12–18 Ch), 5-catheter pack = £5.23; paediatric (6–10 Ch), 5-catheter pack = £5.23

Maersk

PVC, male, female or paediatric. Net price, male (12–24 Ch), 5-catheter pack = £5.00; female (12–16 Ch), 5-catheter pack = £5.00; paediatric (6–10 Ch), 5-catheter pack = £5.00

Pennine

Male, female, or paediatric. Net price, male (12–16 Ch), 10-catheter pack = £3.64; female (10–14 Ch), 10-catheter pack = £3.32; paediatric (6–10 Ch), 10-catheter pack = £3.32

Portex

PVC, male or female, 8–14 Ch. Net price, male, 5-catheter pack = £7.15; female, 5-catheter pack = £6.85

Rüsch

Jacques®, soft red rubber, 8–18 Ch. Net price 1 catheter = £1.40, 5-catheter pack = £5.79

Riplex Jacques®, PVC, male or female, 8–18 Ch. Net price, male, 5-catheter pack = £6.66; female, 5-catheter pack = £6.07

Riplex®, extra-long, PVC, male or female, 8–18 Ch. Net price 5-catheter pack = £6.75

Simpla

Male, female, or paediatric. Net price, male (12–14 Ch), 5-catheter pack = £5.00; female (12–14 Ch), 5-catheter pack = £5.00; paediatric (8–10 Ch), 5-catheter pack = £5.00

SIMS Portex

PVC, male or female, 8–14 Ch. Net price, male, 5-catheter pack = £7.30; female, 5-catheter pack = £7.05

Nélaton catheters (single use)

Astra Tech

Lofric®, PVC, single use, male, female, paediatric, or Tiemann tip. Net price, male (8–24 Ch); female (8–18 Ch); paediatric (6–10 Ch); Tiemann tip (10–20 Ch), 25-catheter pack (all) = £30.00

Coloplast

Conveen Easicath®, single use, male, female, paediatric, or Tiemann tip. Net price, male (8–22 Ch); female (8–16 Ch); paediatric (6–10 Ch); Tiemann tip (10–20 Ch), 25-catheter pack (all) = £25.00

EMS

Aquacath®, single use, male, female, or paediatric. Net price, male (8–18 Ch); female (8–18 Ch); paediatric (6–10 Ch), 25-catheter pack (all) = £25.00

SIMS Portex

Uro-Flo Silky®, single use, male or female, 8–16 Ch. Net price 25-catheter pack = £30.00

Nélaton catheters (with handle)

EMS

Intex®, PVC, female 8–14 Ch. Net price 5-catheter pack = £5.00

Scott catheters (short curved tubular catheter for women and girls)

SIMS Portex

Polyethylene, female, 8–14 Ch. Net price 5-catheter pack = £11.45

CATHETER VALVE

For use with an indwelling catheter after assessment of bladder function by an appropriate medical professional.

It is recommended that the catheter valve is changed every 5–7 days.

Bard

Flip-Flo® catheter valve. Net price 5 = £11.00

EMS

Catheter valve. Net price 5 = £11.00

STOMA APPLIANCES

Stoma appliances are listed in Part IXC of *Drug Tariff* or Part 6 of *Scottish Drug Tariff.*

It is not necessary to state an **order number** on a prescription for one of these products provided the **full details** as given in the BNF are included on the **prescription**.

CLOSED POUCHES AND COLOSTOMY SETS

Closed pouches are suitable for patients with a **colostomy** and well-formed stools

Braun Biotrol range

Biotrol® (Braun Biotrol)

Almarys, one-piece pouch with skin protector adhesive, cover and filter. Net price 30 pouches (clear, starter hole) = £57.30; beige (25, 30, 35, 40, 45, 50 or 60 mm holes) = £57.30

Almarys Petite, one-piece pouch with skin protector adhesive, cover and filter, beige. Net price 30 pouches (starter hole, 25, 30, 35, or 40 mm holes) = £50.70

Biopore, one-piece pouch with adhesive and filter, white. Net price 50 pouches (25, 30, 35, 40, 45 or 50 mm holes) = £61.10

Colo S, one-piece pouch with skin protector adhesive, white. Net price 30 pouches (25, 30, 35, 40, 45, 50, or 60 mm holes) = £63.04

Elite Closed, covered one-piece pouch with skin protector adhesive and filter, white or beige. Net price 30 pouches (starter hole, 25, 30, 35, 40, 45, 50, 60, 70 mm holes) = £66.82; clear (25, 30, 35, 40, 45, 50, 60, 70 mm holes) 30 pouches = £61.77; starter hole, 30 = £62.62

Elite Petite, one-piece pouch with skin protector adhesive and filter, beige. Net price 30 pouches (starter hole, 25, 30, 35, 40 or 45 mm holes) = £56.52

Lockring 2, two-piece pouches with filter and backing, white. Net price 30 pouches (for 35, 50 or 75 mm flanges) = £30.45; paediatric, beige (35 mm hole) 30 pouches = £26.70

Mini S, one-piece pouch with skin protector adhesive and filter, beige. Net price 30 pouches (25, 30, 35, or 40 mm) = £52.01

Integrale, one-piece pouch with skin protector adhesive and filter, white. Net price 30 pouches (starter hole, 25, 30, 35, 40, 45, 50, 60, 70 mm holes) − £66.82

Preference Closed, fabric covered one-piece pouch with skin protector adhesive, porous adhesive collar, and filter, white or beige. Net price 30 pouches (starter hole, 25, 30, 35, 40, 45, 50, 60 mm holes) = £63.24

CliniMed range
Impact® (CliniMed)

Colostomy bag (= pouch), one-piece closed pouch with wafer, filter and disposable liner, opaque. Net price 30 pouches (19, 25, 32, 38, 44 or 51 mm holes) = £61.92

Vogue® **shorter closed bag** (CliniMed)

Colostomy bag (= pouch), one-piece pouch, opaque or clear. Net price 30 pouches (25, 32, 38, 44, 51 mm or 10 mm cut-to-fit holes) = £53.09

Welland (CliniMed)

Oval flange closed bag, one-piece pouch with oval shaped wafer, filter and soft backing, opaque or clear. Net price 30 pouches (10 mm cut-to-fit holes) = £62.18

Softback colostomy bag, one-piece closed pouch with wafer, filter, and soft backing, opaque or clear. Net price 30 pouches (25, 32, 38, 44, 51, 60 mm or 10 mm cut-to-fit holes) = £60.14

Welland colostomy bag (= pouch), one-piece closed pouch with wafer and filter, opaque or clear. Net price 30 pouches (25, 32, 38, 44, 51, 60 mm, or 10 mm cut-to-fit holes) = £58.85

Coloplast range
Assura® (Coloplast)

Maxi, closed pouches, opaque or clear. Net price 30 one-piece pouches (opaque or clear: 20, 25, 30, 35, 40 mm; clear: also 45 or 50 mm holes; 20 mm can be cut to fit up to 55 mm) = £63.57; 30 two-piece pouches, opaque or clear (to fit 40, 50, or 60 mm base plates) = £35.07

Midi, closed pouches with flatus filter, opaque or clear. Net price 30 one-piece pouches (25, 30, 35, 40, 45, or 50 mm holes) = £63.57; 30 two-piece pouches (to fit 40, 50, or 60 mm base plates) = £35.07; base plate (40, 50, or 60 mm), 5 = £13.91

Mini, closed pouches with filter and soft backing. Net price 30 one-piece pouches (clear: 20 mm cut-to-fit hole; 25 or 30 mm holes; opaque: 20 mm cut-to-fit hole; 25, 30, 35, or 40 mm holes) = £51.90

Minicap, closed pouches, opaque. Net price 30 two-piece pouches (to fit 40 or 50 mm base plates) = £28.08

Seal Integral Convexity, one-piece closed pouch. Net price 10 maxi or midi pouches (clear: 15, 18, 21, 25, 28, 31, 35, 38 or 41 mm holes) = £21.19; (opaque: 15–33 mm or 15–43 mm starter holes) = £21.19

Note. Should be used only after assessment of suitability by appropriate medical professional

Conseal® **System** (Coloplast)

Two-piece pouch. Net price 30 bags (to fit 40 or 50 mm base plates) = £36.96; base plate (40 or 50 mm) 5 = £13.66; colostomy plug (40 × 35 or 45 mm, 50 × 35 or 45 mm) 10 = £12.44; discharge bag (40 or 50 mm) 50 = £2.70

K-Flex® (Coloplast)

One-piece closed pouch with karaya skin protector and filter. Net price 30 pouches (clear: 10, 30, or 40 mm holes; opaque: 30 or 40 mm holes) = £66.39

Extra, one-piece closed pouch. Net price, No. 1 (24 mm hole), 100 pouches = £90.10; No. 2 (30 or 40 mm holes), 100 = £110.30; No. 3 (30 mm hole), 100 = £132.30, 50 mm hole, 100 = £133.30

Regular, one-piece closed pouch. Net price, No. 1 (24 mm hole), 100 pouches = £76.00; No. 2 (30 mm hole), 100 = £90.10; No. 3 (30 mm hole), 100 = £108.10; No. 5 (24 mm hole), 100 = £101.30

mc2000® (Coloplast)

One-piece pouch with double seal and filter, opaque or clear. Net price 30 pouches (25, 30, 35, 40, 45, 50, 55, or 60 mm holes) = £68.70

mc2002® (Coloplast)

Two-piece pouch with filter, opaque or clear. Net price 30 pouches (to fit 40 or 60 mm base plates) = £38.82; base plate (40 mm × 15 or 25 mm, 60 × 35 or 45 mm) 5 = £14.33; belt plate (40 or 60 mm) 10 = £5.88

pc3000® (Coloplast)

One-piece pouch, opaque or clear. Net price 30 pouches (25, 30, 35, 40, 45, 50, or 55 mm holes; 25 mm can be cut to fit up to 60 mm) = £64.56

ConvaTec range
Colodress® (ConvaTec)

Colodress, one-piece closed pouch with textured backing, opaque beige. Net price 30 pouches (19, 32, 38, 45, or 50 mm holes; 19 mm can be cut to fit) = £62.34

Colodress Plus, one-piece closed pouch with single-release paper and filter. Net price 30 pouches (opaque or clear: 19, 25, 32, 38, 45, 50, or 64 mm holes; opaque: 19 mm can be cut to fit) = £62.34; Mini pouches, 30 pouches (19, 25, 32, 38, or 45 mm holes) = £56.51

Colodress Plus Lite, one-piece closed pouch, standard, opaque. Net price 30 pouches (25, 32, 38, 45 or 50 mm holes; 19 mm can be cut to fit) = £57.30

Combihesive Natura® (ConvaTec)

Two-piece closed pouch with filter, opaque. Net price 30 pouches (to fit 32, 38, 45, 57 or 70 mm flanges) = £32.07; Mini pouches, 20 pouches (to fit 32, 38, 45 or 57 mm flanges) = £17.58

Consecura® (ConvaTec)

Two-piece closed pouch with filter. Net price 50 pouches (clear or opaque to fit 35, 45 or 55 mm flanges) = £53.45

Naturess® (ConvaTec)

Naturess, closed pouches. Net price 50 pouches (standard opaque pouch: 19 mm starter hole, 25, 32, 38, 45 or 50 mm hole; standard clear pouch: 19 mm starter hole) = £96.39; 50 pouches (small opaque pouch: 19 mm starter hole, 25, 32, 38 or 45 mm holes) = £85.68

Naturess® **A** (ConvaTec)

Naturess A, closed pouches with absorbent pads. Net price 50 pouches (standard opaque pouch: 19 mm starter hole, 25, 32, 38, 45 or 50 mm hole) = £96.39

Surgicare System ® **2** (ConvaTec)

System 2, two-piece closed pouch, white. Net price 30 pouches (to fit 38, 45, 57, or 70 mm flanges) = £31.36

System 2 Combihesive, two-piece closed pouch with textured backing, beige. Net price 30 pouches (to fit 38, 45, 57, or 70 mm flanges) = £31.36; with filter, 30 pouches (to fit 32, 38, 45, 57, or 70 mm flanges) = £32.23 ; Mini pouches, 20 pouches (to fit 32, 38, 45, or 57 mm flanges) = £17.93

Dansac range
Dansac® (Dansac)

Combi Colo F, one-piece pouch with filter, opaque or clear. Net price 100 pouches (standard pouch: 25, 30, 38, 44, 50, or 63 mm holes; small pouch: 25, 30, or 38 mm holes) = £165.04

CombiMicro C + S, one-piece pouch with porous adhesive, filter, skin barrier ring, and fabric backing, opaque or clear. Net price 30 pouches (25, 32, 38, 44, 50, 63 mm or cut-to-fit; 10-38 mm; 38-63 mm holes) = £67.68

Standard Colo, one-piece pouch with filter, clear. Net price 100 pouches (22, 30, 32, or 38 mm holes) = £148.22

Unique, one-piece closed pouch, opaque or clear. Net price 30 pouches (25, 30, 35, 40, 45, 50, 60 mm or cut-to-fit holes) = £59.07; oval flange, opaque or clear, starter hole, net price 30 = £59.07

Unique 2, two-piece closed pouch, opaque or clear. Net price 30 pouches (to fit 36, 43, 55 or 80 mm flange) = £32.73; flange, 36, 43, or 55 mm, net price 5 = £13.39; 80 mm, net price, 5 = £13.66

Unique 2 Mini, two-piece closed pouch with cover, opaque. Net price 30 pouches (to fit 36, 43 or 55 mm flange) = £27.00

Unique 2 MiniCap, two-piece closed pouch, opaque. Net price 30 pouches (to fit 36, 43 or 55 mm flange) = £28.33

Unique 2 Plus, two-piece closed pouch with cover, opaque. Net price 30 pouches (to fit 36, 43, 55 or 80 mm flange) = £31.80

Unique Light, one-piece closed pouch with filter and comfort backing, opaque. Net price 30 pouches (25, 30, 35, 40, 45, 50 or 60 mm holes; 20–60 mm starter hole) = £60.21

Unique Mini, one-piece closed pouch, opaque. Net price 30 pouches (25, 30, 35, or 40 mm holes; 20 mm can be cut to fit up to 50 mm) = £54.39

DePuy range
Schacht® (DePuy)

Colostomy bag (= pouch), one-piece closed pouch. Net price 100 pouches = £34.26

Colostomy appliance. Net price 1 appliance = £29.55

Hollister range
Classic® (Hollister)

All with 25, 32, 38, 44, 51, 64, or 76 mm holes

Adhesive (series 217), one-piece closed pouch with adhesive and filter, clear. Net price 50 pouches = £66.43

Karaya seal (series 716), one-piece pouch with karaya skin protector (without filter), must be worn with belt, clear. Net price 30 pouches = £56.49

Karaya seal with filter (series 211), one-piece closed pouch with karaya skin protector and filter, must be worn with belt, opaque. Net price 30 pouches = £56.49

Karaya 5® Seal (series 331 and 332), one-piece closed pouch with porous adhesive, karaya skin protector seal, and filter, may be worn with belt, opaque or clear. Net price 30 pouches = £66.99

Microporous adhesive (series 314), one-piece compact closed pouch with porous adhesive and filter, may be worn with belt, clear. Net price 50 pouches = £71.88

Compact® (Hollister)

Closed, one-piece pouch with filter and comfort backing. Net price 30 pouches (beige or clear: 13-64 mm cut-to-fit; 25, 32, 38, 44, 51, or 64 mm) = £63.04

Guardian® (Hollister)

All with 25, 38, 51, or 64 mm holes

Guardian (series 451 and 450), two-piece closed pouch with filter, opaque (with double side comfort backing) or clear(with single side comfort backing). Net price 15 pouches = £16.23

Guardian mini-pouch (series 452), two-piece compact closed pouch with filter, opaque. Net price 15 pouches = £15.18

Flanges. Net price 'F' floating flange (25, 38, 51, 64 mm) 5 = £13.10, (102 mm) 5 = £13.73; 'S' stationary flange (25, 38, 51, or 64 mm) 5 = £12.98

Stoma cap, with filter, opaque. Net price 30 (38, 51, or 64 mm) = £29.88

Belt adaptor. Net price 10 = £9.14

HolliGard® (Hollister)

All with 25, 32, 38, 44, 51, 64, or 76 mm holes

Microporous adhesive (series 411), one-piece closed pouch with porous adhesive, HolliGard® seal, and filter, may be worn with belt, opaque. Net price 30 pouches = £69.52

Without adhesive (series 416), one-piece closed pouch with HolliGard® seal and filter, must be worn with belt, clear. Net price 30 pouches = £64.76

Impression C® (Hollister)

Closed, one-piece pouch with wafer, filter and bridge, comfort backing, beige. Net price 10 pouches (19, 22, 25, 29, 32, 35, 38, 41, 44 or 51 mm holes) = £21.94

Impression CPL® (Hollister)

Closed, two-piece pouch with filter and comfort backing, clear or beige. Net price 30 pouches (38, 44, 57 or 70 mm holes) = £31.52

Mini, two-piece closed pouch with filter, opaque. Net price 30 pouches (38, 44, 57 or 70 mm holes) = £27.23

Moderma® (Hollister)

Closed, one-piece pouch with barrier, filter and comfort backing, beige, quiet film. Net price 30 pouches (clear or opaque: 15–50 mm starter hole; opaque: 20, 25, 30, 35, 40, 45 or 50 mm holes) = £58.50

Moderma® L.C (Hollister)

Closed, one-piece pouch with barrier, filter and comfort backing on both sides, beige. Net price 30 pouches (starter hole: 15–50 mm; 20, 25, 30, 35, 40, 45 or 50 mm holes) = £58.50

Premium® (Hollister)

All with 25, 32, 38, 44, 51, 64, or 76 mm holes

Karaya 5® Seal (series 355 and 353), one-piece closed pouch with porous adhesive, karaya skin protector and filter, may be worn with belt, opaque or clear. Net price 15 pouches = £33.79

Synthetic Seal (series 354 and 356), one-piece closed pouch with porous adhesive, synthetic skin protector seal and filter, opaque or clear. Net price 15 pouches = £34.89

Jade-Euro-Med range
Rubber bags screwcap (Jade-Euro-Med)

Black butyl, one-piece closed pouch. Net price 1 day pouch = £27.72; 1 night pouch = £32.33

White rubber, one-piece closed pouch. Net price 1 day pouch = £15.40; 1 night pouch = £17.65

Rubber bags spout (Jade-Euro-Med)

Black butyl, one-piece closed pouch. Net price 1 day pouch or night pouch = £29.27

White rubber, one-piece closed pouch. Net price 1 day pouch or night pouch = £13.84

Marlen range
Ultra® (Marlen)

All with 12, 16, 19, 22, 25, 29, 32, 34, 38, 41, 44, 48, 50, 54, 57, 60, 63, 70, 73, 76 mm or cut-to-fit holes; opaque or clear; flat or shallow convex.

Closed, one-piece pouch. Net price 15 pouches = £28.80

Oakmed range
Option® (Oakmed)

Colostomy Plus, closed, one-piece pouch, clear or opaque. Net price 30 pouches (starter hole, 20, 25, 30, 35, 40, 45, 50, 55 or 60 mm holes) = £57.35

Mini, closed, one-piece pouch, clear or opaque. Net price 30 pouches (10–50 mm cut-to-fit holes) = £50.70
Standard, closed, one-piece pouch, clear or opaque. Net price 30 pouches (starter hole, 20, 25, 30, 35, 40, 45 or 50 mm holes) = £56.00

Pelican range
Pelican® (Pelican)
Closed, one-piece pouch (formerly Simplaseel®). Net price 30 pouches (26, 32, 40, 45, 50 mm holes) = £70.98; 30 casual pouches (32, 40, or 45 mm holes) = £67.02
Mini, closed, one-piece pouch. Net price 30 pouches (opaque or clear: 20–65 mm cut-to-fit holes; opaque: 27, 34, 41, 48 or 55 mm holes) = £52.50
Pelican Select® (Pelican)
Closed, one-piece pouch with skin protector, filter, fabric front and back. Net price 30 pouches, clear or opaque, 20-65 mm (cut-to-fit) = £61.06; opaque (27, 34, 41, 48, or 55 mm holes), 30 = £61.06
Phoenix® (Pelican)
Closed, one-piece closed pouch. Net price (both 32, 40, or 45 mm holes) 100 pouches = £160.46; 100 casual pouches = £149.26
Sassco® (Pelican)
Closed, one-piece closed pouch. Net price 100 pouches (32, 40, or 45 mm holes) = £152.83

Rüsch range
Ostopore® (Rüsch)
Colo AV-opaque, one-piece closed pouch with adhesive and vent. Net price 30 pouches (25, 32, 38, or 45 mm holes) with 2 belt flanges = £40.56
Colo KAV-opaque, one-piece closed pouch with karaya seal skin protector, adhesive, and vent. Net price 30 pouches (25, 32, 38, 45, or 51 mm holes) with 5 belt flanges = £55.22
Colo KAV-transparent, one-piece closed pouch with karaya seal skin protector, adhesive, and vent. Net price 30 pouches (32, 38, 45, or 51 mm holes) with 30 belt flanges = £70.51
Rubber bags (Rüsch)
White rubber, one-piece closed pouch with spout outlet. Net price (both 19, 25, or 28 mm holes), 1 day pouch = £11.51; 1 night pouch = £12.42
Translet® (Rüsch)
Premier colostomy set, 1 adhesive ring with 6 bags. Net price 15 (27, 40, or 57 mm hole) = £63.90; spare bags 10 (18 or 28 cm length) = £4.90; adhesive rings or microporous spare adhesive rings (27, 40, or 57 mm) 5 = £6.54
Royal colostomy set, 1 adhesive ring and 6 odourproof bags. Net price 15 (27, 40, or 57 mm) = £88.80; spare bags (18 or 28 cm length) 10 = £7.76

Salts range
Cohflex® (Salts)
Closed, one-piece pouch with single-release paper, wafer, and filter, fabric front and back, flesh. Net price 30 pouches (all may be cut to fit; 25, 30, 35, 40, 45, 50, 55, 60 mm or 10–60 mm cut-to-fit holes) = £57.30
Coloset® (Salts)
Closed, one-piece pouch. Net price 30 pouches (medium: 713655) = £15.25; (small: 713656) = £10.04; (large: 713658) = £12.65; (medium: 713659) = £11.54
Confidence® (Salts)
One-piece closed pouch, opaque. Net price 30 pouches (13 mm starter hole, 25, 32, 38, 45, or 52 mm holes) = £58.09
One-piece closed pouch with transparent front. Net price 30 pouches (13 mm starter hole) = £55.62; with overlap film, 30 pouches (13 mm starter hole, 25, 32, 38, 45 or 52 mm holes) = £57.30
Mini, closed pouches. Net price 30 pouches (13 mm starter hole, 25, 32, 38, 45 or 52 mm holes) = £45.77

Eakin® (Salts)
Closed, one-piece pouch, clear. 32, 45, or 64 mm holes, net price 20 pouches = £42.57
Second Nature (Salts)
Second Nature, two-piece closed pouch. Net price 30 pouches (opaque: 32, 38, 45 or 57 mm; clear: 45 or 57 mm) = £32.05
Simplicity® (Salts)
Closed, two-piece closed pouch, clear or pink, medium. Net price, clear (40, 50, 60, or 70 mm) 30 = £15.93; pink (40, 50, or 60 mm holes) 30 = £15.77; flange, standard (30, 40, 50, or 60 mm hole) 5 = £2.89
Simplicity 1® (Salts)
Anatomical, closed one-piece pouch. Net price, clear (cut-to-fit), 30 = £63.91; opaque (30, 40, 50, 60 mm, or cut-to-fit holes), 30 = £63.91
Closed, one-piece pouch with porous adhesive, skin protector seal, and filter, fabric front and back. Net price 30 pouches (all may be cut to fit; opaque or pink: 30, 40, 50, or 60 mm holes; opaque, clear or pink: cut-to-fit holes) = £65.60
Paediatric, closed one-piece pouch with single-release paper, porous adhesive, clear. Net price 30 pouches (13 mm cut-to-fit hole) = £44.43
Simplicity 2® (Salts)
Closed, two-piece closed pouch (may also be applied directly to skin). Net price 30 pouches (40, 50, 60, or 70 mm holes, also 30 mm only for direct application to skin) = £33.83; flange (30, 40, 50, or 60 mm) 5 = £14.26
Solo® (Salts)
Solo closed, one-piece pouch with single-release paper, and adhesive flange, clear. Net price (30, 40, 50, or 60 mm holes), 30 pouches = £18.26; with filter, 30 pouches = £27.57
Supasac® (Salts)
Closed, one-piece pouch. Net price 30 (medium) = £23.79

Shannon range
Ostostomy (Shannon)
Adhesive appliance. Net price, 1 (TJS 948B) = £48.25
Appliance. Net price, 1 appliance (TJS 962) = £16.81
Day bag (= pouch). Net price 1 pouch, TJS 948f = £22.13; TJS 948j = £25.32
Disposable bag (= pouch). Net price TJS 948g, 100 pouches = £10.96
Night bag (= pouch). Net price 1 pouch, TJS 948e = £25.32; TJS 948k = £27.61
Outfit. Net price 1 TJS 948A = £74.72, 1 TJS 948NA = £72.36; 1 TJS 948T = £39.62
Easychange® (Shannon)
Appliance. Net price 1 appliance = £4.43
Spare bag (= pouch). Net price 100 pouches = £44.22
Shannon (Shannon)
Disposable bag (= pouch), closed pouches with plasters. Net price 12 pouches = £6.05
Elastic necks. Net price 50 pouches = £22.11

Shaw range
Hainsworth® (Shaw)
Hainsworth® bag (= pouch), one-piece closed pouch. Net price (both 25, 32, 38, or 51 mm holes), 20 pouches with body mould adhesive = £41.11; 20 pouches with Healwell® adhesive = £21.58
Shaw (Shaw)
Colostomy outfit, comprising, 4-inch wide elastic belt with groinstrap (26- to 42-inch), 1 flange and 100 colostomy pouches. Net price one NSI 6 outfit with 11 × 6-inch pouches = £38.10; one NSI 7 outfit with 12× 8-inch pouches = £38.86; one NSI 8 outfit with 11× 6-inch pouches = £41.60
Double seal, one-piece closed pouch. Net price 100 11 × 6-inch pouches = £9.83; 100 12 × 8-inch pouches = £10.76

Stick-on bag (= pouch), one-piece closed pouch with plasters. Net price 10 pouches = £8.18

SIMS Portex range
Adhesive (SIMS Portex)

Stomabag, one-piece closed pouch with adhesive, opaque. Net price (25, 32, 38, 44, 51, or 64 mm holes), 90 pouches = £126.18; with filter, 90 pouches = £141.90
Beta® (SIMS Portex)

Closed, two-piece pouch with filter. Net price, 1 kit comprising 30 pouches and 8 Seal-a-peel sheets (100 × 100 mm) = £52.17; 90 spare pouches = £143.65
Chiron® (SIMS Portex)

Adhesive appliance with spout bag. Net price 1 appliance (Mk I and Mk III) = £68.53
Clearseal bag (= pouch), one-piece closed pouch. Net price 10 pouches (305 × 127 mm: 22 mm hole) = £14.87
Closed bag, one-piece closed pouch. Net price 10 pouches (305 × 127 mm or 230 × 127 mm: 38 mm hole) = £14.87
Disposable bag (= pouch), one-piece closed pouch. Net price 10 pouches (305 × 102 mm or 305 × 127 mm: 19 mm hole) = £9.91
Reinforced, one-piece disposable pouch. Net price 10 pouches = £14.87
Chironseal® (SIMS Portex)

Closed bag (= pouch), one-piece closed pouch. Net price 10 pouches (305 × 102, 305 × 127, 230 × 127, or 305 × 150 mm: 22 or 38 mm holes) = £11.16; 10 pouches (305 × 205 or 305× 255 mm: 22 or 38 mm hole) = £12.81
Reinforced, one-piece disposable closed pouch. Net price 10 pouches (305 × 102 mm: 25 or 38 mm holes or 305 × 127 mm: 38 mm hole) = £14.87
EC1® (SIMS Portex)

Colo Classic, one-piece closed pouch with wafer, comfort backing, and filter, opaque or clear. Net price 30 pouches (25, 32, 38, 44, 51, 64 mm or 15–64 mm cut-to-fit holes) = £67.81
Mirage® (SIMS Portex)

Closed, one-piece pouch, beige or clear. Net price 30 pouches (25, 32, 38, 44, 51 or 64 mm, or 19–44 mm or 19–64 mm cut-to-fit holes) = £57.30; large (19–90 mm cut-to-fit holes) 10 = £20.70
Omni® (SIMS Portex)

Closed, one-piece pouch with wafer, porous adhesive, filter. Net price 30 pouches (opaque: 25, 32, 38, 44, or 51 mm; opaque or clear: 15–44 mm cut-to-fit holes) = £68.79
Redifit® (SIMS Portex)

Continuation bag (= pouch), one-piece closed pouch with karaya skin protector, may be worn with belt, opaque. Net price 20 pouches (32, 38, 44, 51, 64, or 75 mm holes) = £71.89
Non-adhesive bag (= pouch), one-piece closed pouch, opaque, must be worn with belt. Net price 20 pouches with karaya skin protector (44 mm hole) = £71.89; without karaya, 20 pouches (38 mm hole) = £54.56
Rediseal® (SIMS Portex)

Small bag (= pouch), one-piece PVC compact closed pouch, opaque. Net price 10 pouches (38, 44, or 51 mm holes) = £14.04
Serenade® (SIMS Portex)

WC Disposable, two-piece closed pouch. Net price 30 pouches (25, 32, 38, 44, or 51 mm holes) with filter = £33.76; 30 pouches (25, 32, 38, 44, or 51 mm holes) with soft-backing and filter = £35.11; Mini pouches, 30 pouches (15–51 mm) with soft backing and filter = £27.59; base plate (25, 32, 38, 44 or 51 mm), 10 = £27.86
Symphony® (SIMS Portex)

WC Disposable, one-piece closed pouch with wafer and filter. Net price 30 pouches (opaque or clear: 25, 32, 38, 44, or 51 mm holes; opaque: 15–44 mm cut-to-fit holes) = £70.95

Symphony Classic® (SIMS Portex)

WC Disposable, one-piece closed bag with soft backing, beige. Net price 30 pouches (25, 32, 38, 44, 51 mm or 15–51 mm cut-to-fit holes) = £70.95

Ward range
Ward (Ward)

Disposable bag (= pouch), one-piece closed pouch. Net price 10 pouches (12 × 4-inch) with 4 × 3-inch plasters = £8.65; 10 pouches (12 × 5-inch) with 4 × 4-inch plasters = £8.65
Celluloid colostomy cup, with sponge or solid rim. Net price 1 (small, medium, or large) cup = £35.93; with belt fitting, 1 cup = £40.99; 1 pouch with mount outlet = £14.94

DRAINABLE POUCHES AND ILEOSTOMY SETS

Drainable pouches are suitable for patients with an **ileostomy** or a **colostomy** with fluid effluent.

Braun Biotrol range
Biotrol® (Braun Biotrol)

Almarys, one-piece pouch with skin protector adhesive and cover. Net price 30 pouches (beige or clear, starter hole) = £61.50; beige (25, 30, 35, 40, 45, 50 or 60 mm holes) = £61.50
Elite, fabric covered one-piece pouch with skin protector adhesive and clamp closure, white or beige. Net price 30 pouches (starter hole, 20, 25, 30, 35, 40, 45, 50, 60, 70 mm holes) = £68.37; 30 clear pouches (20, 25, 30, 35, 40, 45, 50, 60, 70 mm or cut-to-fit holes) = £63.02; starter hole, 30 = £64.19
Elite Petite, one-piece pouch with skin protector adhesive and fabric backing, beige. Net price 30 pouches (starter hole, 25, 30, 35, 40 or 45 mm holes) = £58.38
Ileo S, one-piece pouch with skin protector adhesive, white. Net price 30 pouches (starter hole, 20, 25, 30, 35, 40, 45, 50, 60, 70 mm holes) = £68.37
Lockring 2, two-piece pouches with backing. Net price 30 pouches (for 35, 50 or 75 mm flanges) = £30.45; paediatric, beige (35 mm hole) 30 pouches = £29.46
Post-op, one-piece pouch with skin protector adhesive, for temporary or permanent colostomies or ileostomies, clear. Net price (cut-to-fit holes) small, 30 pouches = £70.89; large, 30 pouches = £99.58
Preference, fabric covered one-piece pouch with skin protector adhesive, porous adhesive collar, beige. Net price 30 pouches (starter hole, 20, 25, 30, 35, 40, 45, 50, 60 mm or cut-to-fit holes) = £68.37

Bullen range
Lenbul® (Bullen)

Day bag (= pouch), one-piece pouch. Net price 1 pouch with screwcap outlet = £12.52
Night bag (= pouch), one-piece pouch. Net price 1 pouch with screwcap outlet = £13.79

CliniMed range
Vogue® **shorter drainable bag** (CliniMed)

Drainable, one-piece pouch, opaque or clear. Net price 30 pouches (25, 32, 38, 44, 51 mm, or 19 mm cut-to-fit holes) = £53.09
Welland® (CliniMed)

Mini, one-piece with wafer and soft backing, opaque or clear. Net price 30 pouches (10 mm cut-to-fit holes) = £57.22
Softback ileostomy bag (= pouch), one-piece with wafer and soft backing, opaque or clear. Net price 30 pouches (25, 32, 38, 44, 51 mm, or 19 mm cut-to-fit holes) = £62.04

Oval drainable, one-piece pouch with wafer and soft backing, opaque or clear. Net price (10 mm cut-to-fit holes), 30 pouches = £65.33

Post-op, one-piece pouch with soft backing, clear or opaque. Net price (10 mm cut-to-fit hole), 30 pouches = £64.26

Coloplast range
Assura® (Coloplast)

Maxi, one-piece pouch, opaque or clear. Net price 30 pouches (10, 25, 30, 35, or 40 mm holes; 10 mm can be cut to fit up to 55 mm) = £64.29; two-piece pouch, opaque or clear. Net price 30 pouches (to fit 40, 50, or 60 mm base plates) = £35.07

Midi, one-piece pouch, opaque or clear. Net price 30 pouches (10, 25, 30, 35, 40, 45 or 50 mm holes; 10 mm can be cut to fit up to 55 mm) = £64.29; two-piece pouch, opaque or clear. Net price 30 pouches (to fit 40, 50 or 60 mm base plates) = £35.07

Mini, one-piece pouch, opaque. Net price 30 pouches (10 mm hole can be cut to fit up to 55 mm) = £64.29

Seal Integral Convexity, one-piece pouch with soft backing. Net price 10 maxi pouches (clear or opaque: 18, 21, 25, 28, 31, 35, 38 or 41 mm holes; clear: 15 mm hole; opaque: 15–33 mm, 15–43 mm starter holes) = £22.20

Note. Should be used only after assessment of suitability by appropriate medical professional

Ileo B® (Coloplast)

One-piece pouch with zinc oxide adhesive, clear or white. Net price 100 pouches (20 mm hole) = £164.30

Mini, one-piece compact pouch with zinc oxide adhesive, white. Net price 100 pouches (20 mm hole) = £163.30

K-Flex® (Coloplast)

One-piece pouch with karaya skin protector, clear. Net price 30 pouches (10 or 40 mm holes) = £73.74

mc2000® (Coloplast)

One-piece pouch with double seal, opaque or clear. Net price 30 pouches (20, 25, 30, 35, 40, 45, 50, 55, 60 mm holes or clear pouch with cut-to-fit hole) = £72.78

Mini, one-piece compact pouch, opaque. Net price 30 pouches (20, 25, 30, 35, or 40 mm holes) = £68.70

mc2002® (Coloplast)

Two-piece pouch, opaque or clear. Net price 30 open pouches (to fit 40 or 60 mm base plates) = £42.84; 30 closed pouches (to fit 40 or 60 mm base plates) = £38.82

pc3000® (Coloplast)

One-piece pouch, opaque or clear. Net price 30 pouches (20, 25, 30, 35, 40, 45, 50, 55, or 60 mm holes; 20 mm can be cut to fit up to 60 mm) = £66.15

Mini starter hole, one-piece pouch. Net price 30 pouches = £59.91

Sterile post-op bag, one-piece pouch. Net price 20 pouches (2200) = £49.44; (2202) = £32.20

ConvaTec range
Combihesive Natura® (ConvaTec)

Two-piece drainable pouch with or without filter. Net price 10 standard pouches, clear or opaque; small pouches, opaque (to fit 32, 38, 45, 57 or 70 mm flanges) = £10.62

Consecura® (ConvaTec)

Two-piece drainable pouch. Net price 20 pouches (clear or opaque to fit 35, 45 or 55 mm flanges) = £21.24

Ileodress® (ConvaTec)

Ileodress, one-piece pouch with textured backing. Net price 10 standard pouches with clip (opaque or clear: 19, 38, 45, 50, or 64 mm holes; 19 mm can be cut to fit; opaque only: 25 and 32 mm holes) = £21.69; 10 small pouches with clip, opaque (19, 25, 32, 38, 45, 50, or 64 mm holes; 19 mm can be cut to fit) = £21.34

Ileodress Plus, one-piece pouch single-release paper. Net price 10 standard pouches with clip (opaque or clear: 19, 38, 45, 50, or 64 mm holes; 19 mm can be cut to fit; opaque only: 25 and 32 mm holes) = £21.69; 10 small

pouches with clip, opaque (19, 25, 32, 38, 45, or 50 mm holes; 19 mm can be cut-to-fit) = £19.07

Little Ones® (ConvaTec)

Paediatric, one-piece pouch. Net price 15 pouches (8 mm cut-to-fit hole) = £29.85

Naturess® (ConvaTec)

Naturess, one-piece pouch with filter. Net price 20 standard pouches (clear or opaque: 19 mm starter hole; opaque: 25, 32, 38, 45 or 50 mm holes) = £42.00; 20 small pouches (opaque: 19 mm starter hole, 25, 32, 38, 45 or 50 mm holes) = £37.80

Stomadress® (ConvaTec)

One-piece pouch, clear. Net price 10 pouches (8 mm cut-to-fit hole) = £21.00

Surgicare System® 2 (ConvaTec)

System 2, two-piece pouches, white. Net price 10 pouches with clip (to fit 32, 38, 45, 57, or 70 mm flanges) = £10.74

System 2 Combihesive, two-piece pouches with textured backing. Net price 10 standard or small pouches with clip, beige (to fit 32, 38, 45, 57, or 70 mm flanges) = £10.78; 10 standard pouches with clip, clear, to fit 45, 57, or 70 mm flanges = £10.78; to fit 100 mm flanges = £19.15

Dansac range
Dansac® (Dansac)

CombiMicro D + S, one-piece pouch with porous adhesive, skin barrier ring, and fabric backing. Net price 30 pouches (25, 32, 38, 44, 50, 63 mm), opaque = £69.60; clear, 30 pouches = £68.98; cut-to-fit holes: 10–38 mm, 38–63 mm, opaque, 30 = £69.60; clear, 30 pouches = £69.60

CombiMicro Infant, one-piece pouch, opaque or clear. Net price 30 pouches (cut-to-fit holes: 10–25 mm) = £60.15

In Vent, one-piece pouch with filter, opaque. Net price 30 pouches (20, 25, 30, 35, 40, 45, 50 mm holes; 15-60 mm cut-to-fit holes) = £63.00

Unique, one-piece pouch, opaque or clear. Net price 30 pouches (20, 25, 30, 35, 40, 45, 50, 60 mm or cut-to-fit holes) = £60.96; oval flange, opaque or clear, starter hole, 30 = £60.96

Unique 2, two-piece pouch, opaque or clear, regular or large. Net price 10 pouches (to fit 36, 43, 55 or 80 mm flange) = £10.82

Unique Infant, one-piece pouch, clear or opaque. Net price 30 pouches (10 mm can be cut to fit 40 mm) = £58.84

Unique Maxi, one-piece pouch. Net price 10 pouches (10 mm can be cut to fit up to 90 mm) = £21.42

Unique Mini, one-piece pouch. Net price 30 pouches (opaque: 20, 25, 30, or 35 mm holes; opaque or clear: 15 mm can be cut to fit up to 50 mm) = £58.93

DePuy range
Raymed® (DePuy)

Butyl day bag (= pouch), one-piece pouch. Net price 1 pouch with screwcap outlet = £24.69; 1 pouch with tap outlet = £25.94

Schacht® (DePuy)

Ileostomy, one-piece pouches. Net price 50 pouches = £21.00

Ileostomy appliance, odourproof. Net price 1 appliance = £31.03

Hollister range
Classic® (Hollister)

Karaya 5® transparent, one-piece pouch with karaya skin protector seal, may be worn with belt. 30- or 40-cm clear pouch with microporous adhesive (series 322 and 327), net price 30 pouches with 1 clamp (25, 32, 38, 44, 51, 64, or 76 mm hole) = £74.00; 30-cm pouches with regular adhesive (series 722) = £74.00

Karaya 5® opaque, one-piece pouch with karaya skin protector seal and porous adhesive, may be worn with belt. Net price 30 pouches with 1 clamp, 23-cm pouches (series 313: 25, 32, 38, 44, or 51 mm holes) = £74.00; 30-cm pouches (series 311: 25, 32, 38, 44, 51, 64, or 76 mm holes) = £71.96

Karaya 5® seal (series 360), one-piece pouch with porous adhesive and karaya skin protector seal, clear. Net price 15 pouches (25, 32, 38, 44, 51, 64, or 76 mm holes) with 1 clamp = £36.31

Loop ostomy bag (= pouch). Net price 20 pouches (3.5 or 4.5 inch) = £69.21

Loop ostomy gasket. Net price 10 (3.5 or 4.5 inch) = £69.21

Compact® (Hollister)

Drainable, one-piece pouch with comfort backing. Net price 10 pouches (beige or clear: 13-64 mm cut-to-fit; 19, 25, 32, 38, 44, 51 mm) = £22.06

Mini Drainable, one-piece pouch with comfort backing, beige. Net price 10 pouches (13-51 mm cut-to-fit; 19, 25, 32, 38, 44, or 51 mm) = £20.18

Guardian® (Hollister)

All with 25, 38, 51, or 64 mm holes

Guardian (series 461 and 460), two-piece pouch, opaque (with beige non-woven double side backing) or clear (with beige non-woven single side backing). Net price 10 pouches with 1 clamp = £10.81; larger pouch to fit 102-mm flange, 10 pouches (clear) with 1 clamp = £22.63

Guardian mini-pouch, two-piece compact pouch, opaque. Net price (series 464), 10 pouches = £10.55; NHS : with inner film and replaceable filter (series 463), 10 pouches with pack of filters and 1 clamp

NHS *With replaceable filter* (series 462), two-piece pouch with inner film and replaceable filter, clear. 10 pouches with pack of filters and 1 clamp

Impression® (Hollister)

One-piece pouch with Convex wafer, synthetic seal and Microporous II adhesive, opaque or clear. Net price 10 pouches (19, 22, 25, 29, 32, 35, 38, 41, 44 or 51 mm holes) = £23.84

Impression CPL® (Hollister)

Two-piece pouch with comfort backing, beige or clear. Net price 10 pouches (38, 44, 57 or 70 mm holes) = £10.61; (102 mm hole) = £20.40

Mini Drainable, two-piece pouch with comfort backing, beige. Net price 10 pouches (38, 44, 57 or 70 mm holes) = £10.20

Premium® (Hollister)

Karaya 5® seal with filter (series 366), one-piece pouch with porous adhesive, karaya skin protector seal, and replaceable filter, may be worn with belt, clear. Net price 15 pouches (25, 32, 38, 44, 51, or 64 mm holes) with 1 clamp and filter elements = £39.60

Synthetic seal (series 364), one-piece pouch with porous adhesive and synthetic skin protector seal, clear. Net price 15 pouches (25, 32, 38, 44, 51, or 64 mm holes) with 1 clamp = £36.31

Jade-Euro-Med range

Rubber bags screwcap (Jade-Euro-Med)

Black butyl, one-piece pouch. Net price 1 day pouch = £27.72; 1 night pouch = £32.33

White rubber, one-piece pouch. Net price 1 day pouch = £15.40; 1 night pouch = £17.65

Rubber bags spout (Jade-Euro-Med)

Black butyl, one-piece pouch. Net price 1 day or night pouch = £29.27

White rubber, one-piece pouch. Net price 1 day pouch = £13.84; 1 night pouch = £13.84

Marlen range

Ultra® (Marlen)

All with 12, 16, 19, 22, 25, 29, 32, 34, 38, 41, 44, 48, 50, 54, 57, 60, 63, 67, 70, 73, 76 mm or cut-to-fit holes; opaque or clear; small or large

Drainable, one-piece pouch. Net price 15 pouches = £32.25; with convex flange, 15 pouches = £33.00

Oakmed range

Option® (Oakmed)

Mini Ileo, one-piece pouch, opaque or clear. Net price 30 pouches (10–50 mm cut-to-fit holes) = £53.70

Ileostomy, one-piece pouch, opaque or clear. Net price 30 pouches (20, 25, 30, 35, 40, 45 or 50 mm holes) = £57.35

LOP-F7® (Oakmed)

Ileostomy appliance. Net price 1 appliance = £38.68

OPR-F® (Oakmed)

Ileostomy appliance. Net price 1 appliance = £80.69

SR-F® (Oakmed)

Ileostomy set. Net price 1 set = £55.60

Pelican range

Sassco® (Pelican)

Ileostomy bag (= pouch), one-piece pouch. Net price 100 pouches (26 or 32 mm holes) = £175.46

Pelican® (Pelican)

Drainable bag (= pouch), formerly Simplaseel®, one-piece pouch, opaque. Net price 30 pouches (26, 32, 40, 45, or 50 mm holes) = £71.73

Post-op drainable bag (= pouch), one-piece pouch. Net price 10 pouches (20–80 mm cut-to-fit) = £39.48

Paediatric drainable bag (= pouch), one-piece pouch. Net price 30 pouches (7–40 mm cut-to-fit) = £64.26

Pelican Select® (Pelican)

Drainable bag (= pouch), one-piece pouch, with skin protector, clear or opaque. Net price 30 pouches (20–65 mm cut-to-fit; 13, 27, 34, 41, 48 or 55 mm holes) = £62.10

Rüsch range

Birkbeck® (Rüsch)

Rubber, one-piece pouch, black or pink. Net price (both 19, 38, or 54 mm holes), 1 day pouch = £26.66; 1 night pouch = £30.49

Disposable, one-piece plastic pouch. Net price 100 pouches = £15.54

Ileostomy appliance. Net price 1 appliance 'A' (19, 38, or 54 mm) = £93.07; 1 appliance 'B' (19, 38, or 54 mm) = £60.06

Ostopore® (Rüsch)

Ileo KAV-opaque, one-piece pouch with karaya seal skin protector, adhesive, and vent, opaque. Net price 30 pouches (25, 32, or 38 mm holes) with 30 belt flanges and 10 clips = £61.78

Rubber bag (Rüsch)

White rubber, one-piece pouch. Net price, 1 day pouch (38, 44, or 51 mm holes) = £11.94; 1 screwcap pouch (38 mm hole) = £12.89; 1 pouch with vent (38 mm hole) = £14.28

White rubber child bag (= pouch), one-piece pouch. Net price (both 19, 25, or 28 mm holes), 1 day pouch = £11.51; 1 night pouch = £14.08

Salts range

Cohflex® (Salts)

Drainable, one-piece pouch with single-release paper, wafer, and fabric front and back. Net price 30 pouches with integral closure clip (flesh: 25, 30, 35, 40, 45, 50, 55, or 60 mm, flesh or clear, 10–60 mm starter hole) = £61.50

Paediatric drainable, one-piece small pouch with single-release paper, wafer, and fabric backing, opaque/clear/beige. Net price 30 pouches with integral closure clip (10–50 mm cut-to-fit holes) = £54.50

Confidence® (Salts)

Confidence, one-piece pouch, opaque. Net price 30 pouches (13 mm starter hole, 25, 32, 38, 45, or 52 mm holes) = £56.40

Confidence, one-piece pouch, small. Net price 30 pouches (13 mm starter hole, 25, 32, 38, 45 or 52 mm holes) = £45.00

Confidence, one-piece pouch with transparent front. Net price 30 pouches standard (13 mm starter hole) = £54.00; large (13 mm starter hole) = £56.40; with over-lap film (25, 32, 38, 45 or 52 mm holes) = £57.30

Eakin® (Salts)

Drainable, one-piece pouch, white or clear. Net price 20 small or large pouches (32, 45, or 64 mm holes) = £49.19

Fistula, one-piece pouch with or without remote drain-age. Net price 10 infant pouches = £36.05; 10 small pouches = £51.17, 10 medium pouches = £66.19; 10 large pouches = £121.69; 20 wide pouches (90 mm hole) = £101.15

Light White® (Salts)

Drainable, one-piece pouch, white. Net price 30 large, small, or medium pouches (all 25, 32, or 38 mm holes) = £48.48

Drainable self-adhesive, one-piece pouch with adhesive, white. Net price 30 pouches (large: 25, 32, 38, or 44 mm holes; small and medium: 25, 32, or 38 mm holes) = £54.87

Koenig Rutzen® **screwcap** (Salts)

All with screwcap outlet

Black butyl all rubber, one-piece pouch. Net price 1 pouch (large: 25, 29, 32, 35, 38, 44, or 51 mm holes; small: 25, 32, 38, 44, or 51 mm) = £30.26; with bridge (soft-face Maggie Bag), 1 pouch (large: 25, 32, 38, 44, or 51 mm holes; small: 25, 32, or 38 mm) = £40.60

Black butyl reinforced, one-piece pouch. Net price 1 large or small pouch (both 25, 32, or 38 mm holes) = £40.60; with bridge (hard-face Maggie Bag), 1 pouch (large: 25, 32, 38, 44, or 51 mm holes; small: 25, 32, or 38 mm) = £47.32

Koenig Rutzen® **spout** (Salts)

All with spout outlet

Black butyl all rubber, one-piece pouch. Net price 1 large or small pouch (both 25, 32, 38, 44, or 51 mm holes) = £22.63; with bridge, 1 pouch (large: 25, 32, 38, 44, or 51 mm holes; small: 25, 32, or 38 mm) = £29.33

Black butyl reinforced, one-piece pouch. Net price 1 large or small pouch (25, 32, or 38 mm holes) = £30.42; with bridge, 1 pouch (large: 25, 32, 38, 44, or 51 mm holes; small: 25, 32, or 38 mm) = £37.46

Kombo® (Salts)

Kombo drainable, one-piece pouch with karaya skin pro-tector seal and adhesive, medium. Net price 30 pouches (30, 40, 50, 60, or 80 mm holes) = £58.00; with filter, 30 pouches = £69.64

Rubber bags (Salts)

All must be used with flange

Black butyl screw, one-piece bag with screwcap outlet. Net price 1 large or small pouch = £29.93

Black butyl spout, one-piece bag with spout outlet. Net price 1 large or small pouch = £20.91

White screw, one-piece bag with screwcap outlet. Net price 1 large or small pouch = £9.96

White spout, one-piece bag with spout outlet. Net price 1 large or small pouch = £8.31

Salger® (Salts)

Drainable, one-piece pouch. Net price 10 pouches (40 or 57 mm holes) = £11.29

Second Nature® (Salts)

Second Nature, two-piece drainable pouch. Net price 30 pouches (opaque: 32, 38, 45 or 57 mm; clear: 45 or 57 mm) = £31.50; secu-ring® to fit 32, 38, 45 or 57 mm flange, 10 = £9.80; wafer (110 × 100 mm to fit 32, 38 or 45 mm flange; 134 × 124 mm to fit 57 mm flange), 5 = £10.99

Simplicity® (Salts)

Drainable, two-piece pouch, clear. Net price 30 230 × 137 mm pouches (40, 50, or 60 mm holes) = £18.16

Post-op, two-piece pouch, clear. Net price 30 300 ×125-mm pouches (40, 50, or 60 mm holes) = £15.77

Simplicity 1® (Salts)

Anatomical, one-piece pouch. Net price clear (cut-to-fit), 30 = £68.70; opaque (30, 40, 50, 60 mm or cut-to-fit holes), 30 = £68.70

Drainable, one-piece pouch with porous adhesive and skin protector seal, fabric front and back. Net price 30 pouches with integral closure clip (opaque or pink: 30, 40, 50, or 60 mm, all may be cut to fit; opaque, clear or pink: 10–60 mm cut-to-fit hole) = £70.48

Paediatric drainable, one-piece pouch with porous adhe-sive and skin protector seal, clear. Net price 30 pouches (cut-to-fit hole) = £44.43

Simplicity 2® (Salts)

Drainable, two-piece pouch (may also be applied directly to skin). Net price 15 pouches (40, 50, 60, or 70 mm holes, also 30 mm only for direct application to skin) = £18.58

Post-op, two-piece pouch (may also be applied directly to skin). Net price 30 pouches (40, 50, 60, or 70 mm holes, also 30 mm only for direct application to skin) = £37.45

Transverse, two-piece pouch (may also be applied directly to skin). Net price 10 pouches (cut-to-fit hole) = £42.58; 5 flanges = £20.81

NHS United® (Salts)

Soft & Secure drainable, one-piece pouch, opaque or clear. Net price 10 pouches (38, 45, or 57 mm holes) = £8.47

Shaw range

Rubber bags (Shaw)

Black screwcap, one-piece pouch with screwcap outlet. Net price (both 19, 38 or 54 mm holes), 1 day pouch = £23.11; 1 night pouch = £24.49

SIMS Portex range

Adhesive (SIMS Portex)

Stomabag, one-piece pouch with adhesive, opaque. Net price 60 pouches (19, 25, 32, 38, 51 mm or cut-to-fit holes) = £92.30

Cavendish® (SIMS Portex)

Odourproof, one-piece pouch. Net price (all 25, 32, or 38 mm holes), 10 opaque pouches with non-adhesive flange = £31.10; 10 opaque pouches with adhesive flange = £37.46; 10 clear PVC pouches = £31.29

Chiron® **screwcap** (SIMS Portex)

All with screwcap outlet

Butyl rubber day bag (= pouch), one-piece pouch, black. Net price 1 pouch (38, 44, or 51 mm hole) = £31.72

Butyl rubber night bag (= pouch), one-piece pouch, black. Net price 1 pouch (38 or 44 mm holes) =£38.83

Latex rubber day bag (= pouch), one-piece pouch. Net price 1 pouch (38 mm hole) = £16.44

Latex rubber night bag (= pouch), one-piece pouch. Net price 1 pouch (38 mm hole) = £21.75

White rubber day bag (= pouch), one-piece pouch. Net price 1 pouch (38, 44, or 51 mm) = £18.63, child-size pouch (38 mm hole) = £16.28; body-size outlet, 1 pouch (38 mm hole) = £18.26, child-size pouch (38 mm hole) = £14.70

White rubber night bag (= pouch), one-piece pouch. Net price 1 pouch (38 or 51 mm hole) = £21.75; body-size outlet, 1 pouch (38 mm hole) = £17.80

Chiron® **spout** (SIMS Portex)

White rubber bag (= pouch), one-piece pouch. Net price 1 day pouch (38 mm hole) = £16.01; 1 night pouch (38 mm hole) = £17.39

EC1® (SIMS Portex)

Ileo classic, one-piece pouch with wafer and comfort backing, opaque. Net price 30 pouches with 1 clamp

(19, 25, 32, 38, 44 mm or 10–44 mm cut-to-fit holes) = £71.04

Mini classic, one-piece compact pouch with wafer and comfort backing, opaque or clear. Net price 30 pouches with 1 clamp (10–44 mm cut-to-fit holes) = £71.04

Post-op classic, one-piece pouch with wafer and comfort backing, clear. Net price 30 pouches with 1 clamp, 10–64 mm cut-to-fit holes = £73.27; 10–90 mm cut-to-fit holes = £103.68

Mirage® (SIMS Portex)

Drainable, one-piece pouch, beige or clear. Net price 30 pouches (25, 32, 38, 44, 51 mm or 19–44 mm or 19–64 mm cut-to-fit holes) = £61.50; large (beige: 19–90 mm cut-to-fit holes) = £64.25

Mini drainable, one piece pouch. Net price 30 pouches (beige: 25, 32, 38, 44, 51 mm holes; beige or clear: up to 44 mm cut-to-fit holes) = £56.70

Omni® (SIMS Portex)

Drainable, one-piece pouch with porous adhesive wafer and replaceable filter. Net price 20 pouches (opaque: 25, 32, 38, 44 mm; opaque or clear: 10–44 mm cut-to-fit hole) = £47.32; NHS opaque (10–90 mm cut-to-fit hole) = £53.39

Redifit® (SIMS Portex)

Opaque, one-piece pouch with karaya skin protector, may be worn with belt. Net price 20 pouches with 2 closure clips (25, 32, 38, 44, 51, or 64 mm holes) = £69.49; small outline pouches, 20 pouches with 2 closure clips (25, 32, or 38 mm) = £69.49

Clear fronted, one-piece pouch with karaya skin protector, may be worn with belt. Net price 20 pouches with 2 closure clips (25, 32, 44, 51, or 64 mm holes) = £68.80

Ward range
Donald Rose® (Ward)

Bag (= pouch), with celluloid collars, solid, flat or fluid rims. Net price 1 pouch = £19.29

Ileostomy appliance. Net price 1 appliance (first stage) = £47.80; 1 appliance (second stage) = £46.69; 1 appliance (new improved) = £49.55

Rubber bags (Ward)

Bag, rubber. Net price 1 pouch, complete with collar = £20.94; 1 pouch, with tap outlet and skirt = £23.40

Night bag (= pouch), shaped rubber with long vertical spring vulcanite screw outlet. Net price 1 pouch = £19.19

Black rubber bag (= pouch), one-piece pouch with screw-cap outlet. Net price (19, 35, or 54 mm hole), 1 day pouch = £18.04; 1 night pouch = £18.85

White rubber ileostomy bag (= pouch) (with flange, pouch with St. Mark's flange. Net price 1 pouch = £27.27

White rubber ileostomy bag (= pouch), one-piece pouch. Net price 1 day pouch (screwcap or spout outlet) = £12.33; 1 night pouch (screwcap or spout outlet) = £13.86; tap outlet, 1 day pouch = £18.06; 1 night pouch = £20.02

White rubber transverse ileostomy bag (= pouch), one-piece pouch. Net price 1 pouch = £28.82

UROSTOMY POUCHES

Braun Biotrol range
Biotrol® (Braun Biotrol)

Lockring 2, two-piece pouch, clear. Net price 10 pouches (35, 50 or 75 mm holes) = £22.90

Bullen range
Lenbul® (Bullen)

Day bag (= pouch), one-piece pouch. Net price 1 pouch with tap outlet = £14.55; 1 pouch with large opening (for 4-inch flange with tap outlet) = £15.10

Night bag (= pouch). Net price 1 pouch with tap outlet = £16.62; 1 pouch with large opening = £17.25

Coloplast range
Assura® (Coloplast)

Maxi, urostomy pouch with soft backing, clear or opaque. Net price 30 (one-piece) pouches (10–55 mm hole) = £119.34; two-piece pouch, 30 pouches (to fit 40, 50 or 60 mm base plates) = £70.05

Midi, urostomy pouch with soft backing, clear or opaque. Net price 30 (one-piece) pouches (10–55 mm hole) = £119.34; two-piece pouch, 30 pouches (to fit 40 or 50 mm base plates) = £70.05

Paediatric, urostomy pouches with soft backing, clear or opaque. Net price 30 (one-piece) pouches (10–35 mm hole) = £119.34; two-piece pouch, 30 pouches (to fit 40 mm base plate) = £70.05; 5 paediatric (40 mm) = £13.91

Seal Integral Convexity, urostomy pouch, maxi, clear. Net price 10 pouches (15, 18, 21, 25, 28 or 31 mm holes) = £38.00

Note. Should be used only after assessment of suitability by appropriate medical professional

Stoma Urine (Coloplast)

Maxi, one-piece pouch with zinc oxide adhesive. Net price 30 pouches (13-mm hole) = £78.51

Midi, one-piece pouch with zinc oxide adhesive. Net price 30 pouches (13-mm hole) = £78.51

URO 2002® (Coloplast)

Two-piece pouch. Net price 20 small pouches (100 mL, to fit 40 mm base plate) = £56.90; 20 large pouches (375 mL, to fit 40 or 60 mm base plate) = £56.90

Base plate. Net price 5 plates (40 mm, to fit 10–35 mm stoma) or 5 plates (60 mm, to fit 10–55 mm stoma) = £14.69

Night drainage system. Net price 10 pouches (1.65 litre), 1 tube, and 2 connectors = £14.28; hospital pack, 10 pouches (1.65 litre), 5 tubes, and 10 connectors = £17.60

ConvaTec range
Combihesive Natura® (ConvaTec)

Two-piece drainable pouch with Accuseal® tap. Net price 10 standard pouches (clear or opaque for 32, 38, 45 or 57 mm flange; clear for 70 mm flange); 10 small pouches (opaque for 32, 38, 45 or 57 mm flange) = £23.72

Two-piece drainable pouch with standard tap. Net price 10 small or standard pouches (clear for 32, 38, 45 or 57 mm flange) = £23.15; 10 standard pouches (clear for 70 mm flange) = £25.07

Surgicare System® 2 (ConvaTec)

Two-piece pouch, with non-reflux valve, clear. Net price 10 (small or standard) pouches (32, 38, 45, or 57 mm flange) = £23.15; 10 standard pouches (70 mm flange) = £25.07, (100 mm flange) = £37.75

Surgicare System® 2 Combihesive (ConvaTec)

Two-piece pouch with Accuseal® tap, and textured backing, clear. Net price 10 standard pouches (32, 38, 45, or 57 mm flange) = £23.72

Urodress® (ConvaTec)

One-piece pouch with Stomahesive® and tap. Net price 10 pouches (19, 25, 32, 38, or 45 mm holes) = £43.59

Urodress® Deep Convex (ConvaTec)

One-piece pouch, clear, standard. Net price 5 pouches (16, 19, 22, 25, 28, 32, 35 or 38 mm holes) = £19.00

Note. Should be used only after assessment of suitability by appropriate medical professional

Dansac range
Unique® 2 (Dansac)

Two-piece pouch, with 1 Dansac® drain tube adaptor, opaque or clear. Net price 10 pouches (to fit 30, 36, 43 or 55 mm flange) = £23.24

DePuy range
Raymed® (DePuy)

Butyl night bag (= pouch), one-piece pouch. Net price 1 pouch with screwcap outlet = £25.69; 1 pouch with tap outlet = £25.80

Hollister range
Classic® (Hollister)

Karaya 5® seal and regular adhesive with attachment for optional belt, one-piece pouch, clear. Net price 20 pouches (series 741, 23-cm pouch: 19, 25, 32, 38, 44, or 51 mm holes; series 748, 30-cm pouch: 25, 32, 38, 44, or 51 mm holes) including 1 standard drain tube = £66.68

Regular adhesive with attachment for optional belt, one-piece pouch, clear. Net price 20 pouches (series 740, 23-cm pouch: 19, 25, 32, 38, 44, or 51 mm holes; series 747, 30-cm pouch: 25, 32, 38, 44, or 51 mm holes) including 1 standard drain tube = £51.11

Compact® (Hollister)

Urostomy pouch with comfort backing. Net price 10 pouches (13–64 mm cut-to-fit; 13, 16, 19, 25, 32, 38, 44 or 51 mm) = £43.69

First Choice® (Hollister)

Urostomy pouch with synthetic skin barrier and Microporous II adhesive (series 146). Net price 10 pouches (13–64 mm starter hole, 19, 25, 32, 38, 44, or 51 mm holes) = £45.69

Guardian® (Hollister)

Guardian, two-piece pouch with wide-bore tap and non-reflux valve, clear (with beige, non-woven single side backing) (series 470). Net price 10 pouches (25-cm for max. 25, 38, or 51 mm stomas), including 1 drain tube adaptor = £23.98

Impression® (Hollister)

One-piece pouch with Convex wafer, synthetic seal and Microporous II® adhesive, clear. Net price 10 pouches (13, 16, 19, 22, 25, 29, 32, 35, 38 or 44 mm) = £45.69

Impression C® (Hollister)

Closed, one-piece pouch with Convex wafer, comfort backing, clear. Net price 10 pouches (13, 16, 19, 22, 25, 29, 32, 35, 38, 44 or 51 mm holes) = £39.92

Impression CPL® (Hollister)

Two-piece pouch with comfort backing. Net price 10 pouches (38, 44, 57 or 70 mm holes) = £23.36

Lo-profile® (Hollister)

Karaya 5® seal and Microporous II® adhesive with gasket for optional belt, one-piece pouch, with non-reflux valve, clear (series 143). Net price 10 pouches (25-cm pouch: 19, 25, 32, 38, 44, or 51 mm gasket), including 1 Lo-profile drain tube = £49.37

Microporous II® adhesive only (beltless) one-piece pouch with non-reflux valve (series 142). Net price 10 pouches (25-cm pouch: 19, 25, 32, 38, 44, or 51 mm holes), including 1 Lo-profile® drain tube = £42.60

Jade-Euro-Med range
Rubber bags (Jade-Euro-Med)

Black butyl, one-piece pouch, odourless. Net price 1 day pouch (tap outlet) = £30.82; 1 night pouch (tap outlet) = £32.33

White rubber, one-piece pouch. Net price 1 day pouch (tap outlet) = £15.40; 1 night pouch (tap outlet) = £17.65

Marlen range
Ultra® (Marlen)

Urostomy pouch, clear. Net price 10 (small or large; flat or shallow convex) pouches (12 mm starter hole, 12, 16, 19, 22, 25, 29, 32, 34, 38, 41, 44, 48, 50, 54, 57, 60, 63, 67, 70, 73, or 76 mm holes) = £39.24

Oakmed range
Urostomy sets (Oakmed)

Urostomy sets. Net price 1 LOP-U appliance (wire ring retainer with 1.5-inch elastic belt for small flange, 10 one-piece flanges and lightweight bags with 1-inch hole, 30 3.5 × 3.5-inch double-sided adhesive plasters) = £38.68; 1 OPR-U appliance (waterproof canvas retaining shield waistband, 2 one-piece flanges and bags with 1- or 2-inch hole and tap outlet, 30 3.5 × 3.5-inch double-sided adhesive plasters) = £80.69; 1 SR-U appliance (plastic retainer ring shield with 1-inch elastic belt for medium flange, Lenbul® 1.5-inch diameter flange, 1 Lenbul® day and 1 night bag with tap outlet, 30 3.5 × 3.5-inch double-sided adhesive plasters) = £60.60

Rüsch range
Rubber bags (Rüsch)

Black rubber (Birkbeck®), one-piece pouch with tap outlet. Net price 1 day pouch (19 mm hole) = £30.49; 1 night pouch (19 mm hole) = £33.26

Pink rubber, one-piece pouch with tap outlet. Net price 1 day pouch (19 mm hole) = £30.49; 1 night pouch (19 mm hole) = £33.26

White rubber, one-piece pouch with tap outlet. Net price 1 day pouch (19, 25, or 28 mm holes) = £16.56; 1 night pouch (19, 25, or 28 mm holes) = £17.01

White rubber (Glasgow), one-piece pouch. Net price 1 pouch (small or large tap) = £20.23

White rubber transverse, one-piece pouch. Net price 1 left or right pouch (small, medium, or large) = £20.23

Salts range
Koenig Rutzen® (Salts)

All rubber white rubber tap bag (= pouch), one-piece pouch with tap outlet. Net price 1 small or medium pouch (both 25, 32, or 38 mm holes) or 1 large pouch (25, 32, 38, 44, or 51 mm holes) = £16.18

All rubber black butyl bag (= pouch), one-piece pouch with tap outlet and non-reflux valve. Net price 1 medium or large pouch (both 19, 25, 32, or 38 mm holes) = £39.07; special size holes also available to order

All rubber MB black butyl bag (= pouch), one-piece pouch with tap outlet, bridge, and non-reflux valve. Net price 1 small, medium, or large pouch (all 19, 25, 32, or 38 mm holes) = £45.69; special size holes also available to order

Black butyl, reinforced bag (= pouch), one-piece pouch with tap outlet and non-reflux valve. Net price 1 medium or large pouch (both 19, 25, 32, or 38 mm holes) = £47.89; special size holes also available to order

MB black butyl, reinforced bag (= pouch), one-piece pouch with tap outlet and non-reflux valve. Net price 1 medium or large pouch (both 19, 25, 32, or 38 mm holes) = £54.86; special size holes also available to order

Rubber bags (Salts)

Black rubber bag (= pouch) (for use with flange), two-piece pouch with tap outlet. Net price 1 small, medium, or large pouch = £36.89; special size holes also available to order

White rubber bag (= pouch) for use with flange, two-piece pouch with tap outlet. Net price 1 small, medium, or large pouch = £10.78

Light White® (Salts)

Urostomy pouch with Realistic® washer, one-piece pouch, white. Net price 20 large pouches (all 25, 32, or 38 mm holes) = £106.45

Urostomy pouch with Realistic® washer, one-piece pouch, clear. Net price 20 large or small pouches (all 25, 32, or 38 mm holes) = £106.66

Urostomy pouch, one-piece pouch, white. Net price 20 large pouches (25, 32, or 38 mm holes) = £81.19

Urostomy pouch, one-piece pouch, clear. Net price 20 large or small pouches (25, 32, or 38 mm holes) = £81.19

Urostomy pouch, one-piece pouch with adhesive, white. Net price 20 large pouches (25, 32, or 38 mm holes) = £84.89

Urostomy pouch, one-piece pouch with adhesive, clear. Net price 20 large or small pouches (both 25, 32, or 38 mm holes) = £84.89

Simplicity 1® (Salts)

Paediatric Uri-bag, one-piece pouch, 13 mm starter hole. Net price 15 pouches = £41.08

SIMS Portex range

Carshalton® (SIMS Portex)

Bag (= pouch), one-piece pouch. Net price 10 oval or tri-angular pouches (both 25, 32, or 38 mm) with acrylic plaster = £19.73

Set, one-piece pouch. Net price 20 oval or triangular pouches with plasters, bodyplate, clamp, connector, and medium belt (both 25, 32, or 38 mm holes) = £66.17

Chiron® **Non-disposable** (SIMS Portex)

Butyl rubber bag (= pouch), one-piece pouch with stop-cock outlet, odourless, black. Net price 1 day bag (22 mm) = £35.32

Latex rubber bag (= pouch), one-piece pouch with stop-cock outlet. Net price (both 38 mm) 1 day bag = £24.47; 1 night bag = £27.75

Rubber child-size bag (= pouch), one-piece pouch with stopcock outlet, white. Net price 1 = £20.53

Rubber day bag (= pouch), one-piece pouch, white with stopcock outlet. Net price 1 (38 mm) = £24.47

Rubber night bag (= pouch), one-piece, white. Net price 1 (38, 44, or 51 mm) = £27.75

Chiron® (SIMS Portex)

Ileal bladder appliance, set comprises 1 web and elastic belt 25 mm wide, 1 wire pressure frame, 1 St Mark's pat-tern rubber flange (without diaphragm), 2 rubber day pouches with stopcock outlet, 30 double-sided plasters. Net price = £76.62

Mirage® (SIMS Portex)

Urostomy pouch. Net price 10 pouches (beige: 25, 32, 38, 44 mm or up to 44 mm cut-to-fit holes) = £38.00; 10 pouches (clear: up to 64 mm cut-to-fit holes) = £38.00

Mitcham® (SIMS Portex)

Maxi, one-piece pouch. Net price 10 pouches with adhe-sive flange (25, 32, or 38 mm) = £40.22, 10 pouches with nonadhesive flange (25, 32, or 38 mm) = £32.84

Mini, one-piece pouch. Net price 10 pouches with adhe-sive flange (19, 25, or 32 mm) = £40.22, 10 pouches with nonadhesive flange (25 mm or 32 mm) = £32.84

Standard, one-piece pouch. Net price 10 pouches with adhesive flange (19, 25, 32 or 38 mm) = £40.22, 10 pouches with nonadhesive flange (19, 25, 32, or 38 mm) = £32.84, 1 pouch with nonadhesive flange and foam pads (25, 32, or 38 mm) = £5.53

Rediflow® (SIMS Portex)

Adhesive set, may be worn with belt. Net price 20 pouches (19, 25, 32, 38, 44, or 51 mm) = £59.09

Ward range

Ward® (Ward)

Ureterostomy bag (= pouch) with tap outlet. Net price 1 night pouch = £19.70; 1 day pouch (19, 35, or 54 mm hole) = £18.45

ADHESIVE PREPARATIONS, ADHESIVE REMOVERS AND DEODORANTS

Adhesive preparations

Hollister® (Hollister)

Medical adhesive spray (with silicones). Net price 90-g aerosol spray = £14.19

Latex adhesive solution (Salts)

Net price per tube = £1.92. Label: 15

Skin adhesive (Manfred Sauer)

Synthetic. Net price 2 × 28 g tube with long nozzle = £13.95; 45 mL bottle with brush = £13.95

Original Latex. Net price 2 × 28 g tube with long nozzle = £7.95

Adhesive removers

Clear Peel® (CliniMed)

Adhesive remover. Net price 50 mL = £2.10

Hollister® (Hollister)

Adhesive remover spray. Net price 76-g spray = £11.89

Salts 'SPR' Plaster Remover (Rezolve)® (Salts)

Adhesive remover spray. Net price 70-g aerosol spray = £2.86. Label: 15

Deodorants

Atmocol® is used as a deodorising spray when emptying the appliance. The other deodorants listed are placed in the appliance.

Atmocol® (Adams)

Aerosol deodorant. Net price 1 unit (400 sprays) = £1.96

Chironair Odour Control Liquid® (SIMS Portex)

Deodorant solution. Net price 113 g = £5.74

Colostomy Plus® (Shannon)

Deodorant. Net price 1 unit = £2.68

Day-drop® (Loxley)

Deodorant solution. Net price 7.5 mL = £1.07; 15 mL = £1.78; 30 mL = £3.04 (7.5 and 15 mL also available as Lemon Day-drop®)

Dor® (Pelican)

Deodorant solution. Net price 7 mL = £1.84

Forest Breeze® (Shaw)

Deodorant. Net price 1 unit = £3.26

LiMone® (CliniMed)

Deodorant spray. Net price 50 mL = £4.12

NaturCare® (AlphaMed)

Deodorant spray. Net price 50 mL = £3.47

Ostobon® (Coloplast)

Deodorant powder. Net price 22 g = £4.01

Saltair No-Roma® (Salts)

Deodorant solution. Net price 28 mL = £2.28; 227 mL = £7.45

Sween® (Bullen)

Deodorant. Net price 36 mL = £4.08

Translet Plus One® (Rüsch)

Deodorant solution for men. Net price 7 mL = £2.88

Translet Plus Two® (Rüsch)

Deodorant solution for women. Net price 7 mL = £2.88

ADHESIVE DEVICES AND RINGS

Bullen range

Adhesive plaster, double-sided. Net price 10 zinc oxide plasters 3.5 × 3.5 inch = £4.04, 4 × 4 inch = £4.98, 5 × 5 inch = £8.41; 10 acrylic base plasters 3.5 × 3.5 inch = £3.62, 4 × 4 inch = £4.65, 5 × 5 inch = £7.83

Flange retention strips. Net price 100 strips 4 × 1 inch = £3.61, 4 × 2 inch = £4.89

Rüsch range

Ostomy plasters, double-sided. Net price 25 plasters (25 mm hole, or no hole) = £6.49

Salts range

Kidney seals. Net price 10 = £4.30

Reliaseal® (Salts)

Adhesive discs, double-sided, round, hypo-allergic. Net price 10 discs (13, 19, 22, 25, 29, 32, or 38 mm) = £16.68

Secuplast® (Salts)

Plasters, circular. Net price 10 plasters (32, 38, 45 or 57 mm) = £9.50

Transacryl® (Salts)

Adhesive plasters, double-sided. Net price 10 plasters (25, 32, or 38 mm) = £5.46

Zopla® (Salts)

Adhesive plasters, double-sided. Net price (both 25, 32, or 38 mm) 10 square plasters = £4.10; 10 round plasters = £4.76

Shannon range

Adhesive plasters, double-sided. Net price 25 plasters = £14.91

Rings. Net price 5 rubber retaining rings = £5.96; 1 plastic locking ring = £2.22

Easychange® (Shannon)

Adhesive plasters, with rings (spare). Net price 5 plasters = £5.90

Shaw range

Adhesive plasters, double-sided, hole cut-to-size. Net price 10 plasters, 4 × 4 inch = £7.31; 5 × 5 inch = £7.58

SIMS Portex range

Adhesive discs, double-sided. Net price 10 discs (76 mm diameter: 19 or 25 mm opening; 90 mm diameter: 32 or 38 mm opening) = £4.51

Rings, elastic, for use with spout bags. Net price 3 rings = £2.22

Carshalton® (SIMS Portex)

Adhesive plasters. Net price both (25, 32, or 38 mm) 10 acrylic plasters = £4.79; 10 zinc oxide plasters = £7.59

Chiron® (SIMS Portex)

Adhesive plasters, double-sided. Net price 10 plasters (90 mm square: 19 or 35 mm hole) = £6.12, (102 mm square: 19 or 35 mm hole) = £7.03, (127 mm square: 19 or 35 mm hole) = £7.73, (150 mm square and 102 × 76 mm: both 19 mm hole) = £8.66, (90 and 102 mm square: both 25 mm hole) = £8.66, (125 mm square: 25 mm hole) = £9.50

Clearseal plasters. Net price 10 plasters (100 mm square: 19 or 35 mm hole) = £7.03

Kidney seals, adhesive flange retaining strips. Net price 10 strips (small or large) = £4.78

Ward range

Adhesive plasters, double-sided with opening. Net price 10 plasters = £4.39

Waterproof plasters, single-sided. Net price 10 (100 mm × 25 mm) = £1.20; 10 (100 mm × 50 mm) = £1.80

BAG CLOSURES

Clamps

Available from *Braun Biotrol* (Biotrol® for post-op pouches, 1 clamp = £1.01), *CliniMed* (for drainage pouches, 1 clamp = £1.01), *Hollister* (for drainable pouches, 1 clamp = £1.01, 20 = £16.99; for Premium® pouches, 1 clamp = £1.06, 20 = £18.00), *SIMS Portex* (10 clamps = £8.40; Carshalton®, 5 clamps = £9.77)

Clips

Available from *ConvaTec* (10 beige clips = £2.82; for Surgicare System® 2, 10 white clips = £2.82; drainable, 10 curved clips = £5.00); *Pelican* (drainable, 20 = £5.84); *Salts* (5 clips = £1.82; for drainable pouches, 10 clips = £6.40), *SIMS Portex* (for odourproof pouches, 10 = £6.49)

Closing Tape

Available from *Shannon* (1 reel = £1.44)

Fastening Ring

Rubber pouch fastening ring. Available from *Shaw* (1 ring = £1.06)

Ties

Available from *CliniMed* (30 soft-end ties, white or beige for drainable pouches = £2.46), *ConvaTec* (50 soft wire ties = £4.97), *Dansac* (50 soft wire ties = £4.87)

BAG COVERS

Bullen

Bag cover, cloth, for day or night bags. Net price 1 cover = £8.12

CliniMed

Bag cover, cloth for closed or drainable pouches. Net price 5 covers = £8.01

Bag shields, spunbonded polypropylene. Net price 10 shields (small: 25–44 mm; large: 10, 51, or 60 mm) = £3.07

Coloplast

Bag cover, cloth for closed or drainable mc2000® or mc2002® pouches (white or flesh), for mc2000® Mini pouches (decorated: white or flesh), for Ileo B® standard pouches, or for URO2002® pouches (white). Net price 5 covers = £21.80

Cover Care

Bag cover, formerly Surgicare System® 2 pouch covers. Net price 3 covers (for 32/38 mm Mini pouches or 45/57 mm pouches) = £6.53; 3 covers (for standard drainable pouches, urostomy pouches, large urostomy pouches, small closed 38/45 mm pouches: small drainable pouches, combihesive closed pouches, medium closed pouches: 57 and 70 mm) = £6.91

Hollister

Bag cover, non-woven. Net price 5 covers (for closed or non-drainable pouch) = £4.36

Impharm

Ostocover® bag cover, cloth, white or coloured. Net price 3 covers = £6.86

Jade-Euro-Med

Bag cover, cloth. Net price 1 cover = £4.28

Pelican

Bag cover, cotton, for closed pouch. Net price 5 covers, normal = £10.58, casual = £10.52; for drainable pouch, 5 covers = £10.93

Rüsch

Bag cover, cloth for Ostopore® pouches. Net price 5 covers (small or large) = £17.06

Salts

Bag covers, cotton, appliance to be stated. Net price 1 cover = £3.57. Cloth, for Eakin® pouches, 1 cover small or large (both 32, 45 or 64 mm) = £4.15

Shaw

Bag covers, cloth. Net price 1 day pouch cover, cotton = £4.80; lycra = £5.06. 1 night cover, cotton = £5.06; lycra = £5.43

SIMS Portex

Bag cover. Net price 1 day or night cotton pouch cover = £10.57; 5 stomabag covers (white or coloured) = £23.72; for Redifit® pouches, 1 cotton cover (25 and 32 mm, 38, 44, and 51 mm, 64, and 75 mm holes) = £7.54; for Symphony® pouches, 5 polyethylene covers = £4.39

Ward

Bag cover, white linen. Net price 1 cover = £6.36

BELTS

Braun Biotrol

Waist belt for Biotrol® pouches. Net price 1 belt = £4.06

Bullen

Belts. Net price 1.5-inch elastic belt with wire or plastic ring retainer (wire; small, medium, or large) = £9.81; 4-inch belt (wire; small, medium, or large) = £13.95; 1-inch elastic belt with plastic ring shield = £10.38; 1 waterproof canvas retaining shield (small, medium, or large) = £15.05; 1 St Mark's = £40.28

Girdles. Net price 1 Camilla® panty girdle = £18.59; 1 Cloe® roll on girdle = £15.49; 1 Constance® panty girdle = £24.57

J. Chawner

Girdles. Net price 1 ostomy girdle = £31.95; 1 ostomy-panty girdle = £28.90; 1 colostomy belt with understraps = £31.30

Coloplast

Belts. For Ileo B® pouches, net price 1 belt = £7.48; for K-Flex® pouches, 1 belt = £5.71; for Assura® pouches, 1 seal belt = £5.71

ConvaTec

Belt, for Surgicare System® 2. Net price 1 belt = £2.82

Dansac

Belt with plates for Combi® pouches. Net price 1 belt plus 5 plates (50–63 mm) = £35.54

DePuy

Belts. Net price 1 ostomy girdle or panty girdle (white or pink colour) = £29.76; 1 4-inch nightbelt with water-proof backing = £9.86; for Schacht® pouches, 1 36-inch belt = £5.36

Hollister

Belt. Net price 1 adjustable ostomy belt (small, medium, or large) = £6.67; 10 = £55.49

Jade-Euro-Med

Belts. Net price 3-inch belt = £14.44: 3-inch one-piece belt, = £18.84; 4-inch one-piece belt = £19.04; 1-inch web and elastic with button and buckle fastening = £8.01; 2-inch belt = £9.48; 3-inch belt = £10.93: 1 girdle and panti-brief with hole for stoma and suspenders or understrap = £46.75; 1 St Mark's (male or female) = £55.19; 1 St Mark's Coutil ostomy = £37.77

Marlen

Belt. Net price 1 adjustable elastic waist belt = £2.65

Orthotic

Belt. Net price 1 ostomy girdle with hole, zip and suspenders (white) = £31.95

Peacock

Belts. Net price 1 St Mark's belt = £38.15

Respond Plus

1 ostomy girdle/pantie brief, with hole and suspenders,15c = £36.05; zipped pocket, 1 = £4.80

Rüsch

Belts. Net price 5 elastic waistbands (Birkbeck®) = £33.84; 5 elastic waistbands with shields = £44.52; 5 retaining rings (19, 38, or 54 mm) = £8.44. 1 narrow or normal width belts (Ostopore®, waist: 17–34 inch or 28–56 inch) = £5.44. White rubber belting 28 mm = £3.70/metre, 72 mm = £7.64/metre. White sausage belt per metre = £7.61. 1 waist and support strap = £6.28

Sallis

Belts. Net price 1 night belt, 14b = £10.54; 14c = £5.50; 1 day belt, 15a = £29.02. 1 zipped pocket (to fit 15a and 16) = £4.93; 1 St Mark's = £26.61, 1 shield = £9.64

Salts

Belts. Net price 25 mm elastic belt (single), with 2 loops (standard 35 inch or extra-large 42 inch) = £3.30; with suspender ends = £3.87; double elastic with 4 loops = £5.61; with waterproof panel 102 mm = £13.56, 150 mm = £16.51; with 4 loops and retaining ring = £17.82. 1 rubber belt with straps and buckles = £6.48; with 2 fastening studs = £3.80. 25 mm button belt with or without loop = £3.30. 1 baby lycra belt = £13.32; with Velcro fastening (standard 35 inch or extra-large 42 inch) = £3.36. 1 colostomy belt = £67.90. 1 ileostomy girdle (Saltair®) = £43.37; 1 ileostomy elastic night belt (Saltair®) = £13.18. For Eakin® pouches, 1 elastic belt (small or large) = £3.26. For Salger® pouches, 1 elastic adjustable belt with or without Velcro fastening = £3.39

SASH

Belt. Net price 50 mm made to measure stoma hernia support belt, attached to plastic flange with hole over stoma = £30.00

Shannon

Belt. Net price 1 elastic belt with shield and Velcro fastening = £7.32; with button and buckle fastening = £4.45

Shaw

Belts, colostomy, all made to measure. Net price 4 inch elastic web belt = £13.73; with under-strap or suspenders, 6 inch = £18.39, 8 inch = £26.40; with lace fastenings, 6 inch = £24.87; 8 inch = £31.51; 10 inch = £29.97; 12 inch = £32.94; 14 inch (made to measure) = £33.59; with zip panel, 10 inch = £37.82; 12 inch = £40.12; 14 inch = £41.99; elastic with nylon fronts, 10 inch = £35.17; 12 inch = £36.95; 14 inch = £39.31. 1 inch adjustable colostomy/ileostomy belt = £7.96; 4 inch (3 sections) = £20.14; 6 inch (3 sections) = £25.39. 1 colostomy night belt (net or rayon, no hole, for use with dressing pad), = £14.65. 4 inch ostomy belt with groin strap = £15.70; with lace fastenings = £16.68; with wire spring = £15.37; double zip panel = £7.96

SIMS Portex

Belts. Net price 25 mm web and elastic belt (WL002 range) = £10.30; 51 mm = £12.01; 75 mm = £13.45; (WL008) 25 mm = £11.25; 1 belt, child (25 mm) = £8.66, 38 mm = £12.06. 1 web net belt with buckle (short) = £6.95. 1 narrow belt (flange diameter: 32, 38, or 51 mm) = £21.41. 1 Redifit adjustable belt (small, medium, or large) = £8.66. 1 non-slip belt = £17.65; 1 elastic non-slip belt = £12.06. 1 rubber belt ('sausage' or tubular) = £22.49; 1 narrow belt = £6.54. 1 two-way stretch night belt (small, medium, large, or extra-large) = £24.14. 1 stoma belt (small: 17–26 inch or medium: 26–43 inch) = £5.72. 1 Carshalton® belt (small, medium, or large) = £9.13

Ward

Belts. Made to measure, all sizes. Net price 1 day belt = £40.16; 1 night belt = £29.56. 1 nylon elastic colostomy belt, with hook and eye fastening and 2 pairs of suspenders or understraps = £41.48. 1 wide rubberised ileostomy belt with 2 straps and buttonhole ends for use with ileostomy boxes or with celluoid hook ends for use with ileostomy bags = £23.56. 1 belt with understraps or suspenders = £26.49. 1 colostomy belt, with 2 pairs of understraps or suspenders (Gabriel®) = £46.88. 1 web and elastic belt with button and buckle fastening. 1 belt (1 inch) = £7.64; 2 inch = £9.85; 3 inch = £11.19. 1 plastic elastic belt with hook end = £10.66. 1 belt with windows for use with ileostomy bags or colostomy cups or 4 stiched holes for studs of colostomy cups or shields. Net price 35 = £4.27

FILTERS AND BRIDGES

Filters

Available from *Braun Biotrol* (Biotrol®, 50 filters = £11.56), *Coloplast* (Filtrodor®, 50 filters = £18.85; Maclet®, 20 filter washers = £26.46), *ConvaTec* (Surgicare System® 2 for closed pouches, 30 filters = £8.09), *Cuxson* (50 patches = £3.12), *Hollister* (replacement filter elements for series 366 drainable bags, 20 = £2.92, 100 = £14.34), *SIMS Portex* (for Beta® and Omni® bags, 20 = £7.30; Doublesure®, 10 filters = £3.46; for Mirage® bags, 20 = £4.00)

Bridges

Available from *Salts* (20 metal bridges ready fixed to lightweight and LWU disposable bags = £8.74; 30 bridges for use with other disposable bags = £13.11), *SIMS Portex* (20 bridges = £3.10)

FLANGES

Braun Biotrol

Flanges. Net price 5 flanges for Biotrol® Lockring 2 pouches (35, 50 or 75mm) = £12.23

Bullen

Flanges. Net price 1 flange for Lenbul® pouches (1 inch diameter, 2 inch base) = £8.85; 1.5 inch diameter, 3 inch base = £13.46; 2 inch diameter, 4 inch base = £15.71

Coloplast

Flanges for Assura® Seal Integral Convexity pouches. Net price 5 (40 mm flange, 15, 18, 21 mm hole) = £13.42; 5 (50 mm flange, 25, 28, 31 mm hole or 15–33 mm starter hole) = £13.42; 5 (60 mm flange, 35, 38 or 41 mm holes or 15–43 mm starter hole) = £13.42

Note. Should be used only after assessment of suitability by appropriate medical professional

ConvaTec

Flanges for Surgicare System® 2. Net price 10 Accordion® flanges, 100 × 100 mm (70 mm hole) = £38.46; 127 ×127 mm (100 mm hole), 10 = £67.89. Combihesive® flexible flanges, 100 × 100 mm (32, 38, or 45 mm hole), 10 = £26.63; 127 × 127 mm (57 or 70 mm hole), 10 = £28.98. Stomahesive® flexible flanges, 100 mm × 100 mm (32, 38, 45, 57 or 70 mm holes) 10 = £23.71. Stomahesive® flanges, 100 × 100 mm (32, 38, 45, 57 or 70 mm holes) 10 = £23.71; 127 ×127 mm (70 mm hole), 10 = £47.81; 152 × 152 mm (100 mm hole), 10 = £57.40. For Combihesive Natura® pouches, 5 flexible flanges (32, 38, 45, 57 or 70 mm holes) – £13.25. For Consecura® pouches, 10 locking flanges (35, 45 or 55 mm holes) = £25.50

Dansac

Flanges for Unique® 2 urostomy pouches. Net price 5 (30 mm flange, 15 mm hole or cut-to-fit 10–22 mm hole) = £12.92; 5 (36 mm flange, 20, 25 mm hole or cut-to-fit 15–28 mm hole) = £12.92; 5 (43 mm flange, 30 mm hole or cut-to-fit 15–35 mm hole) = £12.92; 5 (55 mm flange, 35, 40 mm hole or cut-to-fit 15–47 mm hole) = £12.92

Convex flanges for Unique 2® pouches. Net price 5 (36 mm flange, 20, 25 mm or cut-to-fot 15-25 mm hole) = £13.42; 5 (43 mm flange, 25, 30 mm or cut-to-fit 15-32 mm hole) = £13.42; 5 (55 mm flange, 35, 40 mm or cut-to-fit 15 44 mm hole) – £13.42

Note. Should be used only after assessment of suitability by appropriate medical professional

DePuy

Flanges. Net price 1 Ileo B® standard rubber flange (0.75, 1.0, 1.25, 1.375, 1.5 inch) = £8.48. For Schacht® pouches, 1 flange (with locking ring) = £5.40; 1 ileo flange (with locking ring) = £5.40. St Mark's flange with inner sheath. Net price 1 flange, all 16 mm deep (76 mm base, 25 or 32 mm diameter; 100 mm base, 35, 38, 45 or 50 mm diameter) = £12.73

Hollister

Flanges for Impression® pouch. Net price 5 Convex flanges with synthetic seal and Microporous adhesive (13, 16, 19, 22, 25, 29, 32, 35, 38, 41, 44 or 51 mm holes) = £13.90; Impression® CPL convex flange (13, 16, 19, 22, 25, 29, 32, 35, 38, 41, 44 or 51 mm holes), 5 = £13.69; Tandem floating flanges with either barrier and adhesive (19, 25, 32, 38, 44, 51 or 57 mm hole) or barrier only (25, 32, 44, 57 cut-to-fit hole), net price 5 = £12.79 or barrier only (89 mm cut-to-fit hole) 5 = £13.26

Jade-Euro-Med

Flanges. Net price 1 St Mark's soft rubber = £13.08; with diaphragm = £13.08

Rüsch

Flange. Net price 2 Birkbeck® white rubber flanges (75 mm base, 16 mm deep, 20 mm diameter); 90 mm base, 16 mm deep, 38 mm diameter; 110 mm base, 16 mm deep, 58 mm diameter = £22.36; St Mark's, in two rubbers with hard centre (76 mm base, 10 or 16 mm deep, 32 or 38 mm diameter), 2 flanges = £33.50; 76 mm base, 13 or 16 mm deep, 25 mm diameter, 2 flanges = £33.50; 102 mm base, 16 mm deep, 44 or 51 mm diameter, 2 flanges = £33.50; in soft honey coloured rubber (51 or 76 mm base, 13 mm deep, 25 mm diameter), 2 flanges = £19.54; (76 mm base, 10 or 16 mm deep, 32 or 38 mm diameter), 2 flanges = £19.54; 102 mm base, 16 mm deep, 44 or 51 mm diameter, 2 flanges = £19.54; with diaphragm, cowl, or dressing retainer at extra cost = £3.24: black, firm rubber (51 mm base, 13 mm deep, 25 mm diameter), 2 flanges = £22.36; 76 mm base, 10 or

16 mm deep, 32 or 38 mm diameter, 2 flanges = £22.36; 102 mm base, 16 mm deep, 44 or 51 mm diameter, 2 flanges = £22.36

Salts

Flange. Net price 1 flange (SF1, soft rubber, 25 mm) = £6.95; SF2, semi-rigid, 25 mm = £11.16; SF3, hard rubber, 25 mm = £7.93; SF4, soft rubber, 38 mm = £7.05; SF5, semi-rigid, 38 mm = £12.09; SF6, semi-rigid, hard rubber = £8.06; SF7, soft rubber, 51 mm = £8.87; SF8R, flexible, recessed, 32 mm = £11.16. 1 baby flange with diaphragm (19 mm) = £9.24. 1 Latex foam diaphragm flange = £39.41; 1 sheath for use with flange = £6.56. For Salger® pouches, 1 polythene flange (40 or 57 mm) = £1.96

Shannon

Flange ring. Net price 1 = £2.23

Shaw

Flange. Net price 1 rubber, adhesive = £5.76; rubber, non-stick = £6.97; with diaphragm = £9.06; non-stick inner diaphragm £2.70; 1 colostomy rubber foam facepiece (face hole diameter: 1.75, 2, 2.5, or 3 inch) = £10.54

SIMS Portex

Flange. Net price 1 rubber flange (16 mm deep, 38 mm diameter) = £16.09; double base hole (38 mm diameter) = £21.33; blue rubber (51 mm base, 13 mm deep, 25 mm diameter or 76 mm base, 10 or 16 mm deep, 38 mm diameter) = £14.56; blue and brown, (76 mm base, 13 mm deep, 25 mm diameter; 10 or 16 mm deep, 38 mm diameter) = £21.13. 1 belt flange (19, 25, 32, 38, 44, 51, or 64 mm) = 27p. For Chiron® pouches, 1 flange (10 or 16 mm deep, 38 mm diameter) = £16.09; 13 mm deep, 25 mm diameter = £16.09; 16 mm deep, 32 mm diameter = £16.09; plastic without diaphragm (13 mm deep, 32 or 38 mm diameter) = £8.05. For Redifit® pouches, 1 belt flange = 65p; St Mark's pattern, 1 flange (51 mm base, 13 mm deep, 25 mm diameter; 76 mm base, 13 mm deep, 25 mm diameter; 76 mm base, 10 or 16 mm deep, 32 or 38 mm diameter; 102 mm base, 16 mm deep, 44 or 51 mm diameter) = £13.71: with dressing retainer or with 16 mm canopy, 38 mm = £17.31

Ward

Flange. Net price 1 plastic/rubber air-filled flange = £17.40; 1 St Mark's standard = £11.45; 1 St Mark's with diaphragm = £14.00

IRRIGATION AND WASH-OUT APPLIANCES

Available from *Astra Tech* (Medena® 5 ileostomy catheters = £4.52), *Braun Biotrol* (Biotrol®, 50 irrigation sleeves = £37.26 or 1 cone = £2.63), *Coloplast* (30 disposable sleeves (1540 or 1560) = £32.43; 1 colotip = £6.15; 1 irrigator bag = £11.64; 1 supporting plate = £5.85; 1 irrigation belt = £5.71); *Dansac* (1 water container = £17.17; 1 clamp = £7.43; 1 cone = £11.03; 1 brush = £7.87; 1 tube = £1.31; 1 belt = £35.54; Irri-drain® with ring holder for silicone ring, 20 = £21.95; silicone ring, 1 = £4.41; Unique® 2 Irri-drain®, 10 (flange: 36, 43 or 55 mm) = £10.80, *Hollister* (irrigator drain for use with Guardian® Two-Piece system, 5 (flange: 38, 51, 64, or 102 mm) = £6.44; 1 stoma cone/irrigator kit = £19.44; 20 irrigator drains = £26.81; 10 replacement cones = £68.95; 1 = £8.43; 1 stoma lubricant = £4.77), *Ward* (1 belt = £8.18)

PRESSURE PLATES, SHIELDS

Coloplast (1 supporting plate = £5.68; Assura® convex inserts for use with two-piece base plates 40, 50, 60 mm, 5 = £1.25), *ConvaTec* (5 System 2® convex inserts for Combihesive®, Stomahesive®, and flexible flanges, 38, 45, or 57 mm) = £1.29, *De Puy* (cotton facepiece with non-slip belt for St. Mark's flange, 45 mm diameter) = £18.00; *Salts* (plastic retaining shield, single = £3.09, double = £4.76, large = £3.77; S S Wire retaining ring, large = £3.09, medium = £2.94, small = £2.86; light white anti-sag ring = £1.23, for belt use = £1.39, for velcro belt fastening = £1.59; convex plate for light white bag (32, 38, or 44 mm), 5 = £13.32; pressure plate for Kombo®, Simplicity®, or Solo® pouches (30, 40, 50, or 60 mm) = £1.92; Eakin® support frame (32, 45, 64, or 90 mm) = £1.20, *Shannon* (faceplate = £7.53), *SIMS Portex* (plastic pressure plates, Surrey model: 25 or 32 mm or Standard model with attached flange for use with lightweight bags: 25, 32, or 38 mm = £7.25; stainless wire pressure frame, hook, lug, to fit 25, 32, 38, 44, or 51 mm flange) = £8.83; cotton facepiece = £21.54; pressure plates (25, 32, or 38 mm) = £5.08, *Ward* (celluloid colostomy cup with sponge or solid rim, small, medium, or large = £35.93, with sponge rubber or solid rim, belt fitting = £40.99; St Mark's shield, celluloid with 4 studs = £7.81)

SKIN PROTECTIVES, FILLERS, AND CLEANSERS

Balspray® (Bullen)
Aerosol. Net price 1 unit = £6.75
Bullen Karaya Gum Powder® (Bullen)
Powder. Net price 70 g = £4.48
Chiron® (SIMS Portex)
Barrier cream (with antiseptic). Net price 52 g = £4.80
CliniShield Wipes® (CliniMed)
Barrier wipes. Net price 50 = £11.88
Comfeel® (Coloplast)
Barrier cream. Net price 60 g = £3.93
Protective film. Net price 30 sachets = £9.00; applicator = £4.26
Dansac® (Dansac)
Soft paste. Net price 50 g = £3.02
Day-Drop® (Loxley)
Barrier Cream. Net price 50 g = £2.15
Derma-gard® (SIMS Portex)
Protective skin wipes. Net price 50 = £14.06
Hollister® (Hollister)
Karaya paste. Net price 128 g = £7.04
Do not apply to severely excoriated skin
Karaya powder. Net price 71 g = £8.11
Premium paste. Net price 57 g = £3.15
Skin gel. Net price 28 g = £6.11. Label: 15
Do not apply to severely excoriated skin
Orabase® (ConvaTec)
Paste, see section 12.3.1
Orahesive® (ConvaTec)
Powder (with adherent properties), see section 12.3.1
Payne® (Payne)
Barrier cream. Net price 50 g = £3.44
Pelican® (Pelican)
Paste (formerlySimpla® gel). Net price 1 pack = £6.44
Preventox® (Manfred Sauer)
Skin protecting film. Net price 50 wipes = £7.95; with roll-on applicator, 50 mL = £6.52
Saltair® (Salts)
Ostomy cleansing soap (soap spirit). Net price 110-mL = £2.59
Salts® (Salts)
Karaya gum powder. Net price per puffer pack = £4.31
Peri-Prep wipes. Net price 50 = £14.02
Stoma paste. Net price 60 g = £3.12
Seel-a-peel® (SIMS Portex)
Paste. Net price 50 mL = £2.75
SIMS Portex® (SIMS Portex)
Karaya gum powder. Net price 100 g = £6.96
Skin shield®Wipes (DePuy)
Barrier wipes. Net price 50 = £8.21
Stomahesive® (ConvaTec)
Paste. Net price 60 g = £6.54. For filling and sealing skin creases

Translet® (Rüsch)
Wipes. Net price 30 = £5.64

SKIN PROTECTORS

Braun Biotrol
Biotrol® skin protectors. Net price 10 × 10 cm or 10 cm diameter, 10 = £16.28
Bullen
Karaya gum washers, regular or extra hard. Net price 10 washers (2 inch diameter: 2 × 0.875 inch or 2 × 1.125 inch hole) = £12.18; 2.5 inch diameter: regular 2.5 × 1.25 inch or extra hard 2.5 × 1.5 inch hole = £14.12; 3 inch diameter: 3 × 0.875 inch, 3 × 1.125 inch, 3 × 1.5 inch, or 3 × 2 inch hole = £16.19
Coloplast
Protective sheets. Net price 10 non-sterile sheets (10 × 10 cm) = £20.16; 5 (15 × 15 cm) = £23.64; 5 (20 × 20 cm) = £43.01; 30 rings (10, 15, 20, 25, 30, 40, or 50 mm) = £34.65
ConvaTec
Wafers. Net price 5 Stomahesive® wafers (100 × 100 mm) = £9.85; 3 (200 × 200 mm) = £24.15; 10 Varihesive® wafers (100 × 100 mm) = £8.53
Dansac
Washers. Net price 25 Dansac® GX-tra seals (20, 30, 40 or 50 mm) = £30.00
DePuy
Schach® rings. Net price 10 foam, colostomy or ileostomy rings = £7.52
Hollister
Skin barrier. Net price 5 Hollister® skin barriers (4 × 4 inch) = £10.06; 5 (8 × 8 inch) = £31.64
Pelican
Protectors (formerly Simplaseel® wafers). Net price 10 (100 × 100 mm) = £18.59
Salts
Protectors. Net price 10 karaya gum washers (small) = £7.40; 10 (large) = £12.06; 5 foam cushions (25, 32, 38, or 51 mm) = £2.45; 5 dri pads (40 mm) = £2.34; 20 Cohesive® washers (small: 50 mm) = £31.16; 10 (large: 95 mm) = £20.80; 10 Realistic® washers (13, 19, 22, 25, 29, 32, or 38 mm) = £15.07; 1 Saltair® twinpack (small) = £9.06; large = £12.68; 10 foam seals (as in twin packs) = £1.84; 5 United® skin barrier wafers (10 × 10 cm) = £9.96; 3 = £23.11; for Salger® pouches, 5 karaya washers with foam (40 or 57 mm) = £12.82
Shannon
Protectors. Net price 1 foam sponge ring = 73p; 10 Kaygee® washers (2.5 inch base: 0.875 or 1.125 inch hole or 2.75 inch base: 0.875 or 1.375 inch hole) = £6.60
Shaw
Protectors. Net price 5 Body Mould® squares (1.0, 1.25, or 1.5 inch hole) = £10.60; 10 washers (1.0 or 1.25 inch hole) = £9.72; 5 rings (1.0, 1.25, or 1.5 inch hole) = £9.72; 12 Healwell® squares (1.0, 1.25 or 1.5 inch hole) = £10.06; 12 rings (1.0, 1.25 or 1.5 inch hole) = £8.69
SIMS Portex
Protectors. Net price 5 foam pads, white (76 mm diameter: 25 mm hole) = £4.73; 76 mm diameter: 29, 32, or 38 mm hole or 90 mm diameter: 32 or 38 mm hole = £6.47; black (25 mm hole) = £6.05: 1 karaya gum sheet (300 × 100 mm) = £6.97: 20 rings (19, 25, 32, 38, or 44 mm) = £23.25; karaya rings (19, 25, 32, 38, or 51 mm) = £25.42: 10 Down's® adhesive karaya gum washers (51 mm base: 22 or 29 mm hole) = £11.32; 70 mm base: 22 or 29 mm hole = £13.96; 10 Redifit® karaya gum washers (25, 32, 38, 44, or 51 mm) = £13.96: 20 Seel-a-peel® squares (100 mm sq) = £39.19; 5 squares (150 mm sq) = £24.13

STOMA CAPS AND DRESSINGS

Available from *Coloplast* (100 Colocap® stomacaps = £110.30; Assura Minicap®, 30 opaque stomacaps, 20 mm starter hole, cut to fit up to 55 mm hole = £32.91), *ConvaTec* (Colodress Plus®, 30 stoma caps (19 mm hole cut-to-size) = £32.21, *Dansac* (50 Dansac® Mini caps (30 or 44 mm) = £54.31; 30 Dansac® Unique Mini caps, 20 mm starter hole, cut to fit up to 50 mm hole; also 30, 40 or 50 mm = £32.10), *Hollister* (50 stoma caps (51 or 76 mm) = £54.97), *Oakmed* (50 Option® stoma caps = £55.52), *Salts* (30 Confidence® stoma caps with filter, 13 mm starter hole = £29.40; 30 stoma caps for Simplicity 1® pouches = £33.09), *SIMS Portex* (20 leisure pouches = £22.88), *Ward* (2 zip fasteners fitted to colostomy belt = £7.76; 1 waterproof front fitted to colostomy belt = £6.40; 1 pair woven understraps with buttonholed ends = £2.97; 1 Donald Rose® ileostomy/colostomy bath belt with internal chamber for dressings and stud fastenings for adjustment = £19.22)

TUBING

Available from *Hollister* (10 urostomy drain tubes = £24.23; 8 tubes for fitting to Lo-Profile® urostomy bags = £22.54; for Premium®urostomy pouches, 10 drain tube adaptors = £19.34), *Salts* (2 night tube adaptors = 93p), *SIMS Portex* (for Carshalton® urostomy pouches, 10 connectors = £4.08), *Ward* (1 metal spring tubing clip = £2.16)

Appendix 9: Wound Management Products and Elastic Hosiery

This appendix includes wound dressings, bandages, and elastic hosiery.

Wound dressings

An overview of the management of *chronic wounds* (including venous ulcers and pressure sores) and the role of different dressings is given below; the notes do not deal with the management of clean surgical wounds which usually heal very rapidly. The correct dressing for wound management depends not only on the type of wound but also on the stage of the healing process. The principal stages of healing are:

    cleansing, removal of debris;
    granulation, vascularisation;
    epithelialisation.

Wound contraction is also important and may begin almost as soon as the wound is clean.

The ideal dressing needs to ensure that the wound remains:

    moist with exudate, but not macerated;
    free of clinical infection and excessive slough;
    free of toxic chemicals, particles or fibres;
    at the optimum temperature for healing;
    undisturbed by the need for frequent changes;
    at the optimum pH value.

As wound healing passes through its different stages, variations in dressing type may be required to satisfy better one or other of these requirements. Depending on the type of wound or the stage of the healing process, the functions of dressings may be summarised as follows:

Type of wound	Role of dressing
Dry, necrotic, black	Moisture retention or rehydration
Yellow, sloughy	If dry, moisture retention or rehydration
	If moist, fluid absorption
	Possibly odour absorption
	Possibly antimicrobial
Clean, exuding (granulating)	Fluid absorption
	Thermal insulation
	Possibly odour absorption
	Possibly antimicrobial
Dry, low exudate (epithelialising)	Moisture retention or rehydration
	Low adherence
	Thermal insulation

Greater understanding of the requirements of a surgical dressing, including recognition of the benefits of maintaining a moist environment for wound healing, has improved the approach towards chronic wound management. A decrease in pain and reduction in healing time is achieved to a marked extent with **alginate**, **foam**, **hydrogel** and **hydrocolloid** dressings and also to an important extent with **vapour-permeable films** and **membranes**; dressings such as dry gauze have little place, and practices such as the use of irritant cleansers may be harmful and are largely obsolete.

Alginate, **foam**, **hydrogel** and **hydrocolloid** dressings are designed to absorb wound exudate and thus to control the state of hydration of a wound. All are claimed to be effective, but as yet there have been few trials able to establish a clear advantage for any particular product. The choice between different dressings may therefore often depend not only on the type and stage of the wound, but also on personal experience, availability of the dressing, patient preference or tolerance and site of the wound.

ALGINATE DRESSINGS

The gelling characteristics of alginate dressings vary according to the product used. Some products only gel to a limited extent to form a partially gelled sheet that can be lifted off; others form an amorphous gel that can be rinsed off with water or physiological saline. A secondary covering is needed. They are highly absorbent and are therefore suitable for moderately or heavily exuding wounds, but not for eschars or for dry wounds.

Algosteril®. Calcium alginate dressing. Net price 5 cm × 5 cm, 1 = 72p; 10 cm × 10 cm, 1 = £1.65 (Beiersdorf)
Uses: moderate to heavily exuding wounds

Comfeel® SeaSorb (formerly Comfeel® Alginate) (Alginate Dressing, Sterile, BP), calcium sodium alginate fibre, sterile, highly absorbent, gelling dressing, 4 cm × 6 cm = 71p; 10 cm × 10 cm = £1.47; 15 cm × 15 cm = £3.10
Uses: heavily exuding wounds including leg ulcers and pressure sores

NHS Comfeel® SeaSorb Filler (formerly Comfeel® Alginate Filler), calcium sodium alginate fibre, highly absorbent, gelling filler, 2 g, 6 = £23.10
Uses: moderately to heavily exuding cavity wounds, fistulas, sinus drainage, decubitus and deep leg ulcers

Kaltogel® (Alginate Dressing, Sterile, BP, type A). Calcium sodium alginate fibre, highly absorbent, quick gelling dressing, net price 5 cm × 5 cm, each = 71p; 10 cm × 10 cm = £1.48 (ConvaTec)
Uses: moderately to heavily exuding wounds including leg ulcers, pressure sores, fungating lesions

Kaltostat® (Alginate Dressing, Sterile, BP, type C). Calcium alginate fibre, flat non-woven pads, 5 cm × 5 cm, net price, each = 73p; 7.5 cm × 12 cm = £1.59; other sizes (NHS) 10 cm × 20 cm, 10 = £37.10; 15 cm × 25 cm, 10 = £64.00; 30 cm × 60 cm, 5 = £123.40; wound packing, 2 g, 5 = £16.40; also (NHS) Kaltostat Fortex®, 10 cm × 10 cm, 10 = £31.40 (ConvaTec)
Uses: haemostatic

Nu-Gel® (Drug Tariff Specification 50). A ready-mixed hydrogel containing alginate, applied directly into wound and covered with secondary dressing. Net price 15 g = £1.75 (J&J)
Uses: dry, sloughy or necrotic, lightly exuding or granulating wounds

Sorbsan® (Alginate Dressing, Sterile, BP, type A). Calcium alginate fibre, highly absorbent, flat non-woven pads, 5 cm × 5 cm, net price, each = 89p; 10 cm × 10 cm = £1.57; other sizes (NHS) 10 cm × 20 cm, 5 = £22.75; surgical packing 30 cm, 5 = £25.25; ribbon, 40 cm (+12.5-cm probe), 5 = £17.00; also (bonded to a secondary absorbent viscose pad) Sorbsan® Plus, 7.5 cm × 10 cm, 1 = £1.43; 10 cm × 15 cm, 1 = £2.53; 10 cm × 20 cm, 1 = £3.23 (Maersk)
Uses: heavily to moderately exuding wounds

NHS Sorbsan® SA. Calcium alginate fibre, highly absorbent flat non-woven pads for wound contact bonded to adhesive semi-permeable polyurethane foam. Net price 9 cm × 11 cm, 5 = £11.20 (Maersk)
Uses: moderately to lightly exuding shallow wounds

Sterigel® (Drug Tariff Specification 50). A ready-mixed hydrogel, applied directly into wound and covered with secondary dressing. Net price 15 g = £1.75 (Seton)
Uses: dry, sloughy or necrotic, lightly exuding or granulating wounds

---

Tegagen® (formerly Tegagel®) (Alginate Dressing, Sterile, BP, type B). Net price each 5 cm × 5 cm = 71p; 10 cm × 10 cm = £1.47 (3M)

Uses: for leg ulcers, pressure sores, second degree burns, post-operative wounds, fungating carcinomas

FOAM DRESSINGS

Foam dressings vary from products that are suitable for lightly exuding wounds to highly absorbent structures for heavily exuding wounds. They may also be used as secondary dressings.

Polyurethane Foam Dressing, BP. Absorbent foam dressing of low adherence; sterile. 7.5 cm × 7.5 cm, net price, each = 87p; 10 cm × 10 cm, each = £1.03; 10 cm × 17.5 cm, each = £1.60; 15 cm × 20 cm, each = £2.16; other sizes (NHS) 10 cm × 25 cm, 35 = £124.15; 25 cm × 30 cm, each = £8.40 (Seton—*Lyofoam*®)

Uses: treatment of burns, decubitus ulcers, donor sites, granulating wounds

Allevyn®. (Drug Tariff title: Polyurethane Foam Film Dressing, Drug Tariff specification 47, type 2) Hydrophilic polyurethane dressing; foam sheets with trilaminate structure, non-adherent wound contact layer, foam based central layer, bacteria and waterproof outer layer. 5 cm × 5 cm, each = 97p; 10 cm × 10 cm, each = £1.92; 10 cm × 20 cm, each = £3.09; 20 cm × 20 cm, each = £5.16; also Allevyn® Adhesive (Drug Tariff title: Polyurethane Foam Film Dressing with Adhesive Margin, Drug Tariff specification 47, type 4), 7.5 cm × 7.5 cm = £1.15; 12.5 cm × 12.5 cm = £2.06; 17.5 cm × 17.5 cm = £4.06; 22.5 cm × 22.5 cm = £5.91; NHS Allevyn® Cavity, circular (5 and 10 cm), tubular (2.5 cm × 9 cm and 4 cm × 12 cm) (S&N Hlth)

Uses: treatment of light to moderately exuding wounds

NHS Cavi-Care®. Soft, conforming cavity wound dressing prepared by mixing thoroughly for 15 seconds immediately before use and allowing to expand its volume within the cavity. Net price 20 g = £16.90 (S&N Hlth)

Uses: in the management of open post-operative granulating cavity wounds (with no underlying tracts or sinuses) such as pilonidal sinus excision, dehisced surgical wounds, hydradenitis suppurativa wounds, peri-anal wounds, perineal wounds, pressure sores

FlexiPore® (formerly Spyroflex®). Sterile, semi permeable, polyurethane foam film adhesive dressing. Net price, 10 cm × 10 cm = £1.73; 20 cm × 20 cm = £5.06; 6 cm × 7 cm = 93p; 10 cm × 30 cm = £3.60; 15 cm × 20 cm = £3.70; NHS 20 cm × 30 cm = £3.75 (TSL)

Uses: treatment of light to moderately exuding wounds, leg ulcers, pressure sores

Lyofoam Extra®. Extra absorbent polyurethane foam dressing, non-adhesive. Net price 10 cm × 10 cm, 1 = £1.72; 17.5 cm × 10 cm, 1 = £2.91; 20 cm × 15 cm, 1 = £3.77; 25 cm × 10 cm, 1 = £3.52; (NHS) 30 cm × 25 cm, 1 = £12.90; with adhesive, 15 cm × 15 cm = £2.06; 22 cm × 22 cm = £4.06; 30 cm × 30 cm = £5.91; sacral, 22 cm × 26 cm = £3.20 (Seton)

Uses: treatment of heavily exuding wounds

Spyrosorb® (Drug Tariff title: Polyurethane Foam Film Dressing, Drug Tariff specification 47, type 1). Sterile, semipermeable, absorbent polyurethane membrane with polyurethane film and hydrophilic adhesive. Net price 10 cm × 10 cm, 5 = £9.90; 20 cm × 20 cm, 5 = £28.25 (S&N Hlth)

Uses: light to moderately exuding wounds

Tielle®. (Drug Tariff title: Polyurethane Foam Film Dressing with Adhesive Margin, Drug Tariff specification 47). Semi-permeable, foamed gel with non-woven wicking layer and polyurethane backing layer. Net price (square) 11 cm × 11 cm = £1.95; 15 cm × 15 cm = £3.25; 18 cm × 18 cm = £4.06; (both rectangular) 7 cm × 9 cm =

£1.05; 15 cm × 20 cm = £3.99; Tielle® Sacrum 18 cm × 18 cm = £2.95 (J&J)

Uses: light to moderately exuding wounds, leg ulcers

HYDROGEL DRESSINGS

Hydrogel dressings are most commonly supplied as an amorphous, cohesive material that can take up the shape of a wound. These dressings are generally used to donate liquid to dry sloughy wounds and facilitate autolytic debridement but they may also have the ability to absorb limited amounts of exudate.

Debrisan®

Beads, dextranomer. Net price 60-g castor = £29.01 (Pharmacia & Upjohn)

Uses: for moist wounds, indolent ulcers and small burns, sprinkle onto wound and cover with appropriate dressing, renew before saturation occurs (usually once or twice daily)

Paste, dextranomer in a soft paste basis. Net price 6 × 10-g pouches = £29.93 (Pharmacia & Upjohn)

Uses: for exudative and infected wounds, decubital ulcers, and leg ulcers, apply firmly and cover with appropriate dressing, renew before saturation occurs (usually twice daily to every 2 days)

NHS Geliperm®. Gel sheets, wet form and tubed granulated gel. Granulate, 20 g, 6 tubes = £19.92, 50 g, 6 tubes = £49.80. Wet, 100 cm × 100 cm, net price, 20 sheets = £42.90, 12 cm × 13 cm, 6 sheets = £29.26; 12 cm × 26 cm, 6 sheets = £52.36 (Geistlich)

Uses: wound and ulcer dressing, burns, donor sites

Intrasite® **Gel** (formerly Scherisorb®) Drug Tariff specification 50. A ready-mixed hydrogel containing modified carboxymethylcellulose polymer applied directly into the wound. Net price 8-g sachet = £1.38; 15-g sachet = £1.85 (S&N Hlth)

Uses: for dry, sloughy or necrotic wounds; lightly exuding wounds; granulating wounds

Iodoflex®

Paste, iodine 0.9% as cadexomer-iodine in a paste basis with gauze backing, net price 5 × 5-g units = £20.40; 3 × 10-g units = £24.50; 2 × 17-g = £25.84 (S&N Hlth)

Uses: for treatment of chronic leg ulcers, apply to wound surface, remove gauze backing and cover; renew when saturated (usually 2–3 times weekly); max. weekly application 150 g

Cautions; Contra-indications: avoid in thyroid disorders, in those receiving lithium, and in pregnancy and breast-feeding; caution in patients with history of thyroid disorders; iodine may be absorbed particularly if large wounds treated

Iodosorb®

Ointment, iodine 0.9% as cadexomer-iodine in an ointment basis, net price 4 × 10 g = £18.05; 2 × 20 g = £18.05 (S&N Hlth)

Uses: for treatment of chronic leg ulcers, apply to wound surface to a depth of approx. 3 mm; renew when saturated (usually 3 times weekly); max. weekly application 150 g

PoM *Powder*, iodine 0.9% as cadexomer-iodine microbeads, net price 3-g sachet = £1.93 (S&N Hlth)

Uses: for treatment of moist wounds, including decubitus ulcers and chronic leg ulcers, apply to wound surface to depth of approx. 3 mm and cover; renew when saturated (usually once daily)

Cautions; Contra-indications: avoid in thyroid disorders, in those receiving lithium, and in pregnancy and breast-feeding; caution in patients with history of thyroid disorders; iodine may be absorbed particularly if large wounds treated

---

Purilon® Gel (Drug Tariff specification 50). Net price 15 g = £1.75 (Coloplast)

Uses: for dry, sloughy or necrotic wounds; lightly exuding wounds; granulating wounds

NHS **Vigilon®**. Semi-permeable hydrogel sheets on a polyethylene mesh support. Sterile, 3 in × 6 in, net price 10 = £78.30, 4 in × 4 in, 10 = £78.30; non-sterile, 4 in × 4 in, 10 = £54.60, 13 in × 24 in, 2 = £95.05 (Seton)

HYDROCOLLOID DRESSINGS

Hydrocolloid dressings are usually presented as an absorbent layer on a vapour-permeable film or foam. Owing to the occlusive nature of their backing they are not considered suitable for the treatment of clinically infected or very heavily exuding wounds, but are suitable for softening eschars or for promoting granulation.

NHS **Biofilm S®**. Hydrocolloid dressing with polyurethane-polyester backing; also in powder form for direct application into wound: 10 cm × 10 cm, net price 10 = £18.04; 20 cm × 20 cm, 5 = £36.24; Biofilm® powder, 10 sachets = £23.29 (Braun Biotrol)

CombiDERM®. Dressing with hydrocolloid adhesive border and absorbent wound contact pad. Net price 10 cm × 10 cm, 1 = £1.25; 14 cm × 14 cm, 1 = £1.74; 15 cm × 18 cm (triangular), 1 = £3.00 (ConvaTec)

Uses: chronic exuding wounds such as leg ulcers, pressure sores; postoperative wounds

Comfeel®. Soft elastic pad consisting of carmellose (carboxymethylcellulose) sodium particles embedded in adhesive mass; smooth outer layer and polyurethane film backing; available as sheets, powder in plastic blister units and paste for direct application into the wound: Ulcer dressing, 10 cm × 10 cm, net price each = £2.11; 15 cm × 15 cm = £4.19; 20 cm × 20 cm = £6.40; other sizes (NHS): 4 cm × 6 cm, 30 = £32.10; powder 6 g, 10 = £3.70; paste 12-g sachet, 10 = £13.70; 50 g, 10 = £52.80 (Coloplast)

Comfeel® Plus. Hydrocolloid dressings containing carmellose (carboxymethylcellulose) sodium and calcium alginate. Contour dressing 6 cm × 8 cm, 1 = £1.67; 9 cm × 11 cm, 1 = £2.89; Ulcer Dressing, 10 cm × 10 cm = £2.15; 15 cm × 15 cm = £4.27; 20 cm × 20 cm = £6.41; NHS Transparent Dressing, 5 cm × 7 cm, 10 = £12.80; 9 cm × 14 cm, 10 = £37.60; 15 cm × 20 cm, 5 = £42.20; NHS Pressure Relieving Dressing, 7 cm × 7 cm, 10 = £37.00; 10 cm × 10 cm, 10 = £37.00; 15 cm × 15 cm, 10 = £76.30 (Coloplast)

DuoDERM® Extra Thin (formerly Granuflex® ExtraThin), 7.5 cm × 7.5 cm, 1 = 61p; 10 cm × 10 cm, 1 = £1.01; 15 cm × 15 cm, 1 = £2.18; NHS 5 cm × 10 cm, 1 = 69p; 5 cm × 20 cm, 1 = £1.38 (ConvaTec)

Granuflex®. Hydrocolloid wound contact layer bonded to plastic foam layer, with outer semipermeable polyurethane film. 10 cm × 10 cm, net price each = £2.14; 15 cm × 15 cm = £4.06; 15 cm × 20 cm = £4.40; 20 cm × 20 cm, 1 = £6.11; NHS 20 cm × 30 cm, 5 = £55.75; also Granuflex® Compression Bandage (NHS), 10 cm × 6.5 m (stretched), 6 = £32.64; also Granuflex® Paste (NHS), net price 30 g = £2.68; also, Granuflex® Bordered Dressing, 10 cm × 10 cm, 1 = £2.55; 10 cm × 13 cm, 1 = £3.01; 15 cm × 18 cm, 1 = £4.69; also (NHS), 6 cm × 6 cm, 5 = £7.38; 15 cm × 15 cm, 5 = £30.98; triangular dressing, 10 cm × 13 cm, 5 = £15.61; 15 cm × 18 cm, 5 = £26.55; also **GranuGel®**, net price 15 g = £1.78 (ConvaTec)

Uses: chronic ulcers, pressure sores, open wounds, debridement of wounds; powders, gel, and pastes used with sheet dressings to fill deep or heavily exuding wounds

Tegasorb®. Hydrocolloid dressing 10 cm × 12 cm (oval), net price each = £2.01; 13 cm × 15 cm (oval), 1 = £3.79; 10 cm × 10 cm, (square) 1= £2.05; 15 cm × 15 cm, (square) 1 = £3.97 (3M)

Uses: chronic wounds such as leg ulcers and pressure sores

Keloid dressing

NHS **Cica-Care®**. Soft, self-adhesive, semi-occlusive silicone gel sheet with backing. Net price, 15 cm × 12 cm, 1 sheet = £22.71 (S&N Hlth)

Uses: temporary management of both existing and new hypertrophic and keloid scars; also for temporary prophylaxis of hypertrophic or keloid scarring in closed wounds

VAPOUR-PERMEABLE FILMS AND MEMBRANES

Vapour-permeable films and membranes allow the passage of water vapour and oxygen but not of water or microorganisms, and are suitable for mildly exuding wounds. They are highly conformable, convenient to use, provide a moist healing environment, and some may permit constant observation of the wound. However, water vapour loss may occur at a slower rate than exudate is generated, so that fluid accumulates under the dressing, which can lead to tissue maceration and to wrinkling at the adhesive contact site (with risk of bacterial entry). Newer versions have increased gaseous permeability; some also contain water-soluble antimicrobials. Despite these advances vapour-permeable films and membranes remain less suitable for large heavily exuding wounds and are probably not suitable for chronic leg ulcers. They are most commonly used as secondary dressings over gels.

Vapour-permeable Adhesive Film Dressing, BP.

(Semi-permeable Adhesive Dressing) Sterile, extensible, waterproof, water vapour-permeable polyurethane film coated with synthetic adhesive mass; transparent. Supplied in single-use pieces. Type 1: 6 cm × 7 cm, net price each = 43p; 10 cm × 12 cm, each = £1.18; 15 cm × 20 cm, each = £2.90 (S&N Hlth—*Opsite® Flexigrid*), Type 2: 12 cm × 12 cm, net price = £1.21 (3M—*Tegaderm®*), Type 3: 10.2 cm × 12.7 cm, net price = £1.28 (J&J—*Bioclusive®*); Type 4, 7.5 cm × 10 cm, net price each = 64p; 10 cm × 14 cm, each = £1.09 (Beiersdorf—*Cutifilm®*); Type 5, 6 cm × 7 cm, net price each = 40p; 10 cm × 14 cm, each = £1.05 (ConvaTec—*Epiview®*)

Uses: postoperative dressing, donor sites, IV sites, superficial decubitus ulcers, amputation stumps, stoma care; protective cover to prevent skin breakdown

NHS **Arglaes®**. Sterile, semi-permeable, self-adhesive, clear, controlled release polyurethane film dressing containing silver. Net price 6 cm × 8 cm, 1 = 99p; 10 cm × 12 cm, 1 = £1.99; 15 cm × 25 cm, 1 = £3.99 (Maersk)

Uses: flat moist wounds including cuts and abrasions; burns and scalds; superficial pressure areas; surgical wounds

NHS **Omiderm®**. Sterile, water-vapour permeable polyurethane film (plain and meshed versions). Net price 5 cm × 7 cm, 20 = £26.09; 8 cm × 10 cm, 20 = £46.12; meshed, 20 = £61.79; 18 cm × 10 cm, 25 = £105.00; meshed, 10 = £61.79; 60 cm × 10 cm, 10 = £154.99; 21 cm × 31 cm, 5 = £79.33; meshed, 5 = £106.30; meshed, 23 cm × 39 cm, 4 = £126.18 (IATRO)

Uses: ulcers; donor sites; superficial and partial thickness burns; meshed: donor sites, skin grafts

---

REDUCED ADHERENCE DRESSING PADS

Perforated film absorbent dressings were developed to overcome the problems of adherence associated with tulle dressings; they are, however, suitable only for wounds with mild to moderate amounts of exudate; they are not, therefore, appropriate for leg ulcers or for other lesions that produce large quantities of viscous exudate.

Knitted viscose primary dressing is an alternative to paraffin gauze for exuding wounds.

Povidone–iodine fabric dressing is a knitted viscose dressing with povidone–iodine incorporated in a hydrophilic polyethylene glycol basis; this facilitates diffusion of the iodine into the wound and permits removal of the dressing by irrigation with water or physiological saline. Although the iodine has a wide spectrum of antimicrobial activity, it is rapidly deactivated by wound exudate and systemic absorption of iodine may occur.

Absorbent Perforated Plastic Film Faced Dressing (Drug Tariff specification 9). Low-adherence dressing consisting of 3 layers:

Melolin®, 5 cm × 5 cm, net price, each = 13p; 10 cm × 10 cm = 21p; 20 cm × 10 cm = 40p (S&N Hlth)

Mepore®, 6 cm × 7 cm, net price, each = 8p; 9 cm × 10 cm = 17p; 9 cm × 15 cm = 28p (SCA Molnlycke)

Release®, 5 cm × 5 cm, net price, each = 12p; 10 cm × 10 cm = 19p; 20 cm × 10 cm = 37p (J&J)

Skintact®, 5 cm × 5 cm, net price, each = 10p; 10 cm × 10 cm = 17p; 20 cm × 10 cm = 33p (Robinson)

Where size not stated, 5 cm size supplied

Uses: dressing for post-operative and low exudate wounds; low adherence property and low absorption capacity

Knitted Viscose Primary Dressing, BP. Warp knitted fabric manufactured from a bright viscose monofilament. 9.5 cm × 9.5 cm (all): net price = 29p (J&J—*N-A Dressing*®); net price = 25p (S&N—*Tricotex*®); silicone-coated, net price = 28p (J&J—*N-A Ultra*®)

Uses: low adherence wound contact layer for use on ulcerative and other granulating wounds with superimposed absorbent pad

Povidone-iodine Fabric Dressing (Drug Tariff specification 43). Knitted viscose primary dressing impregnated with povidone-iodine ointment 10%, 5 cm × 5 cm, net price, each = 26p, 9.5 cm × 9.5 cm = 39p (J&J—*Inadine*®)

Uses: wound contact layer for abrasions and superficial burns; max. 4 dressings at same time

NHS **Ete**®. Wound pad of rayon wadding with rayon silk wound contact layer stitched in chequered pattern (SCA Molnlycke)

Uses: leg wounds, decubitus ulcers, minor burns, donor sites

NHS **Melolite**®. Absorbent fabric pad covered on both sides by polyethylene net (S&N Hlth)

Uses: primary dressing over clean sutured wounds, lacerations, and abrasions

NHS **Mesorb**®. Cellulose wadding pad with gauze wound contact layer and non-woven repellent backing (SCA Molnlycke)

Uses: post-operative use for heavily exuding wounds

NHS **Perfron**®. Absorbent pad consisting of alternate layers of absorbent cotton and crepe cellulose tissue, in sleeve of non-woven viscose fabric with coating of polypropylene (J&J)

Uses: low adherence pad for heavily exuding wounds; laminate structure delays strike through

NHS * **Surgipad**®. Absorbent pad of absorbent cotton and viscose in sleeve of non-woven viscose fabric (J&J)

Uses: for heavily exuding wounds requiring frequent dressing changes

* Except in Sterile Dressing Pack with Non-woven Pads

ODOUR ABSORBENT DRESSINGS

These dressings have an important role in absorbing the odour of infected wounds. Some dressings may also benefit wound healing by binding bacteria, but this effect awaits confirmation.

NHS **Actisorb Plus**®. Knitted fabric of activated charcoal, with one-way stretch, with silver residues, within spun-bonded nylon sleeve. Net price (each) 10.5 cm × 10.5 cm = £2.73 (J&J)

NHS **Carbonet**®. Activated charcoal dressing. 10 cm × 10 cm, net price, each = £2.47; 10 cm × 20 cm = £4.82 (S&N Hlth)

NHS **CliniSorb**® **Odour Control Dressings.** Layer of activated charcoal cloth between viscose rayon with outer polyamide coating. Net price 10 cm × 10 cm, 10 = £15.10; 10 cm × 20 cm, 10 = £20.15; 15 cm × 25 cm, 10 = £32.70 (CliniMed)

NHS **Kaltocarb**®. Dressing in 3 layers: wound-facing layer of calcium alginate fibre; absorbent middle layer of activated charcoal cloth; backing layer of bonded polyester and viscose non-woven material. Net price 7.5 cm × 12 cm, 25 = £51.48; 15 cm × 15 cm, 15 = £67.80 (ConvaTec)

NHS **Lyofoam C**®. Lyofoam sheet with layer of activated charcoal cloth and additional outer envelope of polyurethane foam. 10 cm × 10 cm, net price, each = £2.67; 15 cm × 20 cm = £5.91; 25 cm × 10 cm = £4.96 (Seton)

DRESSING PACKS

The role of dressing packs is very limited. They are used to provide a clean field; packs shown below include cotton wool balls but these are not recommended for use on wounds.

Sterile Dressing Pack (Drug Tariff specification 10; Scottish, 16). Contains gauze and cotton tissue pad, gauze swabs, absorbent cotton wool balls, absorbent paper towel, water repellent inner wrapper. Net price per pack = 69p

Sterile Dressing Pack with Non-woven Pads (Drug Tariff specification 35). Contains non-woven fabric covered dressing pad (*Surgipad*®), non-woven fabric swabs (*Topper 8*®), absorbent cotton wool balls, absorbent paper towel, water repellent inner wrapper. Net price per pack = 74p; also 72p (*Vernaid*®)

TULLE DRESSINGS

Tulle dressings are manufactured from cotton or viscose fibres which are impregnated with white or yellow soft paraffin to prevent the fibres from sticking, but this is only partly successful and the paraffin has the disadvantage of reducing absorbency. Versions containing a reduced amount of soft paraffin (i.e. Paratulle® and Unitulle®) are less liable to interfere with absorption; those containing the traditional amount (such as Jelonet®) have been considered more suitable for skin graft transfer.

Paraffin Gauze Dressing, BP (Tulle Gras). Fabric of leno weave, weft and warp threads of cotton and/or viscose yarn, impregnated with white or yellow soft paraffin; sterile. 10 cm × 10 cm, net price, each = 30p; pack of 10 pieces = £2.10 (most suppliers including Seton—*Paratulle*®; Hoechst Marion Roussel—*Unitulle*®; S&N Hlth—*Jelonet*®)

Uses: treatment of abrasions, burns, and other injuries of skin, and ulcerative conditions; postoperatively as penile and vaginal dressing and for sinus packing; heavier loading for skin graft transfer

MEDICATED TULLE DRESSINGS

Medicated tulle dressings all have disadvantages; they are not generally recommended for wound care. **Framycetin gauze dressing** is associated with a high incidence of hypersensitivity and exposure to large amounts can lead to absorption of framycetin with the consequent risk of systemic effects such as ototoxicity; its use should be limited to specific indications, on a short-term basis. Hypersensitivity is less of a problem with **sodium fusidate dressing**, but the theoretical possibility of developing bacterial resistance may be of special concern where the antibiotic is likely to be needed for systemic use (e.g. in bone infections and in burns). Although resistance and hypersensitivity are less likely with **chlorhexidine gauze dressing**, its efficacy has been questioned.

Chlorhexidine Gauze Dressing, BP. Fabric of leno weave, weft and warp threads of cotton and/or viscose yarn, impregnated with ointment containing chlorhexidine acetate; sterile. 5 cm × 5 cm, net price each = 22p; 10 cm × 10 cm = 46p (Seton—*Serotulle*®; Hoechst Marion Roussel—*Clorhexitulle*®; S&N Hlth—*Bactigras*®)

PoM **Framycetin Gauze Dressing, BP.** Fabric of leno weave, weft and warp threads of cotton, impregnated with ointment containing framycetin sulphate 1% in white soft paraffin containing 10% wool fat; sterile. 10 cm × 10 cm, net price each = 23p; NHS 10 cm × 30 cm, 10 = £8.24 (Hoechst Marion Roussel—*Sofra-Tulle* ®)

Cautions: large areas (risk of ototoxicity); see also cautions in section 13.10.1

Uses: wide range of infected lesions

PoM **Sodium Fusidate Gauze Dressing, BP.** Leno weave cotton gauze impregnated with ointment containing sodium fusidate 2% in white soft paraffin and wool fat. 10 cm × 10 cm, net price = 22p (Leo—*Fucidin Intertulle*®)

SURGICAL ABSORBENTS

Surgical absorbent dressings have many disadvantages, since they adhere to the wound, shed fibres into it, and dehydrate it; they also permit leakage of exudate ('strike through') with an associated risk of infection.

Absorbent Cotton, BP. Carded cotton fibres of not less than 10 mm average staple length, available in rolls and balls. 25 g, net price = 54p; 100 g = £1.24; 500 g = £4.29 (most suppliers). 25-g pack to be supplied when weight not stated

Uses: general purpose cleansing and swabbing, pre-operative skin preparation, application of medicaments; supplementary absorbent pad to absorb excess wound exudate

Absorbent Cotton, Hospital Quality. As for absorbent cotton but lower quality materials, shorter staple length etc. 100 g, net price = 90p; 500 g = £2.84 (most suppliers)

Drug Tariff specifies to be supplied only where specifically ordered

Uses: suitable only as general purpose absorbent, for swabbing, and routine cleansing of incontinent patients; not for wound cleansing

Gauze and Cotton Tissue, BP 1988. Consists of absorbent cotton enclosed in absorbent cotton gauze type 12 or absorbent cotton and viscose gauze type 2.

500 g, net price = £5.53 (most suppliers, including Robinsons—*Gamgee Tissue*® (blue label))

Uses: absorbent and protective pad, as burns dressing on non-adherent layer

Gauze and Cotton Tissue (Drug Tariff specification 14). Similar to above. 500 g, net price = £4.04 (most suppliers, including Robinsons—*Gamgee Tissue*® (pink label))

Drug Tariff specifies to be supplied only where specifically ordered

Uses: absorbent and protective pad, as burns dressing on non-adherent layer

Absorbent Lint, BPC. Cotton cloth of plain weave with nap raised on one side from warp yarns. 25 g, net price = 71p; 100 g = £2.16; 500 g = £9.09 (most suppliers). 25-g pack supplied where no quantity stated

Uses: external absorbent protective dressing

Absorbent Cotton Gauze, BP 1988. Cotton fabric of plain weave, in rolls and as swabs (see below), usually Type 13 light, sterile. 90 cm (all) ×1 m, net price = 83p; 3 m = £1.78; 5 m = £2.75; 10 m = £5.34 (most suppliers). 1-m packet supplied when no size stated

Uses: pre-operative preparation, for cleansing and swabbing

Note. Drug Tariff also includes unsterilised absorbent cotton gauze, 25 m roll, net price = £12.17

Cellulose Wadding, BP 1988. Delignified wood pulp bleached white, in multiple laminate form. 500 g, net price = £2.22 (most suppliers)

Uses: absorbing large volumes of fluid

NHS **Absorbent Muslin, BP 1988.** Fabric of plain weave, warp threads of cotton, weft threads of cotton and/or viscose

Uses: wet dressing, soaked in 0.9% sterile sodium chloride solution

NHS **Absorbent Cotton Ribbon Gauze, BP.** Cotton fabric of plain weave in ribbon form with fast selvedge edges

Uses: post-surgery cavity packing for sinus, dental, throat cavities etc.

Absorbent Cotton and Viscose Ribbon Gauze, BP. Woven fabric in ribbon form with fast selvedge edges, warp threads of cotton, weft threads of viscose or combined cotton and viscose yarn, sterile. 5 m (both) × 1.25 cm, net price = 64p; 2.5 cm = 71p

Uses: post-surgery cavity packing for sinus, dental, throat cavities etc.

Gauze Swab, BP 1988. Consists of absorbent cotton gauze type 13 light or absorbent cotton and viscose gauze type 1 folded into squares or rectangles of 8-ply with no cut edges exposed. Sterile, 7.5 cm square, net price 5-pad packet = 31p; non-sterile, 10 cm square 100-pad packet = £4.99 (most suppliers)

Filmated Gauze Swab, BP 1988. As for Gauze Swab, but with thin layer of Absorbent Cotton enclosed within. Non-sterile, 10 cm × 10 cm, net price 100-pad packet = £6.20 (Vernon-Carus—*Cotfil*®)

Uses: general swabbing and cleansing

Non-woven Fabric Swab (Drug Tariff specification 28). Consists of non-woven fabric folded 4-ply; alternative to gauze swabs, type 13 light. Sterile, 7.5 cm square, net price 5-pad packet = 20p; non-sterile, 10 cm square, 100-pad packet = £2.34 (J & J—*Topper 8*®); 100-pad pack = £2.34 (CliniMed)

Uses: general purpose swabbing and cleansing; absorbs more quickly than gauze

Filmated Non-woven Fabric Swab (Drug Tariff specification 29). Film of viscose fibres enclosed within non-woven viscose fabric folded 8-ply. Non-sterile, 10 cm square, net price 100-pad packet = £5.07 (J & J—*Regal*®)

Uses: general purpose swabbing and cleansing

Bandages and adhesives

According to their structure and performance bandages are used for dressing retention, for support, and for compression.

NON-EXTENSIBLE BANDAGES

Bandages made from non-extensible woven fabrics have generally been replaced by more conformable products therefore their role is now extremely limited.

Open-wove Bandage, BP 1988 . Cotton cloth, plain weave, warp of cotton, weft of cotton, viscose, or combination, one continuous length. Type 1, 5 m (all): 2.5 cm, net price = 28p; 5 cm = 46p; 7.5 cm = 65p; 10 cm = 85p (most suppliers) 5 m × 5 cm supplied when size not stated
Uses: protection and retention of absorbent dressings; support for minor strains, sprains; securing splints

Triangular Calico Bandage, BP 1980. Unbleached calico rt. angle triangle. 90 cm × 90 cm × 1.27 m, net price = £1.02 (most suppliers)
Uses: sling

NHS **Domette Bandage, BP 1988.** Fabric, plain weave, cotton warp and wool weft (hospital quality also available, all cotton). 5 m (all): 5 cm, net price = 54p; 7.5 cm = 81p; 10 cm = £1.08; 15 cm = £1.61 (Robert Bailey, Vernon-Carus)
Uses: protection and support where warmth required

Multiple Pack Dressing No. 1 (Drug Tariff). Contains absorbent cotton, absorbent cotton gauze type 13 light (sterile), open-wove bandages (banded). Net price per pack = £3.10

Multiple Pack Dressing No. 2 (Drug Tariff). As for No. 1 (above) but with larger quantities of cotton and cotton gauze and two sizes of bandages. Net price per pack = £5.19

LIGHT-WEIGHT CONFORMING BANDAGES

Lightweight conforming bandages are used for dressing retention, with the aim of keeping the dressing close to the wound without inhibiting movement or restricting blood flow. The elasticity of **conforming-stretch bandages** (also termed contour bandages) is greater than that of **cotton conforming bandages**.

Cotton Conforming Bandage, BP 1988. Cotton fabric, plain weave, treated to impart some elasticity to warp and weft. 3.5 m (all):
type A, 5 cm, net price = 58p; 7.5 cm = 72p; 10 cm = 88p, 15 cm = £1.21 (S&N Hlth—*Crinx*®)
type B, 5 cm = 59p, 7.5 cm = 76p, 10 cm = 92p, 15 cm = £1.21 (J&J—*Kling*®)
Uses: retention of dressings in difficult positions (e.g. over joints)

Knitted Polyamide and Cellulose Contour Bandage, BP 1988. Fabric, knitted warp of polyamide filament, weft of cotton or viscose, fast edges, one continuous length. 4 m stretched (all): 5 cm = 18p, 7 cm = 23p, 10 cm = 25p, 15 cm = 44p (Parema—*K-Band*®); 5 cm = 15p, 7 cm = 20p, 10 cm = 21p, 15 cm = 37p (Boston —*Texband*®)

Polyamide and Cellulose Contour Bandage, BP 1988 (formerly Nylon and Viscose Stretch Bandage). Fabric, plain weave, warp of polyamide filament, weft of cotton or viscose, fast edges, one continuous length. 4 m stretched (all): Robinsons—*Stayform*®(5 cm = 30p, 7.5 cm = 38p, 10 cm = 43p, 15 cm = 73p); Seton—*Slinky*® (net price 5 cm = 37p, 7.5 cm = 53p, 10 cm = 64p, 15 cm = 91p); S&N Hlth—*Easifix* ® (5 cm = 31p, 7.5 cm = 38p, 10 cm = 44p, 15 cm = 75p)
Uses: retention of dressings

TUBULAR BANDAGES

Tubular bandages are available in different forms, according to the function required of them. Some are used under orthopaedic casts and some are suitable for protecting areas to which creams or ointments (other than those containing potent corticosteroids) have been applied. The conformability of the elasticated versions makes them particularly suitable for retaining dressings on difficult parts of the body, but their use as the only means of applying pressure to an oedematous limb or to a varicose ulcer is not appropriate, since the pressure they exert is inadequate.

Elasticated Tubular Bandage, BP (formerly Elasticated Surgical Tubular Stockinette). Knitted fabric, elasticated threads of rubber-cored polyamide or polyester with cotton or cotton and viscose yarn, tubular. Lengths 50 cm and 1 m, various widths 6.25 cm–12 cm; B. Braun JLB—*Textube*® (formerly called *Lastogrip*®); Salt—*Rediform*®, S&N Hlth—*Tensogrip*®; Seton—*Tubigrip*®; Sigma—*Sigma ETB*®). Where no brand stated by prescriber, net price of stockinette supplied not to exceed: length 50 cm, 6.25 cm = 57p, 6.75 cm = 60p, 7.5 cm = 60p, 8.75 cm = 68p, 10 cm = 68p, 12 cm = 73p; length 1 m, 6.25 cm = £1.04, 6.75 cm = £1.09, 7.5 cm = £1.09, 8.75 cm = £1.14, 10 cm = £1.14, 12 cm = £1.40
Uses: retention of dressings on limbs, abdomen, trunk

Elasticated Surgical Tubular Stockinette, Foam padded (Drug Tariff specification 25). Fabric as for Elasticated Tubular Bandage with polyurethane foam lining. Heel, elbow, knee, small, net price = £2.36, medium = £2.55, large = £2.73; sacral, small, medium, and large (all) = £12.19 (Seton—*Tubipad*®)
Uses: relief of pressure and elimination of friction in relevant area; porosity of foam lining allows normal water loss from skin surface

Elasticated Viscose Stockinette (Drug Tariff specification 46). Lightweight plain-knitted elasticated tubular bandage. Length 1 m (all): net price 3.5 cm (small limb) = 72p; 5 cm (medium limb) = 78p; 7.5 cm (large limb) =£1.04; 10.75 cm (OS limb, head, child trunk) = £1.67; 17.5 cm (adult trunk) = £2.10 (Seton—*Tubifast*®)
Uses: retention of dressings

Elastic Net Surgical Tubular Stockinette (Drug Tariff Specification 26). Lightweight elastic open-work net tubular fabric.
type A : arm/leg, 40 cm × 1.8 cm (size C), net price = 34p; thigh/head, 60 cm × 2.5 cm (size E) = 62p; trunk (adult), 60 cm × 4.5 cm (size F) = 91p; trunk (OS adult) 60 cm × 5.4 cm (size G) = £1.22 (Seton—*Netelast*®)

Cotton Stockinette, Bleached, BP 1988 (formerly Cotton Surgical Tubular Stockinette). Knitted fabric, cotton yarn, tubular. 1 m × 2.5 cm, net price = 25p; 5 cm = 38p; 7.5 cm = 46p; 6 m × 10 cm = £3.15 (J&J, Seton)
Uses: 1 m lengths, basis (with wadding) for Plaster of Paris bandages etc. ; 6 m length, compression bandage

Ribbed Cotton and Viscose Surgical Tubular Stockinette, BP 1988. Knitted fabric of 1:1 ribbed structure, singles yarn spun from blend of two-thirds cotton and one-third viscose fibres, tubular. Length 5 m (all):
type A (lightweight): arm/leg (child), arm (adult) 5 cm, net price = £1.98; arm (OS adult), leg (adult) 7.5 cm = £2.58; leg (OS adult) 10 cm = £3.44; trunk (child) 15 cm = £4.94; trunk (adult) 20 cm = £5.69; trunk (OS adult) 25 cm = £6.83 (Seton)
type B (heavyweight): sizes as for type A, net price £1.91–£6.57 (Sallis—*Eesiban*®)
Drug Tariff specifies various combinations of sizes to provide sufficient material for part or full body coverage
Uses: protective dressings with tar-based and other non-steroid ointments

---

NHS Tubular Gauze Bandage, Seamless.
Unbleached cotton yarn, positioned with applicators. 20 m roll (all): 00, net price = £2.15; 01 = £2.18; 12 = £2.93; 34 = £4.29; 56 = £5.93; 78 = £6.97; T1 = £10.00; T2 = £12.95 (Seton—*Tubegauz®*)
Uses: retention of dressings on limbs, abdomen, trunk

SUPPORT BANDAGES

Light support bandages, which include the various forms of crepe bandage, are used in the prevention of oedema; they are also used to provide support for mild sprains and joints but their effectiveness has not been proven for this purpose. Since they have limited extensibility, they are able to provide light support without exerting undue pressure.

Crepe Bandage, BP 1988. Fabric, plain weave, warp of wool threads and crepe-twisted cotton threads, weft of cotton threads; stretch bandage. 4.5 m stretched (all): 5 cm, net price = 80p; 7.5 cm = £1.12; 10 cm = £1.46; 15 cm = £2.11 (most suppliers)
Uses: light support system for strains, sprains, compression over paste bandages for varicose veins
Cotton Crepe Bandage, BP 1988. Fabric, plain weave, warp of crepe-twisted cotton threads, weft of cotton and/or viscose threads; stretch bandage. 4.5 m stretched (both): 7.5 cm, net price = £2.55; 10 cm = £3.28; other sizes NHS (most suppliers)
Uses: light support system for strains, sprains, compression over paste bandages for varicose ulcers
Cotton, Polyamide and Elastane Bandage. Fabric, cotton, polyamide, and elastane; light support bandage (Type 2). 4.5 m stretched (all): 5 cm, net price = 60p, 7.5 cm = 85p, 10 cm = £1.10, 15 cm = £1.60 (S&N Hlth—*Soffcrepe®*)
Uses: light support for sprains and strains; retention of dressings
NHS Cotton Stretch Bandage, BP 1988. Fabric, plain weave, warp of crepe-twisted cotton threads, weft of cotton threads; stretch bandage, lighter than cotton crepe. 4.5 m stretched (all): 5 cm, net price = 30p; 7.5 cm = 41p; 10 cm = 54p; 15 cm = 76p (most suppliers)
Uses: light support system for strains, sprains, compression over paste bandages for varicose veins
Cotton Suspensory Bandage (Drug Tariff). Type 1: cotton net bag with draw tapes and webbing waistband; net price small, medium, and large (all) = £1.36, extra large = £1.43. Type 2: cotton net bag with elastic edge and webbing waistband; small = £1.48, medium = £1.53, large = £1.59, extra large = £1.66. Type 3: cotton net bag with elastic edge and webbing waistband with elastic insertion; small, medium, and large (all) = £1.61; extra large = £1.67. Type supplied to be endorsed
Uses: support of scrotum
Knitted Elastomer and Viscose Bandage. Knitted fabric, viscose and elastomer yarn, light support bandage (Type 2). 4.5 m stretched (all): 5 cm, net price = 48p, 7 cm = 68p, 10 cm = 89p, 15 cm = £1.28 (Parema—*K-Lite®*)
Uses: light support for sprains and strains

HIGH COMPRESSION BANDAGES

These products are used to provide the high compression needed for the management of gross varices, post-thrombotic venous insufficiency, venous leg ulcers, and gross oedema in average-sized limbs. Their use calls for an expert knowledge of the elastic properties of the products and experience in the technique of providing careful graduated compression. Inappropriate application can lead to uneven and inadequate pressures or to hazardous levels of pressure. In particular, injudicious use of compression in limbs with arterial disease has been reported to cause severe skin and tissue necrosis (in some instances calling for amputation); therefore, unless distal pulses are strong, Doppler testing is required before treatment with compression.

Drug Tariff specification 52
PEC High Compression Bandage (Drug Tariff). Polyamide, elastane, and cotton compression (high) extensible bandage, 3.5 m unstretched (both): 7.5 cm, net price = £2.41; 10 cm = £3.12 (Seton—*Setopress®*)
Uses: high compression for varicose ulcers
VEC High Compression Bandage (Drug Tariff). Viscose, elastane, and cotton compression (high) extensible bandage, 3 m unstretched (both); 7.5 cm, net price = £2.34; 10 cm = £3.02 (S&N—*Tensopress®*)
Uses: high compression for varicose ulcers
High Compression Bandage (Drug Tariff). Cotton, viscose, nylon, and Lycra® extensible bandage, 3 m (unstretched), 10 cm = £3.02 (ConvaTec—*SurePress®*); also available NHS *SurePress®* absorbent padding, net price 6 = £3.00
Uses: high compression for venous leg ulcers

EXTRA-HIGH PERFORMANCE COMPRESSION BANDAGES

These bandages are capable of applying pressures even higher than those of high compression bandages, therefore the same stringent warnings apply. Their use is reserved for the largest and most oedematous limbs.

Elastic Web Bandage, BP (also termed Blue Line Webbing). Characteristic fabric woven ribbon fashion, warp threads of cotton and rubber with mid-line threads coloured blue, weft threads of cotton or combined cotton and viscose; may be dyed skin colour; with or without foot loop. Per m (both) 7.5 cm, net price = 70p; 10 cm = £1.00; with foot loop (Drug Tariff specification 2a) 7.5 cm each = £4.02 (Marlow, Seton)
Uses: provision of support and high compression over large surface
Elastic Web Bandage without Foot Loop (also termed Red Line Webbing) (Drug Tariff specification 2b) (Scott-Curwen). Characteristic fabric woven ribbon fashion, warp threads of cotton and rubber with mid-line threads coloured red, weft threads of cotton or combined cotton and viscose. 7.5 cm × 2.75 m (2.5 m unstretched), net price = £3.18; 7.5 cm × 3.75 m (3.5 m unstretched) = £3.84
Uses: provision of support and high compression over large surfaces
NHS Cotton and Rubber Elastic Bandage, BP. Fabric, plain weave, warp of combined cotton and rubber threads, weft of cotton threads (S&N Hlth)
Uses: provision of high compression and medium support
Heavy Cotton and Rubber Elastic Bandage, BP. Heavy version of above with one end folded as foot loop; fastener also supplied. 1.8 m unstretched × 7.5 cm, net price = £10.79 (Marlow, Seton, S&N Hlth—*Elastoweb®*).
Uses: provision of high even compression over large surface

ADHESIVE BANDAGES

Elastic adhesive bandages are used to provide compression in the treatment of varicose veins and for the support of fractured ribs and clavicles and injured joints. They have also been used with **zinc paste bandage** in the treatment of venous ulcers, but they can cause skin reactions in susceptible patients and may not produce sufficient pressures for healing (significantly lower than those provided by other compression bandages).

Elastic Adhesive Bandage, BP. Woven fabric, elastic in warp (crepe-twisted cotton threads), weft of cotton and/or viscose threads spread with adhesive mass containing zinc oxide. 4.5 m stretched (all): 5 cm, net price = £3.01; 7.5 cm = £4.35; 10 cm = £5.79 (Robinsons—*Flexoplast*®; S&N Hlth—*Elastoplast*® Bandage).
7.5 cm width supplied when size not stated
Uses: compression for chronic leg ulcers; compression and support for fractured ribs, clavicles, swollen or sprained joints

NHS **Half-spread Elastic Adhesive Bandage, BP 1988.** Fabric as for elastic adhesive bandage but only partially spread with adhesive. (S&N Hlth)
Uses: compression for leg ulcers; compression and support for fractured ribs, clavicles, swollen/sprained joints

NHS **Ventilated Elastic Adhesive Bandage, BP.**
Fabric as for elastic adhesive bandage but adhesive spread such that there are regular strips of unspread fabric along length. (S&N Hlth)
Uses: compression for leg ulcers; compression and support for fractured ribs, clavicles, swollen/sprained joints

NHS **Extension strapping, BP.** Woven fabric, elastic in weft, spread with adhesive mass containing zinc oxide, warp threads cotton and/or viscose, weft threads crepe-twisted cotton. (S&N Hlth)
Uses: support of light strains, joints and limbs removed from plaster casts, fractured ribs; traction bandaging

COHESIVE BANDAGES

Cohesive bandages adhere to themselves, but not to the skin, and are useful for providing support for sports use where ordinary stretch bandages might become displaced and adhesive bandages are inappropriate. Care is needed in their application, however, since the loss of ability for movement between turns of the bandage to equalise local areas of high tension carries the potential for creating a tourniquet effect. They should not be used if arterial disease is suspected.

NHS Cohesive extensible bandages
These elastic bandages adhere to themselves and not to the patient's skin, which prevents slipping during use. 3M—*Coban*®, 4.5 m stretched (2.5, 5, 7.5, 10 and 15 cm); J&J—*Secure*® *Forte*, 4.5 m stretched (6, 8 and 10 cm); Robinsons—*Cohfast*®, latex free, 4.5 m stretched (5 and 7.5 cm); 6.3 m stretched (10 cm), S&N Hlth—*Coplus*®, 6.3 m stretched (2.5, 3.8, 5, 7.5, 10 and 15 cm)
Uses: support of sprained joints

MEDICATED BANDAGES

Zinc Paste Bandage remains one of the standard treatments for leg ulcers and can be left on undisturbed for up to a week; it is often used in association with compression for treatment of venous ulcers.
Zinc paste bandages are also used with **coal tar** or **ichthammol** in chronic lichenified skin conditions such as chronic eczema (ichthammol often being preferred since its action is considered to be milder).They are also used with **calamine** in milder eczematous skin conditions (but the inclusion of **clioquinol** may lead to irritation in susceptible subjects).

Zinc Paste Bandage, BP. Cotton fabric, plain weave, impregnated with suitable paste containing zinc oxide; requires additional bandaging. Net price 6 m × 7.5 cm = £3.01 (Seton—*Steripaste*® (15%)); £2.96 (Seton—*Zincaband*® (15%)); £3.03 (S&N Hlth—*Viscopaste PB7*® (10%), *additives: include* hydroxybenzoates)
Zinc Paste and Calamine Bandage (Drug Tariff specification 5). Cotton fabric, plain weave, impregnated with suitable paste containing calamine and zinc oxide; requires additional bandaging. Net price 6 m × 7.5 cm = £3.05 (Seton—*Calaband*®)

Zinc Paste, Calamine, and Clioquinol Bandage, BP. Cotton fabric, plain weave, impregnated with suitable paste containing calamine, clioquinol, and zinc oxide; requires additional bandaging. Net price 6 m × 7.5 cm = £3.05 (Seton—*Quinaband*®, *additives: include* hydroxybenzoates)
Zinc Paste and Coal Tar Bandage, BP. Cotton fabric, plain weave, impregnated with a suitable paste containing coal tar and zinc oxide; requires additional bandaging. Net price 6 m × 7.5 cm = £2.96 (Seton—*Tarband*®, *additives: include* hydroxybenzoates; S&N Hlth—*Coltapaste*®, *additives: include* wool fat)
Uses: see section 13.5
Zinc Paste and Ichthammol Bandage, BP. Cotton fabric, plain weave, impregnated with suitable paste containing zinc oxide and ichthammol; requires additional bandaging. Net price 6 m × 7.5 cm = £2.96 (Seton—*Icthaband*®(15/2%), *additives: include* hydroxybenzoates; S&N Hlth—*Ichthopaste*®(6/2%), *additives:* none as listed in section 13.1)
Uses: see section 13.5

Medicated stocking
Zipzoc®. Sterile rayon stocking impregnated with ointment containing zinc oxide 20%. Net price 4-pouch carton = £13.96; 10-pouch carton = £34.90 (S&N Hlth)
Uses: chronic leg ulcers; can be used under appropriate compression bandages or hosiery in chronic venous insufficiency

SURGICAL ADHESIVE TAPES

Adhesive tapes are useful for retaining dressings on joints or awkward body parts. These tapes, particularly those containing rubber, can cause irritant and allergic reactions in susceptible patients; synthetic adhesives have been developed to overcome this problem, but they, too, may sometimes be associated with reactions. Adhesive tapes that are occlusive may cause skin maceration. Care is needed not to apply these tapes under tension, to avoid creating a tourniquet affect. If applied over joints they need to be orientated so that the area of maximum extensibility of the fabric is in the direction of movement of the limb.

Permeable adhesive tapes

Zinc Oxide Adhesive Tape, BP 1988. (Zinc Oxide Plaster). Fabric, plain weave, warp and weft of cotton and/or viscose, spread with an adhesive containing zinc oxide. 1.25 cm, net price 3 m = 55p, 5 m = 76p; 2.5 cm, 1 m = 35p, 3 m = 81p, 5 m = £1.10; 5 cm × 5 m = £1.86; 7.5 cm × 5 m = £2.81 (most suppliers)
Drug Tariff specifies 1 m × 2.5 cm supplied when size not stated
Uses: securing dressings and immobilising small areas
Permeable Woven Synthetic Adhesive Tape, BP 1988. Non-extensible closely woven fabric, spread with a polymeric adhesive. 5 m (all): 1.25 cm, net price = 63p; 2.5 cm = 92p; 5 cm = £1.60 (Beiersdorf—*Leukosilk*®)
Uses: securing dressings
For patients with skin reaction to other plasters and strapping, requiring use for long periods
Elastic Adhesive Tape, BP 1988 (Elastic Adhesive Plaster). Woven fabric, elastic in warp (crepe-twisted cotton threads), weft of cotton and/or viscose threads, spread with adhesive mass containing zinc oxide. 1.5 m stretched × 2.5 cm, net price = 72p; 4.5 m stretched × 2.5 cm = £1.35 (Robinsons—*Flexoplast*®; S&N—*Elastoplast*®).
Uses: securing dressings
For 5 cm width, see Elastic Adhesive Bandage

Permeable Non-woven Synthetic Adhesive Tape, BP 1988.

Backing of paper-based or non-woven textile material spread with a polymeric adhesive mass. 5 m (all): BioDiagnostics—*Scanpor*® (net price 1.25 cm = 39p, 2.5 cm = 63p, 5 cm = £1.09); Beiersdorf—*Leukopor*® (1.25 cm = 43p, 2.5 cm = 68p, 5 cm = £1.18); 3M—*Micropore*® (1.25 cm = 57p, 2.5 cm = 85p, 5 cm = £1.51); S&N Hlth—*Hypal 2* ® (1.25 cm = 59p, 2.5 cm = 90p, 5 cm = £1.66). Where no brand stated by prescriber, net price of tape supplied not to exceed 39p (1.25 cm), 63p (2.5 cm), £1.09 (5 cm)

Uses: securing dressings; skin closures for small incisions
For patients with skin reaction to other plasters and strapping, requiring use for long periods

Occlusive adhesive tapes

Impermeable Plastic Adhesive Tape, BP 1988.

Extensible water-impermeable plastic film spread with an adhesive mass. 2.5 cm × 3 m, net price = £1.07; 5 m = £1.60; 5 cm × 5 m = £2.03; 7.5 cm × 5 m = £2.95 (Robinsons; Seton; S&N Hlth)

Uses: securing dressings; covering site of infection where exclusion of air, water, and water vapour is required

Impermeable Plastic Synthetic Adhesive Tape, BP 1988.

Extensible water-impermeable plastic film spread with a polymeric adhesive mass. 5 m (both): net price, 2.5 cm = £1.49; 5 cm = £2.84 (3M—*Blenderm*®)

Uses: isolating wounds from external environment; covering sites where total exclusion of water and water vapour required; securing dressings and appliances

ADHESIVE DRESSINGS

Adhesive dressings (also termed 'island dressings') have a limited role for minor wounds only. The inclusion of an antiseptic is not particularly useful and may cause skin irritation in susceptible subjects.

Permeable adhesive dressings

NHS **Elastic Adhesive Dressing, BP.** Wound dressing or dressing strip, pad attached to piece of extension plaster, leaving suitable adhesive margin; both pad and margin covered with suitable protector; pad may be dyed yellow and may be impregnated with suitable antiseptic (see below); extension plaster may be perforated or ventilated

Uses: general purpose wound dressing

Note. Permitted antiseptics are aminacrine hydrochloride, chlorhexidine hydrochloride (both 0.07–0.13%), chlorhexidine gluconate (0.11–0.20%); domiphen bromide (0.05–0.25%)

NHS **Permeable Plastic Wound Dressing, BP.** Consisting of an absorbent pad, which may be dyed and impregnated with a suitable antiseptic (see under Elastic Adhesive Dressing), attached to a piece of permeable plastic surgical adhesive tape, to leave a suitable adhesive margin; both pad and margin covered with suitable protector (most suppliers)

Uses: general purpose wound dressing, permeable to air and water

Vapour permeable adhesive dressings

Vapour-permeable Waterproof Plastic Wound Dressing, BP

(former Drug Tariff title: Semipermeable Waterproof Plastic Wound Dressing). Consists of absorbent pad, may be dyed and impregnated with suitable antiseptic (see under Elastic Adhesive Dressing), attached to piece of semipermeable waterproof surgical adhesive tape, to leave suitable adhesive margin; both pad and margin covered with suitable protector. 8.5 cm ×

6 cm, net price = 30p (S&N Hlth—*Elastoplast Airstrip*®)

Uses: general purpose waterproof wound dressing, permeable to air and water vapour

Occlusive adhesive dressings

NHS **Impermeable Plastic Wound Dressing, BP.**

Consists of absorbent pad, may be dyed and impregnated with suitable antiseptic (see under Elastic Adhesive Dressing), attached to piece of impermeable plastic surgical adhesive tape, to leave suitable adhesive margin; both pad and margin covered with suitable protector (most suppliers)

Uses: protective covering for wounds requiring an occlusive dressing

SKIN CLOSURE DRESSINGS

Skin closure strips are used as an alternative to sutures for minor cuts and lacerations.

Skin closure strips, sterile

Leukostrip®, 6.4 mm × 76 mm, 3 strips per envelope. Net price 10 envelopes = £4.98 (Beiersdorf)

Steri-strip®, 6 mm × 75 mm, 3 strips per envelope. Net price 12 envelopes = £8.08; NHS 3 mm × 75 mm, 12 envelopes = £8.08; 12 mm × 100 mm, 12 envelopes = £10.51 (3M)

Drug Tariff specifies that these are specifically for personal administration by the prescriber

Elastic hosiery

Before elastic hosiery can be dispensed, the quantity (single or pair), article (including accessories), and compression class (I, II or III) must be specified by the prescriber; all dispensed articles must state on the packaging that they conform with Drug Tariff technical specification No. 40, for further details see Drug Tariff.

GRADUATED COMPRESSION HOSIERY

Class 1 Light Support

Hosiery, compression at ankle 14–17 mm Hg, thigh length or below knee with knitted in heel. Net price per pair, circular knit (standard), thigh length = £6.12, below knee = £5.58; light weight elastic net (made-to-measure), thigh length = £16.36, below knee = £12.78

Uses: superficial or early varices, varicosis during pregnancy

Class 2 Medium Support

Hosiery, compression at ankle 18–24 mm Hg, thigh length or below knee with knitted in heel. Net price per pair, circular knit (standard), thigh length = £9.08, below knee = £8.16, (made-to-measure), thigh length = £30.34, below knee = £18.98; net (made-to-measure), thigh length = £16.36, below knee = £12.78; flat bed (made-to-measure, only with closed heel and open toe), thigh length = £30.34, below knee = £18.98

Uses: varices of medium severity, ulcer treatment and prophylaxis, mild oedema, varicosis during pregnancy

Class 3 Strong Support

Hosiery, compression at ankle 25–35 mm Hg, thigh length or below knee with open or knitted in heel. Net price per pair, circular knit (standard), thigh length = £10.76, below knee = £9.26, (made-to-measure) thigh length = £30.34, below knee = £18.98; one way stretch (made-to-measure, only with open heel and open toe), thigh length = £30.34, below knee = £18.98

Uses: gross varices, post thrombotic venous insufficiency, gross oedema, ulcer treatment and prophylaxis

---

ACCESSORIES

Suspender
Suspender, for thigh stockings, net price = 53p, belt (specification 13), = £4.07, fitted (additional price) = 53p

ANKLETS

Class 2 Medium Support
Anklets, compression 18–24 mm Hg, circular knit (standard and made-to-measure), net price per pair = £5.36; flat bed (standard and made-to-measure) = £11.12; net (made-to-measure) = £10.52
Uses: soft tissue support

Class 3 Strong Support
Anklets, compression 25–35 mm Hg, circular knit (standard and made-to-measure), net price per pair = £7.46; one way stretch (standard and made-to-measure) = £7.46
Uses: soft tissue support

KNEE CAPS

Class 2 Medium Support
Kneecaps, circular knit (standard and made-to-measure), net price per pair = £5.36; flat bed (standard and made-to-measure) = £11.12; net (made-to-measure) = £8.74
Uses: soft tissue support

Class 3 Strong Support
Kneecaps, circular knit (standard and made-to-measure), net price per pair = £7.14; one way stretch (standard and made-to-measure) = £7.14
Uses: soft tissue support

Appendix 10: Cautionary and Advisory Labels for Dispensed Medicines

Numbers following the preparation entries in the BNF correspond to the code numbers of the cautionary labels that pharmacists are recommended to add when dispensing. It is also expected that pharmacists will counsel patients when necessary.

Counselling needs to be related to the age, experience, background, and understanding of the individual patient. The pharmacist should ensure that the patient understands how to take or use the medicine and how to follow the correct dosage schedule. Any effects of the medicine on driving or work, any foods or medicines to be avoided, and what to do if a dose is missed should also be explained. Other matters, such as the possibility of staining of the clothes or skin by a medicine should also be mentioned.

For some preparations there is a special need for counselling, such as an unusual method or time of administration or a potential interaction with a common food or domestic remedy, and this is indicated where necessary.

ORIGINAL PACKS. Many preparations are now dispensed in unbroken original packs that bear complete instructions for the patient or provide a leaflet addressed to the patient. These labels or leaflets should not normally be obscured or removed. Where it is known that such instructions are provided with an original pack intended for the patient no label has been listed under the preparation. Label 10 may be used where appropriate. Leaflets are available from various sources advising on the administration of preparations such as eye-drops, eye ointments, inhalers, and suppositories.

SCOPE OF LABELS. In general no label recommendations have been made for injections on the assumption that they will be administered by a health professional or a well-instructed patient. The labelling is not exhaustive and pharmacists are recommended to use their professional discretion in labelling new preparations and those for which no labels are shown.

Individual labelling advice is not given on the administration of the large variety of antacids. In the absence of instructions from the prescriber, and if on enquiry the patient has had no verbal instructions, the directions given under 'Dose' should be used on the label.

It is recognised that there may be occasions when pharmacists will use their knowledge and professional discretion and decide to omit one or more of the recommended labels for a particular patient. In this case counselling is of the utmost importance. There may also be an occasion when a prescriber does not wish additional cautionary labels to be used, in which case the prescription should be endorsed 'NCL' (no cautionary labels). The exact wording that is required instead should then be specified on the prescription.

Pharmacists have traditionally labelled medicines with various wordings in addition to those directions specified on the prescription. Such labels include 'Shake the bottle', 'For external use only', and 'Store in a cool place', as well as 'Discard . . . . days after opening' and 'Do not use after . . . .', which apply particularly to antibiotic mixtures, diluted liquid and topical preparations, and to eye-drops. Although not listed in the BNF these labels should continue to be used when appropriate; indeed, 'For external use only' is a legal requirement on external liquid preparations, while 'Keep out of the reach of children' is a legal requirement on all dispensed medicines.

It is the usual practice for patients to take standard tablets with water or other liquid and for this reason no separate label has been recommended.

The label or labels for each preparation are recommended after careful consideration of the information available. However, it is recognised that in some cases this information may be either incomplete or open to a different interpretation. The Executive Editor will therefore be grateful to receive any constructive comments on the labelling suggested for any preparation.

Recommended label wordings

Wordings which can be given as separate warnings are labels 1–19 and labels 29–33. Wordings which can be incorporated in an appropriate position in the directions for dosage or administration are labels 21–28. A label has been omitted for number 20.

If separate labels are used it is recommended that the wordings be used without modification. If changes are made to suit computer requirements, care should be taken to retain the sense of the original.

(1) Warning. May cause drowsiness

To be used on *preparations for children* containing antihistamines, or other preparations given to children where the warnings of label 2 on driving or alcohol would not be appropriate.

(2) Warning. May cause drowsiness. If affected do not drive or operate machinery. Avoid alcoholic drink

To be used on *preparations for adults that can cause drowsiness*, thereby affecting the ability to drive and operate hazardous machinery; label 1 is more appropriate for children. *It is an offence to drive while under the influence of drink or drugs.*

Some of these preparations only cause drowsiness in the first few days of treatment and some only cause drowsiness in higher doses.

In such cases the patient should be told that the advice applies until the effects have worn off. However many of these preparations can produce a slowing of reaction time and a loss of mental concentration that can have the same effects as drowsiness.

Avoidance of alcoholic drink is recommended because the effects of CNS depressants are enhanced by alcohol. Strict prohibition however could lead to some patients not taking the medicine. Pharmacists should therefore explain the risk and encourage compliance, particularly in patients who may think they already tolerate the effects of alcohol (see also label 3). Queries from patients with epilepsy regarding fitness to drive should be referred back to the patient's doctor.

Side-effects unrelated to drowsiness that may affect a patient's ability to drive or operate machinery safely include *blurred vision, dizziness, or nausea*. In general, no label has been recommended to cover these cases, but the patient should be suitably counselled.

(3) Warning. May cause drowsiness. If affected do not drive or operate machinery

To be used on *preparations containing monoamine-oxidase inhibitors*; the warning to avoid alcohol and dealcoholised (low alcohol) drink is covered by the patient information leaflet.

Also to be used as for label 2 but where alcohol is not an issue.

(4) Warning. Avoid alcoholic drink

To be used on *preparations where a reaction such as flushing may occur if alcohol is taken* (e.g. metronidazole and chlorpropamide). Alcohol may also enhance the hypoglycaemia produced by some oral antidiabetic drugs but routine application of a warning label is not considered necessary.

(5) Do not take indigestion remedies at the same time of day as this medicine

To be used with label 25 on *preparations coated to resist gastric acid* (e.g. enteric-coated tablets). This is to avoid the possibility of premature dissolution of the coating in the presence of an alkaline pH.

Label 5 also applies to drugs such as ketoconazole *where the absorption is significantly affected by antacids*; the usual period of avoidance recommended is 2 to 4 hours.

(6) Do not take iron preparations or indigestion remedies at the same time of day as this medicine

To be used on *preparations containing ciprofloxacin, doxycycline, minocycline, and penicillamine*. These drugs chelate iron and calcium ions and are less well absorbed when given with iron or calcium-containing antacids. If necessary these incompatible preparations may be given about two hours apart.

(7) Do not take milk, iron preparations or indigestion remedies at the same time of day as this medicine

To be used on *preparations containing tetracyclines that chelate iron, calcium, and magnesium* and are thus less available for absorption; if it is necessary to give milk, iron or antacids, the usual period of avoidance is about 2 hours. Doxycycline and minocycline are less liable to form chelates and therefore only require label 6 (see above).

(8) Do not stop taking this medicine except on your doctor's advice

To be used on *preparations that contain a drug which is required to be taken over long periods without the patient necessarily perceiving any benefit* (e.g. antituberculous drugs).

Also to be used on *preparations that contain a drug whose withdrawal is likely to be a particular hazard* (e.g. clonidine for hypertension). Label 10 (see below) is more appropriate for corticosteroids.

(9) Take at regular intervals. Complete the prescribed course unless otherwise directed

To be used on *preparations where a course of treatment should be completed* to reduce the incidence of relapse or failure of treatment.

The preparations are antimicrobial drugs given by mouth. Very occasionally, some may have severe side-effects (e.g. diarrhoea in patients receiving clindamycin) and in such cases the patient may need to be advised of reasons for stopping treatment quickly and returning to the doctor.

(10) Warning. Follow the printed instructions you have been given with this medicine

To be used particularly on *preparations containing anticoagulants, lithium and oral corticosteroids*. The appropriate treatment card should be given to the patient and any necessary explanations given.

This label may also be used on other preparations to remind the patient of the instructions that have been given.

(11) Avoid exposure of skin to direct sunlight or sun lamps

To be used *on preparations that may cause phototoxic or photoallergic reactions* if the patient is exposed to ultraviolet radiation. Many drugs other than those listed (e.g. phenothiazines and sulphonamides) may on rare occasions cause reactions in susceptible patients. Exposure to high intensity ultraviolet radiation from sunray lamps and sunbeds is particularly likely to cause reactions.

(12) Do not take anything containing aspirin while taking this medicine

To be used on *preparations containing probenecid and sulphinpyrazone* whose activity is reduced by aspirin.

Label 12 should not be used for anticoagulants since label 10 is more appropriate.

(13) Dissolve or mix with water before taking

To be used on *preparations that are intended to be dissolved in water* (e.g. soluble tablets) or *mixed with water* (e.g. powders, granules) before use. In a few cases other liquids such as fruit juice or milk may be used.

(14) This medicine may colour the urine

To be used on *preparations that may cause the patient's urine to turn an unusual colour*. These include phenolphthalein (alkaline urine pink), triamterene (blue under some lights), levodopa (dark reddish), and rifampicin (red).

(15)   Caution flammable: keep away from fire or flames

To be used on *preparations containing sufficient flammable solvent to render them flammable if exposed to a naked flame.*

(16)   Allow to dissolve under the tongue. Do not transfer from this container. Keep tightly closed. Discard eight weeks after opening

To be used on *glyceryl trinitrate tablets* to remind the patient not to transfer the tablets to plastic or less suitable containers.

(17)   Do not take more than . . . in 24 hours

To be used on *preparations for the treatment of acute migraine* except those containing ergotamine, for which label 18 is used. The dose form should be specified, e.g. tablets or capsules.

It may also be used on preparations for which no dose has been specified by the prescriber.

(18)   Do not take more than . . . in 24 hours or . . . in any one week

To be used on preparations containing ergotamine. The dose form should be specified, e.g. tablets or suppositories.

(19)   Warning. Causes drowsiness which may continue the next day. If affected do not drive or operate machinery. Avoid alcoholic drink

To be used on *preparations containing hypnotics (or some other drugs with sedative effects) prescribed to be taken at night.* On the rare occasions (e.g. nitrazepam in epilepsy) when hypnotics are prescribed for daytime administration this label would clearly not be appropriate. Also to be used as *an alternative to the label 2 wording* (the choice being at the discretion of the pharmacist) *for anxiolytics prescribed to be taken at night.*

It is hoped that this wording will convey adequately the problem of residual morning sedation after taking 'sleeping tablets'.

(21)   . . . with or after food

To be used on *preparations that are liable to cause gastric irritation,* or *those that are better absorbed with food.*

Patients should be advised that a *small amount of food is sufficient.*

(22)   . . . half to one hour before food

To be used on some preparations *whose absorption is thereby improved.* Most oral antibiotics require label 23 instead (see below).

(23)   . . . an hour before food or on an empty stomach

To be used on *oral antibiotics whose absorption may be reduced by the presence of food and acid in the stomach.*

(24)   . . . sucked or chewed

To be used on *preparations that should be sucked or chewed.*

The pharmacist should use discretion as to which of these words is appropriate.

(25)   . . . swallowed whole, not chewed

To be used on *preparations that are enteric-coated or designed for modified-release.*

Also to be used on *preparations that taste very unpleasant or may damage the mouth* if not swallowed whole.

(26)   . . . dissolved under the tongue

To be used on *preparations designed for sublingual use.* Patients should be advised to hold under the tongue and avoid swallowing until dissolved. The buccal mucosa between the gum and cheek is occasionally specified by the prescriber.

(27)   . . . with plenty of water

To be used on *preparations that should be well diluted* (e.g. chloral hydrate), *where a high fluid intake is required* (e.g. sulphonamides), or *where water is required to aid the action* (e.g. methylcellulose). The patient should be advised that 'plenty' means at least 150 mL (about a tumblerful). In most cases fruit juice, tea, or coffee may be used.

(28)   To be spread thinly . . .

To be used on *external preparations* that should be applied sparingly (e.g. corticosteroids, dithranol).

(29)   Do not take more than 2 at any one time. Do not take more than 8 in 24 hours

To be used on containers of dispensed *solid dose preparations containing paracetamol for adults when the instruction on the label indicates that the dose can be taken on an 'as required' basis.* The dose form should be specified, e.g. tablets or capsules.

This label has been introduced because of the serious consequences of overdosage with paracetamol.

(30)   Contains paracetamol

To be used on containers of dispensed *preparations containing paracetamol when the name on the label does not include the word 'paracetamol'.*

(31)   Contains aspirin and paracetamol

To be used on containers of dispensed *preparations containing aspirin and paracetamol (e.g. benorylate), when the name on the label does not include the words 'aspirin' and 'paracetamol'.*

(32)   Contains aspirin

To be used on containers of dispensed *preparations containing aspirin when the name on the label does not include the word 'aspirin'.*

(33)   Contains an aspirin-like medicine

To be used on containers of dispensed *preparations containing a salicylate derivative.*

Products and their labels

Products introduced or amended since publication of BNF No. 34 (September 1997) are underlined.
Proprietary names are in *italic*.
C = counselling advised; see BNF = consult product entry in BNF

Acamprosate, 21, 25

Acarbose, C, administration, see BNF

Acebutolol, 8

Aceclofenac, 21

Acemetacin, 21, C, driving

Acetazolamide, 3

Acetazolamide m/r, 3, 25

Achromycin, 7, 9, 23, C, posture

Aciclovir susp and tabs, 9

Acipimox, 21

Acitretin, 10 patient information leaflet, 21

Acrivastine, C, driving, alcohol, see BNF

Actinac, 28

Acupan, 2, 14 (urine pink)

Adalat caps, 21, C, administration, see BNF

Adalat LA, 25

Adalat Retard, 21, 25

Adcortyl external preps, 28

Adcortyl with Graneodin, 28

Adipine MR, 21, 25

Adizem preps, 25

AeroBec, 8, C, dose

AeroBec Forte, 8, 10 steroid card, C, dose

Aerocrom, 8

Aerolin Autohaler, C, dose, see BNF

Airomir, C dose, see BNF

Akineton, 2

Albendazole, 9

Alclometasone external preps, 28

Aldomet, 3, 8

Alendronic acid, C, administration, see BNF

Alfuzosin, 3, C, dose, see BNF

Alfuzosin m/r, 3, 25, C, dose, see BNF

Algitec, C, chew thoroughly

Allegron, 2

Allopurinol, 8, 21, 27

Alphosyl HC, 28

Aloxiprin, 12, 21

Alphaderm, 28

Alprazolam, 2

Altretamine, 21

Alupent inhalation, C, dose, see BNF

Alvedon, 30

Alvercol, 25, 27, C, administration, see BNF

Amantadine, C, driving

Aminophylline m/r, see preps

Amiodarone, 11

Amisulpride, 2

Amitriptyline, 2

Amitriptyline m/r, 2, 25

Amorolfine, 10 patient information leaflet

Amoxapine, 2

Amoxil, 9

Amoxil dispersible tabs and sachets, 9, 13

Amoxil Fiztab, 9, 10 patient information leaflet

Amoxil paed susp, 9, C, use of pipette

Amoxycillin, 9

Amoxycillin chewable tabs, 9, 10 patient information leaflet

Amoxycillin dispersible tabs and sachets, 9, 13

Amphotericin loz, 9, 24, C, after food

Amphotericin mixt (g.i.), 9, C, use of pipette

Amphotericin mixt (mouth), 9, C, use of pipette, hold in mouth, after food

Amphotericin tabs, 9

Ampicillin, 9, 23

Ampiclox, 9, 23

Ampiclox Neonatal, 9, C, use of pipette

Amylobarbitone, 19

Amytal, 19

Anafranil, 2

Anafranil m/r, 2, 25

Androcur, 3, 21

Andropatch, C, administration, see BNF

Angettes-75, 32

Angiopine MH, 25

Angitil SR, 25

Anhydrol Forte, 15

Anquil, 2

Antabuse, 2, C, alcohol reaction, see BNF

Antacids, see BNF dose statements

Antepsin, 5, C, administration, see BNF

Anthranol preps, 28

Anticoagulants, oral, 10 anticoagulant card

Antihistamines (see individual preparations)

Antipressan, 8

Anturan, 12, 21

Apsin VK, 9, 23

Arpimycin, 9

Arpicolin, C, driving

Artane, C, before or after food, driving, see BNF

Arythmol, 21, 25

Arthrotec, 21, 25

Asacol tabs, 5, 25, C, blood disorder symptoms, see BNF

Asacol enema and supps, C, blood disorder symptoms, see BNF

Ascorbic acid, effervescent, 13

Ascorbic acid tabs (500mg), 24

Asendis, 2

Aspav, 2, 13, 21, 32

Aspirin and papaveretum dispersible tabs, 2, 13, 21, also 32 (if 'aspirin' not on label)

Aspirin dispersible tabs, 13, 21, also 32 (if 'aspirin' not on label)

Aspirin effervescent, 13, also 32 (if 'aspirin' not on label)

Aspirin e/c, 5, 25, also 32 (if 'aspirin' not on label)

Aspirin m/r, 25, also 32 (if 'aspirin' not on label)

Aspirin supps, 32 (if 'aspirin' not on label)

Aspirin tabs, 21, also 32 (if 'aspirin' not on label)

Aspirin, paracetamol and codeine tabs, 21, 29, also 31 (if 'aspirin' and 'paracetamol' not on label)

Astemizole, C, driving, alcohol, see BNF

Atarax, 2

Atenolol, 8

Ativan, 2 or 19

Atorvastatin, C, muscle effects, see BNF

Atovaquone, 21

Atromid-S, 21

Atrovent inhalations, C, dose, see BNF

Augmentin susp and tabs, 9

Augmentin Duo, 9

Augmentin dispersible tabs, 9, 13

Auranofin, 21, C, blood disorder symptoms, see BNF

Aureocort, 28

Avloclor, 5, C, malaria prophylaxis, see BNF

Avomine, 2

Azapropazone, 11, 21, C, photosensitivity, see BNF

Azatadine, 2

Azathioprine, 21

Azithromycin, 5, 9, 23

Baclofen, 2, 8

Balsalazide, 21, 25

Baratol, 2

Baxan, 9

Beclazone, 8, 10 steroid card (250-microgram only), C, dose

Becloforte preps, 8, 10 steroid card, C, dose

Beclomethasone external preps, 28

Beclomethasone inhalations, 8, 10 steroid card (high-dose preparations only), C, dose

Becodisks, 8, C, dose

Becotide preps, 8, C, dose

Bedranol S.R., 8, 25

Bendogen, 21

Benemid, 12, 21, 27

Benoral susp and tabs, 21, 31

Benoral gran, 13, 21, 31

Benorylate, 21, 31

Benorylate gran, 13, 21, 31

Benperidol, 2

Benzhexol, C, before or after food, driving, see BNF

Benzoin tincture, cpd, 15

Benztropine, 2

Berkolol, 8

Berotec, C, dose, see BNF

Beta-Adalat, 8, 25

Betacap, 15, 28

Beta-Cardone, 8

Betahistine, 21

Betaloc, 8

Betaloc-SA, 8, 25

Betamethasone inj, 10 steroid card

Betamethasone tab, 10 steroid card, 21

Betamethasone external preps, 28

Betamethasone scalp application, 15, 28

Betaxolol tabs, 8

Bethanechol, 22

Bethanidine, 21

Betim, 8

Betnelan, 10 steroid card, 21

Betnesol injection, 10 steroid card

Betnesol tabs, 10 steroid card, 13, 21

Betnovate external preps, 28

Betnovate scalp application, 15, 28

Betnovate-RD, 28

Bettamousse, 28

Bezafibrate, 21

Bezalip, 21

Bezalip-Mono, 21, 25

Biorphen, C, driving

Biperiden, 2

Bisacodyl tabs, 5, 25

Bisoprolol, 8

Blocadren, 8

Bonefos caps and tabs, C, food and calcium, see BNF

Bricanyl inhalations, C, dose, see BNF

Bricanyl SA, 25

Britiazim, 25

Britlofex, 2

Broflex, C, before or after food, driving, see BNF
Bromazepam, 2
Bromocriptine, 21, C, hypotensive reactions, see BNF
Brompheniramine, 2
Brufen, 21
Brufen gran, 13, 21
Brufen Retard, 25, 27
Buccastem, 2, C, administration, see BNF
Budesonide inhalations, 8, 10 steroid card (high-dose preparations only), C, dose
Budesonide m/r, 5, 10 steroid card, 22, 25
Buprenorphine, 2, 26
Burinex K, 25, 27, C, posture, see BNF
Buserelin nasal spray, C, nasal decongestants, see BNF
Buspar, C, driving
Buspirone, C, driving
Butacote, 5, 21, 25, C, blood disorder symptoms, see BNF
Butobarbitone, 19

Cabaser, 21, C, hypotensive reactions, see BNF
Cabergoline, 21, C, hypotensive reactions, see BNF
Cacit, 13
Cacit D3, 13
Cafergot, 18, C, dosage
Calceos, 24
Calcicard CR, 25
Calcichew preps, 24
Calcidrink, 13
Calcisorb, 13, 21, C, may be sprinkled on food
Calcium-500, 24
Calcium carbonate tabs, chewable, 24
Calcium carbonate tabs and gran effervescent, 13
Calcium gluconate tabs, 24
Calcium phosphate sachets, 13
Calcium Resonium, 2
Calcium and ergocalciferol tabs, C, administration, see BNF
Calcort, 5, 10 steroid card
Calmurid HC, 28
Calpol susp, 30
Camcolit 250 tabs, 10 lithium card, C, fluid and salt intake, see BNF
Camcolit 400 tabs, 10 lithium card, 25, C, fluid and salt intake, see BNF
Campral EC, 21, 25
Canesten HC, 28
Canesten spray, 15
Caprin, 5, 25, 32
Carbachol, 22
Carbamazepine chewable, 3, 8, 21, 24, C, blood, hepatic or skin disorder symptoms (see BNF), driving (see BNF, p. 210)
Carbamazepine liq, supps and tabs, 3, 8, C, blood, hepatic or skin disorder symptoms (see BNF), driving (see BNF, p. 210)
Carbamazepine m/r, 3, 8, 25, C, blood, hepatic or skin disorder symptoms (see BNF), driving (see BNF, p. 210)
Carbenoxolone sodium, see preps
Carbimazole, C, blood disorder symptoms, see BNF
Cardene SR, 25
Cardilate MR, 25
Cardinol, 8
Carisoma, 2
Carisoprodol, 2
Carylderm lotion, 15
Catapres, 3, 8
Catapres Perlongets, 3, 8, 25
Caved-S, 24
Cedax, 9

Cedocard Retard, 25
Cefaclor, 9
Cefaclor m/r, 9, 21, 25
Cefadroxil, 9
Cefixime, 9
Cefpodoxime, 5, 9, 21
Ceftibuten, 9
Cefuroxime susp, 9, 21
Cefuroxime sachets, 9, 13, 21
Cefuroxime tab, 9, 21, 25
Celance, C, hypotensive reactions, see BNF
Celectol, 8, 22
Celevac (constipation or diarrhoea), C, administration, see BNF
Celevac tabs (anorectic), C, administration, see BNF
Celiprolol, 8, 22
CellCept, 23
Centyl K, 25, 27, C, posture, see BNF
Cephalexin, 9
Cephradine, 9
Ceporex caps, mixts, and tabs, 9
Cerivastatin, C, muscle effects, see BNF
Cetirizine, C, driving, alcohol, see BNF
Chloral hydrate, 19, 27
Chloral paed elixir, 1, 27
Chloral mixt, 19, 27
Chlordiazepoxide, 2
Chlormethiazole, 19
Chloroquine, 5, C, malaria prophylaxis, see BNF
Chlorpheniramine, 2
Chlorpromazine mixts and supps, 2, 11
Chlorpromazine tabs, 2, 11
Chlorpropamide, 4
Cholestyramine, 13, C, avoid other drugs at same time, see BNF
Cimetidine chewable tabs, C, administration, see BNF
Cimetidine effervescent tabs, 13
Cinnarizine, 2
Cinobac, 9, C, driving
Cinoxacin, 9
Cipramil, C, driving
Ciprofloxacin, 6, 9, 25, C, driving
Ciproxin tabs, 6, 9, 25, C, driving
Cisapride, C, administration, see BNF
Citalopram, C, driving
Citramag, 10 patient information leaflet, 13, C, administration
Citrical, 13
Clarithromycin, 9
Clarithromycin m/r, 9, 21, 25
Clarityn, C, driving, alcohol, see BNF
Clemastine, 2
Clindamycin, 9, 27, C, diarrhoea, see BNF
Clinoril, 21
Clobazam, 2 or 19, 8, C, driving (see BNF, p. 210)
Clobetasol external preps, 28
Clobetasol scalp application, 15, 28
Clofazimine, 8, 14 (urine red), 21
Clofibrate, 21
Clomipramine, 2
Clomipramine m/r, 2, 25
Clonazepam, 2, 8, C, driving (see BNF, p. 210)
Clonidine see *Catapres*
Clonidine m/r, 3, 8, 25
Clopixol, 2
Clorazepate, 2 or 19
Clotrimazole spray, 15
Clozapine, 2, 10 patient information leaflet
Clozaril, 2, 10 patient information leaflet
Coal tar paint, 15
Co-amoxiclav, 9
Co-amoxiclav dispersible tabs, 9, 13
Cobadex, 28
Co-beneldopa, 14 (urine reddish), 21

Co-beneldopa dispersible tabs, 14 (urine reddish), 21, C, administration, see BNF
Co-beneldopa m/r, 5, 14 (urine reddish), 25
Co-Betaloc, 8
Co-Betaloc SA, 8, 25
Co-careldopa, 14 (urine reddish), 21
Co-careldopa m/r, 14 (urine reddish), 25
Co-codamol caps and tabs, 29, 30
Co-codamol dispersible tabs, 13, 29, 30
Co-codaprin dispersible tabs, 13, 21, 32
Co-codaprin tabs, 21, 32
Codafen Continus, 2, 21, 25
Codalax, 14 (urine red)
Co-danthramer, 14 (urine red)
Co-danthrusate, 14 (urine red)
Codeine phosphate syr and tabs, 2
Co-dergocrine, 22
Co-dydramol, 21, 29, 30
Co-fluampicil, 9, 22
Cogentin, 2
Colazide, 21, 25
Colestid, 13, C, avoid other drugs at same time, see BNF
Colestipol preps, 13, C, avoid other drugs at same time, see BNF
Collodion, flexible, 15
Colofac, C, administration, see BNF
Colpermin, 5, 22, 25
Coltec EC, 5, 25
Combivent, C, dose
Co-methiamol, 29, 30
Complement Continus, 25
Concordin, 2, 11
Condyline, 15
Convulex, 8, 25, C, blood or hepatic disorder symptoms (see BNF), driving (see BNF, p. 210)
Co-prenozide, 8, 25
Co-proxamol, 2, 10 patient information leaflet, 29, 30
Coracten, 25
Cordarone X, 11
Corgard, 8
Corgaretic, 8
Corticosteroid external preps, 28
Corticosteroid tabs, 10 steroid card, 21
Corticosteroid injections (systemic), 10 steroid card
Cortisone tab, 10 steroid card, 21
Cortisyl, 10 steroid card, 21
Cosalgesic, 2, 10 patient information leaflet, 29, 30
Co-tenidone, 8
Co-trimoxazole mixts and tabs, 9
Co-trimoxazole dispersible tabs, 9, 13
Coversyl, 22
Creon preps, C, administration, see BNF
Crixivan, C, administration, see BNF
Cromogen Easi-Breathe, 8
Cuplex, 15
Cyclizine, 2
Cyclophosphamide, 27
Cycloserine caps, 2, 8
Cyclosporin , C, administration, see BNF
Cymevene, 21
Cyproheptadine, 2
Cyprostat, 3, 21
Cyproterone, 3, 21
Cystrin, 3

Daktacort, 28
Daktarin oral gel, 9, C, hold in mouth, after food
Dalacin C, 9, 27, C, diarrhoea, see BNF
Dalmane, 19
Dantrium, 2
Dantrolene, 2
Dapsone, 8

Dental Practitioners' Formulary

List of Dental Preparations

The following list has been approved by the appropriate Secretaries of State, and the preparations therein may be prescribed by dental practitioners on form FP14 (GP14 in Scotland).

Sugar-free versions, where available, are preferred.

Aciclovir Cream, BP
Aciclovir Oral Suspension, BP, 200 mg/5 mL
Aciclovir Tablets, BP, 200 mg
Amoxycillin Capsules, BP
Amoxycillin Oral Powder, DPF
Amoxycillin Oral Suspension, BP
Amoxycillin Tablets, Dispersible, DPF
Amphotericin Lozenges, BP
Amphotericin Oral Suspension, DPF
Ampicillin Capsules, BP
Ampicillin Oral Suspension, BP
Artificial Saliva, DPF
Ascorbic Acid Tablets, BP
Aspirin Tablets, Dispersible, BP[1]
Benzydamine Mouthwash, DPF
Benzydamine Oral Spray, DPF
Carbamazepine Tablets, BP
Carmellose Gelatin Paste, DPF
Cephalexin Capsules, BP
Cephalexin Oral Suspension, BP
Cephalexin Tablets, BP
Cephradine Capsules, BP
Cephradine Oral Solution, DPF
Chlorhexidine Gluconate 1% Gel, DPF
Chlorhexidine Mouthwash, DPF
Chlorhexidine Oral Spray, DPF
Chlorpheniramine Tablets, BP
Choline Salicylate Dental Gel, BP
Clindamycin Capsules, BP
Clindamycin Oral Suspension, Paediatric, DPF
Diazepam Oral Solution, BP, 2 mg/5 mL
Diazepam Tablets, BP
Diflunisal Tablets, BP
Dihydrocodeine Tablets, BP, 30 mg
Doxycycline Capsules, BP, 100 mg
Ephedrine Nasal Drops, BP
Erythromycin Ethyl Succinate Oral Suspension, BP
Erythromycin Ethyl Succinate Tablets, BP
Erythromycin Stearate Tablets, BP
Erythromycin Tablets, BP
Fluconazole Capsules, 50 mg, DPF
Fluconazole Oral Suspension, 50 mg/5 mL, DPF

> Preparations in this list which are not included in the BP or BPC are described on next page

Hydrocortisone Cream, BP, 1%
Hydrocortisone Lozenges, BPC
Hydrocortisone and Miconazole Cream, DPF
Hydrocortisone and Miconazole Ointment, DPF
Hydrogen Peroxide Mouthwash, DPF
Ibuprofen Oral Suspension, BP, sugar-free
Ibuprofen Tablets, BP
Lignocaine 5% Ointment, DPF
Menthol and Eucalyptus Inhalation, BP 1980[2]
Metronidazole Oral Suspension, DPF
Metronidazole Tablets, BP
Miconazole Oral Gel, DPF
Mouthwash Solution-tablets, DPF
Nitrazepam Tablets, BP
Nystatin Ointment, BP
Nystatin Oral Suspension, BP
Nystatin Pastilles, DPF
Oxytetracycline Capsules, BP
Oxytetracycline Tablets, BP
Paracetamol Oral Suspension, BP[3]
Paracetamol Tablets, BP
Paracetamol Tablets, Soluble, BP
Penciclovir Cream, DPF
Pethidine Tablets, BP
Phenoxymethylpenicillin Oral Solution, BP
Phenoxymethylpenicillin Tablets, BP
Povidone-iodine Mouthwash, DPF
Probenecid Tablets, BP
Promethazine Hydrochloride Tablets, BP
Promethazine Oral Solution, BP
Sodium Chloride Mouthwash, Compound, BP
Sodium Fluoride Oral Drops, DPF
Sodium Fluoride Tablets, DPF
Sodium Fusidate Ointment, BP
Sodium Perborate Mouthwash, DPF
Temazepam Oral Solution, BP
Temazepam Tablets, DPF
Tetracycline Capsules, BP
Tetracycline Tablets, BP
Thymol Glycerin, Compound, BP 1988[2]
Triamcinolone Dental Paste, BP
Vitamin B Tablets, Compound, Strong, BPC
Zinc Sulphate Mouthwash, DPF

---

1. BP 1993 has directed that when soluble aspirin tablets are prescribed, dispersible aspirin tablets should be dispensed
2. This preparation does not appear in subsequent editions of the BP
3. BP 1993 directs that when Paediatric Paracetamol Oral Suspension or Paediatric Paracetamol Mixture is prescribed and no strength stated Paracetamol Oral Suspension 120 mg/5 mL should be dispensed

Details of DPF preparations

Preparations on the List of Dental Preparations which are specified as DPF are described as follows in the DPF.

Although brand names have sometimes been included for identification purposes preparations on the list should be prescribed by non-proprietary name.

PoM **Amoxycillin Oral Powder** (proprietary product: *Amoxil Sachets SF*), amoxycillin 750 mg and 3 g (as trihydrate) sachet

PoM **Amoxycillin Tablets Dispersible** (proprietary product: *Amoxil Dispersible Tablets*), amoxycillin 500 mg (as trihydrate)

PoM **Amphotericin Oral Suspension** (proprietary product: *Fungilin Suspension*), amphotericin 100 mg/mL

Artificial Saliva, (proprietary product: *Luborant*) consists of sorbitol 1.8 g, carmellose sodium (sodium carboxymethylcellulose) 390 mg, dibasic potassium phosphate 48.23 mg, potassium chloride 37.5 mg, monobasic potassium phosphate 21.97 mg, calcium chloride 9.972 mg, magnesium chloride 3.528 mg, sodium fluoride 258 micrograms/60 mL, with preservatives and colouring agents

Benzydamine Mouthwash (proprietary product: *Difflam Oral Rinse*), benzydamine hydrochloride 0.15%

Benzydamine Oral Spray (proprietary product: *Difflam Spray*), benzydamine hydrochloride 0.15%

Carmellose Gelatin Paste (proprietary product: *Orabase Oral Paste*), gelatin, pectin, carmellose sodium, 16.58% of each in a suitable basis

PoM **Cephradine Oral Solution** (proprietary product: *Velosef Syrup*), cephradine 250 mg/5mL when reconstituted with water

Chlorhexidine Gluconate 1% Gel (proprietary product: *Corsodyl Dental Gel*), chlorhexidine gluconate 1%

Chlorhexidine Mouthwash (proprietary products: *Chlorohex 2000 Mouthwash, Corsodyl Mouthwash*), chlorhexidine gluconate 0.2%

Chlorhexidine Oral Spray (proprietary product: *Corsodyl Oral Spray*), chlorhexidine gluconate 0.2%

PoM **Clindamycin Oral Suspension, Paediatric** (proprietary product: *Dalacin C Paediatric Suspension*), clindamycin 75 mg (as palmitate hydrochloride)/5mL when reconstituted with purified water (freshly boiled and cooled)

PoM **Fluconazole Capsules 50 mg** (proprietary product: *Diflucan*), fluconazole 50 mg

PoM **Fluconazole Oral Suspension 50 mg/5 mL** (proprietary product: *Diflucan*), fluconazole 50 mg/5 mL when reconstituted with water

PoM **Hydrocortisone and Miconazole Cream** (proprietary product: *Daktacort Cream*), hydrocortisone 1%, miconazole nitrate 2%

PoM **Hydrocortisone and Miconazole Ointment** (proprietary product: *Daktacort Ointment*), hydrocortisone 1%, miconazole nitrate 2%

Hydrogen Peroxide Mouthwash consists of hydrogen peroxide solution 6% (≡ approx. 20 volume), BP

Lignocaine 5% Ointment, (proprietary product: *Xylocaine Ointment*), lignocaine 5% in a suitable basis

PoM **Metronidazole Oral Suspension** (proprietary product: *Flagyl S*), metronidazole 200 mg (as benzoate)/5mL

PoM[1] **Miconazole Oral Gel** (proprietary product: *Daktarin Oral Gel*), miconazole 24 mg/mL

1. For exemption, see p. 474

Mouthwash Solution-tablets, consist of tablets which may contain antimicrobial, colouring and flavouring agents in a suitable soluble effervescent basis to make a mouthwash suitable for dental purposes

PoM **Nystatin Pastilles** (proprietary product: *Nystan Pastilles*), nystatin 100 000 units

▼ PoM **Penciclovir Cream** (proprietary product: *Vectavir Cream*), penciclovir 1 %

Povidone-iodine Mouthwash (proprietary product: *Betadine Mouthwash*), povidone-iodine 1%

Sodium Fluoride Oral Drops, see section 9.5.3

Sodium Fluoride Tablets, see section 9.5.3

Sodium Perborate Mouthwash (proprietary product: *Bocasan Mouthwash*), sodium perborate 68.6%

CD[2] **Temazepam Tablets,** temazepam 10 and 20 mg

2. See p. 7 for prescribing requirements for temazepam

Zinc Sulphate Mouthwash, consists of zinc sulphate lotion, BP. Directions for use: dilute 1 part with 4 parts of warm water

Note. May be difficult to obtain

Nurse Prescribers' Formulary

Nurse Prescribers' Formulary Appendix (Appendix NPF). List of preparations approved by the Secretary of State which may be prescribed on forms FP10(CN) and FP10(PN) (forms GP10(CN) and GP10(PN) in Scotland) by Nurses for National Health Service patients

Preparations on this list which are not included in the BP or BPC are described on p. 691

Medicinal preparations

Almond Oil Ear Drops, NPF
Aqueous Cream, BP
Arachis Oil Enema, NPF[1]
Aspirin Tablets, Dispersible, 300 mg, BP
Bisacodyl Suppositories, BP (includes 5-mg and 10-mg strengths)
Bisacodyl Tablets, BP
Cadexomer–Iodine Ointment, NPF
Cadexomer–Iodine Paste, NPF
Cadexomer–Iodine Powder, NPF
Calamine Cream, Aqueous, BP
Calamine Lotion, BP
Calamine Lotion, Oily, BP 1980
Carbaryl Lotion, BP, alcoholic containing at least 0.5%
Carbaryl Lotion, BP, aqueous containing at least 0.5%
Carbaryl shampoos containing at least 0.5%[2]
Catheter Maintenance Solution, Chlorhexidine, NPF
Catheter Maintenance Solution, Mandelic Acid, NPF
Catheter Maintenance Solution, Sodium Chloride, NPF
Catheter Maintenance Solution, 'Solution G', NPF
Catheter Maintenance Solution, 'Solution R', NPF
Clotrimazole Cream 1%, BP
Co-danthramer Capsules, NPF
Co-danthramer Capsules, Strong, NPF
Co-danthramer Oral Suspension, NPF
Co-danthramer Oral Suspension, Strong, NPF
Co-danthrusate Capsules, BP
Co-danthrusate Oral Suspension, NPF
Dextranomer Beads, NPF
Dextranomer Paste, NPF
Dimethicone barrier creams containing at least 10%
Docusate Capsules, NPF
Docusate Enema, NPF
Docusate Enema, Compound, NPF
Docusate Oral Solution, NPF[3]
Docusate Oral Solution, Paediatric, NPF[3]
Emulsifying Ointment, BP
Glycerol Suppositories, BP
Hydrous Ointment, BP
Ispaghula Husk Granules, NPF

Ispaghula Husk Granules, Effervescent, NPF
Ispaghula Husk Powder, NPF
Ispaghula Husk Powder, Effervescent, NPF[1]
Lactitol Powder, NPF
Lactulose Powder, NPF
Lactulose Solution, BP
Lignocaine Gel, BP
Lignocaine Ointment, NPF
Lignocaine and Chlorhexidine Gel, BP
Magnesium Hydroxide Mixture, BP
Magnesium Sulphate Paste, BP
Malathion alcoholic lotions containing at least 0.5%
Malathion aqueous lotions containing at least 0.5%
Malathion shampoos containing at least 1%[2]
Mebendazole Tablets, NPF
Mebendazole Oral Suspension, NPF
Miconazole Oral Gel, NPF
Nystatin Oral Suspension, BP
Nystatin Pastilles, NPF
Olive Oil Ear Drops, NPF
Paracetamol Oral Suspension, BP (includes 120 mg/ 5 mL and 250 mg/5 mL strengths—both of which are available as sugar-free formulations)
Paracetamol Tablets, BP
Paracetamol Tablets, Soluble, BP
Permethrin Cream, NPF
Permethrin Cream Rinse, NPF
Phenothrin Alcoholic Lotion, NPF
Phosphates Enema, BP
Piperazine Citrate Elixir, BP
Piperazine and Senna Powder, NPF
Povidone–Iodine Aqueous Solution, NPF[4]
Senna Granules, Standardised, BP
Senna Oral Solution, NPF
Senna Tablets, BP
Senna and Ispaghula Granules, NPF
Sodium Chloride Solution, Sterile, BP
Sodium Citrate Compound Enema, NPF
Sterculia Granules, NPF
Sterculia and Frangula Granules, NPF
Streptokinase and Streptodornase Topical Powder, NPF
Thymol Glycerin, Compound, BP 1988
Titanium Ointment, NPF
Zinc and Castor Oil Ointment, BP
Zinc Oxide and Dimethicone Spray, NPF

1. This preparation has now been introduced into the BP
2. No longer prescribable under NHS
3. May no longer be available
4. This preparation has now been introduced into the BP as Povidone–Iodine Solution

This list is currently **only** for the purposes of the **Nurse Prescribing demonstration scheme** which involves nurses with a District Nurse (DN) or Health Visitor (HV) qualification.

Appliances and Reagents (including Wound Management Products)

Chemical Reagents
The following as listed in Part IXR of the Drug
Tariff (Part 9 of the Scottish Drug Tariff):
  Detection Tablets for Glycosuria
  Detection Tablets for Ketonuria
  Detection Strips for Glycosuria
  Detection Strips for Ketonuria
  Detection Strips for Proteinuria
  Detection Strips for Blood Glucose
Fertility (Ovulation) Thermometer as listed
  under Contraceptive Devices in Part IXA of the
  Drug Tariff (Part 3 of the Scottish Drug Tariff)
Film Gloves, Disposable, EMA as listed under
  Protectives in Part IXA of the Drug Tariff (Part
  2 of the Scottish Drug Tariff)
Elastic Hosiery including accessories as listed in
  Part IXA of the Drug Tariff (Part 4 of the
  Scottish Drug Tariff)
Hypodermic Equipment
The following as listed in Part IXA of the Drug
  Tariff (Part 3 of the Scottish Drug Tariff):
  Hypodermic Syringes—U100 Insulin
  Hypodermic Syringe Carrying Case[1]
  Screw cap to convert Hypodermic Syringe Car-
    rying Case for use with Pre-set U100 Insulin
    Syringe[1]
  Hypodermic Syringe—Single Use or Single-pa-
    tient Use, U100 Insulin with Needle
  Hypodermic Needles—Sterile, Single-use
  Lancets—Sterile, Single-use
  Needle Clipping Device
Incontinence Appliances as listed in Part IXB of
  the Drug Tariff (Part 5 of the Scottish Drug Tar-
  iff)
Pessaries, Ring as listed in Part IXA of the
  Drug Tariff (Part 3 of the Scottish Drug Tariff)
Stoma Appliances and Associated Products as
  listed in Part IXC of the Drug Tariff (Part 6 of
  the Scottish Drug Tariff)
Urethral Catheters as listed under Catheters in
  Part IXA of the Drug Tariff (Part 3 of the
  Scottish Drug Tariff)
Urine Sugar Analysis Equipment as listed in Part
  IXA of the Drug Tariff (Parts 3 and 9 of the
  Scottish Drug Tariff)

Wound Management and Related Products
  (including bandages, dressings, gauzes, lint,
  stockinette, etc)
The following as listed in Part IXA of the Drug
  Tariff (Part 2 of the Scottish Drug Tariff):
  Absorbent Cottons
  Absorbent Cotton Gauzes
  Absorbent Cotton and Viscose Ribbon Gauze,
    BP 1988
  Absorbent Lint, BPC
  Arm Slings
  Cellulose Wadding, BP 1988
  Cotton Conforming Bandage, BP 1988
  Cotton Crêpe Bandage, BP 1988
  Cotton, Polyamide and Elastane Bandage
  Crêpe Bandage, BP 1988
  Elastic Adhesive Bandage, BP
  Elastic Web Bandages
  Elastomer and Viscose Bandage, Knitted
  Gauze and Cellulose Wadding Tissue, BP 1988[1]
  Gauze and Cotton Tissues
  Heavy Cotton and Rubber Elastic Bandage, BP
  High Compression Bandages (Extensible)
  Knitted Polyamide and Cellulose Contour Band-
    age, BP 1988
  Knitted Viscose Primary Dressing, BP, Type 1
  Multiple Pack Dressing No. 1
  Multiple Pack Dressing No. 2
  Open-wove Bandage, BP 1988, Type 1
  Paraffin Gauze Dressing, BP
  Perforated Film Absorbent Dressing[2]
  Polyamide and Cellulose Contour Bandage, BP
    1988
  Povidone–Iodine Fabric Dressing, Sterile
  Skin Closure Strips, Sterile
  Sterile Dressing Packs
  Stockinettes
  Surgical Adhesive Tapes
  Suspensory Bandages, Cotton
  Swabs
  Titanium Dioxide Elastic Adhesive Bandage,
    BP[1]
  Triangular Calico Bandage, BP 1980
  Vapour-permeable Adhesive Film Dressing, BP
  Vapour-permeable Waterproof Plastic Wound
    Dressing, BP, Sterile
  Wound Management Dressings (including gel,
    colloid and foam)
  Zinc Paste Bandages (including both plain and
    with additional ingredients)

1. May no longer be available
2. Now named Absorbent, Perforated Plastic Film Faced Dressing

In the Drug Tariff Appliances and Reagents which may **not** be prescribed by Nurses are annotated (N)
In the Scottish Drug Tariff Appliances and Reagents which may **not** be prescribed by Nurses are annotated **Nx**

> This list is currently **only** for the purposes of the
> **Nurse Prescribing demonstration scheme**
> which involves nurses with a District Nurse (DN)
> or Health Visitor (HV) qualification.

Details of NPF preparations

Preparations on the Nurse Prescribers' Formulary which are not included in the BP or BPC are described as follows in the pilot edition of the Nurse Prescribers' Formulary which has been produced for the Nurse Prescribing demonstration scheme.

Although brand names have sometimes been included for identification purposes preparations on the list should be prescribed by non-proprietary name.

Almond Oil Ear Drops, almond oil 10 mL supplied in a multidose container fitted with an appropriate applicator

Arachis Oil Enema, (proprietary product: *Fletchers' Arachis Oil Retention Enema*), arachis oil

Cadexomer–Iodine Ointment, (proprietary product: *Iodosorb Ointment*), cadexomer–iodine containing iodine 0.9% in an ointment basis

PoM **Cadexomer–Iodine Paste,** (proprietary product: *Iodoflex*), cadexomer–iodine containing iodine 0.9% in a paste basis

PoM **Cadexomer–Iodine Powder,** (proprietary product: *Iodosorb Powder*), cadexomer–iodine containing iodine 0.9%

NHS **Carbaryl shampoos,** (proprietary product: *Carylderm Shampoo*), carbaryl 1% in a shampoo basis

Catheter Maintenance Solution, Chlorhexidine, (proprietary products: *Uro-Tainer Chlorhexidine*; *Uriflex C*), chlorhexidine 0.02%

Catheter Maintenance Solution, Mandelic Acid, (proprietary product: *Uro-Tainer Mandelic Acid*), mandelic acid 1%

Catheter Maintenance Solution, Sodium Chloride, (proprietary products: *Uro-Tainer Sodium Chloride*; *Uriflex-S*), sodium chloride 0.9%

Catheter Maintenance Solution, 'Solution G', (proprietary products: *Uro-Tainer Suby G*, *Uriflex G*), citric acid 3.23%, magnesium oxide 0.38%, sodium bicarbonate 0.7%, disodium edetate 0.01%

Catheter Maintenance Solution, 'Solution R', (proprietary products: *Uro-Tainer Solution R*, *Uriflex R*), citric acid 6%, gluconolactone 0.6%, magnesium carbonate 2.8%, disodium edetate 0.01%

PoM **Co-danthramer Capsules,** co-danthramer 25/200 (danthron 25 mg, poloxamer '188' 200 mg)

PoM **Co-danthramer Capsules, Strong,** co-danthramer 37.5/500 (danthron 37.5 mg, poloxamer '188' 500 mg)

PoM **Co-danthramer Oral Suspension,** (proprietary product: *Codalax*), co-danthramer 25/200 in 5 mL (danthron 25 mg, poloxamer '188' 200 mg/5 mL)

PoM **Co-danthramer Oral Suspension, Strong,** (proprietary product: *Codalax Forte*), co-danthramer 75/1000 in 5 mL (danthron 75 mg, poloxamer '188' 1 g/5 mL)

PoM **Co-danthrusate Oral Suspension,** (proprietary product: *Normax*), co-danthrusate 50/60 (danthron 50 mg, docusate sodium 60 mg/5 mL)

Dextranomer Beads, (proprietary product: *Debrisan Beads*), dextranomer

Dextranomer Paste, (proprietary product: *Debrisan Paste*), dextranomer in a soft paste basis

Dimethicone barrier creams, (proprietary products: *Conotrane Cream*, dimethicone '350' 22%; *Siopel Barrier Cream*, dimethicone '1000' 10%; *Vasogen Barrier Cream*, dimethicone 20%), dimethicone 10–22%

Docusate Capsules, (proprietary product: *Dioctyl Capsules*), docusate sodium 100 mg

Docusate Enema, (proprietary product: *Norgalax Micro-enema*) docusate sodium 120 mg in 10 g

Docusate Enema, Compound, (proprietary product: *Fletchers' Enemette*), docusate sodium 90 mg, glycerol 3.78 g/5 mL with macragol and sorbic acid

Docusate Oral Solution, docusate sodium 50 mg/5 mL [*Note.* May no longer be available]

Docusate Oral Solution, Paediatric, docusate sodium 12.5 mg/5 mL [*Note.* May no longer be available]

Ispaghula Husk Granules, (proprietary product: *Isogel*), ispaghula husk 90%

Ispaghula Husk Granules, Effervescent, (proprietary product: *Fybogel Granules*), ispaghula husk 3.5 g/sachet

Ispaghula Husk Powder, (proprietary product: *Konsyl*), ispaghula husk 3.4 g or 6 g per sachet

Ispaghula Husk Powder, Effervescent, (proprietary product: *Regulan Powder*), ispaghula husk 3.6 g/6.4-g sachet [*Note.* May no longer be available]

Lactitol Powder, lactitol 10 g/sachet

Lactulose Powder, (proprietary products: *Lactulose Dry, Duphalac Dry*), lactulose 10 g/sachet

Lignocaine Ointment, (proprietary product: *Xylocaine Ointment*), lignocaine 5%

Malathion alcoholic lotions, (proprietary products: *Prioderm Lotion*; *Suleo-M Lotion*), malathion 0.5% in an alcoholic basis

Malathion aqueous lotions, (proprietary products: *Derbac-M Liquid; Quellada M Liquid*), malathion 0.5% in an aqueous basis

NHS **Malathion shampoos,** (proprietary products: *Prioderm Cream Shampoo; Quellada M Cream Shampoo*), malathion 1% in a shampoo basis

PoM[1] **Mebendazole Tablets,** (proprietary products: *Ovex, Vermox*), mebendazole 100 mg

1. For exemption, see p. 294

PoM **Mebendazole Oral Suspension,** (proprietary product: *Vermox*), mebendazole 100 mg/5 mL

PoM[2] **Miconazole Oral Gel,** (proprietary product: *Daktarin Oral Gel*), miconazole 24 mg/mL

2. For exemption, see p. 274

PoM **Nystatin Pastilles,** (proprietary product: *Nystan Pastilles*), nystatin 100 000 units

Olive Oil Ear Drops, olive oil 10 mL supplied in a multidose container fitted with an appropriate applicator

Permethrin Cream, (proprietary product: *Lyclear Dermal Cream*), permethrin 5%

Permethrin Cream Rinse, (proprietary product: *Lyclear Cream Rinse*), permethrin 1%

Phenothrin Alcoholic Lotion, (proprietary product: *Full Marks Lotion*), phenothrin 0.2% in a basis containing isopropyl alcohol

Piperazine and Senna Powder, (proprietary product: *Pripsen Oral Powder*), piperazine phosphate 4 g, sennosides 15.3 mg/sachet

Povidone–Iodine Aqueous Solution, (proprietary product: *Betadine Antiseptic Solution*), povidone–iodine 10%

Senna Oral Solution, (proprietary product: *Senokot Syrup*), sennosides 7.5 mg/5 mL

Senna and Ispaghula Granules, (proprietary product: *Manevac Granules*), senna fruit 12.4%, ispaghula 54.2%

Sodium Citrate Compound Enema, (proprietary products: Fleet *Micro-enema*; *Micolette Micro-enema*; *Micralax Micro-enema; Relaxit Micro-enema*), sodium citrate 450 mg with glycerol, sorbitol and an anionic surfactant

Sterculia Granules, (proprietary product: *Normacol Granules*), sterculia 62%

Sterculia and Frangula Granules, (proprietary product: *Normacol Plus Granules*), sterculia 62%, frangula (standardised) 8%

PoM **Streptokinase and Streptodornase Topical Powder,** (proprietary product: *Varidase Topical*), streptokinase 100 000 units, streptodornase 25 000 units

Titanium Ointment, (proprietary product: *Metanium Ointment*), titanium dioxide 20%, titanium peroxide 5%, titanium salicylate 3%, titanium tannate 0.1%

Zinc Oxide and Dimethicone Spray, (proprietary product: *Sprilon*), dimethicone 1.04%, zinc oxide 12.5% in a pressurised aerosol unit

Index of Manufacturers

'Special-order' manufacturers—see p. 702

Abbott
Abbott Laboratories Ltd,
Abbott House, Norden Rd,
Maidenhead, Berks SL6 4XE.
(01628) 773355

A&H
Allen & Hanburys Ltd,
see GlaxoWellcome.

Adams
Adams Healthcare Ltd
Lotherton Way,
Garforth, Leeds LS25 2JY.
(0113) 2320066

Alcon
Alcon Laboratories (UK) Ltd,
Pentagon Park, Boundary Way,
Hemel Hempstead, Herts
HP2 7UD.
(01442) 341234

Alembic Products
Alembic Products Ltd,
River Lane, Saltney,
Chester, Cheshire CH4 8RQ.
(01244) 680147

ALK
ALK (UK),
8 Bennet Rd, Reading,
Berks RG2 0QX.
(0118) 9313200

Allerayde
Allerayde,
3 Sanigar Court, Whittle Close,
Newark, Notts NG24 2BW.
(01636) 613444

Allergan
Allergan Ltd,
Coronation Rd, High
Wycombe, Bucks HP12 3SH.
(01494) 444722

Alpha
Alpha Therapeutic UK Ltd,
Howlett Way, Thetford,
Norfolk IP24 1HZ.
(01842) 764260

AlphaMed
AlphaMed Ltd,
Bensham House,
340 Bensham Lane,
Thornton Heath,
Surrey CR7 7EQ.
0181-684 0470

Amersham
Amersham International plc,
Amersham Place,
Little Chalfont, Bucks
HP7 9NA.
(01494) 544000

Amgen
Amgen Ltd,
240 Cambridge Science Park,
Milton Rd, Cambridge
CB4 4WD.
(01223) 420305

Anpharm
see Antigen.
(01704) 562999

Antigen
Antigen Pharmaceuticals (UK),
Antigen House,
82 Waterloo Rd, Hillside,
Southport PR8 4QW.
(01704) 562777

APS
Approved Prescription Services
Ltd,
Brampton Rd, Hampden Park,
Eastbourne, East Sussex
BN22 9AG.
(01323) 501111

Ardern
Ardern Healthcare Ltd,
Pipers Brook Farm, Eastham,
Tenbury Wells, Worcs
WR15 8NP.
(01584) 781777

Ashbourne
Ashbourne Pharmaceuticals Ltd,
Victors Barns, Hill Farm,
Brixworth, Northampton
NN6 9DQ.
(01604) 882190

ASTA Medica
ASTA Medica Ltd,
168 Cowley Rd, Cambridge
CB4 4DL.
(01223) 423434

Astra
Astra Pharmaceuticals Ltd,
Home Park, Kings Langley,
Herts WD4 8DH.
(01923) 266191

Astra Tech
Astra Tech Ltd,
Stroudwater Business Park,
Brunel Way, Stonehouse, Glos
GL10 3SW.
(01453) 791763

Athena
Athena Neurosciences
(Europe) Ltd,
1 Meadway Court,
Rutherford Close,
Stevenage, Herts SG1 2EF.
(01438) 730200

Aurum
Aurum Pharmaceuticals Ltd,
48–50 High St, Billingshurst,
West Sussex RH14 9NY.
(01403) 786781

Bailey, Robert
Robert Bailey & Son plc,
Dysart St, Great Moor,
Stockport, Cheshire
SK2 7PF.
0161-483 1133

Baker Norton
Division of Norton Healthcare
see Norton.

Bard
Bard Ltd,
Forest House, Brighton Rd,
Crawley, West Sussex
RH11 9BP.
(01293) 527888

Bartholomew Rhodes
see Ashbourne.
(01604) 882626

Baxter
Baxter Healthcare Ltd,
Caxton Way, Thetford, Norfolk
IP24 3SE.
(01842) 767000

Baxter Hyland
Baxter Healthcare Ltd,
(Hyland-Immuno Division),
Wallingford Rd,
Compton, Newbury,
Berks RG20 7QW.
(01635) 206000

Bayer
Bayer plc,
Pharmaceutical Division,
Bayer House, Strawberry Hill,
Newbury, Berks RG14 1JA.
(01635) 563000

Bayer Consumer Care
see Bayer.

Bayer Diagnostics
Bayer plc,
Diagnostics Division,
Bayer House,
Strawberry Hill,
Newbury, Berks RG14 1JA.
(01635) 563000

Baypharm
see Bayer.

BCM Specials
Boots Contract Manufacturing,
1 Thane Rd West,
Nottingham NG2 3AA.
0500 925935

Becton Dickinson
Becton Dickinson UK Ltd,
Between Towns Rd,
Cowley, Oxford,
Oxon OX4 3LY.
(01865) 748844

Beecham
Beecham Research,
see SmithKline Beecham.

Beiersdorf
Beiersdorf UK Ltd,
Yeomans Drive, Blakelands,
Milton Keynes,
Bucks MK14 5LS.
(01908) 211444

Bell and Croyden
John Bell and Croyden,
54 Wigmore St, London
W1H 0AU.
0171-935 5555

Bencard
see SmithKline Beecham.

Berk
Berk Pharmaceuticals,
see APS.

BHR
BHR Pharmaceuticals Ltd,
41 Centenary Business Centre,
Hammond Close,
Attleborough Fields, Nuneaton,
Warwickshire CV11 6RY.
(01203) 353742

Bio Diagnostics
Bio Diagnostics Ltd,
Upton Industrial Estate,
Rectory Rd, Upton-upon-
Severn, Worcs WR8 0XL.
(01684) 592262

Biocare
Biocare International Inc.
Belvoir House, Chapel St,
Haconby, Lincs
PE10 0UP.
(01778) 570441

Biogen
Biogen Ltd,
Ocean House,
The Ring, Bracknell,
Berks RG12 1AX.
(01344) 867033

Bioglan
Bioglan Laboratories Ltd,
5 Hunting Gate, Hitchin,
Herts SG4 0TJ.
(01462) 438444

Bio-Medical
Bio-Medical Services,
BMS Laboratories Ltd,
River View Rd, Beverley,
North Humberside HU17 0LD.
(01482) 860228

Biorex
Biorex Laboratories Ltd,
2 Crossfield Chambers,
Gladbeck Way, Enfield,
Middx EN2 7HT.
0181-366 9301

Blake
Thomas Blake & Co,
The Byre House, Fearby,
Nr. Masham, North Yorkshire
HG4 4NF.
(01765) 689042

BM Diagnostics
Boehringer Mannheim
(Diagnostics & Biochemicals)
Ltd,
Bell Lane, Lewes,
East Sussex BN7 1LG.
(01273) 480444

BOC
BOC Gases,
Priestly Rd, Worsley,
Manchester M28 2UT.
0800 111333

Boehringer Ingelheim
Boehringer Ingelheim Ltd,
Ellesfield Ave, Bracknell, Berks
RG12 4YS.
(01344) 424600

Boehringer Mannheim
Boehringer Mannheim UK Ltd,
Simpson Parkway, Kirkton
Campus, Livingston, West
Lothian EH54 7BH.
(01506) 412512

Boston
Boston Hospital Products,
Unit 1-3 Waymills,
Whitchurch,
Shropshire SY13 1QN.
(01948) 664487

BPL
Bio Products Laboratory,
Dagger Lane, Elstree, Herts
WD6 3BX.
0181-905 1818

Braun
B. Braun (Medical) Ltd,
Braun House, 13–14
Farmbrough Close, Aylesbury
Vale Industrial Park, Aylesbury,
Bucks HP20 1DQ.
(01296) 393900

Braun Biotrol
B. Braun Biotrol,
Parkway Close,
Parkway Industrial Estate,
Sheffield S9 4WJ.
(0114) 2730346

Bristol-Myers
Bristol-Myers Squibb
Pharmaceuticals Ltd,
141–149 Staines Rd, Hounslow,
Middx TW3 3JA.
0181-572 7422

Britannia
Britannia Pharmaceuticals Ltd,
41–51 Brighton Rd, Redhill,
Surrey RH1 6YS.
(01737) 773741

Bullen
C. S. Bullen Ltd,
3–7 Moss St, Liverpool L6 1EY.
0151-207 6995

Bullen & Smears
Bullen & Smears Ltd,
see Bullen.

Cambridge
Cambridge Laboratories,
Richmond House,
Old Brewery Court,
Sandyford Rd,
Newcastle upon Tyne NE2 1XG.
0191-261 5950

Camp
Camp Ltd,
30–32 Sovereign Rd, Kings
Norton Business Centre,
Birmingham B30 3HN.
0121-451 3016

Centeon
Centeon Ltd,
RPR House,
52 St. Leonards Rd,
Eastbourne, East Sussex
BN21 3YG.
(01323) 410200

Ceretron
Ceretron Ltd,
Tredan House, Church Rd,
Great Bookham,
Surrey KT23 3JG.
0181-813 6668

Chauvin
Chauvin Pharmaceuticals Ltd,
Ashton Rd, Harold Hill,
Romford,
Essex RM3 8SL.
(01708) 383838

J. Chawner
J. Chawner Surgical Belts Ltd,
Unit 1B Mayfields
Southcrest, Redditch B98 7DU
(01527) 404353

Chefaro
Chefaro Proprietaries Ltd,
see Organon.
(01223) 420956

Chiron
Chiron UK Ltd,
Salamander Quay West,
Park Lane, Harefield, Middx
UB9 6NY.
(01895) 824087

Chugai
Chugai Pharma UK Ltd,
Mulliner House, Flanders Rd
Turnham Green,
London W4 1NN.
0181-987 5668

CIBA Vision
CIBA Vision Ophthalmics,
Flanders Rd, Hedge End,
Southampton SO30 2LG.
(01489) 775534

Clement Clarke
Clement Clarke International
Ltd,
Airmed House, Edinburgh Way,
Harlow, Essex CM20 2ED.
(01279) 414969

CliniFlex
CliniFlex Ltd,
see CliniMed.

CliniMed
CliniMed Ltd,
Cavell House, Knaves Beech
Way, Loudwater, High
Wycombe, Bucks HP10 9QY.
(01628) 850100

Colgate-Palmolive
Colgate-Palmolive Ltd,
Guildford Business Park,
Middleton Rd, Guildford,
Surrey GU2 5LZ.
(01483) 302222

Coloplast
Coloplast Ltd,
Peterborough Business Park,
Peterborough PE2 6FX.
(01733) 392000

Concord
Concord Pharmaceuticals Ltd,
Leaden Roding, Dunmow,
Essex CM6 1SD.
(01279) 876911

ConvaTec
ConvaTec Ltd,
Harrington House, Milton Rd,
Ickenham, Uxbridge, Middx
UB10 8PU.
(01895) 678888

Co-Pharma
Co-Pharma Ltd,
Talbot House, Church St,
Rickmansworth, Herts
WD3 1DE.
(01923) 710934

Cortecs
Cortecs plc,
Techbase 3, Newtech Square,
Deeside Industrial Estate,
Deeside, Flintshire CH5 2NT.
(01244) 288888

Cover Care
Cover Care,
5 Ancaster Gardens, Wollaton
Park, Nottingham NG8 1FR.
(0115) 928 7883

Cow & Gate
see Nutricia Clinical
(01225) 768381

Cox
Cox Pharmaceuticals,
A. H. Cox & Co Ltd,
Whiddon Valley, Barnstaple,
Devon EX32 8NS.
(01271) 311257

CP
CP Pharmaceuticals Ltd,
Ash Rd North, Wrexham
Industrial Estate, Wrexham,
Clwyd LL13 9UF.
(01978) 661261

Crawford
Crawford Pharmaceuticals,
Furtho House,
20 Towcester Rd,
Milton Keynes MK19 6AQ.
(01908) 262346

Credenhill
Credenhill Ltd,
10 Cossall Industrial Estate,
Ilkeston, Derbys DE7 5UG.
(0115) 932 0144

Crookes
Crookes Healthcare Ltd,
PO Box 57, Central Park,
Lenton Lane,
Nottingham NG7 2LJ.
(0115) 953 9922

Cupal
Cupal Ltd,
See Seton.

Cussons
Cussons (UK) Ltd,
Kersal Vale, Manchester
M7 0GL.
0161-792 6111

Cutter
see Bayer.

Cuxson
Cuxson, Gerrard & Co Ltd,
Oldbury, Warley, West Midlands
B69 4BF.
0121-544 7117

Daniels
see Martindale

Dansac
Dansac Ltd,
Victory House, Vision Park,
Histon, Cambridge CB4 4ZR.
(01223) 235100

DDC
DDC (London) Ltd,
6 Clifton Gardens,
London W9 1DT.
0171-289 1113

DDD
DDD Ltd,
94 Rickmansworth Rd,
Watford, Herts WD1 7JJ.
(01923) 229251

DDSA
DDSA Pharmaceuticals Ltd,
310 Old Brompton Rd, London
SW5 9JQ.
0171-373 7884

De Vilbiss
De Vilbiss Health Care UK Ltd,
Airlinks, Spitfire Way, Heston,
Middx TW5 9NR.
0181-756 1133

De Witt
E. C. De Witt & Co Ltd,
Tudor Rd, Manor Park,
Runcorn, Cheshire WA7 1SZ.
(01928) 579029

Delandale
Delandale Laboratories Ltd,
see Lorex

Dental Health
Dental Health Products Ltd,
Pearl Assurance House,
Mill St, Maidstone,
Kent ME15 6XH.
(01622) 762269

DePuy
DePuy Healthcare,
Millshaw House, Manor Mill
Lane, Leeds LS11 8LQ.
(0113) 270 6000

Dermal
Dermal Laboratories Ltd,
Tatmore Place, Gosmore,
Hitchin, Herts SG4 7QR.
(01462) 458866

Dexcel
Dexcel Pharma Ltd,
Bishop Crewe House,
North St, Daventry,
Northants NN11 5PN.
(01327) 312266

DF
Duncan, Flockhart & Co Ltd,
see GlaxoWellcome.

Dista
Dista Products Ltd,
see Lilly.

Dominion
Dominion Pharma Ltd,
Dominion House, Lion Lane,
Haslemere, Surrey GU27 1JL.
(01428) 661078

Du Pont
Du Pont Pharmaceuticals Ltd,
Avenue One, Letchworth
Garden City, Herts SG6 2HU.
(01462) 482648

Dumex
Dumex Ltd,
Tring Business Centre,
Upper Icknield Way,
Tring, Herts HP23 4JX.
(01442) 890090

Durbin
B & S Durbin Ltd,
240 Northolt Rd, South Harrow,
Middx HA2 8DU.
0181-422 1303

Dylade
see Fresenius.

Eastern
Eastern Pharmaceuticals Ltd,
Coomb House, 7 St Johns Rd,
Isleworth, Middx TW7 6NA.
0181-569 8174

Eisai
Eisai Ltd,
3 Shortlands,
London W6 8EE.
0181-600 1400

Elan
Elan Pharma Ltd,
see P-D.

Elida Gibbs
Elida Gibbs Ltd,
Coal Rd, Seacroft, Leeds
LS14 2AR.
(0113) 273 7473

Ellis
Ellis, Son & Paramore Ltd,
see Camp

EMS
EMS Medical Ltd,
Unit 3, Stroud Industrial Estate,
Stonedale Rd, Oldends Lane,
Stonehouse, Glos GL10 2DG.
(01453) 791791

Epiderm
Epiderm Ltd,
52 Main St, Middleton,
Matlock, Derbyshire DE4 4LU.
(01629) 826833

Ethical Generics Ltd
Ethical Generics Ltd,
West Point, 46–48 West St,
Newbury, Berkshire RG14 1BD.
(01635) 568400

Ethical Research
Ethical Research Marketing,
3A Landgate, Rye,
East Sussex TN31 7LH.
(01797) 225021

Euroderma
Euroderma Ltd,
The Old Coach House,
34 Elm Rd, Chessington,
Surrey KT9 1AW.
0181-974 2266

Evans
Evans Medical Ltd,
Evans House, Regent Park,
Kingston Rd, Leatherhead,
Surrey KT22 7PQ.
(01372) 364000

Everfresh
Everfresh Natural Foods,
Gatehouse Close, Aylesbury,
Bucks HP19 3DE.
(01296) 25333

Exelgyn
Exelgyn,
PO Box 7,
Bramhall SK7 3FG.
(0800) 7316120

Fabre
Pierre Fabre Ltd
Hyde Abbey House
23 Hyde St, Winchester,
Hampshire SO23 7DR
(01962) 856956

Farillon
Farillon Ltd,
Ashton Rd, Romford,
Essex RM3 8UF.
(01708) 379000

Farley
Farley Health Products,
Mint Bridge Rd, Kendal,
Cumbria LA9 6NL
(01539) 723815

Faulding DBL
Faulding Pharmaceuticals plc,
Queensway,
Leamington Spa CV31 3RW.
(01926) 820820

Ferraris
Ferraris Medical Ltd,
Ferraris House, Aden Rd,
Enfield, Middx EN3 7SE.
0181-805 9055

Ferring
Ferring Pharmaceuticals Ltd,
Greville House, Hatton Rd,
Feltham, Middx TW14 9PX.
0181-893 1543

Fisons
Fisons plc,
Pharmaceutical Division,
Coleorton Hall, Ashby Rd,
Coleorton, Coalville, Leics
LE67 8GP.
(01509) 634000

Florizel
Florizel Ltd,
PO Box 138,
Stevenage SG2 8YN.
(01462) 436156

Flynn
Flynn Pharma Ltd,
7 Serlby Court, Addison Rd,
London W14 8EE.
(01438) 820152

Forley
Forley Ltd,
54 Hillbury Ave, Harrow,
Middx HA3 8EW.
0181-665 9169

Fournier
Fournier Pharmaceuticals Ltd,
22-23 Progress Business
Centre, Whittle Parkway,
Slough SL1 6DG.
(01753) 740400

Fox
C. H. Fox Ltd,
22 Tavistock St, London
WC2E 7PY
0171-240 3111

FP
Family Planning Sales Ltd,
28 Kelburne Rd, Cowley,
Oxford OX4 3SZ.
(01865) 772486

Fresenius
Fresenius Ltd,
6–8 Christleton Court,
Stuart Rd, Manor Park,
Runcorn, Cheshire WA7 1ST.
(01928) 579444

Fry
Fry Surgical International Ltd,
Unit 17, Goldsworth Park
Trading Estate, Woking, Surrey
GU21 3BA.
(01483) 721404

Fujisawa
Fujisawa Ltd,
C P House, 8th Floor,
97–107 Uxbridge Rd,
London W5 5TL.
0181-840 9520

Futuna
Futuna Ltd,
Sound Opinion,
PO Box 775,
Swindon, Wilts SN6 8UG.
(01793) 710170

Gainor Medical
Gainor Medical Europe,
Milton Keynes
Distribution Centre,
Bradbourne Drive, Tilbrook,
Milton Keynes MK7 8BN.
(01908) 365361

Galderma
Galderma (UK) Ltd,
Leywood House,
47 Woodside Rd, Amersham,
Bucks HP6 6AA.
(01494) 432606

Galen
Galen Ltd,
Seagoe Industrial Estate,
Craigavon, Northern Ireland
BT63 5UA.
(01762) 334974

Garnier
Laboratoires Garnier,
Golden Ltd,
PO Box 5, Pontyclun, Glam
CF7 8XW.
(01443) 237456

Geistlich
Geistlich Sons Ltd,
Newton Bank, Long Lane,
Chester CH2 2PF.
(01244) 347534

General Dietary
General Dietary Ltd,
PO Box 38,
Kingston upon Thames, Surrey
KT2 7YP.
0181-336 2323

Generics
Generics (UK) Ltd,
12 Station Close, Potters Bar,
Herts EN6 1TL.
(01707) 644556

Gensia
Gensia Automedics Ltd,
Unit 31, Wellington Business
Park, Dukes Ride, Crowthorne,
Berks RG45 6LS.
(01344) 759300

Genus
see Wyeth

Genzyme
Genzyme Therapeutics,
37 Hollands Rd, Haverhill,
Suffolk CB9 8PU.
(01440) 703522

GlaxoWellcome
GlaxoWellcome UK,
Stockley Park West, Uxbridge,
Middx UB11 1BT.
0181-990 9000

Glenwood
Glenwood Laboratories Ltd,
Jenkins Dale, Chatham,
Kent ME4 5RD.
(01634) 830535

Gluten Free Foods Ltd
Gluten Free Foods Ltd,
Unit 10 Honeypot Business
Park, Parr Rd, Stanmore
Middx HA7 1NL.
0181-952 0052

Goldshield
Goldshield Pharmaceuticals Ltd,
NLA Tower,
12–16 Addiscombe Rd,
Croydon CR0 0XT.
0181-649 8500

Heinz
H.J. Heinz Company Ltd,
Hayes Park, Hayes,
Middx UB4 8AL
0181-573 7757

Henleys
Henleys Medical Supplies Ltd,
Brownfields, Welwyn Garden
City, Herts AL7 1AN.
(01707) 333164

Hillcross
Hillcross Pharmaceuticals,
Talbot St, Briercliffe, Burnley
BB10 2JY.
(01282) 830042

Hoechst Marion Roussel

Hoechst Marion Roussel Ltd,
Broadwater Park, Denham,
Uxbridge, Middx UB9 5HP.
(01895) 834343

Hollister

Hollister Ltd,
Rectory Court, 42 Broad St,
Wokingham, Berks RG40 1AB.
(01189) 895000

Hospital Management & Supplies

Hospital Management and
Supplies Ltd,
Salthouse Rd, Brackmills,
Northampton, NN4 7UF.
(01604) 704600

Houghs

Houghs Healthcare Ltd,
18–22 Chapel St, Manchester
M19 3PT.
0161-224 3271

Hutchings

Hutchings Healthcare Ltd,
Rede House, New Barn Lane,
Henfield, West Sussex BN5 9SJ.
(01273) 495033

Hypoguard

Hypoguard Ltd,
Dock Lane, Melton,
Woodbridge, Suffolk IP12 1PE.
(01394) 387333

IATRO

IATRO Medical Systems,
(Division of SHIVAM Overseas
Ltd)
35 Quaggy Walk, Blackheath,
London SE3 9EJ.
0181-297 9081

ICN

ICN Pharmaceuticals Ltd,
1 Elmwood,
Chineham Business Park,
Crockford Lane,
Basingstoke,
Hants RG24 8WG.
(01256) 707744

IDIS

IDIS Ltd World Medicines,
Millbank House, 171 Ewell Rd,
Surbiton, Surrey.
KT6 6AX.
0181-410 0700

Immuno

Baxter Healthcare Ltd,
Hyland Immuno,
Wallingford Rd,
Compton, Newbury,
Berks RG20 7QW.
(01635) 206000

Impharm

Impharm Nationwide Ltd,
PWS Building, Nelson St,
Bolton BL3 2JW.
(01204) 371155

IMS

International Medication
Systems (UK) Ltd,
Foster Ave, Woodside Park
Estate, Dunstable,
Beds LU5 5TA.
(01582) 475005

Incare

see Hollister.

Innovative

Innovative Technologies Ltd,
Unit B, Tarvin Sands Complex,
Tarvin, Cheshire CH3 8JF.
(01829) 741515

Innovex

see Novex.

Invicta

see Pfizer.

ISIS

ISIS Products Ltd,
Gough Lane, Bamber Bridge,
Preston, Lancs PR5 6AQ.
(01772) 628311

J&J

Johnson & Johnson Ltd,
Foundation Park, Roxborough
Way, Maidenhead,
Berkshire SL6 3UG.
(01628) 822222

J&J Medical

Johnson & Johnson Medical,
Coronation Rd, Ascot, Berks
SL5 9EY.
(01344) 871000

J&J MSD

Johnson & Johnson MSD,
Enterprise House, Station Rd,
Loudwater, High Wycombe,
Bucks HP10 9UF.
(01494) 450778

Jacobs

The Jacobs Bakery Ltd,
Suttons Business Park, Earley,
Reading, Berks RG6 1AZ.
(0118) 9492000

Jade-Euro-Med

Jade-Euro-Med
Unit 14, East Hanningfield
Industrial Estate, Oldchurch
Rd, East Hanningfield,
Chelmsford, Essex
CM3 8BG
(01245) 400413

Janssen-Cilag

Janssen-Cilag Ltd,
PO Box 79, Saunderton,
High Wycombe, Bucks
HP14 4HJ.
(01494) 567567

JHC

JHC Healthcare Ltd,
The Maltings, Bridge St,
Hitchin, Herts SG5 2DE.
(01462) 432533

JLB

B. Braun JLB Ltd,
Unit 2A, St Columb Industrial
Estate, St Columb Major,
Cornwall TR9 6SF.
(01637) 880065

K & K-Greeff

K & K-Greeff Ltd,
Suffolk House, George St,
Croydon CR9 3QL.
0181-686 0544

K/L

K/L Pharmaceuticals Ltd,
25 Macadam Place, South
Newmoor Industrial Estate,
Irvine KA11 4HP.
(01294) 215951

Kendall

The Kendall Co (UK) Ltd,
2 Elmwood, Chineham Business
Park, Crockford Lane,
Basingstoke, Hants RG24 8WG.
(01256) 708880

Kendall-Lastonet

see Kendall.

Kent

Kent Pharmaceuticals Ltd,
Wotton Rd, Ashford, Kent
TN23 6LL.
(01233) 641802

Kestrel

Kestrel Healthcare Ltd,
21a Hyde St, Winchester,
Hants SO23 7DR.
(01962) 866449

Kimal

Kimal Scientific Products Ltd,
Arundel Rd, Uxbridge, Middx
UB8 2SA.
(01895) 270951

Knoll

Knoll Ltd,
9 Castle Quay,
Castle Boulevard, Nottingham
NG7 1FW.
(0115) 912 5000

Kyowa Hakko

Kyowa Hakko UK Ltd,
CP House, 97–107 Uxbridge
Rd, Ealing, London W5 5TL.
0181-840 4600

LAB

Laboratories for Applied
Biology Ltd,
91 Amhurst Park, London
N16 5DR.
0181-800 2252

Laerdal

Laerdal Medical Ltd,
Laerdal House, Goodmead Rd,
Orpington, Kent BR6 0HX.
(01689) 876634

Lagap

Lagap Pharmaceuticals Ltd,
37 Woolmer Way, Bordon,
Hants GU35 9QE.
(01420) 478301

Lamberts

Lamberts (Dalston) Ltd,
P O Box 883, Oxford
OX4 3RR.
(01865) 717300

Larkhall
Larkhall Green Farm,
225 Putney Bridge Rd,
London SW15 2PY.
0181-874 1130

Lederle
see Wyeth

Lennon
see Trinity

Leo
Leo Pharmaceuticals,
Longwick Rd, Princes
Risborough, Bucks
HP27 9RR.
(01844) 347333

LifeScan
LifeScan,
Enterprise House, Station Rd,
Loudwater, High Wycombe,
Bucks HP10 9UF.
(01494) 450423

Lilly
Eli Lilly & Co Ltd,
Dextra Court, Chapel Hill,
Basingstoke, Hants RG21 5SY.
(01256) 315000

Link
Link Pharmaceuticals Ltd,
7/8 Sterling Buildings,
Carfax, Horsham, West Sussex
RH12 1DR.
(01403) 272451

Lipha
see Merck.

Liposome Company
The Liposome Co Ltd,
3 Shortlands, Hammersmith
International Centre,
London W6 8EH.
0181-324 0058

Lorex
Lorex Synthélabo Ltd,
5 Roxborough Way,
Foundation Park,
Maidenhead,
Berks SL6 3UD.
(01628) 501200

Loxley
Loxley Medical,
Unit 5D, Carnaby Industrial
Estate, Bridlington, North
Humberside YO15 3QY.
(01262) 603979

LRC
LRC Products Ltd,
London International House,
Turnford Place, Broxbourne,
Herts EN10 6LN.
(01992) 451111

Lundbeck
Lundbeck Ltd,
Sunningdale House, Caldecott
Lake Business Park, Caldecott,
Milton Keynes MK7 8LF.
(01908) 649966

3M
3M Health Care Ltd,
3M House, Morley St,
Loughborough,
Leics LE11 1EP.
(01509) 611611

Maersk
Maersk Medical Ltd,
Thornhill Rd,
North Moons Moat, Redditch,
Worcs B98 9NL.
(01527) 64222

Manfred Sauer
Manfred Sauer UK,
Mill Lane, Eastry,
Kent CT13 0QJ.
(01304) 620446

Mandeville
Mandeville Medicines,
Stoke Mandeville Hospital,
Aylesbury, Bucks HP21 8AL.
(01296) 394142

Manx
Manx Pharma,
7th Floor Kent House,
Lower Stone St,
Maidstone, Kent ME15 6LH.
(01622) 766389

Marlen
Marlen (UK) Ltd,
Unit F4C,
Keighley Business Centre,
South St, Keighley,
West Yorkshire BD21 1AG.
(01535) 610300

Martindale
Martindale Pharmaceuticals Ltd,
Bampton Rd, Harold Hill,
Romford, Essex RM3 8UG.
(01708) 386660

Matrix
Matrix Pharmaceutical Ltd,
Selborne House, Mill Lane,
Alton, Hants GU34 2QL.

Medac
Medac (UK),
13 Lynedoch Crescent,
Glasgow G3 6EQ.
0141-332 8464

Medasil
Medasil (Surgical) Ltd,
Medasil House, Hunslet Rd,
Leeds LS10 1AU.
(0113) 243 3491

Medic-Aid
Medic-Aid Ltd,
Hook Lane, Pagham, Sussex
PO21 3PP.
(01243) 267321

Medigas
Medigas Ltd,
Enterprise Drive, Four Ashes,
Wolverhampton WV10 7DF.
(01902) 791944

MediSense
MediSense Britain Ltd,
16–17 The Courtyard,
Gorsey Lane, Coleshill,
Birmingham B46 1JA.
(01675) 467044

Medix
see Clement Clarke.

Medo
see Schwarz.

Mepra-pharm
see Co-Pharma.

Merck
E. Merck Pharmaceuticals,
Harrier House, High St,
West Drayton, Middlesex,
UB7 7QG.
(01895) 452200

Milupa
Milupa Ltd,
Milupa House, Uxbridge Rd,
Hillingdon, Middx UB10 0NE.
0181-573 9966

Monmouth
Monmouth Pharmaceuticals,
3/4 Huxley Rd, The Surrey
Research Park, Guildford,
Surrey GU2 5RE.
(01483) 565299

Morson
see MSD.

MSD
Merck Sharp & Dohme Ltd,
Hertford Rd, Hoddesdon, Herts
EN11 9BU.
(01992) 467272

Napp
Napp Laboratories Ltd,
Cambridge Science Park, Milton
Rd, Cambridge CB4 4GW.
(01223) 424444

Nestlé
Nestlé UK Ltd,
St. George's House, Croydon
CR9 1NR.
0181-686 3333

Nestlé Clinical
Nestlé Clinical Nutrition,
Trinity Court, Church St
Rickmansworth,
Hertfordshire WD3 1LD,
(01923) 897772

Network Management
Network Management Ltd,
Victoria House, Victoria Rd,
Aldershot, Hants GU11 1DB.
(01252) 351100

Neutrogena
see J&J

NeXstar
NeXstar Pharmaceuticals Ltd,
The Quorum, Barnwell Rd,
Cambridge CB5 8RE.
(01223) 571400

Nordic
see Ferring.
0181-898 8665

Norgine
Norgine Ltd,
Chaplin House, Moorhall Rd,
Harefield, Middx UB9 6NS.
(01895) 826600

Norma
see Wallace Mfg.

North West

North West Medical Supplies Ltd,
Green Arms Rd, Bolton
BL7 0ND.
(01204) 852383

Norton

Norton Healthcare Ltd,
Gemini House, Flex Meadow,
Harlow, Essex CM19 5TJ.
(01279) 426666

Novartis

Novartis Pharmaceuticals UK,
Frimley Business Park,
Frimley, Camberley,
Surrey GU16 5SG.
(01276) 692255

Novartis Consumer Health

Novartis Consumer Health,
Wimblehurst Rd, Horsham,
West Sussex RH12 4AB.
(01403) 210211

Novex

Novex Pharma Ltd,
Innovex House, Marlow Park,
Marlow, Bucks SL7 1TB.
(01628) 491500

Novo Nordisk

Novo Nordisk Pharmaceutical Ltd,
Novo Nordisk House,
Broadfield Park, Brighton Rd,
Pease Pottage, Crawley, West
Sussex RH11 9RT.
(01293) 613555

Nutricia Clinical

Nutricia Clinical Care,
Nutricia Ltd, White Horse
Business Park, Trowbridge,
Wiltshire BA14 0XQ
(01225) 711677

Nutricia Dietary

Nutricia Dietary Products Ltd,
see Nutricia Clinical
(01225) 711801.

Nycomed

Nycomed (UK) Ltd,
Nycomed House, 2111 Coventry
Rd, Sheldon, Birmingham
B26 3EA.
0121-742 2444

Oakmed

Oakmed Ltd,
54 Adams Ave,
Northampton NN1 4LJ.
(01604) 239250

Octapharma

Octapharma Ltd,
Olton Bridge, 245 Warwick Rd,
Solihull, West Midlands
B92 7AH.
0121-706 8885

Omni Triage

Omni Triage Medical Ltd,
131 Tranmere Rd,
London SW18 3QP.
0171-737 7781

Omnicare

The Omnicare Group Ltd,
Enterprise Drive, Four Ashes,
Wolverhampton WV10 7DF.
0500 823773

Opus

see Trinity.

Oral B Labs

Oral B Laboratories Ltd,
Gatehouse Rd, Aylesbury,
Bucks HP19 3ED.
(01296) 432601

Organon

Organon Laboratories Ltd,
Cambridge Science Park, Milton
Rd, Cambridge, CB4 4FL.
(01223) 423445

Organon-Teknika

see Organon
(01223) 423650

Orion

Orion Pharma (UK) Ltd,
1st Floor, Leat House,
Overbridge Square, Hambridge
Lane, Newbury, Berks
RG14 5UX.
(01635) 520300

Orphan Europe

Orphan Europe (UK),
Bray Business Centre,
Bray-on-Thames, Berks
SL6 2ED.
(01628) 773342

Orthotic

Orthotic Services Ltd
Heartlands House, 19 Catro St,
The Heartlands,
Birmingham B7 4TS.
0121-359 6323

Owen Mumford

Owen Mumford Ltd,
Brook Hill, Woodstock, Oxford
OX20 1TU.
(01993) 812021

Oxford Nutrition

Oxford Nutrition Ltd,
PO Box 110, Witney, Oxon
OX8 7FJ.
(01993) 709752

Oxygen Therapy Co Ltd

The Oxygen Therapy Co Ltd,
Dumballs Rd, Cardiff
CF1 6JE.
0800 373580

Paines & Byrne

Paines & Byrne Ltd,
Yamanouchi House, Pyrford Rd,
West Byfleet,
Surrey KT14 6RA.
(01932) 355405

Parema

Parema Ltd,
Sullington Rd, Shepshed,
Loughborough,
Leics LE12 9JJ.
(01509) 502051

Pari

Pari Medical Ltd,
Enterprise House, Station
Approach, West Byfleet,
Surrey KT14 6NE.
(01932) 341122

Pasteur Mérieux

Pasteur Mérieux MSD Ltd,
Clivemont House,
Clivemont Rd, Maidenhead,
Berks SL6 7BU.
(01628) 785291

Payne

S G & P Payne,
Percy House, Brook St, Hyde,
Cheshire SK14 2NS.
0161-367 8561

P-D

Parke-Davis Medical,
Lambert Court, Chestnut Ave,
Eastleigh, Hants SO53 3ZQ.
(01703) 620500

Pelican

see Simpla
(01222) 747787

Penn

Penn Pharmaceuticals Ltd,
Tafarnaubach Industrial Estate,
Tredegar, Gwent, NP2 3AA.
(01495) 711222

Pennine

Pennine Healthcare,
Pontefract St, Ascot Drive
Industrial Estate,
Derby DE2 8JD.
(01332) 384489

Perstorp

Perstorp Pharma Ltd,
Intec 2, Wade Rd, Basingstoke,
Hants RG24 8NE.
(01256) 477868

Pfizer

Pfizer Ltd,
Sandwich, Kent CT13 9NJ.
(01304) 616161

Pfizer Consumer

Pfizer Consumer Healthcare,
Wilsom Rd, Alton,
Hants GU34 2TJ.
(01420) 84801

Pharmacia & Upjohn

Pharmacia & Upjohn Ltd,
Davy Ave, Knowlhill,
Milton Keynes, MK5 8PH.
(01908) 661101

Pharma-Global

Pharma-Global Ltd,
SEQ Ltd, Nerin House,
26 Ridgeway St, Douglas,
Isle of Man IM1 1EL.
(01624) 613997

Pharmark

Pharmark Ltd,
7 Windermere Rd, West
Wickham, Kent BR4 9AN.
0181-688 5895

Pharmax
Pharmax Ltd,
Bourne Rd, Bexley,
Kent DA5 1NX.
(01322) 550550

Phoenix
Phoenix Pharmaceuticals Ltd,
Glevum Works, Upton St,
Gloucester GL1 4LA.
(01452) 522255

Pickles
J. Pickles & Sons,
Beech House, 62 High St,
Knaresborough, N. Yorks
HG5 0EA.
(01423) 867314

Procter & Gamble
Procter & Gamble (Health &
Beauty Care) Ltd,
The Heights, Brooklands,
Weybridge, Surrey KT13 0XP.
(01932) 896000

Procter & Gamble Pharm.
Procter & Gamble
Pharmaceuticals UK Ltd,
Lovett House, Lovett Rd,
Staines, Middx TW18 3AZ.
(01784) 495000

Quinoderm Ltd
Quinoderm Ltd,
Manchester Rd, Hollinwood,
Oldham, Lancs OL8 4PB.
0161-624 9307

Ranbaxy
Ranbaxy (UK) Ltd,
Suite 28, 140 Park Lane,
London W1Y 3AA.
0171-495 5511

Rand Rocket
Rand Rocket Ltd,
ABCare House, Hownsgill
Industrial Park, Consett,
County Durham DH8 7NU.
(01207) 591099

R&C
Reckitt & Colman Products Ltd,
Dansom Lane, Hull HU8 7DS.
(01482) 326151

Renacare
Renacare Ltd,
Nunn Brook Rd, Huthwaite,
Sutton-in-Ashfield,
Notts NG17 2HU.
(01623) 555809

Rhône-Poulenc Rorer
Rhône-Poulenc Rorer Ltd,
RPR House, 50 Kings Hill Av,
Kings Hill, West Malling,
Kent ME19 4AH.
(01732) 584000

Richborough
see Pfizer.

Rima
Rima Pharmaceuticals Ltd,
214–216 St. James's Rd,
Croydon, Surrey CR0 2BW.
0181-683 1266

Robinsons
Robinson Healthcare,
Hipper House, Chesterfield,
Derbyshire S40 1YF.
(01246) 220022

RoC
Laboratoires RoC UK Ltd,
see J & J

Roche
Roche Products Ltd,
PO Box 8, Welwyn Garden City,
Herts AL7 3AY.
(01707) 366000

Roche Consumer Health
see Roche

Rosemont
Rosemont Pharmaceuticals Ltd,
Rosemont House, Yorkdale
Industrial Park, Braithwaite St,
Leeds LS11 9XE.
(0113) 244 1999

Rowa
Rowa Pharmaceuticals Ltd,
Bantry, Co Cork, Ireland.
(00 353 27) 50077

Rüsch
Rüsch UK Ltd,
PO Box 138, Halifax Rd,
Cressex Business Park,
High Wycombe,
Bucks HP12 3NB.
(01494) 532761

Rybar
see Shire

Sallis
E. Sallis Ltd,
Vernon Works, Waterford St,
Basford, Nottingham
NG6 0DH.
(0115) 978 7841

Salts
Salt & Son Ltd,
Lord St,
Birmingham B7 4DS.
0121-359 5123

Sankyo
Sankyo Pharma UK Ltd,
Sankyo House, Repton Place,
White Lion Rd, Amersham,
Bucks HP7 9LP.
(01494) 766866

Sanofi Winthrop
Sanofi Winthrop Ltd,
One Onslow St, Guildford,
Surrey GU1 4YS.
(01483) 505515

Sara Lee
Sara Lee Household & Personal
Care (UK) Ltd,
225 Bath Rd, Slough SL1 4AU.
(01753) 523971

SCA Mölnlycke
SCA Mölnlycke Ltd,
Southfields Rd, Dunstable, Beds
LU6 3EJ.
(01582) 677400

Schär
Dr Schär,
P O Box 126,
Worcester WR3 7WB.
(01905) 28833

Schein Rexodent
Schein Rexodent,
25-27 Merrick Rd, Southall,
Middx UB2 4AU
0181-235 5005

Schering Health
Schering Health Care Ltd,
The Brow, Burgess Hill,
West Sussex RH15 9NE.
(01444) 232323

Schering-Plough
Schering-Plough Ltd,
Shire Park, Welwyn Garden
City, Herts AL7 1TW.
(01707) 363636

Scholl
Scholl Consumer Products Ltd,
475 Capability Green, Luton,
Beds LU1 3LU.
(01582) 482929

Schwarz
Schwarz Pharma Ltd,
Schwarz House, East St,
Chesham, Bucks HP5 1DG.
(01494) 772071

Scotia
Scotia Pharmaceuticals Ltd,
Scotia House,
Scotia Business Park,
Stirling FK9 4TZ.
(01786) 895100

Searle
Searle Division of Monsanto
plc,
PO Box 53, Lane End Rd, High
Wycombe, Bucks HP12 4HL.
(01494) 521124

Serono
Serono Laboratories (UK) Ltd,
99 Bridge Rd East, Welwyn
Garden City, Herts AL7 1BG.
(01707) 331972

Servier
Servier Laboratories Ltd,
Fulmer Hall, Windmill Rd,
Fulmer, Slough SL3 6HH.
(01753) 662744

Seton
Seton Healthcare,
Seton Healthcare Group plc,
Tubiton House, Medlock St,
Oldham, Lancs OL1 3HS.
0161-652 2222

Seton-Prebbles
see Seton

Seven Seas
Seven Seas Ltd,
Hedon Rd, Marfleet, Hull
HU9 5NJ.
(01482) 375234

Shannon
T. J. Shannon Ltd,
59 Bradford St, Bolton
BL2 1HT.
(01204) 521789

Shaw
A. H. Shaw and Partners Ltd,
Manor Rd, Ossett, West
Yorkshire WF5 0LF.
(01924) 273474

Sherwood Davis & Geck
Sherwood Davis & Geck,
154 Fareham Rd, Gosport,
Hants PO13 0AS.
(01329) 224114

Shire
Shire Pharmaceuticals Ltd,
Fosse House, East Anton Court,
Icknield Way, Andover, Hants
SP10 5RG.
(01264) 333455

SHS
SHS International Ltd,
100 Wavertree Boulevard,
Liverpool L7 9PT.
0151-228 8161

Sigma
Sigma Pharmaceuticals plc,
PO Box 233, Watford, Herts
WD2 4EW.
(01923) 250201

Simpla
see Seton

SIMS Portex
SIMS Portex Ltd,
Hythe, Kent CT21 6JL.
(01303) 260551

Sinclair
Sinclair Pharmaceuticals Ltd,
Borough Rd, Godalming, Surrey
GU7 2AB.
(01483) 426644

S&N Hlth.
Smith & Nephew Healthcare
Ltd,
Healthcare House, Goulton St,
Hull HU3 4DJ.
(01482) 222200

SK&F
see SmithKline Beecham.

SmithKline Beecham
SmithKline Beecham
Pharmaceuticals,
SmithKline Beecham plc,
Mundells, Welwyn Garden City,
Herts AL7 1EY.
(01707) 325111

SmithKline Beecham Health-care
SmithKline Beecham
Consumer Healthcare,
SB House, Brentford,
Middx TW8 9BD.
0181-560 5151

SNBTS
Scottish National Blood
Transfusion Service,
Protein Fractionation Centre,
Ellen's Glen Rd,
Edinburgh EH17 7QT.
0131-664 2317

Solvay
Solvay Healthcare Ltd,
Hamilton House, Gaters Hill,
West End, Southampton
SO18 3JD.
(01703) 472281

Speywood
Speywood Pharmaceuticals Ltd,
1 Bath Rd, Maidenhead,
Berks SL6 4UH.
(01628) 771417

Squibb
see Bristol-Myers.

Stafford-Miller
Stafford-Miller Ltd,
Broadwater Rd,
Welwyn Garden City, Herts
AL7 3SP.
(01707) 331001

STD Pharmaceutical
STD Pharmaceutical Products,
Fields Yard, Plough Lane,
Hereford HR4 0EL.
(01432) 353684

Steeper
Steeper (Orthopaedic) Ltd,
Unit 4D, Mead Rise,
Temple Gate, Bristol BS3 4RP.
(0117) 971 7436

Sterling Health
see SmithKline Beecham
Healthcare

Sterwin
see Sanofi Winthrop

Stiefel
Stiefel Laboratories (UK) Ltd,
Holtspur Lane, Wooburn Green,
High Wycombe, Bucks
HP10 0AU.
(01628) 524966

Storz
Storz Ophthalmics,
154 Fareham Rd, Gosport,
Hants PO13 0AS.
(01329) 224000

Stuart
see Zeneca

Sussex
Sussex Pharmaceutical Ltd,
Charlwoods Rd,
East Grinstead,
Sussex RH19 2HL.
(01342) 311311

Sutherland
Sutherland Health Ltd,
Unit 1, Rivermead, Pipers Way,
Thatcham, Berks RG13 4EP.
(01635) 874488

Syner-Med
Syner-Med (Pharmaceutical
Products) Ltd,
Airport House, Purley Way,
Croydon, Surrey CR0 0XY.
0181-781 1954

Takeda
Takeda UK Ltd,
3 The Courtyard, Meadowbank,
Furlong Rd, Bourne End,
Bucks SL8 5AJ.
(01628) 526614

Terumo
Terumo Europe N.V.
1st Floor Offices,
62 Mount Pleasant Rd,
Tunbridge Wells,
Kent TN1 1RB.
(01892) 526331

Thackraycare
see DePuy

Thames
see Cortecs

Thornton & Ross
Thornton & Ross Ltd,
Linthwaite Laboratories,
Huddersfield HD7 5QH.
(01484) 842217

Tillomed
Tillomed Laboratories Ltd,
Unit 2, Campus 5, Letchworth
Business Park, Letchworth
Garden City, Herts SG6 2JF.
(01462) 480344

Timesco
Timesco of London,
Timesco House
1 Knights Rd, London E16 2AT.
0171-511 1234

Torbet
Torbet Laboratories Ltd,
Pearl Assurance House,
Mill St, Maidstone,
Kent ME15 6XH.
(01622) 762269

Tosara
Tosara Products Ltd,
Baldoyle Industrial Estate,
Grange Rd, Dublin 13.
Dublin 321199

Trinity
Trinity Pharmaceuticals Ltd,
Tuition House,
27–37 St. George's Rd,
Wimbledon, London
SW19 4DS.
0181-944 9443

TSL
Tissue Science Laboratories Ltd,
Greyholme House,
49 Victoria Rd, Aldershot,
Hants GU11 1SJ.
(01252) 333002

Typharm
Typharm Ltd,
14 Parkstone Rd, Poole,
Dorset BH15 2PG.
(01202) 666626

UCB Pharma
UCB Pharma Ltd,
Star House, 69 Clarendon Rd,
Watford, Herts WD1 1DJ.
(01923) 211811

Ultrapharm
Ultrapharm Ltd,
PO Box 18, Henley-on-Thames,
Oxon RG9 2AW.
(01491) 578016

Unigreg
Unigreg Ltd,
Enterprise House,
181–189 Garth Rd, Morden,
Surrey SM4 4LL.
0181-330 1421

Unipath
Unipath Ltd,
Norse Rd, Bedford
MK41 0QG.
(01234) 347161

Universal
Universal Hospital Supplies,
313 Chase Rd,
London N14 6JH.
0181-920 6207

Vernon-Carus
Vernon-Carus Ltd,
Penwortham Mills, Preston,
Lancs PR1 9SN.
(01772) 744493

Vestric
Vestric Ltd,
West Lane, Runcorn,
Cheshire WA7 2PE.
(01928) 717070

Vitaflo
Vitaflo Ltd,
6 Moss St, Paisley PA1 1BJ.
0800 515174

Vitalograph
Vitalograph Ltd,
Maids Moreton House, Maids
Moreton, Buckingham
MK18 1SW.
(01280) 822811

Vygon
Vygon (UK) Ltd,
Bridge Rd, Cirencester,
Glos GL7 1PT.
(01285) 657051

H G Wallace
H G Wallace Ltd,
Colchester, Essex CO2 8JH.
(01206) 795133

Wallace Mfg
Wallace Manufacturing
Chemists Ltd,
Randles Rd, Knowsley
Industrial Park, Merseyside
L34 9HX.
0151-549 1255

Wanskerne
Wanskerne Ltd,
31 High Cross St, St. Austell,
Cornwall PL25 4AN.
(01726) 69500

Ward
Ward Surgical Appliance Co
Ltd,
57A Brightwell Ave, Westcliffe-
on-Sea, Essex SS0 9EB.
(01702) 354064

Warner Lambert
see P-D

WBP
see Boehringer Ingelheim

Whitehall
Whitehall Laboratories Ltd,
Huntercombe Lane South,
Taplow, Maidenhead,
Berks SL6 0PH.
(01628) 669011

Willis
S. R. Willis & Sons Ltd,
176 Albion Rd,
London N16 9JR.
0171-254 7373

Windsor
see Boehringer Ingelheim.

W-L
Warner Lambert UK Ltd,
see P-D.

Wyeth
Wyeth Laboratories,
Huntercombe Lane South,
Taplow, Maidenhead,
Berks SL6 0PH.
(01628) 604377

Wyvern
Wyvern Medical Ltd,
PO Box 17, Ledbury,
Herefordshire HR8 2ES.
(01531) 631105

Yamanouchi
Yamanouchi Pharma Ltd,
Yamanouchi House, Pyrford Rd,
West Byfleet, Surrey
KT14 6RA.
(01932) 345535

Zeal
G. H. Zeal Ltd,
8 Lombard Rd, Merton, London
SW19 3UU.
0181-542 2283

Zeneca
Zeneca Pharma,
King's Court, Water Lane,
Wilmslow, Cheshire SK9 5AZ.
(01625) 712712

'Special-order' Manufacturers

The following **companies** manufacture 'special-order' products: BCM Specials, Martindale, Rosemont.
Hospital manufacturing units also manufacture 'special-order' products, details may be obtained from any of the centres listed below.

It should be noted that when a product has a licence *the Department of Health recommends that the licensed product should be ordered* unless a specific formulation is required.

ENGLAND

East Anglian and Oxford
Mr G. Hanson,
Regional Production
Pharmacist,
Pharmacy Department,
The Ipswich Hospital,
Heath Rd, Ipswich,
Suffolk IP4 5PD.
(01473) 712233 Extn 5603

Mersey
Dr M. G. Lee,
Regional Quality Control
Pharmacist,
Pharmacy Practice Unit,
70 Pembroke Place
Liverpool L69 3BX.
0151-794 8138

North Thames
Mr M. Lillywhite,
Regional Production
Pharmacist,
St. Bartholomew's Hospital,
West Smithfield, London
EC1A 7BE.
0171-601 7477

North Western
Mr M.D. Booth,
Production & Aseptic Services
Manager,
Stockport Pharmaceuticals,
Stepping Hill Hospital,
Stockport, Cheshire SK2 7JE.
0161-419 5657

Northern
Mr P. W. McKenzie,
Regional Technical Services
Pharmacist,
Pharmacy Department,
Newcastle General Hospital,
Westgate Rd,
Newcastle upon Tyne NE4 6BE.
0191-273 8811 Extn 22479

South East Thames
Mr J. Cheetham,
Principal Pharmacist,
Guy's Hospital,
St. Thomas' St,
London SE1 9RT.
0171-955 5000 Extn 5378/3712

South West Thames
Mr S. J. Riley,
Regional Production
Pharmacist,
Pharmacy Department,
Lanesborough Wing,
St. George's Hospital,
Blackshaw Rd, Tooting,
London SW17 0QT.
0181-725 1770

South Western
Mr C. W. Lewis,
Director,
Manorpark Pharmaceuticals,
Blackberry Hill Hospital,
Manor Rd, Bristol BS16 2EW.
(0117) 975 4852

Trent
Mr A. C. Moore,
Regional Production
Representative, Royal
Hallamshire Hospital, Glossop
Rd, Sheffield S10 2JF.
(0114) 271 2325

Wessex
Dr E. Brierley,
Regional Manufacturing Unit,
Queen Alexandra Hospital,
Cosham, Portsmouth,
Hants PO6 3LY.
(01705) 286335

West Midlands
Mr P. G. Williams,
Principal Pharmacist,
Pharmacy Manufacturing Unit,
Burton Hospital NHS Trust,
Belvedere Rd,
Burton-on-Trent DE13 0RB
(01283) 566333 Extn 5138

Yorkshire
Mr E. Holt,
Principal Pharmacist,
Production Unit,
The Royal Infirmary,
Acre St, Lindley, Huddersfield,
West Yorks HD3 3EA.
(01484) 422191 Extn 2421

NORTHERN IRELAND

Mrs S. M. Millership,
Principal Pharmacist,
Central Pharmaceutical
Production Unit,
CSA Distribution Centre,
77 Boucher Cres, Belfast
BT12 6HU.
(01232) 553407

SCOTLAND

Mr J. A. Cook,
Principal Pharmacist—
Regional Production,
Tayside Pharmaceuticals,
Ninewells Hospital,
Dundee DD1 9SY.
(01382) 632273

WALES

Mr C. Powell
Specialist Principal Pharmacist,
Sterile Products Unit,
Pharmacy Department,
University Hospital of Wales,
The Heath, Cardiff CF4 4XW.
(01222) 747747 Extn 3114

Index

Where an entry is followed by more than one page reference, the principal reference is printed in **bold** type. Proprietary (trade) names are printed in *italic* type.

Sandimmun, 381
Sandocal preparations, 413
Sandoglobulin, 531
Sando-K, 402
Sandostatin, 390
Sandrena, 322
Sanomigran, 209
Saquinavir, 276, **279**
Sassco, 653, 656
Saventrine IV, 104
Savlon Dry powder, 514
Scabies, 508
Scandishake, 638
Scandonest, 553
Scanpor, 674
Schacht, 652, 655
Schar, 638
Schering PC4, 355
Scheriproct, 55
Scherisorb, 667
Schistosoma, 295
Schistosomicides, 295
Schizophrenia, 162
Scleritis, 452
Scleroderma, 419
Sclerosants, 121
Scopoderm TTS, 194
Scopolamine see Hyoscine
Scott catheter, 650
Scottish Prescribing Analysis, 1
Scurvy, 419
Sea-legs, 190
SeaSorb, 666
Seborrhoeic dermatitis, 489
Seborrhoeic eczema, 489
Secadrex, 76
Secobarbital see Quinalbarbitone
Seconal Sodium, 162
Second Nature, 653, 657
Secron, 154
Sectral, 76
Secure Forte, 673
Securon preparations, 101–2
Securopen, 243
Sedation, anaesthesia, 540
Sedatives, 155
    see also Anxiolytics
Seel-a-peel, 664
Select-A-Jet Dopamine, 104
Selegiline, 221, **225**
Selenium sulphide, 502
Selsun, 503
Semi-Daonil, 304
Semi-permeable adhesive film, 668
Semitard MC—discontinued
Semprex, 142
Senlax, 51
Senna, 50
Senokot, 50
Senselle, 348
Septicaemia, initial therapy, 235
Septrin, 260
Seravit, Paediatric, 636
Serc, 194
Serdolect, 172
Serenace, 166
Serenade, 654
Serevent, 129
Sermorelin, 331
Serophene, 328
Seroquel, 172
Serotonin re-uptake inhibitor anti-
depressants see Antidepressants
Serotulle, 670
Seroxat, 184
Sertindole, 170, **172**
Sertraline, 183, **184**
Sesame oil, presence of, 2
Setlers preparations, 31
Seton Urisac, 644
Setopress, 672
Sevoflurane, 538, **539**

Sevredol, 200
Sex hormones, 317, 325
    androgens, 325
        antagonists, 327
        malignant disease, 384
    oestrogens, 317
        antagonists, 328, 385
    progestogens, 323
Sexual deviation, 164, 327
Shampoos, 502
Shared care, 4
Shigellosis, 41, 234
Shingles, 274
Shock, 103, 105, 313, 407
    anaphylactic, 146
    cardiogenic, 103
    septic, 313
Short bowel syndrome, ACBS, 641
SHS Modjul Flavour, 638
Sicca syndrome, 475
    ACBS, 641
Sidestream Durable, 135
Sigma ETB, 671
Silastic, 649
Silgrip, 647
Silikon-100, 649–50
Silver sulphadiazine, 504
Simeco, 31
Simethicone see Dimethicone, acti-
vated, 31
Simpla gel, 664
Simplaseel, 656
Simple eye ointment, 461
Simple linctus, 153
    paediatric, 153
Simplene, 457
Simplicity, 653, 657, 660
Simvastatin, 119, **120**
Sinemet preparations, 222–3
Sinequan, 179
Singulair, xi
Sinthrome, 112
Sinusitis, 235
Sinutab preparations, 154, 198
Siopel, 480
Skelid, 336
Skin preparations
    additives, 477
    anaesthetic, 481
    antibacterials, 503
    antipruritic, 481
    antiviral, 508
    barrier, 480
    cleansing, 511
    corticosteroids, 481
    emollient, 478
    ulcers, 515
Skinoren, 495
Skintact, 669
Sleepia, 144
Slinky, 671
Slofenac preparations, 430
Slo-Indo, 431
Slo-Phyllin, 132
Slow-Fe, 392
Slow-Fe Folic, 393
Slow-K, 402
Slow-Sodium, 403
Slow-Trasicor, 79
Slozem, 98
Smallpox vaccine, 529
Smoking, cigarette, 230
Snake bites, 26
    antivenom, 26
Sno Phenicol, 450
Sno Pilo, 456
Sno Pro, 638
Sno Tears, 461
Soap
    soft, 513
        enema, 49
    spirit, 513

Soda mint tablets, 30
Sodium acid phosphate, 415
Sodium alendronate see Alendronic
    acid
Sodium Amytal, 162
Sodium aurothiomalate, 437, **438**
Sodium bicarbonate, 404, 406
    antacid preparations, 30
    capsules, 404
    ear drops, 467
    intravenous infusion, 406
    tablets, 404
    urine alkalinisation, 362
Sodium calcium edetate see Sodium
    calciumedetate
Sodium calciumedetate, 25
    infusion table, 628
Sodium carboxymethylcellulose see
    Carmellose
Sodium cellulose phosphate, 414
Sodium chloride, 402–5
    bladder irrigation, 363
    eye, 449, **461**
    infusion, 405
        glucose and, 405
        hypercalcaemia, 413
        potassium chloride and,
            406
        potassium chloride, glu-
            cose and, 406
    mouthwash, compound, 474,
        475
    nose, 470
    oropharynx, 475
    solution
        eye, 461
        skin cleansing, 512
    tablets, 403
Sodium citrate
    bladder irrigation, 363
    rectal, 53
    urine alkalinisation, 362
Sodium clodronate, 336
    infusion table, 628
Sodium content, antacids, 28
Sodium cromoglicate see Sodium
    cromoglycate
Sodium cromoglycate
    asthma, 140
    eye, 453, **454**
    food allergy, 46–7
    nose, 467, **469**
Sodium feredetate see Sodium iron-
    edetate
Sodium fluoride, 416
Sodium fusidate, **257**, 505
    dressing, 670
    ointment (Fucidin), 505
    see also Fusidic acid
Sodium hyaluronate, 462
Sodium ironedetate, 393
Sodium lactate, 406
    intravenous infusion, 406
    compound, 405
Sodium nitrite, 24
Sodium nitroprusside see Nitro-
    prusside
Sodium perborate, 474
    mouthwash, 475
Sodium picosulphate, 50
    preparations, 50
Sodium stibogluconate, 291
Sodium tetradecyl sulphate, 121
Sodium thiosulphate, 24
Sodium valproate see Valproate
Softcrepe, 672
Sofradex
    ear, 465
    eye, 453
Soframycin, 504
    eye, 451
Sofra-Tulle, 670

COMMITTEE ON SAFETY OF MEDICINES

MEDICINES CONTROL AGENCY

REPORT ON SUSPECTED ADVERSE DRUG REACTIONS

- **Recently introduced products**
  Please report **all** suspected reactions, including minor ones, that could conceivably be attributable to the drug. New products are identified by a black triangle (▼) in the British National Formulary.
- Please also report reactions to vaccines.
- Record all other drugs taken in previous 3 months including self-medication.
- Report suspected drug interactions.

- Established products
  Please report **serious or unusual** suspected reactions to all agents, but not minor reactions. Include reactions that are fatal, life-threatening, disabling, incapacitating, or which result in or prolong hospitalisation.

  See *Adverse Reactions to Drugs* section in the BNF for advice on reporting reactions

Do not be put off reporting because some details are not known

REPORTING DOCTOR

Name and Professional Address _____

Telephone _____ Specialty _____
Signature _____ Date _____

PATIENT'S DETAILS

Surname _____ Other Names _____
Date of birth (or age) _____ Sex: M ☐ F ☐ Weight (kg) _____
Hospital if relevant _____ Hospital Number _____
Consultant in charge or GP Principal _____

SUSPECTED DRUG

Give brand name of drug and batch number if known	Route	Daily dose	Date drug started	Date drug stopped	Therapeutic Indication

SUSPECTED REACTIONS

Was the patient hospitalised because of the reaction?   Yes ☐ No ☐

	Date reaction started	Date reaction ended	Outcome (e.g. fatal, recovered, continuing)

Other drugs taken in the last 3 months including self-medication

Give brand name if known

Write **None** if no other drug has been taken

	Route	Daily dose	Date drug started	Date drug stopped	Therapeutic Indication

Relevant additional information including medical history, investigations, known allergies, suspected drug interactions. For congenital abnormalities state all other drugs taken during pregnancy and the LMP. Please attach additional pages if necessary.

Send to **Medicines Control Agency, CSM FREEPOST, LONDON SW8 5BR**

or if you are in one of the following NHS regions:

to **CSM Mersey, FREEPOST, Liverpool L3 3AB**

or **CSM West Midlands, FREEPOST SW2991, Birmingham B18 7BR**

or **CSM Northern, FREEPOST 1085, Newcastle upon Tyne NE1 1BR**

or **CSM Wales, FREEPOST, Cardiff CF4 1ZZ**

If you would like information about other reports associated with the suspected drug, tick here ☐

FOR OFFICE USE ONLY

COMMITTEE ON SAFETY OF MEDICINES

MEDICINES CONTROL AGENCY

REPORT ON SUSPECTED ADVERSE DRUG REACTIONS

- **Recently introduced products**
  Please report **all** suspected reactions, including minor ones, that could conceivably be attributable to the drug. New products are identified by a black triangle (▼) in the British National Formulary.

- **Established products**
  Please report **serious or unusual** suspected reactions to all agents, but not minor reactions. Include reactions that are fatal, life-threatening, disabling, incapacitating, or which result in or prolong hospitalisation.

- Please also report reactions to vaccines.
- Record all other drugs taken in previous 3 months including self-medication
- Report suspected drug interactions.

See *Adverse Reactions to Drugs* section in the BNF for advice on reporting reactions

Do not be put off reporting because some details are not known

REPORTING DOCTOR

Name and Professional Address _____

Telephone _____ Specialty _____

Signature _____ Date _____

PATIENT'S DETAILS

Surname _____ Other Names _____

Date of birth (or age) _____ Sex: M ☐ F ☐ Weight (kg) _____

Hospital if relevant _____ Hospital Number _____

Consultant in charge or GP Principal _____

SUSPECTED DRUG

Give brand name of drug and batch number if known

	Route	Daily dose	Date drug started	Date drug stopped	Therapeutic Indication

SUSPECTED REACTIONS

Was the patient hospitalised because of the reaction?   Yes ☐ No ☐

	Date reaction started	Date reaction ended	Outcome (e.g. fatal, recovered, continuing)

Other drugs taken in the last 3 months including self-medication

Give brand name if known
Write **None** if no other drug has been taken

	Route	Daily dose	Date drug started	Date drug stopped	Therapeutic Indication

Relevant additional information including medical history, investigations, known allergies, suspected drug interactions. For congenital abnormalities state all other drugs taken during pregnancy and the LMP. Please attach additional pages if necessary.

Send to **Medicines Control Agency, CSM FREEPOST, LONDON SW8 5BR**
or if you are in one of the following NHS regions:

to **CSM Mersey, FREEPOST, Liverpool L3 3AB**
or **CSM West Midlands, FREEPOST SW2991, Birmingham B18 7BR**
or **CSM Northern, FREEPOST 1085, Newcastle upon Tyne NE1 1BR**
or **CSM Wales, FREEPOST, Cardiff CF4 1ZZ**

If you would like information about other reports associated with the suspected drug, tick here ☐

FOR OFFICE USE ONLY

In Confidence
COMMITTEE ON SAFETY OF MEDICINES   MEDICINES CONTROL AGENCY

REPORT ON SUSPECTED ADVERSE DRUG REACTIONS

- **Recently introduced products**
  Please report **all** suspected reactions, including minor ones that could conceivably be attributable to the drug. New products are identified by a black triangle (▼) in the British National Formulary.

- Established products
  Please report **serious or unusual** suspected reactions to all agents, but not minor reactions. Include reactions that are fatal, life-threatening, disabling, incapacitating, or which result in or prolong hospitalisation.

- Please also report reactions to vaccines.
- Record all other drugs taken in previous 3 months including self-medication.
- Report suspected drug interactions.

> See *Adverse Reactions to Drugs* section in the BNF for advice on reporting reactions

Do not be put off reporting because some details are not known

REPORTING DOCTOR

Name and Professional Address _____

Telephone _____ Specialty _____
Signature _____ Date _____

PATIENT'S DETAILS

Surname _____ Other Names _____
Date of birth (or age) _____ Sex: M ☐ F ☐ Weight (kg) _____
Hospital if relevant _____ Hospital Number _____
Consultant in charge or GP Principal _____

SUSPECTED DRUG

Give brand name of drug and batch number if known	Route	Daily dose	Date drug started	Date drug stopped	Therapeutic Indication

SUSPECTED REACTIONS

Was the patient hospitalised because of the reaction?   Yes ☐ No ☐

	Date reaction started	Date reaction ended	Outcome (e.g. fatal, recovered, continuing)

Other drugs taken in the last 3 months including self-medication

Give brand name if known
Write **None** if no other drug has been taken

	Route	Daily dose	Date drug started	Date drug stopped	Therapeutic Indication

Relevant additional information including medical history, investigations, known allergies, suspected drug interactions. For congenital abnormalities state all other drugs taken during pregnancy and the LMP. Please attach additional pages if necessary.

Send to **Medicines Control Agency, CSM FREEPOST, LONDON SW8 5BR**
or if you are in one of the following NHS regions:

to **CSM Mersey, FREEPOST, Liverpool L3 3AB**
or **CSM West Midlands, FREEPOST SW2991, Birmingham B18 7BR**
or **CSM Northern, FREEPOST 1085, Newcastle upon Tyne NE1 1BR**
or **CSM Wales, FREEPOST, Cardiff CF4 1ZZ**

If you would like information about other reports associated with the suspected drug, tick here ☐

FOR OFFICE USE ONLY

In Confidence

COMMITTEE ON SAFETY OF MEDICINES

REPORT ON SUSPECTED ADVERSE DRUG REACTIONS

MEDICINES CONTROL AGENCY

- **Recently introduced products**
  - Estab ished products

  Please report **all** suspected reactions, including minor ones, that could conceivably be attributable to the drug. New products are identified by a black triangle (▼) in the British National Formulary.

  Please report **serious or unusual** suspected reactions to all agents, but not minor reactions. Include reactions that are fatal, life-threatening, disabling, incapacitating, or which result in or prolong hospitalisation.

- Please also report reactions to vaccines.
- Record all other drugs taken in previous 3 months including se f-medication.
- Report suspected drug interactions.

See *Adverse Reactions to Drugs* section in the BNF for advice on reporting reactions

Do not be put off reporting because some details are not known

REPORTING DOCTOR

Name and Professional Address _____

Telephone _____ Specialty _____

Signature _____ Date _____

PATIENT'S DETAILS

Surname _____ Other Names _____

Date of birth (or age) _____ Sex: M ☐ F ☐ Weight (kg) _____

Hospital if relevant _____ Hospital Number _____

Consultant in charge or GP Principal _____

SUSPECTED DRUG

Give brand name of drug and batch number if known	Route	Daily dose	Date drug started	Date drug stopped	Therapeutic Indication

SUSPECTED REACTIONS

Was the patient hospitalised because of the reaction? Yes ☐ No ☐	Date reaction started	Date reaction ended	Outcome (e.g. fatal, recovered, continuing)

Other drugs taken in the last 3 months including self-medication

Give brand name if known

Write **None** if no other drug has been taken

	Route	Daily dose	Date drug started	Date drug stopped	Therapeutic Indication

Relevant additional information including medical history, investigations, known allergies, suspected drug interactions. For congenital abnormalities state all other drugs taken during pregnancy and the LMP. Please attach additional pages if necessary.

Send to **Medicines Control Agency, CSM FREEPOST, LONDON SW8 5BR**

or if you are in one of the following NHS regions:

to **CSM Mersey, FREEPOST, Liverpool L3 3AB**

or **CSM West Midlands, FREEPOST SW2991, Birmingham B18 7BR**

or **CSM Northern, FREEPOST 1085, Newcastle upon Tyne NE1 1BR**

or **CSM Wales, FREEPOST, Cardiff CF4 1ZZ**

If you would like information about other reports associated with the suspected drug, tick here ☐

FOR OFFICE USE ONLY